C0-AUG-177

Pediatric Epilepsy

Diagnosis and Therapy

Second Edition

Pediatric Epilepsy

Diagnosis and Therapy

Second Edition

John M. Pellock, M.D.
Medical College of Virginia/Virginia Commonwealth University
Richmond, Virginia

W. Edwin Dodson, M.D.
Washington University School of Medicine
St. Louis, Missouri

Blaise F.D. Bourgeois, M.D.
Children's Hospital, Harvard Medical School
Boston, Massachusetts

Editors

DEMOS

New York

Demos Medical Publishing, Inc., 386 Park Avenue South, New York, New York 10016

© 2001 by Demos Medical Publishing, Inc. All rights reserved. This book is protected by copyright. No part of it may be reproduced, stored in a retrieval system, or transmitted in any form or by any means, electronic, mechanical, photocopying, recording, or otherwise, without the prior written permission of the publisher.

Library of Congress Cataloging-in-Publication Data

Available from the publisher upon request

Made in the United States of America

ACKNOWLEDGMENTS

The editors sincerely thank several people for their hard work, contributions, and encouragement, which enabled this book to be completed. Drs. Kiffen Penry and Charles Pippenger originally proposed that we accept this project, and since the first edition many have encouraged us to update and expand this text. Dr. Diana Schneider and her staff at Demos have encouraged, helped develop, directed, and even pushed us when necessary to bring this project to its successful and timely completion. We further thank all others for their contribution, patience, and tolerance of our editing styles. Kathleen Yonan in Richmond deserves special acknowledgment and thanks for all of her expert help in communications, typing, copying, and diplomatically keeping the editors dedicated to the task of completing this book.

Dedication

To our families and to the children and families for whom we care

CONTENTS

Epilepsy Surgery and Other Issues

Preface

The second edition of *Pediatric Epilepsy: Diagnosis and Therapy* is intended to meet the same goals as the first edition: to assist all who are involved in caring for children with seizures and epilepsy. Since the preparation of the initial offering, there has been an explosive growth of information concerning epilepsy, including advances in neuroscience, pharmacology, genetics, diagnostic testing, and both medical and surgical treatment options. Clinicians, and especially child neurologists and epileptologists, have become more comfortable with the concept of epilepsy syndrome, and in this edition we have expanded the discussion about the particular syndromes of childhood, along with the difficulties sometimes encountered in making a fixed diagnosis of seizure type or syndrome in very young infants. Yes, the diagnosis of epilepsy has become more complicated, but it continues to enable us to treat those children whose disorders can be categorized with much greater specificity. Additionally, better knowledge of disease process, metabolic disturbances, and genetics allows further understanding. Still, however, for many children who have seizures the cause remains elusive, their diagnosis remains descriptive, and therapy is empirical, but many more options now exist. Our knowledge about clinical pharmacology of antiepileptic drugs has continued to advance. Throughout the text differences are noted between neonates, infants, older children, and adolescent age groups in pharmacokinetic profiles. Furthermore, a better understanding of adverse effects, particularly those life-threatening reactions, allows truly individualized therapy.

This continues to be the only book of its kind and scope. We have tried to balance discussions of practical medical management with the scientific basis of epilepsy and its treatment in a clear and concise manner. The book focuses on the special issues of children with epilepsy and is intended as both a practical guide and a reference for clinicians and investigators. With many more options for the treatment of epilepsy, including new antiepileptic drugs, vagus nerve stimulation, the reemergence of the ketogenic diet, and a better understanding of surgical intervention, hope for a more normal life for all children with epilepsy should be encouraged. Epilepsy surgery, previously reserved for adults and for those treated with extremely refractory epilepsy, has become more accepted.

Each chapter contained in this book has been markedly updated or is a newly written chapter. In the initial section on basic mechanisms of epilepsy, a chapter by Dr. Ruth Ottman on the genetics of epilepsy has been added because of the marked advances seen in this area over the last decade. Major changes have been incorporated since the section on classification, epidemiology, and diagnosis. Dr. Douglas Nordli has expanded the International League Against Epilepsy classification to include special considerations in very young children. Dr. Allen Hauser offers a completely updated epidemiology review, while Dr. Ruben Kuzniecky has greatly expanded the section on neuroimaging. Added to the epilepsy syndrome section are specific chapters enlarging the discussion of encephalopathic epilepsy to include those occurring after infancy (Dr. Shunsuke Ohtahara) and the Lennox-Gastaut syndrome and related disorders (Dr. Tracy Glauser). General principles of therapy have been rewritten and updated concerning mechanisms of action, pharmacokinetics, and general decisions regarding treatment for both chronic and acute management. Still problematic in the treatment of young women are concerns of teratogenicity with antiepileptic drugs, again reviewed by Dr. Mark Yerby. The section on therapy has been markedly enlarged with separate reviews of the benzodiazepines and phenobarbital. Fosphenytoin is added to phenytoin, and oxcarbazepine is added to carbamazepine as new compounds. The ketogenic diet and expanded considerations concerning drug interactions of combination therapy are included. New medications, including felbamate, gabapentin, lamotrigine, topiramate, tiagabine, vigabatrin, and zonisamide, each have separate new chapters along with a review of other new antiepileptic drugs by Drs. Robert Fisher and John Kerrigan. Vitamins and other antiepileptic therapies are reviewed by Dr. Philip Sheridan.

As surgical intervention for the treatment of epilepsy becomes an ever-enlarging field, this section has been markedly expanded, beginning with a discussion on the cost of surgery followed by a comprehensive review of surgical evaluation and treatment for specific epilepsy types. Issues regarding quality of life and cognition and behavior are discussed in the final chapters of this book. To accomplish this more extensive review of pediatric epilepsy, the previous editors asked Dr. Blaise Bourgeois to join them in editing this second edition. We have also added international authors.

We would be remiss in introducing this second edition without acknowledging the contribution of several of the previous authors who have now died. Drs. Kiffen Penry and Fritz Dreifuss, two of the founding fathers of pediatric epilepsy in the United States, have left us to carry on their work. Dr. Eric Lothman died quite prematurely, but his contribution to the understanding of the pathophysiology of seizures and epilepsy remains current even in this edition, and in years to come. In honoring these and others who have encouraged and guided our careers, we hope that this book meets the needs of those who care for children with epilepsy and the children and families who experience seizures. For some, epilepsy will be a transient and distant memory, while for others epilepsy is an ever-present burden. Evaluating and treating these children in the most appropriate and efficient fashion while avoiding adverse cognitive and psychosocial effects is both challenging and rewarding, and it requires state-of-the-art knowledge, such as that presented in this book. Our goal continues to be the perfect result—no seizures, no side effects, and no stigma to limit these children from achieving their full potential.

J.M.P.
W.E.D.
B.F.D.B.

Contributors

Albert P. Aldenkamp, Ph.D., Sterkselseweg, The Netherlands

John E. Annegers, Ph.D., Department of Neurology, University of Texas School of Public Health, Houston, Texas

G. Arunkumar, M.D., Department of Pediatric Neurology, Albuquerque, New Mexico

Joan K. Austin, D.N.S., R.N., Indiana University, School of Nursing, Indianapolis, Indiana

Charles E. Begley, M.D., Department of Neurology, University of Texas School of Public Health, Houston, Texas

Samuel F. Berkovic, M.D., Department of Neurology, Austin Hospital, Heidelberg, Melbourne, Australia

Blaise F.D. Bourgeois, M.D., Department of Neurology, Children's Hospital, Harvard Medical School, Boston, Massachusetts

James C. Cloyd, Pharm. D., Department of Pharmacy Practice, Minnesota Comprehensive Epilepsy Program, University of Minnesota, Minneapolis, Minnesota

Nihal C. DeLanerolle, D.Phil, D.Sc, Department of Neurology, Yale University School of Medicine, New Haven, Connecticut

Robert J. DeLorenzo, M.D., Ph.D., M.P.H., Department of Neurology, Medical College of Virginia, Virginia Commonwealth University, Richmond, Virginia

Darryl C. De Vivo, M.D., Departments of Neurology and Pediatrics, Columbia Presbyterian Medical Center, New York, New York

W. Edwin Dodson, M.D., Departments of Pediatrics, Neurology, and Neurological Surgery, Washington University School of Medicine, St. Louis, Missouri

Michael S. Duchowny, M.D., Department of Neurology, Miami Children's Hospital, Miami, Florida

Kevin Farrell, M.B., The University of British Columbia, Division of Neurology, Department of Pediatrics, B.C.'s Children's Hospital, Vancouver, British Columbia, Canada

Robert S. Fisher, M.D., Ph.D., Barrow Neurological Institute, St. Joseph's Hospital Medical Center, Phoenix, Arizona

James D. Frost, Jr., M.D., Section of Neurophysiology, Department of Neurology, Baylor College of Medicine, and the Methodist Hospital, Houston, Texas

William R. Garnett, Pharm.D., Department of Pharmacy and Pharmaceutics, School of Pharmacy, Virginia Commonwealth University, Medical College of Virginia, Richmond, Virginia

Jamie Gilman, M.D., Neuroscience Center, Miami Children's Hospital, Miami, Florida

Tracy A. Glauser, M.D., Children's Hospital Medical Center, Department of Neurology, Cincinnati, Ohio

W. Allen Hauser, M.D., Columbia University, G.H. Sergievsky Center, New York, New York

Gregory L. Holmes, M.D., Department of Neurology, Harvard Medical School, Children's Hospital, Boston, Massachusetts

Richard A. Hrachovy, M.D., Section of Neurophysiology, Department of Neurology, Baylor College of Medicine, and the Methodist Hospital, Houston, Texas

Michael V. Johnston, M.D., Departments of Neurology and Pediatrics, Johns Hopkins Medical Institutions, and the Kennedy Krieger Institute, Baltimore, Maryland

Peter Kellaway, Ph.D., Department of Neurology, Baylor College of Medicine, Houston, Texas

John F. Kerrigan, III, M.D., Division of Pediatric Neurology, Barrow Neurological Institute, Phoenix, Arizona

Prakash Kotagal, M.D., Section of Pediatric Epilepsy and Neuropharmacology, Cleveland Clinic Foundation, Cleveland, Ohio

Günter Krämer, M.D., Swiss Epilepsy Center, Zurich, Switzerland

Ruben I. Kuzniecky, M.D., Department of Neurology, University of Alabama, Epilepsy Center, Birmingham, Alabama

David J. Leszczyszyn, M.D., Division of Child Neurology, Department of Neurology, MCV Comprehensive Epilepsy Institute, Medical College of Virginia, Virginia Commonwealth University, Richmond, Virginia

Katherine M. Martien, M.D., F.A.A.P., Department of Pediatrics, Massachusetts General Hospital, Boston, Massachusetts

John W. McDonald, M.D., Ph.D., Department of Neurology, Washington University School of Medicine, St. Louis, Missouri

Eli M. Mizrahi, M.D., Baylor College of Medicine, Department of Neurology, Houston, Texas, U.S.A.

Diego A. Morita, M.D., Division of Neurology, Department of Pediatrics, Children's Hospital Medical Center, Cincinnati, Ohio

Lawrence D. Morton, M.D., Division of Child Neurology, Department of Neurology, Medical College of Virginia, Virginia Commonwealth University, Richmond, Virginia

Solomon L. Moshé, M.D., Montefiore Medical Center, Department of Neurology, New York, New York

Edwin C. Myer, M.D., Division of Child Neurology, Department of Neurology, Medical College of Virginia, Virginia Commonwealth University, Richmond, Virginia

Douglas R. Nordli, Jr., M.D., Department of Clinical Neurology and Pediatrics, Children's Memorial Hospital, Chicago, Illinois

Christine O'Dell, M.D., Department of Neurology and Pediatrics, Montefiore/Einstein Epilepsy Management Center, Albert Einstein College of Medicine, Bronx, New York

Jeffrey G. Ojemann, M.D., Department of Neurological Surgery, Washington University School of Medicine, St. Louis, Missouri

Shunsuke Ohtahara, M.D., Department of Child Neurology, Okayama University Medical School, Shikatacho, Okayama, Japan

Ruth Ottman, M.D., Columbia University, G.H. Sergievsky Center, New York, New York

Michael J. Painter, M.D., Departments of Neurology and Pediatrics, University of Pittsburgh School of Medicine, Pittsburgh, Pennsylvania

T.S. Park, M.D., Department of Neurosurgery, St. Louis Children's Hospital, Washington University School of Medicine, St. Louis, Missouri

Phillip L. Pearl, M.D., Children's National Medical Center, Washington, D.C.

Timothy A. Pedley, M.D., Department of Neurology, Columbia Comprehensive Epilepsy Center, and Columbia-Presbyterian Medical Center, New York, New York

John M. Pellock, M.D., Division of Child Neurology, Department of Neurology, MCV Comprehensive Epilepsy Institute, Medical College of Virginia, Virginia Commonwealth University, Richmond, Virginia

Arthur L. Prensky, M.D., Department of Pediatric Neurology, Washington University School of Medicine, St. Louis Children's Hospital, St. Louis, Missouri

N. Paul Rosman, M.D., Division of Pediatric Neurology, The Floating Hospital for Children, New England Medical Center, Boston, Massachusetts

A. David Rothner, M.D., Section of Pediatric Neurology, Cleveland Clinic Foundation, Cleveland, Ohio

Robert S. Rust, M.D., Department of Neurology, Children's Hospital, Boston, Massachusetts

Nancy Santilli, R.N., P.N.P., M.N., Comprehensive Epilepsy Program, University of Virginia, Charlottesville, Virginia

Sanford Schneider, M.D., Division of Child Neurology, Loma Linda University School of Medicine, Loma Linda, California

Philip H. Sheridan, M.D., Developmental Neurology Branch, National Institute of Neurological Disorders and Stroke, National Institutes of Health, Bethesda, Maryland

Shlomo Shinnar, M.D., Ph.D., Department of Neurology and Pediatrics, Montefiore/Einstein Epilepsy Management Center, Albert Einstein College of Medicine, Bronx, New York

Robert S. Sloviter, Ph.D., Neurology Research Center, Helen Hayes Hospital, West Haverstraw, New York

O. Carter Snead, III, M.D., University of Toronto, Hospital for Sick Children, Division of Neurology, Toronto, Canada

Kenneth W. Sommerville, M.D., Abbott Laboratories, Abbott Park, Illinois

Libor Velisek, M.D., Ph.D., Albert Einstein College of Medicine, Bronx, New York

James W. Wheless, M.D., Department of Neurology, University of Texas, Houston, Texas

L. James Willmore, M.D., Department of Neurology, St. Louis University, St. Louis, Missouri

H. Steve White, M.D., Department of Pharmacology and Toxicology, University of Utah , Salt Lake City, Utah

Yasuko Yamatogi, M.D., Department of Child Neurology, Okayama University medical School, Okayama, Japan

Mark S. Yerby, M.D., M.P.H., Oregon Comprehensive Epilepsy Program, Good Samaritan Hospital and Medical Center, Portland, Oregon

Pathophysiology of Seizures and Epilepsy in the Immature Brain: Cells, Synapses, and Circuits

Libor Velíšek, M.D., Ph.D., and Solomon L. Moshé, M.D.

Epidemiologic studies show that the propensity of the young brain to develop seizures is much greater than that of the adult brain. These studies cover not only the U.S. population (1,2) but also populations in France, Great Britain, and Scandinavia; therefore, the results appear to be universal (3).

There are many more provoked seizures in neonates and infants than in adults. Causes may involve trauma, hypoxic-ischemic encephalopathy, hypertension, metabolic abnormalities (amino acid disturbances, hypocalcemia, hypoglycemia, and electrolyte imbalance), infections, drug withdrawal, pyridoxine dependency, and toxins (4). Similarly, genetic predisposition to epilepsy may be expressed in infancy. Genetic factors may be expressed as familial congenital cerebral malformations and seizures such as neurocutaneous syndromes, genetic syndromes, and benign familial epilepsy (4). Additionally, several intractable epileptic syndromes occur only in early infancy or childhood (5). In children, focal brain dysfunction often produces multifocal seizures and status epilepticus suggesting less effective barriers to seizure spread and generalization (6).

This chapter explores several questions. What conditions make a part of the population prone to develop seizures or epilepsy at certain stages of development? Are these conditions acquired or inherited? Are there seizure-provoking factors in epileptic patients? What are the factors that promote interictal activity in an epileptic patient to become a full seizure? Are these factors intrinsic to the neurons, glial cells, or extracellular space in the patient's brain, or are they extrinsic, environmental factors? How do the seizures propagate? How and why do they stop? What are the consequences?

Many factors have the potential to contribute to the increased susceptibility to seizures and the development of epilepsy in the immature brain. In Table 1-1, factors A1–A5 operate in the normal and abnormal brain while factors B1–B3 may be more specific for abnormal brains. The roles of these factors in the pathophysiology of childhood seizures can be studied in animal models of seizures and epilepsy. In these types of studies, however, the investigator needs to correlate the brain development of the animal to that of the human brain. Such correlations are difficult and should be viewed cautiously because not all developmental parameters follow similar curves in animals and humans. Nonetheless, based on comparative ontogenetic studies of the rate of brain growth, a 7- to 8-day-old rat brain may be considered equivalent to the brain of a full-term human infant. Similarly, a rat less than 7 to 8 days old may be considered equivalent

Table 1-1. Factors That Influence the Propensity of the Immature Brain to Develop Frequent Seizures

A. In animals with normal brain development
1. Excitatory processes develop before inhibitory processes
2. Differences in ionic microenvironment
3. Delayed development of circuits that can modify the expression of seizures
4. Seizures begetting seizures as a consequence of frequent seizures early in life
5. High chance of exposure to potentially epileptogenic stimuli (fever, infection, hypoxia)

B. In animals with altered brain development
1. Genetic predisposition
2. High incidence of structural brain anomalies
3. High probability of seizures begetting seizures as a consequence of frequent seizures early in life

to a premature human infant brain (7,8). The rat reaches puberty between 33 and 38 days of age (9). The rat at 2 to 3 weeks, therefore, may be equivalent to a human infant or toddler, whereas at 4 to 5 weeks it may be considered equivalent to a prepubescent child.

There is ample evidence that seizure susceptibility changes with age in experimental animals as it does in humans. In vitro studies of immature cortical neurons from 2- to 3-weeks-old rats indicate that these neurons are more prone to develop epileptiform discharges following a variety of stimuli, such as low extracellular calcium (10), repetitive stimulation (11), and penicillin, bicuculline, or picrotoxin administration (12–15). In vivo studies with several models of seizure induction indicate that in 2- to 3-week-old rats the susceptibility to seizures is higher and seizures spread more easily than in any other age group (16–23) (Figures 1-1 and 1-2). These young rats are also more prone to develop status epilepticus than older rats.

Most of the seizures that are induced experimentally by the administration of chemicals or electric stimulation represent acute seizure models. Kindling is a semichronic model of seizure in the young brain that is induced by repeated electrical stimulation of the brain over 2 to 3 days in developing rats (17,24). Until now there have been only a few successful efforts to develop chronic models of epilepsy in the developing brain that better mimic human epilepsy. Examples of these methods include kindling in kittens (25) and the long-term effects of the administration of tetanus toxin into the hippocampus of young rats (26). The epileptic potential of experimentally induced brain structural abnormalities has not been adequately

explored because these models are expensive, labor-intensive, and time-consuming (27–31).

In this chapter we aim to summarize current information about the differences in the epileptogenicity of young and adult brain and to present possible future research directions in the field of developmental epilepsy.

EXCITATORY PROCESSES PREDOMINATE IN THE NORMAL IMMATURE BRAIN

Physiologic, morphologic, biochemical, and molecular biology studies have been performed to determine differences between the young and adult brain that address the following questions:

1. What are the mechanisms responsible for the enhanced seizure susceptibility of the developing brain?
2. Why is the seizure spread less well confined in the immature brain than in the adult brain?

Physiology

In the rat brain excitatory mechanisms develop faster than inhibitory mechanisms. In vivo microelectrode studies show that inhibition in the paired-pulse paradigm in the area cornu Ammonis 1 (CA_1) of the hippocampus begins after age 18 in rats and then steadily increases to reach adult levels by age 28 days. In contrast, by age 14 days the measures of excitation (i.e., excitability and spike width) are already at fully mature levels (32). These results indicate that in the rat hippocampus excitatory processes are fully mature within two weeks of birth, whereas the inhibitory processes do not reach adult levels until several weeks later (32).

The available data in seizure models support these findings. The intensity of postictal refractoriness (the period that follows a seizure) increases with age (Figures 1-2 and 1-3). In rats younger than 2 to 3 weeks of age, therefore, electrical kindling in the amygdala or hippocampus can be induced with stimuli given at short interstimulus intervals. (18,24,33,34). This is not the case in adult rats (35,36). In younger rats, if two sites are kindled concurrently, both sites develop severe kindled seizures (37,38). In adults, one of them develops kindling while the other site is suppressed (Figure 1-2) (39). The age-specific failure of both inter- and intra-hemispheric mechanisms to suppress the development of multiple kindling foci may represent the same mechanisms that lead to the high incidence of multifocal seizures in the immature central nervous system (CNS) (37,38). In 15-day-old rats, additional kindling stimulation quickly progresses to induce severe seizures (37). In contrast, in adult rats induction of severe seizures requires approximately 250 kindling stimulations (40).

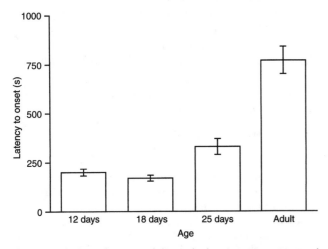

Figure 1-1. Increased susceptibility of the immature 12- and 18-day-old rats to seizures induced by pentylenetetrazol. Male rats aged 12, 18, and 25 days and adults were subcutaneously injected with 100 mg/kg of pentylenetetrazol. Latency to onset of tonic-clonic seizures, which occur throughout development (95), was determined. A shorter latency to onset of seizures indicates increased susceptibility to seizures. Twelve- and 18-day-old rats have the shortest latencies. Modified from (22).

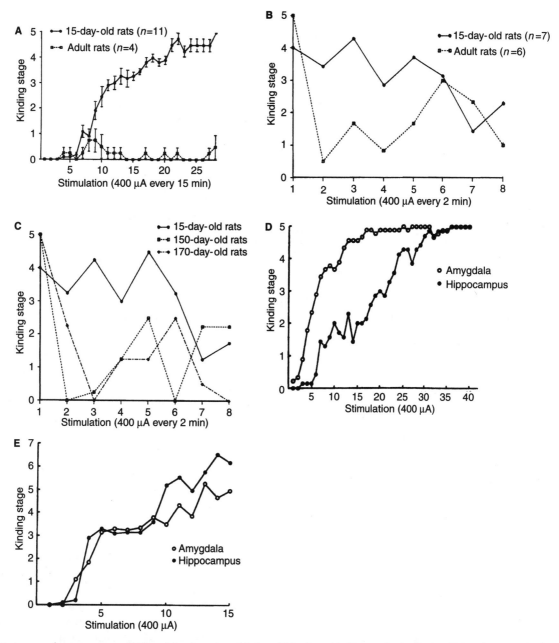

Figure 1-2. Increased seizure susceptibility of the immature 15-day-old brain to kindling-evoked seizures. Electrodes were implanted in the amygdala in A, B, and C and amygdala and hippocampus in D and E. In this composite, the x-axis depicts the severity of kindled seizures using the kindling scale of Racine (260) as modified by Moshé (261) and by Haas and coworkers (37). Kindling stages higher than 4 are secondarily generalized convulsions. Each point represents the mean behavioral kindling stage for the particular stimulation. **A.** Kindling can be induced in 15-day-old rats using a 15-minute interstimulus interval; this stimulation paradigm fails to elicit kindling in adult rats. **B.** The intensity of postictal depression is decreased in 15-day-old rats. In this paradigm, 15-day-old rats and adult rats that had experienced a generalized seizure received seven additional stimuli, each delivered at 2-minute intervals. Fifteen-day-old rats experienced more secondarily generalized seizures than adults, especially during the first 8 minutes. **C.** The intensity of postictal refractoriness increases with age. The same rats were tested at three different ages: 15, 150, and 210 days. **D.** Kindling antagonism in adult rats. Kindling stimuli were delivered in the amygdala and ipsilateral hippocampus on an alternating basis, and each stimulation is plotted separately. Kindling was induced from the amygdala but not the hippocampus. **E.** Lack of kindling antagonism between amygdala and hippocampus in 16- to 17-day-old rats under the same experimental conditions that induce antagonism in adults. Modified from (18, 38, 262).

The increased epileptogenesis may arise from age-specific conditions for excitation and inhibition in the brain (41). Early postnatally, cortical glutamate-mediated excitation utilizes mostly N-methyl-D-aspartic acid (NMDA) receptors. This role of NMDA receptors and diminishes with increasing age in favor of α-amino-3-hydroxy-5-methylisoxazolepropionic acid (AMPA)-receptor–mediated glutamate transmission (42,43). Additionally, early postnatally, γ-aminobutyric acid (GABA) has excitatory effects through GABA$_A$

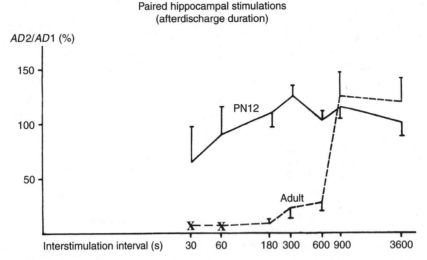

Figure 1-3. Insufficient postictal refractory period in the 12-day-old hippocampus. Twelve-day-old rats and adult rats were implanted with hippocampal stimulating electrodes and cortical recording electrodes. Each of two stimulations consisted of two trains of 121 constant current rectangular pulses (15 s, 8 Hz, 1 ms duration) with intensity twice as high as necessary to induce a hippocampal-cortical evoked potential using a stimulation with a single pulse. Interstimulation intervals were in the range from 30 to 3600 s (1 hour; x-axis). The duration of the afterdischarge (*AD*) was recorded after each stimulation and the results were expressed as $AD2/AD1 \times 100$. The postictal refractory period in 12-day-old rats was shorter than 30 s because already at this interstimulation interval there was no difference between the duration of the *AD*1 and *AD*2. In contrast, in adult rats, the postictal refractory period lasted from 600 to 900 s because at 900 s interstimulation interval, the duration of *AD*2 was equal to the *AD*1.

receptors in several structures such as hippocampus, cerebral cortex, cerebellum, and spinal cord and, therefore, enhances rather than antagonizes glutamate excitatory actions (41,44,45). Thus, early in life, GABAergic inhibition may be mediated solely via GABA$_B$ receptors (41). In the developing brain, therefore, the GABA$_B$ inhibition may be strengthened; this appears to be the case in the substantia nigra pars reticulata, a site critical for control of seizures (46) although this enhancement probably cannot compensate for abundant excitation.

Morphology

Anatomic studies have identified the differential development of morphologically distinct types of synapses that can be assigned to "excitatory" and "inhibitory" functions. The classic study of Schwartzkroin showed that the excitatory type of synapse is already present during the first and second postnatal week in the rabbit hippocampal area CA_1 while the inhibitory type of synapse starts to appear during the third postnatal week (47). Thus, net excitation develops in parallel with the excitatory type of synapses while the development of inhibition follows the occurrence of the inhibitory type of synapses (48). In the area CA_3 of the immature hippocampus, the development of inhibition occurs earlier than in CA_1; however, abundant excitatory axonal collaterals in this area form a complex network that loses its complexity with maturation. Thus, the excessive excitatory wiring in the area CA_3 may contribute to increased epileptogenicity of the

immature hippocampus and to faster, less restrained seizure propagation early in life (49,50). Finally, faster spread of seizures and recruitment of additional areas in the immature nervous system compared with the adult CNS may be the result of extensive direct coupling of the neurons that have been identified in the neocortex of young rats. This coupling is lost with maturation (51).

Biochemistry and Molecular Biology

The developmental hyperexcitability of the all subtypes of glutamate receptors (43,52) may be a consequence of their developmentally regulated subunit composition (53). The subunit composition of AMPA subtype of glutamate receptors changes during development from calcium-permeable isoforms in the immature brain to calcium-impermeable isoforms in adulthood (54). In this scenario, the enhanced calcium influx into the immature neurons via fast excitatory receptor channels may be a powerful source of depolarization. Similarly, there are significant developmental differences in the expression of GABA$_A$-receptor subunit mRNAs, which also suggest age-specific composition of GABA$_A$ receptors (55). The striking correlation between the seizure-specific function and the distribution of certain GABA$_A$-receptor subunit mRNAs in certain brain areas suggests the existence of developmentally regulated GABA$_A$-receptor isoforms that could affect seizures in an opposite way compared with adult GABA$_A$-receptor isoforms (56).

The relatively delayed maturation of other neuromodulatory systems may contribute to the increased epileptogenicity of the immature brain. In adult rats norepinephrine depletion accelerates the rate of kindling, decreases the intensity of postictal refractoriness and permits the development of multiple seizure foci (57–59). In this respect, the norepinephrine-depleted adult rats resemble two-week-old rats in which the norepinephrine transmission has not reached adult levels (17).

DIFFERENCES IN IONIC MICROENVIRONMENT AND GLIAL SUPPORT IN THE NORMAL IMMATURE BRAIN

Setting the Scene

In young children the brain is more vulnerable to insults from the external environment (60,61). These insults may be the result of epileptogenic features of exogenous or endogenous pyrogens, toxins produced by infectious agents, or reactive metabolic by-products of the host tissues. The increased vulnerability of the young brain results from the still developing blood–brain barrier, which, in fact, reflects the development of glial cells (62). Glia have an essential role in maintaining a constant extracellular environment of the nervous system (63). In the mature brain glia contribute to neuronal stability by maintaining ion homeostasis. Almost all ions involved in synaptic transmission undergo age-specific changes reflected by developmental changes in the distribution pattern of ionic channels and the efficacy of energy-dependent ionic transporters in both glia and neurons (64). There is no general rule that the development of ionic channels follows; however, it seems that in the early developmental stages many ionic channels promote calcium permeability (64).

The next questions to consider are: Are the developmental changes in ionic environment powerful enough to affect age-specific seizure susceptibility? How does the maturation of transporter systems affect the development of seizures in the immature brain?

Potassium

Potassium has an important role in the regulation of ionic fluxes early in the development of the nervous system. The intracellular concentration of potassium in neurons increases with maturation, possibly due to an increase in Na^+/K^+-ATPase (adenosine triphosphatase) content and activity. The enzyme Na^+/K^+-ATPase is responsible for the afterhyperpolarization following glutamate-induced excitatory postsynaptic potentials (EPSPs) (65). During afterhyperpolarization it is more difficult to elicit another population spike.

In young rats the afterhyperpolarization is minimal until age 11 days and increases during the first five postnatal weeks. Young neurons, therefore, have more favorable conditions for generating repetitive action potentials than adult neurons. This further increases the the immature brain's susceptibility to seizures.

Extracellular K^+ efflux accompanies repetitive neuronal discharges (66) and increases the extracellular K^+ concentration. In immature brain these discharge-induced changes result in higher extracellular K^+ concentration ($[K^+]_o$) than in adult rat brain (67,68). Excessive neuronal activity causes brain $[K^+]_o$ to reach 14 to 20 mM in the immature rats versus only 10 to 12 mM in adults (14,68). In any age group accumulation of extracellular K^+ causes proportionate depolarization of the neurons and thereby increases neuronal excitability. However, the capability of young CNS to accumulate extracellular K^+ is much larger than that of the adult brain because of the underdevelopment of extracellular K^+ clearance systems. Therefore, repetitive discharges in the young brain tend to depolarize the neurons more than similar discharges in the adult brain because in an environment with repeated epileptiform discharges, high $[K^+]_o$ favors a transition from interictal to ictal state (14,69,70).

In brain there are three principal extracellular K^+ clearance systems. All of these are immature in the young brain and contribute to decreased K^+ removal from the extracellular space. The first clearance system is Na^+/K^+-ATPase with a neuronal (65) and a glial (71) pool. The second system is $K^+ - Cl^-$ transport into astrocytes (72). The density of astrocytes in the rat hippocampus is developmentally regulated. During the first postnatal week in the rat, it is very low in all hippocampal regions, while during the second postnatal week it is sparse only in the stratum pyramidale (73). The third mechanism by which K^+ is removed is the spatial redistribution that hides and dilutes K^+ in the remote and narrow recesses of the extracellular space. Neurons, astrocytes, and oligodendrocytes share this function; however, the maturation of oligodendrocytes in not finished before four weeks of age (73). In the young brain, therefore, the extracellular space is wider (74) and spatial redistribution, measured by extracellular slow potentials (75), is slower, contributing to higher activity-dependent local concentrations of potassium. This spatial redistribution reaches adult level at approximately 4 weeks of age, similar to the maturation of Ca^{2+} and Mg^{2+} equilibration. These findings demonstrate that the sequence of events in the maturation of various glial elements promotes ictogenesis in the immature brain and may support ongoing epileptiform activity (76,77).

The developmental features of potassium concentration and clearance as well as potassium effects on neuronal membrane excitability make potassium a prime contributor to the increased seizure susceptibility of the immature brain. In particular, it seems to promote the transition from interictal to ictal seizure state.

Calcium

Extracellular calcium has age-specific effects on neuronal excitability. Electrophysiologic studies have shown that glutamate, and especially NMDA, receptors in the immature hippocampal pyramidal neurons are regulated by extracellular calcium instead of magnesium as in mature neurons (78–80). Therefore, in the immature brain, activity-dependent changes in extracellular calcium may exert a greater influence on ion flow that results from activation of NMDA receptors. Developmentally immature forms of the AMPA subtype of glutamate-receptor channels lack the GluR2 subunit. Enhanced calcium influx into neurons via these channels may be a powerful source of depolarization (54).

The role of intracellular calcium in seizure susceptibility of the immature brain is less obvious and probably indirect. Intracellular calcium affects neuronal maturation because of calcium-regulated transcription (81); however, the correlation between this calcium effect and seizure susceptibility of the immature brain has not been studied systematically. Furthermore, developmentally regulated intracellular calcium levels (64,82–84) may determine the speed at which the axon reaches its synaptic target. Thus, higher intracellular calcium levels early in the development may affect the complexity of the neuronal network and its excitability by delaying the plug-in of the inhibitory elements.

DELAYED DEVELOPMENT OF CIRCUITS THAT MODIFY THE EXPRESSION OF SEIZURES IN THE NORMAL IMMATURE BRAIN

Spread of Metabolic Activation During Seizures

Defining the roles of brain structures in the initiation and propagation of seizures has been difficult. Although several morphologic and physiologic methods are available, none provide direct answers as to whether seizures propagate directly from one structure to another via a specific pathway or whether these structures are involved indirectly through relay areas. The best approach to defining the involvement of different structures combines electrophysiology and imaging to track down the pathways of seizure spread. Electrophysiology alone is limited because surface electrodes cover only superficial neocortical regions, while depth electrodes record from a small area only. Thus,

many electrodes would be needed to assess the electrical activity throughout the brain; therefore, metabolic imaging techniques are very helpful.

Metabolic studies using the radioactive glucose analogue 2-deoxyglucose (2-DG) have provided significant information about changes in the metabolic activity of several structures both during seizures and during the immediate postictal period. This information reflects only the metabolic activity of the structures; their actual role in seizure generation, propagation, or control, however, can only be estimated. Although 2-DG is an excellent source of qualitative information about brain metabolism changes, 2-DG studies in animals undergoing seizures may not provide absolute quantification because certain assumptions proposed by Sokoloff apply only under normal (resting) conditions (85); therefore, the 2-DG results should be interpreted with caution.

There are several 2-DG metabolic studies demonstrating age-specific metabolic involvement of brain structures during seizures produced by kainic acid, kindling, bicuculline, pentylenetetrazol, and flurothyl (16,86–89). The excitotoxin kainic acid and kindling induce focal seizures, which subsequently generalize. Furthermore, kainic acid–induced seizures progress into status epilepticus (16,90–92). Pentylenetetrazol and flurothyl seizures are believed to be primarily generalized seizures and have age-specific features; these seizures also can progress to status epilepticus (22,93–99).

In young rats until the third week of age, kainic acid–induced status epilepticus produces a rise in metabolism restricted to the hippocampus and lateral septum (16,87). This is paralleled by paroxysmal electroencephalogram (EEG) discharges that are recorded in the hippocampus (16,87,91,100). Starting from the end of the third week, there is a rise in labeling of other structures that are part of or closely linked to the limbic system. These include the amygdala complex, the mediodorsal and adjacent thalamic nuclei, piriform, entorhinal and rostral limbic cortical regions, and areas of projection of the fornix. Therefore, after the third week, the ictal metabolic maps are similar to those observed in adults (87,101). In amygdala kindling in 15-day-old rats, the metabolic activation during severe seizures is restricted to limbic structures (88,89) even when the rats manifest secondarily generalized seizures. There are also age-related differences in seizure-induced metabolic activation of the substantia nigra pars reticulata (SNR). While in the adult rats, there is a significant metabolic activation of the SNR during kindling and kainic acid–induced status epilepticus (102–106); neither kindled seizures nor kainic acid–induced status epilepticus metabolically activate the SNR in young rats (16,107).

A series of studies based on pentylenetetrazol-induced status epilepticus have revealed different age-specific patterns of metabolic activity and blood flow. In 10-day-old rats this model results in a uniform increase in the cerebral metabolism and blood flow throughout the brain. At 21 days, an age when developmentally specific pentylenetetrazol clonic seizures begin to occur (22,95), the pattern of activation changes due to significant decreases of local metabolism and blood flow in the cortex, hippocampus, mammillary body, thalamic nuclei, and white matter. Moderate metabolic and blood flow increases are restricted to a few structures (97,99). In the adult rats this seizure model causes rises in metabolism primarily in the neocortex, cerebellum, and vestibular nuclei (94). The data based on metabolic rate and on blood flow rate are consistent and demonstrate age-specific patterns of brain metabolic activation caused by seizures.

Flurothyl-induced seizures, which cause a 20 percent mortality in 15-day-old rats produces yet a different pattern of brain activation. This seizure model activates glucose metabolism in the brain stem but not the SNR and decreases metabolism in the neocortex. Other structures are not affected (Sperber, personal communication).

Brain Structures Controlling Seizures

Several brain sites play a critical role in the control or activation of seizures. These sites include SNR, superior colliculus, subthalamic nucleus, pedunculo-pontine nucleus, anterior thalamus, and area tempestas (108–116). Thus, far, developmental data are available only for the SNR (56).

In the adult male rat SNR there are two GABA$_A$-sensitive, topographically distinct functional regions localized in the anterior and posterior SNR (SNR$_{anterior}$ and SNR$_{posterior}$, respectively) (117–119). These two SNR regions mediate differential effects on clonic flurothyl seizures. In the SNR$_{anterior}$, bilateral microinfusions of muscimol have anticonvulsant effects, while in the SNR$_{posterior}$, muscimol microinfusions have proconvulsant effects. Similarly, microinfusions of other drugs that act at the GABA receptor, such as bicuculline, ZAPA, and zolpidem, produce site-specific effects on seizures in the SNR (Table 1-2) (118,120). Site-specific effects of flurothyl-induced seizures in the SNR are probably not limited only to GABAergic drugs. Varying the pH of infusions causes differential drug actions in the SNR$_{anterior}$ and SNR$_{posterior}$ (121). In situ histochemistry studies have demonstrated that in adult male rats there are two SNR functional regions with different distributions of GABA$_A$ receptor α1 subunit mRNA (117). This subunit is the most abundant GABA$_A$ receptor subunit in the adult SNR (122). At the cellular level there are few large clusters

Table 1-2. Region- and Age-Specific Effects of Nigral GABA-ergic Drug Microinfusions on Flurothyl Seizures in Male Rats

Drug	15-Day-Old Rats	Adult Rats	
	SNR$_{anterior}$ or SNR$_{posterior}$	SNR$_{anterior}$	SNR$_{posterior}$
Muscimol	Proconvulsant	Anticonvulsant	Proconvulsant
Bicuculline	Proconvulsant	Proconvulsant	No effect
ZAPA	Biphasic effects	Anticonvulsant	Proconvulsant
Zolpidem	Anticonvulsant	Anticonvulsant	No effect
GVG	Anticonvulsant	Anticonvulsant	Proconvulsant

Muscimol is a GABA$_A$ receptor agonist on both low- and high-affinity receptors; bicuculline is a GABA$_A$ receptor antagonist on low-affinity receptors; ZAPA is a GABA$_A$ receptor agonist on low-affinity receptors; zolpidem is an agonist of benzodiazepine I binding site of GABA$_A$ receptor. γ-vinyl GABA is an irreversible inhibitor of the GABA-degradation enzyme, GABA-transaminase. Based on data in (117,118,120).

of labeled cells with high expression of hybridization grains in the SNR$_{anterior}$. In the SNR$_{posterior}$ there is a high density of labeled cells, which have moderate expression of the a1 hybridization grains. The two SNR regions use different output pathways for their effects on seizures as determined by 2-DG studies. In the SNR$_{anterior}$ muscimol infusions decrease glucose utilization in the striatum, sensorimotor cortex, and ventromedial thalamus and increase glucose utilization in superior colliculus (117). In contrast, in the SNR$_{posterior}$ muscimol infusions increase glucose utilization in the dorsal striatum, globus pallidus, and superior colliculus and decrease glucose utilization in thalamus (117). These data support the findings of the topographic and functional segregation of the SNR-linked systems involved in the control of seizures in adult male rats.

The two regions of the SNR, however, do not develop simultaneously. In 15-day-old male rats activation of high-affinity GABA$_A$ receptors mediate only proconvulsant effects (123,124). Thus, the differentiation of the SNR into two functional regions, which was described for adult male rats (119), has not yet developed in 15-day-old male rats (117,118). At this age there is only one functional region within the SNR with respect to the effects of microinfusions of GABA$_A$ergic drug on seizures. These results suggest that the immature, undifferentiated SNR has some similarities with the SNR$_{posterior}$ in terms of the presence of the proconvulsant GABA$_A$ receptor subtype. Similarly, in situ hybridization studies have revealed that the a1 subunit cluster containing cells are uniformly distributed throughout the SNR. Thus, the distribution and density of this receptor subtype resembles the pattern described in the SNR$_{posterior}$ in adult male rats. In 15-day-old male rats muscimol infusions in the SNR also produce specific metabolic changes compared with controls. Regardless of the site of muscimol infusion, glucose utilization increases in the ipsilateral dorsal striatum, globus pallidus, and superior colliculus and does not change in the sensorimotor cortex. In contrast, muscimol infusions decrease glucose utilization in the ipsilateral ventromedial thalamus (117). Thus, the data suggest that in 15-day-old male rats there is only a single output network that resembles the $SNR_{posterior}$ network in adult rats.

When does the differentiation of the two SNR seizure-modifying regions occur? At age 25 days the SNR starts to differentiate; infusions of muscimol in the $SNR_{anterior}$ have no effects on flurothyl seizures, while infusions in the $SNR_{posterior}$ have proconvulsant effects. This maturation of the anticonvulsant SNR region strikingly coincides with sexual maturation (9). In male rats there is a sudden drop in plasma testosterone levels at age 20 to 25 days (125–127) just before the age when the $SNR_{anterior}$ assumes its anticonvulsant characteristics. To test the hypothesis that testosterone plays a role in formation of the anticonvulsant $SNR_{anterior}$, Velíšková studied male rats that were castrated on the day of birth. Later on the rats were exposed to flurothyl following bilateral infusions of muscimol in the $SNR_{anterior}$ or $SNR_{posterior}$. In the $SNR_{anterior}$ in 15-day-old neonatally castrated male rats, muscimol infusions had no effects on seizures; by age 25 days, however, muscimol infusions had anticonvulsant effects. Thus, in neonatally castrated male rats the emergence of the anticonvulsant $SNR_{anterior}$ appeared earlier, suggesting that the depletion of postnatal testosterone accelerated the appearance of the anticonvulsant $SNR_{anterior}$.

The data demonstrate that the age-specific susceptibility to seizures may be influenced by developmental maturation of structures controlling seizures. This maturation is affected by gonadal hormones.

HIGH INCIDENCE OF STRUCTURAL BRAIN ANOMALIES DURING DEVELOPMENT

Childhood epilepsies are often associated with brain anomalies. Among epileptic syndromes of childhood, the catastrophic epilepsies including West and Lennox-Gastaut syndromes are associated with the broadest spectrum of pathoanatomic abnormalities, including neuronal migration disorders and small foci of neuronal necrosis (128). Pre- and perinatal brain alterations, therefore, become a condition *sine qua non* for the development of experimental seizures in the immature brain. Several experimental models have been developed that induce brain injury and malformations that lead to spontaneous seizures. Currently there are data from four models on methylazoxymethanol-induced

migration disorder, neocortical freezing lesions, neuronal migration disorder induced by irradiation in utero, and the double cortex mutation.

Methylazoxymethanol-Induced Neuronal Migration Disorders

Methylazoxymethanol (MAM) is a powerful alkylating agent (129) acting during the G1 and M phases of mitotic cycle of dividing cells. Administration of MAM on embryonic day 15 in the rat interferes with neuroblastic division and neuronal migration toward cortical layers II–V (130) and results in brain malformations in 100 percent of cases (Table 1-3; Figure 1-4) (131). Young rats with MAM-induced neuronal migration disorders express a modest increase in seizure susceptibility. In MAM-exposed rats hyperthermia at age 14 days induced seizures in 14 of 39 rats, while in age-matched controls only one rat of 30 had a seizure (27). The higher seizure susceptibility to hyperthermia in these rats was also associated with a higher mortality rate. At age 14 days rats with MAM-induced lesions have a lower threshold to kainic acid–induced seizures than controls in terms of seizure onset and duration (28,131,132). These effects may be associated with the alterations of AMPA-receptor GluR2 flip and NMDA-receptor NR1 subunit distribution in the dysplastic areas of neocortex and hippocampus (133). Additionally, brain slices from rats exposed in utero to MAM

Table 1-3. Prenatal Brain Abnormalities Induced by Various Teratogens

Model	Age of Application	Results
MAM	E14, E15	Decreased brain size, decreased cortical thickness, loss of normal lamination in layers II–V of the neocortex with abnormally migrated neurons, bilateral ectopias in the pyramidal layer of the hippocampal CA_1, and cell loss in the striatum and thalamus (131)
Irradiation	E16, E17	Diffuse cortical dysplasia, periventricular heterotopia, dispersion of hippocampal pyramidal cell layer, corpus callosum agenesis (29)
Double cortex	Genetic mutation	Layers of gray matter placed inside the forebrain white matter resulting in an inverted migration pattern (31)

E14, E15, E16, and E17 indicate exposure on the respective days of embryonic development.

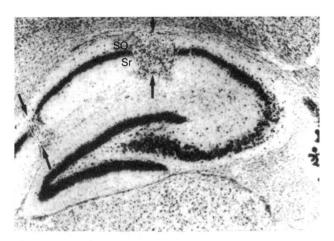

Figure 1-4. Brain section from 15-day-old rat with neuronal migration disorder induced by prenatal treatment with MAM. Coronal section of hippocampus showing areas of neuronal ectopias in the CA_1 subfield *(arrows)*. Ectopic neurons are scattered in the stratum oriens (so) and stratum radiatum (sr). Reprinted from Germano IM, Sperber EF. Transplacentally induced neuronal migration disorders: an animal model for the study of the epilepsies. *J Neurosci Res* 1998; 51:473–488, with permission.

display an increased proportion of bursting cells in the hippocampal CA_1 pyramidal cells compared to controls (134). Spontaneous seizures, however, have not been observed in the MAM model.

Freezing Lesions

A search for a model of perinatal damage resulting in dysplastic cortex rekindled the interest in the neocortical freezing-induced focus used in adult rats by Escueta and coworkers (135,136) and in neonatal rats by Dvořák and Feit (137). In this model a relatively restricted freezing lesion is produced by a cold probe in the neonatal rat neocortex on the first or second day of life (30). The lesion results in the loss of normal cortical lamination and creates a focal microgyrus. Moreover, there are ectopic cell clusters in layer I of the neocortex and in the white matter (30,138). Prominent hyperexcitability of the disorganized neocortical network in the region of focal lesion appears as early as 12 days of age (139). In adult 4- to 6-month-old rats, electrical stimulation of the neocortical afferents supplying the microgyrus leads to epileptiform discharges that propagate over 4 mm in the horizontal direction, while in sham-operated control tissue the horizontal propagation is limited to under 1 mm (30). While the administration of the NMDA-receptor antagonist MK-801 before the lesion can prevent the development of the discharges, it has little or no effect on an already developed focus and on the propagation of ictal discharges (30,140). Discharges from the already developed focus can be inhibited by the AMPA-receptor antagonist NBQX (140a). As in the case with the MAM

model, freezing lesions in developing rats have not yet been observed to cause spontaneous seizures.

Irradiation Lesions

Exposure of 16- or 17-day-old rat embryos to irradiation disrupts neuronal migrations resulting in the creation of numerous dysplastic lesions (29). These rats have a higher susceptibility to the development of electrographic epileptiform discharges after seizure provocation with acepromazine or xylazine. Similarly, in vitro neocortical slices from adult rats exposed to irradiation in utero generate more robust epileptiform activity in bicuculline containing medium than slices from control rats (141). The results suggest that irradiation lesions are epileptogenic as a result of altered GABAergic transmission; however, spontaneous seizures have not been observed.

GENETIC PREDISPOSITION TO SEIZURES AND EPILEPSIES

Although many forms of human epilepsy are genetically determined (142), the mechanisms by which most genetic aberrations alter epileptogenicity still need to be elucidated. There are several animal models of inherited epilepsies. These include one model of genetically determined epilepsy in baboons *(Papio papio)*, three established genetic models of epilepsy in rats, several mutant mouse strains with epileptic disorders (143), and one mouse strain with well-defined brain anomaly of double cortex (31).

Baboons

A subpopulation of Senegalese baboon with genetically determined photosensitive epilepsy was one of the earliest genetic epileptic disturbances studied (144–149). Rhythmic photic stimulation induces progressing myoclonus. The model reflects a quite rare human condition — reflex myoclonus (150). These baboons do not exhibit photosensitivity until prepubertal age. The model is now rarely investigated because of decreased availability of baboons.

Rats

There is a well-established model of generalized tonic-clonic (or brainstem) seizures in the rat induced by intense auditory stimulation. This genetically epilepsy prone rat (GEPR) is susceptible to environmentally induced seizures that cannot be precipitated in otherwise normal animals. Drug studies suggest that decrements in monoaminergic transmission may be

Table 1-4. Strengths and Weaknesses of Absence Seizure Models in Genetically Prone Rats

Positive features	Spontaneous seizures
	Good electroclinical correlation to human absences
	Good response to antiabsence drugs
Negative features	Developmental discrepancy with the onset of human absence seizures

one of the seizure susceptibility determinants; however, non-monoaminergic abnormalities may also play roles in seizure predisposition of the GEPR (151–153).

There are two rat models with spontaneous spike-and-wave discharges akin to human absence seizures: the genetically epilepsy-prone rat from Strasbourg (GAERS) (154) and Wag/Rij strain with spontaneous absence epilepsy from Nijmeegen (155). Both models provide potentially useful information about the mechanisms involved in the generation of absence seizures. The age of onset of these seizures is relatively late, so these models cannot be used for study of absence seizures early in life. Spontaneous seizures in GAERS appear well after four weeks of age, and their incidence increases into adulthood (156). In the Wag/Rij strain, the seizures appear even later, around day 75 of life (157). This is in contrast to human absence epilepsy, which begins in childhood and by puberty spontaneously remits in some instances. On the other hand, the electroclinical correlation between these models and human epilepsies with absence seizures is quite good. Thus, these models may provide an opportunity for better understanding the pathogenesis of spike-and-wave EEG rhythms and associated behaviors.

Mice

Single-locus neurologic mutations in mice provide powerful genetic systems for exploration of the mechanisms that underlie epilepsy. Today most of the efforts have concentrated on the search for the genes responsible for absence epilepsy. A systematic EEG survey of over 110 mapped mouse mutants revealed five mutant genes, located on separate chromosomes, that produce a pattern of spontaneous 6 to 7 Hz spike-and-wave discharges accompanied by behavioral arrest, myoclonic jerks, and uniform responsivity to treatment with ethosuximide (143). These mouse strains have been classified according to the prevalent behavioral feature as lethargic (lh/lh), tottering (tg/tg), ducky (du/du), mocha^{2j} (mh^{2j}/mh^{2j}), and stargazer (stg/stg). These models provide compelling evidence for the genetic heterogeneity of the spike-and-wave trait in the mammalian brain. Developmentally, in strains tg and stg spontaneous seizures appear during a two-day period

between ages 16 and 18 days and increase in frequency to maximal levels within one week. Seizure severity varies across the strains and is genetically linked. The rates for spontaneous seizure are greatest in stg and lowest in du mice (stg > tg > lh > mh^{2j} > du) (158). These data show that a defect at a single gene locus is sufficient to produce a spontaneous, generalized, spike-and-wave seizure disorder. Moreover, the EEG trait is genetically heterogeneous and can arise from several different recessive mutations. To summarize, the cellular mechanisms responsible for these mutations are not heterogeneous, and each mutation gives rise to a distinct syndrome with a characteristic seizure frequency, sensitivity to antiepileptic drugs, and severity of the associated neurologic phenotype (158).

Mice with the mutation of the reeler gene have a significant brain anomaly in which the layers of gray matter are mislocated inside the forebrain white matter. A similar migration defect affects reeler mice and leads to disruption of the normal inside-out pattern of cortical development; instead, an "outside-in pattern" of migration of neocortical neurons is seen (31). This is analogous to the human brain anomaly termed *double cortex*. In both the X-linked genetically induced double cortex malformation in humans (159) and in mice, large ectopias are epileptogenic (31).

HIGH CHANCE OF EXPOSURE TO EPILEPTOGENIC STIMULI DURING DEVELOPMENT

Infants are exposed to potentially epileptogenic stimuli represented by infectious agents that lead to fever and sometimes to cerebral infections. Neonates and infants may also often experience perinatal hypoxia/ischemia. In susceptible subjects these stimuli induce seizures that can occur many times a day and may be difficult to control with currently available antiepileptic drugs (160–166). Several investigators have recently begun studying the effects of high temperature or hypoxia on seizures in rats with normal and abnormal brain. The pertinent questions are: In the experimental models, do stimuli such as fever or hypoxia induce seizures if delivered early in life? If yes, do they increase subsequent seizure susceptibility? Is this change permanent? If the stimuli do not produce acute seizures, do they alter future susceptibility anyway? To date, there are studies using hyperthermia or hypoxia as the seizure-triggering stimuli in the developing brain.

Normal Brain

Hyperthermia-induced seizures in developing rats (167–170), provide a valuable model to assess developmental seizure susceptibility as a result of preexisting alterations such as hypoxia (171). In 10- to 11-day-old rats hyperthermia can be induced by exposure to a stream of heated air, and the seizures are easily quantified by behavioral and electroencephalographic techniques (168). Because of low mortality (11%) and high long-term survival, this model is suitable for long-term studies and appears to be extremely valuable for studying the mechanisms and sequelae of febrile seizures (168). While hyperthermic insult produces seizures in infant rats, these animals do not develop epilepsy.

Other studies have evaluated epileptogenesis following early life hypoxic insult (172–175). In one study, rat pups, exposed to a 3 percent O_2 on day 10 day were either kindled or exposed to corneal electroshock at adulthood at age 70 days. Neither kindled seizure development from the septal nucleus or amygdala nor electroconvulsive shock profiles were significantly altered by hypoxic pretreatment (176). In another study, rat pups were subjected to 6 percent O_2 hypoxia on either the first or tenth day of life. In flurothyl-induced seizures and amygdala kindling, there were no differences between hypoxic rats and rats not exposed to hypoxia (173). In contrast, a study that subjected 5-day-old rats to hypoxia demonstrated a slight transient increased susceptibility to seizures induced by hippocampal stimulation (174). In the hippocampal kindling model, mild or moderate hypoxia on the fifteenth day of life did not change seizure susceptibility, while severe hypoxia associated with ischemia delayed the development of kindled seizures (177). Jensen (172) determined the long-term consequences of exposure to hypoxia in 10-day-old rats. Whereas 10-day-old rats exposed to hypoxia performed normally in the water maze, open field and handling tests, these rats were more susceptible to flurothyl-induced seizures in adulthood. This effect was enhanced if the 10-day-old hypoxic rats also experienced acute seizures during hypoxia. A detailed analysis (178) showed that global hypoxia (3–4%) induces acute seizure activity in young rats during a developmental window between 5 and 10 days of age, with a peak around day 10 to 12. Animals rendered hypoxic between age 10 and 12 days had long-term decreases in seizure threshold. Although there was no apparent histologic damage in these rats suggesting that the neuronal changes are only functional (178), hypoxia-induced seizures and long-term changes in seizure susceptibility could be prevented by excitatory amino acid antagonists.

Hypoxia-induced brain injury has long-term effects on seizure thresholds. Chiba (175) showed that 10-day-old rats exposed to severe 0 percent O_2 hypoxia have increased susceptibility to pentylenetetrazol-induced seizures in adulthood. Moreover, 13 of 20 hypoxic rats developed status epilepticus in adulthood compared with none of the 20 controls. Additionally, the amygdala kindling rate in adult rats that had been subjected to hypoxia at age 10 days was twice faster than in controls. Although none of the hypoxia models induce spontaneous seizures, they do illustrate how hypoxia and hypoxia-induced seizures in young brain can increase seizure susceptibility in adult brain without altering other brain functions.

Thus, the available data suggest that febrile seizures and hypoxia-induced seizures may have model-specific consequences (172,176). This agrees with epidemiologic prospective studies in humans, which suggest that the outcome depends on the underlying disease rather than on the seizure itself (160).

Abnormal Brain

There have been only few attempts study the role of elevated temperature or hypoxia in animals with abnormal brain, although this situation may be relatively frequent in neonates and infants with seizures (179,180). In one study, in which neuronal migration disorders were induced by prenatal administration of the alkylating agent MAM, 14-day-old rat pups had a higher incidence of hyperthermia-induced seizures and a higher mortality rate than controls. Moreover, in rats with the neuronal migration disorder, hyperthermia resulted in hippocampal pyramidal cell loss independent of seizure activity (27). Long-term studies are needed to better understand the long-term effects of these changes.

CONSEQUENCES OF SEIZURES

Brain abnormalities are frequent in human epilepsy. In temporal lobe epilepsy sclerosis of Ammon's horn is frequently found. Catastrophic epileptic syndromes such as West syndrome and Lennox-Gastaut syndrome are associated with a broad spectrum of pathoanatomic abnormalities including dysraphic states, disrupted neuronal migration with pachygyria, neuronal necrosis, and microdysgenesis (128,181). Key questions include: Are repeated seizures or status epilepticus the primary cause for hippocampal damage? Do seizures beget more seizures as a consequence of seizure-induced hippocampal damage? Is seizure-induced hippocampal damage developmentally regulated (182)?

Seizure-Induced Structural Hippocampal Damage

Studies in adult animals have shown that severe or repeated seizures can indeed induce hippocampal damage (183–189). In adult rats, kainic acid, pilocarpine administration, or electric stimulation produce status epilepticus and hippocampal damage. This seizure-induced damage is more pronounced in CA_3 and hilar cells than in CA_1 (104,184,188,189) and is accompanied by sprouting of the mossy fibers of the granule cells in dentate gyrus to the supragranular layers (190–197). Later, 1 to 2 months after the insult, this damage leads to spontaneous seizures and may result in serious behavioral deficits (100,198,199). Thus, the relationship between seizures and hippocampal damage in this model suggests that repeated prolonged seizures can induce hippocampal damage, which further degrades brain function and begets further seizures.

The situation in the developing brain is less straightforward. Several studies in developing animals indicate that severe seizures induced by kainic acid, pilocarpine, or flurothyl do not produce hippocampal damage until the end of the third or beginning of the fourth postnatal week (16, 194, 200–203). Only minor damage was observed in few 15-day-old rats after pilocarpine-induced status epilepticus (202). Additionally, in 15-day-old rats, synaptic reorganization did not occur following kindling, kainic acid, or flurothyl-induced status epilepticus (194). This is in contrast with the much greater propensity of the immature brain to develop status epilepticus than the adult brain (18,204). However, under certain circumstances seizure-induced damage may occur even in young rats.

KA status epilepticus

Adult   Pup

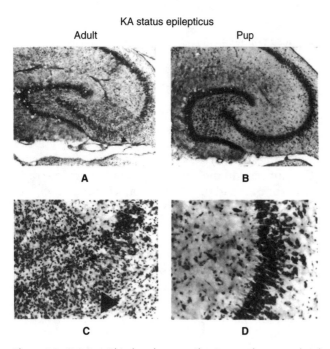

Figure 1-5. Kainic acid-induced status epilepticus produce age-related hippocampal damage. Horizontal sections from adult rat (**A, C**) showing extensive cell loss in the hippocampal CA_3 subfield following status epilepticus. In comparison, in 15-day-old rat, no cell loss is apparent (**B, D**). The severity of status epilepticus was greater in the 15-day-old rats than in the adults. Reprinted from Sperber EF, Haas, KZ, Moshé, SL. Developmental aspects of status epilepticus. *Int Pediatr* 1992; 7:213–222, with permission.

In 15-day-old rats lithium- or pilocarpine-induced status epilepticus may induce serious damage in CA_1, subiculum, neocortex, amygdala, and thalamus (182). In another study that measured neuron-specific enolase as a marker of neuronal damage after lithium- or pilocarpine-induced status epilepticus, the enzyme increased in serum after status epilepticus in 15-day-old rate, but the rise was only 10 percent as high as in adult rats (205). Taken together, these studies indicate that the immature hippocampus is more resistant to the development of seizure-induced damage than in the adult.

The question why the young brain, particularly young hippocampus, although more prone to develop status epilepticus is less vulnerable to seizure-induced damage remains unanswered. One of possible explanations may be that immature neurons are better able to clear depolarization-induced intracellular excess of calcium fast enough to prevent cell damage (97,206–208).

Seizure-Induced Functional Alterations

Do functional alterations occur in the immature brain as a consequence of severe seizures, like those observed in the catastrophic epilepsies in childhood? Although there are only few studies in developing rats with follow-up after severe seizures, an interesting difference between kainic acid–induced and pentylenetetrazol-induced status epilepticus in 10- and 25-day-old rats has been demonstrated (209). When tested at 45 days, only status epilepticus induced by kainic acid caused deficits in shuttle box–conditioned avoidance learning even though pentylenetetrazol-induced status epilepticus of similar duration and intensity. Thus, the development of learning impairment seems to be specific for kainic acid toxin and not a consequence of status epilepticus. In a different study (100), a correlation between age, behavioral, and morphologic deficits was shown. The rats experiencing kainic acid–induced status epilepticus on postnatal days 5 and 10 performed normally in behavioral tasks in adulthood. Rats exposed to kainic acid on day 20 demonstrated behavioral alterations in one task, while the rats exposed on day 30 were incapable of completing all three tests and developed hippocampal lesions. Repeated flurothyl-induced seizures in 15-day-old rats (three times daily for 5 days) impaired the performance of these rats in adulthood in the water maze and auditory location but did not induce gross morphologic deficits in the hippocampus (210).

Furthermore, seizures in the immature rats also have long-term metabolic consequences (99,211–213). An interesting insight on long-term effects of status epilepticus in young brain was recently published (99). In young rats subjected to pentylenetetrazol-induced status epilepticus at either day 10 or day 21, neurons in the neocortex, hippocampus, and thalamic and hypothalamic nuclei were transiently stained with acid fuchsin, with a peak occurring at 24 hours after the seizures. This staining was accompanied by short-term increase and long-term (in adulthood) decrease in the metabolic rate and blood flow rate in the respective structures but not by cell degeneration. Immature neurons in contrast to adult neurons were only transiently stressed by status epilepticus. Although they did not suffer gross morphologic damage, they demonstrated long-term metabolic consequences (99).

These findings may suggest that although status epilepticus early in life does not produce hippocampal damage, it may impair behavior. The consequences of seizures may vary with the seizure type and the agent used to induce the seizures. At the earlier stages of brain development, the seizures must be very severe to induce long-term functional alterations; however, all these studies have been performed in normally developing rats. To better understand the impact of seizures in catastrophic epilepsies similar studies should be performed in rats with abnormal brains (27).

Seizure-Induced Alterations in Seizure Susceptibility

Since the nineteenth century, there was a notion in human epilepsy that "seizures beget seizures" (214). Many animal models of epilepsy support this theory in adults; however, the question of whether seizures beget seizures early in life is less clear.

Prepubescent (30-day-old) and adult rats subjected to kainic acid–induced status epilepticus demonstrate a high incidence of spontaneous recurrent seizures and an increased susceptibility to seizures induced by kindling and flurothyl. However, kainic acid–induced seizures of similar severity in animals (younger than 20 days) have a low rate of spontaneous recurrent seizures in adulthood and do not differ from controls in their susceptibility to kindling- or flurothyl-induced seizures (100,199,204). The long-term consequences of pilocarpine-induced status epilepticus in adult rats are characterized by an acute period of status epilepticus, a silent period, and then chronic spontaneous recurrent seizures. Spontaneous recurrent seizures develop only in the rats exposed to pilocarpine-induced status epilepticus after day 18 of life (215).

Kindling studies in developing rats have demonstrated that rat pups easily kindle beyond stage 5 to severe seizures (stages 6–8) (37,38,216). Similarly in kittens, the development of kindling was progressive and permanent (25). These studies demonstrated that in the young brain, kindling is permanent, although permanent synaptic changes cannot be detected in the dentate gyrus. Thus, early in life there may be a dissociation between seizure-induced damage and permanence of epilepsy. Although permanent changes occur, the kindled seizures need to be triggered by external stimuli and spontaneous seizures are rare (25,37).

Unilateral intrahippocampal injection of tetanus toxin in 9- to 11-day-old rats produces a different picture (26). Within 24 to 72 hours the rat pups develop frequent, prolonged seizures in both the injected and contralateral hippocampus and bilaterally in the neocortex with multiple independent spike foci. One week later, the number of seizures decreases, but interictal spiking persists. In adulthood, some of these rats develop epilepsy and/or epileptiform EEG activity. Analysis of hippocampal slices from the epileptic adult rats shows burst discharges and paroxysmal depolarizing shifts in CA_3 neurons indicative of long-term changes in neuronal membrane properties (26).

The results suggest that in the normal rat, seizures that are triggered before the third week of life can on occasion predispose the brain to seizures in adulthood. It is interesting that on both occasions seizures early in life altered the subsequent seizure susceptibility if the seizures were multiple; however, a bout of status epilepticus does not appear to beget seizures later on.

AGE-SPECIFIC TREATMENTS

Based on clinical experience, it has been accepted that many antiepileptic drugs that are effective against partial seizures in adults may also be effective against partial seizures in infancy and early childhood (217). Developmental neurobiology , however, suggest that the young brain is not just a small version of the adult brain. There are many age-related features, factors, and functions in the young brain that may affect seizure susceptibility and seizure suppression (218). The treatment of seizures therefore should take into account these maturational changes. Additionally, there is concern about the long-term effects of antiepileptic drug treatment on brain development. Thus, the relevant questions are: What are the best age-specific treatments of seizures for the young brain? How aggressive should treatment be in terms of total seizure control if the available drugs also produce undesirable side effects? With this in mind, the consensus conference on the development of antiepileptic drugs in children proposed that studies for screening putative antiepileptic drugs should be performed in immature animals as well as in adult animals to identify agents that may be age-specific. In addition, the long-term effects of these drugs in the developing brain should be carefully assessed (217).

Several developmental studies have demonstrated age-specific short-term (acute) effects of classic antiepileptic drugs, GABAergic drugs, and excitatory amino acid antagonists (219–226) (Table 1-5).

Table 1-5. Age-Specific Effects of Antiepileptic Drugs in Rats

Effective at All Ages	Effective in Developing Brain, Ineffective in Adult Brain	Effective in Adult Brain, Ineffective or Toxic in Developing Brain
Carbamazepine	Vigabatrin	Phenytoin
Phenobarbital	Baclofen	Pyridoxine
Midazolam	MK-801	Clonazepam

Unfortunately for several drugs, the beneficiary acute anticonvulsant effects may be associated with long-term toxicity. Some drugs have acute toxic effects in the young brain at doses that are therapeutic in the adult brain.

Drugs Effective Against Seizures At All Ages

Carbamazepine and antiepileptic drugs enhancing $GABA_A$-mediated inhibition such as phenobarbital and benzodiazepines (i.e., clonazepam and midazolam) are approximately equipotent in both young and adult rats in several seizure models (220,227–230). In 12-day-old rats with pentylenetetrazol-induced seizures, however, phenobarbital and carbamazepine simultaneously suppress tonic-clonic seizures and increase the incidence of clonic seizures (228,229). This suggests that antiepileptic drugs may have differential effects on various seizure types within a single model. Prior acute administration of phenobarbital inhibits kainic acid–induced clonic seizures in both 12-day-old rays and adult rats (227). However, chronic daily administration of phenobarbital after the kainic acid challenge has more detrimental effects on memory, learning, and activity level than kainic acid–induced seizures per se (231).

Drugs Effectiveness Against Seizures in Immature and Adult Brain

Systemic administration of vigabatrin (γ-vinyl GABA); an irreversible inhibitor of the GABA-degrading enzyme GABA transaminase) 24 hours before seizure testing prevents flurothyl-induced seizures in 15-day-old but not adult rats (220). Baclofen (a $GABA_B$ receptor agonist) administered systemically is also much more effective in 15-day-old rate than in adult rats against flurothyl-, pentylenetetrazol-, and kindling-induced seizures (220,232,233).

Most of the excitatory amino acid antagonists, such as MK-801 and 2-amino-7-heptanoic acid are more effective in 12-day-old rats against pentylenetetrazol- and flurothyl-induced seizures than in adult rats (219,222,234), an effect that may be associated with blood–brain barrier maturation. In contrast, MK-801 exacerbates kainic acid–induced seizures in neonatal

and 11- to 12-day-old rats and in higher doses actually induces seizures (235). Repeated administration of MK-801 in neonatal rats leads to a significant decrease in brain size and weight (236,237). In humans MK-801 has significant behavioral effects that caused its withdrawal from clinical trials (238).

There are drugs with acute toxic effects in the young brain after doses that may be therapeutically effective or even inactive in the adult brain. Phenytoin, which is an effective antiepileptic drug in both adult and young patients (239,240), may be toxic in high doses (241,242). High doses of phenytoin per se may be toxic and proconvulsant in young rats (226). Similarly, high doses of pyridoxine may be toxic in 12- and 18-day-old rats (243).

Certain drugs, such as the NMDA receptor antagonist CGP39551, have a stronger anticonvulsant activity in adult rats than in 12-day-old rats (223). The reasons for this differential effect are unresolved (244).

FUTURE RESEARCH DIRECTIONS

The Epileptogenicity of Brain Anomalies

The brain anomalies found in catastrophic epilepsies of childhood are summarized in Table 1-6. This wide variety of anomalies may have a pre-, peri-, or even postnatal origin. As noted previously, there are several experimental models for producing neuronal migration disorders (see Table 1-3). There is a need to evaluate additional severe migration disorders that involve prenatal and perinatal neuronal alterations and alterations of radial glia to determine the epileptic potential and consequences of these malformations.

Chronic Epilepsy and Catastrophic Epilepsy

In the rat, infancy and childhood last a mere five weeks until the onset of puberty. In cats (25), the process is slower, with puberty arriving at 7 to 9 months, and can be studied for months. While the developmental models of seizures and kindling may bear certain similarities to many therapy-responding seizures in

Table 1-6. Brain Anomalies Associated with Catastrophic Epilepsies of Childhood

Syndrome	Brain Anomalies
West syndrome	Neuronal migration disruptions, pachygyria, brain weight reduction, neuronal necrosis, dysgenesis, dysraphic states (128)
Lennox-Gastaut syndrome	All of the above and small foci of neuronal necrosis in the cortical and subcortical structures of forebrain and in the cerebellum (259)

childhood, there are no for models of intractable, catastrophic epilepsies of childhood, such as early infantile epilepsies and West and Lennox-Gastaut syndromes. The available models of severe epilepsy that eventually express spontaneous seizures have an early developmental limit — epilepsy does not occur if the inducing condition (status epilepticus) occurs before age 18 days in the rat. This is later than the ages of West and Lennox-Gastaut syndromes in infants (8). Therefore, in the rat, there should be a search for age-specific seizures within the age window of 10 and 20 days with intractable features that would be similar to catastrophic childhood epilepsies. This is needed to provide a model to screen putative antiepileptics and to determine mechanisms of these therapy-resistant syndromes. In this respect, the tetanus toxin model is promising because it results in the development of spontaneous seizures. NMDA-receptor agonists also produce age-specific, intractable seizures with certain features of the West and Lennox-Gastaut syndromes, although test animals do not develop spontaneous seizures (23,245,246).

Gender Differences in Seizure Susceptibility

Historic data from patients suggest that there may be significant gender-related differences in seizure susceptibility (247). Studied in several animal models of seizures (248–251), the result point to the anticonvulsant action of progesterone and its derivatives and to the proconvulsant action of estrogens. These conclusions, however, are not supported by all studies. For example, Holmes showed that anticonvulsant effects of progesterone in kindling occurred in developing rats but not in the adult rats (252,253). Other studies show that gender differences, reflected in the control of seizures, may be operant before puberty as a result of sexually dimorphic brain organization (254–258).

With the rapid expansion of neurobiology, cell physiology, molecular biology, and neurochemistry, there is hope that appropriate developmental models of epilepsy will be created to treat epilepsies of infancy and childhood.

Acknowledgment

The research of Dr. Solomon L. Moshé, a Martin A. and Emily Fisher Fellow, is supported in part by NIH grant NS-20253. Dr. Libor Velíšek is supported in part by CURE Foundation.

REFERENCES

1. Hauser WA, Kurland LT. The epidemiology of epilepsy in Rochester, Minnesota, 1935–1967. *Epilepsia* 1975; 16:1–66.

2. Hauser W. The prevalence and incidence of convulsive disorders in children. *Epilepsia* 1994; 35:1–6.

3. Hauser WA. Incidence and prevalence. In: Engel J Jr, Pedley TA, eds. *Epilepsy: A Comprehensive Textbook.* Philadelphia: Lippincott-Raven, 1997:47–57.

4. Scher M. Neonatal seizures. In: Wyllie E, ed. *The Treatment of Epilepsy: Principles and Practice.* Baltimore: Williams & Wilkins, 1996:600–621.

5. Shields WD. Investigational antiepileptic drugs for the treatment of childhood seizure disorders: a review of efficacy and safety. *Epilepsia* 1994; 35:S24–S29.

6. Swann JW, Moshé SL. Developmental issues in animal models. In: Engel J Jr, Pedley TA, eds. *Epilepsy: A Comprehensive Textbook.* Philadelphia: Lippincott-Raven, 1997:467–479.

7. Dobbing J, Sands J. Comparative aspects of the brain growth spurt. *Early Hum Dev* 1979; 3:79–83.

8. Gottlieb A, Keydor I, Epstein HT. Rodent brain growth stages. An analytical review. *Biol Neonate* 1977; 32:166–176.

9. Ojeda SR, Urbanski HF. Puberty in the rat. In: Knobil E, ed. *The Physiology of Reproduction.* New York: Raven Press, 1994:363–411.

10. Hamon B, Heinemann U. Developmental changes in neuronal sensitivity to excitatory amino acids in area CA_1 of the rat hippocampus. *Brain Res* 1988; 466:286–290.

11. Schwartzkroin PA. Epileptogenesis in the immature CNS. In: Schwartzkroin PA, Wheal HV, eds. *Electrophysiology of Epilepsy.* London: Academic Press, 1984:389–412.

12. Swann JW, Brady RJ. Penicillin-induced epileptogenesis in immature rats CA_3 hippocampal pyramidal cells. *Dev Brain Res* 1984; 12:243–254.

13. Swann JW, Smith KL, Brady RJ. Age-dependent alterations in the operations of hippocampal neural networks. *Ann NY Acad Sci* 1991; 627:264–276.

14. Hablitz JJ, Heinemann U. Extracellular K^+ and Ca^{2+} changes during epileptiform discharges in the immature rat neocortex. *Brain Res* 1987; 433:299–303.

15. Hablitz JJ, Heinemann U. Alterations in the microenvironment during spreading depression associated with epileptiform activity in the immature neocortex. *Dev Brain Res* 1989; 46:243–252.

16. Albala BJ, Moshé SL, Okada R. Kainic-acid–induced seizures: a developmental study. *Dev Brain Res* 1984; 13:139–148.

17. Moshé SL, Sharpless NS, Kaplan J. Kindling in developing rats: afterdischarge thresholds. *Brain Res* 1981; 211:190–195.

18. Moshé SL, Albala BJ, Ackermann RF, Engel JJ. Increased seizure susceptibility of the immature brain. *Dev Brain Res* 1983; 7:81–85.

19. de Feo M, Mecarelli O, Ricci G. Bicuculline- and allyglycine-induced epilepsy in developing rats. *Exp Neurol* 1985; 90:411–421.

20. de Feo MR, Mecarelli O. Ontogenetic models of epilepsy. In: Avanzini G, Fariello R, Heinemann U,

Mutani R, eds. *Epileptogenic and Excitotoxic Mechanisms.* London: John Libbey, 1993:89–97.

21. Zouhar A, Mareš P, Liššková-Bernášková K, Mudrochová M. Motor and electrocorticographic epileptic activity induced by bicuculline in developing rats. *Epilepsia* 1989; 30:501–510.

22. Velíšek L, Kubová H, Pohl M, et al. Pentylenetetrazol-induced seizures in rats: an ontogenetic study. *Naunyn-Schmiedeberg's Arch Pharmacol* 1992; 346:588–591.

23. Mareš P, Velíšek L. *N*-methyl-*D*-aspartate (NMDA)-induced seizures in developing rats. *Dev Brain Res* 1992; 65:185–189.

24. Baram TZ, Hirsch E, Schultz L. Short-interval amygdala kindling in neonatal rats. *Dev Brain Res* 1993; 73:79–83.

25. Shouse MN, King A, Langer J, et al. The ontogeny of feline temporal lobe epilepsy: kindling a spontaneous seizure disorder in kittens. *Dev Brain Res* 1990; 52:215–224.

26. Lee CL, Hrachovy RA, Smith KL, Frost JD Jr, Swann JW. Tetanus toxin–induced seizures in infant rats and their effects on hippocampal excitability in adulthood. *Brain Res* 1995; 677:97–109.

27. Germano IM, Zhang YF, Sperber EF, Moshé SL. Neuronal migration disorders increase susceptibility to hyperthermia-induced seizures in developing rats. *Epilepsia* 1996; 37:902–910.

28. Germano IM, Sperber EF. Increased seizure susceptibility in adult rats with neuronal migration disorders. *Brain Res* 1997; 777:219–222.

29. Roper SN, Gilmore RL, Houser CR. Experimentally induced disorders of neuronal migration produce an increased propensity for electrographic seizures in rats. *Epilepsy Res* 1995; 21:205–219.

30. Luhman HJ, Raabe K. Characterization of neuronal migration disorders in neocortical structures: I. Expression of epileptiform activity in an animal model. *Epilepsy Res* 1996; 26:67–74.

31. Gonzalez JL, Russo CJ, Goldowitz D, et al. Birthdate and cell marker analysis of scrambler: a novel mutation affecting cortical development with a reeler-like phenotype. *J Neurosci* 1997; 17:9204–9211.

32. Michelson HB, Lothman EW. An in vivo electrophysiological study of the ontogeny of excitatory and inhibitory processes in the rat hippocampus. *Dev Brain Res* 1989; 47:113–122.

33. Velíšek L, Mareš P. Increased epileptogenesis in the immature hippocampus. *Exp Brain Res Series* 1991; 20:183–185.

34. Michelson HB, Williamson JM, Lothman EW. Ontogeny of kindling: the acquisition of kindled responses at different ages with rapidly recurring hippocampal seizures. *Epilepsia* 1989; 30:672.

35. Goddard GV. The kindling model of epilepsy. *Trends Neurosci* 1983; 7:275–279.

36. Racine R. Kindling: the first decade. *Neurosurgery* 1978; 3:234–252.

37. Haas K, Sperber EF, Moshé SL. Kindling in developing animals: expression of severe seizures and enhanced development of bilateral foci. *Dev Brain Res* 1990; 56:275–280.

38. Haas KZ, Sperber EF, Moshé SL. Kindling in developing animals: interactions between ipsilateral foci. *Dev Brain Res* 1992; 68:140–143.

39. Burchfiel JL, Serpa KA, Duffy FH. Further studies of antagonism of seizure development between concurrently developing kindled limbic foci in the rat. *Exp Neurol* 1982; 75:476–489.

40. Pinel JPJ, Rovner LI. Experimental epileptogenesis: kindling-induced epilepsy in rats. *Exp Neurol* 1978; 58:190–202.

41. Ben-Ari Y, Khazipov R, Leinekugel X, Caillard O, Gaiarsa J-L. GABA$_A$, NMDA and AMPA receptors: a developmentally regulated 'ménage á trois.' *Trends Neurosci* 1997; 20:523–529.

42. Tremblay E, Roisin MP, Represa A, Charriaut-Marlangue C, Ben-Ari Y. Transient increased density of NMDA binding sites in the developing rat hippocampus. *Brain Res* 1988; 461:393–396.

43. Tsumoto T, Hagihara H, Sato H, Hata S. NMDA receptors in the visual cortex of young kittens are more effective than those of adult cats. *Nature* 1987; 327:513–514.

44. Mueller A, Chesnut R, Schwartzkroin P. Actions of GABA in developing rabbit hippocampus: an *in vitro* study. *Neurosci Lett* 1983; 39:193–198.

45. Michelson HB, Wong RKS. Excitatory synaptic responses mediated by GABA(A) receptors in the hippocampus. *Science* 1991; 253:1420–1423.

46. Garant DS, Sperber EF, Moshé SL. The density of GABA$_B$ binding sites in the substantia nigra is greater in rat pups than in adults. *Eur J Pharmacol* 1992; 214:75–78.

47. Schwartzkroin PA, Kunkel DD, Mathers LH. Development of rabbit hippocampus: anatomy. *Dev Brain Res* 1982; 2:452–468.

48. Schwartzkroin PA. Development of rabbit hippocampus: physiology. *Dev Brain Res* 1982; 2:469–486.

49. Swann JW, Smith KL, Gomez CM, Brady RJ. The ontogeny of hippocampal local circuits and focal epileptogenesis. *Epilepsy Res Suppl* 1992; 9:115–125.

50. Swann JW. Synaptogenesis and epileptogenesis in developing neural networks. In: Schwartzkroin PA, Moshé SL, Noebells JL, Swann JW, eds. *Brain Development and Epilepsy.* New York: Oxford University Press, 1995:195–233.

51. Peinado A, Yuste R, Katz LC. Extensive dye coupling between rat neocortical neurons during the critical period of circuit formation. *Neuron* 1993; 10:103–114.

52. Swann JW, Smith KL, Brady RJ. Neural networks and synaptic transmission in immature hippocampus. *Adv Exp Med Biol* 1990; 268:161–171.

53. Pellegrini-Giampietro D, Bennett M, Zukin R. Differential expression of three glutamate receptor genes in developing rat brain: an in situ hybridization study. *Proc Natl Acad Sci USA* 1991; 88:4157–4161.

54. Pellegrini-Giampietro DE, Gorter JA, Bennett MV, Zukin RS. The GluR2 (GluR-B) hypothesis: Ca(2+)-permeable AMPA receptors in neurological disorders. *Trends Neurosci* 1997; 20:464–470.

55. Laurie DJ, Wisden W, Seeburg PH. The distribution of thirteen GABA$_A$ receptor subunit mRNAs in the rat brain. III. Embryonic and postnatal development. *J Neurosci* 1992; 12:4151–4172.

56. Moshé SL, Garant DS, Sperber EF, et al. Ontogeny and topography of seizure regulation by the substantia nigra. *Brain Dev* 1995; 17(Suppl):61–72.

57. Corcorán ME, Mason ST. Role of forebrain catecholamines in amygdaloid kindling. *Brain Res* 1980; 190:473–484.

58. McIntyre DC, Edson N. Facilitation of amygdala kindling after norepinephrine depletion with 6-hydroxydopamine in rats. *Exp Neurol* 1981; 74:748–757.

59. Burchfiel JL, Applegate CD, Konkol RJ. Kindling antagonism: a role for norepinephrine in seizure suppression. In: Wada JA, ed. *Kindling 3*. New York: Raven Press, 1986:213–229.

60. Shinnar S, Berg AT, Moshé SL, et al. Risk of seizure recurrence following a first unprovoked seizure in childhood. *Pediatrics* 1990; 85:1076–1085.

61. Moshé S, Shinnar S, Swann J. Partial (focal) seizures in developing brain. In: Schwarzkroin P, Moshé S, Noebels J, Swann JW, eds. *Brain Development and Epilepsy*. New York: Oxford University Press, 1995:34–65.

62. Rodier PM. Developing brain as a target of toxicity. *Environ Health Perspect* 1995; 103(Suppl 6):73–76.

63. Hayakawa K, Konishi Y, Kuriyama M, Konishi K, Matsuda T. Normal brain maturation in MRI. *Eur J Radiol* 1991; 12:208–215.

64. Spitzer NC. Regulation of excitability in developing neurons. In: Schwartzkroin PA, Moshé SL, Noebells JL, Swann JW, eds. *Brain Development and Epilepsy*. New York: Oxford University Press, 1995:144–170.

65. Fukuda A, Prince DA. Postnatal development of electrogenic sodium pump activity in rat hippocampal pyramidal neurons. *Brain Res Dev Brain Res* 1992; 65:101–114.

66. Kohling R, Lucke A, Nagao T, Speckmann EJ, Avoli M. Extracellular potassium elevations in the hippocampus of rats with long-term pilocarpine seizures. *Neurosci Lett* 1995; 201:87–91.

67. Heinemann U, Lux HD. Ceiling of stimulus-induced rises in extracellular potassium concentration in the cat. *Brain Res* 1977; 120:231–249.

68. Swann JW, Smith KL, Brady RJ. Extracellular K$^+$ accumulation during penicillin induced epileptogenesis in the CA$_3$ region of immature rat hippocampus. *Dev Brain Res* 1986; 395:243–255.

69. Haglund MM, Schwartzkroin PA. Role of Na-K pump potassium regulation and IPSPs in seizures and spreading depression in immature rabbit hippocampal slices. *J Neurophysiol* 1990; 63:225–239.

70. Mutani R, Futamachi KJ, Prince DA. Potassium activity in immature cortex. *Brain Res* 1984; 75:27–39.

71. Grisar T. Glial and neuronal Na-K-pump in epilepsy. *Ann Neurol* 1984; 16:128–134.

72. Ballanyi K, Grafe P, ten Bruggencate G. Ion activities and potassium uptake mechanisms of glial cells in guinea pig olfactory cortex slices. *J Physiol (London)* 1987; 382:159–174.

73. Heinemann U, Albrecht D, Beck H, et al. Potassium homeostasis and epileptogenesis in the immature hippocampus. In: Avanzini G, Fariello R, Heinemann U, Mutani R, eds. *Epileptogenic and Excitotoxic Mechanisms*. London: John Libbey, 1993:99–106.

74. Ransom BR, Carlini WG, Connors BW. Brain extracellular space: developmental studies in rat optic nerve. *Ann NY Acad Sci* 1986; 481:87–105.

75. Lothman EW, Somjen GG. Extracellular potassium activity, intracellular and extracellular potential responses in the spinal cord. *J Physiol (London)* 1975; 252:115–136.

76. Nixdorf-Bergweiler BE, Albrecht D, Heinemann U. Developmental changes in the number, size, and orientation of GFAP-positive cells in the CA$_1$ region of rat hippocampus. *Glia* 1994; 12:180–195.

77. Vernadakis A. Neuronal–glial interactions during development and aging. *Fed Proc* 1975; 34:89–95.

78. Brady RJ, Smith KL, Swann JW. Calcium modulation of the N-methyl-D-aspartate (NMDA) response and electrographic seizures in immature hippocampus. *Neurosci Lett* 1991; 124:92–96.

79. Baudry M, Arst D, Oliver M, Lynch G. Development of glutamate binding sites and their regulation by calcium in the rat hippocampus. *Dev Brain Res* 1981; 1:37–48.

80. Mayer ML, Westbrook GL, Guthrie PB. Voltage dependent block by Mg^{2+} of NMDA responses in spinal cord neurons. *Nature* 1984; 309:261–263.

81. Bading H, Ginty DD, Greenberg ME. Regulation of gene expression in hippocampal neurons by distinct calcium signaling pathways. *Science* 1993; 260:181–186.

82. Coulter DA, Huguenard JR, Prince DA. Calcium currents in rat thalamocortical relay neurones: kinetic properties of the transient, low threshold current. *J Physiol* 1989; 414:587–604.

83. Thompson SM, Wong RK. Development of calcium current subtypes in isolated rat hippocampal pyramidal cells. *J Physiol* 1991; 439:671–689.

84. Yaari Y, Hamon B, Lux HD. Development of two types of calcium channels in cultured mammalian hippocampal neurons. *Science* 1987; 235:680–682.

85. Sokoloff L, Reivich M, Kennedy C, et al. The [^{14}C] deoxyglucose method for the measurement of local cerebral glucose utilization: theory, procedures and normal values in the conscious and anesthetized albino rat. *J Neurochem* 1977; 28:897–916.

86. Daval JL, Pereira de Vasconcelos A, el Hamdi G, Werck MC, Nehlig A. Quantitative autoradiographic measurements of functional changes induced by generalized seizures in the developing rat brain: central adenosine and benzodiazepine receptors and local cerebral glucose utilization. *Epilepsy Res Suppl* 1992; 9:83–92; discussion 93.

87. Tremblay E, Nitecka L, Berger M, Ben-Ari Y. Maturation of kainic acid seizure–brain damage syndrome in the rat. I. Clinical, electrographic and metabolic observations. *Neuroscience* 1984; 13:1051–1072.

88. Ackermann RF, Moshé SL, Albala BJ, Engel JJ. Anatomical substrates of amygdala kindling in immature rats demonstrated by 2-deoxyglucose autoradiography. *Epilepsia* 1982; 23:434–435.

89. Ackermann RF, Moshé SL, Albala BJ. Restriction of enhanced ^{14}C-2-deoxyglucose utilization to rhinencephalic structures in immature amygdala-kindled rats. *Exp Neurol* 1989; 104:73–81.

90. Cherubini E, DeFeo MR, Mecarelli O, Ricci GF. Behavioral and electrographic patterns induced by systemic administration of kainic acid in developing rats. *Dev Brain Res* 1983; 9:69–77.

91. Ben-Ari Y, Tremblay E, Berger M, Nitecka L. Kainic acid seizure syndrome and binding sites in developing rats. *Dev Brain Res* 1984; 14:284–288.

92. Velíšková J, Velíšek L, Mareš P. Epileptic phenomena produced by kainic acid in laboratory rats during ontogenesis. *Physiol Bohemoslov* 1988; 37:395–405.

93. Sperber EF, Moshé SL. Age-related differences in seizure susceptibility to flurothyl. *Dev Brain Res* 1988; 39:295–297.

94. Ben-Ari Y, Riche D, Tremblay E, Charton G. Alterations in local glucose consumption following systemic administration of kainic acid, bicuculline or metrazol. *Eur Neurol* 1981; 20:173–175.

95. Vernadakis A, Woodbury DM. The developing animal as a model. *Epilepsia* 1969; 10:163–178.

96. Pereira de Vasconcelos A, el Hamdi G, Vert P, Nehlig A. An experimental model of generalized seizures for the measurement of local cerebral glucose utilization in the immature rat. II. Mapping of the brain metabolism using quantitative [^{14}C]-2-deoxyglucose technique. *Dev Brain Res* 1992; 69:243–259.

97. Pereira de Vasconcelos A, Boyet S, Koziel V, Nehlig A. Effects of pentylenetetrazol-induced status epilepticus on local cerebral blood flow in the developing rat. *J Cereb Blood Flow Metab* 1995; 15:270–283.

98. Nehlig A. Cerebral energy metabolism, glucose transport and blood flow: changes with maturation and adaptation to hypoglycaemia. *Diabetes Metab* 1997; 23:18–29.

99. Nehlig A, Pereira de Vasconcelos A. The model of pentylenetetrazol-induced status epilepticus in the immature rat: short- and long-term effects. *Epilepsy Res* 1996; 26:93–103.

100. Stafstrom CE, Chronopoulos A, Thurber S, Thompson JL, Holmes GL. Age-dependent cognitive and behavioral deficits after kainic acid seizures. *Epilepsia* 1993; 34:420–432.

101. Ben-Ari Y. Limbic seizure and brain damage produced by kainic acid: mechanisms and relevance to human temporal lobe epilepsy. *Neurosci* 1985; 14:375–403.

102. Engel JJ, Wolfson L, Brown LL. Anatomical correlates of electrical and behavioral events related to amygdaloid kindling. *Ann Neurol* 1978; 3:538–544.

103. Campbell KA. Plasticity in the propagation of hippocampal stimulation–induced activity: a [^{14}C]2-deoxyglucose mapping study. *Brain Res* 1990; 520:199–207.

104. Lothman EW, Collins RC. Kainic acid induced limbic seizures: metabolic, behavioral, electroencephalographic and neuropathological correlates. *Brain Res* 1981; 218:299–318.

105. Pereira de Vasconcelos A, Vergnes M, Boyet S, Marescaux C, Nehlig A. Forebrain metabolic activation induced by the repetition of audiogenic seizures in Wistar rats. *Brain Res* 1997; 762:114–120.

106. Wooten GF, Collins RC. Regional brain glucose utilization following intrastriatal injections of kainic acid. *Brain Res* 1980; 201:173–184.

107. Sperber EF, Stanton PK, Haas K, Ackermann RF, Moshé SL. Developmental differences in the neurobiology of epileptic brain damage. *Epilepsy Res Suppl* 1992; 9:67–80; discussion 80–81.

108. Gale K. Subcortical structures and pathways involved in convulsive seizure generalization. *J Clin Neurophysiol* 1992; 9:264–277.

109. Gale K, Pazos A, Maggio R, Japikse K, Pritchard P. Blockade of GABA receptors in superior colliculus protects against focally evoked limbic motor seizures. *Brain Res* 1993; 603:279–283.

110. Iadarola MJ, Gale K. Substantia nigra: site of anticonvulsant activity mediated by γ-aminobutyric acid. *Science* 1982; 218:1237–1240.

111. Maggio R, Gale K. Seizures evoked from area tempestas are subject to control by GABA and glutamate receptors in substantia nigra. *Exp Neurol* 1989; 105:184–188.

112. Redgrave P, Marrow L, Dean P. Anticonvulsant role of nigrotectal projection in the maximal electroshock model of epilepsy. II. Pathways from substantia nigra pars lateralis and adjacent peripeduncular area to the dorsal midbrain. *Neuroscience* 1992; 46:391–406.

113. Redgrave P, Marrow L, Dean P. Topographical organization of the nigrotectal projection in rat: evidence for segregated channels. *Neuroscience* 1992; 50:571–595.

114. Redgrave P, Simkins M, Overton P, Dean P. Anticonvulsant role of nigrotectal projection in the maximal electroshock model of epilepsy. I. Mapping of dorsal midbrain with bicuculline. *Neuroscience* 1992; 46:379–390.

115. Deransart C, Marescaux C, Depaulis A. Involvement of nigral glutamatergic inputs in the control of seizures in a genetic model of absence epilepsy in the rat. *Neuroscience* 1996; 71:721–728.

116. Velíšková J, Velíšek L, Moshé SL. Subthalamic nucleus: a new anticonvulsant site in the brain. *NeuroReport* 1996; 7:1786–1788.

117. Moshé SL, Brown LL, Kubová H, et al. Maturation and segregation of brain networks that modify seizures. *Brain Res* 1994; 665:141–146.

118. Velíšková J, Velíšek L, Nunes M, Moshé S. Developmental regulation of regional functionality of substantia nigra GABA$_A$ receptors involved in seizures. *Eur J Pharmacol* 1996; 309:167–173.

119. Shebab S, Simkins M, Dean P, Redgrave P. Regional distribution of the anticonvulsant and behavioral effects of muscimol injected into the substantia nigra of rats. *Eur J Neurosci* 1996; 8:749–757.

120. Velíšková J, Löscher W, Moshé SL. Regional and age specific effects of zolpidem microinfusions in the substantia nigra on seizures. *Epilepsy Res* 1998; 30:107–114.

121. Velíšek L, Velíšková J, Moshé SL. Site-specific effects of local pH changes in the substantia nigra pars reticulata on flurothyl-induced seizures. *Brain Res* 1998; 782:310–313.

122. Wisden W, Laurie DJ, Monyer H, Seeburg PH. The distribution of 13 GABA$_A$ receptor subunit mRNAs in the rat brain. I. Telencephalon, diencephalon, mesencephalon. *J Neurosci* 1992; 12:1040–1062.

123. Moshé SL, Albala BJ. Nigral muscimol infusions facilitate the development of seizures in immature rats. *Dev Brain Res* 1984; 13:305–308.

124. Xu SG, Garant DS, Sperber EF, Moshé SL. The proconvulsant effect of nigral infusion of THIP on flurothyl-induced seizures in rat pups. *Dev Brain Res* 1992; 68:275–277.

125. Lee VWK, de Kretser DM, Hudson B, Wang C. Variations in serum FSH, LH and testosterone levels in male rats from birth to sexual maturity. *J Reprod Fert* 1975; 42:121–126.

126. Piacsek BE, Goodspeed MP. Maturation of the pituitary-gonadal system in the male rat. *J Reprod Fert* 1978; 52:29–35.

127. Döhler KD, Wuttke W. Changes with age in levels of serum gonadotropins, prolactin, and gonadal steroids in prepubertal male and female rats. *Endocrinology* 1975; 97:898–907.

128. Meencke HJ, Gerhard C. Morphological aspects of aetiology and the course of infantile spasms (West syndrome). *Neuropediatrics* 1985; 16:59–66.

129. Nagata Y, Matsumoto H. Studies on methylazoxymethanol: methylation of nucleic acids in fetal rat brain. *Proc Soc Exp Biol Med* 1969; 132:383–385.

130. Angerine JB, Sidman RL. Autoradiographic study of cell migration during histogenesis of cerebral cortex of mouse. *Nature* 1961; 1192:766–768.

131. Germano IM, Sperber EF. Transplacentally induced neuronal migration disorders: an animal model for the study of the epilepsies. *J Neurosci Res* 1998; 51:473–488.

132. de Feo MR, Mecarelli O, Ricci GF. Seizure susceptibility in immature rats with microencephaly induced by prenatal exposure to methylazoxymethanol acetate. *Pharmacol Res* 1995; 31:109–114.

133. Rafiki A, Chevassus-au-Louis N, Ben-Ari Y, Khrestchatisky M, Represa A. Glutamate receptors in dysplastic cortex: an in situ hybridization and immunohistochemistry study in rats with prenatal treatment with methylazoxymethanol. *Brain Res* 1998; 782:147–152.

134. Baraban SC, Schwartzkroin PA. Electrophysiology of CA_1 pyramidal neurons in an animal model of neuronal migration disorders: prenatal methylazoxymethanol treatment. *Epilepsy Res* 1995; 22:145–156.

135. Escueta AV, Davidson D, Hartwig G, Reilly E. The freezing lesion. II. Potassium transport within nerve terminals isolated from epileptogenic foci. *Brain Res* 1974; 78:223–227.

136. Escueta AV, Davidson D, Hartwig G, Reilly E. The freezing lesion. III. The effects of diphenylhydantoin on potassium transport within nerve terminals from the primary foci. *Brain Res* 1975; 86:85–96.

137. Dvořák K, Feit J. Migration of neuroblasts through partial necrosis of the cerebral cortex in newborn rats. Contribution of the problems of morphological developmental period of cerebral microgyria. *Acta Neuropathol* 1977; 38:203–212.

138. Rosen GD, Sherman GF, Galaburda AM. Birthdates of neurons in induced microgyria. *Brain Res* 1996; 727:71–78.

139. Jacobs KM, Gutnick MJ, Prince DA. Hyperexcitability in a model of cortical maldevelopment. *Cereb Cortex* 1996; 6:514–523.

140. Rosen GD, Sigel EA, Sherman GF, Galaburda AM. The neuroprotective effects of MK-801 on the induction of microgyria by freezing injury to the newborn rat neocortex. *Neuroscience* 1995; 69:107–114.

140a. Luhmann HJ, Raabe K. Characterization of neuronal migration disorders in neocortical structures. *Epilepsy Res* 1996; 26:67–74.

141. Roper SN, King MA, Abraham LA, Boillot MA. Disinhibited in vitro neocortical slices containing experimentally induced cortical dysplasia demonstrate hyperexcitability. *Epilepsy Res* 1997; 26:443–449.

142. Pennacchio LA, Lehesjoki AE, Stone NE, et al. Mutations in the gene encoding cystatin B in progressive myoclonus epilepsy (EPM1) [see comments]. *Science* 1996; 271:1731–1734.

143. Noebels JL, Tharp BL. Absence seizures in developing brain. In: Schwartzkroin PA, Moshé SL, Noebels JL, Swann JW, eds. *Brain Development and Epilepsy.* New York: Oxford University Press, 1995:66–93.

144. Meldrum BS, Horton RW. Convulsive effects of 4-deoxy-pyridoxine and of bicuculline in photosensitive baboons (*Papio papio*) and in rhesus monkeys (*Maccaca mulatta*). *Brain Res* 1971; 35:419–436.

145. Meldrum BS, Horton RW. Neuronal inhibition mediated by GABA and patterns of convulsions in baboons with photosensitive epilepsy. In: Harris P, Mawdsley C, eds. *Epilepsy.* New York: Churchill-Livingstone, 1974:55–64.

146. Meldrum BS, Horton RW, Brierley JB. Epileptic brain damage in adolescent baboons following seizures induced by allyl-glycine. *Brain* 1974; 97:407–418.

147. Meldrum BS, Croucher MJ, Badman G, Collins JF. Anti-epileptic action of excitatory amino acid antagonists in the photosensitive baboon, *Papio papio*. *Neurosci Lett* 1983; 39:101–104.

148. Meldrum BS. GABAergic agents as anticonvulsants in baboons with photosensitive epilepsy. *Neurosci Lett* 1984; 47:345–349.

149. Naquet R, Menini C, Riche D, Silva-Barrat C, Valin A. Photic epilepsy in man and in the baboon, *Papio papio*. In:

Meldrum BS, Ferrendelli JA, Wieser HG, eds. *Anatomy of Epileptogenesis*. London: John Libbey, 1988:107–126.

150. Fisher RS. Animal models of epilepsies. *Brain Res Rev* 1989; 14:245–278.

151. Browning RA, Wang C, Lanker ML, Jobe PC. Electroshock- and pentylenetetrazol-induced seizures in genetically epilepsy-prone rats (GEPRs): differences in threshold and pattern. *Epilepsy Res* 1990; 6:1–11.

152. Browning RA, Wade DR, Marcinczyk M, Long GL, Jobe PC. Regional brain abnormalities in norepinephrine uptake and dopamine beta-hydroxylase activity in the genetically epilepsy prone rat. *J Pharmacol Exp Ther* 1989; 249:229–235.

153. Jobe PC, Mishra PK, Ludvig N, Dailey JW. Scope and contribution of genetic models to an understanding of the epilepsies. *Crit Rev Neurobiol* 1991; 6:183–220.

154. Marescaux C, Vergnes M, Depaulis A. Genetic absence epilepsy in rats from Strasbourg — A review. *J Neural Transm* 1992; 35(Suppl):37–69.

155. Ramakers GMJ, Peeters BWMM, Vossen JMH, Coenen AML. CNQX, a new non-NMDA receptor antagonist, reduces spike wave discharges in the WAG/Rij rat model of absence epilepsy. *Epilepsy Res* 1991; 9:127–131.

156. Vergnes M, Marescaux C, Depaulis A, Micheletti G, Warter JM. Ontogeny of spontaneous petit mal–like seizures in Wistar rats. *Dev Brain Res* 1986; 30:85-87.

157. Coenen AM, Van Luijtelaar EL. The WAG/Rij rat model for absence epilepsy: age and sex factors. *Epilepsy Res* 1987; 1:297–301.

158. Noebels JL. Genetic and phenotypic heterogeneity of inherited spike-and-and wave epilepsies. In: Malafosse A, Genton P, Hirsch E, et al., eds. *Idiopathic Generalized Epilepsies*. London: John Libbey, 1994:215–225.

159. Gleeson JG, Allen KM, Fox JW, et al. Double cortin, a brain-specific gene mutated in human *X*-linked lissencephaly and double cortex syndrome, encodes a putative signaling protein. *Cell* 1998; 92:63–72.

160. Verity CM, Ross EM, Golding J. Epilepsy in the first 10 years of life: findings of the child health and education study. *Br Med J* 1992; 305:857–861.

161. Nelson KB, Ellenberg JH. Predictors of epilepsy in children who have experienced febrile seizures. *N Engl J Med* 1976; 295:1029–1033.

162. Coulter DL. Continuous infantile spasms as a form of status epilepticus. *J Child Neurol* 1986; 1:215–217.

163. Constantinou JE, Gillis J, Ouvrier RA, Rahilly PM. Hypoxic-ischaemic encephalopathy after near miss sudden infant death syndrome. *Arch Dis Childhood* 1989; 64:703–708.

164. Cowan LD, Bodensteiner JB, Leviton A, Doherty L. Prevalence of the epilepsies in children and adolescents. *Epilepsia* 1989; 30:94–106.

165. Liu CC, Chen JS, Lin CH, Chen YJ, Huang CC. Bacterial meningitis in infants and children in southern Taiwan: emphasis on *Haemophilus influenzae* type B infection. *J Formosa Med Assoc* 1993; 92:884–888.

166. Wen DY, Bottini AG, Hall WA, Haines SJ. Infections in neurologic surgery. The intraventricular use of antibiotics. *Neurosurg Clin N Am* 1992; 3:343–354.

167. Morimoto T, Fukuda M, Aibara Y, Nagao H, Kida K. The influence of blood gas changes on hyperthermia-induced seizures in developing rats. *Dev Brain Res* 1996; 92:77–80.

168. Baram TZ, Gerth A, Schultz L. Febrile seizures: an appropriate-aged model suitable for long-term studies. *Dev Brain Res* 1997; 98:265–270.

169. Holtzman D, Obana K, Olson J. Hyperthermia-induced seizures in the rat pup: a model for febrile convulsions in children. *Science* 1981; 213:1034–1036.

170. Olson JE, Scher MS, Holtzman D. Effects of anticonvulsants on hyperthermia-induced seizures in the rat pup. *Epilepsia* 1984; 25:96–99.

171. Olson JE, Horne DS, Holtzman D, Miller M. Hyperthermia-induced seizures in rat pups with preexisting ischemic brain injury. *Epilepsia* 1985; 26:360–364.

172. Jensen FE, Holmes GL, Lombroso CT, Blume HK, Firkusny IR. Age-dependent changes in long-term seizure susceptibility and behavior after hypoxia in rats. *Epilepsia* 1992; 33:971–980.

173. Moshé SL, Albala BJ. Perinatal hypoxia and subsequent development of seizures. *Physiol Behav* 1985; 35:819–823.

174. Maresová D, Mareš P. Effect of hypoxia on hippocampal afterdischarges in young rats. *Exp Brain Res Series* 1991; 20:171–173.

175. Chiba S. Long term effect of postnatal hypoxia on the seizure susceptibility in rats. *Life Sci* 1985; 37:1597–1604.

176. Applegate CD, Jensen F, Burchfiel JL, Lombroso C. The effects of neonatal hypoxia on kindled seizure development and electroconvulsive shock profiles. *Epilepsia* 1996; 37:723–727.

177. Holmes GL, Weber DA. Effects of hypoxic-ischemic encephalopathies on kindling in developing animals. *Exp Neurol* 1985; 90:194–203.

178. Jensen FE. An animal model of hypoxia-induced perinatal seizures. *Ital J Neurol Sci* 1995; 16:59–68.

179. Watanabe K, Takeuchi T, Hakamada S, Hayakawa F. Neurophysiological and neuroradiological features preceding infantile spasms. *Brain Dev* 1987; 9:391–398.

180. Watanabe K, Hara K, Miyazaki S, Hakamada S. The role of perinatal brain injury in the genesis of childhood epilepsy. *Fol Psych Neurol Jap* 1980; 34:227–232.

181. Meencke HJ, Veith G. Hippocampal sclerosis in epilepsy. In: Lüders HO, ed. *Epilepsy Surgery*. New York: Raven Press, 1991:705–715.

182. Wasterlain CG. Recurrent seizures in the developing brain are harmful. *Epilepsia* 1997; 38:728–734.

183. Bekenstein J, Rempe D, Lothman E. Decreased heterosynaptic and homosynaptic paired pulse inhibition in the rat hippocampus as a chronic sequela to limbic status epilepticus. *Brain Res* 1993; 111–120.

184. Nadler JV, Perry BW, Cotman CW. Intraventricular kainic acid preferentially destroys hippocampal pyramidal cells. *Nature* 1978; 271:676–677.

185. Sloviter RS. "Epileptic" brain damage in rats induced by sustained stimulation of the perforant path I. Acute electrophysiological and light microscope studies. *Brain Res Bull* 1983; 10:675–697.

186. Sloviter RS. Decreased hippocampal inhibition and a selective loss of interneurons in experimental epilepsy. *Science* 1987; 235:73–76.

187. Sloviter RS, Dean E, Sollas AL, Goodman JH. Apoptosis and necrosis induced in different hippocampal neuron populations by repetitive perforant path stimulation in the rat. *J Comp Neurol* 1996; 366:516–533.

188. Schmidt-Kastner R, Humpel C, Wetmore C, Olson L. Cellular hybridization for BDNF, trkB, and NGF mRNAs and BDNF-immunoreactivity in rat forebrain after pilocarpine-induced status epilepticus. *Exp Brain Res* 1996; 107:331–347.

189. Schmidt-Kastner R, Heim C, Sontag K-H. Damage of substantia nigra pars reticulata during pilocarpine-induced status epilepticus in the rat: immunohistochemical study of neurons, astrocytes and serum-protein extravasation. *Exp Brain Res* 1991; 86:125–140.

190. Cronin J, Dudek FE. Chronic seizures and collateral sprouting of dentate mossy fibers after kainic acid treatment in rats. *Brain Res* 1988; 474:181–184.

191. Golarai G, Parada I, Sutula T. Mossy fiber synaptic reorganization induced by repetitive pentylenetetrazol seizures. *Soc Neurosci Abstr* 1988; 14:882.

192. Nadler JV, Perry BW, Cotman CW. Selective reinnervation of hippocampal area CA_1 and the fascia dentata after destruction of CA_3–CA_4 afferents. *Brain Res* 1980; 182:1–9.

193. Sutula T, He X, Cavazos J, Scott G. Synaptic reorganization induced in the hippocampus by abnormal functional activity. *Science* 1988; 239:1147–1150.

194. Sperber EF. The relationship between seizures and damage in the maturing brain. In: Heinemann U, Engel J Jr, Avanzini G, et al., eds. *Progressive Nature of Epileptogenesis*. Amsterdam: Elsevier, 1996:365–376.

195. Tauck DL, Nadler JV. Evidence of functional mossy fiber sprouting in hippocampal formation of kainic acid–treated rats. *J Neurosci* 1985; 5:1016–1022.

196. Sperk G, Lassman H, Baran H, Seitelberger F, Hornykiewicz O. Kainic acid–induced seizures: dose relationship of behavioural, neurochemical and histopathological changes. *Brain Res* 1985; 338:289–295.

197. Lassman H, Petsche U, Kitz K, et al. The role of brain edema in epileptic brain damage induced by systemic kainic acid injection. *Neuroscience* 1984; 13:691.

198. Lothman EW, Bertram EH, Kapur J, Stringer JL. Recurrent spontaneous hippocampal seizures in the rat as a chronic sequela to limbic status epilepticus. *Epilepsy Res* 1990; 6:110–118.

199. Holmes GL. The long-term effects of seizures on the developing brain: clinical and laboratory issues. *Brain Dev* 1991; 13:393–409.

200. Holmes GL, Thompson JL. Effects of kainic acid on seizure susceptibility in the developing brain. *Dev Brain Res* 1988; 39:51–59.

201. Nitecka L, Tremblay E, Charton G, et al. Maturation of kainic acid seizure-brain damage syndrome in the rat. II. Histopathological sequelae. *Neuroscience* 1984; 13:1073–1094.

202. Cavalheiro EA, Silva DF, Turski WA, et al. The susceptibility of rats to pilocarpine-induced seizures is age-dependent. *Dev Brain Res* 1987; 465:43–58.

203. Sperber EF, Haas KZ, Stanton PK, Moshé SL. Resistance of the immature brain to seizure-induced synaptic reorganization. *Dev Brain Res* 1991; 60:88–93.

204. Okada R, Moshé SL, Albala BJ. Infantile status epilepticus and future seizure susceptibility in the rat. *Dev Brain Res* 1984; 15:177–183.

205. Sankar R, Shin DH, Wasterlain CG. Serum neuron-specific enolase is a marker for neuronal damage following status epilepticus in the rat. *Epilepsy Res* 1997; 28:129–136.

206. Schanne FAX, Kane AB, Young EE, Farber JL. Calcium dependence of toxic cell death: a final common pathway. *Science* 1979; 205:700–702.

207. Alcantara S, de Lecea L, Del Rio JA, Ferrer I, Soriano E. Transient colocalization of parvalbumin and calbindin D28k in the postnatal cerebral cortex: evidence for a phenotypic shift in developing nonpyramidal neurons. *Eur J Neurosci* 1996; 8:1329–1339.

208. Friedman LK, Sperber EF, Moshé SL, Bennett MV, Zukin RS. Developmental regulation of glutamate and GABA(A) receptor gene expression in rat hippocampus following kainate-induced status epilepticus. *Dev Neurosci* 1997; 19:529–542.

209. de Feo MR, Mecarelli O, Palladini G, Ricci GF. Long-term effects of early status epilepticus on the acquisition avoidance behavior in rats. *Epilepsia* 1986; 27:476–482.

210. Neill JC, Liu Z, Sarkisian M, et al. Recurrent seizures in immature rats: effect on auditory and visual discrimination. *Dev Brain Res* 1996; 95:283–292.

211. Wasterlain CG. Effects of neonatal status epilepticus on rat brain development. *Neurology* 1976; 26:975–986.

212. Wasterlain CG, Dwyer BE. Brain metabolism during prolonged seizures in neonates. In: Delgado-Escueta AV, Wasterlain CG, Treiman DM, Porter RJ, eds. *Status Epilepticus*. New York: Raven Press, 1983:241–260.

213. Wasterlain CG, Shirassaka Y. Seizures, brain damage and brain development. *Brain Dev* 1994; 16:279–295.

214. Gowers WR. *Epilepsy and Other Chronic Convulsive Diseases*. London: J.A. Churchill, 1881.

215. Priel MR, dos Santos NF, Cavalheiro EA. Developmental aspects of the pilocarpine model of epilepsy. *Epilepsy Res* 1996; 26:115–121.

216. Sperber EF, Haas KZ, Moshé SL. Mechanisms of kindling in developing animals. In: Wada JA, ed. *Kindling 4*. New York: Plenum Press, 1990:157–168.

217. Sheridan PH, Jacobs MP. The development of antiepileptic drugs for children. Report from the NIH workshop, Bethesda, Maryland, February 17–18, 1994. *Epilepsy Res* 1996; 23:87–92.

218. Moshé SL. Sex and the substantia nigra: administration, teaching, patient care, and research. *J Clin Neurophysiol* 1997; 14:484–494.

219. Velíšek L, Velíšková J, Ptachewich Y, Shinnar S, Moshé SL. Effects of MK-801 and phenytoin on flurothyl-induced seizures during development. *Epilepsia* 1995; 36:179–185.

220. Velíšek L, Velíšková J, Ptachewich Y, et al. Age-dependent effects of GABA agents on flurothyl seizures. *Epilepsia* 1995; 36:636–643.

221. Velíšek L, Mareš P. Developmental aspects of the anticonvulsant action of MK-801. In: Kamenka J-M, Domino EF, eds. *Multiple Sigma and PCP Receptor Ligands: Mechanisms for Neuromodulation and Neuroprotection?* Ann Arbor: NPP Books, 1992:779–795.

222. Velíšek L, Kusá R, Kulovaná M, Mareš P. Excitatory amino acid antagonists and pentylenetetrazol-induced seizures during ontogenesis: I. The effects of 2-amino-7-phosphonoheptanoate. *Life Sci* 1990; 46:1349–1357.

223. Velíšek L, Vachová D, Mareš P. Excitatory amino acid antagonists and pentylenetetrazol-induced seizures during ontogenesis. IV. Effects of CGP 39551. *Pharmacol Biochem Behav* 1997; 56:493–498.

224. Mareš P, Lišková-Bernášková K, Mudrochová M. Convulsant action of diphenylhydantoin overdose in young rats. *Activ Nerv Sup (Praha)* 1987; 29:30–35.

225. Mareš P, Velíšek L. Comparison of antiepileptic action of valproate and ethosuximide in adult and immature rats. *Pol J Pharmacol Pharm* 1987; 39:505–512.

226. Mareš P, Marešová D, Schickerová R. Effect of antiepileptic drugs on metrazol convulsions during ontogenesis in rats. *Physiol Bohemoslov* 1981; 30:113–121.

227. Velíšek L, Kubová H, Velíšková J, Mareš P, Ortová. M. Action of antiepileptic drugs against kainic acid–induced seizures and automatisms during ontogenesis in rats. *Epilepsia* 1992; 33:987–993.

228. Kubová H, Mareš P. Anticonvulsant action of oxcarbazepine, hydroxycarbamazepine, and carbamazepine against metrazol-induced motor seizures in developing rats. *Epilepsia* 1993; 34:188–192.

229. Kubová H, Mareš P. Anticonvulsant effects of phenobarbital and primidone during ontogenesis in rats. *Epilepsy Res* 1991; 10:148–155.

230. Kubová H, Mareš P, Voríček J. Stable anticonvulsant action of benzodiazepines during development in rats. *J Pharm Pharmacol* 1993; 45:807–810.

231. Mikati MA, Holmes GL, Chronopoulos A, et al. Phenobarbital modifies seizure-related brain injury in the developing brain. *Ann Neurol* 1994; 36:425–433.

232. Velíšková J, Velíšek L, Moshé SL. Age-specific effects of baclofen on pentylenetetrazol-induced seizures in developing rats. *Epilepsia* 1996; 37:718–722.

233. Wurpel JND, Sperber EF, Moshé SL. Baclofen inhibits amygdala kindling in immature rats. *Epilepsy Res* 1990; 5:1–7.

234. Velíšek L, Verešová S, Pôbišová H, Mareš P. Excitatory amino acid antagonists and pentylenetetrazol-induced seizures during ontogenesis: II. The effects of MK-801. *Psychopharmacology* 1991; 104:510–514.

235. Stafstrom CE, Tandon P, Hori A, et al. Acute effects of MK801 on kainic acid–induced seizures in neonatal rats. *Epilepsy Res* 1997; 26:335–344.

236. Facchinetti F, Ciani E, Dall'Olio R, et al. Structural, neurochemical and behavioural consequences of neonatal blockade of NMDA receptor through chronic treatment with CGP 39551 or MK-801. *Dev Brain Res* 1993; 74:219–224.

237. Tandon P, Liu Z, Stafstrom CE, et al. Long-term effects of excitatory amino acid antagonists NBQX and MK-801 on the developing brain. *Dev Brain Res* 1996; 95:256–262.

238. Troupin AS, Mendius JR, Cheng F, Risinger MW. MK-801. In: Meldrum BS, Porter RJ, eds. *New Anticonvulsant Drugs*. London: John Libbey, 1986:191–201.

239. Woodbury DM. Antiepileptic drugs. Phenytoin: introduction and history. In: Glaser GH, Penry JK, Woodbury DM, eds. *Antiepileptic Drugs: Mechanisms of Action*. New York: Raven Press, 1980:305–313.

240. Wyllie E, ed. *The Treatment of Epilepsy: Principles and Practice*. Philadelphia: Lea & Febiger, 1993.

241. Osorio I, Burnstine TH, Remler B, Manon-Espaillat R, Reed RC. Phenytoin-induced seizures: a paradoxical effect at toxic concentrations in epileptic patients. *Epilepsia* 1989; 30:230–234.

242. Stanková L, Kubová H, Mareš P. Anticonvulsant action of lamotrigine during ontogenesis in rats. *Epilepsy Res* 1992; 13:17–22.

243. Veresová S, Kábová R, Velíšek L. Proconvulsant effects induced by pyridoxine in young rats. *Epilepsy Res* 1998; 29:259–264.

244. Chapman AG, Graham JL, Patel S, Meldrum S. Anticonvulsant activity of two orally active competitive *N*-methyl-*D*-aspartate antagonists, CGP 37849 and CGP 39551, against sound-induced seizures in DBA/2 mice and photically induced myoclonus in *Papio papio*. *Epilepsia* 1991; 32:578–587.

245. Velíšek L, Mareš P. Age-dependent anticonvulsant action of clonazepam in the *N*-methyl-*D*-aspartate model of seizures. *Pharmacol Biochem Behav* 1995; 52:291–296.

246. Kábová R, Liptáková S, Šlamberová, Pometlová M, Velíšek L. Age-specific *N*-methyl-*D*-aspartate-induced seizures: perspectives for the West syndrome model. *Epilepsia* 1999; 40:1357–1369.

247. Gowers WR. *Epilepsy and Chronic Convulsive Diseases. Their Causes, Symptoms and Treatment*. New York: William Wood, 1885.

248. Woolley DE, Timiras PS, Woodbury DM. Some effects of sex steroids on brain excitability and metabolism. *Proc West Pharmacol Soc* 1960; 3:11–23.

249. Woolley DE, Timiras PS. The gonad-brain relationship: effects of female sex hormones on electroshock convulsions in the rat. *Endocrinology* 1962; 70:196–209.

250. Pericic D, Manev H, Lakic N. Sex differences in the response of rats to drugs affecting GABAergic transmission. *Life Sci* 1985; 36:541–547.

251. Pericic D, Manev H, Geber J. Sex-related differences in the response of mice, rats and cats to the administration of picrotoxin. *Life Sci* 1986; 38:905–913.

252. Holmes GL, Weber DA, Kloczko N, Zimmerman AW. Relationship of endocrine function to inhibition of kindling. *Dev Brain Res* 1984; 16:55–59.

253. Holmes GL, Weber DA. The effect of progesterone on kindling: a developmental study. *Dev Brain Res* 1984; 16:45–53.

254. Arnold AP, Gorski RA. Gonadal steroid induction of structural sex differences in the central nervous system. *Ann Rev Neurosci* 1984; 7:413–442.

255. Dubrovsky B, Filipini D, Gijsbers K, Birmingham M. Early and late effects of steroid hormones on the central nervous system. *Ciba Foundation Symposium* 1990; 153:240–257.

256. McEwen BS. Gonadal steroid influences on brain development and sexual differentiation. In: Greep R, ed. *Reproductive Physiology IV*. Baltimore: University Park Press, 1983:99–145.

257. McEwen BS. Non-genomic and genomic effects of steroids on neural activity. *Trends Pharmacol Sci* 1991; 12:141–144.

258. McEwen BS. Steroid hormones: Effect on brain development and function. *Horm Res* 1992; 37(Suppl 3):1–10.

259. Caviness VSJ, Hatten ME, McConnell SK, Takahashi T. Developmental neuropathology and childhood epilepsies. In: Schwartzkroin PA, Moshé SL, Noebels JL, Swann JW, eds. *Brain Development and Epilepsy*. New York: Oxford University Press, 1995:94–121.

260. Racine RJ. Modification of seizure activity by electrical stimulation: II. Motor seizures. *Electroencephalogr Clin Neurophysiol* 1972; 32:281–294.

261. Moshé SL. The kindling phenomenon and its possible relevance to febrile seizures. In: Nelson KB, Ellenberg JH, eds. *Febrile Seizures*. New York: Raven Press, 1981:59–63.

262. Moshé SL, Albala BJ. Kindling in developing rats: persistence of seizures into adulthood. *Dev Brain Res* 1982; 4:67–71.

263. Sperber EF, Haas KZ, Moshé SL. Developmental aspects of status epilepticus. *Int Pediatr* 1992; 7:213–222.

CHAPTER 2

Ion Channels, Membranes, and Molecules in Epilepsy and Neuronal Excitability

Robert J. DeLorenzo, M.D., Ph.D., M.P.H

Important advances have been made in molecular neurobiology that enhance understanding the regulation of neuronal excitability in epilepsy and other brain functions. This research typically has involved antiepileptic drugs (AEDs) and other pharmacologic probes that have defined different mechanisms affecting neuronal excitability. The investigation of AEDs in these systems has also shed new light on the molecular basis of epilepsy and on the mechanisms of antiepileptic drug action (1–5).

This chapter provides the scientific background to assist the clinician in keeping abreast of several rapidly advancing fields. It highlights issues that influence neuronal excitability and seizures with emphasis on the mechanisms of sustained repetitive firing (SRF), sodium channels, the gamma-aminobutyric acid (GABA)–chloride channel complex, potassium channels, excitatory transmission, regulation of metabotropic receptors, carbonic anhydrase inhibition, neuromodulators, calcium-mediated regulation of neuronal function, and inhibition of epileptogenesis. In considering these quite different mechanisms, this chapter brings together many of the concepts considered in Chapters 3 and 22.

SUSTAINED REPETITIVE FIRING (SRF)

Sustained high-frequency repetitive firing is an important property of vertebrate and invertebrate neurons that correlates with the excitability state of the neuron (6–11). Many central nervous system (CNS) neurons exhibit SRF. Although no direct evidence has demonstrated the link between SRF and epilepsy, information from in vitro studies on isolated neurons may have some bearing on altered neuronal excitability and anticonvulsant action.

Sustained repetitive firing is a nonsynaptic property of neurons. The relevance of limitation of SRF to AED action is strengthened by several important observations. The therapeutic efficacy of each AED in controlling seizures in animals and humans is similar to that for controlling SRF in isolated, cultured neurons. These results indicate (7) that therapeutic levels of AEDs in cerebrospinal fluid (CSF) correlate with the concentrations that are most effective against SRF. The effects of anticonvulsants in limiting SRF have been shown in a variety of neurons from different regions of the mammalian CNS maintained in culture. This argues that this effect is not unique to specific regions or cell types. Anticonvulsants prevent bursting in the epileptic focus and restrict the spread of epileptic activity from the focus to normal surrounding tissue. Thus, suppression of SRF by anticonvulsants may inhibit excitability by inhibiting the spread of seizure activity. Membrane properties of nonepileptic neurons may be important in understanding drug mechanisms of action and may have a special relationship to the properties of SRF. SRF is an important model for studying the excitability of isolated neurons.

SUSTAINED REPETITIVE FIRING AND SODIUM CHANNEL REGULATION

In studying SRF, several properties of neuronal excitability and seizure phenomenon have been recognized. The AEDs that block SRF have several properties in common. Blocking of SRF is voltage-dependent and the anticonvulsant effect is use-dependent. Research on the role of the sodium channel in regulating SRF indicates that the drug effects on SRF are mediated through a use-dependent blockage of the sodium channel. Phenytoin and carbamazepine can reduce the amplitude of the sodium-dependent action potential in a use-dependent fashion (9). These studies indicate that modulation of sodium channels by anticonvulsants, and possibly endogenous anticonvulsant-like molecules, may play an important role in the regulation of neuronal excitability in seizure discharge. Studies directed at investigating the heterogeneity of sodium channel molecules and their relationship to altered neuronal excitability is an area of important research.

BENZODIAZEPINE RECEPTORS AND MEMBRANE EXCITABILITY

In the 1970s use of radioactively labeled benzodiazepine derivatives allowed the detection of specific nanomolar benzodiazepine receptor sites in brain membrane (12–14). These sites have a very high affinity for the benzodiazepines, binding in low nanomolar concentration ranges. Binding to these receptors is reversible, saturable, and stereospecific. Nanomolar benzodiazepines receptors have now been identified in human brain, where they are widely distributed. The specific membrane protein that accounts for the majority of nanomolar benzodiazepine binding has a molecular weight of approximately 50,000 daltons and has been purified from animal and human brain (15).

High-affinity benzodiazepine binding has also been observed in peripheral, nonneuronal tissue (16). This binding is caused by a different class of benzodiazepine receptor molecules, because both the potency and the tissue distribution of this binding are different from the central type receptor. This second class of high-affinity benzodiazepine binding sites was designated "peripheral type receptor" (16) but was subsequently shown that the peripheral-type benzodiazepine receptor is also present in neuronal tissue. Thus, both peripheral and central high-affinity benzodiazepine receptors exist in brain.

High nanomolar and low micromolar benzodiazepine binding sites have been identified more recently in brain membranes (17,18). In addition, another benzodiazepine receptor that binds in the high nanomolar range has been identified in brain cytosol (18). These novel benzodiazepine binding sites are stereospecific and have potencies for benzodiazepine binding that correlate with the ability of these compounds to inhibit maximal electric shock–induced seizures. Benzodiazepine binding to micromolar benzodiazepine receptors is displaced by phenytoin. These results indicate that high nanomolar and low-micromolar-affinity benzodiazepine receptors may represent important anticonvulsant binding sites in brain membrane that mediate some of the effects of benzodiazepines in high concentration in curtailing status epilepticus, generalized tonic-clonic seizures, and maximal electric shock–induced seizures.

Benzodiazepines are effective in nanomolar concentrations in blocking pentylenetetrazol-induced seizures in animals and in treating absence seizures. In addition, benzodiazepines in high nanomolar and low micromolar ranges inhibit maximal electric shock–induced seizures in animals. Furthermore, benzodiazepines are effective in humans in stopping generalized tonic-clonic seizures and status epilepticus when given in intravenous doses that produce low micromolar serum concentrations. The potency of the benzodiazepines in blocking maximal electric shock–induced seizures, however, correlates in neither time nor consequence with their ability to inhibit pentylenetetrazol-induced seizures or bind to the nanomolar central benzodiazepine receptor (17). Thus, other mechanisms appear to underlie this generalized anticonvulsant property of the benzodiazepines in high concentration ranges. Lower-affinity benzodiazepine binding sites in the high nanomolar and low micromolar ranges have also been described (17,19). These lower-affinity receptor sites come into play in the concentration ranges in which benzodiazepines produce effects on maximal electric shock–induced seizures in animals, in generalized tonic-clonic seizures in man, and on SRF in cultured neurons.

Diazepam and clonazepam reduce SRF in high nanomolar and low micromolar concentrations (7). These concentrations are above therapeutic free-serum concentrations achieved in ambulatory patients treated with benzodiazepines but are within the ranges of free-serum concentrations achieved in patients treated for status epilepticus or acutely for generalized tonic-clonic seizures. In addition to the discrepancy in concentration ranges, the potency of benzodiazepines for suppressing SRF does not correlate with benzodiazepine binding to the nanomolar central receptor or with their ability to inhibit pentylenetetrazol-induced seizures but does correlate with binding to the lower-affinity benzodiazepine binding system.

THE GABA SYSTEM, NEURONAL EXCITABILITY, AND SEIZURE ACTIVITY

Gamma aminobutyric acid is the major inhibitory neurotransmitter in brain. It has been extensively characterized and plays a major role in regulating neuronal excitability by controlling chloride permeability (20–22). Specific binding sites for GABA molecules have been identified in neuronal membrane. Although not all GABA receptors are linked to the chloride channel, a large proportion of these receptors are directly involved in regulating chloride channel function. The major inhibitory effect of GABA on the nervous system is mediated through its ability to regulate chloride channel permeability. GABA binding to the GABA receptor potentiates the opening of the chloride channel allowing chloride ions to flow more easily into the cell. This causes cellular hyperpolarization and inhibits neuronal firing because chloride ions increase the internal electrical negativity of the cell. This is believed to be the major mechanism by which GABA produces its inhibitory effect on neurons.

Functions of GABA on neuronal systems have been closely linked with the effects of the benzodiazepines (20–22). A significant portion of the nanomolar benzodiazepine receptors in brain are associated with the GABA-binding sites and are thereby functionally linked to the chloride channel in neuronal membranes. The GABA–nanomolar benzodiazepine receptor/chloride ionophore macromolecular complex is an important example of the interrelationship between membrane receptors and neuronal excitability (21). The ability of AEDs and the benzodiazepines to modulate chloride conductances is a major molecular mechanism regulating neuronal excitability.

The GABA–Chloride Channel Complex Regulates Seizure Discharge

The chloride channel is surrounded by a GABA receptor, a nanomolar central benzodiazepine receptor, and a receptor site that binds picrotoxin and related convulsants as well as barbiturates and related depressants. This channel and its properties related to the benzodiazepines, GABA, and convulsant and barbiturate molecules have been characterized in detail (23). Picrotoxin binds to the proposed site and modulates benzodiazepine and GABA-receptor binding in a way that inhibits chloride channel permeability, therefore making the cell more excitable. Barbiturate binding potentiates benzodiazepine receptor binding and thus indirectly potentiates the GABA effect on opening the chloride channel and enhancing neuronal inhibition. This complex interaction between GABA, benzodiazepines, picrotoxin and related convulsants, and the barbiturates and related depressants is a prime example of how pharmacologic agents modulate the function of ion channels through specific receptor binding.

Benzodiazepines are an important class of compounds that have antianxiety or anxiolytic effects and sedative, muscle relaxant, and anticonvulsant properties (12,20–22,24). As anticonvulsants, these compounds are effective in blocking both pentylenetetrazol-induced seizures in animals and, at higher concentrations, maximal electric shock–induced seizures. Benzodiazepines are the most commonly prescribed drugs for the initial treatment of generalized

tonic-clonic seizures and status epilepticus in hospital emergency rooms. The anticonvulsant properties of the benzodiazepines, therefore, are not only of academic importance but also have widespread clinical use. The research characterizing this benzodiazepine receptor (13–16,25,26) demonstrates AED receptor–mediated regulation of neuronal excitability. Benzodiazepine binding to the nanomolar receptor site potentiates GABA effects on neuronal inhibition, providing one clear mechanism by which these compounds regulate neuronal excitability. Correlative neuropharmacologic studies have indicated that the anxiolytic and antipentylenetetrazol-induced anticonvulsant activity of these compounds are mediated through the high-affinity benzodiazepine nanomolar receptors. The effects of benzodiazepines on maximal electric shock–induced seizures and on generalized convulsions, however, cannot be clearly explained by these nanomolar actions.

GABA$_A$ and GABA$_B$ Mediated Neuronal Inhibition

As described previously, the best characterized inhibitory effect of GABA on the nervous system is to open chloride channels and hyperpolarize the membrane, an effect that is mediated through GABA$_A$ receptors. In addition to GABA$_A$ receptors, scientists have characterized GABA$_B$ receptors that primarily open potassium channels in the membrane either pre- or postsynaptically. Opening potassium channels also results in hyperpolarization of the cell. Any alteration or decrease in GABA-mediated inhibition through GABA$_A$ or GABA$_B$ receptors can lead to seizures. These data clearly indicate that GABA receptors in the regulation of chloride and potassium channels can regulate seizure discharge.

Potassium Channels

Potassium channels play a major role in regulating neuronal excitability. Although more than 20 types of potassium channels have been identified by biophysical studies, there are four major groups: calcium-activated, voltage-gated, sodium-activated, and inwardly rectifying potassium channels. These different types of potassium channels are regulated by neuromodulators, ions, and second messenger systems. The opening of potassium channels has the effect of hyperpolarizing neurons or reversing depolarizing actions that exist during the transmission of the action potential or the neuroexcitatory input. Following depolarization, several calcium-activated potassium channels play a major role in the after-hyperpolarization that occurs to restore the resting potential of a neuron (27). Electrographic studies on hippocampal neurons from patients undergoing temporal lobectomies have demonstrated alterations in potassium channels in epileptic tissue (28). In addition, compounds that can block potassium channels and prevent the effect of these channels on hyperpolarization are potent convulsants. Fluoraminopyridine and dendrotoxin I are potent convulsants that have been used in numerous animal models to cause seizures (29,30). In addition, compounds that are currently used as antihypertensive drugs, including chromakalim, minoxidil, diazoxide, and penicidil, act as potassium channel openers in muscle membranes and may have potential for use as anticonvulsant compounds (31,32). The possibility of developing new classes of compounds that can activate or potentiate potassium channel activity may play an important role in increasing hyperpolarization following excessive excitatory activity and may serve to reverse the decreased levels of some potassium channels observed in patients with epilepsy.

Some anticonvulsant compounds may also play a role as potassium channel openers. Carbamazepine has been found to enhance potassium conductances in neurons (33). Other potential anticonvulsant compounds are being evaluated but may also potentiate potassium channel activation. Investigation of anticonvulsant drugs regulating potassium channels is a major frontier in the development of new anticonvulsant compounds.

EXCITATORY TRANSMISSION

Glutamate is now widely accepted as the major excitatory neurotransmitter in the brain. Understanding the role of excitatory transmission and its overactivation in epilepsy is an important area for anticonvulsant drug development. Only since the early 1980s has the role of glutamate, aspartate, and other compounds that serve as excitatory transmitters been clearly identified. Several important receptors have been identified in the brain that respond to glutamate and other excitatory neurotransmitters (34). The major glutamate receptors that regulate ion channels include the n-methyl-d-aspartate (NMDA), the quisqualate or AMPA, and the kainate channels. In addition, there are other more recently identified subcategories of excitatory amino acid ion channels regulated by glutamate (35).

NMDA receptor–regulated ion channels are an important class of excitatory amino acid coupled channels in brain that not only play a role in neuronal excitability but also have long-term effects on long-term plasticity changes in brain. NMDA receptor–activated channels are permeable to sodium, potassium, and calcium. They can be voltage blocked by magnesium, which indicates that they can only be in an operative form when the cell is partly depolarized by other excitatory receptor activation. This type of modulation allows for complex regulation of NMDA receptor-activity. For an NMDA channel to be activated, it requires both the excitatory amino acid transmitter glutamate or aspartate to bind to the NMDA-receptor site and for the molecule glycine or D-serine to bind at the neuromodulatory site on the receptor. This channel can be blocked by antagonists of either glutamate or glycine at their respective recognition sites. Regulation of NDMA receptors may play an important role in the development of anticonvulsant drugs. In addition, long-term changes in NMDA channel expression may accompany epileptogenesis. Properties of NMDA-receptor channels are altered in neurons from kindled rats (36). Furthermore, NMDA-receptor antagonists are anticonvulsants in several models of epilepsy (37). Glutamate- and glycine-site competitive antagonists also have anticonvulsant activity (42). NMDA channels can also be inhibited by noncompetitive channel blockers that work when the channel is open. These drugs include dizocilpine (MK-801) and phencyclidine. Although both of these compounds are good anticonvulsants, both have major side effects when used in anticonvulsant doses (39). Nevertheless, the possible role of glutamate/NMDA-channel regulation is an important area for the development of anticonvulsant compounds and those that may prevent epileptogenesis.

AMPA receptors are major excitatory amino acid receptors that play an important role in the fast depolarizing actions of glutamate contributing to the fast excitatory transmission in the CNS. During epilepsy the AMPA receptors are responsible for the early component of the discharges involved in spike discharges and paroxysmal depolarizing shifts. The later elements of these phenomena are primarily related to NMDA receptor activation. Quinoxalinediones (40) were one of the first AMPA receptor antagonists that were found to have anticonvulsant property in several models of epilepsy (41,42). Several classes of AMPA channel inhibitors have also been developed that have anticonvulsant activity. Both indirect AMPA antagonists and noncompetitive allosteric inhibitors of AMPA receptors have anticonvulsant property in several animal models (41). The AMPA receptor has several molecular subtypes that are differentially expressed in different neurons (43). Receptors containing the Glu-R-2 subunit have a much lower permeability to calcium and show a component of their activation that has a linear rectifying current voltage relationship. Receptors lacking the Glu-R-2 subunit are different and show a significant calcium permeability and an inwardly rectifying property (44). Evidence indicates that differential expression of the Glu-R-2 subunit may play an important role in epileptogenesis and altered neuronal excitability. Thus, the ability to selectively modify

AMPA receptors containing Glu-R-2 subunits may play an important role in the development of anticonvulsant compounds.

Kainate channels also play an important role in fast depolarizing actions of glutamate in the CNS. However, only a few drugs have been identified as primary kainate antagonists, although some of the AMPA antagonists also inhibit kainic acid channels (45). At the present time it is not clear whether selective inhibition of kainate channels has any advantage in terms of anticonvulsant development over the development of AMPA channel inhibitors. The possible role of kainate glutamate receptors in modulating seizure discharge and anticonvulsant drug development is an important frontier for further research.

METABOTROPIC RECEPTORS

Metabotropic receptors are glutamate or excitatory amino acid–activated receptors that are not coupled to ion channels. These excitatory amino acid receptors are coupled to second messenger systems in the membrane that have an important role in regulating cellular metabolism and function (46). Metabotropic receptors are coupled to G proteins and enzymes that regulate adenylate cyclase or guanylate cyclase. Regulating these enzymes by metabotropic receptor activation changes levels of cyclic adenosine monophosphate (cAMP) or cyclic guanasine monophosphate (cGMP). Modulating the activation or inhibition of metabotropic receptor activation by excitatory transmission plays an important role in modifying neuronal function over both short- and long-term periods relative to seizure activity. Metabotropic receptors play an important role in producing sustained changes in neuronal excitability that may have implications in epileptogenesis and the development of seizure discharges. Evidence has accumulated for a possible role of glutamate metabotropic receptors in the development of epileptogenesis (47). Inhibition of metabotropic receptor activation during epileptogenesis in several models has blocked the development of long-term epilepsy. Metabotropic receptor inhibitors, therefore, are possible future areas for the development of novel antiepileptic drugs.

CARBONIC ANHYDRASE INHIBITION

Carbonic anhydrase is a major enzyme system that has been found to regulate GABA-mediated inhibitory potentials and therefore has important anticonvulsant or antiepileptic effects (48). GABA-receptor ion channels are permeable to both chloride and bicarbonate ions. Bicarbonate ions normally move outward through the GABA receptor producing a depolarizing effect that is normally smaller than the hyperpolarizing action of the inward movement of chloride ions. The movement of bicarbonate ions out of the neuron following entry of chloride ions can produce a potential depolarizing effect that can be mediated by the GABA-receptor channel. Inhibitors of carbonic anhydrase play a role in blocking this effect. Thus, blocking the depolarization effects mediated by the GABA receptor through bicarbonate ion movement may be an important role of carbonic anhydrase inhibitors in increasing the hyperpolarizing effect of the GABA receptor in the neuron. There may be other actions of carbonic anhydrase inhibitors that go through other mechanisms, but this is another area of research for the development of anticonvulsant drugs.

NEUROMODULATORS

There are many classes of neuromodulators, but two major classes have been widely studied that have significant implications in regulating seizure activity, adenosine and the monoamines. Both adenosine and monoamines influence seizures and epileptogenesis in several models of epilepsy.

Adenosine is released during seizure activity and acts as an endogenous anticonvulsant (49,50). One form of the adenosine receptor (A1 receptor) is coupled to the G protein system in a similar mechanism as is the metabotropic receptor. Activation of the A1 adenosine receptor stabilizes the resting membrane potential presynaptically and blocks glutamate release but not GABA release (51). Several analogues of adenosine acting at the A1 receptor exhibit good anticonvulsant effects in several models of epilepsy (52,53). These compounds, however, have significant adverse cardiovascular effects, and their potential role as anticonvulsants needs further investigation. Another major type of adenosine receptor is the A3 receptor. Selected antagonists of the A3 receptor have also been recently shown to have anticonvulsant activity (54).

Regulation of adenosine receptors, both chronically and during seizure activity, may play important roles in developing new anticonvulsant drugs. The major challenge in this area, however, is to develop compounds that do not have complicating side effects, such as cardiovascular alterations or effects on other aspects of the nervous system.

Monoamines are important classes of neurotransmitters that play important roles in modulating both excitatory and inhibitory neurotransmission. Abnormalities in monoaminergic transmission in several animal models and in human epileptic foci taken from patients following epilepsy surgery have indicated that there may a role for monoamine receptor activation in chronic epilepsy. Pharmacologic manipulation of monoaminergic neurotransmission plays a role in the development of several seizure syndromes, such as the reflex epilepsies (55). Noradrenaline agonists, such as a the $\alpha2$ agonists are protective against seizure activity and antagonists act as convulsant compounds. These effects have been well studied in amygdala kindling in rats and kittens (56,57). Dopamine antagonists have also been shown to be protective in photosensitive epilepsy from animals and humans (58,59). Monoamine oxidase B inhibitors play a role as anticonvulsants in several seizure models. In addition, serotonin antagonists have also been shown to be antiepileptic. Thus, the possible role of monoamines in relation to monoamine receptors in epilepsy is another potential area for development of future anticonvulsant compounds.

CALCIUM REGULATION OF NEURONAL FUNCTION

Calcium plays a major role in modulating normal activity and function of the nervous system (60–62). One of its most widely recognized roles is modulating synaptic neurotransmission. A host of studies have demonstrated the importance of calcium in stimulus-secretion coupling (63). In addition to its important effects on neurotransmission, calcium plays a major role as a second messenger in neuronal and nonneuronal tissues.

Several lines of evidence indicate calcium's importance in regulating neuronal excitability and producing anticonvulsant effects. Because of its importance as a second messenger, it is reasonable to assume that alterations in the normal function of calcium-regulated processes may underlie some of the abnormalities of neuronal excitability seen in seizure disorders.

Accumulating evidence suggests that abnormalities in major calcium-regulated enzymatic processes or ion channels underlie alterations in neuronal excitability and result in seizure activity (64). The role of calcium in antiepileptic drug action and in regulating seizure excitability has been recently reviewed (64,65). Certain anticonvulsants have been shown to regulate the entry of calcium into cells through both voltage-regulated and transmitter-regulated calcium channels. In addition, anticonvulsants inhibit important calcium-mediated enzyme systems that play important roles in cell function and neuronal excitability. These mechanisms may also be significant for some anticonvulsant effects.

Calcium Channels and Neuronal Excitability

The entry of calcium into a cell triggers many biochemical and biophysical actions (60,66). This major second-messenger effect of calcium has been clearly linked to the regulation of neuronal excitability and cell metabolism (60,62). Thus, controlling calcium entry into the cell is the first major step in regulating the effect of calcium as a second messenger.

Depolarization-dependent action potentials are typically mediated by a large sodium current into the cell. Calcium simultaneously enters the cell during depolarization. Recently, the importance of this calcium entry during action potential generation has been more clearly understood. Accumulation of increased concentrations of calcium within a neuron is related to SRF of neurons that can occur in vitro or during epileptic activity. Calcium entry is also regulated by specific excitatory amino acid receptors. This type of calcium channel is opened or closed in response to binding of excitatory amino acids (EAA) to specific calcium channel–linked receptors. The ability of these channels to produce tonic, long-lasting excitability changes in hippocampal neurons and in other cortical neurons has implications for long-term potentiation, memory, and excitability.

In conceptualizing the role of calcium in neuronal excitability and anticonvulsant drug action, one must consider both voltage-regulated and excitatory amino acid–modulated calcium channels. The regulation of calcium channels, like the regulation of the chloride channel, by the benzodiazepines, barbiturates, and convulsant drugs may play an important role in modifying neuronal excitability.

Voltage-Gated Calcium Channels

Voltage-regulated or gated calcium channels affect neuronal excitability. As an action potential arrives at a nerve terminal, depolarization of the nerve terminal membrane causes entry of calcium through voltage-gated calcium channels with subsequent release of neurotransmitters. This is the classic paradigm for calcium-mediated neurotransmitter release and was the initial observation that demonstrated the importance of calcium in neuronal excitability, but little was understood about the specific mechanisms of calcium channels in brain.

Early insight into the neuropharmacology of calcium channels came from studies of smooth muscle and cardiac cells during the 1970s. The dihydropyridine type of calcium channel blocker and related molecules were shown to be effective in blocking calcium channels in peripheral tissue (65,67,68). These compounds were classified as "organic calcium channel blockers" and represented a major advance in pharmacology. Numerous analogues were developed, and specific binding sites for the dihydropyridines and other analogues were identified and characterized. This led to the first molecular characterization of calcium channels and their regulation by specific receptor sites. A major controversy developed based on the observation that the organic calcium blockers, effective in inhibiting calcium entry into nonneuronal tissue, seemed to be ineffective in blocking voltage-gated calcium entry into neurons (69). Numerous investigators demonstrated that calcium entry as a result of neuronal activity was not significantly inhibited by therapeutic or relevant concentrations of the organic calcium channel blockers (65). Because there was at that time no clear evidence for more than one type of calcium channel, this dichotomy was not well understood and was attributed to unusual properties of the neuronal membrane and to specific differences in drug penetration into the nervous system. More recent studies using benzodiazepines and phenothiazines (70,71–73) demonstrated that these compounds in fact could significantly block voltage-gated calcium channels in neurons. These results indicated that calcium channels in brain were distinct from calcium channels in peripheral tissue.

With the development of patch and voltage clamp technology, more sophisticated characterization of calcium channels has been possible. It is now clear that there are at least three, and possibly more, types of calcium channels in neurons (69,74,75). One type of voltage-gated calcium channel is insensitive to dihydropyridines, while a second type of calcium channel is sensitive to these compounds. A third type of brain membrane calcium channel has also been postulated that is different from the first two types of channels. Although a set terminology has not been developed for these different channels, initial classification by Tsien (75) is currently in use and describes these channels as the T, N, and L type channels, respectively.

The heterogeneity of calcium channels provides a major insight into different mechanisms of regulating calcium excitability in the nervous system. These observations also explain the fact that the major voltage-gated calcium channels in brain that were insensitive to dihydropyridines were a different class of channel from those found in peripheral tissues. In certain regions of the nervous system and at certain sites on the cell body, however, there are calcium channels that are sensitive to dihydropyridines and are similar to those calcium channels in nonneuronal tissue. The different types of calcium channels are distributed in characteristic patterns over the surface of a neuron. Some channels may be localized at the synapse, while others may be present at a higher density at the cell body. The heterogeneity and individual function of specific types of calcium channels are important areas for further investigation as in the development of specific drugs to regulate each type of channel.

Several anticonvulsant compounds block or alter calcium entry through voltage-gated calcium channels. Ferrendelli and coworkers (76,77) described the ability of phenytoin, phenobarbital, carbamazepine, but not ethosuximide, to block voltage-dependent calcium entry into isolated nerve terminal preparations. Subsequent studies have demonstrated that benzodiazepines as well as phenytoin and barbiturates can regulate calcium entry into isolated neurons. However, the concentrations of antiepileptic drugs that are required to block calcium entry are in the low micromolar range, concentrations that are approximately one order of magnitude higher than the therapeutic levels of these drugs achieved in spinal fluid. Although these concentrations may be relevant to anticonvulsant actions, they are more likely related to toxic side effects.

Excitatory Amino Acid Receptors and Calcium Channels

L-glutamate was proposed as an excitatory neurotransmitter over 30 years ago (78). Recently, excitatory amino acids (EAA) have been found to play important roles in epilepsy, neuronal excitability, and learning (78–80). The two main excitatory neurotransmitters currently known are glutamate and aspartate (81). Many pathways in the brain use these neurotransmitters, including hippocampal afferents and major cortical output tracts that are widely activated during convulsions.

Excitatory amino acids bind to specific membrane receptors (82,83). Currently, four major types of EAA receptors have been characterized. One major EAA receptor is characterized by binding of the EAA analogue NMDA. The NMDA receptor has now been well studied and represents a specific type of excitatory amino acid receptor. Three types of non-NMDA receptors that bind other analogues of excitatory amino acids but have different properties from the NMDA receptor have also been identified. The non-NMDA receptors bind EAAs but not NMDA. The non-NMDA receptors include binding sites for kainic acid, quisqualate, and 2-amino-4-phosphonobutyrate (2-APB).

Excitatory transmission regulated by EAA receptors plays a major role in synaptic transmission in the CNS. Excitatory amino acids regulate specific ion channels that allow calcium and sodium to enter the cell when the channel is activated by the EAA receptor (82,83). These specific channels are actually opened or gated by the EAA. The currents activated by EAA receptors are both rapid and long-lasting. The postsynaptic localization of these receptors, as well as their presence over the cell body, have been implicated in explaining how EAAs alter neuronal excitability, causing rapid depolarization in some situations and long-lasting neuronal changes in other cells. Thus, this type of calcium entry is activated by specific EAAs and has been implicated in many neuromodulating effects in the brain. Important convulsants, such as kainic acid, alter neuronal excitability by binding to these receptor sites and activating calcium and sodium channels. Compounds that bind to EAA receptors but do not activate the channel can inhibit EAA effects on these receptors. Several of these compounds have potent anticonvulsant actions and are very effective in maximal electric shock–induced seizure models (82).

Because of their potential importance to epileptogenesis (79), EAA receptors and the calcium channels that they regulate have been the focus of extensive research (80,84). These receptor sites are responsible for mediating some of the effects of kainic acid in producing convulsant discharge in the brain. NMDA receptors have been implicated in the phenomenon of long-term potentiation and in long-term alterations of neuronal excitability. The EAA analogue, 2-amino-7-phosphoroheptanoate (APH, AP7), is a potent anticonvulsant in various seizure models. These and other investigations provide strong evidence that EAA receptors and their regulation of calcium channels are important mechanisms in regulating neuronal excitability and, potentially, in AED actions. It is anticipated that several new anticonvulsant compounds will be developed that act specifically through this mechanism.

Modulating the Calcium Signal in Controlling Neuronal Excitability

The discovery of a calcium binding protein, calmodulin (CaM), was the first major breakthrough in understanding the molecular mechanisms that mediate calcium second messenger effects (85,86). Evidence now suggests that many of the effects of calcium on cell function are mediated by calmodulin (71,72,87–89). Several important calcium-regulated processes are mediated by calmodulin and by a major calmodulin target enzyme system, calmodulin kinase II (90–92). Evidence from several laboratories has now confirmed the original calmodulin hypothesis of neurotransmission and substantiated the role of calmodulin in mediating some of the effects of calcium on neuronal excitability. Antiepileptic drugs, including phenytoin, carbamazepine, and the benzodiazepines antagonize calcium-mediated effect and inhibit calmodulin activation of calmodulin kinase II (66,93). Concentrations required to inhibit CaM kinase II are in the low micromolar concentration ranges for antiepileptic drug effects on the protein kinase. This enzyme plays an important role in mediating calcium-dependent protein phosphorylation of membrane and soluble proteins.

CaM kinase II has been implicated by several investigators to be a major molecular mechanism mediating some of the second messenger effects of calcium in the cell. Thus, control of this important calcium-mediated event by phenytoin, carbamazepine, and diazepam may be a major action of these drugs. The precise

relationship of this particular effect to clinically useful anticonvulsant activity or their related side effects remains to be elucidated.

The importance of calmodulin kinase II in regulating neuronal excitability is widely recognized. Injection of CaM kinase II into invertebrate neurons regulates potassium and calcium currents (94). In addition, CaM kinase II levels in hippocampal neurons are chronically altered during the long-term alteration of neuronal excitability that occurs in kindling (95). CaM kinase II activity is inhibited by specific anticonvulsants (64,72), and the subunits of CaM kinase II are a major protein component of the postsynaptic density localizing this important enzyme system directly at the synapse (96,97). Further understanding the role of CaM kinase II in the pathophysiology of epilepsy and in controlling neuronal excitability is clearly important.

Another major molecular mechanism regulating the effects of calcium on neuronal excitability and cell function is the major enzyme system, protein kinase C. Protein kinase C has been implicated in many of the effects of calcium on cell function and has been implicated in some of the effects of calcium in regulating specific ion conductances (62). Although no direct studies have been performed to investigate the effects of anticonvulsant drugs on the C-kinase system, this too is an important area for investigation. Modulation of these calcium target enzyme systems by anticonvulsant drugs is a potential area for new drug development.

Inhibition of Epileptogenesis

More than half of the epilepsies are described as symptomatic or acquired. These types of epilepsy are acquired through environmental stress or injuries to the nervous system that result in the permanent alteration of neuronal function resulting in epilepsy (98,99). Conditions such as stroke, head trauma, metabolic disease, prolonged seizures, tumors, or other neurologic insults can permanently alter the brain and trigger mechanisms of neuronal plasticity that eventually result in the development of epilepsy. Because of the diversity of causes of epilepsy, epilepsy is not considered a disease but rather a condition. In addition to the acquired causes as described previously, other idiopathic forms of epilepsy may have a genetic basis (98,99).

The process of epileptogenesis refers to the development of spontaneous recurrent seizures in a previously normal brain. Symptomatic epilepsy, representing a significant number of patients that develop epilepsy, occurs through the process of epileptogenesis. This an important area to consider for anticonvulsant drug development. Compounds that prevent the development of epileptogenesis may have important clinical ramifications. If specific antiepileptogenic drugs can be administered following a brain injury, symptomatic epilepsy may be prevented. Although these compounds may not be true anticonvulsant drugs, they would be the ultimate antiepileptic drugs by preventing the development of epilepsy. This is a new and important area for future research.

Molecular genetics has set the stage for major advances in studying neurologic diseases, and initial advances have been made in understanding specific mutations that are associated with epilepsy and other neurologic conditions (100). In addition to specific mutations, the permanent alterations in brain function and diminished expression are associated with epileptogenesis. In symptomatic epilepsy normal brain tissue is permanently altered and develops spontaneous recurrent seizures. These changes entail long-lasting changes in gene expression at both transcriptional and posttranscriptional levels in association with the induction of epileptogenesis. Understanding the effects of severe environmental stresses on the multiple sites of transcriptional and posttranscriptional regulation of gene expression is likely to provide important insights into how altered neuronal function and develop and point to novel strategies that will prevent epileptogenesis. This important area for future research represents a frontier in the development of antiepileptic drugs.

REFERENCES

1. Meldrum BS. Current strategies for designing and identifying new anticonvulsant drugs. In: Engel J, Pedley TA, eds. *Epilepsy: A Comprehensive Textbook*. New York: Raven Press, 1997; 2:1405–1416.

2. Levy RH, Mattson RH, Meldrum BS. *Antiepileptic Drugs*. 4th ed. New York: Raven Press, 1995.

3. DeLorenzo RJ, Dashefsky L. Anticonvulsants. In: *Handbook of Neurochemistry*. 1985; 9:363–403.

4. Delgado-Escueta AV, Ward AA, Woodbury DM, Porter RJ, eds. *Advances in Neurology*. New York: Raven Press, 1986; 44:3–55.

5. Nistico G, Morselli P, Lloyd K, Fariello R, Engel, eds. *Neurotransmitters, Seizures, and Epilepsy III*. New York: Raven Press, 1986.

6. Macdonald RL, McLean MJ. Cellular bases of barbiturate and phenytoin anticonvulsant drug action. *Epilepsia* 1982; 23:S7–S18.

7. Macdonald RL, McLean MJ. Anticonvulsant drugs: mechanisms of action. *Advances in Neurology*. New York: Raven Press, 1986; 44:713–736.

8. McLean MJ, Macdonald RL. Multiple actions of phenytoin on mouse spinal cord neurons in cell culture. *J Pharmacol Exp Ther* 1983; 227:779–789.

9. McLean MJ, Macdonald RL. Limitation of high frequency repetitive firing of cultured mouse neurons by anticonvulsant drugs. *Neurology* 1984; 34:288.

10. McLean MJ, Macdonald RL. Carbamazepine and 10,11-epoxycarbamazepine produce use- and voltage-dependent limitation of rapidly firing action potentials of mouse central neurons in cell culture. *J Pharmacol Exp Ther* 1986; 238:727–738.

11. McLean MG, Macdonald RL. Sodium valproate, but not ethosuximide, produces use- and voltage-dependent limitation of high frequency repetitive firing of action potentials of mouse central neurons in cell culture. *J Pharmacol Exp Ther* 1986; 237:727–1001–11.

12. Killiam EK, Suria A. Benzodiazepine. In: Glaser GH, Penry JK, Woodbury DM, eds. *Antiepileptic Drugs: Mechanisms of Action*. New York: Raven Press, 1980:597–616.

13. Braestrup C, Squires RF. Pharmacological characterization of benzodiazepine receptors. *Eur J Pharmacol* 1978; 48:263–270.

14. Mohler H, Okada T. Properties of [^{3}H]-diazepam binding to benzodiazepine receptors in rat cerebral cortex. *Life Sci* 1977; 20:2101–2110.

15. Battersby MK, Richard JG, Mohler N. Benzodiazepine receptor: photoaffinity labeling and localization. *Eur J Pharmacol* 1979; 57:277–278.

16. Mestre M, Carriot T, Belin C, et al. Electrophysiological and pharmacological evidence that peripheral type benzodiazepine receptors are coupled to calcium channels in the heart. *Life Sci* 1985; 36:391–400.

17. Bowling AC, DeLorenzo RJ. Micromolar benzodiazepine receptors: identification and characterization in central nervous system. *Science* 1982; 216:1247–1250.

18. Bowling AC, DeLorenzo RJ. Photoaffinity labeling of a novel benzodiazepine binding protein in rat brain. *Eur J Pharmacol* 1987; 135:97–100.

19. Yang J, Johansen J, Kleinhaus AL, DeLorenzo RJ, Zorumski CF. Effects of medazepam on voltage-gated ion currents of cultured chick sensory neurons. *Eur J Pharmacol* 1987; 143:383–387.

20. Tallman JF, Paul SM, Skolnick P, Gallager DW. Receptors for the age of anxiety: pharmacology of the benzodiazepines. *Science* 1980; 207:274–281.

21. Olsen RW, Wamsley JK, Lee RJ, Lomax P. Benzodiazepine/barbiturate/GABA receptor chloride ionophore complex in a genetic model for generalized epilepsy. *Advances in Neurology* 1986; 33:365–378.

22. Olsen RW, Wong EHF, Stauber GB, King RG. Biochemical pharmacology of the GABA/benzodiazepine receptor/ionophore protein. *Fed Proc* 1984; 43:2773–2778.

23. Ticku MK, Maksay G. Convulsant/anticonvulsant drugs and GABAergic transmission. In: Nistico G, Morselli P, Lloyd K, Fariello R, Engel J, eds. *Neurotransmitters, Seizures and Epilepsy III*. New York: Raven Press, 1986:163–177.

24. Martin IL, Brown CL, Doble A. Multiple benzodiazepine receptors: structures in the brain or structures in the mind? A critical review. *Life Sci* 1980; 32:1925–1933.

25. Mohler H, Battersby MK, Richard JG. Benzodiazepine receptor protein identified and visualized in brain tissue by a photoaffinity label. *Proc Natl Acad Sci USA* 1980; 77:1666–1670.

26. Johansen J, Taft WC, Yang J, Kleinhaus AL, DeLorenzo RJ. Benzodiazepine inhibition of calcium conductance in identified leech neurons. *Proc Natl Acad Sci USA* 1985; 82:3935–3939.

27. Sah P. Ca^{2+}-activated K^+ currents in neurones: types, physiological roles and modulation. *TINS* 1996; 19:150–154.

28. Beck H, Blumke I, Kral T, et. al. Properties of a delayed rectifier potassium current in dentate granule cells isolated from the hippocampus of patients with chronic temporal lobe epilepsy. *Epilepsia* 1996; 37:892–901.

29. Velluti JC, Caputi A, Macadar O. Limbic epilepsy induced in the rat by dendrotoxin, a polypeptide isolated from the green mamba venom. *Toxicon* 1987; 25:649–657.

30. Rutecki PA, Lebeda FJ, Johnston D. 4-aminopyridine produces epileptiform activity in hippocampus and enhances synaptic excitation and inhibition. *J Neurophysiol* 1987; 57:1911–1924.

31. Weston AH, Edward G. Recent progress in potassium channel opener pharmacology. *Biochem Pharmacol* 1992; 43:47–54.

32. Popoli P, Pezzola A, Sagratella S, Zeng YC, Scotti de Carolis A. Cromakalim (BRL 34915) counteracts the epileptiform activity elicited by diltiazem and verapamil in rats. *Br J Pharmacol* 1991; 104:907–913.

33. Zona C, Tancredi V, Palma E, Pirrone GC, Avoil M. Potassium currents in rat cortical neurons in culture are enhanced by the antiepileptic drug carbamazepine. *Can J Physiol Pharmacol* 1990; 68:545–547.

34. Watkins JC, Evans RH. Excitatory amino acid transmitters. *Annu Rev Pharmacol Toxicol* 1981; 21:165–204.

35. Hollman M, Heinemann S. Cloned glutamate receptors. *Annu Rev Neurosci* 1994; 17:31–108.

36. Köhr G, De Koninck Y, Mody I. Properties of NMDA receptor channels in neurons acutely isolated from epileptic (kindled) rats. *J Neurosci* 1993; 13:3612–3627.

37. Croucher MJ, Collins JF, Meldrum BS. Anticonvulsant action of excitatory amino acid antagonists. *Science* 1982; 216:899–901.

38. Meldrum BS, Chapman AG. Competitive NMDA antagonists as drugs. In: Watkins JC, Collingridge GL, eds. *The NMDA Receptor.* Oxford, England: IRL Press, 1994:455.

39. Chapman AG, Meldrum BS. Non-competitive *N*-methyl-*D*-aspartate antagonists protect against sound-induced seizures in DBA/2 mice. *Eur J Pharmacol* 1989; 166:201–211.

40. Honoré T, Davies SN, Drejer J, et al. Quinoxalinediones: potent competitive non-NMDA glutamate receptor antagonists. *Science* 1992; 257:398–401.

41. Chapman AG, Smith SE, Meldrum BS. The anticonvulsant effect of the non-NMDA antagonists, NBQX and GYKI 52466, in mice. *Epilepsy Res* 1991; 9:92–96.

42. Swedberg MDB, Jacobsen F, Honore T. Anticonvulsant, anxiolytic and discriminative effects of the AMPA antagonist 2,3-dihydroxy-6-nitro-7-sulfamoylbenzo(f)quinoxaline (NBQX). *J Pharmacol Exp Ther* 1995; 274:1113–1121.

43. Geiger JRP, Melcher T, Koh D-S, et al. Relative abundance of subunit mRNAs determines gating and Ca^{2+} permeability of AMPA receptors in principal neurons and interneurons in rat CNS. *Neuron* 1995; 13:193–204.

44. Lomeli H, Mosbacher J, Melcher T, et al. Control of kinetic properties of AMPA receptor channels by nuclear RNA editing. *Science* 1994; 266:1709–1713.

45. Bleakman D, Schoepp DD, Ballyk B, et al. Pharmacological discrimination of GluR5 and GluR6 kainate receptor subtypes by (3S,4aR,6R8aR)-6-[21(2)H-tetrazole-5-yl]ethyl]decahydroisoquinoline-3 carboxylic acid. *J Pharmacol Exp Ther* 1996; 49:581–588.

46. Pin J-P, Duvoisin R. The metabotropic glutamate receptors: structure and functions. *Neuropharmacology* 1995; 119:569–577.

47. Akiyama K, Daigen A, Yamada N, et al. Long-lasting enhancement of metabotropic excitatory amino acid receptor-mediated polyphosphoinositide hydrolysis in the amygdala/pyriform cortex of deep prepiriform cortical kindled rats. *Brain Res* 1992; 569:71–77.

48. Staley KJ, Soldo BL, Proctor WR. Ionic mechanisms of neuronal excitation by inhibitory $GABA_A$ receptors. *Science* 1995; 269:977–981.

49. Dragunow M. Purinergic mechanisms in epilepsy. *Prog Neurobiol* 1988; 31:85–108.

50. During MJ, Spencer DD. Adenosine: A potential mediator of seizure arrest and postical refractoriness. *Ann Neurol* 1992; 32:618–624.

51. Yoon K-W, Rothman SM. Adenosine inhibits excitatory but not inhibitory synaptic transmission in the hippocampus. *J Neurosci* 1991; 11:1375–1380.

52. von Lubitz DKJE, Paul IA, Carter M, Jacobson KA. Effects of N6-cyclopentyl adenosine and 8-cyclopentyl-1,3-dipropylxanthine on *N*-methyl-*D*-aspartate induced seizures in mice. *Eur J Pharmacol* 1993; 249:265–270.

53. Zhang G, Franklin PH, Murray TF. Activation of adenosine A1 receptors underlies anticonvulsant effect of CGS21680. *Eur J Pharmacol* 1994; 255:239–243.

54. von Lubitz DKJE, Carter MF, Deutsch SI, et al. The effects of adenosine A3 receptor stimulation on seizures in mice. *Eur J Pharmacol* 1995; 275:23–29.

55. Horton R, Anlezark GM, Meldrum B. Noradrenergic influences on sound-induced seizures. *J Pharmacol Exp Ther* 1980; 214:437–442.

56. Pelletier MR, Carcoran ME. Infusions of 2 nonadrenergic agonists and antagonists into the amygdala: Effects on kindling. *Brain Res* 1993; 632:29–35.

57. Shouse MN, Langer J, Bier M, et al. The 2-adrenoceptor agonist clonidine suppresses seizures, whereas the 2-adrenoceptor antagonist idazoxan promotes seizures in amygdala-kindled kittens: a comparison of amygdala and pontine microinfusion effects. *Epilepsia* 1996; 37:709–717.

58. Anlezark GM, Blackwood DHR, Meldrum BS, Ram VJ, Neumeyer JL. Comparative assessment of dopamine agonist aporphines as anticonvulsants in two models of reflex epilepsy. *Psychopharmacology (Berlin)* 1983; 81:135–139.

59. Mervaala E, Andermann F, Quesney FL, Krelina M. Common dopaminergic mechanism for epileptic photosensitivity in progressive myoclonus epilepsies. *Neurology* 1990; 40:53–56.

60. Rubin RP. The role of calcium in the release of neurotransmitter substances and hormones. *Pharmacol Rev* 1972; 22:389–428.

61. Rasmussen H, Goodman DBP. Relationships between calcium and cyclic nucleotides in cell activation. *Physiol Rev* 1977; 57:421–509.

62. Rasmussen H. The calcium messenger system. *NEJM*, 1986, 314(17):1094–1101.

63. Katz B, Miledi R. Further study of the role of calcium in synaptic transmission. *J Physiol (London)* 1970; 207:789–801.

64. DeLorenzo RJ. A molecular approach to the calcium signal in brain: relationship to synaptic modulation and seizure discharge. *Advances in Neurology* 1986; 44:435–464.

65. Taft WC, DeLorenzo RJ. Regulation of calcium channels in brain: implications for the clinical neurosciences. *Yale J Biol Med* 1987; 60:99–106.

66. Douglas WW. Stimulus-secretion coupling: The concept and clues from chromaffin and other cells. *Br J Pharmacol* 1986; 34:451–474.

67. Bolger GT, Gengo P, Koockowski R. Characterization of binding of the calcium channel antagonist, [³H]nitrendipine, to guinea pig ileal smooth muscle. *J Pharmacol Exp Therap* 1983; 225:291–299.

68. Gould RJ, Murphy KMM, Snyder SH. [³H]nitrendipine-labeled calcium channels discriminate inorganic calcium agonists and antagonists. *Proc Natl Acad Sci USA* 1982; 79:3656–3660.

69. Miller RJ. Multiple calcium channels and neuronal function. *Science* 1987; 235:46–52.39.

70. Leslie SW, Friedman MB, Coleman RR. Effects of chlordiazepoxide on depolarization-induced calcium influx into synaptosomes. *Biochem Pharmacol* 1980; 29:2439–2443.

71. DeLorenzo RJ. Role of calmodulin in neurotransmitter release and synaptic function. *Ann NY Acad Sci* 1980; 356:92–109.

72. DeLorenzo RJ. The calmodulin hypothesis of neurotransmission. *Cell Calcium* 1981; 2:365–385.

73. DeLorenzo RJ, Taft WC, Andrews WT. Regulation of voltage-sensitive calcium channels in brain by micromolar affinity benzodiazepine receptors. In: Katz B, Rahamimoff R, eds. *Calcium, Neuronal Function and Neurotransmitter Release.* Boston: Martinus Nijhoff, 1985:375–394.

74. Nowyck MC, Fox AP, Tsien RW. Three types of neuronal calcium channel with different calcium agonist sensitivity. *Nature* 1985; 316:440–443.

75. Tsien R. Calcium currents in heart cells and neurons. In: Kaczmarek L, Levitan I, eds. *Neuromodulation: The Biochemical Control of Neuronal Excitability.* New York: University Press, 1987:206–242.

76. Ferrendelli JA, Daniels-McQueen S. Comparative actions of phenytoin and other anticonvulsant drugs on potassium- and veratridine-stimulated calcium uptake in synaptosomes. *J Pharmacol Exp Therap* 1982; 220:29–34.

77. Ferrendelli JA, Kinocherf DA. Phenytoin: effects on calcium flux and cyclic nucleotides. *Epilepsia* 1977; 17:331–336.

78. Rothman S, Olney J. Excitotoxicity and the NMDA receptor. *Trends Neurosci* 1987; 10:299–301.

79. Choi D, Dichter M. Excitatory amino acid neurotransmitters and excitotoxins. *Curr Neurol* 1989; 9:1–26.

80. Turski L, Cavalheiro E, Turski W, Meldrum B. Excitatory neurotransmission within substantia nigra pars reticulata regulates threshold for seizures produced by pilocarpine in rats. *Neuroscience* 1986; 18(1):61–77.

81. Czuczwar S, Frey H, Loscher W. *N*-methyl-*d*, L-Aspartic acid-induced convulsions in mice and their blockade by antiepileptic drugs and other agents. In: Nistico G, Morselli P, Lloyd K, Fariello R, Engel J, eds. *Neurotransmitters, Seizures and Epilepsy III.* New York: Raven Press, 1986:235–246.

82. Watkins J, Olverman H. Agonists and antagonists for excitatory amino acid receptors. *Trends Neurosci* 1987; 10(7):265–272.

83. Mayer ML, Westbrook GL. The physiology of excitatory amino acids in the vertebrate central nervous system. *Prog Neurobiol* 1987; 28:197–276.

84. Meldrum B, Chapman A. Excitatory amino acid antagonists and anticonvulsant agents: receptor subtype involvement in different seizure models. In: Nistico G, Morselli P., Lloyd K, Fariello R, Engel J, eds. *Neurotransmitters, Seizures, and Epilepsy III,* New York: Raven Press, 1986:223–245.

85. Cheung WY. Calmodulin role in cellular regulation. *Science* 1980; 207:19–27.

86. Klee CB, Crouch TH, Richmand PG. Calmodulin. *Annu Rev Biochem* 1980; 49:489–515.

87. DeLorenzo RJ, Freedman SD, Yohe WB, Maurer SC. Stimulation of Ca^{2+}-dependent neurotransmitter release and presynaptic nerve terminal protein phosphorylation by calmodulin and a calmodulin-like protein isolated from synaptic vesicles. *Proc Natl Acad Sci USA* 1979; 76:1838–1842.

88. DeLorenzo RJ. Calmodulin in neurotransmitter release and synaptic function. *Fed Proc* 1982; 41:2275.

89. DeLorenzo RJ. Calcium-calmodulin protein phosphorylation in neuronal transmission: a molecular approach to neuronal excitability and anticonvulsant drug action. In: Delgado-Escueta AV, Wasterlain CG, Treiman DM, and Porter RJ, eds. *Advances in Neurology,* Vol. 34, Status epilepticus. New York: Raven Press, 1983:325–338.

90. Goldenring JR, Gonzalez B, McGuire JS, Jr, DeLorenzo RJ. Purification and characterization of a calmodulin-dependent kinase from rat brain cytosol able to phosphorylate tubulin and microtubule-associated proteins. *J Biol Chem* 1983; 258:12632–12640.

91. Bennett MK, Erondu NE, Kennedy MB. Purification and characterization of a calmodulin-dependent protein

kinase that is highly concentrated in brain. *J Biol Chem* 1983; 258:12735–12744.

92. Schulman H, Greengard P. Stimulation of brain membrane protein phosphorylation by calcium and an endogenous heat-stable protein. *Nature* 1978; 271:478–479.

93. DeLorenzo RJ, Burdette S, Holderness J. Benzodiazepine inhibition of the calcium-calmodulin protein kinase system in brain membrane. *Science* 1981; 213:546–649.

94. Sakakibara M, Alkon DL, DeLorenzo RJ, et al. Modulation of calcium-mediated inactivation of ionic currents by Ca^{2+}/calmodulin- dependent protein kinase II. *J Biophys* 1986; 50:319–327.

95. Goldenring JR, Wasterlain CG, Oestreicher A, et al. Kindling induces a long-lasting change in the activity of a hippocampal membrane calmodulin-dependent protein kinase system. *Brain Res* 1986; 377:47–53.

96. Goldenring JR, McGuire JS Jr, DeLorenzo RJ. Identification of the major postsynaptic density protein as homologous with the major calmodulin-binding subunit of a calmodulin-dependent protein kinase. *J Neurochem* 1984; 42:1077–1084.

97. Kennedy MR, Bennett MK, Erondu NE. Biochemical and immunochemical evidence that the "major PSD protein" is a subunit of a calmodulin-dependent protein kinase. *Proc Natl Acad Sci USA* 1983; 80:7357–7361.

98. Hauser WA, Hesdorffer DC. *Epilepsy: Frequency, Causes, and Consequences*. New York: Demos, 1990.

99. DeLorenzo RJ, Towne AR. Epilepsy. *Curr Neurol* 1989; 2:27–76.

100. DeLorenzo, RJ and Morris, TA. Long-term modulation of genetic expression in epilepsy and other neurological diseases. *The Neuroscientist*, Vol. 5, No. 1, 1999, in press.

CHAPTER 3

Metabolic and Pharmacologic Consequences of Seizures

Michael V. Johnston, M.D., and John W. McDonald, M.D., Ph.D.

The massive neuronal discharge associated with seizure activity is closely linked to a marked rise in cerebral metabolic activity. Generally, the brain withstands the metabolic challenge of seizures quite well because enhanced cerebral blood flow is capable of delivering adequate fuel unless there is a catastrophic reduction in perfusion. Nevertheless, prolonged seizures or status epilepticus can produce an imbalance between metabolic activity and cerebral perfusion and may cause permanent brain injury. Even patients with shorter but very frequent seizures appear to suffer from a metabolic disturbance of brain activity manifested by temporary encephalopathy.

Until recently, there was little direct experimental information about the mechanisms by which prolonged seizures cause neuronal dysfunction or injury. Because many individuals with generalized convulsive seizures become cyanotic and have periods of apnea, traditional theories emphasized the role of systemic hypoxemia and other metabolic disturbances in seizure-related brain injury. However, clinical experience and experimental evidence from animal models indicate that prolonged seizures alone are sufficient to damage the brain, especially sensitive areas such as the hippocampus (1). In contrast to hypoxic-ischemic brain damage, energy depletion does not appear to play a primary role in seizure-induced neuronal injury (2). Estimates from animal experiments indicate that during seizures energy utilization increases by more than 200 percent and tissue adenosine triphosphate (ATP) levels remain at more than 95 percent of control, even during prolonged status epilepticus (3,4). The regional histological pattern of brain injury produced by status epilepticus is also different from that produced by hypoxia-ischemia or hypoglycemia. Despite the fact that energy substrates are depleted earlier in the course of hypoxia and hypoglycemia, histological evidence of injury appears more rapidly after seizures (2). These observations indicate that there must be a more direct mechanistic link between prolonged seizures and neuronal injury than is provided by the energy failure theory.

A more attractive hypothesis currently gaining support is that seizure-related brain injury is initiated by excessive stimulation of neuronal receptors for excitatory amino acid (EAA) neurotransmitters. According to this theory, a seizure initiates release of EAA neurotransmitters such as glutamate and aspartate from nerve terminals into the synaptic cleft, where they bind to specific neuronal receptors and cause postsynaptic excitation. Under normal circumstances, activation of EAA receptors mediates as much as half of the neuronal communication in the brain (5). In the developing brain, EAA receptors appear to serve an additional role as regulators of neuronal development. However, during a prolonged seizure, if the EAA neurotransmitter release continues unabated to raise the synaptic concentration of glutamate, excessive EAA receptor stimulation may damage and eventually kill neurons.

An important component of the theory holds that EAAs cause intracellular calcium overload, which intoxicates neurons (3,6,7). Calcium and sodium are allowed to enter neurons through pores or ionophores controlled by EAA receptors. The concentration of calcium within the neuron is normally 10,000 times lower than in the extracellular fluid, and calcium entry is tightly controlled. The neuron has several mechanisms for protecting itself from excessive calcium influx, including sequestration of calcium within mitochondria and endoplasmic reticulum and energy-dependent pumps that move calcium outward across the cell membrane. Continued bombardment of the neuron by EAA neurotransmitters can overwhelm these protective mechanisms, allowing calcium to poison the metabolic machinery of the neuron. The EAA theory proposes that excitatory neurotransmitters are a major direct link between excessive seizure activity and neuronal injury; however, metabolic derangements such as hypoxia may play a contributing destructive role by reducing the efficiency of energy-dependent protective mechanisms and hastening EAA-stimulated metabolic exhaustion (8).

PHARMACOLOGY OF EXCITATORY AMINO ACID RECEPTORS

Glutamate, the primary EAA neurotransmitter, is released from presynaptic nerve terminals, but the synaptic concentration is quickly reduced by an active reuptake process mediated by a specific, energy-dependent reuptake pump. Impairment in the activity of the EAA reuptake pump may play an important role in EAA neurotoxicity in disease states. In experimental hypoxia-ischemia, synaptosomal uptake of glutamate is transiently reduced, contributing to the marked elevations in extracellular glutamate concentrations that may reach the micromolar range (9). Metabolic disorders may contribute to EAA neurotoxicity by this mechanism.

The excitatory responses to glutamate are mediated by several receptor subtypes that may be classified into two broad categories as either N-methyl-D-aspartate (NMDA) or non-NMDA type EAA receptors (10,11) (Figures 3-1 and 3-2). NMDA maximally activates a glutamate receptor that is linked to an ion channel. Together the receptor and its channel are referred to as the NMDA receptor/channel complex (see Figure 3-1). The NMDA channel is permeable to cations such as sodium and calcium, and at normal membrane potential the channel is blocked by magnesium ions (12). Partial depolarization of the membrane potential is necessary for the magnesium block to be removed. As a result, the NMDA receptor/channel complex is not generally involved in ordinary rapid impulse flow.

Several antagonists of the NMDA receptor/channel complex have been developed, some of which block the NMDA receptor (competitive NMDA antagonists) and others that block the associated cation channel (noncompetitive antagonists). Drugs such as 3 (2-carboxylpiperazin-4-yl) propyl-1-phosphonic acid (CPP), CGS-19755, and 2-amino-5-phosphonovaleric acid (AP5) are competitive blockers at the NMDA receptor (13). The channel binding site is commonly referred to as the phencyclidine receptor. Two major noncompetitive channel-blocking drugs are MK-801 and phencyclidine (14–16). The NMDA

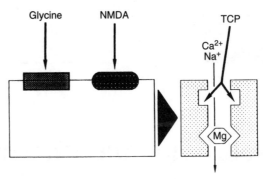

Figure 3-1. Current understanding of the components of the NMDA receptor/channel complex, based on biochemical and electrophysiological evidence, is outlined in this schematic diagram. The NMDA recognition site is coupled to a cationic channel that is permeable to Ca^{2+} and Na^+. NMDA-receptor activation is modulated by several regulatory sites. Activation of a closely associated glycine recognition site is required for channel activation and markedly enhances responses to NMDA. Physiological concentrations of Mg^{2+} block the NMDA-associated ionophore, and membrane depolarization relieves this blockade. Thus, NMDA receptor/channel activation requires activation of both NMDA and glycine receptor and concurrent membrane depolarization. NMDA-receptor channel activation also can be modulated by Zn^{2+} and polyamines (not illustrated). Noncompetitive NMDA receptor antagonists such as phencyclidine and its thienyl derivative TCP block NMDA responses by binding within the NMDA-operated ionophore (6–8). Cerebral events that impair the mechanisms that regulate Ca^{2+} homeostasis can produce a prolonged elevation of intracellular Ca^{2+} concentration and cytotoxicity.

receptor/channel complex also includes several regulatory sites. One receptor is specific for the simple amino acid glycine (17). Unlike the inhibitory glycine site in the spinal cord, this site is not sensitive to strychnine, and activation facilitates opening of the NMDA channel by glutamate. Recognition sites for zinc and polyamines also appear to regulate NMDA receptor/channel complex activity (6).

Non-NMDA receptors have been identified that are preferentially activated by the glutamate analogues quisqualic acid and kainic acid (11). Kainic acid was identified a number of years ago as a very potent neurotoxic and convulsant agent in the adult brain (18,19). Two types of non-NMDA receptor have been identified: one that is linked to an ion channel that fluxes sodium and to a lesser extent calcium, and another that is linked to stimulation of phosphoinositide (PPI) turnover or downregulation of cyclic-AMP production. The ion-channel linked receptors are called alpha-amino-3-hydroxy-5-methyl-4-isoxazole pupionate (AMPA) receptors after a glutamate analogue that selectively stimulates them (20). The receptors linked to several messengers are called metabotropic receptors. Antagonists have been identified that block the quisqualate receptor linked to the ion channel and the phosphoinositol-linked (metabotropic) receptor (21). A marked increase in glutamate release, which occurs during a prolonged seizure, is likely

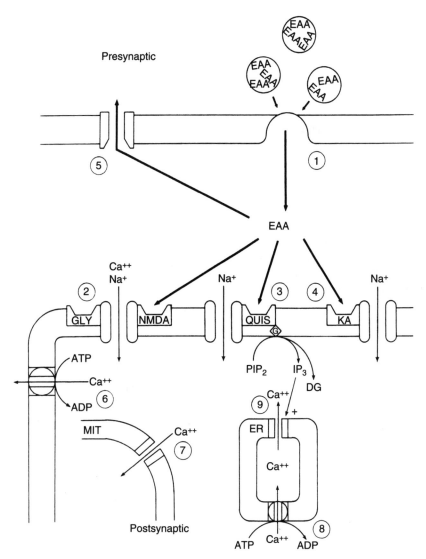

Figure 3-2. This schematic diagram outlines the synaptic components that contribute to EAA-mediated synaptic transmission, second messenger generation, and calcium homeostasis. **1**: EAAs such as glutamate are released from presynaptic terminals in a calcium-dependent process by presynaptic depolarization. **2–4**: Glutamate in the synaptic cleft depolarizes the postsynaptic membrane by binding to at least three subsets of EAA receptors. Activation of (2), the NMDA receptor/channel complex, (3), quisqualate receptors, and (4), kainate receptors, produced calcium (Ca^{2+}) and sodium (Na^+) entry through receptor-associated ionophores. Furthermore, activation of a subset of quisqualate receptors that are linked to phospholipase C produces phosphoinositol hydrolysis and generation of the second messengers inositol triphosphate and diacylglycerol. **5**: The excitatory action of synaptically released EAA is terminated by a presynaptic, high-affinity, energy-dependant transport process.

to result in the activation of all types of glutamate receptors.

DEVELOPMENTAL CHANGES IN GLUTAMATE NEUROTOXICITY

The immature brain is quite sensitive to neurotoxicity from glutamate and certain of its analogues (18,22). Olney discovered a number of years ago that feeding monosodium glutamate to neonatal mice produced characteristic lesions in the hypothalamus. More recently, it has become clear that the receptors that mediate glutamate neurotoxicity respond differently

in the immature brain compared with the adult brain. These observations have important implications for the EAA neurotransmitter hypothesis of epileptic brain injury in children.

In adults, kainic acid is the most potent neurotoxic analogue of glutamate, but in neonatal rodents, NMDA is the most toxic analogue (22,25). Although kainic acid produces seizures in the immature brain, it produces little cytotoxicity (26). In contrast, NMDA injected into the seven-day-old rat brain produces prolonged seizures and extensive neurotoxicity. At seven days of age, the relative neurotoxicity of several glutamate analogues in NMDA >>> quisqualate > kainic = zero, whereas in the adult kainic acid >>

NMDA $\geq$ quisqualate. The severity of brain injury produced by direct injection of NMDA into the seven-day-old rat brain is approximately 60 times greater than in the adult. There is relatively sharp peak of sensitivity to NMDA neurotoxicity at seven days of age in the rat with less sensitivity at times before and after, suggesting a potentially important effect of age on sensitivity to EAA-mediated injury. The shift in sensitivity to NMDA neurotoxicity parallels developmental changes in genetic expression of NMDA subunits that make up the receptor channel complex (27,28).

The susceptibility of the developing brain to NMDA-induced brain injury parallels the susceptibility to hypoxic-ischemic brain injury. Olney's studies suggest that the acute neurohistological picture of NMDA-induced injury in the seven-day-old rat brain is virtually identical to that from a hypoxic-ischemic injury at the same age (25). NMDA may induce metabolic changes similar to hypoxia-ischemia. Studies using ^{31}P magnetic resonance spectroscopy in brain slices indicate that NMDA produces a rapid exhaustion of phosphocreatine stores and nucleotide triphosphate levels following its application (29). The noncompetitive antagonist MK-801 protects against hypoxic-ischemic damage in the seven-day-old rat brain (30). These studies suggest that overactivation of NMDA receptors may be a final common pathway for hypoxic-ischemic injury, as well as other types of developmental brain injury.

EVIDENCE THAT EAA NEUROTRANSMITTERS PLAY A ROLE IN SEIZURE-RELATED INJURY

The link between excessive EAA neurotransmitter activity and epileptic brain injury was initially strengthened by Meldrum's pioneering studies in subhuman primates (1). These studies showed that seizures alone could damage the brain and that the EAA analogue kainic acid produced sustained seizures and brain injury with a regional histological pattern resembling epileptic brain injury (31,32). Two recent models have provided additional, more direct experimental evidence.

In experiments conducted by Sloviter, electrical stimulation of the perforant pathway that projects into the hippocampus from the entorhinal cortex leads to neuronal degeneration in hippocampal zones innervated by perforant pathway fibers (33). The perforant pathway is the major excitatory glutamatergic afferent pathway into the hippocampus. The acute neuropathological changes produced by the persistent stimulation resemble the histopathology seen when glutamate analogues or other convulsant substances are injected into the hippocampus (34).

The pathology replicates the typical "epileptic" pattern of injury with damage to dentate basket cells, hilar cells, and CA3 and CA1 pyramidal cells of the hippocampus. CA2 neurons are typically spared. Electron microscopy shows acutely swollen dendritic segments distributed in a laminar pattern corresponding to the neuronal-receptive fields of EAA pathways in the perforant projection. Somatostatin-containing neurons are especially vulnerable, whereas γ-aminobutyric acid (GABA) neurons are relatively spared (35).

In a second model of epileptic brain injury developed by Collins and Olney, persistent focal seizure activity is induced by focal application of the GABA receptor–blocking drug bicuculline onto the cerebral cortex (36). The seizure activity causes acute neurodegenerative changes in specific thalamic regions innervated by the corresponding corticothalamic pathway. This model also produces acute neuropathological changes, which resemble glutamate-like neuronal degeneration. Using this model, Olney's group demonstrated that ketamine and MK-801, two powerful blockers of the action of NMDA-type EAA receptors, completely abolish the thalamic damage caused by the focal seizure activity (37). MK-801 reduced but did not prevent the electrical seizure activity itself, suggesting that the neuroprotective action resulted from blockade of NMDA-type EAA receptor activation rather than from a reduction in neurotransmitter release. The results of these experiments along with the electrical stimulation studies support the hypothesis that EAA receptor stimulation plays an important role in seizure-induced neuronal injury. They also suggest that the neurotoxic effects of seizures can be dissociated from effects of excessive electrical activity.

EAA MECHANISMS IN SEIZURES AND INJURY IN THE IMMATURE BRAIN

The immature brain, especially the seven-day-old rat brain, is quite sensitive to NMDA-mediated neurotoxicity, but the potential contribution of this mechanism to damage from seizures has not been clearly delineated. The models of prolonged direct electrical stimulation of the perforant pathway and of bicuculline-induced focal seizures described for adult animals have not been examined in the infant. However, both perforant pathway stimulation and the lithium-pilocarpine model of status epilepticus have been shown to produce neurotoxicity in the hippocampus of 15-day-old rodents (38).

Experimental work does indicate that there is a dissociation between the direct neurotoxic effect of NMDA and indirect neurotoxicity from the seizures it produces. In experiments in which NMDA was injected into one side of the seven-day-old rat brain, bihemispheric high-voltage epileptiform discharges are produced, but damage is confined to the side of the injected hemisphere (37). Also, in our experiments anticonvulsants such as phenytoin, diazepam, and pentobarbital markedly reduced NMDA-induced seizure activity but did not reduce the neurotoxic effects of injected NMDA. MK-801 and other NMDA antagonists produce significant levels of neuroprotection at doses that do not block behavioral seizures. EAA-mediated neurotoxicity is a plausible mechanism for seizure-related injury in the developing brain, but further experimental work is needed to define its role. Activation of non-NMDA receptors also could contribute to seizure-related injury because phosphoinositide turnover and release of free fatty acids are stimulated by seizures (39). An important implication of this hypothesis is that the distribution and severity of pathological injury in the developing brain would be expected to differ from the pattern in the adult.

EAA mechanisms also could play a role in epileptogenesis and seizure expression. In an in vitro model of electrographic seizures in hippocampal slices, NMDA antagonists such as AP4 and MK-801 prevented the progressive development of seizures but did not block previously induced seizures (40). This suggested that the process of establishing a long-lasting seizure-prone state depended on NMDA receptor/channel complex, whereas the expression of seizures was not. This suggests an important distinction between antiepileptogenic and anticonvulsant pharmacological agents.

It is also possible that EAA receptors play a role in other more subtle developmental sequelae of seizures. In addition to their role in transmembrane signaling, EAA neurotransmitters participate in a variety of neurodevelopmental events. These include promotion of neuronal survival, growth, and differentiation of neurons; regulation of neuronal circuitry and cytoarchitecture; regulation of activity-dependent synaptic plasticity; and certain forms of learning and memory (41). Excitotoxic amino acids may act as neurotrophic factors promoting neuronal survival growth and differentiation during development. The NMDA receptor/channel complex appears to play a critical role in visually determined plasticity in the visual cortex (42). Drugs that block the NMDA receptor/channel complex may block the physiologically determined ocular dominance shifts that normally occur with monocular deprivation. The NMDA receptor/channel complex also appears to play a critical role in the formation of long-term potentiation, an electrical model of learning and memory (43). Disturbances in these normal developmental mechanisms by excessive EAA neurotransmitters released during repeated seizures could potentially be a mechanism for a variety of neurobehavioral disturbances in patients with seizures. Seizure-induced disturbances in EAA mechanisms involved in memory in the hippocampus might be responsible for disturbances in learning and memory in patients with frequent or prolonged seizures. This encephalopathic disturbance might occur in the absence of permanent injury.

ONTOGENY OF EAA SYNAPTIC MARKERS

Synaptic markers of EAA neurotransmitters undergo marked changes during postnatal development. Recent studies of the ontogeny of NMDA and quisqualate-sensitive receptor subtypes during postnatal development indicate that NMDA-type and quisqualate-type glutamate receptors have a unique ontogenetic profile in the hippocampal formation (44). When receptors for NMDA-sensitive ^{3}H-glutamate binding, strychnine-insensitive glycine binding, and ^{3}H-N-(1[2-thienyl]cyclohexyl)3,4-piperidine (TCP) binding to the channel were examined independently, all were found to be overexpressed relative to the adult in the neonatal period. NMDA-sensitive binding exceeded adult levels by 50 to 120 percent in all regions of the hippocampus examined, with peak densities occurring between postnatal days 10 and 28. The ontogenetic profiles of the glycine modulatory site and the phencyclidine receptor were similar to each other but were delayed with respect to the timing of the NMDA recognition site. The physiological relevance of overexpression of NMDA recognition sites relative to other components of the NMDA receptor/channel complex are unclear. However, the temporal expression of NMDA recognition sites correlates with the development of synaptogenesis.

The ontogeny of NMDA receptor binding also appears to correlate with physiological changes. Postsynaptic excitation appears to predominate over inhibition during the first postnatal weeks of hippocampal development, as does enhanced seizure susceptibility. In *CA3* of the hippocampus, superfusion with NMDA elicits recurrent synchronized burst activity, and the epileptogenic effect of NMDA increases from postnatal days 1 to 10 (45). Also, the susceptibility to epileptiform activity increases from postnatal days 4 to 6 to postnatal day 14 (46). This activity is blocked by specific NMDA receptor antagonists (47). There is also a parallel between the developmental expression of NMDA recognition sites and the development of long-term potentiation; however, the development of NMDA receptors tends to lag behind the development of sensitivity to NMDA neurotoxicity, which transiently peaks on day seven.

EXCITATORY AMINO ACID MECHANISMS IN THE PATHOGENESIS OF PARTIAL EPILEPSY

Whether excitotoxic mechanisms actually play a role in the pathogenesis of childhood temporal lobe epilepsy associated with hippocampal damage is the subject of vigorous debate (38). Although the laboratory evidence discussed earlier suggests that this is possible, human epidemiologic data suggest that prolonged seizures are usually harmless in children (48). Although a history of febrile status epilepticus is frequently obtained in patients undergoing temporal lobectomy surgery for partial complex seizures, magnetic resonance imaging studies suggest that many patients have hippocampal anomalies that predated onset of seizures (49). However, recent serial MR imaging has identified a few children who acquired hippocampal sclerosis following very prolonged focal febrile seizures (50). Although a great deal remains to be done to define these relationships, this evidence suggests that EAA pathways also may have a role in the pathogenesis of certain forms of chronic epilepsy.

Partial complex seizures following hippocampal injury or malformation are sometimes progressive, suggesting that a vicious cycle is created in which further seizures lead to progressive injury and synaptic reorganization, which beget more seizures. EAA mechanisms could contribute to progressive metabolic disturbances and injury that could perpetuate this process. Abnormal recurrent sprouting of excitatory mossy fibers in the hippocampus that have lost their targets

in *CA*3 region has been implicated in this process (26). Loss of inhibitory interneurons in the hippocampus may also contribute to this process (26). Our autoradiographic studies of tissue resected from patients with temporal lobe epilepsy shows a reduction in binding to the phencyclidine site of the NMDA receptor/channel complex and a relative increase in associated NMDA receptor sites (51). Other studies have found elevations in the non-NMDA receptors in human hippocampal tissue (52). Recent studies of human hippocampal AMPA and NMDA messenger RNA levels in temporal lobe epilepsy patients also found elevated levels for AMPA GluR1 and NMDAR2 subunits (53). These results are consistent with our autoradiographic receptor studies suggesting that alterations in glutamate receptor levels and subunit composition contribute to neuronal hyperexcitability and seizure generation. The relative relationship between increased NMDA receptor sites compared with channel sites resembles the patterns seen in the immature rat brain.

These observations suggest a hypothetical mechanism for progressive epileptic change in certain patients with complex partial seizures (Figure 3-3). In this hypothesis, a severe insult such as prolonged status epilepticus or hypoxia-ischemia leads to EAA release and a glutamate-type of injury to dendritic

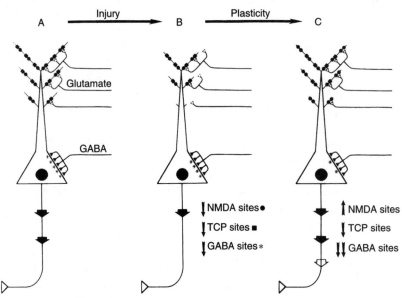

Figure 3-3. A speculative proposal of the mechanisms that contribute to the progressive epileptic changes observed in patients with complex partial seizures. **A**: Schematic illustration of a typical pyramidal cell from Ca$_{1-3}$ hippocampal subfields. Glutamatergic input (*open triangles*) from the perforant path originates in the entorhinal cortex and synapses on distal pyramidal cell dendrites and GABAergic interrneurons. A severe focal cerebral insult causes overactivation of EAA receptors and produces excitotoxic injury localized mainly to dendritic regions of the pyramidal cells. **B**: The dendritic region of surviving pyramidal cells is stunted and the number of functional NMDA recognition sites (*solid circles*) and corresponding TCP channels (*solid squares*) are reduced. Moderate loss of functional GABA$_A$ sites occurs. As a result of impaired EAA synaptic transmission, the level of pyramidal cell excitation is reduced, as depicted by the large arrow of the merging axon. In response to reduced pyramidal cell excitation, a series of compensatory synaptic alterations take place. **C**: Dendritic zones regenerate, EAA neurotransmission is enhanced by up-regulating NMDA recognition sites, and the level of functional inhibition is reduced by down-regulating GABA$_A$ sites. These changes in turn would compensate for the reduced pyramid cell excitation that results from cerebral injury by increasing excitatory tone. However, these compensatory changes could produced enhanced susceptibility to seizure and seizure-related excitotoxicity by lowering the seizure threshold. The compensatory epileptogenic events lead to a cycle of repeated seizures and injury.

regions of the hippocampus and to other susceptible regions. This form of injury causes loss of some pyramidal neurons, but those that remain have stunted, injured dendritic arbors (31). Perhaps in response to a reduced surface area of dendrites, postsynaptic NMDA receptor/channel complexes adjust by up-regulating their NMDA receptors. This would compensate for the reduced dendritic surface area available for excitatory input to the neuron. In addition, a reduction in the number of inhibitory GABA receptors might also serve to increase excitatory tone.

An increased ratio of NMDA receptors per channel might sensitize the neuron to enhance excitability and further injury from physiological amounts of synaptic glutamate. Potentially, the seizure threshold might be lower, and further dendritic injury might result from excitatory events that are only mildly superphysiological. This additional injury in turn leads to a cycle of repeated seizures and injury. An important implication of this model is that pharmacological attempts could be made to prevent further EAA-mediated injury and thereby halt the progression of the disorder. Based on studies suggesting that there is a distinction between epileptogenesis and epileptic expression, drugs might be developed that would reduce the progressive epileptic process, although they themselves might not be good antiseizure agents (40,54).

CONCLUSION

Although seizures dramatically raise the brain's metabolic activity during the ictal event, they generally do not have any long-term damaging effect. However, data from animal models of status epilepticus and supraphysiological stimulation of specific excitatory pathways indicate that neuronal injury in sensitive areas such as the hippocampus can occur through a glutamate-mediated excitotoxic mechanism. Developing animals appear to be less affected by this mechanism than adults. However, recent studies in children suggest that hippocampal sclerosis occasionally may be caused by prolonged febrile status epilepticus. Analysis of hippocampal tissue removed at surgery from patients with temporal lobe epilepsy indicate that levels of neuronal glutamate receptors are elevated. This may contribute to epileptogenicity and a progressive cycle of further excitotoxic injury. A better understanding is needed of the factors that contribute to epileptic excitotoxicity.

REFERENCES

1. Meldrum BS, Brierly JB. Prolonged epileptic seizures in primates. Ischemic cell change and its relationship to ictal physiological events. *Arch Neurol* 1973; 28:10–17.

2. Auer RN, Siesjo BK. Biological differences between ischemic, hypoglycemia and epilepsy. *Ann Neurol* 1988; 24:699–707.

3. Siesjo BK. Cell damage in the brain: A speculative synthesis. *J Cereb Blood Flow Metab* 1981; 1:155–185.

4. Ingvar M, Siesjo BK. Local blood flow and glucose consumption in the rat brain during sustained bicuculline-induced seizures. *Acta Neurol Scand* 1983; 68:129–144.

5. Fonnum F. Glutamate: a neurotransmitter in mammalian brain. *J Neurochem* 1984; 38:1–11.

6. Choi DW. Ionic dependence of glutamate neurotoxicity. *J Neurosci* 1987; 7:369–379.

7. Rothman SM, Olney JW. Glutamate and the pathophysiology of hypoxic-ischemic brain damage. *Ann Neurol* 1986; 19:105–111.

8. Novelli A, Reilly JA, Lysko PG, Henneberry RC. Glutamate becomes neurotoxic via the *N*-methyl-*D*-aspartate receptor when intracellular energy levels are reduced. *Brain Res* 1988; 451:205–212.

9. Silverstein FS, Buchanan K, Johnston MV. Perinatal hypoxia-ischemia disrupts striatal high affinity ^{3}H-glutamate uptake into synaptosomes. *J Neurochem* 1986; 47:1614–1619.

10. Watkins JC, Evans RH. Excitatory amino acid transmitters. *Annu Rev Pharmacol Toxicol* 1981; 21:165–204.

11. Monahan DT, Bridges RJ, Cotman CW. The excitatory amino acid receptors: their classes, pharmacology and distinct properties in the function of the central nervous system. *Annu Rev Pharmacol Toxicol* 1989; 24:365–402.

12. Ascher P, Nowak I. Electrophysiological studies of NMDA receptors. *Trends Neurosci* 1987; 10:284–286.

13. Boast CA, Gerhardt SC, Pastor G, et al. The NMDA antagonists CGS-19755 and CPP reduce ischemic brain damage in gerbils. *Brain Res* 1988; 442:345–348.

14. Gill R, Foster C, Woodruff GN. Systemic administration of MK-801 protects against ischemia-induced hippocampal neurodegeneration in the gerbil. *J Neurosci* 1987; 7:3343–3349.

15. Kemp JA, Foster AC, Wong EHF. Non-competitive antagonists of excitatory amino acid receptors. *Trends Neurosci* 1987; 19:294–299.

16. McDonald JW, Silverstein FS, Johnston MV. Neuroprotective effects of MK-801, TCP, PCP, CPP against NMDA neurotoxicity. *Brain Res* 1989; 290:33–40.

17. Johnson JW, Ascher P. Glycine potentiates the NMDA response in cultured mouse brain neurons. *Nature* 1987; 325:529–531.

18. Olney JW, Ho OL, Rhee V. Cytotoxic effects of acid and sulfate containing amino acids on the infant mouse central nervous system. *Exp Brain Res* 1971; 14:61–76.

19. Zaczek R, Nelson MF, Coyle JT. Effects of anesthetics and anticonvulsants on the action of kainic acid in the rat hippocampus. *Eur J Pharmacol* 1979; 52:323–327.

20. McDonald JW, Trescher WH, Johnston MV. Susceptibility of brain to AMPA induced neurotoxicity transiently peaks during early postnatal development. *Brain Res* 1992; 583:54–70.

21. Honore T, Davies SN, Drejer J, et al. Quinoxaline-diones: Potent competitive non-NMDA glutamate receptor antagonists. *Science* 1988; 241:701–703.

22. McDonald JW, Silverstein FS, Johnston MV. Neurotoxicity of NMDA is markedly enhanced in developing rat central nervous system. *Brain Res* 1988; 459:200–203.

23. Campochiaro P, Coyle JT. Ontogenetic development of kainate neurotoxicity: correlates with glutamate innervation. *Proc Natl Acad Sci USA* 1978; 75:2025–2029.

24. Silverstein FS, Chen RC, Johnston MV. The glutamate agonist quisqualic acid is neurotoxic in striatum and hippocampus of immature rat brain. *Neurosci Lett* 1986; 71:13–18.

25. Ikonomidou C, Mosinger JL, Shahid Salles I, Labruyere J, Olney JW. Sensitivity of the developing rat brain to hypobaric/ischemic damage parallels sensitivity to *N*-methyl-*D*-aspartate neurotoxicity. *J. Neurosci* 1989; 9:2809–2818.

26. Holmes GL. Epilepsy in the developing brain: lessons from the laboratory and clinic. *Epilepsia* 1997; 38:12–30.

27. Burgard EC, Hablitz JJ. Developmental changes in NMDA and non-NMDA receptor-mediated synaptic potentials in rat neocortex. *J Neurophysiol* 1993; 69:230–240.

28. Sheng M, Cummings J, Rolau LA. Changing subunit composition of heteromeric NMDA receptors during development of rat cortex. *Nature* 1994; 368:144–147.

29. Jacquin T, Gillet B, Fortine G, et al. Metabolic action of NMDA in newborn rat brain ex vivo: ^{31}P magnetic resonance spectroscopy. *Brain Res* 1989; 497:296–304.

30. McDonald JW, Silverstein FS, Johnston MV. MK-801 protects the neonatal brain from hypoxic-ischemic damage. *Eur J Pharmacol* 1987; 140:359–361.

31. Olney JW, Collins RC, Sloviter RS. Excitotoxic mechanism of epileptic brain damage. In: Delgado-Escueta AV, Ward AA Jr, Woodbury DM, Porter RJ (eds.). *Basic Mechanisms of the Epilepsies: Molecular and Cellular Approaches.* New York: Raven Press, 1986:857–877. (*Advances in Neurology;* vol 44).

32. Nadler JV, Perry BW, Cotman CW. Intraventricular kainic acid preferentially destroys hippocampal pyramidal cells. *Nature* 1978; 271:676–677.

33. Sloviter RS. "Epileptic" brain damage in rats induced by sustained electrical stimulation of the perforant path. I. Acute electrophysiological and light microscope studies. *Brain Res Bull* 1983; 10:685–697.

34. Loney JW, DeGubareff T, Sloviter RS. "Epileptic" brain damage in rats induced by sustained electrical stimulation of the perforant path. II. Ultra-structural analysis of acute hippocampal pathology. *Brain Res Bull* 1983; 10:699–712.

35. Sloviter RS. Decreased hippocampal inhibition and a selective loss of interneurons in experimental epilepsy. *Science* 1987; 235:73–76.

36. Clifford DB, Zorumski CF, Olney JW. Ketamine and MK-801 prevent degeneration of thalamic neurons induced by focal cortical seizures. *Exp Neurol* 1989; 105:272–279.

37. McDonald JW, Silverstein FS, Cardona D, et al. Systemic administration of MK-801 protects against NMDA and quisqualate mediated neurotoxicity in perinatal rat. *Neuroscience* 1990; 36:589–599.

38. Wasterlain CG. Recurrent seizures in the developing brain are harmful. *Epilepsia* 1997; 38:728–734.

39. Iadarola M, Nicoletti F, Naranjo J, Putnam F, Costa E. Kindling enhances stimulation of inositol phospholipid hydrolysis elicited by ibotenic acid in rat hippocampal slices. *Brain Res* 1986; 374:174–178.

40. Stasheff SF, Anderson WW, Clark S, Wilson WA. NMDA antagonists differentiate epileptogenesis from seizure expression in an in vitro model. *Science* 1989; 245:648–651.

41. Mattson MD. Neurotransmitters in the regulation of neurocytoarchitecture. *Brain Res Rev* 1988; 13:179–212.

42. Kleinschmidt A, Bear MF, Singer W. Blockade of "NMDA" receptors disrupts experience dependent plasticity of kitten striate cortex. *Science* 1987; 238:355–358.

43. Nicoll RA, Kauer JA, Malenka RC. The current excitement in long term potentiation. *Neuron* 1988; 1:97–103.

44. McDonald JW, Johnston MV, Young AB. Differential ontogenetic development of three receptors comprising the NMDA receptor channel complex in the rat hippocampus. *Exp Neurol* 1990; 110:237–247.

45. King AE, Cherubini E, Ben-Ari Y. NMDA induces recurrent synchronized burst activity in immature hippocampal CA_3 neurons in vitro. *Dev Brain Res* 1989; 46:1–8.

46. Swann FW, Brady RJ. Penicillin-induced epileptogenesis in immature rat CA_3 hippocampal pyramidal cells. *Dev Brain Res* 1984; 12:243–254.

47. Brady RJ, Swann JW. Ketamine selectively suppresses synchronized after discharges in immature hippocampus. *Neurosci Lett* 69:143–149.

48. Camfield PR. Recurrent seizures in the developing brain are not harmful. *Epilepsia* 1997; 38:735–737.

49. Fernandez G, Effenberger O, Vinz B, et al. Hippocampal malformation as a cause of familial febrile convulsions and subsequent hippocampal sclerosis. *Neurology* 1998; 50:909–917.

50. VanLandingham KE, Heinz ER, Cavazos JE, Lewis DV. MRI evidence of hippocampal injury after prolonged focal febrile convulsions. *Ann Neurol* 1998; 43:413–426.

51. McDonald JW, Garofolo EA, Hood TA, Sackelleres C, Johnston MV. Altered excitatory and inhibitory amino acid receptor binding in hippocampus for patients with temporal lobe epilepsy. *Ann Neurol* 1991; 29:529–541.

52. Hosford DA, Crain BJ, Cao Z, et al. Increased AMPA-sensitive quisqualate receptor binding and reduced NMDA receptor binding in epileptic human hippocampus. *J Neurosci* 1991; 11:428–434

53. Mathern GW, Pretorius JK, Kornblum HI, et al. Human hippocampal AMPA and NMDA mRNA levels in temporal lobe epilepsy patients. *Brain* 1997; 120:1937–1959.

54. McNamara, JO, Russell, PD, Rigsbee, I, Bonhaus, DW. Anticonvulsant and antiepileptic actions of MK-801 in the kindling and electroshock models. *Neuropharmacology* 1988; 22:563–568.

CHAPTER 4

The Pathology of the Epilepsies: Insights from Pathology to Mechanisms of Causation of Temporal Lobe Epilepsy

Nihal C. de Lanerolle, D.Phil., D.Sc.

Epilepsy is now well recognized not as a single disease entity but as a variety of syndromes, all characterized symptomatically by paroxysmal abnormal electrical activity of the brain and recurrent behavioral seizures. Underlying these syndromes are a variety of etiologies and pathologies. This understanding of symptomatic epileptic syndromes was formalized in the International Classification of the Epilepsies (1). Over the years an extensive literature has accumulated on the pathologies of the epilepsies, and it is not possible in the space of this chapter to review this literature in its entirety. A general review of the different pathologies can be found in other publications (2,3). In the past 10 years, however, there has been a major effort in centers around the world to investigate the pathology of temporal lobe epilepsy (TLE). This chapter reviews this recent body of work and assesses what can be learned about the mechanisms underlying the causation of epilepsy.

THE HIPPOCAMPAL PATHOLOGY OF TEMPORAL LOBE EPILEPSY

Early Studies of Temporal Lobe Pathology

Studies on the pathology of TLE have a long history, beginning perhaps with a paper by Bouchet and Cazauvielh (4). These early studies, discussed in several papers, most notably in an excellent review by Gloor (5), show that in TLE pathological alterations may be found in several regions of the temporal lobe — the hippocampus, amygdala, entorhinal cortex, and even the temporal neocortex.

Before discussing the pathology of the hippocampus, a few comments on the findings in associated temporal lobe regions (amygdala, entorhinal and temporal neocortex) are in order. The pathology of the amygdala in TLE has received relatively little study for a variety of reasons, including its complex anatomy and the difficulty of obtaining intact, reliably oriented specimens through surgical resections. However, early studies (6) and more recent studies (7,8) indicate that there may be neuronal loss and/or gliosis of this structure. The degree of neuronal loss is estimated to be approximately 60 percent of controls (7,8). Although Hudson and coworkers (8) describe some patients as having only amygdala sclerosis, this is not corroborated by Wolf and coworkers (8), who found no such cases. In a study of 55 brains of epileptic patients obtained post mortem, Margerison and Corsellis (9) reported that patchy nerve cell loss and gliosis were present in the amygdala in 27 percent of their cases. However, they observed that in no instance was there amygdaloid damage without a hippocampal lesion. Moreover, there were 21 of 55 cases in which hippocampal damage was not accompanied by an amygdaloid lesion. Thus, the amygdala lesion by itself may not be sufficient to cause epilepsy, although it may be a contributing factor. Two parallel studies by Feindel and Rasmussen (10,11) suggest an important role for the amygdala in the pathogenesis of epilepsy. These authors compared the surgical outcomes of temporal lobectomies in patients with only the amygdala and a small part of the hippocampal uncal region removed with those in whom, additionally, a greater part of the hippocampus was removed. The incidence of good outcomes in the two groups was the same. Although the inference can be made from these studies that the amygdala removal was common to the two groups, it was not exclusive to either. From the description of the surgical resection in the amygdala excision procedure (10) it appears that uncal hippocampal regions such as the band of Giacomini and terminal part of the dentate gyrus in the medial surface of the uncus, anterior portions of the pes hippocampus, and parts of the entorhinal cortex may have been removed as well. Given the importance of entorhinal afferents in driving the hippocampus and the anterior hippocampal region in the human as the main pathway for entorhinal afferents to and efferents from the hippocampus, a primary role for the hippocampus can still be argued. There is still no definitive study in which the amygdala, exclusively, has been surgically removed.

The entorhinal cortex has major afferents to the hippocampus and receives efferents from the hippocampus. It has been implicated as a major player in a network of areas supporting temporal lobe seizures (12), and its removal during anterior temporal lobectomy is thought to be essential for the control of complex partial seizures (13). However, little pathological change was noted in this region until recent work on the entorhinal cortex shows that there is selective loss of layer III neurons in the medial entorhinal cortex (14). The implication of such cell loss for epileptogenesis remains speculative.

Although volumetric studies of the temporal lobe has often demonstrated a decreased volume of the entire temporal lobe on the epileptogenic side, pathological observations of surgically excised temporal neocortex during temporal lobectomy for epilepsy rarely show any definitive changes (de Lanerolle, unpublished data). However, there are reports that in some patients developmental abnormalities such as dysgenesis and heterotopias may be observed. Overall, the pathological changes in the temporal neocortex, as described to date, are minor.

Early histopathological studies of the hippocampus of persons with TLE observed the presence of "sclerosis." The term *sclerosis*, as originally used, is a descriptive term for a hippocampus that is shrunken and hardened (indurated) and which, upon histological examination, shows neuronal loss and gliosis (for a fuller discussion of sclerosis see reference 15). This histological pattern is most characteristic in CA_1 or the Sommer sector (Figure 4-1). The first autopsy study to correlate TLE (based on clinical semiology) with sclerosis was by Stauder (16), who reported that all patients with TLE always had hippocampal sclerosis (16). Subsequent studies by Sano and Malmud and Margerison and Corsellis have reported hippocampal sclerosis in about 60 percent of patients with TLE, with varying proportions showing bilateral or unilateral sclerosis (9,17).

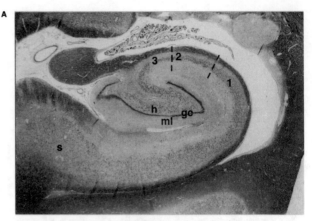

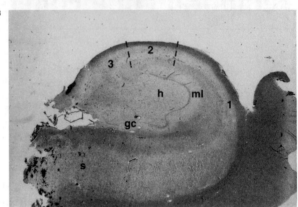

Figure 4-1. A. Photomicrograph of a coronal section of an autopsy hippocampus stained with cresyl violet for Nissl substance. Note the abundance of granule cells (gc) in the dentate gyrus and pyramidal and other neurons in the fields of Ammon's horn. **B.** A photomicrograph of a coronal section of the hippocampus of an MTLE patients also stained with cresyl violet. Note the extensive loss of neurons. Abbreviations: 1, 2, and 3 = Ammon's horn or CA fields; *h* = hilus or CA4; *ml* = dentate molecular layer; *s* = subiculum. (Pictures courtesy of Dr. Jung Kim).

The general consensus, therefore, is that sclerosis of the hippocampus is correlated with TLE. However, whether sclerosis is the cause or effect of seizures is a point of continuing debate (5,15). A fact of relevance for pediatric epilepsy is that sclerosis of the hippocampus is clearly linked to a history of febrile seizures, childhood status epilepticus (18–20) or birth trauma (20). Prolonged complicated seizures or status epilepticus during a febrile episode is shown to be associated with sclerosis in the hippocampus (21,22). Nevertheless, sclerosis is reported in infants dying of status epilepticus not resulting from a febrile episode (21). Status epilepticus by itself between the ages of 3 months and 7 years can be associated with sclerosis (5). While hippocampal sclerosis is a prominent feature in the pathology of TLE, it is by no means the only feature. It is not found in approximately 15 percent of patients in whom an extrahippocampal mass lesion (e.g., a tumor, hamartoma, arteriovenous malformation) may be the cause of the seizure (18,20,23,24).

Although much less is known about how such lesions cause seizures, recent studies are beginning to shed some light.

Recent Studies of Hippocampal Pathology

In the past decade or so, there has been a great increase in the number of studies that have examined hippocampi surgically removed for the control of medically refractory seizures. This increase in investigative activity has stemmed from the en bloc resection of the hippocampus and the availability of many new anatomical and physiological techniques that can be applied to the study of human brain seizure foci. These studies point to a variety of pathological features that characterize the hippocampal seizure focus.

Principal Neuron Loss in Adult and Pediatric Populations

To describe more precisely the nature of hippocampal sclerosis, several studies have attempted to quantitatively estimate the degree of neuron loss in epileptic hippocampi. Mouritzen Dam made cell counts in the hippocampi obtained at autopsy from 20 TLE patients and compared them with those from 20 nonepileptic controls (25,26). She reported that epilepsy patients showed neuron loss in all areas of the hippocampus and dentate granule cell layer, the most severely affected regions being the granule cell layer and Ammon's horn area H_3 (hilus). Sagar and Oxbury examined 32 surgically excised hippocampi from patients with TLE using the same counting methods as Mouritzen Dam, correlating cell counts in the dentate gyrus, Ammon's horn areas H_3 (hilus), H_2 (CA_3 and CA_2) and H_1 (CA_1) with the age of onset of the first (febrile) convulsion (27). They observed that cell loss is found in the dentate and all Ammon's horn areas, with the cell counts being lower when the first convulsion occurs at age 3 years or less. In those patients showing cell loss in all areas, the first convulsion was observed to last more than 30 minutes or repetitive convulsions occurred during the first day.

Babb and coworkers analyzed a larger series ($n = 45$) of surgically excised hippocampi along with other parts of the temporal lobe (28). Their findings confirmed previous findings of significant reductions in neurons in the dentate gyrus and all fields of Ammon's horn in patients with TLE compared with controls. In contrast, the subiculum, entorhinal cortex, and other temporal neocortical areas did not show cell loss. Their study also makes clear for the first time that the degree of hippocampal neuron loss may depend on the particular neural substrate causing seizures: in patients with extra-hippocampal lesions compared to autopsy controls, they found no statistically significant decrease

in Ammon's horn and only a relatively small decrease in the fascia dentata (28). Furthermore, in a study correlating pyramidal cell densities with presurgical stereoencephalography derived from hippocampal depth electrode recordings, patients who consistently exhibited anterior hippocampal focal changes in stereoencephalography, accompanying onset of ictus, had cell densities that were selectively reduced in the anterior hippocampus compared to the posterior hippocampus, whereas in those with more regional onset, cell densities were reduced both anteriorly and posteriorly (28).

At the Yale Epilepsy Center, hippocampi have been removed from patients with medically refractory TLE under four circumstances (29,30): (1) as a result of anteromedial temporal lobe resection (AMTR) with hippocampectomy in patients with hippocampal/ temporal lobe atrophy; (2) as a result of AMTR with hippocampectomy in patients with a medial temporal lobe mass (also resected) and poor temporal lobe specific memory; (3) as a result of AMTR with partial hippocampectomy in patients with a medial temporal lobe mass (also resected) and intact temporal lobe specific memory; and (4) if the preoperative localizing data are nonconcordant, patients are studied with invasive monitoring and subsequently undergo AMTR with hippocampectomy, if a medial temporal (amygdala, hippocampal or parahippocampal) seizure focus is detected. Cell counts of those hippocampi compared with counts from autopsy samples from neurologically normal subjects reveal three patterns of cell loss, which are expressed in different patient groups (3,31).

Among patients in whom the hippocampus was shown to be atrophied on imaging and evaluated to be the focus of seizure initiation, there is significant (>50%) loss of dentate granule cells and pyramidal cells in most areas of Ammon's horn with some variability in the extent of cell loss between individual cases (32). A subset of these patients (referred to as CA_1 group) had only cell loss in CA_1 but not the area dentata. These patients most closely resemble those with typical mesial temporal sclerosis. In hippocampal tissue removed from patients with an extrahippocampal temporal lobe mass lesion, with or without loss of memory ($n = 44$) (referred to as mass-associated temporal lobe epilepsy, MaTLE), there was an uniform loss of about 25 percent of neurons in all fields. Likewise, in a group of patients ($n = 15$) in whom there was no hippocampal sclerosis or a mass lesion (referred to as paradoxical temporal lobe epilepsy, PTLE), there was also about 25 percent neuron loss in all fields of the hippocampus. The surgical outcome after hippocampectomy with AMTR in the MTLE, CA_1 only, and MaTLE patients was excellent (>90%), whereas in PTLE it was poorer (about

60%). Thus, there seem to be different pathological substrates even among patients with TLE.

Correlation coefficient analyses of cell numbers between different CA fields also support distinguishing the aforementioned groups (31). In PTLE there is a strong positive correlation ($r > 0.5$, Spearman rank correlation coefficient) between neuron numbers in area CA_4 with those in CA_3, CA_2, and CA_1, but there is no correlation between dentate granule cell numbers and CA field neuron numbers. In MaTLE there is a strong positive correlation ($r > 0.7$) between dentate granule cells and CA fields as well as between the CA fields. In MTLE there is a correlation between CA fields, which was weaker ($r = 0.4$ to 0.6) than in the other groups. Additionally, there was a weak correlation ($r = 0.38$) between the dentate and CA_4 but not other CA fields. These three patterns of cell loss suggest different underlying pathogenic mechanisms.

Regional protein content assessed from Coomassie blue stained sections from the different patient groups (MTLE, MaTLE, PTLE and autopsy) show that in spite of moderate regional cell losses of about 25 percent in MaTLE and PTLE hippocampi, they possess similar high regional gray matter protein densities as autopsy cases (33). Likewise, compared to the very marked loss of neurons in MTLE hippocampi, corresponding changes in regional variations of protein density are greatly attenuated (e.g., 60% neuron loss in hilus but only a 10% protein loss). This smaller loss in protein density in MTLE suggests that there may be an increase in neuropil due to remodeling despite loss of cell bodies. Such changes are indeed observed and discussed further here.

Hippocampal neuron loss in pediatric epilepsy patients has been most closely analyzed by Mathern and coworkers (34,35). In one study, eight surgical patients (aged 5.5 months—11.5 years) were examined (35,36). Four of these patients had developed intractable epilepsy shortly after birth, whereas the other four had developed normally for periods ranging from 10 to 120 months and then developed seizures. They were all medically intractable, and their epileptogenic regions were determined to be large areas of extrahippocampal developmental or dysgenic lesions (i.e., cortical dysplasia). Neuron density measurements in all children with seizures, showed a decrease in hippocampal neurons (approximately 23%) in the fascia dentata, CA_4 (deep portions of hilus), and CA_2. A second study compared 28 pediatric patients (18 hemispherectomies, 6 multilobar resections, and 4 temporal lobectomies), median age 34 months, and 23 autopsies, median age 19 months (34). The patients were classified into three categories: (1) extratemporal, in which the congenital or acquired pathologies were outside the temporal neocortex; (2) temporal, in which the pathologies extended into the temporal neocortical region; and (3) hippocampal, in which no region other than the hippocampus was implicated. In children with hippocampal seizures there was a decrease in neuron density (50%) in the granule cell layer and all areas of the hippocampus compared with autopsy controls (see Figure 7 in ref. 34). Children with extratemporal pathologies showed only a decrease in hilar cell densities. However, in children with extrahippocampal (congenital and acquired) pathologies, presumably both extratemporal and temporal pathology groups, there was loss in granule cells but not in other regions compared with controls (see Figure 6 in ref. 34). Compared with extra/temporal group, children with temporal lesions showed greater decreases (approximately 20–30%) in neuron densities in hilus, CA_3, and CA_2 (least damage in CA_3 and CA_2). The results of these two series of studies are somewhat conflicting, particularly in relation to neuron loss in the extrahippocampal (extratemporal and temporal) pathologies. In the first series alone (eight cases), a loss of neurons in the fascia dentata was reported. This seems to be supported by the lumped data for temporal and extratemporal pathologies but not when either group is compared individually with controls. A third study included 19 pediatric patients (age 1.2 ± 0.4 year) with large extrahippocampal regions of cortical dysplasia in neocortex involving the temporal lobe that had multilobar or hemispheric resections (37). This pediatric patient group had a decrease in granule cells compared with autopsy controls but no cell loss in any other regions.

Although it is unclear to what extent the same patients are included in the three studies (34–37), a point that clearly emerges from these studies is that CA_1 cell loss is found only in children with a hippocampal seizure focus, not in those with any extrahippocampal pathology.

Comparison of these data to findings in adults reveal that both children and adults with a hippocampal seizure focus show extensive ($\geq 50\%$) cell loss in all areas (dentate and CA fields) of the hippocampus, excluding the subiculum (31,38). Children with extrahippocampal temporal lobe lesions show much less cell loss than those with a hippocampal seizure focus, as is also the case in adults with extrahippocampal temporal lobe lesions [children: 20–30% (34); adults: approximately 25 percent (31)].Whereas this neuron loss in children is limited to the hilus, CA_3, CA_2, and perhaps dentate granule cells, in adults the loss of neurons is uniform across all hippocampal areas. Extratemporal lesions (frontal, parietal, occipital) in children do not produce measurable cell loss in any hippocampal area in contrast to adults, who show about a 25 percent loss uniformly across all hippocampal areas.

Comparison of pediatric and adult cell count data suggests that in patients with a hippocampal seizure focus there is a pathogenic mechanism different from other groups that results in a loss of neurons throughout the area dentata and hippocampus very early in the course of the disease. With extrahippocampal pathologies, hippocampal cell loss may be a progressive consequence of seizure spread through the hippocampus. The closer the pathology is to the hippocampus (e.g., pediatric temporal group compared with extratemporal group), the earlier and more extensive the cell loss. In adults with extrahippocampal lesions, the uniform cell loss of approximately 25 percent observed throughout the area dentata and hippocampus may simply be the consequence of a longer (several years) period of seizure spread through the hippocampal formation.

Interneuron Loss in Adult Hippocampi

The aforementioned quantitative studies of neuron density do not distinguish between principal neurons (dentate granule cells and pyramidal cells) and interneurons. These studies most likely are biased toward estimating the principal neurons (granule cells and pyramidal cells). Immunocytochemical staining, with antibodies specific to neuroactive substances contained in interneurons, provides a means for assessing interneuron disposition even though quantitation cannot be done reliably. Immunocytochemical studies have demonstrated that in the MTLE patient group, but not in the MaTLE and PTLE groups, somatostatin (SOM), neuropeptide Y (NPY), and substance P (SP) neurons in the hilus are selectively lost (39,40). The loss of these interneurons is observed even in the absence

of detectable pyramidal neuron loss in the hilus (30). Gamma-aminobutyric acid (GABA)-containing interneurons in the area dentata, however, appear to be unaffected in all patient groups (40,41). In Ammon's horn the populations of SOM, NPY, SP, and GABA neurons in the MTLE group are not lost (in contrast to the hilus) even in the face of a great loss of pyramidal neurons (42). Thus, the selective loss of SOM, NPY, and SP neurons in the hilus is a reliable diagnostic feature of the MTLE hippocampus.

Axonal Sprouting in Adult Hippocampi

There is much evidence of the growth of new fiber systems, or sprouting, in TLE, as suggested by the protein changes previously discussed (33). The most prominent of these is the growth of a recurrent collateral into the dentate inner molecular layer from the granule cell mossy axon, most evident in MTLE hippocampi (39,43–45). Studies that visualize this sprouting by immunohistochemical staining of the peptide dynorphin (DYN) located within the mossy axon find this recurrent collateral system only in MTLE, not in MaTLE or PTLE (44,46) (Figure 4-2). However, using the Timm-stain method to visualize the zinc within this pathway, Mathern and coworkers found a small amount of Timm-positive silver grains, even in the MaTLE patients, more visible among the granule cell bodies (47). The amount of label is much less than in MTLE cases. Quantitation of this mossy fiber pathway by computerized densitometry confirmed that it was significantly greater in MTLE than in patients with extrahippocampal mass lesions (48). However, mossy fiber sprouting is not inevitable in MTLE, as a small

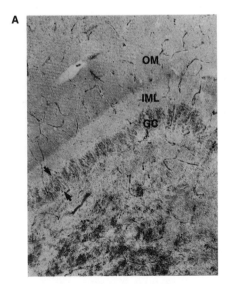
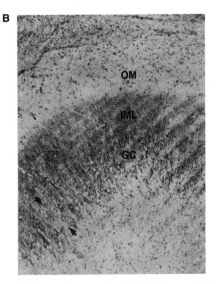

Figure 4-2. Photomicrographs of dynorphin-like (DYN) immunoreactivity in the fascia dentata of an MaTLE **(A)** and MTLE **(B)** hippocampus. In **(A)** DYN is found in granule cells (GC), which appear darker than background. The inner molecular layer (IML) is devoid of immunoreactivity. In **(B)** the MTLE hippocampus granule cells are more dispersed than in (A) and DYN is found throughout the IML which gives it a darker hue. Abbreviation: OM = outer molecular layer. (Adapted from de Lanerolle et al., *Epilepsy Research Supplement* 9, Chapter 20).

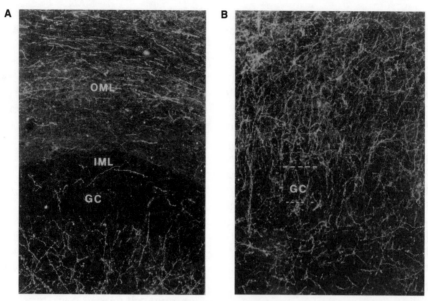

Figure 4-3. Dark field photomicrographs of neuropeptide Y (NPY) immunoreactive fibers in the molecular layer of the dentate gyrus in an MaTLE **(A)** and MTLE **(B)** hippocampus, respectively. Note the increase in NPY fibers throughout the molecular layer in the MTLE patient. Abbreviations: GC = granule cell layer; IML = inner molecular layer; OML = outer molecular layer.

proportion do not show labeling in the inner molecular layer [MTLE/DYN-negative group in (46)], and this difference is related to the excitable state of the granule cells.

At least four other examples of axonal sprouting are observed in the MTLE hippocampus compared with other patient groups and autopsy controls (39,40), and they are seen in the dentate molecular layer. The most striking is the increase in neuropeptide Y (NPY) immunoreactive axons throughout the dentate molecular layer in MTLE compared with MaTLE, PTLE, and autopsy groups in which NPY fibers are sparse in the inner and middle molecular layers (Figure 4-3). These NPY axons in MTLE synapse on granule cell dendrites in the inner molecular layer as well as smaller, unidentified dendrites in the inner and outer molecular layer (49). Like NPY, the somatostatin (SOM) fibers in MTLE show an increase throughout the molecular layer (39), and ultrastructural studies show that there are a greater number of immunoreactive axons and terminals in the inner as well as outer molecular layer. In the inner molecular layer, the SOM terminals synapse with granule cell apical dendrites only in MTLE, suggesting a more direct regulation of granule cells by SOM (49). Substance P immunoreactive fibers and terminals also show evidence of sprouting in MTLE, extending their normal territory of granule cell innervation to cover more of the proximal region of the apical dendrites and forming distinctive synapses on granule cell somata and the proximal dendrites (30). Evidence of sprouting was also observed in the distribution of acetylcholinesterase in the sclerotic hippocampus (30).

Interneuron Loss and Axonal Sprouting in Pediatric Patients

The distribution of the neuropeptidergic systems (DYN, NPY, SOM, and SP) has not been systematically studied in pediatric patients. In the Yale Epilepsy Surgery Program of over 300 patients in whom hippocampal tissue was removed, only 30 were under the age of 16 years, and of this group, five were under 12 years old (5.5 years, 5 years, 3 years, 1.6 year, and 11 years). Of this group of five, two had neuronal loss only in area CA_1 with no loss of peptidergic interneurons in the hilus or evidence of sprouting. Two others had peptidergic interneuron loss (NPY, SOM, SP) in the hilus but no evidence of sprouting. The CA_1 field in these cases had only minimal injury. The fifth patient (11 years old) had an extrahippocampal mass lesion, and the hippocampal organization was similar to MaTLE patients (i.e., no sprouting or other evidence of reorganization). In these youngest of our patients no sprouting of peptidergic systems was recognizable. Additionally, these pediatric data suggest that adult pathologies, such as CA_1 only damage and MaTLE, could develop at a very early point in the disease, and these may be relatively stable. The two patients (aged 5 years and 1.6 year) had only hilar interneuron loss but no sprouting. This suggests that interneuron loss may be an early event in the pathogenesis of MTLE.

In studies of children undergoing surgery for control of intractable seizures, Mathern and coworkers found that all patients showed mossy fiber sprouting (Timm stain), but those with a hippocampal seizure focus had greater sprouting than those with extrahippocampal foci. The pediatric patients thus resemble their adult counterparts (34,35).

Dentate Granule Cell Morphology

In addition to questions about possible loss of neurons in a hippocampal seizure focus, pathologists have been interested in whether the morphology of surviving neurons is altered in ways that favor increased excitability. The earliest work along these lines were by the Scheibels, who who analyzed Golgi-silver impregnated neurons in hippocampi removed from patients with mesial sclerosis (50–52). They identified four features of dendritic morphology that they thought indicated pathological changes in these neurons: a "closed parasol" formation, a "windblown look," development of apical dendrites from the "wrong" or axonal end of the cell, and loss of dendritic spines with dendritic nodulation. A more recent study that has compared granule cells from sclerotic hippocampi (MTLE) with those from nonsclerotic hippocampi (MaTLE) found that all of the features identified by the Scheibels were in fact features also seen in granule cells in nonepileptogenic hippocampi (53). This study determined that the main characteristics of MTLE granule cells was an increase in the dendrite length in the inner molecular layer as well as an increase in branching and segmentation (53). In addition, the axons of some granule cells from sclerotic hippocampi had collaterals that traveled into the inner molecular layer of the dentate gyrus (54,55) (Figure 4-4) and synapsed on granule cell

dendrites (55). These studies document the presence of granule cell recurrent collaterals initially proposed on the basis of Timm-stain studies (see below). On the basis of a small sample (8 neurons), it was reported that within sclerotic hippocampi (MTLE) granule cells that had recurrent collaterals also had fewer dendritic branches but a much higher spine density in the inner molecular layer than cells without recurrent collaterals (56).

Neurotransmitter Receptor Expression

The effectiveness of neurotransmitter systems in the hippocampus in altering neuronal excitability depends, among other factors, on the availability of receptors. The distribution and localization of several neurotransmitter receptor systems in the hippocampus have been reported.

In MTLE patients but not in other groups, the distribution of the GABA$_A$ benzodiazepine receptors, studied by receptor autoradiography, shows reduction in ligand binding in the dentate molecular layer and all areas of Ammon's horn (57). The loss of receptors is related to the loss of neurons. However, even on a per neuron basis, the ligand density tends to be lower in MTLE than in autopsy, MaTLE or PTLE groups, and is significantly lower in CA_1 and CA_3 regions. Hand and coworkers showed with [³H]-flumazenil binding that the density of receptors per neuron was reduced (>50%) in only CA_1. However, the binding affinity was increased in the dentate gyrus (59%),

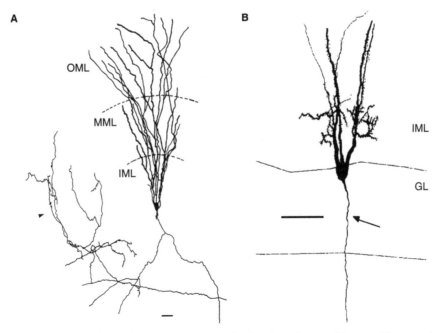

Figure 4-4. **A.** A biocytin-filled granule cell from a human MTLE patient showing the trajectory of its axon. The axon shows recurrent branches extending into the molecular layer. Scale bar = 20 μm. (Adapted from M. Isokawa, *Brain Res* 1997; 744:341). **B.** A granule cells from an MTLE patient (intracellularly filled with Lucifer Yellow and photoconverted) showing many new branches in the inner molecular layer region. Scale bar = 50 μm. (Adapted from von Campe et al., *Hippocampus* 1997; 7:481).

hilus (63%), and subiculum (65%) (58). Other studies have also confirmed that GABA$_A$ ligand binding is reduced in fields CA_1 and CA_4 (59); CA_4, CA_3, and CA_1 (60) but not in the dentate gyrus. The distribution of GABA$_B$ receptors in human epileptogenic hippocampus has not been studied to date.

Several studies have examined the distribution of glutamate excitatory receptor subtypes by receptor autoradiography in hippocampi from epilepsy patients (59,61–63). Brines and coworkers showed that for the N-methyl-D-aspartate (NMDA), α-amino-3-hydroxy-5-methyl-4-isoxazolepropionate (AMPA)—sensitive quisqualate receptors, and kainic acid receptors, MaTLE and autopsy binding densities were, in general, indistinguishable (63). In contrast, MTLE in comparison to autopsy and MaTLE groups, had regional differences when binding densities were adjusted for the number of neurons. Thus, the NMDA-sensitive sites were increased in the hilus and area CA_1 of MTLE, and AMPA/quisqualate-sensitive sites were increased in the hilus, CA_1, and CA_3 of the MTLE group. Kainate preferring sites were most prominently increased throughout the dentate molecular layer in MTLE compared to its restriction to the inner molecular layer in other groups. The differences between this study and earlier ones (59,61,62) are discussed in Brines and coworkers (63).

Immunohistochemical localization of glutamate receptor protein subunits also shows further changes in receptor organization in MTLE patients compared with MaTLE, PTLE, and autopsy controls. In MTLE, there is a distinctive increase in GluR$_1$ expression at the mossy cell dendrite excrescences in the hilus and pyramidal cell dendritic excrescences in area CA_3, where mossy fiber terminals synapse. Expression of GluR$_2$ is upregulated in the dentate molecular layer (64–67). Measurements of messenger RNA (mRNA) localization by in situ hybridization indicates decreased message levels for GluR$_1$ and GluR$_2$ in all Ammon's horn fields in sclerotic (MTLE) hippocampi but not in MaTLE or autopsy cases. However, when these tissue levels were corrected for changes in neuron densities, MTLE patients had increased mRNA levels per neuron compared with tissue from autopsies. The increase in GluR$_1$ and GluR$_2$ mRNA per neuron in the hilus correlates well with the increase in protein levels detected by immunocytochemistry (67). In contrast, GluR$_3$ mRNA was increased in all CA fields in MaTLE patients but not in MTLE (68). NMDA receptor subunit localization studies demonstrate no changes in NMDAR$_1$ (65,68) but show an increase in NMDAR$_2$ in the inner molecular layer of MTLE (sclerotic) hippocampi (69). However, another study by the same authors reports an increase in NMDAR$_2$ mRNA in dentate granule cells of mass lesion patients (MaTLE) but not in MTLE (sclerotic) hippocampi (68).

The distribution of metabotropic glutamate receptors has been described in normal (autopsy) hippocampi (70), but there are no published studies on hippocampi from patients with TLE. Our preliminary studies (de Lanerolle and Paz, unpublished) with receptor subunit specific antibodies reveal changes in the expression of mGluR$_1\alpha$ in the area dentata. In MaTLE, mGluR$_1\alpha$ immunoreactivity was found on granule cell bodies, with light staining in the inner molecular layer and darker staining in the outer ML. In MTLE, however, there was uniform staining throughout the dentate molecular layer. Additionally, only in the MTLE hilus were occasional cells whose cell bodies and proximal dendrites were immunostained. These cells were of varied morphology resembling pyramidal and multipolar neurons. These studies, together, point to changes in glutamate receptors in the MTLE hippocampus.

The distribution of vasoactive intestinal peptide (VIP) receptors studied with [^{125}I]-VIP as a ligand revealed that in MTLE patients there were significant increases in the levels of ligand binding in all CA fields and the subiculum compared with other patient groups and autopsy controls (71) (Figure 4-5). Binding densities in all CA fields were negatively correlated with neuron numbers in patient hippocampi.

In pathological specimens from MaTLE and PTLE the localization of the dopamine D$_2$ receptor is confined to the middle part of the dentate molecular layer, whereas in MTLE, the receptors are most dense on the granule cell bodies and in the inner molecular layer (Figure 4-6). Additionally, ligand binding is increased in all CA fields of the MTLE (72,73).

Calcium Binding Proteins

Calcium binding proteins are often thought of as cytosolic proteins that can buffer neurons from calcium overload caused by excessive glutamatergic stimulation and prevent their death (74). Although this view, however, may be an oversimplification of their role (75–77), neurons possessing calcium binding proteins (calbindin-D28k, parvalbumin, and calretinin) should be selectively preserved in an epileptogenic focus. Several studies have examined this proposition and found that this is not the case (78,81–84). The presence of calbindin-D28k in surviving cells may be no more important than simply as a marker of these cells (3,28,47). Similarly, there is no evidence that parvalbumin or calretinin offer selective advantage from injury to a large population of neurons (79,80).

Neurotrophins and Other Growth-Promoting Factors

The neurotrophins, nerve growth factor (NGF), brain-derived neurotrophic factor (BDNF), and neurotrophin

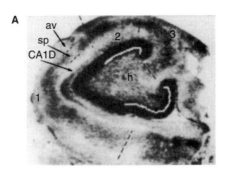
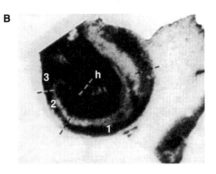

Figure 4-5. Autoradiograms of human hippocampi showing [^{125}I]-VIP binding *(black areas)*. **A.** The hippocampus of a MaTLE patient. **B.** The hippocampus of a MTLE patient. The white line in **(A)** demarcates the position of the granule cell layer. CA_1 to CA_3 are fields of Ammon's horn. The dashed lines indicate the limits of these areas. (Abbreviations: av = alveus; h = hilus or CA_4; CA_1D = apical dendrite region of CA_1 corresponding to strata radiatum and lacunosum moleculare; s = subiculum; sp = stratum pyramidale. (Adapted from de Lanerolle et al., *Brain Res* 1995; 686:184).

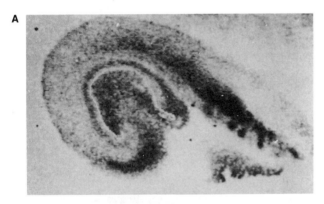
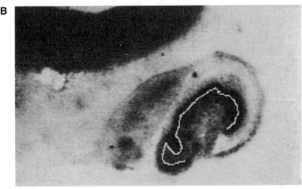

Figure 4-6. Autoradiograms of human hippocampi showing [^{125}I]Iodosulpride (a dopamine D_2 receptor specific ligand) binding*(black areas)*. **A.** A MaTLE patient. Ligand binding is in the middle molecular layer, CA_3, and subiculum. **B.** A MTLE patient. There is increased binding in the granule cell layer, inner molecular layer, and the hilus in contrast to MaTLE.

3 (NT3) promote axonal sprouting and support neuron survival (85). The expression of these growth factors in surgically removed hippocampi has been examined by in situ hybridization studies in a small group of patients (7 sclerotic or MTLE and 2 MaTLE) and autopsy controls (86). These studies show that dentate granule cell mRNA levels of NGF, BDNF, and NT3 were significantly increased in MTLE compared with

autopsy and MaTLE cases. The granule cell BDNF and NGF—but not NT3—levels were inversely correlated with granule cell density. Also, granule cell BDNF and NT3 mRNA levels correlated positively with mossy fiber collateral sprouting into the inner molecular layer of the dentate gyrus. These relationships suggest that there may be a causal link between granule cell sprouting (perhaps neurotrophins promoting growth) and granule cell responses to excessive excitation, but these causal links remain to be defined experimentally. The neurite growth-associated protein GAP-43 is also increased within axonal processes throughout the dentate molecular layer of MTLE hippocampi but not controls (87), correlating well with the increased peptidergic and mossy fiber sprouting into this area (39).

In addition to neuronally produced growth factors, reactive astrocytes make and release a variety of cell adhesion and extracellular matrix (ECM) molecules that determine the formation of new synapses and neural pattern formation (88). ECM molecules of the tenascin gene family are a group of structurally related glycoproteins that are glia-derived (89). The distribution of the glycoprotein tenascin/cytotactin (TN-C) in TLE shows about a fourfold increase of TN-C in sclerotic (MTLE) hippocampi compared with autopsy controls and MaTLE and a loss of TN-C boundaries. TN-C was an ECM component. In sclerotic (MTLE) hippocampi, TN-C immunoreactivity was increased in all hippocampal subfields (dentate and CA_1 to CA_4), obliterating TN-C boundaries seen in controls. Within the dentate gyrus, TN-C expression was markedly increased throughout the molecular layers (inner molecular layer and outer molecular layer) and correlated with a similar astrocyte GFAP increase and GAP-43 increase in the same areas (inner molecular layer and outer molecular layer) (87). Based on the known functions of TN-C, the loss of TN-C borders in the dentate gyrus may facilitate sprouting of neuronal processes into new territories.

Sodium Pump and Cytochrome Oxidase

The enzyme Na^+/K^+-ATPase (sodium pump) is composed of homologous isoforms of which $\alpha2$ and $\alpha3$ isoforms are differentially expressed in the central nervous system. This enzyme establishes the transmembrane ion gradients that underlie electrical excitability. To evaluate the role of sodium pumps in human TLE, their distribution has been examined by autoradiography (90) and in situ hybridization for mRNA (Brines, unpublished). In MTLE, specific binding of ^{3}H-ouabain is decreased in the hilus, CA_3, and CA_1 subfields, as is the mRNA for the isoforms. In all epilepsy groups sodium pump is increased in the dentate molecular layer, CA_2, and subicular region. MTLE had moderate increases in ouabain in CA_4 and CA_3 as well, indicating an upregulation of sodium pump in all hippocampal areas.

The sodium pump requires ATP to function. Cytochrome-c-oxidase activity (the principal source of ATP) determined histochemically showed reduced activity in all hippocampal fields in both MaTLE and MTLE groups compared to autopsy controls (33). These data suggest that although sodium pump protein in surviving neurons is upregulated in TLE, sodium pump capacity may be limited by the reduced levels of the cytochrome-c-oxidase and, presumably, ATP availability.

Changes in Chemical Phenotype

The MTLE hippocampus shows several instances in which hippocampal neurons change pharmacological phenotypes. This was first observed in some hilar neurons in the MTLE group that expressed dynorphin, an opioid peptide not expressed in MaTLE, PTLE, or autopsy controls (39,46). Some hilar neurons in just the MTLE group express in their somata the glutamate receptor subunit protein $GluR_1$. Both these cell types resemble mossy cells (46,67). Neurons resembling large aspiny hilar neurons were reported to be immunoreactive for tyrosine hydroxylase in the MTLE group (91). Additionally, adrenocorticotropic (ACTH) immunoreactive neurons were reported within the subiculum of the MTLE group but not the autopsy controls. Staining for ACTH in the MaTLE and PTLE groups was slight (92). The functional significance of these abnormal expression patterns of neuroactive substances remains to be elucidated.

Astrocyte Biology

Gliosis is prominent in the epileptogenic hippocampus (93). Numerous studies have attempted to define the role of glia that accumulate in the hippocampus in focal epilepsy (94–96). Traditionally, such glial accumulations have been considered to be a reactive response to neuron loss, the glia serving as scavengers of dead neurons. Based on the more recent understandings of the properties and functions of astroglia, they have been ascribed a variety of possible roles in the epileptic hippocampus — maintenance of ionic and pH composition of the extracellular environment, regulation of the extracellular space, removal of synaptically released, excitatory neurotransmitters and synthesis of transmitters. However, the direct study of hippocampal astrocytes from hippocampal seizure foci has only just begun (97). Electrophysiological study of astrocytes in primary cultures established from surgically removed hippocampi revealed that these astrocytes have many neuron-like features. The resting membrane potential of astrocytes from MTLE hippocampi (seizure focus) was significantly depolarized (approximately −55 mV) compared with MaTLE and PTLE hippocampal astrocytes (approximately −75 mV) or neocortical astrocytes (−80 mV). MTLE astrocytes also displayed much larger tetrodotoxin (TTX)-sensitive Na^+ currents with an approximately 66-fold higher Na^+ channel density compared with astrocytes from the neocortex or hippocampi of other patient groups. As a consequence of such higher channel density, astrocytes in MTLE were capable of generating action potentials, but spontaneous firing was not observed.

Table 4-1 is a summary of anatomical and neurochemical changes in the dentate gyrus.

MECHANISMS OF CAUSATION, INSIGHTS FROM PATHOLOGY

Studies of the pathology of the hippocampus in TLE suggest that there are multiple causes of seizures within this group (30). In MaTLE patients, the mass lesion itself may serve as the focus of seizure initiation, as its removal produces excellent seizure control (98). How such mass lesions generate epileptiform activity is still unclear although several suggestions — excitability related to astrocytic function (99) and excitability related to perilesional or lesional alterations in neurotransmitters and/or receptors (100,101) have been made. In the PTLE group the location of the seizure focus is uncertain. However, surgical removal of anteromedial temporal lobe structures including the hippocampus results in seizure control in some PTLE patients (approximately 60% compared with >90% in MTLE). The similarity of organization of the hippocampus in this group with that of autopsy controls (reviewed earlier in this chapter) would favor the position that the hippocampus may not play a significant role in epileptogenesis. The contribution of other regions such as amygdala and entorhinal cortex to epileptogenesis in PTLE remains to be determined. It is also possible that surgery interrupts

Table 4-1. Summary of Anatomical and Neurochemical Changes in Dentate Gyrus

	GC Layer	Hilus/PML	IML	OML	References
Neurons					
Granular	—	0	0	0	(3)
NPY	0	—	0	0	(39)
SOM	0	—	0	0	(39)
SP	0	—	0	0	(39)
Fibers					
DYN	+ ?	0	+	0	(39,44)
NPY	0	0	+	+	(39)
SOM	0	0	+	+	(39)
SP	0	—	+	+	(399)
Ach	0	0	—	+	(115)
GAD	0	0	+	+	(40)
Receptors					
NPY	0	0	+	0	
SOM	+	0	+	+	(116)
Dopamine D_2	+	+	+	0	(73)
VIP	+	+	+	+	(71)
GABA (Benzo.)	+ (affinity)	+ (affinity)	0	0	(58)
NMDA	0	+	0	0	(63)
AMPA/Quis.	0	+	—	—	(63)
Kainate	0	0	+	+	(63)
$GluR_1$	0	+	0/+	0/+	(66,67)
$GluR_2$	0	+	+	+	(64,67)
NMDA R_1	0	0	0	0	(70)
NMDA R_2	0	0	+	0	(68)
Growth Factors					
NGF (in situ)	+	0	0	0	(86)
BDNF (in situ)	+	0	0	0	
NT3 (in situ)	+	0	0	0	
GAP 43	0	0	+	+	(87)
TN-C	0	0	+	+	(87)
GFAP	+	+	+	+	(87)
Na^+/K^+ ATPase					(33)
Cytochrome oxidase					(33)
Calcium Binding Proteins					
Calbindin	—	0	0	0	
Parvalbumin	0	—	0	0	(79)
Calretinin (neurons)	0	+	+	+	(81)
Calretinin (fibers)	0	0	+	+	(81)

Abbreviations: 0 = no change; + = increase; − = decrease; GC = granule cell layer; IML = inner molecular layer; in situ = in situ hybridization histochemistry; OML = outer molecular layer; PML = subgranular polymorphic layer of hilus.

the spread of seizures through the hippocampus from extratemporal epileptogenic regions, as yet unidentified in PTLE.

In the MTLE group, the hippocampus has a high probability of being the seizure focus. Its surgical removal with entorhinal cortex, temporal pole, and amygdala results in good seizure control (102). A significant proportion of MTLE patients have a history of febrile convulsions (103,104), and these patients have more severe sclerosis than MTLE patients without a history of febrile seizures (3,27). In a recent study of two families in which 13 of 23 members experienced febrile seizures, it has been proposed that a subtle preexisting hippocampal malformation may facilitate febrile convulsions and contribute to the development of hippocampal sclerosis (105). Whereas the MTLE hippocampus shows a variety of organizational features distinctive from the causes of TLE, the central unanswered question is which of these changes are causative and which are secondary? Two major hypotheses have dominated discussions, each based on the premise that a single feature of the MTLE hippocampus can explain epileptogenesis within such a region.

The "mossy fiber sprouting hypothesis" (45,106) is based on the evidence of aberrant mossy fiber recurrent collaterals from granule cell mossy fiber axons into the inner molecular layer of the dentate and synapses onto dentate granule cell dendrites (44). Synapses carrying glutamate would cause hyperexcitability of granule cells and, therefore, seizures (107). Unfortunately, this hypothesis is inconsistent with several recent pathological observations. In PTLE patients, who lack mossy axon recurrent collateral sprouting, approximately 60 percent become seizure-free after AMTR. Although mossy fiber sprouting is common in MTLE, it is not consistently present; therefore, hyperexcitability is possible without recurrent collaterals. Furthermore, cyclohexamide, a protein synthesis inhibitor, blocks pilocarpine- and kainate-induced mossy fiber sprouting in rats but not the development of spontaneous seizures (108,109). Finally, in the stargazer (stg) single locus mouse mutation showing generalized spike-wave epilepsy, spontaneous repetitive discharges appear 4 to 6 weeks before the appearance of mossy fiber sprouting (110).

The "dormant basket cell hypothesis" was put forward on the basis of the anatomical observation that inhibitory GABA neurons, especially the basket cells on the granule cell/hilus border (111) and in area CA_1 appear to be intact even in an epileptogenic hippocampus (111,112). This is also correlated with loss in a population of hilar interneurons, the mossy cells. The theory suggests that the inhibitory basket cell neurons, which are normally activated by mossy cells, would be rendered "dormant" by the loss of the latter. Thus, the granule cells would be more excitable. To date, there is no direct evidence for mossy cell excitation of inhibitory neurons. Furthermore, in human MTLE, loss of mossy cells in the hilus is incomplete.

The pathology of the MTLE hippocampus, as previously reviewed, strongly suggests a complex and multifactorial pathophysiological mechanism in epileptogenesis and seizure maintenance. The majority of these changes center around the dentate gyrus, the principal gateway for inputs to the hippocampus. The critical factors in such a pathophysiology appear to include the selective loss of hilar subgranular interneurons that normally contain the neuropeptides NPY, SP, and SOM (113). This loss of interneurons is seen in all MTLE patients with or without extensive principal neuron loss and whether or not mossy fiber recurrent collateral sprouting is present. This early loss of interneurons, most of which carry inhibitory neurotransmitters, may be an early cause of granule cell hyperexcitability. Experimental confirmation of such a function of these subgranular interneurons in the human hippocampus has yet to be carried out. The plastic responses—sprouting and receptor changes—may be later responses of the hippocampus

to neuronal hyperexcitability. Interestingly, many of these plastic changes [NPY, SOM, and SP sprouting; dopamine D2, NPY, and SOM receptor upregulation in the dentate; mossy fiber sprouting with the expression of DYN, along with the relative sparing of GABA neurons and even some evidence of GABA fiber sprouting (40)] may contribute to increasing the inhibition of granular neurons. Changes in neurotrophic factors and ECM molecules are in keeping with increased axonal sprouting. The elaboration of these putative, inhibitory mechanisms may account for the suppression of seizure activity during interictal periods. However, the periodic occurrence of seizures must imply an excitatory mechanism that can override these presumed inhibitory mechanisms.

The identification of such overriding excitatory mechanisms at seizure foci is of critical importance. Some of the parameters of such mechanisms can be inferred from the studies on human tissue as well as in vivo studies on patients carried out for the diagnosis and removal of seizure foci. In vivo dialysis studies showed that there is a significant elevation in extracellular glutamate levels in the epileptogenic hippocampus just before and during a seizure (114). Such elevated glutamate levels could by themselves overexcite neurons at the focus. In addition, the increased expression of glutamate receptors at critical synapses in the hippocampus may favor enhanced glutamatergic excitation of hippocampal pathways. Included in this environment is an accumulation of astroglia with properties that might contribute to the excitability of the region. Metabolic alterations within the hippocampus may further add to its hyperexcitability due to the decrease in cytochrome-c-oxidase levels in the epileptogenic hippocampus. Insufficient ATP could reduce sodium pump activity and increase neuronal excitability. The temporal combination of several excitatory mechanisms may trigger the seizure.

Critical questions that remain unanswered are: What mechanisms caused the extracellular glutamate to increase at seizure onset? Is there a single causative mechanism that results in all the processes favoring excitation and, if so, what triggers the mechanism? Is there synchrony in these excitatory processes at the time of a seizure? Although experimental systems will be necessary to study and test some of these issues, only continued study of human seizure foci will yield insight to these critical questions.

Acknowledgments. I thank Ms. Illona Kovacs for her excellent technical assistance and Dr. Michael Brines, my collaborator over many years, for stimulating discussions and insight, which resulted in much of the data gathered in my laboratory; Dr. Dennis Spencer for providing the human tissue and his continuing support of this work; and Dr. Spencer and Dr.

Carole LaMotte for critical reading of an earlier draft of this paper. The work was supported by NIH grants NS06208 and NS30619 to NdeL.

REFERENCES

1. Dreifuss FE, Martinez-Lage M, Roger J, Seino M, Dam M. Proposal for classification of epilepsies and epileptic syndromes. *Epilepsia* 1985; 26:268–278.

2. Kim JH. Pathology of seizure disorders. *Neuroimag Clin North Am* 1995; 5:527–545.

3. Kim JH, Guimaraes PO, Shen M-Y, Masukawa LM, Spencer DD. Hippocampal neuronal density in temporal lobe epilepsy with and without gliomas. *Acta Neuropathol* 1990; 80:41–45.

4. Bouchet C, Cazauvievlh Y. De l'épilepsie considérée dans ses rapports avec l'aliénation mentale. Recherche sur la nature et le siége de ces deux maladies. *Arch Gén Méd* 1825; 9:510–542.

5. Gloor P. Mesial temporal sclerosis: historical background and an overview from a modern perspective. In: Lüders H, ed. *Epilepsy Surgery.* New York: Raven Press, 1991:6889–6703.

6. Gloor P. The role of the amygdala in temporal lobe epilepsy. In: Aggleton JP, ed. *The Amygdala. Neurobiological Aspects of Emotion, Memory, and Mental Dysfunction.* New York: Wiley-Liss, 1992:505–538.

7. Hudson LP, Munoz DG, Miller L, et al. Amygdaloid sclerosis in temporal lobe epilepsy. *Ann Neurol* 1993; 33:622–631.

8. Wolf HK, Aliashkevich AF, Blümcke I, Wiestler OD, Zentner J. Neuronal loss and gliosis of the amygdaloid nucleus in temporal lobe epilepsy. A quantitative analysis of 70 surgical specimens. *Acta Neuropathol* 1997; 93:606–610.

9. Margerison JH, Corsellis JAN. Epilepsy and the temporal lobes. *Brain* 1966; 89:499–530.

10. Feindel W, Rasmussen T. Temporal lobectomy with amygdalectomy and minimal hippocampal resection: review of 100 cases. *Can J Neurol Sci* 1991; 18:603–605.

11. Rasmussen T, Feindel W. Temporal lobectomy: review of 100 cases with major hippocampectomy. *Can J Neurol Sci* 1991; 18:601–602.

12. Lothman EW, Bertram EH, Stringer JL. Functional anatomy of hippocampal seizures. *Prog Neurobiol* 1991; 37,1–82.

13. Goldring S, Edwards I, Harding GW, Bernardo KL. Results of anterior temporal lobectomy that spares the amygdala in patients with complex partial seizures. *J Neurosurg* 1992; 77, 185–193.

14. Du F, Whetsell WO Jr, Abou-Khalil B, et al. Preferential neuronal loss in layer III of the entorhinal cortex in patients with temporal lobe epilepsy. *Epilepsy Res* 1993; 16:223–233.

15. Meencke HJ, Veith G. Hippocampal sclerosis in epilepsy. In: Lüders HO, ed. *Epilepsy Surgery.* New York: Raven Press, 1991:705–715.

16. Stauder KH. Epilepsie und schläfenlappen. *Arch Psychiatr* 1935; 104:181–212.

17. Sano K, Malamud N. Clinical significance of sclerosis of the cornu armonis. *Arch Neurol Psychiatr* 1953; 70:40–53.

18. Cavanagh JB, Meyer A. Aetiological aspects of Ammon's horn sclerosis associated with temporal lobe epilepsy. *Br Med J* 1956; 2:1403–1407.

19. Falconer MA, Serafetinides EA, Corsellis, JAN. Etiology and pathogenesis of temporal lobe epilepsy. *Arch Neurol* 1964; 10:233–248.

20. Bruton CJ. *The Neuropathology of Temporal Lobe Epilepsy.* Oxford: Oxford University Press, 1988.

21. Zimmerman HM. The histopathology of convulsive disorders in children. *J Pediatr* 1940; 13:859–890.

22. Maher J, McLachlan RS. Febrile convulsions. Is seizure duration the most important predictor of temporal lobe epilepsy? *Brain* 1995; 118:1521–1528.

23. Gastaut H, Toga M, Roger J, Gibson WC. A correlation of clinical, electroencephalographic and anatomical findings in nine autopsied cases of "temporal lobe epilepsy." *Epilepsia* 1959; 1:56–85.

24. Kim JH, Kraemer DL, Spencer DD. The neuropathology of epilepsy. In: Hopkins A, Shovron S, Cascino G, eds. *Epilepsy.* London: Chapman & Hall, 1995:243–267.

25. Mouritzen Dam A. Epilepsy and neuron loss in the hippocampus. *Epilepsia* 1980; 21:617–629.

26. Mouritzen Dam A. Hippocampal neuron loss in epilepsy and after experimental seizures. *Acta Neurol Scand* 1982; 66:601–642.

27. Sagar, HJ, Oxbury JM. Hippocampal neuronal loss in temporal lobe epilepsy: correlation with early childhood convulsions. *Ann Neurol* 1987; 22:334–340.

28. Babb TL, Brown WJ, Pretorius J, et al. Temporal lobe volumetric cell densities in temporal lobe epilepsy. *Epilepsia* 1984; 25:729–740.

29. Spencer DD, Pappas CT. Surgical decisions regarding medically intractable epilepsy. *Clin Neurosurg* 1992; 38:548–566.

30. de Lanerolle NC, Magge SN, Phillips MF, et al. Adaptive changes of epileptic human temporal lobe tissue: properties of neurons and glia. In: Wolf P, ed. *Seizures and Syndromes in Epilepsy.* London: John Libbey, 1994:431–448.

31. de Lanerolle NC, Kim JH, Brines ML. Cellular and molecular alterations in partial epilepsy. *Clin Neurosci* 1994; 2:64–81.

32. Bronen RA, Cheung G, Charles JT, et al. Imaging findings in hippocampal sclerosis: correlation with pathology. *AJNR* 1991; 12:933–940.

33. Brines ML, Tabuteau H, Sundaresan S, et al. Regional distribution of hippocampal Na$^+$,K$^+$-ATPase, cytochrome oxidase, and total protein in temporal lobe epilepsy. *Epilepsia* 1995; 36:371–383.

34. Mathern GW, Babb TL, Mischel PS, et al. Childhood generalized and mesial temporal epilepsies demonstrate different amounts and patterns of hippocampal neuron loss and mossy fiber synaptic reorganization. *Brain* 1996; 119:965–987.

35. Mathern GW, Leite JP, Pretorius JK, et al. Severe seizures in young children are associated with hippocampal neuron losses and aberrant mossy fiber sprouting during fascia dentata postnatal development. In: Heinemann U, Engel J Jr, Avanzini G, et al., eds. *Progressive Nature of Epileptogenesis (Epilepsy Res. Suppl 12)*. Amsterdam: Elsevier Science BV, 1996: 33–43.

36. Mathern GW, Leite JP, Pretorius JK, et al. Children with severe epilepsy: evidence of hippocampal neuron losses and aberrant mossy fiber sprouting during postnatal granule cell migration and differentiation. *Dev Brain Res* 1994; 78:70–80.

37. Mathern GW, Kuhlman PA, Mendoza D, Pretorius JK. Human fascia dentata and hippocampal neuron densities differ depending on the epileptic syndrome and age at first seizure. *J Neuropathol Exp Neurol* 1997; 56:199–212.

38. Babb TL, Lieb JP, Brown WJ, Pretorius J, Crandall PH. Distribution of pyramidal cell density and hyperexcitability in the epileptic human hippocampal formation. *Epilepsia* 1984; 25:721–728.

39. de Lanerolle NC, Kim JH, Robbins RJ, Spencer DD. Hippocampal interneuron loss and plasticity in human temporal lobe epilepsy. *Brain Res* 1989; 495:387–395.

40. Mathern GW, Babb TL, Pretorius JK, Leite JP. Reactive synaptogenesis and neuron densities for neuropeptide Y, somatostatin, and glutamate decarboxylase immunoreactivity in the epileptogenic human fascia dentata. *J Neurosci* 1995; 15:3990–4004.

41. Babb TL, Pretorius JK, Crandall PH. Glutamate decarboxylase-immunoreactive neurons are preserved in human epileptic hippocampus. *J Neurosci* 1989; 9:2562–2574.

42. de Lanerolle NC, Brines ML, Kim JH, et al. Neurochemical remodelling of the hippocampus in human temporal lobe epilepsy. In: Engel JJ, Wasterlain C, Cavalheiro EA, Heinemann U, Avanzini G, eds. *Molecular Neurobiology of Epilepsy*. Amsterdam: Elsevier Science Publishers, BV, 1992:205–220.

43. Sutula T, Cascino G, Cavazos J, Pavada I, Ramirez L. Mossy fiber synaptic reorganization in the epileptic human temporal lobe. *Ann Neurol* 1989; 26:321–330.

44. Houser CR, Miyashiro JE, Swartz BE, et al. Altered patterns of dynorphin immunoreactivity suggest mossy fiber reorganization in human hippocampal epilepsy. *J Neurosci* 1990; 10:267–282.

45. Babb TL, Pretorius JK, Kupfer WR, et al. Aberrant synaptic reorganization in human epileptic hippocampus: evidence for feedforward excitation. *Dendron* 1992; 1:7–25.

46. de Lanerolle NC, Williamson A, Meredith C, et al. Dynorphin and the kappa 1 ligand [^{3}H]-U69,539 binding in the human epileptogenic hippocampus. *Epilepsy Res* 1997; 28:189–205.

47. Mathern GW, Babb TL, Armstrong DL. Hippocampal sclerosis. In: Engel J, Pedley TA, eds. *Epilepsy: A Comprehensive Textbook*. Philadelphia: Lippincott-Raven, 1997:133–155.

48. Mathern GW, Pretorius JK, Babb TL. Quantified patterns of mossy fiber sprouting and neuron densities in hippocampal and lesional seizures. *J Neurosurg* 1995; 82:211–219.

49. Philips MW. Synaptic and pathway remodeling of the human hippocampus in temporal lobe epilepsy. New Haven: Yale University, 1993. Thesis.

50. Scheibel ME, Scheibel AB. Hippocampal pathology in temporal lobe epilepsy. A Golgi survey. In: Brazier MAB, ed. *Epilepsy. Its Phenomenon in Man*. New York: Academic Press, 1973:315–337.

51. Scheibel ME, Crandall PH, Scheibel AB. The hippocampal-dentate complex in temporal lobe epilepsy. A Golgi study. *Epilepsia* 1974; 15:55–80.

52. Scheibel A, Paul L, Fried I. Some structural substrates of the epileptic seizure state. In: Jasper H, Gelder NV, ed. *Basic Mechanisms of Neuronal Hyperexcitability*. New York: Liss, 1983.

53. von Campe G, Spencer DD, de Lanerolle NC. Morphology of dentate granule cells in the human epileptogenic hippocampus. *Hippocampus* 1997; 7:472–488.

54. Isokawa M, Levesque MF, Babb TL, Engel JJ. Single mossy fiber axonal systems of human dentate granule cells studied in hippocampal slices from patients with temporal lobe epilepsy. *J Neurosci* 1993; 13:1511–1522.

55. Frank JE, Pokorny J, Kunkel DD, Schwartzkroin PA. Physiologic and morphologic characteristics of granule cell circuitry in human epileptic hippocampus. *Epilepsia* 1995; 36:543–558.

56. Isokawa M. Preservation of dendrites with the presence of reorganized mossy fiber collaterals in hippocampal dentate granule cells in patients with temporal lobe epilepsy. Brain Res 1997; 744:339–343.

57. Johnson EW, de Lanerolle NC, Kim JH, et al. "Central" and "peripheral" benzodiazepine receptors: opposite changes in human epileptic tissue. *Neurology* 1992; 42:811–815.

58. Hand KSP, Baird VH, Van Paesschen W, et al. Central benzodiazepine receptor autoradiography in hippocampal sclerosis. *Br J Pharmacol* 1997; 122:358–364.

59. McDonald JW, Garofalo EA, Hood T, et al. Altered excitatory and inhibitory amino acid receptor binding in hippocampus of patients with temporal lobe epilepsy. *Ann Neurol* 1991; 29:529–541.

60. Burdette DE, Sakurai SY, Henry TR, et al. Temporal lobe central benzodiazepine binding in unilateral mesial temporal lobe epilepsy. *Neurology* 1995; 45:934–941.

61. Geddes JW, Cahan LD, Cooper SM, et al. Altered distribution of excitatory amino acid receptors in temporal lobe epilepsy. *Exp Neurol* 1990; 108:214–220.

62. Hosford DA, Crain BJ, Cao Z, et al. Increased AMPA-sensitive quisqualate receptor binding and reduced NMDA receptor binding in epileptic human hippocampus. *J Neurosci* 1991; 11:428–434.

63. Brines ML, Sundaresan S, Spencer DD, de Lanerolle NC. Quantitative autoradiographic analysis of glutamate receptor subtypes in human temporal lobe epilepsy:

upregulation in reorganized epileptogenic hippocampus. *Eur J Neurosci* 1997; 9:2035–2044.

64. Blümcke I, Wolf HK, Hof PR, Morrison JH, Wiestler OD. Regional distribution of the AMPA glutamate receptor subunits GluR2(4) in human hippocampus. *Brain Res* 1995; 682:239–244.

65. Blümcke I, Beck H, Scheffler B, et al. Altered distribution of the α-amino-3-hydroxy-5-methyl-4-isoxazole propionate receptor subunit GluR2(4) and the *N*-methyl-*D*-aspartate receptor subunit NMDAR1 in the hippocampus of patients with temporal lobe epilepsy. *Acta Neuropathol* 1996; 92:576–587.

66. Lynd-Balta E, Pilcher WH, Joseph SA. Distribution of AMPA receptor subunits in the hippocampal formation of temporal lobe epilepsy patients. *Neuroscience* 1996; 72:15–29.

67. de Lanerolle NC, Eid T, von Campe G, et al. Glutamate receptor subunits GluR1 and GluR2/3 distribution shows reorganization in the human epileptogenic hippocampus. *Eur J Neurosci* 1998; 10:1687–1703.

68. Mathern GW, Pretorius JK, Kornblum HI, et al. Human hippocampal AMPA and NMDA mRNA levels in temporal lobe epilepsy patients. *Brain* 1997; 120:1937–1959.

69. Mathern GW, Leite JP, Babb TL, et al. Aberrant hippocampal mossy fiber sprouting correlates with greater NMDAR2 receptor staining. *NeuroReport* 1996; 7:1029–1035.

70. Blümke I, Behle K, Malitschek B, et al. Immunohistochemical distribution of metabotropic glutamate receptor subtypes mGluR1b, mGluR2/3, mGluR4a and mGluR5 in human hippocampus. *Brain Res* 1996; 736:217–226.

71. de Lanerolle NC, Gunel M, Sundaresan S, et al. Vasoactive intestinal polypeptide and its receptor changes in human temporal lobe epilepsy. *Brain Res* 1995; 686:182–193.

72. de Lanerolle NC, Tompkins JR, Spencer DD. Hippocampal dopamine receptor changes in human temporal lobe epilepsy. *Soc Neurosci Abstr* 1990; 16:308.

73. Tompkins J. Alterations in D2 receptor concentrations in human temporal lobe epilepsy. M.D., New Haven: Yale University, 1990. Thesis.

74. Scharfman EE, Schwartzkroin PA. Protection of dentate hilar cells from prolonged stimulation by intracellular calcium chelation. *Science* 1989; 246:257–260.

75. Dalgarno D, Klevit RE, Levine AB, Williams RJP. The calcium receptor and trigger. *Trends Pharmacol Sci* 1984; 5:266–271.

76. Köhr G, Lambert CE, Mody I. Calbindin D-28K (CaBP) levels and calcium currents in acutely dissociated epileptic neurons. *Exp Brain Res* 1991; 85:543–551.

77. Bainbridge KG, Celio MR, Rogers JH. Calcium binding proteins in the nervous system. *Trends Neurosci* 1992; 15:303–308.

78. Sloviter RS, Sollas AL, Barbaro NM, Laxer KD. Calcium-binding protein (Calbindin-D28K) and parvalbumin immunocytochemistry in the normal and epileptic human hippocampus. *J Comp Neurol* 1991; 308:381–396.

79. Zhu Z-Q, Armstrong DL, Hamilton WJ, Grossman RG. Disproportionate loss of CA4 parvalbumin-immunoreactive interneurons in patients with Ammon's horn sclerosis. *J Neuropathol Exp Neurol* 1997; 56:988–997.

80. de Lanerolle NC, Brines ML, Williamson A, Kim JH, Spencer DD. Neurotransmitters and their receptors in human temporal lobe epilepsy. In: Ribak CE, Gall CM, Mody I, eds. *The Dentate Gyrus and Its Role in Seizures*. Amsterdam: Elsevier Science Publishers BV, 1992:235–250.

81. Blümcke I, Beck H, Nitsch R, et al. Preservation of calretinin-immunoreactive neurons in the hippocampus of epilepsy patients with Ammon's horn sclerosis. *J Neuropathol Exp Neurol* 1996; 55:329–341.

82. Nitsch R, Leranth C. Substance P-containing hypothalamic afferents to the monkey hippocampus: An immuno-histochemical, tract tracing, and co-existence study. *Exp Brain Res* 1994; 101:231–240.

83. Kosaka T, Katsumara H, Hawal K, Wu J-Y, Heizmann CW. GABAergic neurons containing the Ca^{2+}-binding protein parvalbumin in the rat hippocampus and dentate gyrus. *Brain Res* 1987; 419:119–130.

84. Nitsch R, Ohm TG. Calretinin immunoreactive structures in the human hippocampal formation. *J Comp Neurol* 1995; 360:475–487.

85. Persson H. Neurotrophin production in the brain. *Semin Neurosci* 1993; 5:227–237.

86. Mathern GW, Babb TL, Micevych PE, Blanco CE, Pretorius JK. Granule cell mRNA levels for BDNF, NGF, and NT-3 correlate with neuron losses or supragranular mossy fiber sprouting in the chronically damaged and epileptic human hippocampus. *Mol Chem Neuropathol* 1997; 30:53–76.

87. Scheffler B, Faissner A, Beck H, et al. Hippocampal loss of tenascin boundaries in Ammon's horn sclerosis. *Glia* 1997; 19:35–46.

88. Faissner A, Götz B, Scholze A. The tenascin gene family-versatile glycoproteins implicated in neural pattern formation and regeneration. *Semin Dev Biol* 1995; 6:139–148.

89. Götz B, Scholze A, Clement A, et al. Tenascin-C contains distinct adhesive, anti-adhesive, and neurite outgrowth promoting sites for neurons. *J Cell Biol* 1996; 132:681–699.

90. Brines ML, Dare AO, de Lanerolle NC. The cardiac glycoside ouabain potentiates excitotoxic injury of adult neurons in rat hippocampus. *Neurosci Lett* 1995; 191:145–148.

91. Zhu Z-Z, Armstrong DL, Grossman RG, Hamilton WJ. Tyrosine hydroxylase-immunoreactive neurons in the temporal lobe in complex partial seizures. *Ann Neurol* 1990; 27:564–572.

92. Lynd-Balta E, Pilcher WH, Joseph SA. Adrenocorticotropic hormone immunoreactivity in the hippocampal formation of temporal lobe epilepsy patients. *Epilepsia* 1996; 37:1081–1087.

93. Foerster O, Penfield W. The structural basis of traumatic epilepsy and results of radical operations. *Brain* 1930; 53:99–119.

94. Trachtenberg MC, Pollen DA. Neuroglia: biophysical properties and physiologic function. *Science* 1970; 167:1248–1252.

95. Grossman RG, Rosman LJ. Intracellular potentials of excitable cells in epileptogenic cortex undergoing fibrillary gliosis after local injury. *Brain Res* 1971; 28:181–201.

96. Glotzner FL. Membrane properties of neuroglia in epileptogenic gliosis. *Brain Res* 1973; 55:159–171.

97. O'Connor ER, Sontheimer H, Spencer DD, de Lanerolle NC. Astrocytes from human hippocampal epileptogenic foci exhibit action potential-like responses. *Epilepsia* 1998; 39:347–354.

98. Spencer DD, Spencer SS, Mattson RH, Williamson PD. Intracerebral masses in patients with intractable partial epilepsy. *Neurology* 1984; 34:432–436.

99. Magge S. Characterization of human astrocytes cultured from tumor related neocortical seizure foci. New Haven: Yale University, 1993. Thesis.

100. Wolf HK, Birkholz T, Wellmer J, et al. Neurochemical profile of glioneuronal lesions from patients with chronic pharmacoresistant focal epilepsies. *J Neuropathol Exp Neurol* 1995; 54:689–697.

101. Wolf HK, Roos D, Blümcke I, Pietsch T, Wiestler OD. Perilesional neurochemical changes in focal epilepsies. *Acta Neuropathol* 1996; 91:376–384.

102. Spencer SS, Schwarcz SS, Spencer DD. The treatment of epilepsy with surgery. *Merrit Putnam Q* 1988; 5:3–17.

103. Cendes F, Andermann F, Dubeau F. Early childhood prolonged febrile convulsions, atrophy and sclerosis of mesial structures, and temporal lobe epilepsy: a MRI volumetric study. *Neurology* 1993; 43:1083–1087.

104. Kuks JB, Cook MJ, Fish DR, Stevens JM, Shorvon SD. Hippocampal sclerosis in epilepsy and childhood febrile seizures. *Lancet* 1993; 342:1391–1394.

105. Fernández G, Effenberger O, Vinz B, et al. Hippocampal malformation as a cause of familial febrile convulsions and subsequent hippocampal sclerosis. *Neurology* 1998; 50:909–917.

106. Tauck D, Nadler J. Evidence of functional mossy fiber sprouting in hippocampal formation of kainic acid treated rats. *J Neurosci* 1985; 5:1016–1022.

107. Dudek FE, Obenaus A, Schweitzer JS, Wuarin JP. Functional significance of hippocampal plasticity in epileptic brain: electrophysiological changes of the dentate granule cells associated with mossy fiber sprouting. *Hippocampus* 1994; 4:259–265.

108. Drake CT, Terman GW, Simmons ML, et al. Dynorphin opioids present in dentate granule cells may function as retrograde inhibitory neurotransmitters. *J Neurosci* 1994; 14:3736–3750.

109. Simmons ML, Terman GW, Drake CT, Chavkin C. Inhibition of glutamate release by presynaptic k1-opioid receptors in the guinea pig dentate gyrus. *J Neurophysiol* 1994; 72:1697–1705.

110. Qiao X, Noebels JL. Developmental analysis of hippocampal mossy fiber outgrowth in a mutant mouse with inherited spike-wave seizures. *J Neurosci* 1993; 13:4622–4635.

111. Sloviter RS. Decreased hippocampal inhibition and a selective loss of interneurons in experimental epilepsy. *Science* 1987; 235:73–76.

112. Sloviter RS. Permanently altered hippocampal structure, excitability, and inhibition after experimental status epilepticus in the rat: the "dormant basket cell" hypothesis and its possible relevance to temporal lobe epilepsy. *Hippocampus* 1991; 1:41–66.

113. Kosaka T, Wu J-Y, Berroit R. GABAergic neurons containing somatostatin-like immunoreactivity in the rat hippocampus and dentate gyrus. *Exp Brain Res* 1988; 71:388–398.

114. During MJ, Spencer DD. Extracellular hippocampal glutamate and spontaneous seizure in the conscious human brain. *Lancet* 1993; 341:1607–1610.

115. Green R, Blume H, Kupperschmid S, Mesulam M-M. Alterations of hippocampal acetylcholinesterase in human temporal lobe epilepsy. *Ann Neurol* 1989; 26:351–367.

116. Robbins RJ, Brines ML, Kim JH, et al. A selective loss of somatostatin in the hippocampus of patients with temporal lobe epilepsy. *Ann Neurol* 1991; 29:325–332.

CHAPTER 5

Genetic Influences on Risk for Epilepsy

Ruth Ottman, Ph.D.

An inherited contribution to the etiology of epilepsy has been suspected for centuries. Until recently, however, little progress has been made in identifying the specific genetic influences on susceptibility to seizures. This slow progress is partly due to underlying complexity in the genetic contributions. The epilepsies are etiologically and clinically heterogeneous, and genetic influences appear to have primary importance in only a subset of patients. Moreover, many different genetic mechanisms may influence risk for epilepsy in different families or different syndromes. Some of these mechanisms involve major effects of single genes, producing simple patterns of inheritance in families (autosomal or *X*-linked, dominant or recessive). Other mechanisms probably involve the combined effects of multiple genes and environmental factors, each with a smaller effect on susceptibility to seizures.

The important genetic mechanisms clearly differ across some clinically defined epilepsy syndromes, but the relationship between clinical syndrome and genetic mechanism is not straightforward. Risk for a single syndrome is sometimes influenced by different genetic mechanisms in different families; conversely, a single genetic mechanism may influence risk for different syndromes within the same family.

Approximately 25 percent of prevalent epilepsy is associated with an antecedent central nervous system (CNS) injury (e.g., head trauma, stroke, or brain infection) and accordingly is classified as "symptomatic" (1). The remainder without identified cause is assigned into two broad classes by the current International Classification of Epileptic Syndromes (2): "idiopathic," reserved for syndromes of presumed genetic origin, and "cryptogenic" for syndromes presumed to be nongenetic but with insufficient evidence to assign a specific etiology. The current system of classification is problematic, however, because idiopathic and cryptogenic epilepsies are not easily distinguishable in terms of the importance of genetic susceptibility. For most of the syndromes currently classified as "idiopathic," clear evidence of a genetic basis, either from linkage studies or from demonstration of a specific mode of inheritance, is lacking. Similarly, in syndromes classified as "cryptogenic," a genetic contribution to etiology cannot be ruled out.

EVIDENCE OF A GENETIC CONTRIBUTION TO EPILEPSY

Most people with epilepsy do not have affected relatives, and for most of those who do have a family history, the familial distribution is inconsistent with a simple Mendelian model. When all types of epilepsy are considered together, however, the risk of developing epilepsy is clearly increased in the relatives of affected people compared with the general population. The best estimates of the extent of this familial aggregation are derived from the Rochester–Olmsted County Record Linkage Project (3,4). In that study, in the families of probands with idiopathic or cryptogenic epilepsy with onset before age 16, the risk of developing epilepsy by age 40 was 3.6 percent in siblings and 10.6 percent in offspring, compared with 1.7 percent in the Rochester population. Overall, the risk of epilepsy was increased 2.5-fold in siblings [95% confidence interval (CI) 1.3–4.4] and 6.7-fold in offspring (95% CI 1.8–17.1). The risk of epilepsy was not increased in more distant relatives, such as nieces, nephews, and grandchildren.

Familial aggregation does not necessarily indicate a genetic etiology; it could result instead from shared environmental exposures in members of the same family. However, four lines of evidence clearly indicate a genetic contribution to the familial aggregation of epilepsy. First, concordance rates in monozygotic twins are consistently higher than in dizygotic twins

Table 5-1. Concordance Rates for Epilepsy in Monozygotic and Dizygotic Twins

	Concordance Rate (%)	
Authors (reference)	Monozygotic Twins	Dizygotic Twins
Lennox and Lennox (5)		
Total	44	7
Brain Injured	11	7
Intact	70	6
Inouye (6)	54	7
Harvald and Hauge (7)	37	10
Corey et al. (8)	19	7
Silanpaa et al. (9)	10	5

Table 5-2. Linkage and Gene Identification in Human Epilepsies (as of July 2000)

Syndrome	Chromosomal Location	Gene
Benign familial neonatal convulsions	20q13	KCNQ2
	8q24	KCNQ3
Juvenile myoclonic epilepsy	6p	?
	15q14	?
Childhood absence epilepsy	8q24	?
Benign familial infantile convulsions	19q	?
Familial autosomal recessive idiopathic myoclonic epilepsy of infancy	16p13	?
Familial adult myoclonic epilepsy	8q24	?
Autosomal dominant partial epilepsy with auditory features	10q22-24	?
Autosomal dominant nocturnal frontal lobe epilepsy	20q13	CHRNA4
	15q24	?
Benign epilepsy of childhood with centrotemporal spikes	15q14	?
Familial partial epilepsy with variable foci	22q11-12	?
Generalized epilepsy with febrile seizures plus	19q13	SCN1B
	2q24	SCN1A
Autosomal dominant febrile convulsions	8q13	?
	19p	?
	5q14-15	?
Progressive myoclonus epilepsy (Unverricht-Lundborg type)	21q22	Cystatin B
Progressive epilepsy with mental retardation	8p23	CLN8
Progressive myoclonus epilepsy (Lafora type)	6q24	EPM2A
Myoclonic epilepsy with ragged red fibers	Mit	tRNA^{Lys}
Myoclonic epilepsy lactic acidosis and strokelike episodes	Mit	tRNA^{Leu}

(5–9) (Table 5-1). The observed concordance rates vary substantially across studies, probably reflecting differences in the methods used to ascertain twin pairs or the definitions of epilepsy employed. Second, seizures are part of the phenotype of many human genetic disorders resulting from either single gene mutations or chromosomal abnormalities (10). Although these disorders account for only about 1 percent of epilepsy, they do illustrate that a wide variety of genetic mechanisms can raise susceptibility to seizures. Third, in experimental animals several genes that raise seizure susceptibility have been identified, and these genes may have homology to human epilepsy susceptibility genes (11). Fourth, positional cloning techniques have been used to chromosomally localize, and subsequently identify, genes that raise risk for a growing list of human epilepsy syndromes (Table 5-2). Research in this area is moving extremely rapidly, so that it is quite likely that by the time this chapter appears in print the list of syndromes in Table 5-2 will be out of date.

The epilepsies with well-established genetic causes constitute only a small proportion of the total. In the majority, the genetic mechanisms underlying familial aggregation of epilepsy are unclear. However, linkage findings, even before identification of the specific causative genes, provide powerful evidence of the genetic influences on epilepsy. They are derived from analysis of statistical association, within families, between a disease phenotype and a genetic marker allele. The analysis must be performed within families because the specific marker allele associated with the disorder generally varies from family to family, in accordance with the distribution of the marker alleles in the population. Such a within-family association is unlikely to be artifactual because most genetic markers have no clinical or social effects, and marker information is based on laboratory analysis of biological samples performed independently of disease status. Thus, finding genetic linkage provides strong evidence that the disease susceptibility is influenced by a gene. Otherwise the condition would not cosegregate with a genetic marker allele. Finding genetic linkage also indicates that the susceptibility gene is located near the marker on the same chromosome.

The first locus for benign familial neonatal convulsions (BFNC), an autosomal dominant syndrome with complete penetrance, was found on chromosome 20q (12). A second locus for the same syndrome was later found on chromosome 8q (13). The gene on chromosome 20q was identified as a novel voltage-gated potassium channel, KCNQ2 (14), and the gene on chromosome 8q was identified as another member of the same family of potassium channels, KCNQ3 (15).

Juvenile myoclonic epilepsy (JME) has an uncertain mode of inheritance, with reduced penetrance and a range of phenotypic expressions within families. Greenberg and coworkers (16) found evidence for linkage of JME to the HLA region of chromosome 6. Two subsequent studies confirmed the linkage (17,18), but others found evidence against it (19,20) and instead found evidence for linkage to chromosome 15q (21). Another recent study suggested that a JME susceptibility gene maps to chromosome 6p but lies some distance centromeric to HLA (22). The lack of consistency in the linkage findings in JME may be partly explained by uncertainty about the phenotype that is produced by the susceptibility gene because the studies reporting positive linkage findings have used several alternative schemes to define which relatives were considered affected.

As shown in Table 5-2, evidence for linkage has also been reported in childhood absence epilepsy, benign familial infantile convulsions, familial autosomal recessive idiopathic myoclonic epilepsy of infancy, and familial adult myoclonic epilepsy (23–26).

Until recently, most *localization-related (partial or focal)* epilepsies were presumed to be nongenetic. However, evidence for linkage has been obtained for four forms of localization-related epilepsy. First, a gene for autosomal dominant partial epilepsy with auditory features (ADPEAF) was localized to chromosome 10q in a single large pedigree (27). Subsequently, evidence for linkage was reported for an overlapping region of chromosome 10q in a large family with autosomal dominant lateral temporal epilepsy, a phenotype clinically similar to ADPEAF (28). Further molecular studies are needed to determine whether these two entities are the same. Second, autosomal dominant nocturnal frontal lobe epilepsy (ADNFLE) was localized to chromosome 20q (29). The ADNFLE gene was identified as the neuronal nicotinic acetylcholine receptor $\alpha4$ subunit (CHRNA4) (30). This locus has been excluded in some families with the same syndrome, suggesting that at least one other gene causing ADNFLE remains to be identified. Evidence for linkage to chromosome 15 has been reported in one of these families (31). Third, a gene for benign epilepsy of childhood with centrotemporal spikes was localized to chromosome 15q14 in the region of the alpha 7 subunit of the neuronal nicotinic acetylcholine receptor (32). Fifth, evidence for linkage to chromosome 22q11 was reported for a family with familial partial epilepsy with variable foci (33).

Evidence for linkage has been reported on chromosomes 8q, 19q, and 5q in three different families with apparently autosomal dominant forms of febrile convulsions (34–36). In a related disorder, generalized epilepsy with febrile seizures plus (GEFS+), linkage was reported on chromosome 19q13, and the gene was identified as *SCN1B*, the voltage-gated sodium channel $\beta1$ subunit (37). In another family with GEFS+, the gene was localized to chromosome 2q and identified as the α-1 subunit of the voltage-gated sodium channel, *SCN1A* (38).

Causative genes have been identified in five progressive epilepsy syndromes with mental retardation. Progressive myoclonus epilepsy of Unverricht-Lundborg type, an autosomal recessive disorder with complete penetrance, was localized to chromosome 21q (39), and the gene was subsequently identified as cystatin B, a protease inhibitor (40). The gene for Lafora's disease, another autosomal recessive form of progressive myoclonus epilepsy, was identified as a novel protein phosphatase gene on chromosome 6q24 (41). An autosomal recessive gene for progressive epilepsy with mental retardation was localized to chromosome 8p (42), and the gene was identified as a neuronal ceroid lipofuscinase (43). Two forms of progressive epilepsy, myoclonic epilepsy with ragged red fibers (MERRF) and myoclonic epilepsy with lactic acidosis and strokelike episodes (MELAS), have been shown to be caused by mutations in mitochondrial genes (44,45).

MATERNAL TRANSMISSION

Risk of epilepsy is approximately twice as high in offspring of affected women as in offspring of affected men (46). This *maternal effect* is inconsistent with any conventional genetic model (46,47). Models involving X-linkage are rejected as an explanation because the risks are nearly the same in male and female offspring. Studies have indicated that the maternal effect cannot be explained either by (1) intrauterine exposure to seizures or anticonvulsants in offspring of women with epilepsy, (2) perinatal complications that occur with increased frequency in women with epilepsy, or (3) patterns of selective fertility (48–51). The possible roles of unidentified environmental exposures, mitochondrial genes, imprinted nuclear genes, or expanded repeat mutations remain to be investigated.

COMPLEXITY IN THE GENETIC CONTRIBUTIONS TO EPILEPSY

Etiologic and Genetic Heterogeneity

Important genetic and nongenetic influences clearly differ among some epilepsy syndromes, and in some cases also among different families that have the same syndrome. For example, locus heterogeneity (i.e., a single syndrome caused by mutations at different genetic loci in different families) has been demonstrated in BFNC through identification of two different susceptibility genes (KCNQ2 on chromosome 20q and KCNQ3 on chromosome 8q) (14,15).

One approach to studying etiologic and genetic heterogeneity is to examine how different clinical characteristics of epilepsy, such as different seizure types, age at onset, and etiology, affect the risk of seizures in relatives of people with epilepsy. The results of such studies can provide important information about which patients are most likely to have a genetic susceptibility. The risk of having seizures has consistently been found to be higher in relatives of patients with idiopathic or cryptogenic epilepsy than in relatives of those with symptomatic epilepsy (52–58). In the classic twin study conducted by Lennox and Lennox (5), the difference in concordance rates between monozygotic and dizygotic twins was greater for twins with idiopathic or cryptogenic epilepsy than for those with identified etiologic factors (Table 5-1). Similarly, Ottman and coworkers (56–57) found that epilepsy following a postnatal CNS lesion caused by conditions such as head trauma, stroke, or brain infection was not associated with increased familial risk. This suggests that the genetic contributions to postnatal symptomatic epilepsy are minimal.

Relatives of patients with early age at onset of epilepsy have also been found to have a higher risk of seizures than relatives of those with later onset (52,53,58). The risks of seizures in relatives are also higher when there is a previous family history of epilepsy than when there is no such history (59,60).

Most of the epileptic syndromes classified as "idiopathic" (presumed genetic) are generalized (2), and until recently most localization-related epilepsies were believed to be nongenetic. However, in most studies the difference in familial risk for generalized versus localization-related epilepsies is small (61). Recent findings indicate that the risk of epilepsy is higher in the parents and siblings of probands with generalized epilepsy than in those of probands with localization-related epilepsy, but this is not true in offspring (56). Similarly, in an earlier study of offspring of epilepsy patients in Rochester (62), the risk of unprovoked seizures was higher in offspring of probands with generalized epilepsy only for the subset of probands who had *absence* seizures.

Genetic contributions are commonly assumed to be different for each clinically defined epilepsy syndrome. If this were true, we would expect that among relatives of probands with specific syndromes, risk would be increased only for the same syndromes as in the probands. Several recent studies suggest that there is a tendency for clinical characteristics to cluster within families. Berkovic and coworkers (63) studied the syndrome classifications of twin pairs concordant for epilepsy and found that in most cases the syndrome

classifications were also concordant. Both Tsuboi (64) and Beck-Mannagetta and Janz (65) found that the distribution of seizure types in affected relatives was skewed toward the same types of seizures as in the probands, although different seizure types were seen also. In a study of 72 families of probands with idiopathic generalized epilepsy syndromes (IGEs), each of which contained three or more affected individuals, multiple different IGEs were seen in 75 percent of families, but there were very few cases of localization-related epilepsy (66).

Our work, however, suggests that some genetic mechanisms raise the risk for both generalized and localization-related epilepsies (67). Risk for all epilepsy in parents and siblings was greater if the proband had generalized epilepsy than if the proband had localization-related epilepsy, but the increased familial risk was not restricted to the same type of epilepsy as in the proband. The difference between these results and those found earlier may be attributed to a different distribution of epilepsy syndromes in the probands. In our study, very few of the probands had IGEs, whereas in the others, many or all of the probands had IGEs. The genetic influences on IGEs do appear to raise risk for IGEs specifically (although they may be shared across different IGEs such as JME, pyknolepsy, etc.). The genetic influences on other forms of epilepsy may have less specific effects than those on IGEs, raising the risk for multiple different syndromes.

Pleiotropy

Some of the genetic influences on idiopathic or cryptogenic epilepsy may have broad phenotypic effects, raising risk for other disorders as well. Evidence is strong for a shared genetic influence on epilepsy and febrile convulsions. Hauser and coworkers (68) found that the risk of *epilepsy* was increased to the same extent in the relatives of probands with febrile convulsions as in relatives of probands with epilepsy. Similarly, the risk of *febrile convulsions* was increased to the same extent in the relatives of probands with epilepsy as in the relatives probands with febrile convulsions.

Previous studies also support the possibility of a shared genetic susceptibility to epilepsy and cerebral palsy. In the National Collaborative Perinatal Project, incidence of cerebral palsy was associated with the mother's history of epilepsy (69), and incidence of nonfebrile seizure disorders in children *without cerebral palsy* was associated with a history of motor deficits in siblings (70). Similarly, Rimoin and Metrakos reported an increased prevalence of convulsions and epileptiform electroencephalogram (EEG) abnormalities in the relatives of children with hemiplegia (71).

Ottman and coworkers (57) found that the risk for idiopathic or cryptogenic epilepsy was increased in the relatives of probands with epilepsy associated with cerebral palsy, and, conversely, the risk of epilepsy associated with cerebral palsy was increased in the relatives of probands with idiopathic or cryptogenic epilepsy.

Gene–Environment Interaction

The effects of some genotypes on the risk for epilepsy may involve interaction with specific environmental exposures (72–73). For example, a genotype that raises the risk for epilepsy might increase susceptibility to the effect of an environmental risk factor such as head injury. In this case, the influence of the genotype on risk would be greater in persons who were exposed to the environmental factor than in those who were unexposed. Recent results do not appear to support this possibility because they suggest that the genetic contributions are minimal for epilepsy occurring in the context of an identified postnatal environmental insult (57,74). However, the postnatal environmental risk factors for epilepsy that have been evaluated in many previous studies (i.e., severe head trauma, stroke, brain tumor, brain surgery, and brain infection) have strong effects, each raising the risk for epilepsy at least 10-fold (75). Other risk factors with milder effects may show different patterns of gene–environment interaction. For example, in a study by Schaumann and coworkers (74), seizure risk was increased in the relatives of probands with alcohol-related seizures. The possibility of interaction between alcohol exposure and genetic susceptibility on risk for epilepsy would be interesting to explore.

OTHER SYNDROMES OF INTEREST FOR GENETIC STUDIES

In the following syndromes, family studies have indicated an important genetic influence on susceptibility, and additional research is under way.

Childhood Absence (Pyknolepsy)

In the 1960s, Metrakos and Metrakos (60) examined the distribution of seizures and EEG abnormalities in families of children with "centrencephalic epilepsy," most of whom would be classified today as having idiopathic childhood absence epilepsy. They concluded that this type of epilepsy and its associated three per second generalized spike-wave EEG trait were caused by an autosomal *dominant* gene with reduced and age-dependent penetrance. In contrast, Boreki and coworkers (76) used data collected by Doose

and coworkers (77) to perform segregation analysis of epilepsy in families of probands with "primary generalized minor motor epilepsies," many of which probably would also be classified today as childhood absence. They concluded that the data were most consistent with an autosomal *recessive* susceptibility allele, which, however, accounted for only 9.3 percent of the variability. Susceptibility genes have not yet been identified in this syndrome, although linkage was reported (23).

Benign Rolandic Epilepsy with Centrotemporal Spikes

Several investigators have suggested an autosomal dominant etiology for benign rolandic epilepsy with associated central temporal spikes or sharp waves in the EEG (78–80). While this syndrome is clearly highly familial, its mode of inheritance remains to be determined.

Febrile Convulsions

Febrile convulsions have been studied extensively from a genetic point of view (81–84). In a segregation analysis of susceptibility to febrile convulsions, Rich and coworkers found significant genetic heterogeneity (84). In the families of probands with only a single febrile convulsion, the data were most consistent with a *polygenic* mode of inheritance, whereas in families of probands with multiple febrile convulsions, the data were consistent with an *autosomal dominant* mode of inheritance. As previously noted, evidence has been obtained for linkage to three different chromosomes in families with apparently autosomal dominant inheritance (34–36). In families with idiopathic epilepsy syndromes, it is of great interest to determine whether susceptibility genes raise risk for febrile convulsions in addition to epilepsy.

CONCLUSIONS

Although evidence is mounting for an important genetic influence on susceptibility to epilepsy, for the majority of patients the specific genetic influences remain to be identified. Identification of genes influencing susceptibility to epilepsy holds great promise for future studies. It could facilitate early identification of susceptible individuals, early treatment, and perhaps prevention of the disorder in some individuals. It is also a first step in investigating the physiologic effects of susceptibility genes, leading to better understanding of pathogenesis and to development of new strategies for treatment and prevention.

REFERENCES

1. Hauser WA, Annegers JF, Kurland LT. Prevalence of epilepsy in Rochester, Minnesota: 1940–1980. *Epilepsia* 1991; 32:429–445.

2. Commission on Classification and Terminology of the International League Against Epilepsy. Proposal for revised classification of epilepsies and epileptic syndromes. *Epilepsia* 1989; 30:389–399.

3. Annegers JF, Hauser WA, Anderson VE. Risk of seizures among relatives of patients with epilepsy: families in a defined population. In: Anderson VE, Hauser WA, Sing C, Porter R, eds., *The Genetic Basis of the Epilepsies.* New York: Raven Press, 1982:151–159.

4. Annegers JF, Hauser WA, Anderson VE, et al. The risks of seizure disorders among relatives of patients with childhood onset epilepsy. *Neurology* 1992; 32:174–179.

5. Lennox WG. *Epilepsy and Related Disorders.* Vol. 1. Boston: Little, Brown, 1960:532–574.

6. Inouye E. Observations on forty twin index cases with chronic epilepsy and their co-twins. *J Nerv Ment Dis* 1960; 130:401–416.

7. Harvald B, Hauge M. Hereditary factors elucidated by twin studies. In: Neel JV, Shaw MW, Schull WJ, eds. *Genetics and the Epidemiology of Chronic Diseases.* Washington D.C.: Public Health Service Publication No. 1163, 1965:61–76.

8. Corey LA, Berg K, Pellock JM, et al. The occurrence of epilepsy and febrile seizures in Virginian and Norwegian twins. *Neurology* 1991; 41:1433–1436.

9. Silanpaa M, Koskenvuo M, Romanov K, et al. Genetic factors in epileptic seizures: evidence from a large twin population. *Acta Neurol Scand* 1991; 84:523–526.

10. Anderson VE, Hauser WA. Genetics of epilepsy. *Prog Med Genet* 1985; 6:9–52.

11. Noebels JL. Targeting epilepsy genes. *Neuron* 1996; 16:241–244.

12. Leppert M, Anderson VE, Quattlebaum T, et al. Benign neonatal convulsions linked to genetic markers on chromosome 20. *Nature* 1989; 337:647–648.

13. Lewis TB, Leach RJ, Ward K, et al. Genetic heterogeneity in benign familial neonatal convulsions: identification of a new locus on chromosome 8q. *Am J Hum Genet* 1993; 53:670–614.

14. Singh NA, Charlier C, Stauffer D, et al. A novel potassium channel gene, KCNQ2, is mutated in an inherited epilepsy of newborns. *Nat Genet* 1998; 18:25–37.

15. Charlier C, Singh NA, Ryan SG, et al. A pore mutation in a novel KQT-like potassium channel gene in an idiopathic epilepsy family. *Nat Genet* 1998; 18:53–55.

16. Greenberg DA, Delgado-Escueta AV, Widelitz H, et al. Juvenile myoclonic epilepsy may be linked to the BF and HLA loci on human chromosome 6. *Am J Med Genet* 1988; 31:185–192.

17. Weissbecker KA, Durner M, Janz D, et al. Confirmation of linkage between juvenile myoclonic epilepsy locus and the HLA region of chromosome 6. *Am J Med Genet* 1991; 38:32–36.

18. Durner M, Sander T, Greenberg DA, et al. Localization of idiopathic generalized epilepsy on chromosome 6p in families ascertained through juvenile myoclonic epilepsy patients. *Neurology* 1991; 41:1651–1655.

19. Whitehouse WP, Rees M, Curtis D, et al. Linkage analysis of idiopathic generalized epilepsy (IGE) and marker loci on chromosome 6p in families of patients with juvenile myoclonic epilepsy: no evidence for an epilepsy locus in the HLA region. *Am J Hum Genet* 1993; 53:652–662.

20. Elmslie FV, Williamson MP, Rees M, et al. Linkage analysis of juvenile myoclonic epilepsy and microsatellite loci spanning 61 cm of human chromosome 6p in 19 nuclear pedigrees provides no evidence for a susceptibility locus in this region. *Am J Hum Genet* 1996; 59:653–663.

21. Elmslie FV, Rees M, Williamson MP, et al. Genetic mapping of a major susceptibility locus for juvenile myoclonic epilepsy on chromosome 15q. *Hum Mol Genet* 1997; 6:1329–1334.

22. Liu AW, Delgado-Escueta AV, Serratosa JM, et al. Juvenile myoclonic epilepsy locus in chromosome 6p21.2-p11: linkage to convulsions and electroencephalography trait. *Am J Hum Genet* 1995; 57:368–381.

23. Fong GC, Shah PU, Gee MN, et al. Childhood absence epilepsy with tonic-clonic seizures and electroencephalogram 3–4-Hz spike and multispike-slow wave complexes: linkage to chromosome 8q24. *Am J Hum Genet* 1998; 63:1117–1129.

24. Guipponi M, Rivier F, Vigevano F, et al. Linkage mapping of benign familial infantile convulsions (BFIC) to chromosome 19q. *Hum Mol Genet* 1997; 6:473–477.

25. Zara F, Gennaro E, Stabile M, et al. Mapping of a locus for a familial autosomal recessive idiopathic myoclonic epilepsy of infancy to chromosome 16p13. *Am J Hum Genet* 2000; 66:1552–1557.

26. Mikami M, Yasuda T, Terao A, et al. Localization of a gene for benign adult familial myoclonic epilepsy to chromosome 8q23.3-q24.1. *Am J Hum Genet* 1999; 65:745–751.

27. Ottman R, Risch N, Hauser WA, et al. Localization of a gene for partial epilepsy to chromosome 10q. *Nat Genet* 1995; 10:56–60.

28. Poza JJ, Saenz A, Martinez-Gil A, et al. Autosomal dominant lateral temporal epilepsy: clinical and genetic study of a large Basque pedigree linked to chromosome 10q. *Ann Neurol* 1999; 45:182–188.

29. Phillips HA, Scheffer IE, Berkovic SF, et al. Localization of a gene for autosomal dominant nocturnal frontal lobe epilepsy to chromosome 20q13.2. *Nat Genet* 1995; 10:117–118.

30. Steinlein OK, Mulley JC, Propping P, et al. A missense mutation in the neuronal nicotinic acetylcholine receptor alpha 4 subunit is associated with autosomal dominant nocturnal frontal lobe epilepsy. *Nat Genet* 1995; 11:201–203.

31. Phillips HA, Scheffer IE, Crossland KM, et al. Autosomal dominant nocturnal frontal-lobe epilepsy: genetic heterogeneity and evidence for a second locus at 15q24. *Am J Hum Genet* 1998; 63:1108–1116.

32. Neubauer BA, Fiedler B, Himmelein B, et al. Centrotemporal spikes in families with rolandic epilepsy. Linkage to chromosome 15q. *Neurology* 1998; 51:1608–1612.

33. Xiong L, Labuda M, Li DS, et al. Mapping of a gene determining familial partial epilepsy with variable foci to chromosome 22q11-q12. *Am J Hum Genet* 1999; 65:1698–1710.

34. Wallace RH, Berkovic SF, Howell RA, et al. Suggestion of a major gene for familial febrile convulsions mapping to 8q13-21. *J Med Genet* 1996; 33:308–312.

35. Johnson E, et al. Evidence for a novel gene for familial febrile convulsions, FEB2, linked to chromosome 19p in an extended family from the Midwest. *Hum Mol Genet* 1998; 7:63–67.

36. Nakayama J, Hamano K, Iwasaki N, et al. Significant evidence for linkage of febrile seizures to chromosome 5q14-q15. *Hum Mol Genet* 2000; 9:87–91.

37. Wallace RH, Wang DW, Singh R, et al. Febrile seizures and generalized epilepsy associated with a mutation in the Na$^+$-channel β-1 subunit gene *SCN1B*. *Nat Genet* 1998; 19:366–3780.

38. Escayg A, MacDonald BT, Meisler MH, et al. Mutations of SCN1A, encoding a neuronal sodium channel, in two families with GEFS+2. *Nat Genet* 2000; 24:343–345.

39. Lehesjoki A, Koskiniemi M, Sistonen P, et al. Localization of a gene for the progressive myoclonus epilepsy to chromosome 21q22. *Proc Nat Acad Sci USA* 1991; 88:3696–3699.

40. Pennacchio LA, Lehesjoki AE, Stone NE, et al. Mutations in the gene encoding cystatin B in progressive myoclonus epilepsy (EPM1) (see comments). *Science* 1996; 271:1731–1734.

41. Minassian BA, Lee JR, Herbrick J-A, et al. Mutations in a gene encoding a novel protein tyrosine phosphatase cause progressive myoclonus epilepsy. *Nat Genet* 1998; 20:171–174.

42. Tahvanainen E, Ranta S, Hirvasniemi A, et al. The gene for a recessively inherited human childhood progressive epilepsy with mental retardation maps to the distal short arm of chromosome 8. *Proc Natl Acad Sci USA* 1994; 90:7267–72670.

43. Ranta S, Zhang Y, Ross B, et al. The neuronal ceroid lipofuscinoses in human EPMR and mnd mutant mice are associated with mutations in CLN8. *Nat Genet* 1999; 23:233–236.

44. Chomyn A. The myoclonic epilepsy and ragged-red fiber mutation provides new insights into human mitochondrial function and genetics. *Am J Hum Genet* 1998; 62:745–751.

45. Hirano M, Pavlakis SG. Mitochondrial myopathy, encephalopathy, lactic acidosis, and strokelike episodes (MELAS): current concepts. *J Child Neurol* 1994; 9:4–13.

46. Ottman R, Hauser WA, Susser M. Genetic and maternal influences on susceptibility to seizures: an analytic review. *Am J Epidemiol* 1985; 122:923–939.

47. Ottman R. A simple test of the multifactorial-polygenic model with sex-dependent thresholds. *J Chron Dis* 1987; 40:165–170.

48. Ottman R, Annegers JF, Hauser WA, et al. Higher seizure risk in offspring of mothers than of fathers with epilepsy. *Am J Hum Genet* 1988; 43:257–264.

49. Schupf N, Ottman R. The likelihood of pregnancy in individuals with idiopathic/cryptogenic epilepsy: social and biologic influences. *Epilepsia* 1994; 35:750–756.

50. Schupf N, Ottman R. Reproduction among individuals with idiopathic/cryptogenic epilepsy: risk factors for reduced fertility within marriage. *Epilepsia* 1996; 37:833–840.

51. Schupf N, Ottman R. Reproduction among individuals with idiopathic/cryptogenic epilepsy: risk factors for spontaneous abortion within marriage. *Epilepsia* 1997; 38:824–829.

52. Anderson VE, Rich SS, Hauser WA, et al. Family studies of epilepsy. In: Anderson VE, Hauser WA, Leppik IE, Noebels JL, Rich SS, eds. *Genetic Strategies in Epilepsy Research* (Epilepsy Res Suppl 4). Amsterdam: Elsevier Science Publishers BV, 1991:89–103.

53. Lennox WG. The genetics of epilepsy. *Am J Psychiatr* 1947; 103:457–462.

54. Tsuboi T, Endo S. Incidence of seizures and EEG abnormalities among offspring of epileptic patients. *Hum Genet* 1977; 36:173–189.

55. Harvald B. On the genetic prognosis of epilepsy. *Acta Psychiatr Neurol* 1951; 26:339–357.

56. Ottman R, Lee JH, Risch N, et al. Clinical indicators of genetic susceptibility in epilepsy. *Epilepsia* 1996; 37:353–361.

57. Ottman R, Annegers JF, Hauser WA, et al. Relations of genetic and environmental factors in the etiology of epilepsy. *Ann Neurol* 1996; 39:442–449.

58. Eisner V, Pauli LL, Livingston S. Hereditary aspects of epilepsy. *Bull Johns Hopkins Hosp* 1959; 105:245–271.

59. Kimball OP, Hersh AH. The genetics of epilepsy. *Acta Genet Med Gemellol* 1955; 4:131–142.

60. Metrakos K, Metrakos JD. Genetics of convulsive disorders II. *Neurology* 1960; 11:474–483.

61. Ottman R. Genetics of the partial epilepsies: a review. *Epilepsia* 1989; 30:107–111.

62. Ottman R, Annegers JF, Hauser WA, et al. Seizure risk in offspring of parents with generalized versus partial epilepsy. *Epilepsia* 1989; 30:157–161.

63. Berkovic SF, Howell RA, Hay DA, Hopper JL. Epilepsies in twins: genetics of the major epilepsy syndromes. *Ann Neurol* 1998; 43:435–445.

64. Tsuboi T. Genetic aspects of epilepsy. *Folia Psychiatr Neurol Jpn* 1980; 34:215–225.

65. Beck-Mannagetta G, Janz D. Syndrome-related genetics in generalized epilepsy. In: Anderson VE, Hauser WA, Leppik IE, Noebels JL, Rich SS, eds. *Genetic Strategies in Epilepsy Research* (Epilepsy Res Suppl 4). Amsterdam: Elsevier Science Publishers BV, 1991:105–111.

66. Italian League Against Epilepsy Genetic Collaborative Group. Concordance of clinical forms of epilepsy in families with several affected members. *Epilepsia* 1993; 34:819–826.

67. Ottman R, Lee JH, Hauser WA, Risch N. Are generalized and partial epilepsies genetically distinct? *Arch Neurol* 1998; 55:339–344.

68. Hauser WA, Annegers JF, Kurland LT. The risk of seizure disorders among relatives of children with febrile convulsions. *Neurology* 1985; 35:1268–1273.

69. Nelson KB, Ellenberg JH. Maternal seizure disorder, outcome of pregnancy, and neurologic abnormalities in the children. *Neurology* 1982; 32:1247–1254.

70. Nelson KB, Ellenberg JH. Antecedents of seizure disorders in early childhood. *Am J Dis Child* 1986;140:1053–1061.

71. Rimoin DL, Metrakos JD. *The Genetics of Convulsive Disorders in the Families of Hemiplegics*. Proc 2nd Intl Congr Hum Genet, Rome. Amsterdam: Excerpta Medica Foundation, 1963; 1655–1658.

72. Ottman R. An epidemiologic approach to gene-environment interaction. *Genet Epidemiol* 1990; 7:177–185.

73. Ottman R. Gene-environment interaction: definitions and study designs. *Prev Med* 1996; 25:764–770.

74. Schaumann BA, Annegers JF, Johnson SB, et al. Family history of seizures in posttraumatic and alcohol-associated seizure disorders. *Epilepsia* 1994; 35:48–52.

75. Hauser WA, Hesdorffer DC. *Epilepsy: Frequency, Causes and Consequences*. New York: Demos Publications, 1990:53–92.

76. Boreki IB, Baier WK, Doose H, et al. Familial transmission of primarily generalized minor seizures. *Am J Hum Genet* 1987; 41(Suppl):A251.

77. Doose H, Baier WK. Genetic factors in epilepsies with primarily generalized minor seizures. *Neuropediatrics* 1987; 18(Supp 1):1–64.

78. Bray PF, Wiser WC. Hereditary characteristics of familial temporal-central focal epilepsy. *Pediatrics* 1965; 36:207–211.

79. Heijbel J, Blom S, Rasmuson M. Benign epilepsy of childhood with centrotemporal EEG foci: a genetic study. *Epilepsia* 1975; 16:285–293.

80. Rodin EA, Whelan JL. Familial occurrence of focal temporal electroencephalographic abnormalities. *Neurology* 1960; 10:542–545.

81. Schumann SH, Miller LJ. Febrile convulsions in families: findings in an epidemiologic survey. *Clin Pediatr* 1966; 5:604–608.

82. Fukuyama YK, Kagarva K, Tanaka K. A genetic study of febrile convulsions. *Eur Neurol* 1979; 18; 166–182.

83. Tsuboi T. Genetic aspects of febrile convulsions: twin and family study. *Hum Genet* 1987; 75:7–14.

84. Rich SS, Annegers JF, Hauser WA, et al. Complex segregation analysis of febrile convulsions. *Am J Hum Genet* 1987; 41:249–257.

CHAPTER 6

Classification of Epilepsies in Childhood

Fritz E. Dreifuss, M.D., F.R.C.P., and Douglas R. Nordli, Jr., M.D.

HISTORICAL BACKGROUND

Early discussions on epilepsy rarely differentiated between epilepsies in childhood and those in adult life. The history of classification of the epilepsies might be defined in three major eras: the philosophical era before the twentieth century, and this included patient observation and to a large degree philosophical speculation as to the nature of the disease; the era of the localizationalists and pathologists, which occurred in the first half of the twentieth century; and the molecular era, including neurochemistry and particularly receptor pharmacology, the physiology of excitatory and inhibitory systems, and molecular biology.

The Philosophical Era

In 1861 Reynolds (1) described convulsions in children by the name *eclampsia*. So-called eclamptic seizures in those days referred to seizures characteristic of the childhood age group that encompassed febrile convulsions and convulsions of the basis of specific systemic diseases. Although Poupart had described absence in a young girl in 1705 (2), different seizure types were not particularly related to different age groups until much later. In 1772 Tissot (3) classified epileptic seizures but made a more specific contribution that is often lost and that was further elaborated by Sachs (4) in the first English language pediatric neurology textbook, that is, the concept that epilepsy is composed of an ongoing predisposing condition or diathesis, but that the individual epileptic seizures, or expression of the epileptic process, is triggered by a concatenation of factors that might be considered as precipitating or triggering factors. The latter are not always recognized, and epilepsy therefore has been defined as a liability to unprovoked seizures, which is probably a procrustean attempt to exclude febrile convulsions from the epilepsy rubric.

Sachs divided childhood epilepsies into the eclamptic and the epileptic. The epileptic seizures were further divided into partial and generalized as well as lesional and idiopathic. He believed that idiopathic seizures on a heritable basis had an ultimately bad prognosis and that symptomatic seizures had an even worse prognosis. He thought that symptomatic epilepsies were the result of neonatal abnormalities, including brain hemorrhage. Freud (5) wrote about epilepsy in his text on the infantile cerebral palsies and related childhood seizures to major brain disturbances leading to the conditions included under the heading of cerebral palsy. Smith (6), in his book on diseases in children published over 100 years ago, stated that eclampsia in children was relatively benign except when severe and protracted, when it might be the cause of certain lesions, and he separated this from epilepsy occurring in older children, which he regarded as symptomatic. Sachs, agreeing with Tissot in defining an underlying predisposition and a precipitating cause, also stated that the prognosis largely depended on the underlying cause of the epilepsy and was otherwise not inherent in the convulsions, a somewhat different conclusion than had been arrived at by Gowers (7), who studied predominantly adults and who believed that the periodicity or repetitiveness of a convulsive disorder carried within it the seeds of a progressive disorder.

The Localizationalist and Pathologist Era

The period of the localizationalists and pathologists began with the experiments of Fritsch and Hitzig and of Ferrier and formed the basis of Hughlings Jackson's localizational endeavors, which in turn inspired the beginning of epilepsy surgery 100 years ago by Victor Horsley. The landmark activities of Penfield, Erickson, and Jasper during the past 50 years more clearly defined the nature of epileptic seizures and their localization in the nervous system. The development of electroencephalography and, in more recent times, electoencephalography with simultaneous visulation of epileptic seizures on a split-screen TV has contributed to understanding epilepsy. This allowed the elaboration of the 1981 classification of epileptic seizures (8), which represented an advance made possible by objective methods of documenting seizures. The addition of other factors, such as anatomic substrate, cause, and age, based on information other than intensive monitoring, were then incorporated into the definition of individual epileptic syndromes (9).

The Molecular Era

Modeling of the epilepsies using various animal models; sophisticated neurophysiological, neurochemical, and pharmacological techniques; tissue slice preparations with the application of excitatory and inhibitory neurotransmitters and both extracellular and intracellular recordings; and the individual neuronal culture preparations have advanced the study of the epilepsies immensely. With these studies has come the realization of epilepsy as a system disease, and the model of secondary epileptogenesis, both kindling and mirror focus examinations, have yielded interesting information. Through the study of molecular biology, researchers now tentatively believe that some human epileptic syndromes may be heritable, a concept that may ultimately alter our understanding of the idiopathic label.

CLASSIFICATION OF EPILEPTIC SEIZURES AND THE EPILEPSIES

Rationale for Classification

The classification of epileptic seizures is quite important for lending uniformity to descriptions for communication, collaborative pharmacological and epidemiological research endeavors, and understanding the function of the central nervous system (CNS). The introduction of the newer antiepileptic drugs with rather specific spectra of activities has further mandated diagnostic accuracy. The division of seizures into those that are generalized from the beginning and those that have an onset with a definable localization in the cortex has enlivened neurologic investigation because there appears to be a distinction between those seizures that arise from six-layered isocortex and remain relatively localized and those whose elaboration involves regions of the brain, disturbances of which interfere with consciousness, memory, and learning. These distinctions now have application in differences in medicinal and surgical management. As an example, it is vital to distinguish between absence seizures and complex partial seizures, which may be

difficult to do on clinical grounds and is pivotal in applying appropriate treatment.

Furthermore, it is increasingly apparent that the cause of a seizure disorder is of primary importance. Whereas the seizure type is the product of the area of the nervous system involved, the causative factors have implications reaching in genetics, higher cortical function, and intelligence. The cause determines prognosis, response to medication, and natural history. The seizure is only the symptom that brings the patient to the physician. The epileptic syndrome, of which the seizure is the symptom, is the determinant of the prognosis and is the product of the underlying disease. Therefore, family history, age of onset, rate of progression, presence or absence of neurologic abnormalities, presence or absence of interictal electroencephalograph (EEG) abnormalities, and the response to medication all contribute to the diagnosis of the syndrome.

Apart from usefulness in communication, classification, and identification, etiologic factors are essential for appropriate therapy, not only in terms of using the most appropriate antiepileptic agent but also in gauging the natural history of the condition, prognosticating the duration of therapy, or determining whether antiepileptic drugs are indeed essential for managing the particular condition. Moreover, the identification of individual syndromes has allowed the application of molecular biology to the ultimate elucidation of the so-called idiopathic epilepsies in that syndromes can, on occasion, be sufficiently discretely identified and that their genetic localization can be determined on the human genome (10,11).

Seizures are categorized as either partial or generalized (Table 6-1). Partial (focal or localization-related) seizures arise in specific loci in the cortex, which carry with them identifiable signatures, either subjective or observational. These may range from disorders of sensation or thought to convulsive movement of a part of the body. Simple partial seizures are those in which consciousness is preserved. These arise from the six-layered isocortex and may remain localized sufficiently long to allow specific symptoms to be discerned. At other times, they spread quite rapidly and become more elaborate in their manifestations and ultimately may generalize. Complex partial seizures are those in which consciousness is impaired; they may follow simple partial seizures or may begin as complex partial seizures with impaired consciousness at the onset. With impairment of consciousness any activity manifested during the seizures occurs in the form of automatisms. The implication of complex partial seizures is that they involve elaboration elements of the limbic system, thus leading to early bilateral dysfunction. This may involve temporal or frontal lobe structures.

Table 6-1. Seizure Categories (8)

I. Partial (Focal, Local) Seizures

Partial seizures are those in which, in general, the first clinical and EEG changes indicate initial activation of a system of neurons limited to part of one cerebral hemisphere. A partial seizure is classified primarily on the basis of whether or not consciousness is impaired during the attack. When consciousness is not impaired, the seizure is classified as a simple partial seizure. When consciousness is impaired, the seizure is classified as a complex partial seizure. Impairment of consciousness may be the first clinical sign, or simple partial seizures may evolve into complex partial seizures. In patients with impaired consciousness, aberrations of behavior (automatisms) may occur. A partial seizure may not terminate, but instead progress to a generalized motor seizure. Impaired consciousness is defined as the inability to respond normally to exogenous stimuli by virtue of altered awareness and/or responsiveness.

There is considerable evidence that simple partial seizures usually have unilateral hemispheric involvement and only rarely have bilateral hemispheric involvement; complex partial seizures, however, frequently have bilateral hemispheric involvement.

Partial seizures can be classified into one of the following three fundamental groups:

Simple partial seizures (consciousness not impaired)

With motor symptoms

With somatosensory or special sensory symptoms

With autonomic symptoms

With psychic symptoms

Complex partial seizures (with impairment of consciousness)

Beginning as simple partial seizures and progressing to impairment of consciousness

With no other features

With features as in A.1-4

With automatisms

With impairment of consciousness at onset

With no other features

With features as in A.1-4

With automatisms

Partial seizures secondarily generalized

II. Generalized Seizures (Convulsive or Nonconvulsive)

Generalized seizures are those in which the first clinical changes indicate initial involvement of both hemispheres. Consciousness may be impaired, and this impairment may be the initial manifestation. Motor manifestations are bilateral. The ictal EEG patterns initially are bilateral and presumably reflect neuronal discharge, which is widespread in both hemispheres.

1. Absence seizures

2. Atypical absence seizures

Myoclonic seizures

Clonic seizures

Tonic seizures

Tonic-clonic seizures

Atonic seizures

III. Unclassified Epileptic Seizures

Includes all seizures that cannot be classified because of inadequate or incomplete data and some that defy classification in hitherto described categories. This includes some neonatal seizures, e.g., rhythmic eye movements, chewing, and swimming movements.

Generalized seizures involve large volumes of brain from the outset and are usually bilateral in their initial manifestations and associated with early impairment of consciousness. They may range from absence seizures characterized only by impaired consciousness to generalized tonic-clonic seizures (GTCS) in which widespread convulsive activity takes place. Myoclonic seizures, tonic seizures, and clonic seizures may also occur as generalized attacks.

The limitation of the classification of epileptic seizures to description of individual seizure types is that the terminology used in daily communication between colleagues usually consists of description of syndromes. This is also true of diagnostic entries in hospital records and communication between collaborators conducting clinical trials. An epileptic syndrome is an epileptic disorder characterized by a cluster of signs and symptoms customarily occurring together (Table 6-2). Some syndromes are very specific, for example, benign rolandic epilepsy, juvenile myoclonic epilepsy, the Lennox-Gastaut syndrome, and the infantile spasm syndrome.

Table 6-2. Features of Epileptic Syndromes

Seizure type(s)

Age of onset
Etiology
Anatomy
Precipitating factors
Severity
EEG, both ictal and interictal
Duration of epilepsy
Associated clinical features
Chronicity
Diurnal and circadian cycling
Occasionally prognosis

CLASSIFICATION OF EPILEPSIES AND EPILEPTIC SYNDROMES

Epilepsies may be classified according to seizure type and EEG findings, for example, either partial or generalized, or according to cause, that is, idiopathic, genetic, or symptomatic. They may be classified by anatomic localization, for example, frontal, rolandic, occipital, or temporal lobe epilepsies. Finally, they may be classified according to precipitating factors. Age of onset may be of importance, as may certain diurnal influences such as the progressive myoclonus epilepsies. In tackling the problem of classifying the epilepsies, these factors are taken into account and the proposed classification is outlined in Table 6-3.

DEFINITIONS

Benign Childhood Epilepsy with Centrotemporal Spikes

Benign childhood epilepsy with centrotemporal spikes is a syndrome of brief, simple, partial, hemifacial motor seizures, frequently with somatosensory symptoms, which have a tendency to evolve into GTCS (12–17). Both seizure types are often related to sleep. Onset is between 3 and 13 years of age (peak, 9–10), and recovery before ages 15 to 16. Genetic predisposition

Table 6-3. International Classification of Epilepsies and Epileptic Syndromes (9)

1.0   Localization-related (focal, local, partial) epilepsies and syndromes
1.1   Idiopathic (with age-related onset). At present, two syndromes are established, but more may be identified in the future.
       Benign childhood epilepsy with centro-temporal spike
       Childhood epilepsy with occipital paroxysms
1.2   Symptomatic. This category comprises syndromes of individual variability,
       which is mainly based on anatomical localization, clinical features, seizure types, and etiological factors (if known).
1.2.1 Epilepsy is characterized by simple partial seizures with the characteristics of seizures:
           Arising from frontal lobes
           Arising from parietal lobes
           Arising from temporal lobes
           Arising from occipital lobes
           Arising from multiple lobes
           Locus of onset unknown
1.2.2 Characterized by complex partial seizures, that is, attacks with alteration of consciousness often with automatisms.
       Characterized by seizures:
           Arising from frontal lobes
           Arising from parietal lobes
           Arising from temporal lobes
           Arising from occipital lobes
           Arising from multiple lobes
           Locus on onset unknown
1.2.3 Characterized by secondarily generalized seizures with seizures:
           Arising from frontal lobes
           Arising from parietal lobes
           Arising from temporal lobes
           Arising from occipital lobes
           Arising from multiple lobes
           Locus on onset unknown
Seizures arising from the temporal lobe. General characteristics: Features strongly suggestive of the diagnosis when present include:
Simple partial seizures typically characterized by autonomic and/or psychic symptoms and certain sensory phenomena such as olfactory, gustatory, auditory (including illusions), and vertiginous seizures. Most common is an epigastric, often rising, sensation.

Table 6-3. (*Continued*)

Complex partial seizures often but not always beginning with motor arrest, typically followed by oro-alimentary automatism. Reactive automatisms frequently follow. Postictal confusion usually occurs. The duration is typically more than 1 minute followed by amnesia. There is frequently a history of febrile seizures and a family history of seizures is common. Memory deficits may occur. Hypometabolism seen in temporal lobe lesions. Unilateral or bilateral temporal spikes are common on EEG. Onset is frequently in childhood or young adulthood. Seizures may progress to generalized tonic-clonic seizures.

Hippocampal (mesiobasal limbic or primary rhinencephalic psychomotor) epilepsy. This is the most common form, and the symptoms are those described in the previous paragraphs except that auditory and vertiginous symptoms may not occur. Seizure occur in clusters at intervals or randomly. They last an average of 2 minutes. Generalized tonic-clonic seizures may occur as a consequence of progressing propagation of seizure discharges. The interictal EEG typically shows medial or mesial anterior temporal sharp waves. Seizures are characterized by rising epigastric discomfort, nausea, marked autonomic signs and other symptoms including borborygmi, belching, pallor, fullness of the face, flushing of the face, arrest of respiration, pupillary dilatation, fear, panic, and olfactory-gustatory hallucinations.

Lateral temporal epilepsy. Seizures characterized by auras of auditory hallucinations or illusions or dreamy states, visual perceptual hallucinations or language disorder in case of language dominant hemisphere focus. The symptoms may progress to complex partial seizures if propagation to mesial temporal structures occur. The surface EEG shows unilateral or bilateral midtemporal or posterior temporal spikes which are most prominent in the lateral derivations.

Arising from the frontal lobe. General characteristics. Features that are strongly suggestive of the diagnosis when present include: frequent short attacks with impairment of consciousness; complex partial seizures arising from the frontal lobe have minimal or no postictal confusion; they are sometimes mistaken for psychogenic seizures; rapid secondary generalizaton is common; status epilepticus is a frequent complication; motor manifestations are prominent; automatisms are complex stereotyped and gestural at onset; urinary incontinence is common during frontal lobe complex partial seizures; and drop attacks frequently occur.

Supplementary motor seizures. Here the seizure patterns are postural, simple focal tonic, with localization, speech arrest, fencing postures, and complex focal features.

Cingulate. Seizure patterns are complex partial with complex motor gestural automatisms at the onset. Vegetative signs are common as are changes in mood and affect.

Anterior frontopolar region. Seizure patterns include initial loss of contact, versive movements of head and eyes, axial clonic jerks and falls and autonomic signs. Secondary generalization is especially common.

Orbitofrontal. Seizure patterns are complex partial with initial motor and gestual automatisms, olfactory hallucinations, and illusions and autonomic signs.

Dorsolateral. The seizure patterns may be tonic or less commonly clonic with versive eye and head movements and speech arrest.

Opercular (perisylvian, insular). Characteristics include mastication, salivation, swallowing, laryngeal symptoms, epigastric aura with fear, and vegetative phenomenon. Simple partial seizures, particularly partial clonic facial seizures, are common. If secondary sensory change occurs, numbness may be a symptom, particularly in the hands. Bilateral movement of the upper extremites may be seen.

Epilepsies of the motor cortex (perirolandic). These are mainly characterized by simple partial seizures, and their localization depends on the side and topography of the are involved. In cases of the lower perirolandic area, there may be speech arrest, vocalization of dysphasia, tonic-clonic movements of the face on the contralateral side, or swallowing. Generalization of the seizure frequently occurs. In the rolandic area, partial motor seizures without march or jacksonian seizures, particularly beginning in the contralateral upper extremities, occur. The nature of the attack is impaired by the characteristics of the seizure propagation, which impart the motor pattern or speech disturbances. In the case of seizures involving the paracentral lobule, tonic movements of the ipsilateral foot may occur, as well as the expected contralateral leg movements. Posticatal or Todd's paralysis is frequent. *Note*: Some epilepsies are difficult to assign to specific lobes. Such epilepsies include central epilepsy, which would include pre- and postcentral symptomatology, as in perirolandic seizures. Such overlap to adjacent anatomical regions is also seen in opercular epilepsy.

Parietal lobe epilepsies. Seizures are predominantly sensory attacks with many characteristics. Positive phenomena consist of tingling and a feeling of electricity, which may be confined or may spread in a jacksonian manner. There may be a desire to move a body part or a sensation as if a part were being moved. Muscle tone may be lost. The parts most frequently involved are those with the largest cortical representation, for example, the hand, arm, and face. There may be tongue sensations of crawling, stiffness, or coldness, and facial sensory phenomena many occur bilaterally. Occasionally, an intrabdominal sensation of sinking, choking, or nausea may occur, particularly in cases of inferior and lateral parietal lobe involvement. Rarely, there may be pain, and this may take the form of a superficial burning dysesthesia or a vague, very severe episodic painful sensation. Partial lobe visual phenomena may occur as photopsias or as hallucinations of a formed variety. Metamorphopsia with distortions, foreshortings, and elongations may occur, and are more frequently seen with nondominant hemisphere discharges. Negative phenomena include numbness, feelings as if a body part were absent, and a loss of awareness of a part or a half of the body; this is known as asomatognosia. This is particularly the case in right-sided attacks. Severe vertigo of disorientation in space may be indicative of inferior parietal lobe seizures. Dominant parietal seizures result in a variety of receptive or conductive speech disturbances. Some well-lateralized genital sensations may occur with paracentral involvement. Some rotatory or postural motor phenomena may occur. Seizures of the paracentral lobule have a tendency to become secondarily generalized.

(continued overleaf)

Table 6-3. (*Continued*)

Occipital lobe epilepsy. The clinical seizure manifestations usually, but not exclusively, include visual manifestations. Elementary visual seizures are characterized by fleeting visual manifestations that may be either negative (scotoma, hemianopsia, amaurosis) or, more commonly, positive (sparks or flashes, phospheres). Such sensations appear in a visual field contralateral to the discharge in the specific visual cortex, and spread to the whole visual field. Perceptive illusions, in which the objects appear to be distorted, may occur. The following varieties can be distinguished: A change in size — macropsia or micropsia — or a change in distance, an inclination of objects in a given plan of space and distortion of objects or a sudden change of shape (metamorphopsia). Visual hallucinatory seizures are occasionally characterized by complex visual perceptions, e.g., colorful scenes of varying complexity. In some cases, the scene is distored or made smaller and, in rare instances, the subject sees his own image (autoscopy). Such illusional and hallucinatory visual seizures involve epileptic discharge in the temporo-parieto-occipital junction. The initial signs may also include clonic and/or tonic contraversion of eyes and head or eyes only (oculoclonic or oculogyric deviation), palpebral jerks, and forced closure of eyelids. Sensation of ocular oscillation or of the whole body may occur, as may headache or migraine with the seizures. The discharge may spread to the temporal lobe, producing seizure manifestations or either lateral posterior temporal or hippocamo-amygdalar epilepsies. When the primary focus is located in the supracalcarine area, the discharge can spread forward on the suprasylvian convexity or the mesial surface, mimicking those of parietal lobe or frontal motor seizures. There is an occasional tendency to become secondarily generalized.

1.3   Unknown as to whether the syndrome is idiopathic or symptomatic
2.0   Generalized epilepsies and syndromes
2.1   Idiopathic (with age-related onset-listed in order of age)
      Benign neonatal familial convulsions
      Benign neonatal convulsions
      Benign myoclonic epilepsy in infancy
      Childhood absence epilepsy (pyknolepsy)
      Juvenile absence epilepsy
      Juvenile myoclonic epilepsy (impulsive petit mal)
      Epilepsy with grand mal (GTCS) seizures on awakening
      Other generalized idiopathic epilepsies, if they do not belong to one of the above syndromes, can still be classified as generalized idiopathic epilepsies.
2.2   Cryptogenic or symptomatic (in order of age)
      West syndrome (infantile spasms, Blitz-Nick-Salaam Krämpfe)
      Lennox-Gastaut syndrome
      Epilepsy with myoclonic-astatic seizures
      Epilepsy with myoclonic absences
2.3   Symptomatic
2.3.1 Nonspecific etiology
      Early myoclonic encephalopathy
2.3.2 Specific syndromes
      Epileptic seizures may complicate many
      disease states. Under this heading are included those diseases in which seizures are a presenting or predominant feature.
3.0   Epilepsies and syndromes undetermined whether focal of generalized
3.1   With both generalized and focal seizures
      Neonatal seizures
      Severe myoclonic epilepsy in infancy
      Epilepsy with continuous spike-waves during slow wave sleep
      Acquired epileptic aphasia (Landau-Kleffner syndrome)
3.2   Without unequivocal generalized or focal features. All cases with generalized tonic-clonic seizures in which clinical and EEG findings do not permit classification as clearly localization-related such as in many cases of sleep-grand mal.
4.0   Special syndromes
4.1   Situation-related syndromes (Gelegenheitsanfalle)
      Febrile convulsions
      Isolated seizures or isolated status epilepticus
      Seizures occurring only when there is an acute metabolic or toxic event due to, for example, alcohol, drugs, eclampsia, nonketogenic hyperglycemia, uremia, etc.

is frequent, and there is male predominance. The EEG has blunt high-voltage centrotemporal spikes, often followed by slow waves that are activated by sleep and tend to spread or shift from side to side.

Childhood Epilepsy with Occipital Paroxysms

The syndrome of childhood epilepsy with occipital paroxysms is, in general respects, similar to the previous one (18). The seizures start with visual symptoms (amaurosis, phosphenes, illusions, or hallucinations) and are often followed by a hemiclonic seizure or automatisms. In 25 percent of the cases, the seizures are immediately followed by migrainous headache. The EEG has paroxysms of high-amplitude spike waves or sharp waves recurring rhythmically on the occipital and posterior temporal areas of one or both hemispheres, but only when the eyes are closed. During seizures, the occipital discharge may spread to the central or temporal region. At present, no definite statement on prognosis is possible.

Benign Neonatal Familial Convulsions

Benign neonatal familial convulsions are rare, dominantly inherited disorders manifesting mostly on the second and third days of life, with clonic or apneic seizures and no specific EEG criteria (19). History and investigations reveal no etiological factors. Approximately 14 percent of these patients later develop epilepsy.

Benign Neonatal Convulsions

Benign neonatal convulsions are very frequently repeated clonic or apneic seizures occurring around the fifth day of life. They have no known cause or concomitant metabolic disturbance (20). Interictal EEG often shows alternating sharp theta waves. There is no recurrence of seizures, and psychomotor development is not affected.

Benign Myoclonic Epilepsy in Infancy

Benign myoclonic epilepsy in infancy is characterized by brief bursts of generalized myoclonus that occur during the first or second year of life in otherwise normal children who often have a family history of convulsions or epilepsy (21). The EEG shows generalized spike waves occurring in brief bursts during the early stages of sleep. These attacks are easily controlled by appropriate treatment. They are not accompanied by any other types of seizures, although GTCS may occur during adolescence. The epilepsy may be accompanied by a relative delay of intellectual development and minor personality disorders.

Childhood Absence Epilepsy (Pyknolepsy)

This syndrome of childhood absence epilepsy (pyknolepsy) occurs in children of school age (peak manifestation, age 6 to 7) with a strong genetic predisposition in otherwise normal children (22–26). It appears more frequently in girls than in boys and is characterized by very frequent (several to many per

day) absences. The EEG reveals bilateral, synchronous symmetrical spike waves, usually three per second, on a normal background activity. GTCS often develop during adolescence. Otherwise, absences may remit or, more rarely, persist as the only seizure type.

Juvenile Absence Epilepsy

The absences of this syndrome are the same as in pyknolepsy, but absences with retropulsive movements are less common (27). Age of manifestation is around puberty. Seizure frequency is lower than in pyknolepsy, with absences occurring less frequently than every day, mostly sporadically. Association with GTCS is frequent, and they precede the absence manifestations more often than in childhood absence epilepsy, often occurring on awakening. Not infrequently, the patients also have myoclonic seizures. Sex distribution is equal. The spike-wave rate is often faster than three per second. Response to therapy is excellent.

Juvenile Myoclonic Epilepsy (Impulsive Petit Mal)

Juvenile myoclonic epilepsy appears around puberty and is characterized by seizures with bilateral, single or repetitive arrhythmic, irregular myoclonic jerks, predominantly in the arms (28–32). Some patients may suddenly fall from a jerk. No disturbance of consciousness is noticeable. The disorder may be inherited, and sex distribution is equal. Often, there are GTCS and, less often, infrequent absences. The seizures usually occur shortly after awakening, and are often precipitated by sleep deprivation. Interictal and ictal EEG have rapid, generalized, often irregular spike waves and polyspike waves; there is no close phase correlation between EEG spikes and jerks. Frequently, the patients are photosensitive. Response to appropriate drugs is good.

Epilepsy with GTCS on Awakening

Epilepsy with GTCS on awakening is a syndrome with onset mostly in the second decade of life. The grand mal seizures are presumably mainly GTCS and occur exclusively or predominantly (over 90% of the time) shortly after awakening, regardless of the time of day, or in a second seizure peak in the evening period of relaxation. If there are other seizures, they are mostly absences or myoclonic, as in juvenile myoclonic epilepsy. Seizures may be precipitated by sleep deprivation and other external factors. Genetic predisposition is relatively frequent. The EEG shows idiopathic generalized epilepsy. There is a significant correlation with photosensitivity.

West Syndrome (Infantile Spasms, Blitz-Nick-Salaam Krampfe)

West syndrome usually consists of a characteristic triad: infantile spasms, arrest of psychomotor development, and hypsarhythmia, although one element may be missing (33–37). Spasms may be flexor, extensor, lightning, or nods but most commonly are mixed. Onset peaks between four and seven months and is always before one year. Boys are more commonly affected, and the prognosis is generally poor. West syndrome may be separated into two groups. The symptomatic group is characterized by the previous existence of brain damage signs (psychomotor retardation, neurologic signs, radiologic signs, or other types of seizures) or by a known cause. The smaller, idiopathic group is characterized by the absence of previous signs of brain damage and of known cause. The prognosis is partly based on early therapy with adrenocorticotropic hormone (ACTH) or oral steroids; however, it principally depends on whether the infantile spasms are symptomatic or idiopathic.

Lennox-Gastaut Syndrome

Lennox-Gastaut syndrome manifests itself in children from one to eight years of age but appears mainly in preschool-age children (38–40). The most common seizure types are tonic-axial, atonic, and absence seizures, but other types such as myoclonic, GTCS, or partial are frequently associated with this syndrome. Seizure frequency is high, and status epilepticus is frequent (stuporous states with myoclonias, tonic, and atonic seizures). The EEG usually has abnormal background activity, slow spike-waves of less than three per second, and often multifocal abnormalities. During sleep, bursts of fast rhythms (around 10/s) appear. In general, there is mental retardation. Seizures are difficult to control, and the development is mostly unfavorable. In 60 percent of cases, the syndrome occurs in children suffering from a previous encephalopathy, but it is primary in other cases.

Epilepsy with Myoclonic-Astatic Seizures

Manifestation begins between the ages of seven months and six years, mostly from two to five years, with (except if beginning in the first year) twice as many boys affected (41,42). There is frequently hereditary predisposition and usually a normal developmental background. The seizures are myoclonic, astatic, myoclonic-astatic, absences with clonic and tonic components, and tonic-clonic. Status epilepticus frequently occurs. Tonic seizures develop late in the course of unfavorable cases. The EEG is initially often irregular with fast spike waves or poly-spike waves. Course and outcome are variable.

Epilepsy with Myoclonic Absences

The syndrome of epilepsy with myoclonic absences is clinically characterized by absences accompanied by severe bilateral rhythmical clonic jerks, often associated with a tonic contraction (43). They are always accompanied on the EEG by bilateral, synchronous, and symmetrical discharge of rhythmical spike waves at three per second, similar to childhood absence. These seizures occur many times a day. Awareness of the jerks may be maintained. Associated seizures are rare. Age of onset is about seven years, and there is a male preponderance. Prognosis is less favorable than in pyknolepsy because of resistance to therapy for the seizures, mental deterioration, and possible evolution to other types of epilepsy such as Lennox-Gastaut syndrome.

Early Myoclonic Encephalopathy

The principal features of early myoclonic encephalopathy are onset before three months of age; initially fragmentary myoclonus, then erratic partial seizures; and massive myoclonias or tonic spasms (44). The EEG is characterized by suppression-burst activity, which may evolve into hypsarhythmia. The course is severe, psychomotor development is arrested, and death may occur in the first year. Familial cases are frequent and suggest the influence of one or several congenital metabolic errors, but there is no constant genetic pattern. The status of early infantile epileptic encephalopathy with suppression bursts, described by Ohtahara and coworkers in relation to early myoclonic encephalopathy, is at present unclear, especially in view of its ictal features and its frequent evolution into a syndrome indistinguishable from West syndrome.

Neonatal Seizures

Neonatal seizures differ from those of older children and adults (45). The most frequent neonatal seizures are described as subtle because the clinical manifestations are frequently overlooked. These include tonic, horizontal deviation of the eyes with or without jerking; eyelid blinking or fluttering; sucking, smacking, or other buccal-lingual oral movements; swimming or pedaling movements; and occasionally apneic spells. Other neonatal seizures occur as tonic extension of the limbs, mimicking decerebrate or decorticate posturing. These occur particularly in premature infants. Multifocal clonic seizures characterized by clonic movements of a limb, which may migrate to other body parts or other limbs, or focal clonic seizures, which are much more localized, may occur. In the latter, the infant is usually not unconscious. Rarely, myoclonic seizures may occur, and the EEG pattern is frequently that of suppression-burst activity. The tonic seizures have a poor prognosis because they frequently accompany intraventricular hemorrhage. The myoclonic seizures also carry a poor prognosis because they are frequently a part of the early myoclonic encephalopathy syndrome.

Severe Myoclonic Epilepsy in Infancy

Severe myoclonic epilepsy in infants is a recently defined syndrome (46). Characteristics include a family history of epilepsy or febrile convulsions, normal development before onset, seizures beginning during the first year of life in the form of generalized or unilateral febrile clonic seizures, secondary appearance of myoclonic jerks, and often partial seizures. EEGs show generalized spike waves and polyspike waves, and early photosensitivity and focal abnormalities occur. Psychomotor development is retarded from the second year of life on, and ataxia, pyramidal signs, and interictal myoclonus appear. This type of epilepsy is very resistant to all forms of treatment.

Epilepsy with Continuous Spike Waves During Slow Sleep

Epilepsy with continuous spike waves during slow sleep results from the association of various seizure types, partial or generalized, occurring during sleep, and atypical absences when awake (47). Tonic seizures do not occur. The characteristic EEG pattern consists of continuous diffuse spike waves during slow-wave sleep, which occurs after the onset of seizures. Duration varies from months to years. The prognosis is guarded because of the appearance of neuropsychological disorders despite the usually benign evolution of seizures.

Acquired Epileptic Aphasia (Landau-Kleffner Syndrome)

The Landau-Kleffner syndrome is a childhood disorder associating an acquired aphasia, multifocal spikes, and spike-and-wave discharges (48). Epileptic seizures and behavioral and psychomotor disturbances occur in two-thirds of the patients. There is verbal auditory agnosia and rapid reduction of spontaneous speech. The seizures are mostly generalized convulsive or partial motor and are rare and remit before the age of 15 years, as do the EEG abnormalities.

Kozhevnikov's Syndrome

Two types of Kozhevnikov's syndrome are now recognized, but only one of these two types is included among the epileptic syndromes of childhood because the other one is not specifically related to this age group (49). The first type represents a particular form of rolandic partial epilepsy in both adults and children and is related to a variable lesion of the motor cortex. Its principal features are motor partial seizures, always well localized; often late appearance of myoclonias in the same site where there are somatomotor seizures; an EEG with normal background activity and focal paroxysmal abnormalities (spikes and slow waves); occurrence at any age in childhood and adulthood; frequently demonstrable cause (tumoral, vascular); and no progressive evolution of the syndrome (clinical, EEG, or psychological) except the evolutive character of the causal lesion. The childhood disorder Rasmussen syndrome (50), which is suspected to be of viral etiology, has onset between 2 and 10 years (peak, 6 years) with seizures that are motor partial seizures but are often associated with other types. Fragmentary motor seizures appear early in the course of the illness and are initially localized but later become erratic and diffuse and persist during sleep. A progressive motor deficit follows, and mental deterioration occurs. The EEG background activity shows asymmetric and slow diffuse delta waves, with numerous ictal and interictal discharges that are not strictly limited to the rolandic area.

Conditions of childhood in which epilepsy plays a prominent presenting role include the following.

Malformations

Conditions such as Acardi syndrome, lissencephaly-pachygyria, and the individual phacomatoses fall into this category.

Proven or Suspected Inborn Errors of Metabolism

In the neonate, these include nonketotic hyperglycenemia and D-glyceric acidemia with early myoclonic encephalopathy. In the infant, this includes phenylketonuria, Tay-Sachs disease, Sandhoff disease, early infantile ceroid lipofuscinosis, and pyridoxine dependency. In later childhood, late infantile ceroid lipofuscinosis, juvenile Gaucher's disease, the juvenile form of ceroid lipofuscinosis, and the Lafora variety of progressive myoclonic epilepsy may present. In adolescence, progressive myoclonic epilepsy of the Lundborg type, Ramsay-Hunt syndrome, and cherry-red-spot myoclonus syndrome (siadidosis with isolated deficiency in neurominidase) are forms of progressive myoclonic epilepsy. The mitochondrial encephalopathies with abnormalities in lactate-pyruvate metabolism frequently present as progressive myoclonic epilepsies including the Ramsay-Hunt syndrome (51).

Applying the International League Against Epilepsy Seizure Classification scheme (Table 6-3) to neonatal and infantile seizures (see Chapter 11 on neonatal seizures and reference 52) can be difficult. Partial seizures in the immature lack declarative focal features: contralateral dystonic hand posture, ipsilateral hand automatisms, and contralateral hand and eye version rarely occur (52–54). Automatisms, when expressed, tends to be elementary and feature simple mouthing movements or swallowing motions. Tonic postures are often nonspecific and may relate to primitive subcortical reflexes that are disinhibited during a seizure (53). Preverbal children, of course, cannot volunteer auras and cannot cooperate with testing to determine alteration of consciousness or amnesia. For all these reasons, accurately diagnosing a partial seizure in an infant, unless there is focal limb clonus, can be very difficult. Even if a partial seizure can be diagnosed, it is nearly impossible to distinguish simple from complex.

Accordingly, many different seizures in the immature are classified under III. Unclassified Epileptic Seizures (see Table 6-1). This may result in a loss of valuable diagnostic and prognostic information and will undoubtedly thwart the refinement of further classification schemes. Classifying these seizures in semiologically descriptive terms therefore may be more useful. (See Chapter 11 on neonatal seizures for more information.)

A similar semiologic classification of infantile seizures has been suggested: astatic, behavioral arrest, clonic, infantile spasms/myoclonic, tonic, and versive (52). These terms are used to describe the most profound alterations seen during a seizure. The following list summarizes the features for, each type:

1. **Astatic** seizures result in sudden loss of postural stability and most often result in a head drop.
2. **Behavioral arrest** seizures have an abrupt alteration in the ongoing motor activity, often coupled with nonspecific movements, perhaps representing primitive automatisms and autonomic changes (e.g., change in color, respiration, oxygen saturation, or heart rate).
3. **Clonic** seizures are similar to those encountered in older children and adults and feature sustained rhythmic jerking of a portion of the body.
4. **Infantile spasms** may be difficult to resolve from myoclonic jerks without detailed polygraphic recordings. When these movements are coupled with a sustained tonic phase and recur in clusters, they are termed *spasms*.
5. **Tonic** seizures feature a sustained tonic posture of the limbs and may be focal, diffuse-symmetric, or diffuse-asymmetric.
6. **Versive** seizures feature sustained horizontal deviation of the eyes.

Our experience suggests that this classification scheme can be reliably applied (52). This scheme intentionally avoids describing seizures as partial or generalized based solely on clinical observations. We believe that this determination needs to be made, in the majority of cases, by analyzing other complementary information including, in some cases, concurrent ictal EEG recordings. In many cases, however, it is not difficult to use this seizure classification system in conjunction with other clinical characteristics to arrive at an epilepsy syndrome. For example, a child with infantile seizures, developmental delay, and hypsarhythmia has West syndrome, or 2.2a. A child with behavioral arrest seizures, a temporal lobe mass, and focal EEG findings would fit into 1.2, or symptomatic localization-related epilepsy.

CONCLUSION

These early attempts at a classification of epileptic syndromes in childhood will be elaborated as increasing knowledge of the cause of these syndromes develops. This will occur from a recognition of the syndromes and in turn will lead to information from applying molecular genetic and neurochemical analysis to them. The future development of antiepileptic drugs is predicated to some degree on this information, as is the rational development of the individual therapeutic plan for each patient with a seizure disorder.

REFERENCES

1. Reynolds JR. *Epilepsy: Its Symptoms, Treatment and Relation to Other Chronic Convulsive Diseases.* London: Churchill, 1861.
2. Temkin O. *The Falling Sickness. A History of Epilepsy from the Greeks to the Beginnings of Modern Neurology.* 2nd ed. Baltimore: Johns Hopkins Press, 1971.
3. Tissot SA. *Traite de l'epilepsia faisant le tome troisieme du traite des nerfs et de leurs maladies.* Paris: PF Didot, 1772.
4. Sachs B. *A Treatise on the Nervous System of Children for Physicians and Students.* New York: William Wood, 1985.
5. Freud S. *Infantile Cerebral Paralysis.* Coral Gables: University of Miami Press, 1968.
6. Smith JL. *A Treatise on the Disease of Infancy and Childhood.* Philadelphia: Lea Brothers, 1886.
7. Gowers WR. *Epilepsy and Other Chronic Convulsive Disorders.* London: Churchill, 1881.
8. Commission Classification and Terminology of the International League Against Epilepsy. Proposal for revised clinical and electroencephalographic classification of epileptic seizures. *Epilepsia* 1981; 22:489–501.
9. Commission on Classification and Terminology of the International League Against Epilepsy: Proposal

for revised classification of epilepsies and epileptic syndromes. *Epilepsia* 1989; 30:389–399.

10. Greenberg DA, Delgado-Escueta AV, Maldonado HM, Widelizt H. Segregation analysis of juvenile myoclonic epilepsy. *Genet Epidemiol* 1988; 5:81–94.

11. Leppert M, Anderson VE, Quattlebaum T, et al. Benign familial neonatal convulsions linked to genetic markers on chromosome 20. *Nature* 1988; 337:647–648.

12. Nayrac P, Beaussart M. Les pointe-ondes prerolandique: expression EEG tres particuliere. *Rev Neurol (Paris)* 1958; 99:201–206.

13. Beaussart M. Benign epilepsy of children with rolandic (centro-temporal) paroxysmal foci. *Epilepsia* 1972; 13:795–811.

14. Beaumanoir A, Ballist T, Varfis G, et al. Benign epilepsy of childhood with rolandic spikes. *Epilepsia* 1974; 15:301–315.

15. Loiseau P, Beaussart M. The seizures of benign childhood epilepsy with rolandic paroxysmal discharges. *Epilepsia* 1973; 14:381–389.

16. Lombroso CT. Sylvian seizures and midtemporal spike foci in children. *Arch Neurol* 1967; 17:52–59.

17. Heijbel J, Blom S, Rasmuson M. Benign epilepsy of childhood with centrotemporal EEG foci: A genetic study. *Epilepsia* 1975; 16:285–293.

18. Gastaut H. A new type of epilepsy: Benign partial epilepsy of childhood with occipital spike waves. In: *Advances in Epileptology: The XIIIth Epilepsy International Symposium.* New York: Raven Press, 1982:18–25.

19. Bjerre I, Corelius E. Benign familial neonatal convulsions. *Acta Paediatr Scand* 1968; 57:557–561.

20. Brown JK. Convulsions in the newborn period. *Dev Med Child Neuol* 1973; 15:823–846.

21. Dravet C, Bureau M. Roger J. Benign myoclonic epilepsy in infants. In: Roger J, Dravet C, Bureau M, et al., eds. *Epileptic Syndromes in Infancy, Childhood and Adolescence.* London: John Libbey Eurotext, 1985; 121–129.

22. Drury I, Dreifuss FE. Pyknoleptic petit mal. *Acta Neurol Scand* 1985; 72:353–362.

23. Loiseau P. Childhood absence epilepsy. In: Roger J, Dravet C, Bureau M, et al., eds. *Epileptic Syndromes in Infancy, Childhood and Adolescence.* London: John Libbey Eurotext, 1985:106–120.

24. Penry JK, Porter RJ, Dreifuss FE. Simultaneous recording of absence seizures with videotape and electroencephalography: a study of 374 seizures in 48 patients. *Brain* 1975; 98:427–440.

25. Currier RD, Kooi KA, Saidman LJ. Prognosis of pure petit mal. A follow-up study. *Neurology* 1963; 13:959–967.

26. Livingston S, Torres I, Pauli LL, et al. Petit mal epilepsy. Results of a prolonged follow-up study of 117 patients. *JAMA* 1965; 194:113–118.

27. Wolf P. Juvenile absence epilepsy. In: Roger J, Dravet C, Bureau M, et al., eds. *Epileptic Syndromes in Infancy, Childhood and Adolescence.* London: John Libbey Eurotext, 1985:242–246.

28. Janz D. Christian W. Impulsive-petit mal. *Dtsch Z Nervenh* 1957; 176:346–386.

29. Delgado-Escueta AV, Enrile-Bascale F: Juvenile myoclonic epilepsy of Janz. *Neurology* 1984; 34:285–294.

30. Tsuboi T. *Primary Generalized Epilepsy with Sporadic Myoclonias of Myoclonic Petit Mal Type.* Stuttgart: Theime, 1977:19–35.

31. Asconape J, Penry JK. Some clinical and EEG aspects of benign juvenile myoclonic epilepsy. *Epilepsia* 1984; 25:108–114.

32. Dreifuss FE. Juvenile myoclonic epilepsy: Characteristics of a primary generalized epilepsy. *Epilepsia* 1989; 30(Suppl 4):S1–S7.

33. West WJ. On a peculiar form of infantile convulsions. *Lancet* 1841; 1:724–725.

34. Jeavons PM, Bower BD. Infantile spasms: A review of the literature and a study of 112 cases. In: *Clinics in Developmental Medicine,* No. 15, London: Spastics Society and Heinemann, 1964.

35. Jeavons PM, Bower BD. Infantile spasms. In: Vinken PJ, Bruyn GW, eds. *Handbook of Clinical Neurology,* vol. 15. Amsterdam: North Holland, 1974:219–234.

36. Kellaway P, Hrachovy RA, Frost JD, et al. Precise characteristics and quantification of infantile spasms. *Ann Neurol* 1979; 6:214–218.

37. Lombroso CT. A prospective study of infantile spasms: Clinical and therapeutic correlations. *Epilepsia* 1983; 24:135–158.

38. Lennox WG, Davis JP. Clinical correlates of the fast and the slow spike and wave electroencephalogram. *Trans Am Neurol Assoc* 1949; 74:194–197.

39. Lennox WG. The slow-spike-wave EEG and its clinical correlates. In: Lennox WG, ed. *Epilepsy and Related Disorders,* vol. 1. Boston: Little, Brown, 1966:156–170.

40. Gastaut H, Roger J, Soularyrol R, et al. Childhood epileptic encephalopathy with diffuse slow spike-waves (otherwise known as "petit mal variant") or Lennox syndrome. *Epilepsia* 1966; 7:139–179.

41. Doose H, Gerken H, Leonhardt R, et al. Centrencephalic myoclonic-astatic petit mal. *Neuropediatrics* 1970; 2:59–78.

42. Doose H, Gundel A. 4–7 cps rhythms in the childhood EEG. In: Anderson VE, Hauser WA, Penry JK, et al. (eds.). *Genetic Basis of the Epilepsies.* New York: Raven Press, 1982:83–93.

43. Tassinari CA, Bureau M. Epilepsy with myoclonic absences. In: Roger J, Dravet C, Bureau M, et al., eds. *Epileptic Syndromes in Infancy, Childhood and Adolescence.* London: John Libbey Eurotext, 1985:121–129.

44. Ohtahara S, Ishida T, Oka E, et al. On the age-dependent epileptic syndromes: the early infantile encephalopathy with suppression-burst. *Brain Dev* 1976; 8:270–288.

45. Volpe JJ. Neonatal seizures. In: Volpe JJ, ed. *Neurology of the Newborn.* Philadelphia: Saunders, 1981:111–137.

46. Dravet C, Bureau M, Roger J. Severe myoclonic epilepsy in infants. In: Roger J, Bureau M, Dravet C, et al., eds. *Epileptic Syndromes in Infancy, Childhood and Adolescence.* London: John Libbey Eurotext, 1985:58–67.

47. Tassinari CA, Bureau M, Dravet C, et al. Epilepsy with continuous spike and waves during slow sleep. In: Roger J, Dravet C, Bureau M, et al., eds. *Epileptic Syndromes*

in Infancy, Childhood and Adolescence. London: John Libbey Eurotext, 1985.

48. Landau WM, Kleffner FR. Syndrome of acquired aphasia with convulsive disorder in children. *Neurology* 1957; 7:523–550.

49. Kojewnikow L. Eine besondere Form von corticaler Epilepsie. *Neurol Centralb* 1895; 14:47–48.

50. Rasmussen TE, Olszewski J, Lloyd-Smith D. Focal cortical seizures due to chronic localized encephalitides. *Neurology* 1958; 8:435–445.

51. Berkovic SF, Andermann F, Carpenter S, et al. Progressive myoclonus epilepsies: Specific cases and diagnosis. *N Engl J Med* 1986; 315:296–305.

52. Nordli DR, Bazil CW, Scheuer ML, Pedley TA. Recognition and classifiction of seizures in infants. *Epilepsia* 1997; 38:553–560.

53. Duchowny MS. Complex partial seizures of infancy. *Arch Neurol* 1987; 44:911–914.

54. Wyllie E, Chee M, Granstrom ML, et al. Temporal lobe epilepsy in early childhood. *Epilepsia* 1993; 34:859–868.

CHAPTER 7

Epidemiology of Epilepsy in Children

W. Allen Hauser, M.D.

As a group, the convulsive disorders are among the most frequently occurring neurologic conditions in children. In the United States approximately 5 percent of children and adolescents can be expected to experience a convulsion of some type by the age of 20 (1). This proportion may be very different in other cultures — higher, for example, in the Japanese and lower in the Chinese or the Asian Indians. The greatest proportion of these children experience convulsions only in association with a febrile illness. Only about a quarter of those experiencing seizures actually meet criteria for "epilepsy" — condition characterized by *recurrent unprovoked seizures* (2).

Despite efforts of organizations such as the International League Against Epilepsy (ILAE) to develop standardized definitions for the convulsive disorders for epidemiologic uses (3), there remain differences in definitions that preclude direct comparison across studies. Furthermore, total population studies of the epidemiology of the convulsive disorders or epilepsy seldom provide sufficient detail regarding the specifics of seizure type and etiology in children. Population-based studies dealing specifically with children are few and suffer from the difficulties with definitions and differences in methodology, which in many situations preclude direct comparisons.

In this chapter I concentrate on contemporary studies targeted toward children while integrating data from total population studies. I concentrate on studies of incidence (newly diagnosed cases) because these are more useful in the assessment of etiology and outcome than prevalence studies. In addition, there is less variation in definitions of seizures and epilepsy in incidence studies than in prevalence studies, allowing some comparison across geographic areas.

DEFINITIONS

For purposes of this chapter, epilepsy is considered a condition characterized by recurrent unprovoked seizures. Few of the studies cited limit inclusion to children with recurrent unprovoked seizures. Rather, authors include various combinations of the following categories as epilepsy, so one must read papers carefully if cross-study comparisons are to be made. Other definitions and, where appropriate, incidence are as follows:

Seizure

A seizure is the clinical manifestation of an abnormal and excessive activity of a set of cortical neurons.

Acute Symptomatic Seizure

Acute symptomatic seizures occur in close temporal association with a systemic or central nervous system (CNS) insult. Approximately 5 percent of children with infections of the CNS have acute symptomatic seizures at the time of infection (4). About 10 percent of children who suffer traumatic brain injury experience early seizures (5,6). By age 20, 1 percent of all children may have experienced acute symptomatic seizures (7). Their inclusion as epilepsy probably doubles the reported incidence of epilepsy.

Febrile Seizure

A febrile seizure is a convulsive episode occurring in association with an acute febrile illness. This is actually a subcategory of acute symptomatic seizure differing only in that all children have the exposure. Some authors place restrictions for inclusion in this category based on age or clinical symptomatology.

In the United States and northern European countries, between 2 percent and 4 percent of all children can be expected to experience a convulsion with a febrile illness by the age of 5 years (8–10), but there is a striking variation in the frequency of occurrence of febrile convulsions worldwide (11–19). The very high frequency reported from Nigeria may be related to misclassification of children suffering from cerebral malaria (20). These children have temperature elevation but probably do not have febrile seizures as defined in Western countries. The high frequency in Japan has been attributed to sleeping arrangements: children tend to sleep with or in close proximity to parents, thus allowing recognition of symptoms. This would not seem to explain all the geographic difference because similar sleeping accommodations are common in China and India — areas in which incidence is of low. It is possible that a selective genetic predisposition for febrile convulsions and the electroencephalogram (EEG) pattern exist in the Japanese.

Most contemporary studies segregate febrile seizures from epilepsy, but a few series have included selected cases, primarily those with "complex" features. Because such cases comprise about 20 percent of all febrile convulsion cases, their inclusion may double the apparent incidence or prevalence of unprovoked seizures or epilepsy.

Neonatal Seizures

Neonatal seizures are those that occur in the first 28 days of life. This definition, which is derived from concepts of mortality statistics, is conceivably in flux. Infants less than 32 weeks gestational age (a group with improving survivorship) are incapable of developing integrated cerebral electrical activity. In some studies of premature infants, convulsive events occurring between birth and 44 weeks gestational age have been considered a neonatal seizure. From the standpoint of this classification, most neonatal seizures, particularly those that occur in the first few days of life, would fall into the acute symptomatic category. Epidemiologically, in full-term infants there seems little unique about seizures after the first 7 days of life when compared with seizures identified after the first month of life.

Definitional difficulties are superimposed upon differences in risk within economic groups and geographic areas. Among full-term infants, the reported frequency ranges from slightly over 1 per 1,000 to 8 per 1,000 live births (21–23). The incidence is lower in developed countries than in developing countries; incidence may be higher in infants born to mothers of low socioeconomic class. The frequency is higher among those with low birth weight and may be higher in children with intracerebral hemorrhage and those who are small for gestational age. There are definite temporal trends in incidence in recent years, with a reduced frequency among full-term infants in most but not all industrialized countries (2,24,25). There also are differences in causes over time. Metabolic insults such as hypoglycemia and hypocalcemia were important in the 1950s and 1960s, while in most contemporary studies hypoxic-ischemic insults account for the majority of cases.

Among survivors of neonatal seizures (about 75% of the total), one-third to one-half can be expected to have an adverse neurologic outcome. Approximately one-third might be expected to experience subsequent unprovoked seizures, most in those with neonatal seizures attributable to anoxic insults. Because the majority of these children experiencing anoxia are expected to have associated neurologic disability, their epilepsy may be intractable. Children with "benign familial neonatal seizures" (26) and those experiencing "fifth day" seizures (27) may have a slight increase in risk for later seizures, but long-term prognosis in general is quite good. While most epidemiologic studies of epilepsy exclude such cases unless they have subsequent unprovoked seizures, their inclusion will substantially increase the reported incidence of epilepsy, particularly that in the first year of life.

Unprovoked Seizure

Unprovoked seizures occur in the absence of an identified acute precipitant. In studies in the United States and Iceland, approximately 25 percent of newly diagnosed unprovoked seizures in children occur as a single event and will never meet criteria for epilepsy (see next section). Half of newly identified unprovoked seizures in childhood in Japan (11) and Spain (83) occurred as isolated events without recurrence.

Epilepsy

Epilepsy is defined as the occurrence of multiple unprovoked seizures separated by more than 24 hours. Although this is the focus of this chapter, it becomes apparent that there are only a few studies providing information on this limited group.

THE EPIDEMIOLOGY OF EPILEPSY

Incidence cohorts are necessary if one wishes to understand the geographic distribution, causes, and prognosis of epilepsy. A number of recent studies of the incidence have used similar methodology and definitions that allow some comparison. These studies form the basis for most of the following discussion.

Incidence

Information about the incidence of epilepsy in children is derived from studies of total populations that provide age-specific information about incidence (28–30) and from studies limited to children. Even in studies limited to children, there are difficulties in comparisons across studies because of the inclusion of different age groups as "children," differences in inclusion criteria, and, for the total population studies that provide age-specific incidence, different age grouping. In general, the incidence of epilepsy (recurrent unprovoked seizures) in children seems relatively similar in studies in the same countries, although there may be some variation across the developed countries (Table 7-1). Incidence is lowest in the United Kingdom and Canada, intermediate in the United States and Japan, and for the most part high in Scandinavia and Italy. The incidence using these same definitions is higher by a factor of 20 percent to 50 percent in developing countries.

In addition, there seem to be some differences in age distribution with maxima in the teenage years.

The incidence of "all unprovoked seizures" should be somewhat higher than the incidence of epilepsy. All recent studies reporting the incidence of "all unprovoked seizures" have been conducted in developed countries, primarily Europe (Table 7-2). There is a reasonable similarity in incidence with the exception of a study in Finland representing the only outlier.

Several studies have reported the frequency of all afebrile seizures. Interpretation of these data is difficult because there seems to be wide variation even in studies in the same country during the same time period (Table 7-3). The study in the developing country (Ecuador) seems to show a clearly higher incidence than those from other areas, fitting perceptions that the incidence of seizures (and epilepsy?) is higher in developing countries.

Some studies have used other definitions of "epilepsy" (Table 7-4). In general, these studies seem consistent with studies from the same geographic area, taking into consideration the age structure studied.

Table 7-1. Incidence of Epilepsy

Study	Incidence (per 100,000)	Gender	Age Group	Etiology	Seizure Type	Definition
1970 British birth cohort (31)	57 AAS 50 AUS 43 RUS		0–10	72% unknown 30% developmental delay	50% GTC	
1958 British birth cohort (32)	41		0–10	75% unknown	70% partial	RUS
	35		0–23			RUS
Houston 1995 (33)	68		0–4			RUS
	60		5–14			
Rochester 1980–1984 (34)	62		0–14	74% unknown	55% partial	RUS
Nova Scotia 1977–1985 (35)	41	M = F	0–14		53% partial	RUS
Copparo 1964–1978 (36)	95	M > F	0–14		80% generalized	RUS
Piedmontese district 1978 (37)	83	M > F	0–14	60% unknown		RUS
Modina 1968–1973 (38)	82	M > F	5–14			RUS
Stockholm 1990–1992 (39)	53			70% unknown 35% neurologic handicap	52% partial	RUS
Faroes 1970–1980 (40)	85	M > F	0–20		51% partial	RUS
Sweden 1974 (41)	82	M > F	0–15	81% unknown	52% partial	RUS
Iceland 1997 (42)	65 AUS 53 RUS	M > F	0–15	80% unknown	53% partial	
Ethiopia 1990 (43)	94		0–9			RUS
	74		10–19			
	86		0–19			
Yelandur 1990 (44)	62	M > F	0–19			RUS
Tanzania 1989 (45)	80	M = F	0–9			RUS
	111		10–19			
Chili 1984–1988 (46)	124	M > F	0–14		65% generalized	RUS
Tokyo birth cohort 1972 (11)	54	M > F	0–14		85% generalized	RUS

AAS = all afebrile seizures; AUS = all unprovoked seizures; RUS = recurrent unprovoked seizures; GTC = generalized tonic-clonic seizures.

Table 7-2. Incidence of All Unprovoked Seizures

Study	Incidence (per 100,000)	Gender	Age Group	Etiology	Seizure Type	Definition
1970 British birth cohort (31)	57 AAS 50 AAS 43 RUS		0–10	72% unknown 30% developmental delay	50% GTC	
Sweden (47) 1985–1987 (7)	73 inc	*F > M*	0–15	3% known	60% generalized (incidence 44)	AUS
Finland 1966 birth cohort (48)	80 first attendance 132	*M > F*	0–14	36% other handicap	58% primary generalized	AUS
Iceland 1998 (42)	65 AUS 53 RUS	*M > F*	0–15	80% unknown	53% partial	
Germany (49)	72	*M > F*	0–8	60% unknown	80% generalized	AUS

AAS=all afebrile seizures; AUS = all unprovoked seizures; RUS = recurrent unprovoked seizures; GTC=generalized tonic-clonic seizures.

Table 7-3. Incidence of All Afebrile Seizures

Study	Incidence (per 100,000)	Gender	Age Group	Etiology (afebrile)	Seizure Type	Definition
1970 British birth cohort (31)	57 AAF 50 AUS 43 RUS		0–10	72% unknown 30% development delay	50% GTC	
Oakland (50)	152	*M > F*	0–6			AAF
Great Britain general practice (51)	154 1974–1983 61 1984–1993		0–20 0–20			AAF AAF
Martinique 1995 (52)	82	*M > F*	0–15		60% generalized	AAF
Ecuador 1984 (53)	219	*M > F*	0–19			AAF
Geneva 1990 (54)	69	*M > F*	0–20			AAF

AAS = all afebrile seizures; GTC=generalized tonic-clonic seizures.

Table 7-4. Incidence of "Epilepsy" Using Other Definitions

Study	Incidence (per 100,000)	Gender	Age Group	Cause	Seizure Type	Definition
Okayama (55)	145	*M > F*	0–10			AUS + some FS
Great Britain general practices 1995 (56)	63		5–9			AUS or first AUS + some FS
	54		10–14			
	101		15–19			

AUS = all unprovoked seizures; FS=febrile seizures; AUS=all unprovoked seizures.

While there are a number of studies that report global incidence, there are few studies that provide data on gender, age, etiology, or seizure type. The following sections summarize results available from studies that report such data. See also Tables 7-1 to 7-4.

Age-Specific Incidence

In all studies providing separate information regarding the incidence by detailed age groups, the incidence is highest in the first year of life. The most recent studies report incidence in the first year of life of about 100 per 100,000 children. Incidence falls after age 1 year, although the rate of the fall varies. In Canada, for example, incidence appears to be stable from ages 1 through 10 years at about 40 per 100,000, and in early adolescence incidence is similar that reported in the adult years of life (20 per 100,000).

For many studies, incidence is provided only for 5- or 10-year age groups. In developing countries, incidence may be higher in adolescence than in early childhood (Figure 7-1). In developed countries, incidence

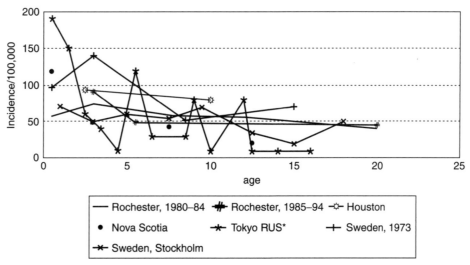

*RUS = recurrent unprovoked seizures.

Figure 7-1. Incidence of epilepsy* in children in developed countries.

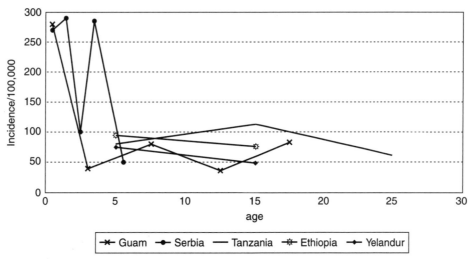

*RUS = recurrent unprovoked seizures.

Figure 7-2. Incidence of epilepsy* in children in developing countries.

is lower in the second decade of life than in the first decade (Figure 7-2). The exception is a recent British study from which one can calculate age-specific incidence. The incidence seems highest in the late teenage years. This study uses a unique definition of "epilepsy." Nonetheless, internal comparisons should be consistent assuming that there is no bias in identification related to age group. This suggests that the observation may be valid.

Gender-Specific Incidence

For most recent studies, when reported, gender-specific incidence in children is higher in males although seldom significantly so. This seems to be true regardless of study definition. Only the Swedish study demonstrates a clearly higher incidence in females (47).

Race

One may make broad comparisons across studies of different races but these are unreliable because of different definitions. In one study of children using broad definitions of epilepsy, the incidence in African American children was higher than that of Caucasian children. This study does not control for socioeconomic status.

Seizure Type

Most recent studies of epilepsy in developed countries report a slight predominance of partial seizure disorders over seizure disorders that are generalized from onset. One must consider the age distribution being studied. Generalized onset seizures seem to predominate in the first year of life, after which partial seizures tend to predominate. Some studies that seem to be exceptions this, notably those from Tokyo and Copparo, where 80 percent to 85 percent of new cases were considered generalized. Because both areas would be expected to have access to modern diagnostic techniques, the predominance is puzzling. When reported, studies in developing countries seem to have a predominance of generalized epilepsy. Whether this represents misclassification related to limited evaluation of incidence cases is not certain. An excess of generalized onset seizures may account for the higher incidence in some countries such as Chile. Studies of "all unprovoked seizures" and studies using more inclusive definitions (e.g., all afebrile seizures) tend to report a preponderance of generalized seizures. It is likely that in children both single unprovoked seizures without recurrence and acute symptomatic seizures are predominantly generalized. This could account for the apparent difference in distribution by seizure type based on study inclusion.

Etiology

When reported, between 60 percent and 80 percent of all new cases in children have no apparent cause. A small proportion of new cases can be attributed to trauma, infection, postnatal vascular lesions, or CNS degenerative conditions. Approximately 20 percent of cases are associated with neurologic handicaps presumed present from birth, mental retardation (MR), cerebral palsy (CP), or a combination thereof. Because most of cases of MR or CP are without obvious cause, a more appropriate estimate for the proportion with identified cause may be 3 percent, as reported in the recent study from Sweden.

Familial (genetic) predisposition certainly plays a role in the risk for developing epilepsy (58–60). The offspring or sibling of a person with epilepsy has a threefold increase in risk of developing epilepsy. Familial aggregation consistent with mendelian inheritance is rare, however. There are childhood-onset syndromes with a clear gene localization for which the patterns of inheritance are understood: benign familial neonatal seizures, benign infantile epilepsy, and Baltic myoclonic epilepsy are examples. A localization on chromosome 6 for juvenile-onset epilepsies remains controversial, and the mode of inheritance is not understood. A linkage for the EEG pattern (not the epilepsy) has been reported for rolandic epilepsy with central temporal spikes.

It is important to point out factors that are *not* causal for epilepsy. Once cases of CP are accounted for, there

has been no evidence of an association between adverse prenatal and perinatal factors and the development of epilepsy. The concept of "birth trauma" or "pregnancy complications" being a cause of epilepsy has not been supported in a variety of studies performed over the past 15 years (61–64). From a similar standpoint, febrile seizures are not "causal" for epilepsy. They are more likely a marker for a preexisting susceptibility—in some cases genetic, in other cases "structural."

Time Trends in Incidence

One of the more intriguing observations from longitudinal studies has been the reduction of the incidence of epilepsy over time that has been observed in two studies. In the studies from a British general practice that includes all afebrile seizures, incidence under age 20 has fallen from 154 per 100,000 from 1975 to 1984 to 61 per 100,000 from 1985 to 1994 (52). In studies in Rochester, Minnesota, the incidence of epilepsy has fallen by about 40 percent between 1935 and 1975 (Table 7-5). This trend seems to have reversed after 1975. The fall in the middle decades of this century is largely unexplained. The increase may be related to increased survivorship of very low birth weight infants.

Epilepsy Syndromes

Considerable emphasis has been placed on epilepsy syndromes in recent years (66). The classification to date is most useful in children, but even in epidemiologic studies in children, a substantial proportion of cases fall into nonspecific categories. Syndrome classification has generally not been useful for classification in population-based studies, although its failure may occur primarily in adults (34,67).

Only two population-based incidence studies of all ages provide a classification of all cases according to epilepsy syndromes. In Bordeaux, France, data on the incidence of seizure and epilepsy syndromes is not presented separately for children (68). One percent had juvenile myoclonic epilepsy, and 1 percent had awakening grand mal. Approximately 1 percent had West syndrome, and 2 percent had pyknolepsy. The

Table 7-5. Incidence of All Unprovoked Seizures in Rochester, Minnesota by Decade

Decade	Age Group		
	0–4	0–9	0–14
1935–1944	129	104	91
1945–1954	124	101	87
1955–1964	85	74	63
1965–1974	73	69	59
1975–1984	93	79	72

incidence of idiopathic localization-related epilepsy was 1.7 per 100,000 (7% of all cases, adults and children). These rates are proportional to those reported for studies in children alone. The incidence of epileptic syndromes for the period between 1980 and 1984 has been presented for the population of Rochester, Minnesota (34). Again, approximately 20 percent of childhood cases fell into nonspecific categories and about one-third were considered localization-related cryptogenic epilepsies without further localization. Despite limitations in these and other population-based studies, some information regarding the frequency of epilepsy syndromes is available.

West Syndrome

The incidence of West syndrome has been evaluated in several geographic areas and appears consistent across studies. Incidence ranges from 2 to 7 per 10,000 live births (Table 7-6). One would expect that the prevalence series would underestimate the incidence, but the highest incidence was estimated from prevalence extrapolation from prevalence series. In all studies reporting gender-specific incidence, there is a male preponderance.

West syndrome underscores the need for population-based incidence cohorts. The clinical perception of the syndrome is that the prognosis is poor. Population-based studies in Iceland and Rochester, Minnesota, suggest a different distribution

Table 7-6. Incidence of West Syndrome (Infantile Spasms)

Study	Incidence per 10,000 Live Births	Gender
Tokyo (11)	1.3	
Oklahoma* (69)	1.9	
Rochester 1955–1984 (70)	2	M > F
1970 British birth cohort (31)	2	M > F
US birth cohort 1965 (58)	2.5	
Iceland 1980–1990 (71)	3	M > F
Denmark (72)	3	
Okayama (73)	3.3	
Finland 1992* (74)	3.2	
Finland (75)	4	M > F
Finland 1976–1993 (76)	4.1	M > F
Finland 1966* (77)	5	
Faeroes 1980 (40)	3% of new cases under age 20 (about 6/10,000)	
Sweden 1985 (47)	6	
Kiel (49)	4.8	
Oakland (50)	1.6	
Atlanta* (78)	7	
Lithuania* (79)	7.5	

*Estimated from prevalence data.

Table 7-7. Incidence of Lennox-Gastaut Syndrome

Study	Incidence per 10,000 Live Births	Gender
1958 British birth cohort (32)	1	
Tokyo (11)	2	
Finland 1992 (74)	2	M > F
Finland 1976–1993 (76)	2.8	M > F
Faroes (40)	3	0–19
Keil-Doose syndrome (49)	3	8 and under

of idiopathic versus symptomatic cases and an excellent prognosis in idiopathic cases.

Lennox-Gastaut Syndrome

The incidence of Lennox-Gastaut syndrome is between 2 and 5 per 10,000 live births (Table 7-7). There probably is no true variation in frequency worldwide. The syndrome accounts for 2 percent to 3 percent of new cases of epilepsy in children (11,54,73,80). In Kiel, Doose syndrome accounts for about 3 per 100,000 cases age 8 and under.

Severe Myoclonic Epilepsy of Infancy (Dravet Syndrome)

Based on one case identified in the National Perinatal Collaborative Project (54,000 live births) and on five cases identified from clinics in western Texas, the cumulative risk through age 7 have been estimated to be approximately 1 in 40,000.

Pyknolepsy and Juvenile Absence Epilepsy

Epilepsies that are characterized by absence seizures are separated into pyknolepsy and juvenile absence epilepsy. The syndromes seem distinct, but they may be difficult to distinguish both clinically and epidemiologically, and they are combined in most epidemiologic studies. In Sweden, Finland, and Rochester, Minnesota, absence epilepsy comprised approximately 8 percent of all childhood-onset epilepsy, and the incidence was about 7 per 100,000 (Table 7-8). Incidence was somewhat lower in the Faeroes and another Finnish study (less than 2 per 100,000) and highest in Copparo (15 per 100,000). Overall, there seems to be considerable consistency for this combined epilepsy syndrome category.

Juvenile Myoclonic Epilepsy

Juvenile myoclonic epilepsy (JME) has received a considerable amount of attention and is perceived as a frequent epilepsy syndrome in children. Most of the

Table 7-8. Incidence of Absence Epilepsy

Study	Incidence per 100,000	Percent Total	Age Group
Faeroes (40)	1.9	2.2% RUS	0–19
Finland (82)	2	1.3% AUS	0–15
Stockholm (39)	4	8% RUS	0–15
Tokyo (11)	4	7% RUS	0–14
Rochester (34)	5	8% RUS	0–14
Iceland (42)	5	8% AUS	0–15
Nova Scotia (35)	6	14% RUS	0–14
Sweden (47)	7	9% AUS	0–15
Kiel (49)	8	11% AUS	0–8
Copparo (36)	15	17% RUS	0–14

RUS = recurrent unprovoked seizures; AUS = all unprovoked seizures.

Table 7-9. Incidence of Juvenile Myoclonic Epilepsy

Study	Incidence per 100,000	Percent Total	Age Group
Stockholm (39)	0.5	1% RUS	0–15
Iceland (42)	0.6	1% AUS	0–15
Rochester (34)	1	0.75 % RUS	0–14
Finland (23)	2	1.3% AUS	0–15
Faeroes (40)	3.2	3.8% RUS	0–19
Northern Sweden (47)	5.9	8% AUS	0–15
Gothenburg	6.3		0–15

RUS = recurrent unprovoked seizures; AUS = all unprovoked seizures.

studies reporting this syndrome in children have been performed in Scandinavian countries (Table 7–9) In Sweden, five children under the age of 15 had a diagnosis of JME with an incidence of 6 per 100,000. In the studies in Iceland and Rochester, Minnesota, most cases were identified between the ages of 15 and 24. If these age groups are included, the incidence under age 25 is approximately 6 per 100,000. In both Rochester and Iceland, between 5 percent and 10 percent of newly diagnosed epilepsy in children may meet criteria for this syndrome. This contrasts with the study in Bordeaux, France, in which 30 percent of cases started at age 5.

Benign Rolandic Epilepsy

Benign rolandic epilepsy is among the more common childhood epilepsy syndromes, and this appears to be confirmed, at least in the studies in Scandinavia and Italy (Table 7–10). In studies in Italy and Iceland, this syndrome accounts for approximately 25 percent of incidence cases of epilepsy in children from birth through age 15 (38,76). In Sweden, the incidence in those under age 15 is 10.7 per 100,000,

Table 7-10. Incidence of Benign Rolandic Epilepsy

Study	Incidence per 100,000	Percent Total	Age Group
Rochester (34)	3	5% RUS	0–14
Sweden (47)	11	14% AUS	0–15
Iceland (42)	16	25% AUS	0–15
Modina (38)	20	25% AUS	4–15
Kiel (49)	8	11% AUS	0–8
Stockholm (39)	5	11% RUS	0–15

RUS = recurrent unprovoked seizures; AUS = all unprovoked seizures.

and this syndrome accounts for about 14 percent of childhood epilepsy. Benign rolandic epilepsy accounts for less than 5 percent of childhood-onset epilepsy in Rochester, Minnesota.

Prevalence

There are numerous studies of the prevalence of epilepsy worldwide (Table 7–11). As mentioned earlier, prevalence provides little information beyond that which is useful for planning health service needs. Data are virtually useless for prognosis or etiology. Furthermore, differences in methodology and definitions frequently preclude the ability to make comparisons across studies. Nonetheless, a presentation regarding the epidemiology of epilepsy would not be complete without some discussion of prevalence.

The definitions of prevalence vary as extensively as the definitions of incidence. Prevalence in various studies worldwide are presented along with the dizzying array of definitions used in various studies. In Table 7–10 I have attempted to stratify studies according to my perception of order of conservativeness of definition. In this context, conservative means the most restrictive and therefore theoretically associated with the lowest prevalence. When definitions are comparable, there seems to be little variation in the prevalence of epilepsy (Table 7–10) (83–88). When compared with studies in the United States and Europe, the prevalence of epilepsy in children may be higher in South America and lower in some parts of Asia (89–91).

Prevalence Seizure Type

Most prevalence studies find a preponderance of generalized onset seizures. This appears to be true regardless of study site, although the proportion with partial seizures is higher in studies from developed countries.

Etiology

Even fewer prevalence studies report etiology in children. When reported, between 60 percent and 80

Table 7-11. Prevalence of Epilepsy

Study	Prevalence per 1,000	Gender	Age	Etiology	Seizure Type	Inclusion	Definition
Rural Iceland 1993 (92)	3.4	M > F	0–14	80% unknown		RUS	Seizure or medications in past year
Kenya 1992 (93)	2.9 5.5	M > F	6–9 10–19		All generalized	Epilepsy RUS??	Current seizures
1970 British birth cohort (31)	2.8		At age 10		50% GTC	RUS	Seizures within 2 years
Tanzania 1989 (45)	3.5 11.1	M > F	0–9 10–19			RUS	Seizures within 2 yrs
Spain 1987 (94)	3.7 active 5.7 lifetime	M > F	6–14			RUS	Seizure or medication within 3 years
Tunisia (95)	4.8 5.7	M > F	0–9 10–19		93% generalized	RUS	Seizures or medication within 3 years
Serbia (96)	4.2	M > F	0–6	35% symptomatic	70% generalized	RUS	Seizures or medication within 3 years
Faeroes 1980 (40)	6.5	M > F	0–19		51% partial LR 50%	RUS	Seizure in 5 yrs
Lithuania 1995 (79)	4.5	M > F	0–15	60% unknown	Generalized 30%	RUS	Seizures in 5 years
Guatemala (97)	7.7 4.6		0–9 10–19			AUS	Seizures in 5 years
Tokyo 1984 (11)	2.8	M > F	9–14			RUS	Seizures in 5 years
Tokyo 1984 (11)	3.4	M > F	9–14			RUS	Seizures or medications in 5 years
Finland 1992 (32)	3.94	M > F	0–15	64% unknown; 17% (1+) intractable; 38% handicap	Equal generalized and partial 13% unclassified or multiple	RUS+ status epilepticus	Seizures or medication in last 5 years
Rochester 1980 (98)	3.9	M > F	0–14	80% unknown	Generalized = partial	RUS	Seizures or medication in 5 years
Yelandur 1990 (42)	4.6 4.9 lifetime	M > F	0–20			RUS	Seizures or medication in 5 years
Pakistan 1987 (99)	9.3 9.9		0–9 10–19			RUS	Seizures or medication in 5 years
Turkey (100)	10.7 7.3	M > F	0–9 10–19			RUS	Seizures or medication in 5 years
Chile 1986 (46)	17	M > F	0–14		Generalized	RUS	Seizures or medication in 5 years

(continued overleaf)

Table 7-11. (*Continued*)

Study	Prevalence per 1,000	Gender	Age	Etiology	Seizure Type	Inclusion	Definition
Oklahoma 1983 (69)	4.71	M > F B > W	0–19	69% unknown 25% developmental delay or motor handicap	Generalized > partial	RUS	Seizures or medication in 5 years
Guam (101)	4.2	M > F	0–19		Generalized	RUS	Seizures or medication in 5 years
Mississippi (102)	5.9 active 8.3 total	M > F	0–19			RUS	Med+seizure in 3 years or no medication and seizure within 5 years
Kentucky (87)	9.3 11.0 12.8		6–16			RUS AUS AAS	Lifetime
Nigeria (103)	6	M > F	0–19			RUS	Seizures or medication in 5 years
Copparo 1978 (36)	4.7 13.9	M > F	0–9 10–19			RUS	Seizures or medication in 5 years
Kashmir 1986 (104)	3.2	M > F	<14		Generalized > partial	RUS	Seizures or medication in 5 years
Calicut, India (105)	22	M > F	8–12	Perinatal diarrhea		RUS	Seizures in 5 years
Bombay Parsi (106)	4.6 3.4	M > F	0–5 10–19		Partial 54%, Generalized 26%	RUS	Seizures in 5 years
Sicily (107)	3.5 3.6	M > F	0–9 10–19	54% unknown	Gen > partial (4:1)	RUS	Seizure within 1 year or within 5 years if on medication
1959 British birth cohort (32)	4.1	M > F	11	Mental retardation 1.3%		RUS	Lifetime
Piedmont 1978 (37)	4.5 (1965–1976)	M = F	0–14	60% unknown		RUS	Lifetime
Sillanpaa 1979 (108)	6.8		4–15		55% partial	RUS	Lifetime
Modina 1968–1973 (38)	4.6 4.5	M > F	5–9 10–14		Partial > generalized	RUS	Lifetime

Study	Rate	Sex	Age	Clinical features	Seizure type	Definition	Time frame
Atlanta 1986 (109)	6 Black > white	m > f	10	Mental retardation 25% Cerebral palsy 15%	58% partial 8% status epilepticus	RUS	Lifetime
Rochester 1980 (98)	7.1	M > F	0–14	85% unknown	Generalized > partial	AUS	Seizures or medication in 5 years
Keil (49)	4.3		0–8			AUS	Seizure or medication in 5 years
Keil (49)	6.3	M > F	0–8			AUS	Lifetime
Okayama 1975 (73)	8.3	M > F	0–10	70% unknown	Unknown 23% Partial 44% Generalized 31%	AUS + some FC	Lifetime
Great Britain general practice of 6000, 1993 (51)	4.8					AAS	Seizure in prior 2 years
Great Britain computerized medication records (56)	3.2 4.1 5.2		5–9 10–14 15–19			AAS and some FS	Current medication
Rochester 1980 (98)	4.0	M > F	0–14	80% unknown	Generalized = partial	RUS	Lifetime
Yelandur 1993 (44)	4.9	M > F	0–20			RUS	Lifetime
Tokyo 1975 (11)	8.2	M > F	9–14			RUS	Lifetime
Ecuador (53)	3.7 8.1 6.2	M > F	0–9 10–19 0–20		Generalized > partial	AAF	Seizures or medications in 1 year
Great Britain general practice of 6000, 1983 (51)	8.1 20.7 14.9	F > M	0–9 10–19 0–20			AAS	Lifetime
Great Britain general practice of 6000, 1993 (51)	5.1 14.7 10.2	F > M	0–9 10–19 0–20			AAS	Lifetime
Ecuador 1984 (53)	7.4 13.9 10.5	M > F	0–9 10–19 0–20		Generalized > partial	AAS	Lifetime

RUS = recurrent unprovoked seizures; AUS = all unprovoked seizures; AAS = atypical absence seizure; FC = febrile convulsion.

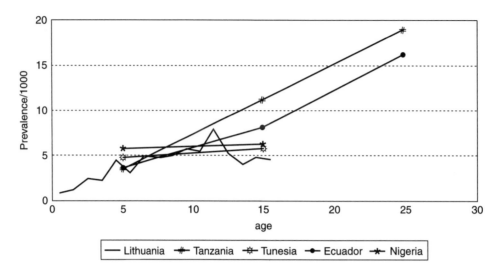

Figure 7-3. Prevalence of epilepsy in children in developed countries.

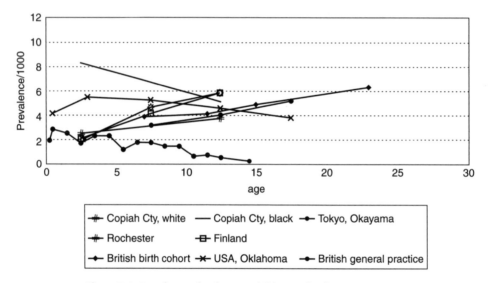

Figure 7-4. Prevalence of epilepsy in children in developing countries.

percent of cases are of unknown cause. Epilepsy associated with neurologic handicap present from birth (e.g., MR or CP) is the most common antecedent, but few studies provide such data. Several studies report the frequency of developmental delay (independent of MR) and other handicap that occurs in up to 25 percent of cases.

Gender

Except for the British general practice study, which used broad definitions of epilepsy, there is a male excess in all studies, although it seldom reaches statistical significance. When age or gender breakdown is provided, females have a higher prevalence in the teenage years in some studies.

Race

Prevalence by racial subgroups can be compared in some studies in the United States. Prevalence is higher in African Americans compared with Caucasians. These studies do not address whether this is a racial factor or a socioeconomic phenomenon.

Cumulative Incidence

A concept more useful than prevalence in terms of epidemiologic measurements is "cumulative incidence," which is the risk of developing a convulsive disorder through to a specific age. Cumulative incidence of epilepsy and lifetime prevalence of epilepsy at age 20 should be similar if there is no mortality attributable to epilepsy (mortality is negligible

Table 7-12. Cumulative Incidence of Epilepsy

Study	Cumulative Incidence (%)	Gender	By Age	Etiology	Seizure Type	Definition
Serbia	0.7		6	65% unknown	70% generalized	RUS
Rochester Minn 1965–1984 (29)	0.67%		15			RUS
	0.84					AUS
	1.06					AAS
Swedish birth cohort 1960 (110)	1.5		14		58% generalized	AUS
Finland birth cohort 1966 (77)	1.7	*M > F*	13	65% unknown	60% generalized	AUS
Finland birth cohort 1987 (111)	0.74	Male	7			AUS
	0.62	Female				
Tokyo (11)	1.6		15			AUS
	0.82					RUS
NCPP (57)	1		7			AAS
British general practice of 6000 (51)	1		20			AAS

RUS = recurrent unprovoked seizures; AUS = all unprovoked seizures.

in children without handicap). Cumulative incidence alone is reported from several studies (Table 7–12) and has been reported in or may be calculated from data provided in many papers reporting incidence. The cumulative incidence for all convulsive disorders through age 20 is slightly more than 4 percent in Rochester, Minnesota; that for epilepsy is slightly more than 1 percent; and that for all afebrile seizures is about 2 percent. These proportions should be similar to the lifetime prevalence for these same definitions. It is the cumulative incidence, not prevalence, that is important for comparisons of risk for epilepsy.

SUMMARY

These descriptive studies provide insights into the frequency of the burden of epilepsy and other convulsive disorders in childhood. No study answers all questions, and there still is much to learn. Despite differences in methods and definitions, there are some facts that can be gleaned from these studies. The burden of epilepsy appears to be greater in developing countries. It is greater in males. In the United States, it may be greater in African Americans. Partial seizures seem to predominate, at least in developed countries. The well-defined epilepsy syndromes are important but are less frequent than assumed, even in children. More than 60 percent of cases have no known cause. There are definite time trends that are largely unexplained. There is much to be learned in terms of basic epidemiology before a major effort can be mounted to address risks and prevention.

REFERENCES

1. Hauser WA, Annegers JF, Rocca WA. Descriptive epidemiology of epilepsy: contributions of population based studies from Rochester, Minnesota. *Mayo Clin Proc* 1996; 71:576–586.

2. Hauser WA, Rich SS, Lee JR, Annegers JF, Anderson VE. Risk of recurrent seizures after two unprovoked seizures. *N Engl J Med* 1998; 338:429–434.

3. Commission on Epidemiology and Prognosis, International League Against Epilepsy. Guidelines for epidemiologic studies on epilepsy. *Epilepsia* 1993; 34:592–596.

4. Annegers JF, Nicolosi A, Beghi E, Hauser WA, Kurland LT. The risk of unprovoked seizures after encephalitis and meningitis. *Neurology* 1988; 38:1407–1410.

5. Hauser WA, Tabaddor K, Factor P, Feiner C. Seizures and head injury in an urban community. *Neurology* 1984; 34:746–758.

6. Annegers JF, Grabow JD, Groover RV, et al. Seizures after head trauma: a population study. Neurology 1980; 30:683–689.

7. Annegers JF, Hauser WA, Lee JR, Rocca WA. Incidence of acute symptomatic seizures in Rochester, Minnesota 1935–1984. *Epilepsia* 1995; 36:327–333.

8. Forsgren L, Sidenvall R, Blomquist HK, Heijbel J. A prospective incidence study of febrile convulsions. *Acta Paediatr Scand* 1990; 79:550–557.

9. Verburgh ME, Bruijnzeels MA, van der Wouden JC, et al. Incidence of febrile seizures in The Netherlands. *Neuroepidemiology* 1992; 11:169–172.

10. Verity CM, Golding J. Risk of epilepsy after febrile convulsions: a national cohort study. *Br Med J* 1991; 303:1373–1376.

11. Tsuboi T. Prevalence and incidence of epilepsy in Tokyo. *Epilepsia* 1988; 29:103–110.

12. Ohtahara S, Ishido S, Oka E, et al. Epilepsy and febrile convulsions in Okayama prefecture: a neuroepidemiologic study. In Fukuyama Y, Arima M, Maehawa K, Yamaguchi K, eds. *Child Neurology: Proceedings of the IYDP Commemorative International Symposium on Developmental Disabilities, Tokyo.* Amsterdam: Elsevier, 1981.

13. Hauser WA. The natural history of febrile seizures. In: Nelson KB, Ellenberg J, eds. *Febrile Seizures.* New York: Raven Press, 1982:5–18.

14. Stanhope JM, Brody JA, Brink E. Convulsions among the Chamorro people of Guam, Mariana Islands. I. Seizure disorders. *Am J Epidemiol* 1972; 95:292–298.

15. Fukuyama Y, Kagawa K, Tanaka K. A genetic study of febrile convulsions. *Eur Neurol* 1978; 18:166–182.

16. Fu Z, Lavine L, Wang Z, et al. Prevalence and incidence of febrile seizures (FBS) in China. *Neurology* 1987; 37(Suppl 1):149.

17. Hauser WA, Ortega R, Zarelli M. The prevalence of epilepsy in a rural Mexican village. *Epilepsia* 1990; 31:604.

18. Gracia F, Loo de Lar S, Castillo L, et al. Epidemiology of epilepsy in Guaymi Indians from Bocas del Toro Province, Republic of Panama. *Epilepsia* 1990; 31:718–724.

19. Bharucha NE, Bharucha EP, Bharucha AE. Febrile seizures. *Neuroepidemiology* 1991; 10:138–142.

20. Akpede GO, Sykes RM, Abiodun PO. Convulsions with malaria: febrile or indicative of cerebral involvement? *J Trop Pediatr* 1993; 39:350–355.

21. Airede KI. Neonatal seizures and a 2 year neurological outcome. *J Trop Pediatr* 1991; 37:3313–3317.

22. Eriksson M, Zetterstrom R. Neonatal convulsions. Incidence and causes in the Stockholm area. *Acta Paediatr Scand* 1979; 68:807–811.

23. Tudehope DI, Harris A, Hawes D, Hayes M. Clinical spectrum and outcome of neonatal convulsions. *Austral Paediatr J* 1988; 24:249–253.

24. Kawakami T, Yoda H, Shima Y, Akamatsu H. Incidence and causes of neonatal seizures in the last 10 years (1981–1990). *No To Hattatsu* 1992 24:525–529.

25. Goldberg HJ. Neonatal convulsions—a 10 year review. *Arch Dis Child* 1983; 58:976–978.

26. Leppert M, Singh N. Benign familial neonatal epilepsy with mutations in two potassium channel genes. *Curr Opin Neurol* 1999; 12:143–147.

27. Pryor DS, Don N, Macourt DC. Fifth day fits: a syndrome of neonatal convulsions. *Arch Dis Child* 1981; 56:753–758.

28. Rwiza HT, Kilonzo GP, Haule J, et al. Prevalence and incidence of epilepsy in Ulanga, a rural Tanzanian district: a community-based study. *Epilepsia* 1992; 33:1051–1056.

29. Hauser WA, Annegers JF, Kurland LT. Incidence of epilepsy and unprovoked seizures in Rochester, Minnesota: 1935–1984. *Epilepsia* 1993; 34:453–468.

30. Ólafsson E, Hauser WA, Ludvigsson P, Gudmundsson G. Incidence of epilepsy in rural Iceland: a population-based study. *Epilepsia* 1996; 37:951–955.

31. Verity CM, Ross EM, Golding J. Epilepsy in the first 10 years of life: findings of the child health and education study. *Br Med J* 1992; 305:857–861.

32. Ross EM, Peckham CS, West PB, Butler NR. Epilepsy in childhood: findings from the National Child development Study. *Br Med J* 1980; 207–210.

33. Annegers JE, Dubinsky S, Coan SP, Newmark ME, Roht L. The incidence of epilepsy and unprovoked seizures in multiethnic, urban health maintenance organizations. *Epilepsia* 1999; 40: 502–506.

34. Zarelli M, Beghi E, Rocca WA, Hauser WA. Incidence of epileptic syndrome in Rochester Minnesota: 1980–1984. *Epilepsia* 1999 (in press).

35. Camfield CS, Camfield PR, Gordon K, Wirrell E, Dooley JM. Incidence of epilepsy in childhood and adolescence: a population-based study in Nova Scotia from 1977 to 1985. *Epilepsia* 1996; 37:19–23.

36. Granieri E, Rosati G, Tola R, et al. A descriptive study of epilepsy in the district of Copparo, Italy 1964–1978. *Epilepsia* 1983; 24:502–514.

37. Benna P, Ferrero P, Bianco C, et al. Epidemiologic aspects of epilepsy in the children of a Piedmontese district (Alba-Bra). *Pan Med* 1984; 26:113–118.

38. Cavazzuti GB. Epidemiology of different types of epilepsy in school age children of Modena, Italy. *Epilepsia* 1980; 21:57–62.

39. Braathen G, Theorell K. A general hospital population of childhood epilepsy. *Acta Paediatr* 1995; 84:1143–1146.

40. Joenson P. Prevalence, incidence and classification of epilepsy in the Faroes. *Acta Neurol Scand* 1986; 74:150–155.

41. Blom S, Heijbe J, Bergfors PG. Incidence of epilepsy in children: a follow-up study three years after the first seizure. *Epilepsia* 1978; 19:345–350.

42. Hauser WA, Ólafsson E, Ludvigsson P, Hesdorffer D, Gudmundsson G. Incidence of unprovoked seizures in Iceland. *Epilepsia* 1997; 38(Suppl 8):136.

43. Tekle-Haimanot R, Forsgren L, Ekstedt J. Incidence of epilepsy in rural central Ethiopia. *Epilepsia* 1997; 38:541–546.

44. Mani KS, Rangan G, Srinivas HV, et al. The Yelandur study: a community based approach to epilepsy in rural South India—epidemiological aspects. *Seizure* 1998; 7:281–288.

45. Rwiza HT, Kilonza GP, Haule J, et al. Prevalence and incidence of epilepsy in Ulanga, a rural Tanzanian district: a community-based study. *Epilepsia* 1992; 33:1051–1060.

46. Lavados J, Germain I, Morales A, et al. A descriptive study of epilepsy in the District of El Salvador, Chile 1984–1988. *Acta Neurol Scand* 1992; 91:718–729.

47. Sidenvall R, Forsgren L, Blomquist HK, Heijbel J. A community-based prospective incidence study of epileptic seizures in children. *Acta Paediatr* 1993; 82:60–65.

48. Wendt LV, Rantakallio P, Saukkonen AL, Makinen H. Epilepsy and associated handicaps in a one year birth cohort in Northern Finland. *Eur J Pediatr* 1985; 144:149–151.

49. Doose H, Sitepu B. Childhood epilepsy in a German city. *Neuropediatrics* 1983; 14:220–224.

50. Van den Berg BJ, Yerushalamy J. Studies on convulsive disorders in young children. I. Incidence of febrile and nonfebrile convulsions by age and other factors. *Pediatr Res* 1969; 3:298–304.

51. Cockerell OC, Eckle I, Goodridge DM, Sander JW, Shorvon SD. Epilepsy in a population of 6000 re-examined: secular trends in first attendance rates,

prevalence, and prognosis. *J Neurol Neurosurg Psychiatry* 1995; 58:570–576.

52. Jallon P, Smadja D, Cabre P, Le Mab G, Bazin M, Epimart group. EPIMART: prospective incidence study of epileptic seizures in newly referred patients in a French Caribbean Island (Martinique). *Epilepsia* 1999; 40:1103–1109.

53. Placencia M, Shorvon SD, Paredes V, et al. Epileptic seizures in an Andean region of Ecuador. *Brain* 1992; 115: 771–782.

54. Jallon P, Goumaz M, Haenggeli C, Morabia A. incidence of first epileptic seizures in the Canon of Geneva, Switzerland. *Epilepsia* 1997; 38:547–582.

55. Ohtahara S, Oka E, Ohtasuka Y, et al. An investigation on the epidemiology of epilepsy. In: *Frequency, Causes and Prevention of Neurological, Psychiatric and Muscular Disorders*. Annual Report of Research. Ministry of Health and Welfare, Japan 1993:55–60.

56. Wallace H, Shorvon S, Tallis R. Age specific incidence and prevalence rates of treated epilepsy in an unselected population of 2,052,922 and age-specific fertility rates of women with epilepsy. *Lancet* 1998; 352:1970–1973.

57. Ellenberg JH, Hirtz DG, Nelson KB. Age at onset of seizures in young children. *Ann Neurol* 1984; 15:127–134.

58. Annegers JF, Hauser WA, Anderson VE, Kurland LT. The risks of seizure disorders among relatives of patients with childhood onset epilepsy. *Neurology* 1982; 32:174–179.

59. Beck-Mannagetta G, Janz D, Hoffmeister U, Behl I, Scholz G. Morbidity risk for seizures and epilepsy in offspring of patients with epilepsy. In: Beck-Mannagetta G, Anderson VE, Doose H, Janz D, eds. *Genetics of the Epilepsies*. Berlin: Springer-Verlag, 1989:119.

60. Anderson E, Hauser WA. Genetics. In: Laidlow R, Richens A, Chadwick D, eds. *Textbook of Epilepsy*. 4th ed. Edinburgh, London, Madrid, Melbourne, New York and Tokyo: Churchill-Livingstone, 1993:47–75.

61. Rocca WA, Sharbrough FW, Hauser WA, Annegers JF, Schoenberg BS. Risk factors for absence seizures: a population-based case-control study in Rochester, Minnesota. *Neurology* 1987; 37:1309–1314.

62. Rocca WA, Sharbrough FW, Hauser WA, Annegers JF, Schoenberg BS. Risk factors for complex partial seizures: a population-based case-control study. *Ann Neurol* 1987; 21:22–31.

63. Rocca WA, Sharbrough FW, Hauser WA, Annegers JF, Schoenberg BS. Risk factors for generalized tonic-clonic seizures: a population-based case-control study in Rochester, Minnesota. *Neurology* 1987; 37:1315–1322.

64. Nelson KB, Ellenberg JH. Antecedents of seizure disorders in early childhood. *Am J Dis Child* 1986; 40:1053–1061.

65. Annegers JF, Hauser WA, Lee JR, Rocca WA. Secular trends and birth cohort effects in unprovoked seizures: Rochester, Minnesota 1935–1984. *Epilepsia* 1995; 36:575–579.

66. Commission on Classification and Terminology of the International League Against Epilepsy. A revised proposal for the classification of epilepsy and epileptic syndromes. *Epilepsia* 1989; 30:268–278.

67. Manford M, Hart YM, Sander JW, Shorvon SD. The National General Practice Study of Epilepsy. The syndromic classification of the International League Against Epilepsy applied to epilepsy in a general population. *Arch Neurol* 1992; 49:801–808

68. Loiseau J, Loiseau P, Guyot M, et al. Survey of seizure disorders in the French Southwest. I. Incidence of epileptic syndromes. *Epilepsia* 1990; 31:391–396.

69. Cowan LD, Bodensteiner JB, Leviton A, Doherty L. Prevalence of the epilepsies in children and adolescents. *Epilepsia* 1989; 30:94–106.

70. Hauser WA, Annegers JF, Gomez M. The incidence of West syndrome in Rochester, Minnesota. *Epilepsia* 1991; 32:83.

71. Ludvìgsson P, Ölafsson E, Sigurdardottir S, Hauser WA. Epidemiologic features of infantile spasms in Iceland. *Epilepsia* 1994; 35:802–805.

72. Howitz P, Platz P. Infantile spasms and HLA antigens. *Arch Dis Child* 1978; 3:680–682.

73. Oka E, Ishida S, Ohtsuka Y, Ohtahara S. Neuroepidemiological study of childhood epilepsy by application of International Classification of Epilepsies and Epileptic Syndromes (ILAE, 1989). *Epilepsia* 1995: 36:658–661.

74. Eriksson KJ, Koivikko MJ. Prevalence, classification and severity of epilepsy and epileptic syndromes in children. *Epilepsia* 1997: 38:1275–1282.

75. Riikonen R, Donner M. Incidence and aetiology of infantile spasms from 1960–1976: a population study in Finland. *Dev Med Child Neurol* 1979; 21:333–343.

76. Rantala H, Putkonen T. Occurrence, outcome and prognostic factors of infantile spasms and Lennox-Gastaut syndrome. *Epilepsia* 1999; 40:286–289.

77. Wendt LV, Rantakallio P, Saukkonen AL, Makinen H. Epilepsy and associated handicaps in a one year birth cohort in Northern Finland. *Eur J Pediatr* 1985; 144: 149–151.

78. Trevathan E, Murphy CC, Yeargin-Allsopp M. Prevalence and descriptive epidemiology of Lennox-Gastaut syndrome among Atlanta children. *Epilepsia* 1997; 38:1283–1288.

79. Endziniene M, Pauza V, Miseviciene I. Prevalence of childhood epilepsy in Kaunas, Lithuania. *Brain Dev* 1997; 19:379–387.

80. Cavazzuti GB. Epidemiology of different types of epilepsy in school age children of Modena, Italy. *Epilepsia* 1980; 21:57–62.

81. Hurst DL. Epidemiology of severe myoclonic epilepsy of infancy. *Epilepsia* 1990; 31:397–400.

82. Eriksson KJ, Koivikko MJ. Prevalence, classification and severity of epilepsy and epileptic syndromes in children. *Epilepsia* 1997: 38:1275–1282.

83. Ochoa Sangrador C, Palencia Luaces R. Study of the prevalence of epilepsy among schoolchildren in Valladolid, Spain. *Epilepsia* 1991; 32:791–797.

84. Ohtahara S, Oka E, Ohtasuka Y, et al. An investigation on the epidemiology of epilepsy. In: *Frequency, Causes and Prevention of Neurological, Psychiatric and Muscular Disorders*. Annual Report of Research. Ministry of Health and Welfare, Japan, 1993:55–60.

85. Hauser WA, Annegers JF, Kurland LT. Prevalence of epilepsy in Rochester, Minnesota: 1940–1980. *Epilepsia* 1991; 32:429–445.

86. Ortega-Avila R, Zarrelli M, Hauser WA. Prevalence of epilepsy in a rural Mexican village. *Epilepsia* 1991; 31:604.

87. Pisani F, Trunfio C, Oteri G, et al. Prevalence of epilepsy in children of Reggio Calabria, Southern Italy. *Acta Neurol* (Napoli) 1987; 9:40–43.

88. Baumann RJ, Marx MB, Leonidakis MG. An estimate of the prevalence of epilepsy in a rural Appalachian population. *Am J Epidemiol* 1977; 106:42–52.

89. Gomez JG, Arciniegas E, Torres J. Prevalence of epilepsy in Bogota, Columbia. *Neurology* 1978; 28:90–94.

90. Chiofalo N, Kirschbaum A, Fuentes A, et al. Prevalence of epilepsy in children of Melipilla, Chile. *Epilepsia* 1979; 20:261–266.

91. Garcia-Pedroza F, Rubio-Donnadieu F, Garcia Ramos G, et al. Prevalence of epilepsy in children: Tlalpan, Mexico City, Mexico. *Neuroepidemiology* 1983; 2:16–23.

92. Ólafsson E, Hauser WA. Prevalence of epilepsy in rural Iceland. *Epilepsia* 1999 (in press).

93. Snow RW, Williams RE, Rogers JE, Mungíala VO, Peshu N. The prevalence of epilepsy among a rural Kenyan population. Its association with premature mortality. *Trop Geogr Med* 1994; 46:175–179.

94. Sangrador OC, Luaces PR. Study of the prevalence of epilepsy among school children in Valladolid, Spain. *Epilepsia* 1991; 32:791–797.

95. Attia-Romdhane N, Mrabet A, Ben Hamida M. Prevalence of epilepsy in Kelibia, Tunisia. *Epilepsia* 1993; 34:1028–1032.

96. Pavlovic M, Jarebinski M, Pekmezovic T, Levic Z. Seizure disorders in pre-school children in a Serbian district. *Neuroepidemiology* 1998; 17:105–110.

97. Mendizabal JF, Salguero LF. Prevalence of epilepsy in a rural community of Guatemala. *Epilepsia* 1996; 37:373–376.

98. Hauser WA, Annegers JF, Kurland LT. Prevalence of epilepsy in Rochester, Minnesota: 1940–1980. *Epilepsia* 1991; 32:429–445.

99. Aziz H, Ali SM, Frances P, Khan MI, Hasan KZ. Epilepsy in Pakistan: a population-based epidemiological study. *Epilepsia* 1994; 35:950–958.

100. Aziz H, Guvener A, Akhtar SW, Hasan KZ. Comparative epidemiology of epilepsy in Pakistan and Turkey: population-based studies using identical protocols. *Epilepsia* 1997; 38:716–722.

101. Stanhope JM, Brody JA, Brink E. Convulsions among the Chamorro people of Guam, Mariana Islands. *Am J Epidemiol* 1972; 95:292–298.

102. Haerer AF, Anderson DW, Schoenberg BS. Prevalence and clinical features in a biracial United States population. *Epilepsia* 1986; 27:66–75.

103. Osuntokun BO, Adeuja OG, Nottiidge VA, et al. Prevalence of the epilepsies in Nigerian Africans: a community-based study. *Epilepsia* 1987; 28:272–279.

104. Koull R, Razdan S, Motta A. Prevalence and pattern of epilepsy (Lath/Mirgi/Laran) in rural Kashmir, India. *Epilepsia* 1988; 29:116–122.

105. Hackett RJ, Hackett L, Bhakta P. The prevalence and associated factors of epilepsy in children in Calicut district, Kerala, India. *Acta Paediatr* 1997; 86:1257–1260.

106. Bharucha NE, Bharucha EP, Bharucha AE, Bhise AV, Schoenberg BS. Prevalence of epilepsy in the Parsi community of Bombay. *Epilepsia* 1988; 29:111–115.

107. Reggio A, Failla G, Patti F, et al. Prevalence of epilepsy. A door-to door study in the Sicilian community Riposto. *Ital J Neurol Sci* 1996; 17:147–151.

108. Sillanpaa M. Epilepsy in children: prevalence, disability and handicap. *Epilepsia* 1992; 33:444–449.

109. Murphy CC, Trevathan E, Yeargin-Allsopp M. Prevalence of epilepsy and epileptic seizures in 10 year old children: results from the metropolitan Atlanta development disabilities study. *Epilepsia* 1995; 36:866–872.

110. Hagberg G, Hansson O. Childhood seizures. *Lancet* 1976; II:208

111. Gissler M, Jarvelin MR, Louhiala P, Hemminki E. Boys have more health problems in childhood than girls: follow-up of the 1987 Finnish birth cohort. *Acta Paediatr* 1999; 88:310–314.

CHAPTER 8

An Approach to the Child with Paroxysmal Phenomena with Emphasis on Nonepileptic Disorders

Arthur L. Prensky, M.D.

Epilepsy is a symptom. It occurs with excessive electrical discharge of cerebral neurons. Any acute or chronic insult to the brain can produce seizures. During infancy and childhood, seizures may assume many different clinical forms (1). When a child presents with what may be his first seizure, the physician is obligated to define the nature of the event and, if necessary, to search for a specific cause. The most common type of seizure in children is associated with moderate to high fever (2). These seizures rarely result in epilepsy or cause neurologic damage (see Chapter 12), and, unless there is reason to suspect sepsis or an infection of the central nervous system (CNS), the child does not require an extensive evaluation if prior development has been normal. Even if an initial seizure occurs in the absence of fever, a search for a specific cause is often not fruitful, as many occur in patients in whom there is no detectable evidence of brain damage or systemic illness. Some of these children have family members who have been diagnosed with epilepsy. This suggests a genetic predisposition for the patient's seizure.

EVALUATION OF THE FIRST SEIZURE

There are two populations of children whose seizures are more likely to be associated with an identifiable insult to the brain: those who have other neurologic signs or a history of abnormal development and those who have partial seizures that arise from a specific region of the cerebral cortex. However, in infants and young children, in particular, it is not unusual for a generalized seizure to be the first sign of an acute or chronic metabolic disorder or an infection of the brain or meninges. All children who have had their first seizure, with or without fever, should be evaluated with a complete history and physical examination to determine if prior development is suspicious, if there are focal neurologic signs or evidence of increased intracranial pressure, or if there is indication of other organ involvement. It is the history and physical examination, along with the age of the child at the time of the initial seizure, that determines the extent of the subsequent laboratory evaluations.

A seizure that occurs just after birth or within the newborn period is more often associated with a definable structural or metabolic disorder that affects the nervous system than an initial seizure that occurs later in infancy or childhood (3–5) (see Chapter 11). A single seizure occurring in the newborn period deserves to be thoroughly investigated. Table 8-1 indicates what would be considered a reasonable evaluation for an otherwise normal newborn with one well-defined seizure. The laboratory studies done at this age are extensive because a seizure may be the first and only sign of a treatable metabolic or infectious disorder affecting the brain or of acute or subacute structural damage such as periventricular leukomalacia or intraventricular hemorrhage. Sophisticated neuroimaging may reveal structural pathology that occurred much earlier in intrauterine life (6). This information may be helpful when giving the family a prognosis. Newborns are subject to infections and intoxications afflicting their parents. Certain tests such as those for acquired immune deficiency syndrome (AIDS) or screening for drugs usually require parental consent. Such consent should always be sought when a newborn has an unexplained seizure.

Table 8-1. The Evaluation of a Neonatal Seizure

A. With a history that suggests a probable cause (intrauterine insult, hypoxia, etc.):
   1. Serum chemistries: glucose, calcium magnesium, electrolytes, BUN, or creatinine
   2. Serum pH, pO$_2$ (arterial or capillary)
   3. Urine screen for toxic substances
   4. Lumbar puncture: CSF protein, glucose, cells, smear and culture
   5. A cranial ultrasound or noncontrasted CT scan of brain
   6. EEG

B. Without a probable cause also include:
   1. TORCH titers
   2. Quantitative urine and serum amino acids
   3. Serum and urine organic acids
   4. AIDS testing
   5. Drug screen

BUN = blood urea nitrogen; CSF = cerebrospinal fluid; CT = computed tomography; EEG = electroencephalo- gram; TORCH = toxoplasmosis, other (congenital syphilis and viruses), rubella, cytomegalovirus, and herpes simplex virus; AIDS = acquired immune deficiency syndrome

Older children and adolescents who are otherwise normal when they present with their first generalized seizure constitute a different situation. If the history is benign and the examination is normal, an encephalogram (EEG) is the only test that is indicated, and even that examination is helpful only in a minority of instances. A normal EEG would not contraindicate the diagnosis of a seizure if the history were sufficiently clear. An abnormal interictal EEG helps if the diagnosis made by history were uncertain. Many children who have had a seizure have a normal EEG in the interictal period or they show nonspecific abnormalities such as diffuse slowing. The history is always the most critical part of making the diagnosis of a seizure unless the episode itself is observed by the doctor. Just as the EEG rarely assists in the diagnosis of a seizure disorder, it also is not entirely reliable in predicting if there will be further episodes (see Chapter 9); however, the initial EEG may define a focus or occasionally show a specific pattern that has some predictive value and helps to plan the child's treatment. It is very important to obtain a history from an adolescent when separated from their parents. This may help to determine whether they are at risk for a social disease or if they have a drug history that could have resulted in a convulsion.

The evaluation of the initial seizure should be much more extensive if the child's history or physical examination is not entirely normal. The following questions need to be answered in the history: Was the event a seizure? Was the seizure focal or generalized? Is there a history of neurologic illness? Has the seizure occurred during the course of an acute or subacute systemic or neurologic illness, that is, were there prior or continuing symptoms such as fever, diarrhea, vomiting, headache, or change in level of consciousness or alterations of comprehension, speech, vision, balance, or strength? Does the child have other chronic disorders that might make his seizure more likely to be the result of structural damage to the brain such as congenital heart disease, hypertension, sickle cell anemia, immunodeficiencies, or collagen vascular disease? A family history is also critical and should emphasize whether other members of the family have had epilepsy, febrile seizures, or other types of neurologic disorders.

The child who presents with a first seizure deserves a thorough neurologic examination and general physical examination with special attention to signs of neuroectodermal diseases, including screening with a Woods lamp. Emphasis should be placed on whether the child has focal neurologic signs such as visual loss, weakness of one part of the body, reflex changes, or disturbances of balance or coordination that might suggest an area of brain damage that could also be the source of the seizure. Signs of elevated intracranial pressure should also be looked for (a bulging fontanel, split sutures, papilledema, slow pulse, and high blood pressure for age), as should signs of meningeal irritation (a stiff neck, Koernig's signs, Brudzinski's sign). Finally, any recent changes in the child's intellectual capacities or language should be documented. The child with a generalized seizure who has a benign history and physical examination need have little more done than a serum glucose, calcium, and magnesium, and a routine EEG. If the history or physical findings suggest the possibility of focal brain damage or elevated intracranial pressure, a computed tomography (CT) or magnetic resonance imaging (MRI) scan is indicated. The latter is more sensitive, especially if one suspects there may be migrational abnormalities that have affected the cortex (7).

The ways in which a child's history and physical examination may influence the further evaluation of a child with a first seizure are outlined in Table 8-2.

At times, more sophisticated metabolic studies are indicated to define the cause of an epileptic disorder. For example, infants or children whose seizures are poorly controlled with medication should have their cerebrospinal fluid (CSF) glycine levels determined. Type II hyperglycinemia may result in an intractable epilepsy, which can be diagnosed only by evaluation of glycine levels in the spinal fluid. Any infant or young child with poorly controlled seizures should also be tested for pyridoxine dependency by being placed on 25–150 mg of pyridoxine daily for at least one month to see if that affects seizure control. Pyridoxine dependency cannot always be diagnosed by a single intravenous injection of the vitamin during an EEG. If

Table 8-2. The Basis for Laboratory Studies

History and Physical Examination	Seizure Type	Type of Evaluation
1. Normal	Generalized	Routine EEG; serum glucose, calcium, magnesium
2. Normal	Partial (focal)	Routine or sleep-deprived EEG; brain scan (CT or MRI); serum glucose, calcium, magnesium
3. Suggests a chronic neurologic insult not previously evaluated with focal physical findings	Generalized or partial	Routine or sleep-deprived EEG; brain imaging (CT or MRI); serum glucose, calcium, magnesium
4. Presence of mental retardation or slow development without focal signs	Generalized or partial	Routine EEG; serum glucose, calcium; serum and urine amino acids; chromosome studies, if otherwise indicated; TORCH titers, if under age 12 months. If seizure is partial, brain imaging is indicated.
5. Normal other than for presence of fever ± vomiting or diarrhea		
a. Seen acutely	Generalized or partial	Lumbar puncture; serum glucose, calcium, electrolytes, BUN; EEG
b. Seen some days later when well	Generalized	Fasting glucose, calcium; EEG
6. Normal other than for a clouded sensorium	Generalized or partial	Brain imaging (CT or MRI). If scan is normal, a lumbar puncture, glucose, calcium, electrolytes. If these are normal, liver chemistries including a serum ammonia, urine ketones, drug screen; EEG; AIDS testing.
7. Presence of increased ICP ± focal signs	Generalized or partial	Brain imaging with contrast enhancement (CT or MRI); calcium, electrolytes, urinalysis; lumbar puncture if scan is normal; EEG. If no cause is found, an MRI may be indicated at a later date.
8. Presence of focal signs of recent onset	Generalized or partial	Contrasted brain scan (CT or MRI); lumbar puncture if scan is normal; EEG; glucose, calcium, electrolytes. If CT scan normal, cardiac evaluation; screen for hemoglobinopathies and coagulation defects, sedimentation rate, antinuclear antibodies, serum cholesterol, triglycerides. Anticardiolipin antibodies if an infarct is seen on imaging.

EEG = electroencephalogram; CT = computed tomography; MRI = magnetic resonance imaging; TORCH = toxoplasmosis, other (congenital syphilis and viruses), rubella, cytomegalovirus, and herpes simplex virus; BUN = blood urea nitrogen; AIDS = acquired immune deficiency syndrome; ICP = increased cranial pressure

the child's seizures always occur in the early morning, especially after the child has skipped or postponed breakfast, the child must be hospitalized and fast to rule out hypoglycemia. The fast should continue until he or she either develops elevated ketone bodies in the urine or hypoglycemia. During that time, the child's clinical condition and serum glucose must be evaluated at regular intervals. After fasting for relatively short periods of time, some young children (aged 2–8 years) drop their blood glucose to very low levels causing a seizure (8). Associated metabolic disorders involving organic and fatty acids should be investigated if the child becomes hypoglycemic.

DISORDERS THAT IMITATE EPILEPSY

Physicians are often asked to distinguish between many forms of epilepsy and other transient disturbances of neurologic function. Nonepileptic neurologic disorders can produce recurrent, paroxysmal changes of movement, consciousness, or behavior that are similar to those exhibited by a child with epilepsy. Some disorders that mimic seizures are more likely to occur in children who have epilepsy, to be associated with epileptiform EEGs, or to be relieved by antiepileptic drugs. This makes their differentiation from epilepsy even more difficult; however, many of these disorders

Table 8-3. Imitators of Epilepsy

Symptoms/Signs	Relative Incidence with Age		
	Neonate and Infant 0–2 Years	Early Childhood 2–8 Years	Late Childhood 8–18 Years
A. Unusual movements			
Masturbation	+++	+	+
Shuddering	+++	+	+
Benign sleep myoclonus	+++	+	+
Startle responses	++	++	+
Paroxysmal torticollis	+	++	
Self-stimulating behaviors		+++	++
Tics		+	+++
Chorea		+	++
Paroxysmal choreoathetosis or dystonia		++	±
Pseudoseizures		+	++
Unusual eye movements	+++	++	+
B. Loss of tone or consciousness			
Syncope		++	+++
Drop attacks		±	±
Narcolepsy/cataplexy		±	+
Attention deficits		+++	+++
C. Disorders of respiration			
Apneic attacks	+++		
Breathholding	+++	+	
Hyperventilation		±	+
D. Perceptual disturbances			
Dizziness		+++	++
Headache		+++	+++
Abdominal pain		+++	+
E. Behavioral disorders			
Headbanging	+	+++	±
Night terrors	+	+++	±
Sleepwalking		+++	+
Nightmares		++	++
Rage		+++	++
Confusion		+	+++
Fear		+	+++

are benign and do not carry the prognosis or stigmata attached to many of the epilepsies. They require no treatment and disappear spontaneously. Others are best treated by medications other than antiepileptic drugs. Thus, it is extremely important to distinguish between repeated paroxysmal events that mimic a seizure and the recurrent seizures that define epilepsy.

Epilepsy and the disorders that imitate it present at all ages and in many different forms. There are several excellent reviews of nonepileptiform disorders based on cause (9–14). This discussion considers disorders based on their symptoms and signs and the age at which they are most likely to be confused with seizures, as well as whether they occur when the patient is awake or asleep (Table 8-3).

DISORDERS THAT OCCUR DURING SLEEP

Movement Disorders

Benign Neonatal Myoclonus

Benign neonatal myoclonus is the most common quasi-epileptic disorder (15,16). It usually occurs during sleep and begins early in infancy, often in the first weeks or months of life; however, it can be seen in older infants and even in young children. The disorder occurs during non-rapid eye movement (NREM) sleep. Rapid, forceful jerks may occur in the distal extremities such as the hands or feet or the more proximal muscles moving the entire limb or the trunk. The jerking usually recurs every 2 to 3 seconds, and episodes may last as long as 30 minutes, although most subside in 1 to 3 minutes only to recur repeatedly during the night. The movements migrate from one muscle group to another. Movements occur on both sides of the body. The involvement usually is synchronous, but it need not be. However, prolonged, repetitive involvement of the same muscles or repetitive synchronous involvement of the same muscle groups on the right and left sides of the body are more likely to be a true seizure. The movements of benign neonatal myoclonus are not stimulus-sensitive, and the EEGs taken during sleep do not record epileptiform activity while the events are going on. The source of the myoclonic movements is thought to be in the brain stem. The movements stop if the child is awakened. When alert, the infant is seen to be developing normally and to have a normal neurologic examination.

Benign neonatal myoclonus is extremely disturbing to parents, but the movements rarely interfere with the infant's sleep and normally do not require treatment. If absolutely essential, the movements can generally be reduced by giving a small dose of clonazepam before bed. The prognosis for these infants is a good one. If the movements begin in early infancy, they tend to disappear in 3 to 4 months. Those few children who develop sleep myoclonus later in infancy may continue to exhibit the movements into the second year of life. There is no indication that benign neonatal myoclonus is associated with a higher incidence of epilepsy or abnormal neurologic development later in life.

Head Banging and Other Rhythmic Parasomnias

Repetitive episodes of head banging can occur as an infant is falling asleep and may be mistaken for a seizure as, unlike diurnal episodes of stereotyped movements, they are not associated with emotional disturbances such as anxiety or frustration (17,18). Other rhythmic movements of the neck and trunk, such as head rolling, body rocking, and leg banging, can occur in children during stage 2 of sleep. These movements are unassociated with EEG abnormalities and can easily be differentiated from seizures by video-EEG or polysomnographic monitoring. If the movements are violent enough to require treatment, they can usually be modified by giving clonazepam before bedtime. Periodic leg movements do not appear to quantitatively alter the quality of sleep in adults (19).

Nocturnal Paroxysmal Dystonia

Nocturnal paroxysmal dystonia is a rare entity that occurs in older children and adults (20). There are brief attacks of dystonic posturing or ballistic or choreic movements in sleep. The attacks usually involve all limbs. The EEG fails to show epileptiform changes during the attack. Despite a normal sleep recording, these attacks are believed by some to be epileptic and to arise from areas of the frontal lobe that cannot be accessed by scalp tracings. Many patients who have this disorder also have, or eventually develop, other forms of diurnal seizures. This disorder indicates how difficult it may be to separate unusual seizures from nonepileptic disorders when a scalp EEG cannot be relied on to pick up paroxysmal transients.

Hypnogogic Paroxysmal Dystonia

Hypnogogic paroxysmal dystonia is an extremely rare disorder in which the patient's sleep is interrupted for brief periods of time (usually under one minute) several times each night by severe dystonic movements of the limbs sometimes accompanied by screaming (21). While it is conceivable that this is an epileptic variant, the few patients whose attacks have been recorded have had no paroxysmal changes in their EEG, although the episodes can be decreased by the use of the antiepileptic drug carbamazepine.

Disorders of Respiration

Apnea

Disturbances of breathing during sleep are common in infants and children. Periods of apnea without other signs are rarely epileptic when they occur during sleep, but the abrupt cessation of respiration can be the only sign of a seizure (22,23). The associated electrical abnormality is usually focal and in the temporal area; however, apnea has been described as the only manifestation of diffuse epileptiform discharges as well. Apnea is sometimes the only sign of a seizure in young infants.

Usually disorders leading to periods of apnea during sleep are classified as central, obstructive, or mixed (24). Most premature infants have apneic events that can be central, secondary to delayed maturation of the centers that control breathing, or obstructive, resulting from partial constriction of the upper airway. Polysomnography uses airflow monitors and strain gauges to relate movement of the chest and abdominal musculature to effective rhythmic inspiration and expiration. In obstructive apnea, movements of chest and/or abdominal musculature continues while the flow of air is markedly decreased or stopped. This is followed by a significant drop in the oxygen saturation of the blood. In central apnea, muscle movements decrease coincident with the drop in airflow. More sophisticated measures of pCO_2 and transesophageal pressure may identify more subtle disorders of breathing during sleep (25).

Central apnea has been reported with tumors of the brain stem or compression of the medulla or upper cord by a mass, bony deformities of the upper spine or foramen magnum (26), partial herniation of the brain, or a Chiari malformation. Metabolic or infectious disorders that damage the respiratory center in the medulla may result in loss of automatic control of respiration during sleep (Ondine's curse) producing long periods of apnea sufficient to cause further brain damage or even death.

Obstructive or mixed forms of apnea are frequently seen in young children with cranial-facial deformities that narrow the oropharynx or with adenotonsillar hypertrophy (27,28). Aspiration may cause similar problems and is more likely to occur in infants or children with significant neurologic damage. However, gastroesophageal reflux can occur in children who are neurologically normal and produce significant repeated periods of apnea in sleep as well as in the waking child.

Behavioral Disorders

The behavioral parasomnias noted in children that are often mistaken for epileptic activity include sleepwalking (somnambulism), night terrors (pavor nocturnus) and nightmares (29,30). The violent behaviors in non-REM sleep in older adults that can result in injury to themselves or to others are rarely seen in children (31).

Sleepwalking

Sleepwalking usually begins between 5 and 10 years of age and can persist into adult life (32). Approximately 15 percent of all children sleepwalk at least one time. Repeated episodes are much less frequent. Sleepwalking is often confused with automatisms seen with complex-partial seizures. The cause of the disorder is not known, but there is a definite increase in the prevalence of sleepwalking in the family members of children who suffer from the problem. Episodes of sleepwalking usually occur 1 to 3 hours after sleep begins. The child arises and walks about the room or the house in a trance and then walks back to bed. Semipurposeful behavior such as undressing and dressing may occur during the attack. The child's eyes are open and the child rarely walks into objects. The child often mumbles, but there is no purposeful speech. Sleepwalkers can sometimes be directed back to bed, but they often become agitated if restrained. Physical violence is not a part of the attack. The child has no memory of the event the next morning. Attacks sometimes increase with stress.

Usually no treatment is required other than providing for the safety of the child, and the disorder subsides spontaneously over a period of several years.

If the attacks are very frequent or prolonged, sedation with benzodiazepines may be of some help.

Night Terrors (Pavor Nocturnus)

Night terrors are most commonly seen in children between 5 and 10 years of age. The disorder also occurs in the first 3 hours of sleep in stages 3 or 4 of slow-wave sleep. It may be confused with complex partial seizures. The cause is not known, but there is a familial predisposition. Night terrors do not appear to be related to the presence or development of epilepsy or other neurologic or psychiatric disorders. Approximately 3 percent of all children have this disorder. The child often screams and then sits up. The child continues to scream and appears to be terrified. There are signs of increased sympathetic activity such as excessive sweating and dilated pupils. The attack can last up to 10 minutes, after which the child falls back to sleep. When awakened, the child has no recollection of the event. The EEG is generally normal. Rare cases of frontal lobe epilepsy have been mistaken for night terrors (33).

Nightmares

Night terrors must be distinguished from nightmares. The latter usually occur later in the night during REM sleep. The EEG is normal. The child may be restless during the dream but usually does not scream. The child often recalls the nightmare and develops a fear of sleeping alone.

Complex partial seizures that occur during sleep are usually associated with automatisms other than walking. The patient may appear anxious, but screaming and sympathetic overactivity are not seen unless someone tries to interrupt the seizure. The child may be incontinent. If the event is recorded, the EEG is usually abnormal.

DISORDERS THAT OCCUR WHEN AWAKE

Simple Paroxysmal Movement Disorders

Myoclonus

Rapid, forceful but isolated or nonrhythmic jerks that occur when the infant or child is awake are considered myoclonic. Whether such movements are epileptic may be a matter of semantics. Myoclonus, like other transient, paroxysmal movements, can originate in areas of brain other than the cortex (34) and can occur in the absence of paroxysmal activity in the EEG at the time the movement is seen. The physiologic processes that regulate large groups of subcortical cells causing them to fire synchronously and repeatedly may be similar to those seen in the recognized epilepsies. However, if the patient has no other neurologic signs, a repeatedly normal EEG, and a benign course in which he fails to develop other seizure types and the movements remain static and eventually disappear, the disorder is usually considered nonepileptic.

Benign myoclonic patterns are usually seen in infants in the first year of life and almost always disappear spontaneously within 18 months. The jerks may be limited to head flexion, or there may be bilateral synchronous jerks of the arms (35). At times they can occur repetitively in brief clusters (36). Lombroso and Fejerman (37) described infants who had bursts of flexor or, less often, extensor movements of neck, trunk, and arms resembling those seen in infantile spasms. Their EEG tracings were always normal and the children continued to develop normally. There was no increased incidence of epilepsy later in childhood.

Spasmodic Torticollis

Infants with spasmodic torticollis are subject to repeated episodes lasting minutes to days during which the head suddenly tilts to one side and the face may rotate to the opposite side (38,39). They are often irritable and uncomfortable at the time but alert and responsive. Brief episodes may occur many times each day while an attack lasts. The attacks usually start in the first months of life. The EEG at the time of the attack shows no epileptiform abnormalities. The cause is not known. This type of torticollis may be related to labyrinthine imbalance in an infant, although there is no associated nystagmus. Others consider it a form of dystonia. Instances of familial occurrence have been reported. Some children come from families with a strong history of migraine, and they develop typical migraine headaches later in life. Attacks of torticollis can also occur intermittently in the presence of gastroesophageal reflux (Sandifer's syndrome). These episodes are usually not paroxysmal and tend to last longer (40). Inflammatory, developmental, and neoplastic disease of the cervical cord, spine, and neck also tend to produce sustained torticollis but not a series of brief episodes. If no secondary cause can be discovered, spasmodic torticollis of infancy usually subsides in the first three years of life. No treatment is indicated.

Paroxysmal Kinesogenic Choreoathetosis

Children with paroxysmal kinesogenic choreoathetosis have abrupt attacks of choreoathetosis and/or dystonia (41–43). These episodes are usually related to startle, stress, or movement. Many brief attacks lasting seconds to several minutes can occur each day. The child is conscious and often uncomfortable during the episode. The disorder can be familial or sporadic.

Kinesthetic choreoathetosis, in which the attacks are associated with the onset of movement, is generally a familial disease. The EEG is normal during the episode or shows movement artifacts. This form of choreoathetosis responds to antiepileptic drugs, particularly carbamazepine. Some authorities have postulated that paroxysmal choreoathetosis is a form of subcortical epilepsy (44). Others have suggested that it is related to benign familial chorea. Sporadic cases sometimes follow such insults as hypoxia, hypoglycemia, and thyrotoxicosis.

Paroxysmal Dystonic Choreoathetosis

Dystonic movements may involve the trunk, limbs, jaw, or tongue. The response is rarely generalized. The character of the movement usually is the same from one attack to another; however, the parts of the body that are involved vary from individual to individual. Unlike kinesogenic choreoathetosis, the movements and abnormal postures generally last for 1 to 2 hours. They are precipitated by movement or startle but are accentuated by alcohol, caffeine, fatigue, or stress (45). Most cases are sporadic, but there is a familial form inherited as an autosomal dominant recently linked to chromosome 2q (46). While most cases are first noted in older children and adolescents, paroxysmal dystonia has been described as a transient disorder in infants (47). Dystonic postures can be associated with gastroesophageal reflux, but these, like paroxysmal torticollis, generally do not last for 1 to 2 hours.

Other Movements

Neurologically impaired children may have many repetitive movements that can be mistaken for seizures. A recent study of a group of these children by Donat and Wright (48) recorded head shaking and nodding, lateral and vertical nystagmus, staring, tongue thrusting, chewing movements, periodic hyperventilation, tonic postures, tics, and excessive startle reactions. Many have been treated for epilepsy unnecessarily because of these symptoms. In addition, self-stimulatory behaviors (discussed later) such as rhythmic hand shaking and body rocking are seen more often in retarded children.

Jitteriness

Jitteriness occurs in newborns and young infants (49). It can be so severe when a neonate is handled or is irritable or crying that it is sometimes mistaken for a clonic seizure; however, purely clonic generalized seizures are extremely rare in the neonate. Furthermore, the jittery infant is usually alert. The movements of a jittery child have more of an oscillatory quality to them than the clonic jerks seen during a seizure. The tremors seen in jitteriness either occur spontaneously or can be provoked by stimulation. They diminish or stop when the extremity is repositioned. However, jittery neonates are much more likely to develop seizures than the normal infant, and they often have abnormal EEGs with epileptiform transients. Jitteriness sometimes has a specific, often treatable cause. The movements are often seen in response to metabolic encephalopathies caused by hypoxia, hypoglycemia, hypocalcemia, and narcotic withdrawal. If possible, the underlying cause of jitteriness should be treated. The movements themselves usually decrease rapidly with time and require no specific therapy. If they are so severe that it is not possible to care for the baby, the baby may have to be sedated for a brief period.

Shuddering

Older infants and children can suffer from paroxysmal bouts of shivering during which spontaneous activity decreases and the upper extremities are adducted and flexed at the elbows or, less often, abducted and extended (50,51). The head an knees are also frequently flexed. Aside from artifact, there are no EEG abnormalities during the attacks and the incidence of epilepsy is no higher in these children than in the general population. Antiepileptic medications do not modify the attacks. Shuddering episodes gradually decrease in frequency and intensity in the first decade of life. Many children who have episodes of shuddering come from families in which many members have an essential tremor, and the two disorders may be related.

Rumination

Rumination appears to be secondary to poor esophageal peristalsis (52). During a typical attack, the neck is hyperextended and there are repetitive swallowing movements and tongue thrusting. Because episodes usually occur during or directly following infant feedings, while they are alert and often uncomfortable, the event is usually easily distinguished from a seizure. The disorder improves with time.

Startle Responses

Startle disease (hyperekplexia) is a rare familial disorder that occurs in major and minor forms (53,54). In the major form, the infant becomes stiff when handled. The episodes of hypertonia may be severe causing apnea, bradycardia, and, rarely, sudden death. Anecdotal reports suggest that forced flexion of the neck or hips interrupts the hypertonic episode. Stiffness decreases during the first year of life. During the same period, the infant develops violent, repetitive jerks upon falling asleep. Many of these children have

paroxysmal abnormalities in their EEGs. When they are recorded during a startle response, there are bilateral centroparietal sharp waves followed by a train of slow waves. This complex is considered as evoked by sensory stimuli and not an epileptiform transient. Older children, juveniles, and adults suddenly stiffen and fall. This is most likely to occur when they are startled, and this is what is usually misinterpreted as an epileptic disorder.

The symptoms of hyperekplexia (stiffness, jerking, and falling) respond to antiepileptic drugs such as clonazepam or valproic acid. Despite these features, the disorder is not considered a form of stimulus-sensitive epilepsy. It more likely represents a defect in inhibitory regulation of brain stem centers by the cerebrum. The disorder remains stable or improves with age. Children who have these symptoms do not develop typical seizures more frequently than the average child.

Recently, the gene for this disorder has been localized to chromosome 5q 33-q35 (55). Mutations that involve the gene that encodes the alpha-1 subunit of the glycine receptor result in exaggerated startle responses (56). Genetic analysis helps to distinguish difficult cases of hyperekplexia from epilepsy or psychogenic disorders. It should prove most useful in those cases that were considered sporadic.

Chorea

Choreic movements are rapid, purposeless movements that are not repetitive or rhythmic (57). They can involve any muscles but are more prominent in the distal musculature. In most disorders, the abnormal movements are bilateral but not synchronous. Hemichorea is limited to only one side of the body. It is seen, at times, with vascular and inflammatory disorders.

In alert children, single movements such as chorea and tics can be confused with myoclonus, although, unlike myoclonic jerks, these movements almost always disappear in sleep (Table 8-4). At times, choreiform movements and multifocal myoclonic jerks are indistinguishable and have to be categorized by the diseases with which they are associated. Multifocal myoclonus is more likely to occur in patients who have progressive degenerative disease of the brain or who are in the course of an acute encephalopathy. Acute chorea can occur with metabolic disorders but is more likely to be seen as the patient recovers from an encephalopathic illness. It also occurs as a sequel to beta-hemolytic streptococcal infections (Sydenham's chorea) (58) and as a result of drug ingestions. Lupus erythematosus can be associated with unilateral or bilateral chorea, as can the antiphospholipid syndrome (59). Mass lesions or cerebrovascular accidents are more likely to produce a hemichorea. Usually this form of chorea is easily

Table 8-4. Tics, Chorea, and Myoclonus

	Tic	Chorea	Multifocal or Myoclonus
Common age of onset (years)	(5–10)	(5–15)	Any age
Clinical picture	Stereotyped, repetitive movements of one or more muscle groups most often located in the face, neck, or upper trunk. They may be rhythmic for brief periods, but usually are irregular.	Rapid, jerky, arrhythmic movements that randomly migrate from one muscle group to another. May be unilateral. Movements tend to involve the limbs, tongue, and mouth more than other areas. Almost never synchronous.	Focal: repetitive and rhythmic jerks. Multifocal: lightning fast movements that can involve multiple muscle groups and move from one part of the body to another. May be synchronous.
Intent	Purposeless	Purposeless. Patient may consciously integrate the jerk into a willed movement.	Purposeless
Voluntary inhibition	Possible for brief periods	Rare	None
Sleep	Improves markedly or disappears	Improves markedly or disappears	Slight or no improvement
Stress or startle	May worsen	No change	May worsen
Level of consciousness	Alert	Alert or obtunded	Alert or obtunded or comatose
Associated neurological problems	Compulsive behaviors, attention deficit, learning disabilities, echolalia, coprolalia	Hypotonia, mild encephalopathic changes	Focal: none or mild encephalopathic changes Multifocal: often evidence of acute or chronic, severe diffuse brain dysfunction
EEG	Normal or background slowing unrelated to the movements	Normal, slow, or epileptiform, but unrelated to the movements	Slow or epileptiform. Spikes can occasionally be linked to the movement.
Brain scan	Normal	Normal or hypodense areas in the corpus striatum or subthalamic region	Often normal. Acute: occasionally evidence of cerebral edema. Chronic: occasional evidence of diffuse atrophy.
Treatment	Haloperiodol, clonidine	Benzodiazepines, haloperidol	Antiepileptics, especially clonazepam

distinguished clinically from seizures. However, the EEG often fails to distinguish between diffuse chorea and multifocal myoclonus, as it is possible for both to occur in the presence of an EEG with slow background activity without epileptiform transients or with unrelated paroxysmal bursts. The presence of multifocal spikes throughout the record favors the diagnosis of myoclonus, especially when the spike is linked to the jerk. Both types of movements may respond favorably to clonazepam. Chorea may also respond to haloperidol or pimozide (58).

Tics

Tics are rarely mistaken for myoclonus. They usually involve only one or, at most, several muscle groups and only in the most severe cases are they migratory (60,61). The movements are usually repetitive and stereotyped. Tics occur sometime during childhood in approximately 20 percent of the pediatric population, but they are usually "simple" in that they are always characterized by the same movement involving only one or two muscle groups. The face and neck muscles are most commonly involved, but a simple tic can involve muscles of respiration. Eye blinking, facial twitches, shrugging of the shoulders, head turning, sniffing, grunting, and repetitive clearing of one's throat are common forms of simple tics. In some children, simple tics may be caused or worsened by anxiety or stress. If left alone, most simple tics subside within weeks to months, although they sometimes recur for another brief period of time. The EEG is usually normal and has no epileptiform activity.

Multiple types of tics or tics that involve quite complicated movements of a number of muscle groups are known as complex tics. When they are chronically associated with vocal tics, the diagnosis of Gilles de la Tourette's disease can be made. This is an organic brain disorder with a definite genetic component. It is inherited as an autosomal dominant with variable penetrance and variable expression. No gene has been associated with the disorder as yet. There is a much higher family incidence of simple and complex tics in relatives of these children when compared with the general population (62). Based on response to therapy, the syndrome may be the result of abnormal metabolism of dopamine in the brain. While the disorder may stabilize or improve slightly in adolescence or early adult life, it fluctuates in childhood and can be sufficiently severe to modify normal activity. If so, it needs to be treated. The movements usually respond to small amounts of haloperidol, clonidine, or risperidone (63). Both tics and chorea can be associated with each other and with neuropsychiatric disorders, particularly obsessive compulsive disease. When this is seen following clinically apparent streptococcal infections or with high antistreptolysin-O (ASO titers), it is known as the PANDAS syndrome (64).

Ocular Movements

Spasmus Nutans

Classically, spasmus nutans consist of a triad of signs: nystagmus, head nodding, and a head tilt (65). Head nodding and intermittent nystagmus are often the first abnormalities noted by the parents. The nystagmoid movements are often more pronounced in one eye than in the other. Both symptoms can fluctuate in intensity and may come and go during the course of the day, resulting in some confusion as to whether the infant is having seizures. Infants with spasmus nutans have a somewhat higher incidence of EEG abnormalities than other children their age, but they are alert, in contact with the environment, and no more likely to develop epilepsy than the average child. The pathophysiology of spasmus nutans is not known. A small subgroup of these infants have mass lesions in the area of the optic chiasm or third ventricle (65). A child who is diagnosed as having spasmus nutans should have a CT scan or MRI. If the scan is normal, no further treatment is necessary. The majority of children with this disorder no longer have signs by five years of age; however, some may have nystagmoid eye movements that persist into adult life, and these children cannot be differentiated from those who have congenital nystagmus (66).

Opsoclonus

Opsoclonus is a very rare disorder of eye movement in which there are rapid conjugate saccadic oscillations separated by intervals (67). They are generally multidirectional, although they usually vary in intensity and direction. They can easily be mistaken for a seizure although the child remains alert and responsive. Generally, opsoclonus is seen in the presence of other neurologic signs such as ataxia and myoclonus. Children who suddenly develop these three signs in early life (Kinsbourne's encephalopathy) may have a neural crest tumor (68), but malignancies are rare even with long-term observation. However, even after children are observed over many years, these malignancies are rare. Unfortunately, children with this disorder frequently have persistent neurologic signs and do not develop normally (69).

Loss of Tone or Consciousness

Attention Deficits and Daydreaming

Children with typical absence attacks have brief episodes in which their activity suddenly ceases and there is a brief loss of contact with the environment. Posture is maintained. Automatisms occur, but they are unusual. Normal activity is usually resumed immediately. Atypical attacks are more indicative of complex-partial seizures during which the episodes last longer, automatisms are more common, incontinence can occur, and the child may be sleepy at the end of the seizure. Few problems mimic absence or complex partial seizures. The most common is daydreaming (70). This is a common occurrence in children who have attention deficit disorders. They can be unaware of their immediate surroundings for a few seconds or as long as a minute. They may not react to voice or visual stimuli but generally respond to touch. They may have no recollection of what transpired around them during the time their thoughts were elsewhere, but often they say they were thinking of something else at the time. Automatisms are rare, but some children have nervous habits such as picking at their nails or rubbing their hands, and these may continue while they stare ahead. The history can sometimes differentiate between daydreaming and absence seizures. Children who daydream never interrupt their own public recitations to stare ahead and lose track of time. A child who stops speaking in the middle of a sentence and has an episode of absence almost invariably has a seizure disorder. In some instances, video-EEG analysis of the spells is needed to arrive at the correct diagnosis (70).

Drop Attacks

One form of generalized epilepsy only involves sudden loss of tone (71). There may not be a recognizable loss of consciousness. These attacks must be distinguished from other disorders that produce a similar clinical picture (66). Some of the causes of sudden drop attacks are listed on Table 8-5.

Table 8-5. Causes of Sudden Loss of Posture

Generalized epilepsy
Syncope
Basilar migraine
Basilar insufficiency
Cataplexy
Compression of the upper cervical cord
Hyperventilation syndrome
Vestibular disorders
Psychogenic illness: hysteria, malingering

Table 8-6. Causes of Syncope

A. Secondary to known precipitating events
  1. Neurocardiogenic
    a. Vasovagal
      1. Fear
      2. Pain
      3. Unpleasant sights (situational)
    b. Reflex
      1. Cough
      2. Micturition
      3. Swallowing
      4. Carotid sinus pressure
  2. Decreased venous return
    a. Orthostatic (with change to an erect position)
    b. Soldier's syncope (standing at attention)
    c. With Valsalva's maneuver
  3. Decreased blood or red cell volume
B. No clear precipitating event by history
  1. Cardiac
    a. Arrhythmia
    b. Obstructive outflow
  2. Cerebrovascular insufficiency
  3. No known cause

These episodes can occur at any age but are more likely to be confused with epilepsy in later childhood and adolescence. Many disorders in which posture is suddenly lost are much more common in elderly patients. Certainly, this is true of basilar insufficiency and the peculiar vestibular disorders that suddenly throw people to the ground. Cataplexy is also much more likely to occur in adults. Compression of the upper cervical cord that presents with sudden drop attacks is exceedingly rare at any age. Basilar insufficiency and cervical cord compression are often associated with ictal and interictal neurologic signs that point to an insult of the brain stem or the cord. Hyperventilation leading to a loss of tone and consciousness can easily be recognized by observing the attack, and the patient or family often give a history of a period of intense overbreathing preceding the loss of posture and consciousness. An adolescent hysteric has many other symptoms of an emotional disorder that help to make the diagnosis. The malingerer may not fall abruptly and when "unconscious" may resist the limbs or eyelids being moved. The ultimate diagnosis of psychogenic drop attacks may depend on recording the attack with EEG telemetry. The three diagnoses that are most often confused with recurrent postural seizures in children and adolescents are syncope, narcolepsy/cataplexy, and basilar migraine. The latter two problems are relatively rare in the pediatric population, whereas syncope is a common event at all ages.

Syncope

Most syncopal episodes in children are neurogenic (72) (Table 8-6). There is reflex slowing of the heart producing a sinus bradycardia and/or a significant drop in systolic and, to a lesser degree, diastolic blood pressure. This may be precipitated by well-defined physical events that overactivate the autonomic nervous system, especially the parasympathetic division. Coughing, micturition, swallowing, and carotid sinus pressure are among the more common reflex causes of neurogenic syncope. Vasovagal syncope is also neurogenic, but the physical stimuli are less well defined and include such sensations as heat, pain, and fear. The

physiologic basis for neurogenic syncope is yet to be defined completely and may involve the CNS (73,74). A second major cause of syncope in children results from decreased blood volume or decreased return of venous blood to the heart.

The majority of syncopal events that are neurogenic in origin or due to decreased blood volume or venous return can be diagnosed by clinical history even if the decrease in blood flow to the brain is sufficiently severe or prolonged to result in tonic or myoclonic muscle activity shortly after the loss of consciousness (75). Most of these children faint in response to one or more limited provocations, that is, micturition, the sight of blood, or a warm, crowded environment, or, in the case of decreased venous return, assumption of upright posture or prolonged standing (76). Many patients realize they are going to faint before losing consciousness. Nausea or vague epigastric sensations are experienced by patients with either syncope or seizures (77). However, other warning signs differ. Patients suffering from syncope are more likely to feel light-headed or dizzy than they are to complain of vertigo. Their visual sensations are also more simple than the visual auras of epileptic children. Vision begins to dim and objects lose their color becoming gray or brown. Brief syncopal episodes are almost never followed by confusion lasting more than seconds after arousal. Drowsiness is less common after a syncopal episode than a seizure and is almost always less prolonged. After an ictal event, a deep sleep from which the patient can hardly be aroused suggests a seizure. Headache may also follow a brief syncope or a seizure, but it is usually more severe after the latter. Unfortunately, if the syncope is prolonged, lasting minutes, and is severe and the brain is deprived of oxygen for a relatively long period of time, the postictal signs of syncope and seizures may be indistinguishable.

Of course, the most serious causes of syncope often occur without warning and produce significant brain hypoxia, which may result in a confused child after consciousness returns. Disorders of cardiac conduction are the most common cause of this type of syncope (78,79), although rarely lesions of the brain stem or upper cord can cause transient cardiac arrhythmias or arrest. Because cardiogenic syncope can sometimes result in sudden death, it is this group of disorders that must be eliminated as a possible cause of fainting when children repeatedly lose consciousness. One clue to a cardiac cause for syncope is when a child faints while exercising (80). Neurogenic syncope can also occur with exercise, but the proportion of children who have cardiac conduction disorders increases in the group that faints during exercise when compared with children who faint at rest.

The physical examination may be of little help in distinguishing syncope from seizures because it is often normal in patients with either symptom. Seizures are more likely to be associated with signs of CNS injury. At times, the cause of syncope can be suspected by obtaining supine blood pressure and noting its change when the child rapidly assumes the standing position. In normal children, the blood pressure remains stable (±5 points) or transiently increases slightly with an increase in the pulse rate of 8 to 20 beats. A drop in blood pressure of 15 or more points or a sinus bradycardia when rapidly standing confirms the history of possible orthostatic hypotension. Auscultation of the heart may also assist in the diagnosis. An irregular rhythm or a murmur may suggest that a cardiac abnormality is the cause of the faint. Provocative office tests such as carotid sinus massage and ocular pressure are not recommended.

The laboratory evaluation of children who faint has become a complicated and argumentative issue regardless of age (81). In the absence of a suspicious history or neurologic findings, an interictal EEG does not differentiate syncope from seizures even if there are paroxysmal transients in the tracing. Neuroimaging is not of value unless a lower brain stem or cervical cord lesion is suspected. If repeated episodes of fainting have occurred with a typical history, we still obtain a routine 12-channel electrocardiogram (EKG). Further testing is not usual unless the time of day in which the fainting takes place suggests the possibility of hypoglycemia. If there is no history of a provocative event or an aura, a more extensive cardiac evaluation is indicated. This may include prolonged ambulatory recording of the EKG, stress testing, and

possibly an echocardiogram. These are expensive and stressful tests, and their yield, even in high-risk patients by history, is probably under 20 percent of those tested.

This raises the question of whether these children would benefit from tilt-table testing and at what point such a test should be attempted. Studies in pediatric patients and young adults thought to have neurocardiogenic syncope show that they have a statistically significant increase in either bradycardia, systolic hypotension, or asystole with head-up tilting for up to 60 minutes when compared with asymptomatic controls. Drugs such as isoproterenol increase the rate of positive responses and further separate the two groups (82,83). However, there are still many false-positives in the control group and 10 to 15 percent false-negatives in the neurocardiogenic group. Furthermore, positive responses in another group of young adults could only be reproduced 54.5 percent of the time (84). It is not likely that a head-up tilt test has any more relevance to differentiating syncope from seizures than the EEG. Furthermore, it is not very likely that tilt-table testing adds useful information to that population of patients who have a good history to suggest neurocardiogenic syncope (85). This leaves those children who have recurrent syncope without a definable cause, especially if it occurs during exercise. Most of these patients will have neurocardiogenic syncope (86). A positive response to the head-up tilt test may establish the diagnosis and eliminate the need for further expensive, stressful tests. We suggest that if a routine EKG and echocardiogram, ambulatory monitoring, and an exercise tolerance test fail to establish the diagnosis, a positive head tilt-up test might suggest appropriate therapy and allow the gradual resumption of full activity by the child. That would be particularly important for children who are interested in resuming competitive sports.

Narcolepsy and Cataplexy

Children who have cataplexy suddenly drop to the ground with loss of muscle tone in response to an unexpected touch or emotional stimulus such as laughter. The attacks are brief, and it is not clear if some patients lose consciousness during them, but that is unlikely. Most children with cataplexy also suffer from narcolepsy, a state of excessive daytime drowsiness punctuated by periods during which the patient rapidly falls asleep, frequently under unusual circumstances such as while engaged in conversation (87). This sometimes leads to confusing narcoleptic attacks with episodes of absence, although the narcoleptic patient appears to be in a state of normal sleep and continues to sleep for many minutes unless aroused by an external stimulus. In addition to cataplexy and narcolepsy, the narcoleptic syndrome includes transient episodes of inability to move when awakening (sleep paralysis) and brief hallucinatory episodes on arousal. The four components of the syndrome do not appear simultaneously, and some may never occur in a narcoleptic patient. Narcolepsy and cataplexy are the two that are most commonly associated. These four phenomena are consistent with abnormal REM sleep, probably as a result of yet undescribed defects in the reticular activating system.

The EEG clearly differentiates between cataplexy and narcolepsy and a tonic or absence seizure if recorded during an attack. In the interictal period, a multiple sleep latency test using the EEG can be helpful. The child is allowed to go to sleep on five different occasions during the day. If REM sleep occurs within 10 minutes of the onset of sleep on two of these occasions, the tracing is compatible with the diagnosis of narcolepsy. The symptoms of narcolepsy can sometimes be ameliorated by the use of stimulant drugs such as fluoxetine (88) or carbamazepine (89).

Basilar Migraine

The basilar migraine variant generally begins in adolescence but may occur in children in the first years of life (90,91). It is more common in females. Some attacks begin with sudden loss of consciousness. Upon recovery, the child often experiences a severe occipital or vertex headache; however, most patients have symptoms of other abnormalities of brain stem function such as dizziness or vertigo or bilateral visual loss. Diplopia, dysarthria, and bilateral paresthesias occur less often. Frequently, there is a family history of migraine. Close relatives may have had similar attacks. Up to one-third of children with basilar migraine have paroxysmal interictal EEGs, some with occipital spike and wave complexes (92). A diagnosis must be made on clinical grounds. Many children with basilar migraine respond to antiepileptic drugs and others respond to agents that block the transport of calcium into the cell.

Disorders of Respiration

Apnea

Sudden apneic attacks that occur when the infant is awake are even more likely to be thought of as possible seizures, especially if the infant also suddenly develops a fixed stare or begins to flail about. However, these kinds of attacks are exactly what one sees with some infants who have gastroesophageal reflux 93). Each of these signs—apnea, staring, and flailing—may occur alone or in combination. Of the three, episodic apnea is the most frequent sign of reflux. The problem is the result of incompetence of the upper and lower esophageal sphincters, which leads to the reflux and sometimes to the aspiration of stomach contents.

This occurs most often when infants are in a flat position just after they are fed. The flailing movements are generally thought to be a response to pain resulting from the acid nature of the stomach contents. The episodes are not associated with EEG abnormalities. Proof of reflux is often difficult to obtain, although in many infants it can be seen during a barium swallow. Lesser degrees of reflux can, at times, be diagnosed by the use of radioisotopes or the measurement of esophageal pH. The presence of reflux does not necessarily mean that the physician has found the cause of the child's symptoms unless the disorder coincides with the time of reflux. The presence of significant reflux in a symptomatic infant is sufficient reason to start therapy. Treatment usually involves positioning the baby in a more upright posture after feeding (94), thickening feedings, and finally, in rare instances, fundal plication (95).

Breathholding

Breathholding also involves attacks of respiratory arrest that can be mistaken for seizures, but the episodes occur in a very different setting (96,97). There are two forms of breathholding spells: pallid and cyanotic. Cyanotic spells were the first to be described. They usually begin in the second or third year of life. Almost invariably, the child has been frightened or frustrated or has had a minor injury and begins to cry vigorously. Then the child suddenly stops breathing, often on inspiration. After several seconds, the child turns blue and loses consciousness. The child is often limp at this time. The period of unconsciousness is brief, usually lasting less than one minute, although it can be more prolonged. When the child regains consciousness he or she is alert and frequently resumes normal activities immediately.

Pallid breathholding attacks often follow minor trauma. Crying is minimal or absent. The child quickly loses consciousness and is limp. The attacks last over one minute and may result in a seizure caused by cerebral ischemia (98).

Both cyanotic and pallid forms of breathholding result from reflex changes that decrease cerebral blood flow. The exact mechanism may vary from one child to another. If there is a reflex cessation of respiration in inspiration, venous return to the thorax may be decreased, resulting in a decreased cardiac output. Other children experience changes in heart rate and rhythm and a decrease in blood pressure.

Neither type of breathholding attack is associated with an epileptic discharge. These attacks are not associated with an increased incidence of epileptic seizures later in life, even if generalized clonic jerks occur during the attack. The diagnosis is usually made by the history. Breathholding attacks usually occur less than two to three times a month in susceptible children. The episodes invariably cease by five to six years of age. Occasionally children have pallid attacks several times a week or even daily. The frequency of the episodes in these children may sometimes be reduced with the use of atropine-like agents, but the optimal treatment is behavioral modification directed at reducing the parents' emotional reactions to the episodes.

Recently, it has been suggested that severe breathholding spells may be inherited as an autosomal dominant trait with variable penetrance (99).

Hyperventilation

Hyperventilation is defined as physiologically inappropriate overbreathing (100). Acute hyperventilation is often associated with a feeling of intense anxiety or even panic. Patients may feel they are suffocating or choking during the attack. Other symptoms of acute anxiety may occur, including dry mouth, globus hystericus, chest pain, palpitations, and tachycardia. If the patient becomes severely alkalotic, he may complain of headache, tinnitus, dizziness or vertigo, tingling of the face and hands, or carpopedal spasm. The patient may lose consciousness. This may be followed by a generalized seizure. The diagnosis is usually made by the history of symptoms and signs that precede the loss of consciousness. In the past, the diagnosis was assumed confirmed if (1) the attack were seen and aborted by having the patient rebreath into a paper bag, and (2) the symptoms could be reproduced by the hyperventilation provocation test. Recently, however, studies have shown that patients' symptoms may have nothing to do with their pCO$_2$. Hyperventilation may be a consequence and not a cause of these attacks (101).

Perceptual Disturbances

Pain

Ictal pain is usually unilateral; it occurs most often in the arm, and it may be the only manifestation of a seizure (102). The focus is often in the contralateral rolandic area. Headache may be the only symptom of a seizure, although this is extremely rare. The pain is unilateral, but the source of the activity in the brain is not certain. Pain also follows complex partial seizures (103), and in our experience, it rarely may be the only symptom of a complex partial seizure. Children who have this type of headache often have signs of cerebral injury, do not get relief from sleep, and do not have a family history of migraine.

Paroxysmal recurrent headaches are characteristic of migraine. When children with migraine headaches

have an aura, it usually is visual. The headaches are apt to be throbbing and are sometimes unilateral. They are often relieved by a brief period of sleep. They are frequently associated with gastrointestinal disturbances. There is a strong family history of migraine in approximately 80 percent of the patients (104).

Epilepsy and migraine coexist in many children. Between 3 percent and 7 percent of children with migraine have epilepsy. Most have complex-partial seizures. A large percentage of migraineurs (perhaps as high as 20%) have interictal records that are paroxysmal. Approximately 60 percent of children who have migraine headaches obtain significant relief with antiepileptic medication (104). Because migraine occurs in 4 percent to 12 percent of children, depending on age, and epilepsy occurs in less than 1 percent, the most recurrent paroxysmal headaches are likely to be migrainous, even in those children who have complex-partial seizures. Furthermore, migraine headaches can be clinically defined by their associated symptoms and family history. When that is not possible, the criteria for diagnosing a headache as an ictal event should rely heavily on recording a paroxysmal change in the EEG taken at the time of the event.

Recurrent abdominal pain (105), usually periumbilical, with or without vomiting, pallor, or an idiopathic fever, can be caused by migraine and perhaps, in rare cases, by epilepsy. Most children who have this problem do not have either disorder. Children with recurrent abdominal pain frequently see a physician to rule out epilepsy. The range of interictal paroxysmal EEGs in children with this syndrome is 7 percent to 76 percent in different series. Approximately 15 percent of these children do have epileptic seizures, and more than 40 percent have recurrent headaches. Approximately 20 percent have a family history of migraine (106). Even those children who have other epileptic seizures do not generally have isolated abdominal pain that is epileptic in origin. Children with abdominal pain usually do not respond to antiepileptic drugs, but approximately 20 percent, in our experience, do respond to antimigrainous drugs such as beta-blockers or tricyclic antidepressants. Children with recurrent abdominal pain who do not have other seizures at the time they first present are unlikely to develop epilepsy. However, they are at greater risk for developing migraine later in life (107). In the majority, the attacks recede and are infrequent and/or have disappeared by the end of puberty. This is another pain syndrome in which the few cases that have been definitely diagnosed as the result of epilepsy have had EEG recordings at the time of the attack. The tracing becomes paroxysmal coincident with the onset of clinical symptoms.

Vertigo and Ataxia

Benign Paroxysmal Vertigo

Sudden or repeated attacks of dysequilibrium in children are sometimes confused with epilepsy. Children with benign paroxysmal vertigo (108–110) have repeated attacks of vertigo lasting minutes to hours. These episodes can occur as often two or three times a week, but many children have only one attack every two to three months. The onset is sudden. During the attack, the child is often unable to walk unaided and maybe nauseated. Nystagmus need not be present. There is no hearing loss or tinnitus. The child is alert, responsive, and distressed. Interictally, the examination and the EEG are normal. There is no change in the audiogram. Caloric tests of vestibular function are usually normal, but a minority of children have evidence of canal paresis indicating dysfunction of the vestibular end organ in the ear. Many of these children have a family history of migraine, and some already have migraine headaches. A substantial number develop migraine later in life. The association between these attacks of vertigo in childhood and migraine is so strong that some have defined benign paroxysmal vertigo as a migraine variant. No treatment is indicated. The attacks do not seem to respond to either antiepileptic or antimigrainous medicines. The disorder usually subsides by six to eight years of age. The term *benign paroxysmal vertigo* is also used to describe positional vertigo in adults (111). This disorder is associated with positional nystagmus and appears to be labyrinthine in origin.

Vestibulocerebellar Ataxia

There are several forms of paroxysmal ataxia that may be mistaken for a seizure. One form is associated with nystagmus, but tests of the semicircular canals are normal. The disorder frequently responds to Diamox. It is an autosomal dominant disorder that has been mapped to chromosome 19p (112). In other families, similar symptoms and signs start in adult life and do not localize to chromosome 19p (113). These patients often do not respond to Diamox. In both disorders, the patients remain oriented and there is no other seizure history.

Behavioral Disorders

Stereotyped Movements

Stereotyped movements are patterned repetitive movements that recur frequently, often many times each day, in the same form (114,115). These movements can be seen in normal children but are much more common in children who are mentally retarded or autistic. Head banging, head rolling, and body rocking often occur when the older infant or child is awake. Head banging is often part of a temper tantrum. Head rolling and body rocking are forms of self-stimulation

that seem to result in pleasurable sensations. Flapping the hands or arms is a movement that also seems to relieve anxiety. The normal infant or child may stop these repetitive movements if touched or diverted by other stimuli. None of these behaviors have any direct association with future epileptic attacks and occur without a significant change in the EEG (when it is technically possible to record the patient). They are more apt to occur in irritable, excessively active, or retarded children. The movements decline rapidly toward the end of the second year of life. No treatment is necessary unless they persist until the child is 30 to 36 months of age. At that time, the movements may be reduced by behavioral modification techniques. There is no specific drug that is effective in treating these disorders without producing significant sedation, although recently it has been suggested, on the basis of a small series, that clomipramine may reduce the movements (116).

Masturbation

Infants who are masturbating are usually sitting with their legs held tightly together, sometimes straddling the bars of their crib or playpen, rocking back and forth (117). The behavior can almost always be aborted by a distracting stimulus and usually disappears spontaneously in several months. Masturbatory movements in older children are less likely to be confused with seizure activity. They usually lay prone on a flat surface such as a rug or bed and rub their genitals back and forth against the fibers. The children are alert and usually stop on command. Furthermore, they can demonstrate the movements when required to do so. What the parents usually mistake as the seizure is the detached look and lack of responsiveness that the children get during the period of climax. The history preceding the climax makes the diagnosis. At times, home video-EEG documentation of these events may allow the physician to determine the nature of the behavior (118).

Acute Confusion

Episodic confusion is not usually seen in children unless accompanied by other signs of acute disease such as fever, vomiting, or obtundation. Metabolic disorders that produce recurrent episodes of ketosis, acidosis, hypoglycemia, or hyperammonemia can also be the cause of recurrent confusional states. Children who have this problem should be screened for a metabolic disorder or drug ingestion (see Table 8-2).

Repeated attacks of confusion, usually associated with delirium, may also occur in children with migraine (119,120). There is often no associated headache, and there is no clinical or laboratory evidence of an infection or a metabolic disturbance. There may be a history of recent trauma. The attack lasts for hours but is almost always over within a day. There is usually a family history of migraine, and the patient may have had typical migraine headaches on other occasions. Confusional migraine is much more likely to occur in adolescence than in the first decade of life. Nonconvulsive status epilepticus may present as an acute confusional state at any age and can only be diagnosed by the EEG (121).

Panic or Fear

Ictal fear is extremely unusual (122). It is usually a brief event and often precedes or is accompanied by other evidence of a complex partial seizure. It is not related to a clear stressor and can be overwhelming. Panic attacks can occur as an acute event during the course of a more chronic anxiety disorder or in patients who are depressed or schizophrenic. They can also occur without there being an underlying emotional disorder. These episodes can begin in childhood, but their frequency increases in late adolescence and adult life (123). Attacks last minutes to hours and are accompanied by many symptoms such as palpitations, sweating, dizziness or vertigo, and feelings of unreality. These attacks may suggest a seizure. Only an EEG at the time of the attack differentiates ictal fear from a nonepileptic panic attack if the history is not clear. Recent studies suggest that individuals who do not have seizures but do suffer from panic disorder may have excessive neuronal activity in the right temporal region. Nonictal panic does not respond to antiepileptic drugs. The underlying disorder must be treated with psychiatric care. Cognitive therapy can be a combination of drugs such as buspirone or fluoxetine.

Rage

Rage attacks are not unusual in epileptic children, especially those who have frontal or temporal lobe lesions, but they are usually not part of the ictal event. Rage is also more common in hyperactive children and in others who have conduct or personality disorders. Ictal rage is unprovoked and not focused on a particular object or individual. It is also rare. Interictal rage or rage reactions without seizures usually occur in response to frustration, stress, or threatening situations. It is not the only evidence of a behavioral problem. It is often preceded by a period of whining, screaming, and crying. The anger is frequently directed at the source. The child may remember the attack. Behavior can frequently be modified during the episode. This type of rage does not respond to antiepileptic drugs, with the possible exception of carbamazepine, and is best treated by behavior modification. Propranolol and stimulant drugs may also help (124). The event can rarely be recorded by EEG because of artifact.

Pseudoseizures

Pseudoseizures are psychogenic seizures defined as episodes that resemble an epileptic seizure but are unassociated with EEG abnormalities (125,126). Implicit in the definition is the idea that individuals who have pseudoseizures do not consciously produce or control them, and thus are not malingerers. The definition of a pseudoseizure has always been an uncomfortable one because there are a number of unusual symptoms that are presumed to be epileptic, but they are not always associated with EEG abnormalities. Pseudoseizures are usually characterized by myoclonus or changes in sensation or behavior. The discharges are thought to arise from the deep frontotemporal region. The issue is further clouded by the fact that a significant percentage of children who have pseudoseizures also have epilepsy and usually have true complex partial or generalized motor seizures. Pseudoseizures do not respond to antiepileptic drugs, but at least 20 percent of those who have these seizures are children with true epilepsy that is poorly controlled. This factor complicates the differential diagnosis.

No particular behavior or movement before, during, or after the ictal state differentiates a seizure from a pseudoseizure. The onset of pseudoseizures often builds over minutes; the symptoms at the onset frequently suggest anxiety or a panic attack, that is, dyspnea, paresthesias, light-headedness, and palpitations; the ictal movements are often asymmetric and without rhythm, such as thrashing or flailing arm movements; the patient may scream or weep (127). However, none of these may occur, and the seizure may still represent a psychologically determined event rather than epilepsy.

The diagnosis of pseudoseizures has been aided considerably in recent years by the development of techniques that allow the EEG to be recorded for long periods of time. EEG telemetry or monitoring by videotape allow the patient's brain waves to be recorded during the episodes in question. Of the two techniques, EEG telemetry is more satisfactory because the physician can also see and evaluate the clinical event (128). There are a number of clues that help distinguish seizures from pseudoseizures (Table 8-7). Pseudoseizures can sometimes be induced by suggestion, usually by giving the patient a saline infusion (129). In our experience, this technique is not suitable for younger children or moderately to severely retarded patients. Suggestion may also induce true seizures in patients who have both pseudoseizures and epilepsy.

The separation of epileptic seizures from pseudoseizures is often difficult and expensive, requiring prolonged EEG recordings and possible hospitalization. However, the distinction is extremely important because pseudoseizures can be sometimes be

Table 8-7. Seizures and Pseudoseizures

	Epileptic Seizures	Pseudoseizures
Type of movement	Clonic jerks that are usually flexor, rhythmic, and in phase in all involved extremities. Sudden drops to the ground.	Movements are often lateral as well as flexor and extensor. Often out of phase in the involved limbs. Some movements have a tremor-like quality. Others are flailing. There are unusual movements such as pelvic thrusts. Sudden drops to the ground.
Automatisms	Simple, such as lip smacking, picking at clothes. Complex, such as dressing, undressing, walking in circles.	Not usually seen or when noted, may not be stereotyped.
Consciousness	Usually out of contact with the environment	May be responsive during the attack
Language	Initial scream, groans, mumbling	Yelling and vulgar language sometimes occur
Incontinence	Frequent	Rare
Self-injury	Rare	Rare
Postictal confusion, headache, drowsiness	Frequent	Rare
Precipitating events	Can be present, specific stressful situations may increase seizure incidence	Incidence can be increased by specific stressful situations
Frequency	Usually single episodes	May occur in clusters
EEG	Often epileptiform transients	Often epileptiform transients
Interictal		
Ictal	Almost always a sudden, paroxysmal discharge, coincident with the attack	No paroxysmal changes
Elevated prolactin after ictus	Yes	No
Response to antiepileptics	Usually	Rare. There may be a placebo effect.

treated effectively as an emotional disturbance; thus, antiepileptic drugs are not overused.

In this chapter we have presented some of the clinical conditions that can be mistaken for epilepsy or an isolated seizure in an infant, young child, or adolescent. The large number of these conditions that encompass motor function, respiration, sensory experience, and behavior, both when awake and asleep in all ages from infancy into adult life, is testimony to the variety of ways in which epilepsy can present. Many families are often perplexed by—or often ignore—unusual behaviors their child is experiencing and postpone seeing a physician because their notion of epilepsy involves a sudden fall to the ground with stiffening and jerking of the limbs. It is important to recognize how many experiences that are out of the normal flow of events during the day or during sleep can be epileptic and how many nonepileptic disorders can mimic those events and confuse the physician.

REFERENCES

1. Tharp BR. An overview of pediatric seizure disorders and epileptic syndromes. *Epilepsia* 1987; 28(Suppl): 36–45.

2. Arnold ST, Dodson WE. Epilepsy in children. *Baillieres Clin Neurol* 1996; 5:783–802.

3. Nelson KB, Ellenberg JH. Predisposing and causative factors in childhood epilepsy. *Epilepsia* 1987; 28(Suppl): 16–24.

4. Painter MJ, Gaus LM. Neonatal seizures: Diagnosis and treatment. *J Child Neurol* 1991; 6:101–108.

5. Lombroso CT. Neonatal seizures: a clinician's overview. *Brain Dev* 1996; 18:1–28.

6. Kuzniecky RI. Neuroimaging in pediatric epilepsy. *Epilepsia* 1996; 37(Suppl 1):S10–S21.

7. Jack CR, Jr. Magnetic resonance imaging in epilepsy. *Mayo Clin Proc* 1996; 71:695–711.

8. Chaussain JL. Glycemic response to 24 hour fast in normal children and children with ketotic hypoglycemia. *J Pediatr* 1974; 82:438–443.

9. Gomez MR, Klass DW. Seizures and other paroxysmal disorders in infants and children. *Curr Probl Pediatra* 1972; 2:3–37.

10. Rabe EF. Recurrent paroxysmal nonepileptic disorders. *Curr Prob Pediatr* 1974; 4:3–31.

11. Pedley TA. Differential diagnosis of episodic symptoms. *Epilepsia* 1983; 24(Suppl):31–44.

12. Rothner AD. "Not everything that shakes is epilepsy." *Cleve Clin J Med* 1989; 56(Suppl 2):206–213.

13. Murphy JV, Dehkharghani F. Diagnosis of childhood seizure disorders. *Epilepsia* 1994; 35(Suppl 2):S7–S17.

14. Williams J, Grant M, Jackson M, et al. Behavioral descriptors that differentiate between seizure and nonseizure

events in a pediatric population. *Clin Pediatr* 1996; 35:243–249.

15. Coulter DL, Allen RJ. Benign neonatal sleep myoclonus. *Arch Neurol* 1982; 39:191–192.

16. Resnick TJ, Moshé SL, Perotta L, et al. Benign neonatal sleep myoclonus: relationship to sleep states. *Arch Neurol* 1986; 43:266–268.

17. Dyken ME, Rodnitzky RL. Periodic, aperiodic, and rhythmic motor disorders of sleep. *Neurology* 1992; 42(7 Suppl 6):68–74.

18. Dyken ME, Lin-Dyken DC, Yamada T. Diagnosing rhythmic motor movement disorder with video-polysomnography. *Pediatr Neurol* 1997; 16:37–41.

19. Mendelson WB. Are periodic leg movements associated with clinical sleep disturbance? *Sleep* 1996; 19:219–223.

20. Meierkord H, Fish DR, Smith SJM, et al. Is nocturnal paroxysmal dystonia a form of frontal lobe epilepsy? *Mov Disord* 1992; 7:38–42.

21. Godbout R, Montplaisir J, Rouleau I. Hypnogenic paroxysmal dystonia: epilepsy or sleep disorder? A case report. *Clin Electroencephalogr* 1985; 16:136–142.

22. Watanabe K, Hara K, Hakamada S, et al. Seizures with apnea in children. *Pediatrics* 1982; 79:87–90.

23. Donati F, Schaffler L, Vassella F. Prolonged epileptic apneas in a newborn: a case report with ictal EEG recording. *Neuropediatrics* 1995; 26:223–225.

24. Thach BT. Sleep apnea in infancy and childhood. *Med Clin North Am* 1985; 69:1289–1315.

25. Guilleminault C, Pelayo R, Leger D, et al. Recognition of sleep-disordered breathing in children. *Pediatrics* 1996; 98:871–882.

26. Yglesias A, Narbona J, Vanaclocha V, et al. Chiari type I malformation, glossopharyngeal neuralgia and central sleep apnoea in a child. *Dev Med Child Neurol* 1996; 38:1126–1130.

27. Kahn A, Groswasser J, Sottiaux M, et al. Mechanisms of obstructive sleep apneas in infants. *Biol Neonate* 1994; 65:235–239.

28. Deutsch ES. Tonsillectomy and adenoidectomy. Changing indications. *Pediatr Clin North Am* 1996; 43:1319–1338.

29. Vela-Bueno A, Soldatos CR. Episodic sleep disorders (parasomnias). *Semin Neurol* 1987; 7:269–276.

30. Woody RC. Sleep disorders in children. *Semin Neurol* 1988; 8:71–77.

31. Moldofsky H, Gilbert R, Lue FA, et al. Sleep-related violence. *Sleep* 1995; 18:731–739.

32. Masand P, Popli AP, Weilburg JB. Sleepwalking. *Am Fam Physician* 1995; 51:649–654.

33. Scheffer IE, Bhatia KP, Lopes-Cendes I, et al. Autosomal dominant frontal epilepsy misdiagnosed as sleep disorder. *Lancet* 1994; 343:515–517.

34. Rothwell JC. Brainstem myoclonus. *Clin Neuroscience* 1995–96; 3:214–218.

35. Shuper A, Mimouni M. Problems of differentiation between epilepsy and non-epileptic paroxysmal events in the first year of life. *Arch Dis Child* 1995; 73:342–344.

36. Ricci S, Cusmai R, Fusco L, et al. Reflex myoclonic epilepsy in infancy: a new age-dependent idiopathic epileptic syndrome related to startle reaction. *Epilepsia* 1995; 36:342–348.

37. Lombroso CT, Fejerman N. Benign myoclonus of early infancy. *Ann Neurol* 1977; 1:138–143.

38. Snyder CH. Paroxysmal torticollis in infancy. *Am J Dis Child* 1969; 117:458–460.

39. Cohen HA, Nussinovitch M, Ashkenasi A, et al. Benign paroxysmal torticollis in infancy. *Pediatr Neurol* 1993; 9:488–490.

40. Ramenofsky ML, Buyse M, Goldberg MJ, et al. Gastroesophageal reflux and torticollis. *J Bone Joint Surg* (Am) 1978; 60:1140–1141.

41. Kertesz A. Paroxysmal kinesogenic choreoathetosis. *Neurology* 1967; 17:680–690.

42. Lance JW. Familial paroxysmal dystonic choreoathetosis and its differentiation from related syndromes. *Ann Neurol* 1977; 2:285–293.

43. Kinast M, Erenberg G, Rothner AD. Paroxysmal choreoathetosis: report of five cases and review of the literature. *Pediatrics* 1980; 65:74–77.

44. Lombroso CT. Paroxysmal choreoathetosis: an epileptic or non-epileptic disorder? *Ital J Neurol Sci* 1995; 16:271–277.

45. Bressman SB, Fahn S, Burke RE. Paroxysmal non-kinesigenic dystonia. *Adv Neurol* 1988; 50:403–413.

46. Fink JK, Hedera P, Mathay JG, et al. Paroxysmal dystonic choreoathetosis linked to chromosome 2q: clinical analysis and proposed pathophysiology. *Neurology* 1997; 49:177–183.

47. Angelini L, Rumi V, Lamperti E, et al. Transient paroxysmal dystonia in infancy. *Neuropediatrics* 1988; 19:171–174.

48. Donat JF, Wright FS. Episodic symptoms mistaken for seizures in the neurologically impaired child. *Neurology* 1990; 40:156–157.

49. Parker S, Zuckerman B, Bauchner H, et al. Jitteriness in full-term neonates: prevalence and correlates. *Pediatrics* 1990; 85:17–23.

50. Vanasse M, Bedard P, Andermann F. Shuddering attacks in children: an early clinical manifestation of essential tremor. *Neurology* 1976; 26:1027–1030.

51. Holmes GL, Russman BS. Shuddering attacks. *Am J Dis Child* 1986; 140:72–73.

52. Herbst JJ. Gastroesophageal reflux. *J Pediatr* 1981; 98:859–870.

53. Andermann F, Keene DL, Andermann E, et al. Startle disease or hyperekplexia: further delineation of the syndrome. *Brain* 1980; 103:985–997.

54. Andermann F, Andermann E. Startle disorders of man: hyperekplexia, jumping and startle epilepsy. *Brain Dev* 1988; 10:213–222.

55. Ryan SG, Sherman SL, Terry JC, et al. Startle disease, or hyperekplexia: a response to clonazepam and assignment of the gene (STHE) to chromosome 5q by linkage analysis. *Ann Neurol* 1992; 31:663–668.

56. Elmslie FV, Hutchings SM, Spencer V, et al. Analysis of GLRA1 in hereditary and sporadic hyperekplexia: a novel mutation in a family cosegregating for hyperekplexia and spastic paraparesis. *J Med Genet* 1996; 33:435–436.

57. Shannon KM. Chorea. *Curr Opin Neurol* 1996; 9:298–302.

58. Garvey MA, Swedo SE. Sydenham's chorea. Clinical and therapeutic update. *Adv Exp Med Biol* 1997; 418:115–120.

59. Cervera R, Asherson RA, Font J, et al. Chorea in the antiphospholipid syndrome. Clinical, radiologic, and immunologic characteristics of 50 patients from our clinics and the recent literature. *Medicine* 1997; 76:203–212.

60. Golden GS. Tourette syndrome: recent advances. *Pediatr Neurol* 1986; 2:189–192.

61. Tics and fits. The current status of Gilles de la Tourette syndrome and its relationship with epilepsy. *Seizure* 1995; 4:259–266.

62. Spencer T, Biederman J, Harding M, et al. The relationship between tic disorders and Tourette's syndrome revisited. *J Am Acad Child & Adolesc Psychiatry* 1995; 34:1133–1139.

63. Lombroso PJ, Scahill L, King RA, et al. Risperidone treatment of children and adolescents with chronic tic disorders: A preliminary report. *J Amer Acad Child & Adolescent Psych* 1995; 34:1147–52.

64. Swedo SE, Leonard HL, Mittleman BB, et al. Identification of children with pediatric autoimmune neuropsychiatric disorders associated with streptococcal infections by a marker associated with rheumatic fever. *Am J Psychiatry* 1997; 154:110–112.

65. King RA, Nelson LB, Wagner RS. Spasmus nutans. *Arch Ophthalmol* 1986; 104:1501–1504.

66. Jayalakshmi P, McNair Scott TF, Tucker SH, et al. Infantile nystagmus: a prospective study of spasmus nutans, congenital nystagmus, and unclassified nystagmus of infancy. *J Pediatr* 1970; 77:177–187.

67. Averbuch-Heller L, Remler B. Opsoclonus. *Semin Neurol* 1996; 16:21–26.

68. Moe PG, Nellhaus G. Infantile polymyoclonia-opsoclonus syndrome and neural crest tumors. *Neurology* 1970; 20:756–764.

69. Pohl KR, Pritchard J, Wilson J. Neurological sequelae of the dancing eye syndrome. *Eur J Pediatr* 1996; 155:237–244.

70. Carmant L, Kramer U, Holmes GL, et al. Differential diagnosis of staring spells in children: a video-EEG study. *Pediatr Neurol* 1996; 14:199–202.

71. Meissner I, Weibers DO, Swanson JW, et al. The natural history of drop attacks. *Neurology* 1986; 36:1029–1034.

72. Pratt JL, Fleisher GR. Syncope in children and adolescents. *Pediatr Emerg Care* 1989; 5:80–82.

73. Somers VK, Abboud FM. Neurocardiogenic syncope. *Adv Intern Med* 1996; 41:399–435.

74. Benditt DG. Neurally mediated syncopal syndromes: pathophysiological concepts and clinical evaluation. *Pacing Clin Electrophysiol* 1997; 20(2 pt 2):572–584.

75. Lempert T. Recognizing syncope: pitfalls and surprises. *J R Soc Med* 1996; 89:372–375.

76. Thomas JE, Schirger A, Fealey RD, et al. Orthostatic hypotension. *Mayo Clin Proc* 1981; 56:117–125.

77. Benke T, Hochleitner M, Bauer G. Aura phenomena during syncope. *Eur Neurol* 1997; 37:28–32.

78. Beder SD, Cohen MH, Riemenschneider TA. Occult arrhythmias as the etiology of unexplained syncope in children with structurally normal hearts. *Am Heart J* 1985; 109:309–313.

79. Ruckman RN. Cardiac causes of syncope. *Pediatr Rev* 1987; 9:101–108.

80. Driscoll DJ, Jacobsen SJ, Porter CJ, et al. Syncope in children and adolescents. *J Am Coll Cardiol* 1997; 29:1039–1045.

81. Linzer M, Yang EH, Estes NA III, et al. Diagnosing syncope. Part 1: Value of history, physical examination, and electrocardiography. Clinical efficacy assessment project of the American College of Physicians. *Ann Intern Med* 1997; 126:989–996.

82. Berkowitz JB, Auld D, Hulse JE, et al. Tilt table evaluation for control pediatric patients: comparison with symptomatic patients. *Clin Cardiol* 1995; 18:521–525.

83. Carlioz R, Graux P, Haye J, et al. Prospective evaluation of high-dose or low-dose isoproterenol upright tilt protocol for unexplained syncope in young adults. *Am Heart J* 1997; 133:346–352.

84. Ruiz GA, Scaglione J, Gonzalez-Zuelgaray J. Reproducibility of head-up tilt test in patients with syncope. *Clin Cardiol* 1996; 19:215–220.

85. Lerman-Sagie T, Lerman P, Mukamel M, et al. A prospective evaluation of pediatric patients with syncope. *Clin Pediatr* 1994; 33:67–70.

86. Grubb BP, Temesy-Armos PN, Samoil D, et al. Tilt table testing in the evaluation and management of athletes with recurrent exercise-induced syncope. *Med Sci Sports Exer* 1993; 25:24–28.

87. Kotagal S, Hartse KM, Walsh JK. Characteristics of narcolepsy in preteenaged children. *Pediatrics* 1990; 85:205–209.

88. Frey J, Darbonne C. Fluoxetine suppresses human cataplexy: a pilot study. *Neurology* 1994; 44:707–709.

89. Vaughn BV, D'Cruz OF. Carbamazepine as a treatment for cataplexy. *Sleep* 1996; 19:101–103.

90. Bickerstaff ER. Basilar artery migraine. *Lancet* 1961; 1:15–17.

91. Lapkin ML, Golden GS. Basilar artery migraine. A review of 30 cases. *Am J Dis Children* 1978; 132:278–281.

92. De Romanis F, Buzzi MG, Assenza S, et al. Basilar migraine with electroencephalographic findings of occipital spike-wave complexes: a long-term study in seven children. *Cephalalgia* 1993; 13:192–196.

93. Spitzer AR, Boyle JT, Tuchman DN, et al. Awake apnea associated with gastroesophageal reflux: a specific clinical syndrome. *J Pediatr* 1984; 104:200–205.

94. Meyers WF, Herbst JJ. Effectiveness of positioning therapy for gastroesophageal reflux. *Pediatrics* 1982; 69:768–772.

95. Fonkalsrud EW, Ament ME. Gastroesophageal reflux in childhood. *Curr Probl Surg* 1996; 33:1–70.

96. Lombroso CT, Lerman P. Breathholding spells (cyanotic and pallid infantile syncope). *Pediatrics* 1967; 39:563–581.

97. Livingston S. Breathholding spells in children: differentiation from epileptic attacks. *JAMA* 1970; 212:2231–2235.

98. Gauk EW, Kidd I, Prichard JS. Mechanism of seizures associated with breathholding spells. *N Engl J Med* 1963; 268:1436–1441.

99. DiMario FJ Jr, Sarfarazi M. Family pedigree analysis of children with severe breathholding spells. *J Pediatr* 1997; 130:647–651.

100. Evans RW. Neurologic aspects of hyperventilation syndrome. *Semin Neurol* 1995; 15:115–125.

101. Hornsveld HK, Garssen B, Dop MJ, et al. Double-blind placebo-controlled study of the hyperventilation provocation test and the validity of the hyperventilation syndrome. *Lancet* 1996; 348:154–158.

102. Blume WT, Young GB. Ictal pain: unilateral, cephalic and abdominal. In: Andermann F, Lugaresi E, eds. *Migraine and Epilepsy*. London: Butterworths, 1987:238–248.

103. D'Alessandro R, Sacquengna T, Pazzaglia P, et al. Headache after partial complex seizures. In: Andermann F, Lugaresi E, eds. *Migraine and epilepsy*. London:Butterworths, 1987:273–328.

104. Prensky AL, Sommer D. Diagnosis and treatment of migraine in children. *Neurology* 1979; 29:506–510.

105. Abu-Arafeh I, Russell G. Prevalence and clinical features of abdominal migraine compared with those of migraine headache. *Arch Dis Child* 1995; 72:413–417.

106. Prensky AL. Migraine and migrainous variants in pediatric patients. *Pediatr Clin North Am* 1976; 23:461–471.

107. Hammond J. The late sequelae of recurrent vomiting of childhood. *Dev Med Child Neurol* 1974; 16:15–22.

108. Watson P, Steele JC. Paroxysmal disequilibrium in the migraine syndrome of childhood. *Arch Otolaryngol* 1974; 99:177–179.

109. Finkelhor BK, Harker LA. Benign paroxysmal vertigo of childhood. *Laryngoscope* 1987; 97:1161–1163.

110. Parker W. Migraine and the vestibular system in childhood and adolescence. *Am J Otol* 1989; 10:364–371.

111. Hughes CA, Proctor L. Benign paroxysmal positional vertigo. *Laryngoscope* 1997; 107:607–613.

112. Vehedi K, Joutel A, Van Bogart P, et al. A gene for hereditary paroxysmal cerebellar ataxia maps to chromosome 19p. *Ann Neurol* 1995; 37:289–293.

113. Damji KF, Allingham RR, Pollock SC, et al. Periodic vestibulocerebellar ataxia, an autosomal dominant ataxia with defective smooth pursuit, is genetically distinct from other autosomal dominant ataxias. *Arch Neurol* 1996; 53:338–344.

114. Smith EA, Van Houten R. A comparison of the characteristics of self-stimulatory behaviors in "normal" children and children with developmental delays. *Res Dev Disabil* 1996; 17:253–268.

115. Tan A, Salgado M, Fahn S. The characterization and outcome of stereotypical movements in nonautistic children. *Mov Disord* 1997; 12:47–52.

116. Lewis MH, Bodfish JW, Powell SB, et al. Clomipramine treatment for stereotype and related repetitive movement disorders associated with mental retardation. *Am J Mental Retard* 1995; 100:299–312.

117. Finkelstein E, Amichai B, Jaworowski S, et al. Masturbation in prepubescent children: a case report and review of the literature. *Child Care Health Dev* 1996; 22:323–326.

118. Bye AM, Nunan J. Video EEG analysis of non-ictal events in children. *Clin Exp Neurol* 1992; 29:92–98.

119. Gascon G, Barlow C. Juvenile migraine presenting as an acute confusional state. *J Pediatr* 1970; 45:628–635.

120. Shaabat A. Confusional migraine in childhood. *Pediatr Neurol* 1996; 15:23–25.

121. Primavera A, Giberti L, Scotto P, et al. Nonconvulsive status epilepticus as a cause of confusion in later life: a report of 5 cases. *Neuropsychobiology* 1994; 30:148–152.

122. McLachlan RS, Blume WT. Isolated fear in complex partial status epilepticus. *Ann Neurol* 1980; 8:639–641.

123. Ollendick TH, Mattis SG, King NJ. Panic in children and adolescents: A review. *J Child Psychol Psychiatry* 1994; 35:113–134.

124. Williams DT, Mehl R, Yudofsky S, et al. The effect of propranolol on uncontrolled rage outbursts in children and adolescents with organic brain dysfunction. *J Am Acad Child Adolesc Psychiatry* 1982; 2:129–135.

125. Williams DT, Spiegel H, Mostofsky DI. Neurogenic and hysterical seizures in children and adolescents: differential diagnostic and therapeutic considerations. *Am J Psychiatry* 1978; 135:82–86.

126. Holmes GI, Sackellares JC, McKiernan J, et al. Evaluation of childhood pseudoseizures using EEG telemetry and video tape monitoring. *J Pediatr* 1980; 97:554–558.

127. Lesser RP. Psychogenic seizures. *Neurology* 1996; 46:1499–1507.

128. Metrick ME, Ritter FJ, Gates JR, et al. Nonepileptic events in childhood. *Epilepsia* 1991; 32:322–328.

129. Walczak TS, Williams DT, Berten W. Utility and reliability of placebo infusion in the evaluation of patients with seizures. *Neurology* 1994; 44:394–399.

CHAPTER 9

The Use of Electroencephalography in the Diagnosis of Epilepsy in Childhood

Douglas R. Nordli, Jr., M.D., and Timothy A. Pedley, M.D.

The electroencephalogram (EEG) is often the single most informative laboratory test in evaluating children with seizures. At the most rudimentary level, it helps in differentiating epileptic from nonepileptic behavior. Because many conditions, including breathholding spells, movement disorders, syncope and cardiac arrhythmias, sleep disorders, migraine, and various psychiatric syndromes, may mimic epilepsy, EEG findings are often essential in making an accurate diagnosis.

EEG, however, offers much more. More detailed analysis of epileptiform abnormalities assists in distinguishing partial from generalized seizures and in identifying epileptic syndromes, which are indispensable cornerstones of rational therapy. EEG aids in recognizing subclinical and nonconvulsive seizures, in documenting antiepileptic drug (AED) toxicity, and probably in selecting patients for AED withdrawal after remission of seizures. Finally, EEG is critical in evaluating patients with medically refractory seizures for focal resective and other surgical procedures.

EEG TECHNIQUE

To record the EEG, a technician places electrodes, usually gold or silver discs, at standard locations on the scalp using collodion adhesive or a conducting paste. Potential differences between pairs of electrodes are then amplified, and the net signal from each amplifier is displayed on a monitor (digital EEG machines) or written on paper (historical EEG machines) to provide a graphic record of EEG voltage changes over time. In practice, modern EEG machines display activity from 20 or more channels (1 pair of electrodes = 1 amplifier channel) simultaneously to provide a comprehensive survey of cerebral electrical activity.

Much of the value of EEG lies in determining the *spatial distribution* of voltage fields on the scalp. To do this, electrodes are grouped in logical arrangements called montages. Montages typically allow comparisons between symmetric areas of the two hemispheres and between parasagittal and temporal areas in the same hemisphere. Most laboratories use as minimum a series of standard montages recommended by the American EEG Society (1). In addition to these, special montages may have to be designed to address issues posed by a particular patient. Creative use of rationally designed montages significantly enhances the utility of the EEG.

A technician typically records spontaneous EEG activity for approximately 30 minutes. However, the yield of positive findings is greatly increased by several activating procedures: hyperventilation, photic stimulation, and sleep. All three are useful in children with suspected seizures or epilepsy.

Hyperventilation

Hyperventilation for at least 3 minutes, preferably 5 minutes if absence seizures are strongly suspected, should be performed whenever possible. Overbreathing can be achieved even with preschool children if the technician incorporates playful strategies such as blowing a pinwheel or "having a race" to see who can breathe faster. The effect of hyperventilation on EEG activity in children is usually dramatic, with high-voltage, generalized, rhythmic slow waves appearing promptly (Figure 9-1). The mechanisms underlying this age-related normal phenomenon are not known, but changes in cerebral blood flow and the neuronal metabolic milieu are probable factors. What is more important, however, is the empiric observation that a

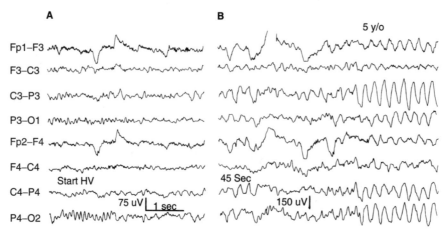

Figure 9-1. Effects of hyperventilation in a 5-year-old child. **A.** EEG at onset of overbreathing effort; **B.** 45 seconds later. There is a moderate buildup of generalized rhythmic slow-wave activity, maximal over the posterior head regions.

brief period of vigorous overbreathing potently activates generalized epileptiform discharges, especially 3-Hz spike-wave activity. Sometimes focal slow-wave activity associated with structural lesions may appear or be accentuated during hyperventilation. The only responses to hyperventilation that can be unambiguously categorized as abnormal are asymmetric changes and epileptiform discharges.

Photic Stimulation

Photic stimulation is performed using stroboscopic flashes of high-intensity white light at rates of 1 to 30 flashes per second. Stimulation is intermittent, with each frequency delivered for 10 to 20 seconds. A normal physiologic response is entrainment of EEG activity over the occipital lobes at the flash frequency (photic driving) (Figure 9-2A). In some normal children, photic stimulation produces no effect, and in others, the photic driving may be asymmetric. A photoparoxysmal response characterized by generalized bursts of irregular spikes, spike-wave discharges, and multiple spike-wave discharges (Figure 9-2B) occurs in some patients with idiopathic generalized epilepsy. However, it also occurs in a significant percentage of normal children without seizures, presumably as an asymptomatic marker of a genetic trait. Doose and Gerken (2) propose a multifactorial mode of inheritance.

Sleep and Sleep Deprivation

Light sleep substantially increases the percentage of EEGs showing epileptiform activity in patients with epilepsy. The occurrences of both focal and generalized discharges are increased in non–rapid eye movement (non-REM) sleep, but rapid eye movement (REM) sleep has a differential effect. Generalized epileptiform activity diminishes markedly or disappears altogether in REM, whereas focal spikes and sharp waves are either unaffected or actually increase in abundance (3).

Sleep deprivation also activates epileptiform activity independent of its sleep-inducing effect (4,5). Kellaway and Frost (6) have speculated that sleep deprivation and spontaneous or sedated sleep activate abnormalities via different mechanisms.

Scheduling the EEG at the time a child normally naps facilitates sleep recordings. Older children may be partially sleep-deprived with benefit. If children do not sleep spontaneously, they may be given chloral hydrate (30–60 mg/kg).

Special Electrodes

Some cortical areas (mesial temporal, orbital frontal, and interhemispheric regions) are relatively inaccessible to conventional recording electrodes. If one of these areas is suspected of being the epileptogenic focus, supplemental electrode placements can augment standard ones. Thus, surface placement of anterior temporal, mandibular notch, and supraorbital electrodes are useful in documenting inferior frontal and mesiobasal temporal epileptiform discharges (7).

More invasively, sphenoidal electrodes, which are fine wires inserted transcutaneously through the mandibular notch so that the tips lie near the foramen ovale at the base of the skull, are commonly used in monitoring units evaluating patients for resective surgery (8). Nasopharyngeal electrodes, which are flexible wires that are inserted through the nose to lie in the posterior pharynx, have been widely used in the past, but subsequent studies have cast doubt on their superiority over surface locations, especially anterior and inferior temporal leads, in recording mesial temporal lobe discharges (7,9,10).

Invasive electrodes should not be used in children except in special circumstances. Maximal information can be obtained routinely using standard scalp

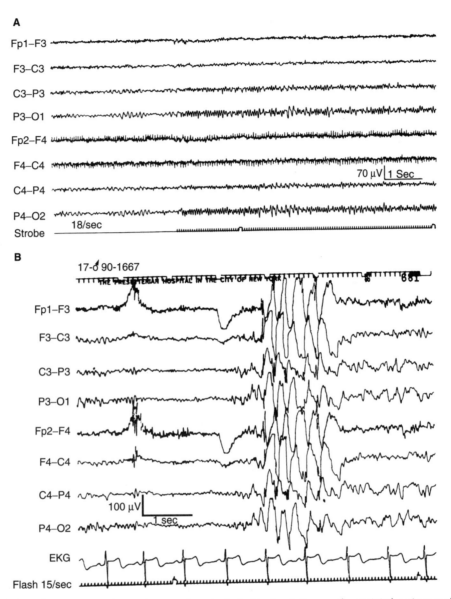

Figure 9-2. A. Normal physiologic response is entrainment of cerebral electrical activity over the occipital regions at the frequency of light stimulation (driving response). **B**. Photoparoxysmal response in another child occurring during stroboscopic light stimulation. Bursts of spikes and irregular spike-wave discharges occur during and immediately after the light stimulus. In this case, there were no clinical manifestations during the photoparoxysmal response and no clinical history of photosensitivity.

electrodes supplemented, as necessary, with additional special placements.

SPECIFIC EEG FINDINGS

Epileptiform Activity and Epileptogenicity

The only EEG finding that indicates a susceptibility to epileptic seizures is epileptiform activity, that is, spikes, sharp waves, or spike-wave discharges (Figure 9-3).

Although epileptiform discharges indicate an increased risk of seizures, they vary in degree of epileptogenicity, that is, the association with active epilepsy. Epileptogenicity is at least partly age-related. In adults, epileptiform discharges have a high association with seizures and occur only rarely in normal individuals. The situation is more complicated in children, largely because of the occurrence of genetic patterns that may not be associated with clinical seizures. Nonetheless, even in children, epileptiform discharges are uncommon in normal individuals, approximating perhaps 2 percent in the prevalence studies of Petersen and coworkers (11). From another perspective, Trojaborg (12) found that 83 percent of children whose EEGs contained focal spikes had seizures.

Another variable that relates to epileptogenicity is location of the discharge. The likelihood of epilepsy

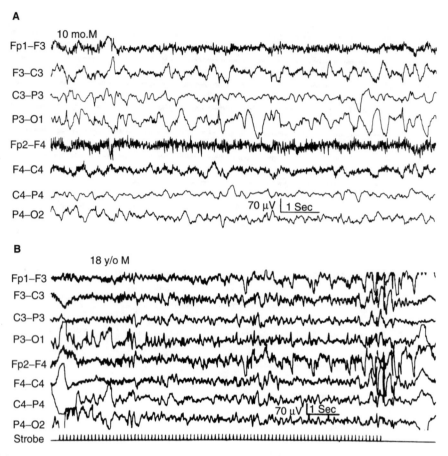

Figure 9-3. A. Focal left parietal spikes (discharge is at P3 in channels 3 and 4) in a 10-month-old boy with simple partial seizures involving his right arm and face. **B**. Generalized 4- to 5-Hz spike-wave activity in an 18-year-old male with idiopathic generalized tonic-clonic seizures.

is highest when epileptiform discharges are multifocal or when they involve the temporal lobe: 76 percent and 90 percent, respectively (13). Risk of epilepsy is considerably lower (approximately 50 percent) when epileptiform activity involves the central-midtemporal (rolandic) or occipital regions (13).

All epileptiform activity decreases in abundance with age or the passage of time, and less than 10 percent persists indefinitely (13). In general, there is no useful correlation in individual patients between the amount of epileptiform activity in the EEG and the number and intensity of clinical seizures.

NONSPECIFIC EEG ABNORMALITIES

Abnormalities other than epileptiform discharges are also common in the EEGs of patients with epilepsy. Nonepileptiform abnormalities are termed *nonspecific* because they occur in many other conditions as well, or sometimes even in normal subjects. Examples of nonspecific abnormalities include focal or generalized slow-wave activity (Figure 9-4) or, less often, asymmetries of frequency or voltage. Unlike epileptiform discharges, such findings do not provide support for

a diagnosis of epilepsy because of their varied clinical associations and because they do not reflect an epileptogenic disturbance of neuronal function. Nonspecific findings are important, however, in providing general information about cerebral function. Thus, evaluation of nonspecific EEG abnormalities may help identify associated static or reversible encephalopathies, underlying focal cerebral lesions, or progressive neurologic syndromes.

PEDIATRIC EPILEPTIC SYNDROMES

Electroencephalography is crucial for accurate classification of different forms of epilepsy. The following are brief descriptions of EEG findings in the more common epileptic syndromes encountered in childhood.

Infantile Spasms (West's Syndrome)

The EEG is always abnormal, grossly so if obtained when seizures are well established. Gibbs and Gibbs (14) identified the most characteristic pattern, hypsarrhythmia, which consists of high-voltage, irregular slow waves occurring asynchronously and randomly

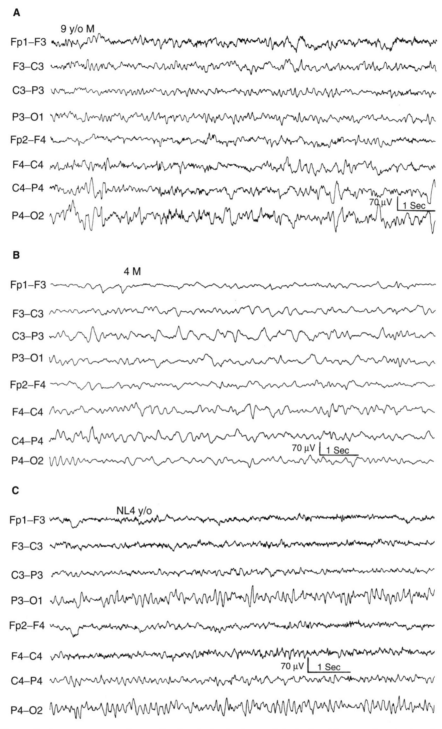

Figure 9-4. A. This EEG sample demonstrates continuous focal arrhythmic slow activity in the right central-parietal region (channels 6–8). **B**. In contrast, this EEG sample shows excessive generalized arrhythmic slow activity. The EEG of a normal 4-year-old is shown for comparison **(C)**.

over all head regions intermixed with spikes and polyspikes from multiple independent loci (Figure 9-5). Variations of the pattern (modified hypsarrhythmia) are common (15), and abnormalities other than hypsarrhythmia occur in up to 10 percent to 15 percent of children with infantile spasms. These other abnormalities, however, are more likely to occur in older infants or if the EEG is performed later in the course of the disorder. Like infantile spasms, hypsarrhythmia is age-specific. It is usually most pronounced in slow-wave sleep and may disappear completely in REM.

Ictal recordings show various patterns (16), but the most common accompaniment to a spasm is one or more generalized, high-voltage slow or sharp-slow

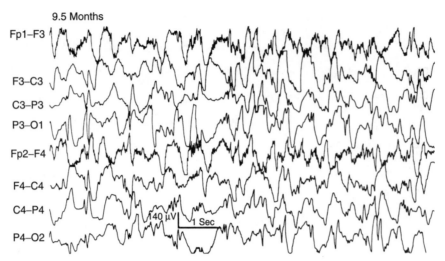

Figure 9-5. Hypsarrhythmia in a 9.5-month-old infant with infantile spasms. There is extremely high-voltage slow-wave activity diffusely, multifocal spikes, and lack of normal organization and patterns.

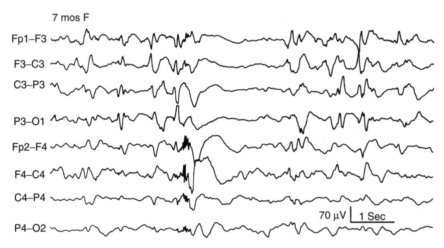

Figure 9-6. Electrodecremental event in a 7-month-old child characterized by transient flattening of background activity *(middle of figure)* Such events frequently accompany the massive spasms of West's syndrome.

waves followed by abrupt voltage attenuation of background activity lasting from 1 to several seconds, the so-called *electrodecremental event* (Figure 9-6) (17). Type of spasm does not correlate well with a particular EEG ictal pattern, and neither do all spasms have EEG correlates. EEG and clinical improvement usually parallel one another, but they may be dissociated.

Childhood Absence Epilepsy

EEGs are rarely normal in untreated children with childhood absence epilepsy (petit mal epilepsy), and hyperventilation is particularly effective in provoking the characteristic EEG abnormality. In fact, repeated normal EEGs in a child with lapse attacks argue strongly against a diagnosis of childhood absence epilepsy. Each absence seizure is accompanied by generalized, symmetric, stereotyped 3- to 4-Hz spike-wave

activity (Figure 9-7A). Background activity is otherwise normal or near normal. Sleep produces striking effects on appearance of the epileptiform activity (Figure 9-7B). Classic features are lost, and instead epileptiform bursts are fragmented, are of shorter duration, and contain more single spikes and multiple spikes.

Spike-wave paroxysms begin abruptly, producing immediate alteration in the child's responsiveness (18). Conversely, when the 3-Hz spike-wave discharge ends, the child's behavior becomes normal at once (18). Detailed analysis of motor and cognitive effects reveals differences in their time course and evolution in relation to the ictal discharge (19). Even short bursts of 3-Hz spike-wave activity produce some functional impairment that may go unrecognized clinically. Thus, childhood absence epilepsy is one instance in which follow-up EEGs are often necessary to gauge how

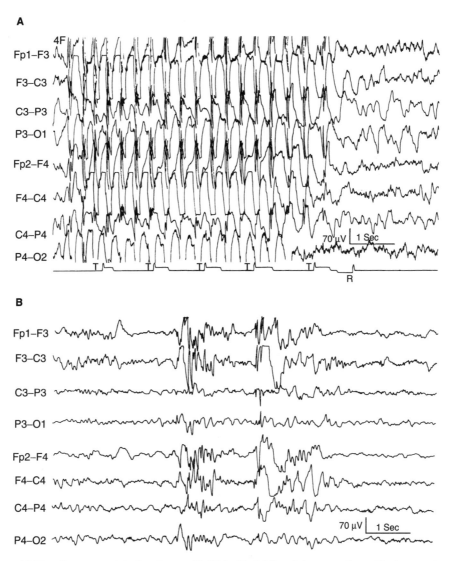

Figure 9-7. A. Stereotyped 3-Hz spike-wave activity in a 4-year-old child with childhood absence epilepsy. The bottom channel records a test tone (T) that the child has been trained to respond to by pressing a button (R). During the generalized spike-wave activity, the child's ability to respond is impaired (absence attack). Normal responsiveness returns immediately upon cessation of the discharge. **B**. EEG from same child showing alteration in spike-wave morphology during sleep. The epileptiform activity has become fragmented and contains multiple spikes (polyspikes). The well-formed 3-Hz spike-wave complexes seen during wakefulness no longer occur. Such changes, although varying in degree, are typical of generalized epileptiform abnormalities.

effective treatment is; clinical reports alone may be inadequate.

Lennox-Gastaut Syndrome

The name *Lennox-Gastaut syndrome* (childhood epileptic encephalopathy) has been applied to a heterogeneous group of children with severe seizures, mental retardation, and a characteristic EEG pattern. EEG findings are most typical between 2 and 7 years of age and are remarkably consistent despite widely different underlying causes, including progressive degenerative or metabolic disease, cerebral malformations, perinatal asphyxia, severe head injury, anoxic encephalopathy, and central nervous system infection (20).

EEGs show generalized, bisynchronous sharp-and-slow wave complexes occurring repetitively, often in extended runs, at 1.5 to 2.5 Hz (Figure 9-8). Within the same record and among patients, the sharp-slow waves vary somewhat in distribution, voltage, and repetition rate. Sleep usually activates epileptiform activity markedly; hyperventilation does so less consistently. Multifocal spikes or sharp waves also occur, especially in older children. Electrodecremental or tonic seizure patterns (Figure 9-9) lasting 2 to 4 seconds occur frequently during sleep, sometimes as often as hundreds of times per night. Clinical correlates of these nocturnal seizure discharges are minimal, most often being slight stiffening of the axial muscles. Background activity is almost always moderately to severely abnormal

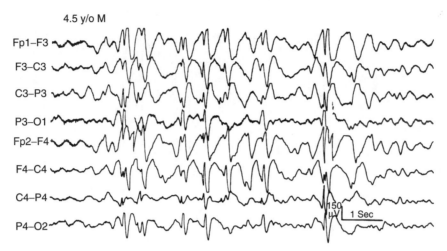

Figure 9-8. Generalized sharp and slow-wave complexes (slow spike-and-wave discharges) occurring repetitively at about 2-Hz in a child with Lennox-Gastaut syndrome.

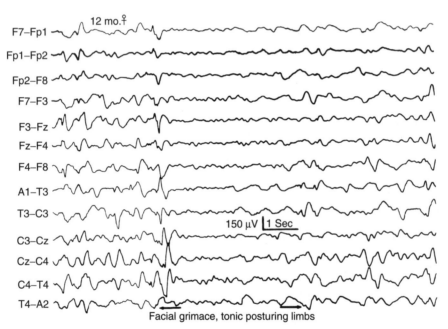

Figure 9-9. Tonic seizure during sleep in a child with severe mental retardation and uncontrolled tonic, atonic, and atypical absence seizures The EEG correlate is an electrodecremental event, Sometimes a low voltage 16- to 25-Hz rhythmic discharge (tonic seizure pattern) occurs during this type of clinical event.

because of excessive slowing and poor development of normal patterns for age.

A history of West's syndrome is present in up to one-third of children with Lennox-Gastaut syndrome (21), suggesting that EEG manifestations of severe encephalopathies reflect, in part, an age-dependent continuum with particular patterns emerging from interaction of maturational and pathologic factors.

Benign Focal Epilepsy with Central-Midtemporal Spikes

The syndrome of benign focal epilepsy with central-midtemporal spikes, which is also referred to

as central-temporal epilepsy, sylvian seizures, and rolandic epilepsy, is an idiopathic localization-related epilepsy with highly characteristic EEG and clinical features (22–24).

EEG findings are distinctive and diagnostic. Focal di- or triphasic sharp waves of almost invariant morphology occur in the central and midtemporal. regions (Figure 9-10). Epileptiform discharges are usually of high voltage (>100 μV), tend to occur in clusters, and activate dramatically during sleep, when they may seem almost continuous. Discharges may be unilateral in a single EEG, but they are almost always bilaterally present with prolonged or repeated

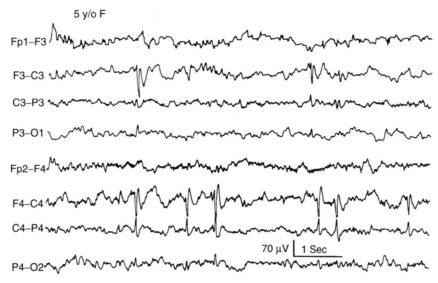

Figure 9-10. Stereotyped di- and triphasic sharp wave discharges occur independently in the central regions bilaterally in this child with idiopathic partial seizures (benign rolandic epilepsy).

recordings. Lateralization may switch in serial tracings (22,23). Generalized spikes and spike-wave activity occasionally occur, usually during sleep (23,25,26), and "benign" occipital spikes or multifocal spikes may coexist, especially in younger patients (22,25).

There is no correlation between EEG findings and seizure occurrence or frequency. As a rule, EEG abnormalities are much more impressive than clinical seizure activity. Indeed, when central-midtemporal spikes are recorded in children without seizures who have EEGs for other reasons, only about half eventually develop typical seizures (13). Furthermore, in symptomatic children, EEG abnormalities persist long after seizures cease. Thus, EEG does not provide assistance in making decisions about when or how long to treat.

Genetic studies indicate that the EEG trait is controlled by an autosomal dominant gene with age-dependent penetrance (27,28).

Benign Focal Epilepsy with Occipital Spikes

Gastaut (29) has described another form of idiopathic localization-related epilepsy in children, in which visual symptoms, either amblyopia or hallucinations, are a common early feature of ictal events. The EEG shows stereotyped, high-voltage (200–300 μV) sharp-wave discharges over one or both occipital regions. Epileptiform activity is attenuated by eye opening and is activated by sleep. Discharge morphology resembles that of central-midtemporal spikes. Background activity is normal. This electroclinical entity is more heterogeneous than benign focal epilepsy with central-midtemporal spikes. Nonetheless, outcome is usually benign in a typical case, with complete resolution of clinical and EEG findings in most children by 18 years

of age. Like central-midtemporal spikes, occipital spikes do not correlate with clinical seizure activity or prognosis, and they often persist after seizures cease. Generalized spike-wave discharges and central-midtemporal spikes may coexist.

Juvenile Myoclonic Epilepsy

Janz and Christian (30) described juvenile myoclonic epilepsy (JME) or "impulsive petit mal" as a subtype of idiopathic generalized epilepsy. Interictal EEGs show generalized 4- to 6-Hz "atypical" spike-wave activity, short bursts of polyspikes, and polyspike-wave discharges (Figure 9-11). An incrementing run of 10- to 16-Hz polyspikes, maximal over the frontal-central areas, followed by a generalized burst of spikes or spike-wave activity accompanies bilateral myoclonic jerks (30,31). If absence seizures occur, the EEG shows 3.5- to 4-Hz generalized spike-wave paroxysms. Photoparoxysmal responses are common in JME, occurring in approximately one-third of patients (32).

Acquired Epileptic Aphasia

Acquired epileptic aphasia, which is also known as the Landau-Kleffner syndrome, is not primarily an epileptic disorder, although epileptiform activity is part of the diagnostic criteria. Seizures occur in approximately 70 percent of cases but usually are infrequent. EEGs show abundant high-voltage epileptiform activity, which may be temporal, bitemporal, or generalized. Considerable slow activity accompanies epileptiform discharges. In the early stages, EEG abnormalities may occur only during sleep, and throughout the illness slow-wave sleep produces marked activation, sometimes with almost continuous generalized

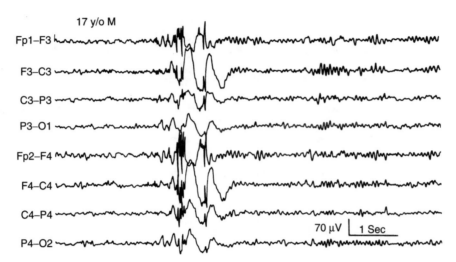

Figure 9-11. Generalized multiple spike-wave (polyspike-wave) discharge followed by a single spike-wave complex in a child with juvenile myoclonic epilepsy.

spike-wave activity. Review of the original case (33) and subsequent cases (34–37) of acquired epileptic aphasia does not support any single EEG feature or combination of features as being distinctive of this syndrome. AED treatment does not clearly alter the natural evolution of EEG abnormalities, clinical findings, or outcome.

Epilepsia Partialis Continua

Epilepsia partialis continua manifests as several different subtypes, but one variant — Rasmussen's syndrome — occurs primarily in children as a reasonably distinct entity (38). EEG findings are variable, and their topography is often difficult to characterize precisely (38,39). Most often, interictal EEGs show excessive arrhythmic or rhythmic delta activity that is usually bilateral but accentuated over a large area contralateral to the partial seizures. Epileptiform discharges are rarely well localized and often sporadic, especially early in the illness. As the disease progresses, more abundant pleomorphic spikes and sharp waves appear over an extensive area or bilaterally. It is usually difficult to recognize distinct ictal discharges with scalp recordings; in any event, correlation of EEG changes with muscle jerks is always poor to nonexistent.

NEONATAL EEG

EEGs of neonates pose special problems in interpretation. From 26 to 40 weeks of gestation, there are explosive maturational changes in the brain that result in rapid changes in neuronal orientation, alignment, and layering accompanied by substantial dendritic development, extensive synaptogenesis, glial proliferation, and onset of myelination. These biological developments underlie rapid and predictable sequences of EEG changes that are sufficiently consistent as to allow

accurate determination of conceptional age in healthy newborns to within 2 weeks.

EEGs in newborns are sufficiently different from those of older children and adults that one must take considerable caution not to overinterpret the significance of certain normal or inconsistent findings, all of which may be only transiently present. Thus, isolated spikes, or sharp transients, are common normal components of the newborn's EEG, and their significance depends on their location and abundance and the infant's state and conceptional age. Tharp (40), Lombroso (41), and Hrachovy and coworkers (42) give complete discussions of neonatal EEG interpretation.

Just as there are special considerations that relate generally to EEG interpretation in the newborn, some cautionary notes are indicated about using EEG in diagnosing and treating newborns with seizures. EEG background activity characterized in terms of expected developmental features provides important information about the extent to which cortical physiology is normally maintained or disturbed (Figure 9-12). Background activity often deteriorates transiently following a seizure because of associated hypoxia or other metabolic stresses. Interictal background activity, therefore, is extremely variable, reflecting the severity of any encephalopathy underlying or associated with seizures and the timing of the EEG in relation to seizure activity. In some infants, specific patterns or evolution of findings on repeated EEGs provide helpful and reliable prognostic information. When using EEG background activity to help predict long-term neurologic outcome, interpretation should be based on interictal tracings to avoid problems related to reversible postictal abnormalities. Identifying and visually quantifying spikes is important, but in newborns these results are less an indication of specific susceptibility to seizures (epileptogenicity) than a measure of the underlying encephalopathy. In general, one should be

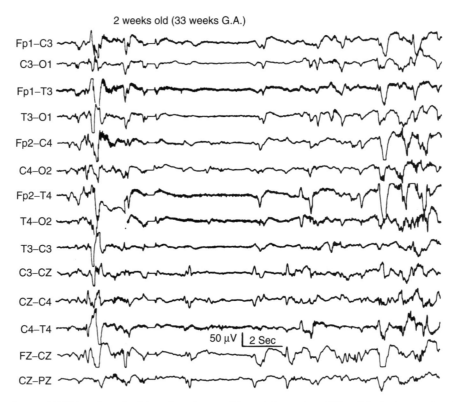

2 weeks old (33 weeks G.A.)

Figure 9-12. Severely abnormal EEG in a 2-week-old newborn born at 33 weeks' gestation. EEG activity is depressed and poorly differentiated bilaterally, with intermittent low-voltage activity and random sharp transients punctuated by higher voltage mixed-frequency burst activity. Note the positive sharp transients occurring at Cz (channels 10–11 and 13–14) *(middle portion of figure)*. Such positive rolandic discharges have a high correlation with periventricular leukomalacia.

extremely conservative in using interictal spikes or sharp waves to diagnose neonatal seizures.

To establish that an observed behavior is an epileptic seizure, one must record an associated ictal discharge. This can be done using conventional EEG recording if the technician makes copious and temporally accurate notations on the tracing. Better still, however, are simultaneous EEG, polygraphic, and video recordings, which provide objective documentation of the relationship among EEG activity, other physiologic variables, and behavior. Kellaway and colleagues at Baylor College of Medicine have exploited this methodology creatively to identify epileptic and nonepileptic paroxysmal behaviors and to propose a new classification of neonatal seizures (43–45). Such data indicate that one must be cautious in inferring an epileptic basis for all paroxysmal clinical events and that concurrent EEG recordings are usually necessary to distinguish epileptic seizures from similar phenomena caused by different mechanisms (43,46).

Focal or multifocal clonic seizures, focal tonic seizures, some generalized myoclonic seizures, and ictal apnea are consistently associated with EEG ictal patterns. In contrast, staring, ocular movements, excessive salivation, and various autonomic phenomena occurring in isolation, such as changes in heart rate and blood pressure, may be accompanied by EEG discharges but often are not. Motor automatisms, including various oral-buccal-lingual movements; progression movements such as stepping, pedaling, or swimming; and complex asynchronous motor activities such as thrashing and writhing, are not consistently accompanied by EEG seizure patterns. Generalized tonic seizures in the newborn also have no EEG correlate. These latter events presumably arise either from nondetectable (at the scalp) epileptic mechanisms or, more likely, from nonepileptic dysfunction of motor systems at subcortical and brainstem levels (release phenomena) (43).

Ictal discharges are almost always focal or multifocal in newborns, with variable spread to ipsilateral regions and the contralateral hemisphere (Figure 9-13). Repetitive rapid spiking is unusual at this age, especially in premature babies, and most seizure patterns consist of rhythmic sequences at almost any frequency or slowly repetitive (0.5–2 Hz) sharp waves. Seizures may occur simultaneously in the same hemisphere or in different hemispheres and progress independently.

LONG-TERM MONITORING

It is often desirable to record EEG activity for longer periods than conventional EEG recordings allow to

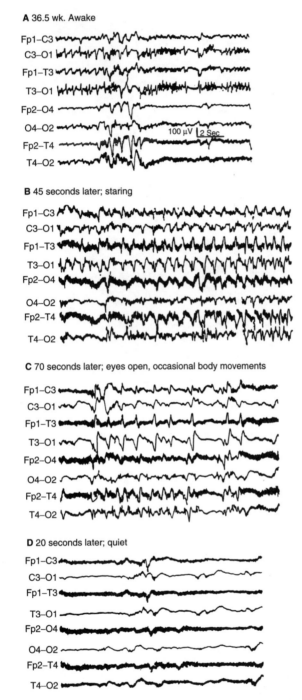

A 36.5 wk. Awake

Fp1–C3
C3–O1
Fp1–T3
T3–O1
Fp2–O4
O4–O2
Fp2–T4
T4–O2

100 µV | 2 Sec

B 45 seconds later; staring

Fp1–C3
C3–O1
Fp1–T3
T3–O1
Fp2–O4
O4–O2
Fp2–T4
T4–O2

C 70 seconds later; eyes open, occasional body movements

Fp1–C3
C3–O1
Fp1–T3
T3–O1
Fp2–O4
O4–O2
Fp2–T4
T4–O2

D 20 seconds later; quiet

Fp1–C3
C3–O1
Fp1–T3
T3–O1
Fp2–O4
O4–O2
Fp2–T4
T4–O2

Figure 9-13. EEG of a newborn with a postconceptional age of 36.5 weeks demonstrating onset of a repetitive sharp wave discharge from the left occipital region (**A**). Forty-five seconds later the discharge involves the entire left hemisphere and is associated with staring (**B**). Simultaneously, there is a buildup of spiking in the right temporal area that evolves independently from the seizure pattern on the left (**B, C**). The baby's eyes remain open, and there are occasional irregular body movements (**C**). Just over 2 minutes after the seizure begins, clinical and EEG seizure activity subside, and EEG background is severely depressed bilaterally (**D**).

increase the likelihood of detecting epileptiform activity or capturing intermittent behavioral events. Two methods of long-term monitoring are now widely available; they have greatly improved diagnostic accuracy and reliability of seizure classification. Both have value in providing continuous recordings through one or more complete wake-sleep cycles and in documenting ictal episodes. Each has additional specific advantages and disadvantages (47–49). Which method one selects depends on the question posed by a particular patient. Gumnit (50) has provided a useful overview.

Ambulatory Monitoring

Multichannel cassette records allow relatively inexpensive continuous EEG recording in the outpatient setting. In terms of EEG information alone, ambulatory cassette recordings are only slightly less accurate in yield of epileptiform abnormalities than recordings made in intensive monitoring units (51). For this purpose, both methods are substantially more useful than routine EEG. Ambulatory EEG is often especially helpful in the pediatric setting, where the young child is often more comfortable in his familiar and unrestricted home environment (52). Limitations include the relatively limited coverage of cortical areas and the absence of video documentation. Thus, ambulatory cassette recordings are inadequate for detailed localization of epileptogenic foci, and very discrete foci may be missed. Furthermore, negative ambulatory EEG recordings are not usually helpful when the question is one of nonepileptic paroxysmal events. Here the video image of the child is frequently indispensable in recognizing and definitively characterizing the event.

Most makers of ambulatory EEG equipment have also converted to digital technology. This technique has all of the advantages of digital technology (see below), allows more channels to be recorded, and offers automated computerized detection of interictal and ictal discharges. These technical advantages have greatly expanded the role of ambulatory monitoring.

Intensive Closed Circuit Television–EEG Monitoring

Closed circuit television (CCTV)–EEG monitoring in a specialty equipped inpatient unit is the procedure of choice to document pseudoseizures, establish precise electrical–clinical correlations, and localize epileptogenic foci for resective surgery Emphasis in intensive monitoring units usually is on behavioral events, not interictal activity.

Demonstrating that an electrical seizure discharge accompanies undiagnosed disturbances in behavior is unequivocal proof of an epileptic mechanism. Unfortunately, the converse is not true without qualifications. Various physiologic and technical considerations conspire to obscure some ictal discharges and thus lead potentially to false-negative results. When the epileptogenic focus lies deep to the surface and the ictal discharge remains localized to this area, scalp recordings may be negative. For example, epileptiform discharges confined to mesiobasal limbic structures may go undetected at the scalp. This means that simple partial seizures manifesting as autonomic, cognitive, affective, or special sensory changes (auras) have EEG correlates in only approximately 15 percent of cases (53). As another confounding variable, consider epileptogenic foci whose physical geometry is such that electrical activity is not ideally oriented for detection by scalp electrodes. Discharges arising from orbital frontal or mesial parasagittal areas may not result in long current loops (dipoles) whose vectors are orthogonal to the surface, the optimal orientation for scalp detection of electrical events. Finally, seizures may be associated with sufficient muscle activity that high-voltage noncerebral electrical activity [electromyography (EMG), movement artifact] prevents detection of low-voltage EEG changes. This is frequently the case with frontal lobe seizures in which early onset of movement makes it difficult to determine whether EEG change has occurred. In the absence of an unambiguous ictal discharge, postictal slowing is usually indicative of a preceding epileptic event if similar changes are not seen in the preseizure record.

To enhance detection of ictal discharges, especially their earliest manifestations, and to provide a comprehensive analysis of the epileptogenic region, most laboratories supplement usual EEG recording sites with additional placements, including extratemporal electrodes, nasopharyngeal and sphenoidal electrodes, and supraorbital electrodes. Because of the many additional recording sites, it is not unusual for monitoring units to record simultaneously from 32, 64, or even more channels. The need for many recording channels is even more urgent when intracranial electrodes are used. These may be depth probes, subdural strips, or subdural grids, each containing multiple recording contacts. Intracranial electrodes are required in patients being evaluated for resective surgery when extensive surface (including sphenoidal) recordings do not provide definitive localization of the epileptogenic zone (54–57) or when other clinical data conflict with EEG findings (58).

A variety of ictal patterns may be seen in children. For the most part, these are similar to those encountered in adults. Focal ictal discharges are often characterized by sustained runs of rhythmic delta or theta-alpha activity that evolve in frequency and voltage. Generalized convulsive seizures may be characterized by runs of diffuse rhythmic fast activity during tonic phases or runs of spike-wave discharges during clonic phases. Some patterns, however, are peculiar to children. Examples of these are runs of rhythmic positive sharp waves in some infantile focal seizures and electrodecremental events (Figure 9-6) during infantile spasms. Seizures in infants and young children usually are focal and secondarily generalize less often than in adolescents and adults. Bilaterally synchronous generalized ictal discharges occur only very rarely in infants less then 13 months old (59).

MAGNETOENCEPHALOGRAPHY

Magnetoencephalography (MEG) detects and measures magnetic activity of the cortex using superconductive quantum interference devices (SQUIDs). Neuronal aggregates that are current sources of brain electrical activity also generate magnetic fields. Models depicting the head as a homogeneously conducting sphere demonstrate that measurements of magnetic fields can provide three-dimensional localization of a neuronal source. MEG differs from EEG in ways that are potentially very useful. For example, MEG is more accurate than EEG in localizing dipoles of neuronal activity oriented parallel to the surface. Furthermore, MEG is relatively unaffected by overlying tissue and bone that significantly attenuate volume conduction of electrical potentials between cortex and scalp. Finally, MEG appears to arise solely from intracellular currents in active neurons (60, 61). Thus, for some current sources, MEG may offer greater spatial resolution than EEG.

Several investigators have used MEG to map epileptogenic foci, and results have compared favorably with EEG localization (61–64). Applications are currently limited by the complex technology required to detect the extraordinarily weak magnetic fields of the brain. Until now, most investigators have used only a single SQUID, which is then moved from place to place on the head. Multichannel recording is clearly feasible, however, and reports are appearing of recording devices with 20 or more channels. There is promise, therefore, of using MEG as a complement to EEG to improve source localization in studying epileptiform activity in people with epilepsy.

Digital technology has quickly changed how EEG signals are collected and stored in many laboratories across the country. One difference is that digital signals are not contaminated by sources of noise encountered with analog technologies. The EEG signal is electronically stored and may be reviewed in any desired montage, sensitivity, or filter setting. The digital format also allows for quantitative methods of EEG analysis, including Fourier (spectral cross-correlation) and cross-spectral analysis. In addition, interpolation techniques may be applied to estimate the electric potentials at intermediate scalp positions from known values at each electrode position. Topographic or spatial maps are another way of displaying EEG data that differs from the conventional display by producing maps of electrical potentials that loosely resemble images seen with MR or CT. Finally, source dipole localization has been proposed as a method to find the intracranial sources generating scalp potentials. Most of these techniques are still research tools and have not yet come into common clinical practice.

CONCLUSIONS

In this chapter we have indicated the role of EEG in evaluating children with known or suspected seizures. EEG is an important, perhaps *the* most important, adjunct to history and examination. But, as with any laboratory test, care and judgment must be used in relating EEG findings to other clinical data. Indeed, the full potential of EEG can only be realized when interpretations are placed in the full clinical context.

EEG interpretation in infants and children is complicated by two important considerations. First, many normal potentials are high-voltage, occur paroxysmally, and have spikey waveforms. Unusual benign variants are common. Thus, EEGs of children are easy to overinterpret or misinterpret. The second issue is that the developing brain has unique neuroanatomic, biochemical, and neurophysiologic features. The various EEG abnormalities in childhood epilepsy and the their clinical expression result from the interaction of developmental features with genetic or acquired pathology.

The EEG examination should always be framed to answer a particular question. There is no evidence that routine follow-up EEGs every 6 or 12 months serve any useful purpose. Dialogue between the clinician and laboratory is essential, especially if special recording circumstances are necessary to obtain maximal information. Questions that the EEG may help answer include:

1. Does the child have epilepsy?
2. Are seizures of localized or generalized onset?
3. Does the child fit a specific electroclinical syndrome?
4. Is clinical deterioration the result of unrecognized seizures, a progressive neurological syndrome, or drug toxicity?
5. Is the child a candidate for surgery?
6. Can AEDs be safely withdrawn?

REFERENCES

1. American EEG Society. Guidelines in EEG and evoked potentials. Guideline seven: a proposal for standard montages to be used in clinical EEG. *J Clin Neurophysiol* 1986; 3(Suppl 1):26–33.
2. Doose H, Gerken H. On the genetics of EEG anomalies in childhood. IV. Photoconvulsive reaction. *Neuropaediatrie* 1973; 4:162–171.
3. Dinner DS. Sleep and pediatric epilepsy *Cleve Clin J Med* 1989; 56(Suppl 2):S234–S239.
4. Ellingson RJ, Wilken V, Bennett DR. Efficacy of sleep deprivation as an activation procedure in epilepsy patients. *J Clin Neurophysiol* 1984; 1:83–101.
5. Rowan AJ, Veldhuizen RJ, Nagelkerke NJD. Comparative evaluation of sleep deprivation and sedated sleep EEGs as diagnostic aids in epilepsy. *Electroencephalogr Clin Neurophysiol* 1982; 54:357–364.
6. Kellaway P, Frost JD. Biorhythmic modulation of epileptic events. In: Pedley TA, Meldrum BS, eds. *Recent Advances in Epilepsy*. Edinburgh: Churchill-Livingstone, 1983:139–154.
7. Sadler RM, Goodwin J. Multiple electrodes for detecting spikes in partial complex seizures. *Can J Neurol Sci* 1989; 16:326–329.
8. Binnie CD, Marston D, Polkey CE, Amin D. Distribution of temporal spikes in relation to the sphenoidal electrode. *Electroencephalogr Clin Neurophysiol* 1989; 73:403–409.
9. Sperling MR, Engel J. Electroencephalographic recording from the temporal lobes: a comparison of ear, anterior temporal, and nasopharyngeal electrodes. *Ann Neurol* 1985; 17:510–513.
10. Sperling MR, Mendius JR, Engel J. Mesial temporal spikes: a simultaneous comparison of sphenoidal, nasopharyngeal, and ear electrodes. *Epilepsia* 1986; 27:81–86.
11. Petersen I, Eeg-Olofsson O, Sellden U. Paroxysmal activity in EEG of normal children. In: Kellaway P Petersen I, eds. *Clinical Electroencephalography of Children*. Stockholm: Alinquist and Wiksell, 1968:167–188.
12. Trojaborg W. Changes of spike foci in children. In: Kellaway P, Petersen I, eds. *Clinical Electroencephalography of Children*. Stockholm: Almquist and Wiksell, 1968:213–226.
13. Kellaway P. The incidence, significance, and natural history of spike foci in children. In: Henry CE, ed. *Current Clinical Neurophysiology, Update on EEG and Evoked Potentials*. New York: Elsevier North-Holland, 1980:151–175.
14. Gibbs RA, Gibbs EZ. *Atlas of Electroencephalography. Vol 2. Epilepsy*. Cambridge: Addison Wesley, 1952.
15. Hrachovy RA, Frost JD, Kellaway P. Hypsarrhythmia: variations on the theme. *Epilepsia* 1984; 25:317–325.
16. Kellaway P, Hrachovy RA, Frost JD, Zion T. Precise characterization and quantification of infantile spasms. *Ann Neurol* 1979; 6:214–218.
17. Hrachovy R, Frost JD. Infantile spasms. *Cleve Clin J Med* 1989; 56(Suppl 1):S10–S16.
18. Browne TR, Penry JK, Porter RJ, Dreifuss FE. Responsiveness before, during and after spike-wave paroxysms. *Neurology* 1974; 24:659–665.

19. Dalby MA. Epilepsy and 3 per second spike and wave rhythms. A clinical, electrographic and prognostic analysis of 346 patients. *Acta Neurol Scand* 1969; 45(Suppl 40):1–83.

20. Markand ON. Slow spike-wave activity in EEG and associated clinical features often called "Lennox" or "Lennox-Gastaut" syndrome. *Neurology* 1977; 27:746–757.

21. Roger J, Dravet C, Bureau M. The Lennox-Gastaut syndrome. *Cleve Clin J Med* 1989; 56(Suppl 2):S172–S180.

22. Lerman P, Kivity S. The benign focal epilepsies of childhood. In: Pedley TA, Meldrum BS, eds. *Recent Advances in Epilepsy.* Vol 3. Edinburgh: Churchill-Livingstone, 1986:137–156.

23. Loiseau P, Duche B. Benign childhood epilepsy with centrotemporal spikes. *Cleve Clin J Med* 1989;56:S17–S22.

24. Beaumanoir A, Ballis T, Varfis G, Ansari K. Benign epilepsy of childhood with rolandic spikes. *Epilepsia* 1974; 15:301–315.

25. Beaussart M. Benign epilepsy of childhood with rolandic (centrotemporal) paroxysmal foci. *Epilepsia* 1972; 13:795–811.

26. Petersen J, Nielsen CJ, Gulann NC. Atypical EEG abnormalities in children with benign partial (rolandic) epilepsy. *Acta Neurol Scand* 1983; 94(Suppl):57–62.

27. Bray FP, Wiser WC. Hereditary characteristics of familial temporal central focal epilepsy. *Pediatrics* 1965; 36:207–211.

28. Heijbel J, Blom S, Rasmuson M. Benign epilepsy of childhood with centrotemporal EEG foci: a genetic study. *Epilepsia* 1975; 16:285–293.

29. Gastaut H. A new type of epilepsy: benign partial epilepsy of childhood with occipital spike-waves. *Clin Electroencephalogr* 1982; 13:13–22.

30. Janz D, Christian W. Impulsiv-Petit mal. *Dtsch Z Nervenheilk* 1957; 176:348–386.

31. Delgado-Escueta AV, Enrile-Bascal FE. Juvenile myoclonic epilepsy of Janz. *Neurology* 1984; 34:285–294.

32. Wolf P, Goosses R. Relation of photosensitivity to epileptic syndromes. *J Neurol Neurosurg Psychiatry* 1986; 49:1368–1391.

33. Landau WM, Kleffner F. Syndrome of acquired aphasia with convulsive disorder in children. *Neurology* 1957; 7:523–530.

34. Holmes GL, McKeever M, Saunders Z. Epileptiform activity in aphasia of childhood: an epiphenomenon? *Epilepsia* 1981; 22:631–639.

35. Sato S, Dreifuss FE. Electroencephalographic findings in a patient with developmental expressive aphasia. *Neurology* 1973; 23:181–184.

36. Gascon G, Victor D, Lombroso L, Goodglass H. Language disorder, convulsive disorder and electroencephalographic abnormalities. *Arch Neurol* 1973; 28:156–162.

37. Sawhney INS, Suresh N, Dhand UK, Chopra JS. Acquired aphasia with epilepsy—Landau-Kleffner syndrome. *Epilepsia* 1988; 29:283–287.

38. Rasmussen T, Andermann E. Update on the syndrome of "chronic encephalitis" and epilepsy. *Cleve Clin J Med* 1989; 56(Suppl 2):S181–S184.

39. Bancaud J. Kojewnikow's syndrome (epilepsia partialis continua) in children. In: Roger J, Dravet C, Bureau M, Dreifuss FE, Wolf P, eds. *Epileptic Syndromes in Infancy, Childhood, and Adolescence.* London: John Libbey, 1985:286–298.

40. Tharp BR. Pediatric electroencephalography. In: Aminoff M, ed. *Electrodiagnosis in Clinical Neurology.* New York: Churchill-Livingstone, 1986:67–117.

41. Lombroso CT. Neonatal electroencephalography In: Neidermeyer E, Lopes da Silva E, eds.*Electroencephalography: Basic Principles: Clinical Applications, and Related Fields.* Baltimore: Urban & Schwarzenberg, 1987:72 5–62.

42. Hrachovy RA, Mizrahi EM, Kellaway P. Neonatal EEG. In: Daly DD, Pedley TA, eds. *Current Practice of EEG.* 2nd ed. New York: Raven Press, 1990.

43. Mizrahi EM, Kellaway R. Characterization and classification of neonatal seizures. *Neurology* 1987; 37:1837–1844.

44. Kellaway P, Mizrahi EM. Clinical, electroencephalographic, therapeutic, and pathophysiologic studies of neonatal seizures. In: Wasterlain CG, Vert P, eds. *Neonatal Seizures. Pathophysiology and Pharmacologic Management.* New York: Raven Press, 1989.

45. Mizrahi EM. Clinical and neurophysiologic correlates of neonatal seizures. *Cleve Clin J Med* 1989; 56(Suppl 1):S100–S104.

46. Volpe JJ. Neonatal seizures: current concepts and revised classification. *Pediatrics* 1989; 84:422–428.

47. Binnie CD. Telemetric EEG monitoring in epilepsy In: Pedley TA, Meldrum BS, eds. *Recent Advances in Epilepsy.* Edinburgh: Churchill-Livingstone. 1983:155–178.

48. Binnie CD, Rowan AJ, Overweg, et al. Telemetric EEG and video monitoring in epilepsy. *Neurology* 1981; 31:298–303.

49. Kaplan P, Lesser R. Long-term monitoring. In: Daly DD, Pedley TA, eds. *Current Practice of EEG.* 2nd ed. New York: Raven Press, 1990.

50. Gumnit RJ. Intensive neurodiagnostic monitoring: role in the treatment of seizures. *Neurology* 1986; 36:1340–1346.

51. Bridgers SL, Ebersole JS. The clinical utility of ambulatory cassette EEG monitoring. *Neurology* 1985; 35:166–173.

52. Stores G. Ambulatory diagnostic monitoring of seizures in children. In: Gumnit RJ, ed. *Intensive Neurodiagnostic Monitoring.* New York: Raven Press, 1987:157–167. Advances in Neurology, vol. 46.

53. Devinsky O, Kelley K, Porter RJ, Theodore WH. Clinical and electroencephalographic features of simple partial seizures. *Neurology* 1988; 38:1347–1352.

54. Lüders H, Hahn J, Lesser RP, et al. Basal temporal subdural electrodes in the evaluation of patients with intractable epilepsy. *Epilepsia* 1989; 30:131–142.

55. Spencer SS, Spencer DD, Williamson PD, Mattson R. Combined depth and subdural electrode investigation in uncontrolled epilepsy. *Neurology* 1990; 40:74–79.

56. Wyler AR, Richey ET, Hermann BP Comparison of scalp to subdural recordings for localizing epileptogenic foci. *J Epilepsy* 1989; 2:91–96.

57. Sperling MR, O'Connor MJ. Comparison of depth and subdural electrodes in recording temporal lobe seizures. *Neurology* 1989; 39:1497–1504.

58. Sammaritano M, De Lotbiniere A, Andermann F, et al. False lateralization by surface EEG of seizure onset in patients with temporal lobe epilepsy and gross focal cerebral lesions. *Ann Neurol* 1987; 21:361–369.

59. Nordli DR, Bazil CW, Scheuer ML, Pedley TA. Recognition and classification of seizures in infants. *Epilepsia* 1997; 38:553–560.

60. Williamson SJ, Kaufman L. Analysis of neuromagnetic signals. In: Gevins AS, Remon A, eds. Methods of analysis of brain electrical and magnetic signals.

1987:405–448. Handbook of Electroencephalography and Clinical Neurophysiology, revised series, vol. 1.

61. Salustri C, Chapman RM. A simple method for 3-dimensional localization of epileptic activity recorded by simultaneous EEG and MEG. *Electroencephalogr Clin Neurophysiol* 1989; 73:473–478.

62. Ricci GB, Romani GL, Modena I, et al. Magnetic recording (MEG) in epilepsy. *Electroencephalogr Clin Neurophysiol* 1981; 52:S95.

63. Barth DS, Baumgartner C, Sutherling WW. Neuromagnetic field modeling of multiple brain regions producing interictal spikes in human epilepsy *Electroencephalogr Clin Neurophysiol* 1989; 73:389–402.

64. Rose DF, Sato S, Smith PD, et al. Localization of magnetic interictal discharges in temporal lobe epilepsy. *Ann Neurol* 1987; 22:348–354.

CHAPTER 10

Neuroimaging in Pediatric Epilepsy

Ruben I. Kuzniecky, M.D.

The impact of modern neuroimaging in the investigation and diagnosis of patients with neurologic diseases has been enormous. The impact in the management of patients with seizures and epilepsy cannot be overemphasized considering the high sensitivity and exquisite degree of anatomic resolution and metabolic information now available with different imaging techniques (1–5). For example, the diagnosis of mesial temporal sclerosis was exclusively based on pathological specimens until a decade ago. Since then magnetic resonance imaging (MRI) clearly is able to demonstrate this entity in vivo (6). The impact of these techniques extends beyond the detection of epileptic lesions by contributing to the proper classification of certain epileptic disorders and by delineating underlying genetic conditions. Modern neuroimaging techniques have directly and indirectly advanced our understanding of the basic pathophysiologic processes associated with the epilepsies (7).

This chapter compares the different imaging modalities and their specific role in children with seizures and epilepsy. It also discusses some of the special technical requirements and problems encountered when imaging the pediatric brain. The use of specific imaging modalities in neonates is briefly discussed.

TECHNICAL CONSIDERATIONS

Sedation

Appropriate and safe sedation is of paramount importance in the imaging of children (8). Our experience suggests that it is better not to initiate an examination without appropriate sedation because it is likely that motion artifact renders the examination invalid. This is particularly the case with MRI studies, which are highly sensitive to motion artifact. There are a number of sedation protocols using different drugs and routes of administration. Oral chloral hydrate (50–100 mg/kg) is widely popular, but intravenous (IV) sodium pentobarbital is used in many centers. Proper physiologic monitoring with MR-compatible equipment is now available and should include heart and respiratory rate, blood pressure, and O_2 and CO_2 concentrations following accepted guidelines. In many medical centers, properly certified sedation teams have been successful by being cost-effective and providing optimal safety.

Scanning Techniques

Although the techniques for scanning children are similar to those used in adults, there are a few technical aspects to be considered. Computed tomography (CT) studies should be done with thin slices (≤5 mm) in all children. When examining a newborn, appropriate windowing should be done because of the high water content.

MRI studies should include a T1-weighted sagittal sequence to examine the midline structures. Axial images are done using the saggital scout. It is important to obtain T1 and T2 information because of the maturational changes occurring during the first 18 months of life (9). This is discussed further under the MRI section. In general, T1 images provide optimal anatomic delineation, whereas T2 images provide the best sensitivity for water- and iron-containing lesions. The use of gradient echo images (for calcifications) and Gd-DTPA contrast agents is generally more limited and should be guided by the possible pathology.

To complete the study, we routinely acquire a three-dimensional (3D) sequence yielding 1–1.5 mm images without gaps. This sequence is extremely useful for studying the hippocampal structures and detecting small areas of focal cortical dysplasia. These images can be reconstructed in any plane with multiple angulations in a relatively short time. We now routinely obtain inversion recovery sequences because they provide improved T1-weighted contrast and fluid attenuated inversion recovery (FLAIR) sequences in view of their excellent T2 contrast without cerebrospinal fluid (CSF) distortion. It remains to be determined whether FLAIR can replace standard T2-weighted sequences in children.

IMAGING MODALITIES

Skull X-ray

Skull x-ray has a very limited role in the neuroimaging of children with epilepsy. In head trauma, skull x-ray may reveal linear fractures, but CT provides excellent bone and intracranial information. Skull x-ray can assess bone flaps and visualize the position of grids, strips, and depth electrodes after implantation. Its complementary role to MRI in patients with intracranial calcifications is marginal. A new use for skull x-ray has been created, however—the screening of patients suspected of having noncompatible cranial MR material before MRI. Because of its limited diagnostic role in epilepsy, it is not discussed further.

Cranial Ultrasound

Ultrasonography (US) is a noninvasive, inexpensive, portable, real-time, and multiplanar imaging modality that is well suited for the study of infants during the perinatal period. Except for special circumstances, US is the imaging modality of choice to study premature infants (10). Ultrasound can provide an accurate delineation of the main brain structures; it can permit an accurate diagnosis of various lesions; and it may aid in the identification of etiologic and pathogenic factors associated with seizures. Ultrasound can be used routinely in preterm infants through the anterior and posterior fontanels, and the examination can be performed in the neonatal unit with monitoring and adequate temperature control.

Ultrasound signals represent variations in acoustic reflections of tissues and tissue interfaces so that echogenic structures and sonolucent structures may be separated from one another and from the more uniform brain substance. Ultrasound is operator-dependent and requires a window for adequate imaging. Cranial ultrasound is most effective for viewing echogenic structures, intraventricular, periventricular, and intracerebral lesions (hemorrhage), as well as sonolucent structures such as CSF- and other fluid-containing lesions, for example, hydrocephalus (11).

Ultrasound is useful in its application to preterm infants with seizures. It is useful in the diagnosis of neonatal hypoxic-ischemic encephalopathy, suspected developmental malformations, infections, microcephaly, and hemorrhagic manifestations of anoxic-ischemic injury (11). Ultrasound can also effectively image the evolution of ischemic injury and the progression or resolution of hemorrhages or their consequences (12) (Figure 10-1).

Ultrasound has also been used in the study of developmental anomalies of the ventricular system, including hydrocephalus, anomalies of the corpus callosum, and other malformations. Although useful, ultrasound is not considered the procedure of choice for the delineation of developmental abnormalities of the CNS. Magnetic resonance imaging is the procedure of choice for the study of these malformations. In infants with macrocephaly and seizures, ultrasound can provide an assessment of ventricular size for hydrocephalus or other pathologic entities associated with enlarged head size. However, CT and MRI provide important additional information in such cases.

Although US is extremely useful, MRI often is necessary for a definitive diagnosis. Because US is limited to a well-defined population of infants, it is not discussed further.

Computed Tomography

Computed tomography uses ionizing radiation and can generate excellent hard tissue imaging contrast with moderately good soft tissue resolution. The strength of CT is its low cost, ready accessibility, and easy use, which provides a relatively reliable imaging modality for unstable patients. Additionally, last generation CT scans can generate images of the brain in seconds.

The role of CT scan in the study of patients with epilepsy has been profoundly altered by the development of MRI. However, CT is still the technique of

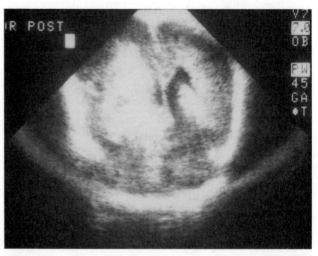

Figure 10-1. Coronal ultrasound of a neonate demonstrating ventricularmegaly and the presence of hemorrhage in the ventricles and parenchyma.

choice in the investigations of patients with seizures and epilepsy under certain conditions. In the neonate and young infant, CT is often of secondary or adjunctive importance, but it serves a significant backup role to ultrasound. This is particularly true if the ultrasound window is lost with age. CT can accurately detect hemorrhage, infarctions, gross malformations, ventricular system pathologies, and lesions with underlying calcification (13–15).

The sensitivity of CT in patients with epilepsy has been reported to be approximately 30 percent (16–20). However, most studies are difficult to compare because of divergent patient selection criteria or technical differences. Nevertheless, CT has high sensitivity for the detection of hemispheric pathology such as tuberous sclerosis, Sturge-Weber syndrome, or cerebral infarction. Unfortunately, CT has overall a low sensitivity because of poor resolution in the temporal fossa. Thus, it is not surprising that CT is unable to detect mesial temporal sclerosis, the most common pathology in temporal lobe epilepsy (TLE) (21,22)

CT is the diagnostic imaging tool of choice in children with epilepsy if an MRI is not available. However, studies have shown that CT may fail to detect abnormalities in up to 40 percent of patients with epileptogenic structural lesions such as small tumors and vascular malformations (6). Contrast CT studies may provide useful information if the plain CT suggests an abnormality. In addition, CT may add information about bony involvement. CT is the technique of choice in the perioperative state because it can rapidly detect recent hemorrhage, hydrocephalus, and major structural changes (5). Although highly diagnostic, the role of CT in the diagnosis of tuberous sclerosis or Sturge-Weber syndrome or other conditions with intracranial calcifications is complementary because MRI provides more information (noncalcified tubers) (23–25).

Magnetic Resonance Imaging

Magnetic resonance imaging is the imaging procedure of choice in the investigation of children with epilepsy (18,26–29). The advantages of MRI include the use of nonionizing radiation, high sensitivity and higher specificity than CT, multiplanar imaging capability, improved contrast of soft tissue, and high anatomic resolution.

Before we discuss the role of MRI in epilepsy, we should consider the important issue of brain maturation and myelination. MRI interpretation in the infant should be rendered with consideration of the normal development and maturational changes observed through the first two years of life. In the newborn, the sylvian and posterior interhemispheric fissures are prominent and the cisterna magna and basilar cisterns are large. These normal findings should not be

misinterpreted as atrophy. In addition, maturational changes are extremely important and can be studied with MRI (9). Briefly, from birth to 6 months, the white matter is hyperintense relative to the gray matter on T2-weighted images. Between 6 and 18 months of age, the white matter slowly becomes hypointense (like the adult brain) in the same sequence. This means that during the first 6 months of life, T2-weighted images are the sequences necessary to detect cortical abnormalities and T1-contrast images are necessary to study brain maturation. After the sixth month the role of each sequence in assessing maturation and structure is reversed, with T2-weighted images necessary for maturational assessment. Failure to acquire both sequences and to understand the normal maturational process may result in improper image interpretation or underdetection of pathology (30). Furthermore, the process of myelination takes place in an organized pattern, and deviations of these patterns should be appropriately recognized.

The sensitivity of MRI in detecting abnormalities in infants and children is dictated by the pathologies underlying childhood epilepsies (Table 10-1) and by the MRI techniques and experience of the interpreting physician. Developmental malformations constitute the most common underlying pathology in infants and young children with epilepsy (7,18). Of all new cases of infantile spasms presenting to our institution over a 12-month period, developmental malformations accounted for 40 percent (Figure 10-2). In the past, reports suggested that MRI was relatively insensitive to the detection of developmental pathology in infants with West syndrome (31). However, studies indicate that this could be related to the lack of use of both T1- and T2-weighted sequences, critical for proper diagnosis during the maturational process as described previously (30). Because of the difficulties described, it is recommended that children with persistent seizures and a normal MRI (performed before age 2 years) should have a repeat MRI study before age 5 years.

MRI is the imaging technique of choice in the investigation of patients with developmental disorders.

Table 10-1. Pathologic Substrates of Childhood Epilepsy

Developmental malformations
Tumors
Hippocampal sclerosis
Prenatal and perinatal destructive injury
Neurocutaneous disorders
Infammatory
Infectious
Metabolic disorders
Vascular malformations
Degenerative disorders

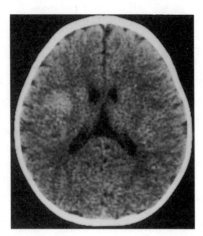

Figure 10-2. Axial noncontrast CT scan in an 8-month-old baby with infantile spasms. There is an area of abnormality involving the right frontal region in the form of a developmental malformation.

MRI can accurately define generalized malformations such as lissencephaly, band heterotopia, and periventricular nodular heterotopia (Figure 10-4). It can also define hemimegalencephaly, schizencephaly, and focal subcortical heterotopia. The range and complexity of cortical developmental malformations is great, and appropriate classification is of utmost importance (32).

In our experience, focal cortical dysplasia (FCD) is the most common developmental pathology in children with extratemporal lobe seizures. These lesions often

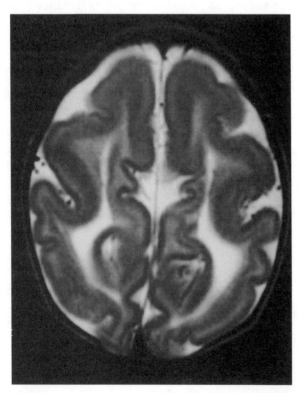

Figure 10-3. Six-month-old girl with infantile spasms and developmental delay. Axial MRI demonstrates lissencephaly with agenesis of the corpus callosum. Note the thick underlying cortex and smooth brain.

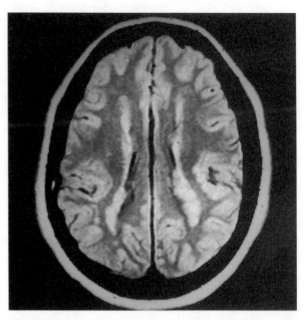

Figure 10-4. Periventricular nodular heterotopia. Axial T2-weighted image demonstrating the presence of abnormal gray matter in the periventricular white matter regions bilaterally. Patient is a 16-year-old female with epilepsy and minimal mental retardation.

are localized to the central and precentral cortical region (33,34). These lesions may range from severe cortical disorganization to subtle malformations of the cortical mantle. The MRI features often consist of an abnormal cortical mantle with abnormal gray-white matter architecture and thick cortex. The presence of T2-weighted abnormalities in the underlying white matter correlates with balloon cells typical of type 2 cortical dysplasia (7). Because some of these lesions are focal and small in nature, the MRI examination should be targeted to the clinically suspected regions using both 3D-volume techniques and inversion recovery sequences. Less commonly, focal polymicrogyria (PMG) is detected in children with focal epilepsy. The lesions may be localized to any lobe, but there is a tendency for perisylvian and rolandic areas. Although pathologically there are small gyri, MRI may give the impression of a thickened cortex. The use of thin T1-weighted images is helpful in detecting the underlying small gyri or irregular inner and outer cortical surface typical of this condition. Further diagnostic improvement may be achieved by using surface coils or thin partition reconstruction (35). Other common pathologies in children with epilepsy include Sturge-Weber syndrome, which most often is unilateral but may also be bilateral. Tuberous sclerosis is a multifocal disease that can be diagnosed by clinical and imaging criteria.

The second major pathologic entity encountered in children with intractable epilepsy is mesial temporal sclerosis (MTS). MTS is pathologically characterized by the presence of a firm atrophic hippocampus and the histologic presence of neuronal loss and

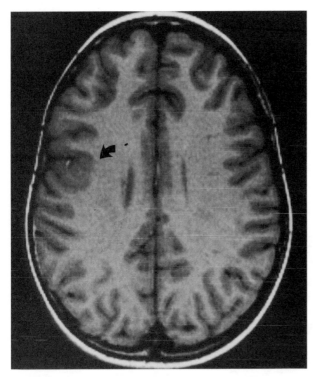

Figure 10-5. Axial T1-weighted MRI in a 9-year-old child with intractable frontal lobe seizures. There is an area of focal thickening that represents focal cortical dysplasia (*arrow*). The patient has been almost seizure-free since surgery.

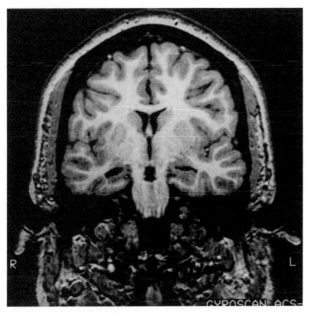

Figure 10-6. Mesial temporal lobe sclerosis. Coronal T1-weighted angulated scan through hippocampal region. Note evidence of right hippocampal atrophy and signal intensity changes typical of MTS.

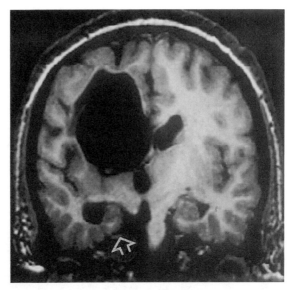

Figure 10-7. Associated porencephaly and ipsilateral hippocampal sclerosis. Coronal T1-weighted MRI of a 16-year-old child with congenital hemiplegia and intractable seizures. Note porencephaly affecting right frontal region and associated right hippocampal atrophy (*arrow*).

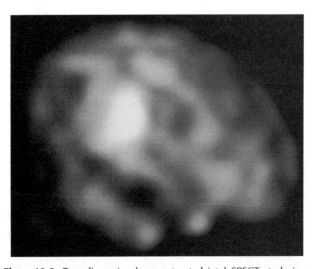

Figure 10-8. Two-dimensional reconstructed ictal SPECT study in a child with intractable focal seizures. Area of hyperperfusion is seen in the right premotor area corresponding to an area of cortical dysplasia and seizure onset.

gliosis in some of the hippocampal subfields. Until the advent of MRI, this entity was not diagnosed preoperatively; however, MRI is capable of detecting this abnormality with high sensitivity and specificity when hippocampal neuronal loss is at least 50 percent. The MRI features of hippocampal sclerosis include (1) hippocampal atrophy, (2) increased signal on T2-weighted images, and (3) decreased signal on inversion recovery sequences (Figure 10-6). The detection of these abnormalities should be carried out with optimized imaging techniques, including angulated coronal sections obtained perpendicular to the long axis of the hippocampal structures using volumetry or qualitative assessment (3,36) (Figure 10-6). A recent study from our laboratory indicates that a combination of techniques (anatomic resolution and signal alteration) is highly sensitive (37). MTS can also be detected in conjunction with other pathologic conditions (dual pathology).

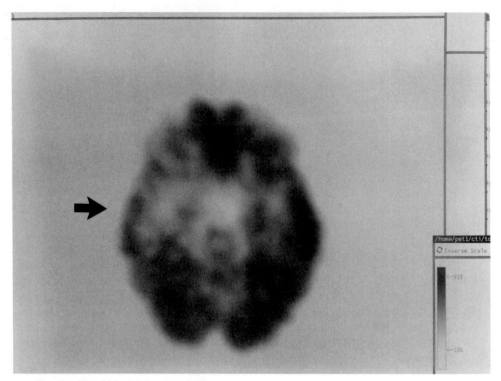

Figure 10-9. Temporal lobe epilepsy. Axial reconstructed FDG-PET scan. There is an area of hypometabolism involving the right posterior temporal and parietal regions compared with the opposite side.

Early destructive injuries constitute another major group of pathologies underlying diffuse or focal injury in children with seizures. The MRI appearance is dependent on the type and time of injury to the brain. Early injuries (first six months of gestation) result in porencephaly. Late gestational, perinatal, or postnatal injuries result in encephalomalacia or ulegyria (38). MRI can distinguish both conditions based on imaging features (8). Of importance, however, is the fact that porencephaly may be associated with ipsilateral MTS (dual pathology) and that MRI can aid in the definition of the epileptic syndrome in these children (Figure 10-7). Encephalomalacias may be diffuse, as in anoxic injuries, or may be localized to the distribution of a cerebral artery branch. Ulegyria, which is less common, typically is localized to the posterior head regions (occipital lobe) with primary involvement of the sulci depth. Although porencephaly is common in children with epilepsy, it is not necessarily the cause of seizures (39). Recent data suggest, in fact, that most patients with porencephaly and seizures have temporal lobe seizures and associated MTS that may be detected with optimized techniques (40).

Other pathologies that are commonly associated with childhood epilepsy include developmental tumors (ganglioglial) and less common neurocutaneous syndromes (incontinentia pigmenti, neurofibromatosis type I, etc.). In general, these disorders are diagnosed on the basis of other features and are not discussed here.

Single Photon Emission Computed Tomography

Single photon emission computed tomography (SPECT) has been used in the study and diagnosis of seizures for several years. SPECT is more readily available than positron emission tomography (PET) and is considerably less expensive. Before we discuss the use of SPECT and PET in childhood epilepsy, it is important to succinctly comment on the metabolic changes that are known to occur during maturation in the first decade of life (41,42). At birth, metabolic function is high in the thalamus, central region, and cerebellar vermis. At three months, activity increases in the striatum, occipitoparietal regions, and cerebellar cortex, with the frontal lobes remaining relatively hypometabolic. At 12 months of age, metabolic activity reaches adult values. From age 2 years to age 6 to 7 years, values double those seen in adults; then glucose consumption decreases progressively to adult values, which are reached by 15 years of age. These physiologic parameters should be considered when interpreting studies in children.

Numerous studies using dynamic and static SPECT techniques in the interictal state have been published (43–46). Although decreased blood flow changes have been reported with variable frequencies, correlative studies have demonstrated that approximately 50 percent of patients with well-documented TLE demonstrate interictal temporal hypoperfusion in the corresponding epileptogenic temporal region (47). However, almost as many patients with TLE do not show abnormalities on interictal SPECT studies. Furthermore, 5 percent to 10 percent of patients may demonstrate hypoperfusion in the contralateral temporal region, which raises the possibility of false lateralization. Although interictal studies may confirm lateralization in patients with MRI and EEG abnormalities, the studies tend to be noncomplementary and therefore not cost-effective. However, interictal scans may be useful as baseline studies for comparison with ictal or postictal SPECT studies in selected cases.

In contrast to interictal studies, ictal studies in TLE are accurate in the localization of the epileptogenic focus. In previous series, increased perfusion abnormalities were reported in up to 97 percent of patients, with very few patients showing inconclusive results (48,49). The ictal patterns are variable, but two types have been consistently demonstrated. The most common pattern consists of primarily unilateral global temporal hyperperfusion with relative decrease perfusion in other cortical areas in the ipsilateral temporal lobe and contralateral hemisphere (50). The other pattern consists of hyperperfusion circumscribed to the mesial structures. This usually is associated with decreased lateral cortical perfusion or relative neocortical temporal hypoperfusion. When compared with the interictal study, the *switch-over* phenomenon is observed. The yield of postictal studies decreases with the time of injection, as suggested by our experience and others. Ictal injections therefore are necessary within the first minute following electrographic and clinical onset in TLE.

Interictal studies are less likely to provide useful information in patients with extratemporal lobe epilepsy. Harvey and coworkers (51) reported bilateral or poorly localized areas of hypoperfusion in 30 percent of their patients. However, only 9 percent of these patients demonstrated focal hypoperfusion defects in correspondence with the clinical, EEG, and MRI data. Conversely, ictal SPECT in extratemporal lobe epilepsy is very useful. Harvey and coworkers reported localization by ictal SPECT in 91 percent of children with frontal lobe epilepsy. In the majority of patients, the areas of hyperperfusion corresponded to the EEG and clinical patterns. Others have also reported good concordance between ictal hyperperfusion patterns and clinical and EEG findings in patients with frontal lobe seizures (Figure 10-11).

We have observed that in extratemporal lobe epilepsy, especially if seizures last less than 20 seconds, blood flow changes are extremely dynamic (52). Delayed injections may not demonstrate perfusion changes, particularly if the injections are given toward the late part of the seizure or in the early postictal phase. This is related to the known connectivity of the frontal lobes and to the rapid dynamic blood flow changes that occur in this type of seizure (52). In our experience, ictal injections should be performed within the first 5 to 10 seconds of ictal onset to obtain accurate localizing information.

Ictal SPECT has also been useful in studying seizure spread patterns. In TLE, ipsilateral basal ganglia hyperperfusion may be seen. This correlates with contralateral dystonic arm posturing (53). Conversely, in extratemporal lobe epilepsy, the patterns of spread are more complex. In mesial frontal seizures, the areas of activation often involve ipsi- or bilateral basal ganglia and contralateral cerebellum (52). In dorsolateral frontal seizures, the ipsilateral basal ganglia and contralateral cerebellum most commonly are activated. No cerebellar activation is seen in parietal or occipital lobe seizures.

The main limitation of ictal SPECT is related to the logistics of timely injections. This may be partially overcome by studying seizure frequency and patterns. The recent availability of stable compounds certainly increases the utility of ictal SPECT.

Positron Emission Tomography

Positron emission tomography has been used for more than a decade in the investigation of patients with seizure disorders (54,55). Most studies have used 2-deoxy-2(^{18}F)fluoro-D-glucose (FDG) in the interictal state. In TLE, interictal studies show hypometabolic areas in the epileptogenic regions. These findings have been observed in approximately 80 percent of patients with TLE. The changes, however, are more extensive than the structural and EEG abnormalities and may involve the ipsilateral suprasylvian and parietal regions. The high sensitivity of MRI in detecting MTS and other pathologies in temporal lobe surgical candidates has diminished the role of PET in the presurgical investigation of such patients. Nevertheless, when MRI is normal, PET may be indicated to aid in the localization (Figure 10-9).

In extratemporal lobe epilepsy, interictal PET-FDG studies are less useful, especially if the MRI is normal and the scalp EEG is nonfocal. However, PET has been reported to be more sensitive in neonates and infants with focal seizures because it is likely that in those cases a developmental malformation is present (56). This is particularly true in patients with infantile spasms and focal features on EEG. When a single region of metabolic abnormality corresponding to the EEG abnormality is detected, surgical treatment is effective in controlling seizures and improving developmental outcome. PET has also improved the understanding of the pathophysiology of infantile spasms by demonstrating activation of cortical regions, brain stem, and lenticular nuclei.

The role of PET in other pediatric epileptic conditions has also been reported. In the Lennox-Gastaut syndrome, PET has demonstrated different metabolic patterns underscoring the heterogeneity of this syndrome (56). In some patients with hemimegalencephaly, PET has shown bilateral metabolic abnormalities. These findings may explain the poor outcome following surgery in those particular patients (57). Finally, in patients with Sturge-Weber syndrome, PET may provide a sensitive measure of the extent of cerebral involvement, especially during the first year of life.

New Techniques

New imaging techniques are being applied to the study of patients with epilepsy. These techniques include magnetic resonance spectroscopy (MRS), magnetic resonance relaxometry (MRR), functional magnetic resonance imaging (FMRI), and receptor PET studies. However, limited data in children with epilepsy are available.

MRS can provide noninvasive biochemical measurements of specific brain metabolites (58–61). In epilepsy, two major techniques have been applied. Phosphorous or ^{31}P spectroscopy is designed to measure phospholipid metabolism and high-energy phosphate compounds. Studies in our laboratory (62) and others (63) have demonstrated a consistent abnormality in the epileptogenic region characterized by abnormal phosphocreatine to inorganic phosphate ratios.

Hydrogen or ^{1}H spectroscopy has demonstrated abnormalities of N-acetyl-aspartate (NAA), a mitochondrial neuronal compound, creatine (Cr), and choline (Cho) in patients with epilepsy. A consistent abnormality in NAA to Cr ratios has been found by several groups in correspondence with the epileptogenic focus in temporal and extratemporal lobe epilepsy (64–66) and in children (67). The abnormal ratios may represent a drop in NAA as a result of neuronal loss and associated increases in Cr resulting from gliosis (Figure 10-13). The sensitivity of MRS appears higher than MRI (58). Hydrogen or ^{1}H spectroscopy has also demonstrated bitemporal abnormalities in up to 40 percent of patients, but the significance of these findings is not clear. More recently, Ng and colleagues (68) have demonstrated an increase in lactate concentrations in the postictal state in the epileptogenic temporal lobe.

MRR for the evaluation of abnormal T1 and T2 signal has been applied to epilepsy. In hippocampal sclerosis, visually assessed hippocampal T2-weighted signal hyperintensity has typically been reported in 50 percent to 65 percent of cases, with a range from 8 percent to 70 percent. Increased sensitivity for the detection of hippocampal pathology has been reported using T2 relaxation time as a quantitative measurement of tissue pathology in the hippocampal gray matter. In patients with TLE, approximately 80 percent have abnormal ipsilateral T2 relaxation time, with up to 30 percent having abnormal contralateral hippocampal T2 values in addition to the ipsilateral abnormality; this may represent the bilateral hippocampal abnormalities described in pathology studies of hippocampal sclerosis (59). The use of T2 relaxometry in other cortical regions is beginning to be explored.

FMRI has also been preliminarily applied to the study of seizure disorders. FMRI utilizes very rapid scanning techniques that theoretically can demonstrate alterations in blood oxygenation. This technique has been applied to map functional areas before cranial surgery (69). Because blood flow changes occur during seizures, it is theoretically possible to use this technique to demonstrate these abnormalities. Jackson and colleagues (70) demonstrated focal blood flow changes in a child with partial seizures using FMRI techniques. Detection of alterations in oxygenation in the epileptic focus may be possible using similar MR principles. FMRI has been applied to lateralized speech for surgery and motor function with the advantage of being noninvasive. However, FMRI is difficult in children because of motion artifact.

Recent PET studies using specific neuroreceptor ligands have reported a variety of findings in epilepsy. Opiate receptor studies with ^{11}C-carfentanil (μ-opiate receptor) have shown increased binding in the lateral neocortex of TLE patients without mesial temporal involvement (71). Other opiate receptor studies have confirmed the specificity of μ-opiate bindings in TLE. In addition, benzodiazepine labeling studies with ^{11}C-flumazenil, a central benzodiazepine receptor antagonist, have shown reduced binding in the epileptogenic focus (72). Flumazenil-labeled PET studies are more sensitive than FDG studies (56), but no prospective study has been carried out. Finally, a single study reported increased binding of ^{11}C-doxepin, a histamine (H_1) receptor in patients with partial seizures (73).

Practical Neuroimaging in Pediatric Epilepsy

Not all patients with epilepsy need neuroimaging studies. Neuroimaging studies may not be necessary in patients with well-defined idiopathic generalized epilepsies such as childhood absence epilepsy (pyknolepsy). In addition, patients with typical idiopathic benign partial epilepsy with centro-temporal spikes may not require an imaging study. However, there are reports of patients with apparent generalized epilepsies or benign partial seizures in which structural abnormalities are seen on MRI (74). In general, the clinical course and atypical features of such patients identify those who require imaging studies. Similarly, patients with uncomplicated febrile convulsions and a normal neurologic examination do not require imaging studies.

Conversely, all patient with symptomatic generalized or focal seizures should have a structural neuroimaging study. Because MRI is far superior to CT scan in the detection of structural lesions, MRI should be the imaging procedure of choice in the evaluation of children with seizures, especially if focal features are present on neurologic examination or EEG. In addition, MRI is indicated if seizures persist in the presence of a previously normal CT scan or when there are progressive neurologic changes.

PET and SPECT are not indicated in the majority of patients with seizures. When surgical treatment is contemplated, PET and SPECT may be indicated. PET may provide localizing information when the MRI is normal in any patient considered for focal resective treatment. In particular, PET may be useful in children with refractory infantile spasms when the MRI is normal and surgical treatment is contemplated. Ictal SPECT is extremely useful in the localization of extratemporal foci, particularly if the MRI is normal or when the area of epileptogenesis is not well-localized. MRS, MRR, and FMRI are at present research tools.

CONCLUSIONS

Neuroimaging techniques continue to improve the diagnosis and management of children with epilepsy. These modern techniques have the major advantage of being noninvasive and multimodal. The role and indications of each of these techniques in patients with epilepsy is rapidly changing. Advances in imaging are likely to improve the care of patients with seizures and epilepsy.

ACKNOWLEDGMENTS

I thank Dr. Martina Bebin for providing clinical material.

REFERENCES

1. Cascino GD, Jack JCR, Parisi JE, et al. Magnetic resonance imaging–based volume studies in temporal lobe epilepsy: pathological correlations. *Ann Neurol* 1991; 30:31–36.

2. Jackson G. New techniques in MR. *Epilepsia* 1994; 36:S2–S13.

3. Jackson GD, Berkovic SF, Duncan JS, Connelly A. Optimising the diagnosis of hippocampal sclerosis using magnetic resonance imaging. *Am J Neuroradiol* 1993; 14:753–762.

4. Kuzniecky R, Cascino GD, Palmini A, et al. Structural imaging. In: Engel JJ (ed.). *Surgical Treatment of the Epilepsies.* 2nd ed. New York: Raven Press, 1993:197–200.

5. Kuzniecky R, Jackson G. Neuroimaging in epilepsy. In: Kuzniecky R, Jackson G (eds.). *Magnetic Resonance in Epilepsy.* New York: Raven Press, 1995:27–48.

6. Kuzniecky R, De La Sayette V, Ethier R, et al. Magnetic resonance imaging in temporal lobe epilepsy: pathological correlations. *Ann Neurol* 1987; 22:341–347.

7. Kuzniecky R. Magnetic resonance imaging in developmental disorders of the cerebral cortex. *Epilepsia* 1994; 35:S44–S56.

8. Barkovich AJ. *Pediatric Neuroimaging.* 2nd ed. New York: Raven Press, 1995.

9. Barkovich A, Kjos B, Jackson D, Norman D. Normal maturation of the neonatal and infant brain: MR imaging at 1.5 T. *Radiology* 1988; 166:173–180.

10. Dubowitz LMS, Bydder GM, Mushin J. Developmental sequence of periventricular leukomalacia. Correlation of ultrasound, clinical, and nuclear magnetic resonance functions. *Arch Dis Child* 1985; 60:349–355.

11. Baarsma R, Laurini R, Baerts O, Okken A. Reliability of sonography in non-hemorrhagic periventricular leukomalacia. *Pediatr Radiol* 1987; 17:189–191.

12. Carson S, Hertzberg B, Bowie J, Burger P. Value of sonography in the diagnosis of intracranial hemorrhage and periventricular leukomalacia: a postmortem study of 35 cases. *Am J Neuroradiol* 1990; 11:677–684.

13. Chiron C, Dulac O, Palacios L, et al. Magnetic resonance imaging in epileptic children treated with γ-vinyl GABA (vigabatrin). *Epilepsia* 1989; 30(Supp 1):736 (Abstract).

14. El Gammal T, Adams RJ, King DW, et al. Modified CT techniques in the evaluation of temporal lobe epilepsy prior to lobectomy. *Am J Neuroradiol* 1987; 8:131–134.

15. Kishikawa H, Ohmoto T, Nishimoto A. Brain tumor with seizures in children. *Brain Develop* (Tokyo) 1980; 12:19–26.

16. Duncan R, Patterson J, Hadley DM, et al. CT, MR and SPECT imaging in temporal lobe epilepsy. *J Neurol Neurosurg Psychiatry* 1990; 53:11–15.

17. Heinz ER, Heinz TR, Radtke R, et al. Efficacy of MRI vs CT in epilepsy. *Am J Neuroradiol* 1988; 9:1123–1128.

18. Kuzniecky R, Murro A, King D, et al. Magnetic resonance imaging in childhood intractable partial epilepsies: Pathologic correlations. *Neurology* 1993; 43:681–687.

19. Schörner W, Meencke WJ, Sander B. Temporal-lobe epilepsy: comparison of CT and MR imaging. *Am J Neuroradiol* 1987; 8:773–781.

20. Theodore WH, Katz D, Kufta C, et al. Pathology of temporal lobe foci: Correlation with CT, MRI, and PET. *Neurology* 1990; 40:797–803.

21. Babb TL, Pretorius JK. Pathological substrates of epilepsy. In: Wylie E (ed.). *The Treatment of Epilepsy: Principles and Practice.* Philadelphia: Lea & Febiger, 1993:55–70.

22. Corsellis AN. The incidence of Ammon's horn sclerosis. *Brain* 1957; 80:193–203.

23. Curatolo P, Cusmai R. Magnetic resonance imaging in the Bourneville syndrome: Relations with EEG. *Neurophysiol Clin* 1988; 18:459–467.

24. Curatolo P, Cusmai R. The value of MRI in tuberous sclerosis. *Neuropediatrics* 1987; 18(3):32–36.

25. Conzen MA, Oppel F. Tuberous sclerosis in neurosurgery. An analysis of 18 patients. *Acta Neurochir* 1990; 106:3–4.

26. Guerrini R, Dravet C, Battaglia A, et al. Focal anomalies of the cortical development and epilepsy: electroclinical features in the bilateral opercular malformations. *Boll Lega Ital Epilessia* 1990; 71:109–111.

27. Gulati P, Jena A, Tripathi RP, Gupta AK. Magnetic resonance imaging in childhood epilepsy. *Indian Pediatr* 1991; 28:761–765.

28. Grattan-Smith JD, Harvey AS, Desmond PM, Chow CW. Hippocampal sclerosis in children with intractable temporal lobe epilepsy: a clinical and MRI correlative study. *Epilepsia* 1993; 34:127.

29. Kotagal P, Lüders H. Recent advances in childhood epilepsy. *Brain Dev* 1994; 16:1–15.

30. Sankar R, Curran J, Kevill J, et al. Microscopic cortical dysplasia in infantile spasms: evolution of white matter abnormalities. *Am J Neuroradiol* 1995; 16:1265–1272.

31. Chugani HT, Shield WD, Shewmon DA, et al. Infantile spasms: I. PET identifies focal cortical dysgenesis in cryptogenic cases for surgical treatment. *Ann Neurol* 1990; 24:406–413.

32. Barkovich A, Kuzniecky R, Dobbyns W, et al. A classification scheme for malformations of cortical development. *Neuropediatrics* 1996; 27:59–63.

33. Kuzniecky R, Andermann F. Congenital bilateral perisylvian syndrome: imaging findings in a multicenter study. *Am J Neuroradiol* 1994; 15:139–144.

34. Palmini A, Andermann F, Olivier A, et al. Focal neuronal migration disorders and intractable partial epilepsy: a study of 30 patients. *Ann Neurol* 1991; 30:741–749.

35. Barkovich J, Rowley H, Andermann F. MR in partial epilepsy: Value of high resolution volumetric techniques. *Am J Neuroradiol* 1995; 16:339–343.

36. Jack JC. MRI-based hippocampal volume measurements in epilepsy. *Epilepsia* 1994; 35:S21–S29.

37. Kuzniecky R, Bilir E, Gilliam F, et al. Multimodality MRI in mesial temporal sclerosis: relative sensitivity and specificity. *Neurology* 1997; 49:774–778.

38. Aicardi J, Goutieres F, Hodebourg de Verbois A. Multicystic encephalomalacia of infants and its relation to abnormal gestation and hydranencephaly. *J Neurol Sci* 1972; 15:357–373.

39. Ho S KR, Gilliam F, Faught E, Bebin M, Morawetz R. Congenital porencephaly and hippocampal sclerosis. Clinical correlates. *Neurology* 1997; 49:1382–1388.

40. Ho S, Kuzniecky R, Gilliam F, et al. Congenital porencephaly: MR features and relationship to hippocampal sclerosis. *Am J Neuroradiol* 1998; 19:135–141.

41. Chiron C, Raynaud C, Maziere B, et al. Changes in regional CBF during brain maturation in children and adolescents. *J Nucl Med* 1992; 33:696–703.

42. Chugani H, Phelps M, Mazziotta B, et al. PET study of human brain functional development. *Ann Neurol* 1987; 22:487–497.

43. Andersen AR, Waldemar G, Dam M, et al. SPECT in the presurgical evaluation of patients with temporal lobe epilepsy—A preliminary report. *Acta Neurochir Suppl (Wien)* 1990.

44. Grunwald F, Durwen HF, Bockisch A, et al. Technetium-99m-HMPAO brain SPECT in medically intractable temporal lobe epilepsy: a postoperative evaluation. *J Nucl Med* 1991; 32:388–394.

45. Stefan H, Kuhnen C, Biersack HJ, Reichmann K. Initial experience with 99m Tc-hexamethyl-propylene amine oxime (HM-PAO) single photon emission computed tomography (SPECT) in patients with focal epilepsy. *Epilepsy Res* 1987; 1:134–138.

46. Duncan R, Patterson J, Hadley D, Wyper D. 99mTc-HMPAO SPECT in temporal lobe epilepsy. *Acta Neurol Scand* 1990; 81:287–293.

47. Berkovic SF, Newton MR, Chiron C, Dulac O. Single photon emission tomography. In: Engel JJ (ed.). *Surgical Treatment of the Epilepsies*. 2nd ed. New York: Raven Press, 1993:233–243.

48. Newton M, Berkovic S, Austin M, Reutens D, McKay W. A postictal switch in blood flow distribution characterizes human temporal lobe seizures. *J Neurol Neurosurg Psychiatry* 1992; 55:891–894.

49. Rowe CC, Berkovic SF, Sia STB, et al. Localization of epileptic foci with single photon emission computed tomography. *Ann Neurol* 1989; 26:660–668.

50. Harvey AS, Bowe JM, Hopkins IJ, et al. Ictal 99mTc-HMPAO single photon emission computed tomography in children with temporal lobe epilepsy. *Epilepsia* 1993; 34:869–877.

51. Harvey AS, Hopkins IJ, Bowe JM, et al. Frontal lobe epilepsy: clinical seizure characteristics and localization with ictal 99mTc-HMPAO SPECT. *Neurology* 1993; 43:1966–1980.

52. Laich E, Kuzniecky R, Mountz J, et al. Supplementary sensorimotor area epilepsy: seizure localization, cortical propagation and subcortical activation pathways using ictal SPECT. *Brain* 1997; 120:855–864.

53. Newton M, Berkovic S, Austin M, et al. Dystonia, clinical lateralization, and regional blood flow changes in temporal lobe seizures. *Neurology* 1992; 42:371–377.

54. Engel JJ, Kuhl DE, Phelps ME, Mazziotta JC. Interictal cerebral glucose metabolism in partial epilepsy and its relation to EEG changes. *Ann Neurol* 1982; 12:510–517.

55. Henry TR, Sutherling WW, Engel JJ, et al. Interictal cerebral metabolism in partial epilepsies of neocortical origin. *Epilepsy Res* 1991; 10:174–182.

56. Chugani H. The role of PET in childhood epilepsy. *J Child Neurol* 1994; 9:S82–S88.

57. Messa C, Grana G, Lucignani G, Fazio F. Functional imaging using PET and SPECT in pediatric neurology. *J Nucl Biol Med* 1994; 38:85–88.

58. Hetherington H, Kuzniecky R, Pan J, et al. Proton MRS in human temporal lobe epilepsy at 4.1 T. *Ann Neurol* 1995; 38(3):396–404.

59. Jackson GD, Connelly A, Gadian DG, et al. 1H MRS and T2 relaxometry of the contralateral temporal lobe after epilepsy surgery. *Epilepsia* 1993; 34(6):144.

60. Connelly A, Jackson G, Duncan J, Gadian D. Proton MRS in temporal lobe epilepsy. *Neurology* 1994; 44:1411–1417.

61. Breiter N, Arroyo S, Mathews V, Lesser R, Barker P. Proton MRS in patients with seizure disorders. *Am J Neuroradiol* 1994; 15:377–384.

62. Kuzniecky R, El Gavish GA, Hetherington HP, Evanochko WT, Pohost GM. In vivo ^{31}P nuclear magnetic resonance spectroscopy of human temporal lobe epilepsy. *Neurology* 1992; 42:1586–1590.

63. Hugg JW, Matson GB, Duyn JH, et al. Lateralization of human focal epilepsy by ^{31}P magnetic resonance spectroscopic imaging. *Neurology* 1992; 42:2011–2018.

64. Hugg JW, Laxer KD, Matson GB, Maudsley AA, Weiner MW. Neuron loss localizes human temporal lobe epilepsy by in vivo proton magnetic resonance spectroscopic imaging. *Ann Neurol* 1993; 34:788–794.

65. Gadian DG, Connelly A, Duncan JS. ^{1}H magnetic resonance spectroscopy in the investigation of intractable epilepsy. *Acta Neurol Scand* 1993; 152:116–122.

66. Cendes F, Andermann F, Preul PC, Arnold DL. Lateralization of temporal lobe epilepsy based on regional metabolic abnormalities in proton MRS. *Ann Neurol* 1994; 35:211–216.

67. Cross H, Connelly A, Jackson G, et al. Proton MRS in children with temporal lobe epilepsy. *Ann Neurol* 1995; 39:107–113.

68. Ng T, Comair Y, Xue M, et al. Temporal lobe epilepsy: presurgical localization with proton chemical shift imaging. *Radiology* 1994; 193:465–471.

69. Connelly A, Jackson GD, Frackowiak RSJ, et al. Functional mapping of activated human primary cortex with a clinical MR imaging system. *Radiology* 1993; 188:125–130.

70. Jackson GD, Connelly A, Cross JH, Gadian DG. Functional magnetic resonance imaging of focal seizures. *Neurology* 1994; 44:850–856.

71. Frost JJ, Mayberg HS, Fisher RS, et al. μ-opiate receptors measured by positron emission tomography are increased in temporal lobe epilepsy. *Ann Neurol* 1988; 23:231–237.

72. Savic I, Persson A, Roland P, et al. In-vivo demonstration of reduced benzodiazepine receptor binding in human epileptic foci. *Lancet* 1988; 2(8616):863–866.

73. Iinuma K, Yokoyama H, Otsuki T, et al. Histamine H1 receptors in complex partial seizures. *Lancet* 1993; 341:238.

74. Aicardi J. *Epilepsy in Children*. New York: Raven Press, 1986.

CHAPTER 11

Neonatal Seizures

Eli M. Mizrahi, M.D., and Peter Kellaway, Ph.D.

Neonatal seizures are an important clinical problem because they indicate the presence of central nervous system (CNS) dysfunction, require urgent attention in determination of etiology and assessment for therapy, and may be associated with increased risk for long-term neurologic sequelae. Recent studies indicate that seizures occur in from 1.8 to 3.5 per 1,000 live births (1–3) and may occur with greater frequency in premature or low-birth-weight infants than in full-term and normal weight infants (1,4–6). Although the neonatal period is defined as up to 28 days post-term (e.g., 44 weeks conceptional age), most neonatal seizures occur within the first week of life, and the majority of them occur within the first few days of life (1,7,8).

CLINICAL DIAGNOSIS

Although the clinical recognition of seizures initiates a series of diagnostic and therapeutic steps, the characterization and classification of the seizures themselves may not always be emphasized. However, detailed characterization and accurate classification are the first critical elements in effective assessment and rational management (Figure 11-1).

Neonatal seizures have been classified according to their most prominent clinical feature by a number of investigators (9–12). In addition, seizures have been classified according to their relationship to electrographic seizure activity [i.e., electroclinical, electrical only, or clinical only (12–14) and according to their pathophysiology (epileptic vs. nonepileptic) (7,12)]. A current classification of neonatal seizures relating clinical seizures to associated electroencephalographic (EEG) seizure activity, presumed pathophysiology, and the characterization of clinical events is given in Table 11-1.

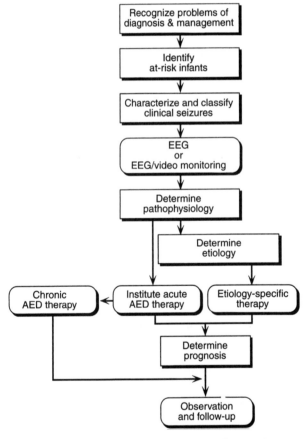

Figure 11-1. Steps in diagnosis and management of neonatal seizures. The steps in diagnosis and management are an orderly progression of considerations and actions designed to accurately recognize and classify seizures (clinically and electroencephalographically), determine pathophysiology (epileptic versus nonepileptic seizures), determine the need for antiepileptic drugs and etiology-specific therapy and assess prognosis.

Electroencephalography has a critical role in the diagnosis and management of neonatal seizures (13,15,16), and more recently EEG-video monitoring

Table 11-1. Clinical Characteristics, Classification, and Presumed Pathophysiology of Neonatal Seizures

Classification	Characterization
Focal clonic	Repetitive, rhythmic contractions of muscle groups of the limbs, face, or trunk May be unifocal or multifocal May occur synchronously or asynchronously in muscle groups on one side of the body May occur simultaneously but asynchronously on both sides Cannot be suppressed by restraint **Pathophysiology:** epileptic
Focal tonic	Sustained posturing of single limbs Sustained asymmetrical posturing of the trunk Sustained eye deviation Cannot be provoked by stimulation or suppressed by restraint **Pathophysiology:** epileptic
Generalized tonic	Sustained symmetrical posturing of limbs, trunk, and neck May be flexor, extensor, or mixed extensor/flexor May be provoked or intensified by stimulation May be suppressed by restraint or repositioning **Presumed pathophysiology:** nonepileptic
Myoclonic	Random, single, rapid contractions of muscle groups of the limbs, face, or trunk Typically not repetitive or may recur at a slow rate May be generalized, focal, or fragmentary May be provoked by stimulation **Presumed pathophysiology:** may be epileptic or nonepileptic
Spasms	May be flexor, extensor, or mixed extensor/flexor May occur in clusters Cannot be provoked by stimulation or suppressed by restraint **Pathophysiology:** epileptic
Motor automatisms Oral signs	Random and roving eye movements or nystagmus (distinct from tonic eye deviation) May be provoked or intensified by tactile stimulation **Presumed pathophysiology:** nonepileptic
Oral-buccal-lingual movements	Sucking, chewing, tongue protrusions May be provoked or intensified by stimulation **Presumed pathophysiology:** nonepileptic
Progression movements	Rowing or swimming movements Pedalling or bicycling movements of the legs May be provoked or intensified by stimulation May be suppressed by restraint or repositioning **Presumed pathophysiology:** nonepileptic
Complex purposeless movements	Sudden arousal with transient increased random activity of limbs May be provoked or intensified by stimulation **Presumed pathophysiology:** nonepileptic

With permission from Mizrahi EM, Kellaway P. *Diagnoses and Management of Neonatal Seizures.* New York: Lippincott-Raven, 1998: 181.

Table 11-2. Most Frequently Identified Causes of Neonatal Seizures*

Hypoxia-ischemia
Intracranial hemorrhage
   Intraventricular
   Intracerebral
   Subdural
   Subarachnoid
Infection of the central nervous system
   Meningitis
   Encephalitis
   Intrauterine
Infarction
Metabolic
   Hypoglycemia
   Hypocalcemia
   Hypomagnesemia
Chromosomal anomalies
Congenital abnormalities of the brain
Neurodegenerative disorders
Inborn errors of metabolism
Benign neonatal convulsions
Benign familial neonatal convulsions
Drug withdrawal or intoxication

*Listed in relative order of frequency. A detailed list of etiologies is given in Table 11.3. Not listed is "unknown" cause, which is encountered in approximately 10% of cases.
Adapted with permission from Mizrahi EM, Kellaway P. *Diagnosis and Management of Neonatal Seizures.* New York: Lippincott-Raven, 1998.

has emerged as an important applied diagnostic tool in the neonatal intensive care unit (NICU) (17). The EEG is best performed when the infant is actually experiencing clinical seizures. Although the ictal EEG can provide evidence for the occurrence of seizures of epileptic origin, the interictal EEG can also provide valuable information concerning the degree and distribution of brain dysfunction. Serial EEGs can increase the likelihood of capturing seizures and can provide objective data concerning the course of brain dysfunction and, ultimately, prognosis through assessment of the character of the background EEG.

SEIZURE PATHOPHYSIOLOGY

The differentiation of epileptic from nonepileptic seizures can be determined by the clinical features of the events, the response of the suspected seizures to stimulation and restraint, and the presence or absence of concomitant electrical seizure activity in the EEG (Table 11-1) (12,13).

Epileptic neonatal seizures are generated by hypersynchronous discharges of a critical mass of cortical neurons. Such seizures include focal clonic, focal tonic (asymmetric tonic posturing and ocular deviation), and certain myoclonic events. These typically cannot be provoked by tactile or proprioceptive stimulation and cannot be suppressed by restraint of the involved limbs or by repositioning the infant. In addition, the clinical events are consistently associated with electrocortical seizure activity.

Other clinical seizure types are generated by nonepileptic mechanisms. These types include generalized tonic posturing and motor automatisms such as oral-buccal-lingual movements, movements of progression, and random eye movements. They can be provoked by stimulation, are suppressed by restraint or repositioning, and have no electrocortical signature. As a group, these seizures are thought to be a reflection of exaggerated reflexes referred to as "brainstem release phenomena" (7,12). In this chapter, the term *seizure* is used to refer to both types of clinical seizures, and the terms *epileptic* and *nonepileptic* are used to specify each type, respectively.

ETIOLOGY

Although different types of clinical seizures may suggest varying etiologies, the occurrence of any type of clinical seizure requires an immediate and thorough evaluation for the full range of etiologies that may be encountered in this age group. The prompt identification of a treatable cause of seizures and rapid institution of etiologic-specific therapy may decrease the likelihood of long-term neurologic sequelae and may effectively control seizures without the need for antiepileptic drugs (AEDs).

In evaluating an infant with neonatal seizures, emphasis is usually placed on the identification of major categories of etiologic factors: hypoxia-ischemia; metabolic disturbances (e.g., hypoglycemia, hypomagnesemia, hypocalcemia); CNS, systemic or intrauterine infections; structural brain lesions (e.g., hemorrhage, infarction, malformations); familial disorders (18–20); and inborn errors of metabolisms (including amino acidurias, urea cycle defects, organic acidurias, mitochondrial disorders, paroxysmal disorders, and metabolic substrate deficiencies) (21–25). Table 11-2 lists the most frequently identified etiologies in a relative order of frequency of occurrence, and Table 11-3 provides a more comprehensive list of possible etiologies and risk factors for seizures.

The evaluation to determine etiology of seizures is individualized. However, basic clinical and laboratory data are typically obtained for each affected infant, based on the major and most frequent categories of potential etiologies—hypoxia-ischemia, metabolic disorders, infection, and structural brain abnormalities

Table 11-3. Etiologic and Risk Factors of Neonatal Seizures

Hypoxia-ischemia
   Antepartum
   Intrapartum
   Postnatal
Infection
   Septicemia
   Meningitis
      Group B β-streptococcus
      Escherichia coli
      Other
   Meningoencephalitis
      Herpes simplex
      Toxoplasmosis
      Coxsackie B
      Rubella
      Cytomegalovirus
      Syphilis
   Human immunodeficiency virus
Intracranial hemorrhage
   Subarachnoid hemorrhage
   Subdural hemorrhage
   Intraventricular hemorrhage
   Intracerebral hemorrhage
Infarction
   Arterial
   Venous
   Polycythemia
   Hypercoaguable state
Congenital anomalies
   Cerebrocortical dysgeneses
      Agyria
      Pachygyria
      Polymicrogyria
      Lissencephaly, type I
         Sporadic
         Miller-Dieker Syndrome
      Lissencephaly, type II
   Perisylvian syndrome
      Microdysgenesis
      Aicardi syndrome
   Hydranencephaly
   Holoprosencephaly
Acute metabolic disturbances
   Hyponatremia and hypernatremia
      Inappropriate fluid therapy
      Sodium bicarbonate therapy in prematures
      Inappropriate antidiuretic hormone
   Hypoglycemia
      Transient
         Small for gestational age
         Prematurity
         Hyperinsulinemia, infant of diabetic mother
         Perinatal asphyxia or trauma (hemorrhage)
         Meningitis
         Postexchange transfusion
      Persistent
         Galactosemia
         Fructosemia

Table 11-3. (*Continued*)

         Leucine sensitivity
         Glycogen storage disease (glucose-6-phosphatase deficiency)
         Infantile gigantism (3.8–5.3 kg)
         Beckwith macroglossia (associated macroglasia)
         Pancreatic islet tumor
         Anterior pituitary hypoplasia
   Hypocalcemia
      Early (secondary)
         Perinatal asphyxia trauma (hemorrhage)
         Small for gestational age
         Infant of diabetic mother
         Postexchange transfusion
         DiGeorge syndrome
         Septicemia
         Maternal hyper- or hypoparathyroidism
      Late (primary)
         Diet—low calcium/phosphorus ratio
   Hypomagnesemia
      Associated with hypocalcemia
      Magnesium malabsorption syndrome
Inborn errors of metabolism
   Aminoaciduria
      Phenylketonuria
      Maple syrup urine disease
      Hyperglycinemia
      Congenital lysinuria
   Urea cycle defects
      Carbamyl phosphate synthetase deficiency
      Ornithine carbamyl transferase deficiency
      Citrullinemia
      Argininosuccinic aciduria
      Transient hyperammonemia of preterm and associated with perinatal asphyxia
   Organic acidurias
      Propionic acidemia
      Methylmalonic acidemia
      Methyl malonyl-coA mutase deficiency
      Biotinidase deficiency
   Pyridoxine
      Deficiency
      Dependency (autosomal recessive)
Neurodermatoses
   Incontinentia pigmenti
   Neurofibromatosis
   Sturge-Weber disease
   Tuberous sclerosis
Toxins
   Endogenous
      Bilirubin encephalopathy
   Exogenous
      Mercury (systemic exposure)
      Hexachlorophene (systemic exposure)
      Medication injected during labor
   Maternal drug dependency
      Cocaine
      Narcotics
      Barbiturates
Genetic
   Benign familial neonatal seizures
   Chromosomal anomalies

Table 11-3. (*Continued*)

Peroxysmal disorders
 Zellweger syndrome
 Neonatal adrenoleukodystrophy
Mitochrondrial disorders
 Leigh syndrome
Congenital malignancies
Unknown
 Benign neonatal convulsions

Adapted from Goddard et al., 1982; Kellaway and Mizrahi, 1987. Adapted and reprinted with permission from Mizrahi EM, Kellaway P. *Diagnosis and Management of Neonatal Seizures*. New York: Lippincott-Raven, 1998.

(Figure 11-2). Of these, the diagnosis of hypoxic-ischemic encephalopathy (HIE) may be the most difficult because precise definitions vary and all pertinent data may not be available. The diagnosis of HIE is based on a number of factors: perinatal history, serial Apgar scores, umbilical blood gas determinations, acid–base balance, the presence of multisystem impairment, and the neurologic examination (8,26–29). Metabolic disorders, such as hypocalcemia, hypomagnesemia, and hypoglycemia are assessed with appropriate serum assays. The presence of infection — viral or bacterial — is determined through a thorough clinical and laboratory evaluation that includes lumbar puncture and blood and urine cultures (30,31).

Neuroimaging is important in the diagnosis of structural brain abnormalities that may be associated with seizures. Head ultrasound is a valuable modality because it can be performed at bedside, but this technique is limited in range and resolution. Computerized tomography (CT) may be the next best neuroimaging technique because it can be performed quickly, but it too may be limited in resolution and in its ability to identify some types of lesions. Magnetic resonance imaging (MRI) can provide high resolution but may require more time to complete a study. In general, CT may be superior to MRI in identification of hemorrhage and intracranial calcifications; a CT performed early after occurrence of infarction may not clearly identify such a lesion but may show it later; CT may identify gross congenital brain anomalies, although MRI can delineate more subtle abnormalities (8,32–34).

Finally, many neonatal seizures may not be associated with a single etiologic factor, and thus it may only be possible to identify a group of etiologic and risk factors present at the time of seizure occurrence.

THERAPY

Effective therapy requires accurate diagnosis. Accurate diagnosis requires precise characterization and classification of seizure type and correct interpretation of the EEG findings. The immediate goals of therapy are seizure control and the identification and treatment of the etiological factor or factors responsible for the seizures. Unfortunately, in many cases the causative agent may not be determined, and even when identified there may be no known effective treatment. Similarly, currently available AEDs may be ineffective. In addition, not all seizures warrant AED treatment because they may not be epileptic in character or, when epileptic, they may be too brief or infrequent to justify treatment. There are several other factors that should be considered in the treatment of neonatal seizure: etiology, seizure duration and severity, the natural history of specific neonatal seizure disorders, and the impact seizures and AEDs may have on the developing brain.

Table 11-4. Etiology-Specific Therapy for Neonatal Seizures of Metabolic Origin

	Acute Therapy	Maintenance Therapy
Glucose, 10% solution[a]	2 ml/kg, IV	Up to 8 mg/kg/min, IV
Calcium gluconate, 10% solution[a]	2 ml/kg IV over 10 min	8 m/kg/day IV[b]
(9.4 mg of elemental Ca/ml)	(18 mg of elemental Ca/kg)	(75 mg of elemental Ca/kg/day)
Magnesium sulfate, 50% solution[a]	0.25 ml/kg, IM	0.25 ml/kg IM repeated every 12
(50 mg of elemental Mg/ml)		hrs until normomagnesemia
Pyridoxine[c]	100 mg, IV	

IV = intravenous; IM = intramuscular.
[a]Diagnosis of hypoglycemia, hypocalcemia, and hypomagnesium is dependent on neonate's gestational age (with preterm infants tending to tolerate lower levels). Administration of metabolic correcting solutions requires careful monitoring of infant's systemic homeostasis, including electrocardiogram monitoring during administration of calcium.
[b]After restoration of normocalcemia, tapering dosage may help in preventing rebound hypocalcemia.
[c]Although often cited as a treatable cause of refractory neonatal seizures, pyridoxine dependency or deficiency is exceedingly rare. Neither electroencephalographic nor clinical criteria for the diagnosis has been established.
Modified with permission from Mizrahi EM, Kellaway P. *Diagnosis and Management of Neonatal Seizures*. New York: Lippincott-Raven, 1998.

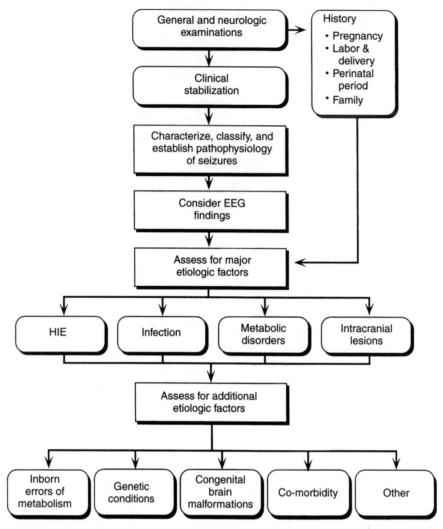

Figure 11-2. Steps in initial management and evaluation of cause. The evaluation of each neonate with seizures is individualized, based upon risk factors and initial clinical findings; however, infants are typically evaluated for the presence of major causative factors, with additional assessment when no cause can be identified. (With permission from Mizrahi EM, Kellaway P. *Diagnosis and Management of Neonatal Seizures.* New York: Lippincott-Raven, 1998.)

Phases of Acute Therapy

There are three phases of therapy, which should be individualized for each infant. They are initial medical management, etiology-specific therapy, and acute AED therapy (Figure 11-3).

Initial Medical Management

The usual principles of general medical management and cardiovascular-respiratory stabilization apply to neonates with seizures, particularly when seizures occur in the critically ill; when the seizures are frequent or prolonged; or when there are clinically significant changes in respiration, heart rate, and blood pressure as a consequence of seizures or vigorous AED therapy. While not all neonates require aggressive measures to support respiration and circulatory perfusion, early

anticipation of these clinical problems may minimize potential difficulties later.

Etiology-Specific Therapy

When potentially treatable causes of seizures are identified, etiology-specific therapy should be initiated as soon as possible to limit ongoing CNS injury. Etiology-specific therapy may also contribute to the control of seizures because some seizures may not be responsive to AED therapy unless the underlying causes are successfully treated. In some cases, etiology-specific therapy may be the only treatment needed, such as the correction of hypocalcemia, hypomagnesemia, or hypoglycemia (Table 11-4). In other cases, however, AEDs must be administered for seizure control the primary.

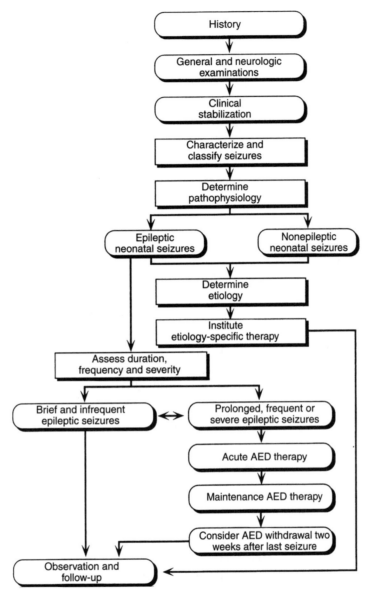

Figure 11-3. Steps in initiation and maintenance of therapy. The major issues in therapy of neonatal seizures are whether etiology-specific therapy can arrest seizures; whether the seizures are epileptic or nonepileptic in origin; and if they are epileptic in origin, whether they are of sufficient duration and frequency to warrant antiepileptic drug therapy. (With permission from Mizrahi EM, Kellaway P. *Diagnosis and Management of Neonatal Seizures.* New York: Lippincott-Raven, 1998.)

Table 11-5. Dosages of First-Line, Second-Line Antiepileptic Drugs in the Treatment of Neonatal Seizures

| Drug | Dose | | Average Therapeutic Range | Apparent Half-Life (Hours) |
	Loading	Maintenance		
Diazepam	0.25 mg/IV (bolus) 0.5 mg/kg (rectal)	May be repeated 1–2 times		31–54
Lorazepam	0.05 mg/kg (IV) (over 2–5 min)	May be repeated		31–54
Phenobarbital	20 mg/kg IV (up to 40 mg)	3–4 mg/kg in 2 doses	20–40 µg/L	100 after day 5–7
Phenytoin*	20 mg/kg IV (over 30–45 min)	3–4 mg/kg in 2–4 doses	15–25 µg/L	100 (40–200)

*Not FDA approved for neonates.
Reprinted with permission from Mizrahi EM, Kellaway P. *Diagnosis and Management of Neonatal Seizures.* New York: Lippincott-Raven; 1998: Based upon data from references 8,9,34c.

First-Line AED Therapy

The AEDs typically used in the acute treatment of neonatal seizures are phenobarbital, phenytoin, and a benzodiazepine (diazepam or lorazepam) given intravenously. The dosages are phenobarbital, 20 mg/kg as a loading dose, followed by additional increments of 10 mg/kg as required to achieve serum levels between 20 and 40 µg/mL; phenytoin, 20 mg/kg as a loading dose to achieve serum levels between 15 and 20 µg/mL; diazepam, 0.1 to 0.3 mg/kg in repeated doses; and lorazepam, 0.05 mg/kg in repeated doses (35–38) (Table 11-5). Acute administration of each of these AEDs may carry some risk of adverse reactions—CNS depression, hypotension, bradycardia, and respiratory depression (all of which may be associated with phenobarbital, diazepam, lorazepam) and cardiac arrhythmia (phenytoin)—thus requiring appropriate monitoring of infants during therapy.

There is a relative consensus as to which AEDs are first- and second-line drugs; phenobarbital is almost universally accepted as the first-line AED and phenytoin as the second (36,39). There is less of a consensus, however, as to the use of additional AEDs if the initial drugs fail to control the seizures. Typically, a benzodiazepine (diazepam or lorazepam) is given in this situation. There is also emerging discussion regarding the effectiveness of the use of initial benzodiazepine treatment before administration of first-line, longer-acting AEDs.

There have been few controlled studies of the relative efficacy of various AEDs in the initial treatment of neonatal seizures. However, the effectiveness of a loading dose of phenobarbital to achieve therapeutic serum levels in previously untreated neonates has been reported. Utilizing loading doses of 14 to 20 mg/kg,

three groups of investigators obtained response rates of 32 percent to 36 percent (40–43). Gal and colleagues reported a higher rate (86%) with higher loading doses (44). Painter and Gaus (45) have suggested that differences in seizure definition and dosing schedules may have been responsible for the discrepancy between these findings. In addition, Painter and colleagues recently compared the effectiveness of acute administration of phenobarbital versus phenytoin in seizure control (46,47) and found no significant difference between them. Neither proved as efficacious as is generally believed.

Regardless of the initial AED used, monotherapy is most appropriate. Doses of the initial AED may be increased to a level at which seizures cease or there is evidence of clinical toxicity, such as excessive sedation. A second AED should be added when seizures have not been controlled by the maximum tolerated dose of the initial AED.

Adjuvant and Alternative Therapy for Refractory Seizures

Because neonatal seizures may be resistant to traditional AEDs, other medications have been tried with varying success (37,46,48). However, the true efficacy of these agents is difficult to assess because some trials have not been well controlled. In addition, reports of the effectiveness of these medications have included a limited number of patients and involved infants who had already received and failed with other AEDs or who were receiving other AEDs concurrently. In addition, some AEDs were given orally rather than parenterally, limiting assessment of the immediate effect of these medications on seizure control. Because of the preliminary nature and limitations of these trials, few safety data are available. Adjuvant and

Table 11-6. Intravenous Dosages of Adjuvant and Alternative Antiepileptic Drug (AEDs) in the Treatment of Neonatal Seizure

AED	Dose — Loading	Dose — Maintenance	Range of Therapeutic Serum Levels	Comments and References
Clonazepam	0.1 mg/kg	Infusion over 5 min	28–117 mg/ml	
Lidocaine	4 mg/kg/hr (first day) or 2 mg/kg	Reduction by 1 mg/kg/hr/day on subsequent days or 6 mg/kg/hr	2.8–10.5 mg/L	Narrow therapeutic range: can be a convulsant at higher levels (51,52)
Midazolam	0.15 mg/kg	0.1–0.4 mg/kg/hr		Water-soluble, without polyethylene glycol and sodium benzoate additives Short half-life (0.8 hr) (54)
Paraldehyde	400 mg/kg or 200 mg/kg IV	200 mg/kg or 16 mg/kg/hr	>10 µg/L	Clearance decreased by phenobarbital and in asphyxia Efficacy linearly dependent upon serum levels (59,60)

Reprinted with permission from Mizrahi EM, Kellaway P. *Diagnosis and Management of Neonatal Seizures.* New York: Lippincott-Raven, 1998.

Table 11-7. Oral Dosages of Adjuvant and Alternative Antiepileptic Drugs in the Treatment of Neonatal Seizure

AED	Dose Loading	Dose Maintenance	Range of Therapeutic Serum Levels	Comments and References
Carbamazepine	5 mg/kg q 12 h	5 mg/kg q 12 h	10–40 μmol/L	Investigated as alternative maintenance AED No data on efficacy (61)
Lamotrigine	4.4 mg/kg/day	4.4 mg/kg/day		Other AEDs discontinued just before administration (48a) Based on a single case report
Primidone	15–25 mg/kg	12–20 mg/kg/day	3–18 μg/L	Elevation of phenobarbital levels if given concurrently Difficult to achieve initial high primidone levels (63,64)
Valproate	20–26 mg/kg	5–10 mg/kg q 12 h	40–50 μg/L	Use associated with hyperammonemia Used with caution as adjunctive agent in polytherapy (65)
Vigabatrin	50 mg/kg	50 mg/kg/day		Incomplete data in the neonate (66) Greater experience in infantile spasms (9)

Reprinted with permission from Mizrahi EM, Kellaway P. *Diagnosis and Management of Neonatal Seizures.* New York: Lippincott-Raven, 1998.

Table 11-8. Clinical Criteria to Initiate Therapy of Neonatal Seizures

Seizure Type	Clinical Characteristics	Therapy	Consensus or Controversy
Focal clonic	Brief and infrequent	AEDs optional	Controversy
	Prolonged and recurrent	AEDs	Consensus
Focal tonic	Brief and infrequent	AEDs optional	Controversy
	Prolonged and recurrent	AEDs	Consensus
Myoclonus	Brief and infrequent	AEDs optional	Controversy
	Provoked by stimulation	No AEDs	Consensus
Generalized tonic posturing or motor automatisms	Suppressed by restraint, provoked by stimulation	No AEDs	Consensus
	Not suppressed by restraint or provoked by stimulation	AEDs optional	Controversy

AED = antiepileptic drug.

alternative AEDs reported to be useful in neonatal seizure therapy are listed in Tables 11-6 and 11-7, discussed subsequently, and in more detail elsewhere (13). In the tables and discussions that follow, the AEDs are grouped according to routes of administration and are listed alphabetically within each group.

Intravenous AEDs

Clonazepam. André and colleagues (49) administered clonazepam, either 0.1 mg/kg or 0.2 mg/kg, to infants with seizures refractory to phenobarbital. All neonates continued to receive phenobarbital, and some received additional AEDs after clonazepam administration.

They concluded that infants receiving the lower dose of clonazepam appeared to respond more favorably (7 of 8) compared with those receiving the higher dose (7 of 10) because improvement of seizure frequency or seizure cessation occurred more quickly in the low-dose group.

Lidocaine. A number of investigators have used lidocaine as an add-on AED in neonates with otherwise refractory seizures (45,50,51). Administered intravenously, it was given in a schedule of decreasing dosages—4 mg/kg/hr, Day 1; 3 mg/kg/hr, Day 2; 2 mg/kg/hr, Day 3; 1 mg/kg/hr, Day 4; discontinuation, Day 5 —to achieve serum levels between 2.8 and 10.5 mg/mL (52). Radvany and colleagues reported seizure control in 19 of 26 neonates (pretreated with phenobarbital) within the first 20 minutes of infusion of lidocaine and within 13 hours in another. Other dosing schedules yielded similar results (2 mg/kg as a loading dose, followed by 6 mg/kg/hr) (51). Although promising, lidocaine has a narrow therapeutic range because serum levels between 0.5 and 4 mg/l may be anticonvulsant, but levels of 7.5 mg/l may induce seizures (45,51,52).

Midazolam. Midazolam is a short-acting benzodiazepine, which initially was given to neonates for sedation (53). Sheth and colleagues (54) administered midazolam to six neonates with seizures refractory to high-dose phenobarbital (serum levels >40 mg/mL): a loading dose of midazolam, 0.15 mg/kg, followed by maintenance doses between 0.1 and 0.4 mg/kg/hr given as a constant intravenous (IV) infusion (no serum levels were reported). Four infants became seizure-free immediately after receiving the loading dose, and the other two infants became seizure-free within the first hour of initiation of midazolam. After the initial response, four of the infants showed no further seizure activity on EEG, and two infants showed a reduction in such activity. The investigators suggest that midazolam has advantages over diazepam and lorazepam because midazolam is water-soluble; does not contain polyethylene glycol and sodium benzoate found in the other drugs (55,56); is faster-acting than lorazepam; and with a short half life (0.8 hours) the titration of midazolam is easier (57,58).

Paraldehyde. Koren and colleagues (59) treated 14 neonates with paraldehyde, given as a single 400 mg/kg bolus to achieve serum levels between 6 and 17.5 mg/dl (mean 11.8 mg/dl). They reported that this regimen reduced the number of seizures by more than 50 percent or completely abolished them. Recommended dosing schedules include 400 mg/kg IV bolus, followed—if seizures persist—by an additional 200 mg/kg dose given over 1 hour, or 200 mg/kg followed by 16 mg/kg/hr to achieve serum levels above 10 mg/dl (59,60). Paraldehyde must be used with caution in neonates with lung disease, and its clearance may be decreased by concomitant administration of phenobarbital and in neonates with birth asphyxia. The drug is administered as a 5% dextrose solution, and the use of plastic tubing is avoided because it can be dissolved by the drug. In addition, it must be shielded from light to prevent precipitation in exposed tubing. Despite these cautions, paraldehyde is considered a relatively safe and effective AED for neonatal seizures. Unfortunately, it is no longer available in the United States.

Oral AEDs

Carbamazepine. Mackintosh and coworkers (61) investigated the pharmacokinetics of carbamazepine in neonates. They administered carbamazepine suspension (10 mg/mL) orally, 5 mg/kg every 12 hours, resulting in peak serum concentrations; between 10 and 40 mg/L, 2 to 12 hours after the first dose (mean, 6.7 ± 1.4 hours). The investigators suggested that the drug can be safely administered to neonates, but no data on efficacy were presented.

Lamotrigine. Lamotrigine was given to a 17-day old, full-term neonate with refractory seizures of undetermined etiology after phenobarbital, phenytoin, midazolam, clonazepam, vigabatrin, pyridoxine, and biotin had failed. Lamotrigine in a single daily dose of 4.4 mg/kg/day was given for 3 days and then in divided daily doses every 12 hours. Seizures remitted 75 minutes after the first dose was given (62).

Primidone. Primidone has been given to neonates with refractory seizures as adjuvant therapy and has been considered by some to be a good third-line AED (45,63). Powell and colleagues (64) gave neonates loading doses between 15 and 25 mg/kg followed by maintenance doses of 12 to 20 mg/kg/day, achieving primidone levels between 3 and 18 mg/L (64). They reported that seizure control was achieved in 13 of 20 infants within 48 hours of initiation of therapy.

Valproate. Gal and colleagues (65) studied neonates with refractory seizures, all of whom were receiving multiple AEDs. Valproate was given as a loading dose of 20 to 25 mg/kg orally, followed by 5 to 10 mg/kg every 12 hours. Standard valproate syrup (25 mg/5 ml) diluted in an equal volume of infant formula was administered either orally or through feeding tubes. Seizures were reported to be controlled in five of the six infants studied. However, valproate was discontinued in three infants because of hyperammonemia. Overall, two of the six infants did achieve seizure control without valproate toxicity. To date, there have been no reports of the use of the new IV preparation of valproate in neonates.

Vigabatrin. Although the experience with vigabatrin in neonates with refractory seizures is anecdotal or preliminary, there are reports of favorable responses (66). Dosing has been according to regimens used for the treatment of infantile spasms (approximately 50 mg/kg/day) (67).

Emerging AED Therapy — Fosphenytoin
The U.S. Food and Drug Administration recently approved fosphenytoin as an AED for parenteral use

in adults. Its efficacy and safety in neonates is currently under investigation, and as of this writing it has not been approved for use in neonates. However, there are important features of fosphenytoin that differentiate it from phenytoin and should be considered if fosphenytoin is eventually approved for use in the newborn.

Fosphenytoin is a prodrug of phenytoin. After fosphenytoin is absorbed, phenytoin is cleaved from the prodrug by phosphatase enzymes. This conversion is rapid and complete in adults. The conversion of the prodrug by phosphatase enzymes in neonates is currently being studied to confirm the presence of the enzyme, identify its characteristics, and determine the rate and degree to which conversion is accomplished. Thus, generalizations concerning the data obtained in adults must be considered cautiously in relation to neonates.

Although phenytoin and fosphenytoin may both produce similar systemic toxicity, including cardiac depression, with fosphenytoin there is less potential for adverse reaction at the infusion site because of the absence of the vehicles needed for parenteral sodium phenytoin (propylene glycol and sodium benzoate). The absence of these vehicles is thought to substantially reduce the potential for irritation of blood vessels and skin at the site of infusion. An additional potential advantage of the use of fosphenytoin is the ability to administer fosphenytoin intramuscularly.

The use of fosphenytoin in neonates with seizures has been recently investigated. Findings indicate that the conversion half-life of fosphenytoin and resultant plasma total and free (unbound) phenytoin concentration-time profiles following IV administration in neonates are similar to values in older children and adults, although the range of values was greater in neonates (68–71).

DECISION MAKING IN THE INITIATION OF AED THERAPY

The initiation of AED therapy requires the consideration of seizure type, pathophysiology, duration and severity of seizures, natural history of the seizure disorder, and anticipated potentially adverse effects of the seizures themselves and the selected AEDs on the infant. Not all neonatal seizures require AED therapy, including those of nonepileptic origin; those of epileptic origin responsive to etiologic-specific treatment; and, perhaps, those epileptic seizures that are brief, infrequent, and self-limited.

Typically, clinicians consider beginning AED therapy without the benefit of EEG and must first decide if the clinical seizures are of epileptic or nonepileptic origin based on bedside observation (Tables 11-8 and 11-9). If the seizures are of epileptic origin, they must be assessed for duration, severity, and etiology. Additional information can be obtained from the EEG.

AED Therapy Based on Features of the Clinical Seizure

When clinical seizures are encountered without the availability of concurrent EEG, management decisions are based solely on the clinical features of the seizures (Table 11-9) (13,72).

1. *Focal clonic or focal tonic seizures that are prolonged and recurrent*. Focal clonic seizures are repetitive and rhythmic muscle contractions that cannot be

Table 11-10. A Balanced Regimen of Antiepileptic (AED) Therapy of Neonatal Seizures

1. Decision to treat with AEDs has been made.
2. Initiate acute therapy to eliminate clinical seizures with first-line AED (phenobarbital).
3. If clinical or EEG seizures persist
   a. First increase phenobarbital
   b. If seizures persist, add phenytoin
   c. If seizures still persist, add benzodiazepines
4. If clinical seizures are controlled but electrical seizures persist ("decoupling"), increase phenobarbital and phenytoin to high-therapeutic levels.
5. After seizure control is obtained or the degree of control is considered acceptable, establish maintenance AED therapy.
6. Withdraw AEDs two weeks following the last clinical seizure and at a time when no electrical seizure activity is present on EEG.
7. Clinical follow-up for seizure recurrence.

EEG = electroencephalogram.

Table 11-9. Electroencephalogram (EEG) Criteria to Initiate Therapy of Neonatal Seizures

Seizure Type	Therapy	Consensus or Controversy
Clinical seizures in the absence of EEG seizure activity	No AEDs	Controversy
EEG seizures in the absence of clinical seizures	AEDs	Consensus

AED = antiepileptic drug.

arrested by restraint or repositioning. Similarly, focal tonic seizures, such as sustained posturing of a limb, cannot be altered by these maneuvers. The focal tonic seizures characterized by eye deviation can be differentiated from the random eye movements of nonepileptic motor automatisms because the epileptic tonic eye deviation is sustained and cannot be evoked by stimulation. These clinical features help to designate them as epileptic in origin. Once the clinical focal clonic or focal tonic seizures are considered epileptic, duration and severity must be considered; when sustained and prolonged, they are treated vigorously with AEDs.

2. *Focal clonic or focal tonic seizures that are brief and infrequent.* The specific features of these seizures of epileptic origin are the same as those just described and provide the basis for their designation as epileptic in origin. Although AEDs may be used in attempts to control them, because these seizures may be brief, occur infrequently, and have a short natural history with relatively rapid spontaneous resolution, the use of AEDs may not always be required. In these circumstances, the potential adverse effects of AEDs may be greater than the potential risk of these brief and infrequent seizures on the developing brain (73). As yet, however, there are no quantitatively based criteria for the differentiation of "brief" and "infrequent" seizures from "prolonged" and "recurrent" seizures. In addition, the issues of whether AEDs or seizures adversely affect the immature brain have not yet been completely resolved (74–76).

3. *Generalized tonic posturing and motor automatisms that can be provoked or intensified by stimulation and suppressed by restraint.* Generalized tonic posturing and motor automatisms (including ocular signs, oral-buccal-lingual movements, movements of progression, and complex purposeless movements, which are more traditionally referred to as "subtle seizures") may be presumed to be of nonepileptic origin. This designation is based on clinical features of the seizures and their response to stimulation and restraint. The differentiation from epileptic seizures can be made at the bedside based on the features of the spontaneous events and the response of the infant to clinical maneuvers: the spontaneous events can be suppressed by restraint or repositioning of the limbs or trunk, and events can be evoked or intensified by tactile or proprioceptive stimulation that are similar in character to spontaneous events. Traditionally, these clinical events have been treated with AEDs, often in high doses, and in some instances

their frequency and severity have diminished. Although this finding has been used to support the notion that these events are epileptic seizures, this effect of AEDs is most likely not the result of specific antiepileptic properties but rather because the drugs used are also CNS depressants. Overall, if generalized tonic posturing and motor automatisms demonstrate characteristic clinical features, they can be presumed to be of nonepileptic origin and do not require AED therapy (12,77). Although the clinical events may be initially quite dramatic, their natural course is one of gradual and spontaneous resolution without AED therapy.

4. *Generalized tonic posturing and motor automatisms that may not be responsive to stimulation or may not be suppressed by restraint.* For some infants, the clinical features of spontaneous, generalized tonic posturing and motor automatisms may be typical of nonepileptic events, but they may not respond in a characteristic way to the clinical maneuvers of restraint, repositioning, or stimulation. This may be due to techniques of stimulation or restraint or to other undefined factors. In these instances, the decision to initiate AED is more difficult. Some clinicians may withhold AEDs with the understanding that the clinical features of the spontaneous events are sufficient evidence of the nonepileptic origin of the events. However, others may initiate AED treatment with the belief that clinical observation and maneuvers alone cannot provide data to indicate underlying pathophysiology. Monitoring studies using EEG-video have shown that these seizure types are nonepileptic in origin and therefore are also not treated with AEDs (12).

AED Therapy Based on EEG or EEG-Video Monitoring

Bedside EEG and EEG-video monitoring are invaluable tools in the diagnosis of neonatal seizures (13,78,79). When available and appropriately applied, they provide additional data in assessing whether AED therapy should be initiated (Table 11-9)—as well as increased, continued, or discontinued.

1. *Clinical seizures may be present in the absence of EEG seizure activity.* These clinical seizure types include generalized tonic posturing and motor automatisms. As discussed previously, the clinical features of the spontaneous events and the response of the events to clinical maneuvers suggest that they are nonepileptic origin. The lack of EEG seizure activity at the time of the clinical seizures provides additional supportive data. These clinical events are not treated with AEDs.

2. *EEG seizure activity may occur in the absence of any associated clinical seizures.* This may occur in neonates who are pharmacologically paralyzed; in neonates with seizure discharges of the depressed brain type (13,78); or in neonates with epileptic seizures already treated with AEDs (see next section). Although electrical seizures occurring in the absence of any clinical seizure activity are treated with AEDs, these electrical seizures may be highly resistant to therapy despite high doses of several AEDs. High-dose polypharmacy may be used in attempts to abolish EEG seizure activity. However, adverse effects of these medications will emerge. This raises the question of the relative value of vigorous AED therapy compared with the potential for respiratory, cardiac, or cardiovascular or CNS depression.

RESPONSE OF CLINICAL AND EEG SEIZURES TO ACUTE AED THERAPY

There is a characteristic response of clinical epileptic seizures to AEDs. In untreated infants, clinical epileptic seizures occur in a time-locked relationship to EEG seizure activity. An initial response to AED administration is the cessation of clinical seizures; however, the EEG seizure activity may persist. This initial response to AED treatment has been referred to as "decoupling" of the clinical from the electrical seizure (12,80–82). The response of the electrical seizures to either increasing doses of an AED or the addition of other AEDs is variable and may prove to be highly resistant to additional AED therapy.

This decoupling response to AED raises an important clinical question: Is the endpoint of AED therapy the cessation of both clinical and electrical seizure activity? Vigorous attempts to eliminate electrical seizure activity may require the administration of high doses and/or multiple AEDs. Regardless of the degree of success in seizure control (which is often incomplete), high-dose and/or polypharmacy may be associated with CNS depression, systemic hypotension, and respiratory depression. Thus, the clinician must consider several factors, including the potential risks of aggressive AED treatment, the potential benefits of therapy, the likelihood of success, and whether electrical seizure activity is harmful to the developing brain.

RISK VERSUS BENEFIT OF ACUTE AED THERAPY

Risk of Recurrent Seizures

Primary Risks

There is no clear consensus as to what, if any, sequelae may be associated with the occurrence of epileptic

seizures in the developing brain (74–76). Some animal studies indicate that there are changes in the CNS at a cellular or molecular level or even of brain circuitry. These may be transient or their influence may be limited when animal performance is tested. In addition, these issues have not been comprehensively addressed in human trials.

Secondary Risks

There are few conclusive clinical investigations of the adverse systemic effects of seizures. However, infants with prolonged seizures may experience changes in respiration, heart rate, or blood pressure and may also have increased metabolic requirements during seizures. These findings may contribute to further compromise an infant who is already ill.

Risk of AED Therapy

Primary Risks

There also is an equal lack of consensus concerning the possible adverse effects of AEDs on the developing brain. Although experimental data suggest some alterations in cell growth and energy substrate utilization with AEDs (83–86), the applicability of these findings to human neonates has been questioned and the relative risks considered small compared with the overall potential gain (8).

Secondary Risks

There also have been few studies of adverse effects of acute AED therapy. However, aggressive treatment may result in CNS depression, hypotension, bradycardia, and respiratory depression (87) and may create the potential for secondary CNS hypoxia or ischemia.

Balanced Treatment Regimens

A balanced AED acute treatment regimen that may minimize perceived risks and maximize therapeutic effectiveness includes acute therapy that is initiated to eliminate clinical seizures with the first-line AED of phenobarbital (Table 11-10). If clinical or EEG seizures persist, phenobarbital dose is increased; then, if necessary, phenytoin is added and, if required, a benzodiazepine. If clinical seizures are controlled but electrical seizures persist, phenobarbital and then phenytoin doses are increased to obtain high therapeutic serum levels. Maintenance therapy is established after seizure control is attained or reaches acceptable levels based on trials of initial therapy.

CHRONIC THERAPY

Maintenance Therapy

Not all neonates require chronic therapy after acute seizures have been controlled. In fact, guidelines for selection of individuals for maintenance therapy are controversial. When a therapeutic effect is obtained acutely, infants are typically placed on maintenance doses of AEDs—either phenobarbital alone or with phenytoin if it had been required to control the clinical seizures acutely (the maintenance dose of each is 3–4 mg/kg/day). Serum levels are monitored; however, the presence of clinical toxicity rather than the finding of elevated serum drug levels should determine adjustment of doses.

The maintenance of stable chronic levels of either phenobarbital or phenytoin may be difficult. When maintenance doses of phenobarbital of 5 mg/kg/day are used, there may be drug accumulation within 5 to 10 days of life (41) because of the relatively slow elimination rate of phenobarbital during this period. This effect may be enhanced in asphyxiated infants who may have concomitant hepatic or renal dysfunction (8,44,88,89). Eventually, however, elimination rates increase with time. Thus, maintenance dosing requirements are relatively lower early in the course of therapy but increase later. There also may be problems in maintenance of therapeutic levels of phenytoin because of its nonlinear kinetics and the rapid decrease in elimination rates during the first weeks of life (90,91).

Discontinuation of Therapy

The discontinuation of AEDs after a period of clinical seizure control is highly individualized because no specific practice guidelines have been established. Most clinicians use personal judgment and clinical experience. Maintenance schedules range from 1 week up to 12 months after the last seizure (92). Specific clinical and EEG predictors of recurrent seizures following AED withdrawal have not been identified (93,94). However, there has been increasing clinical interest in short-term therapy, with AED withdrawal 2 weeks following the infant's last clinical seizure (95). The natural history of the specific neonatal seizure disorder may be the best determinant of the timing of AED discontinuation. For example, seizures that are the consequence of acute disorders, such as hypocalcemia, may not require AED therapy after the disorder has been successfully treated. Overall, the decision to withdraw AEDs is primarily based on the clinical course of individual infants, the presence or absence of clinical seizures, and the absence of electrical seizures recorded by the EEG performed before AED discontinuation.

PROGNOSIS

The purported objectives of rapid diagnosis, accurate identification of etiology, and successful AED treatment are to prevent adverse sequelae of seizures and improve long-term outcomes of affected neonates. However, there are few comprehensive studies that define conclusively a relationship between cessation of seizures and prognosis in terms of subsequent neurologic deficit, behavioral or intellectual status, or the development of post-neonatal epilepsy. It may be assumed, however, that easily controlled seizures are the result of transient, successfully treated, or benign CNS disorders of neonates, whereas medically refractory neonatal seizures may be the result of more sustained, less treatable, or more severe brain disorders. Overall, it appears that the primary factor that predicts outcome is the underlying cause of the seizures rather than specific characteristics of the epileptic events themselves (12,96–101).

REFERENCES

1. Lanska MJ, Lanska DJ, Baumann RJ, et al. A population-based study of neonatal seizures in Fayette County, Kentucky. *Neurology* 1995; 45:724–732.

2. Ronen GM, Penney S. The epidemiology of clinical neonatal seizures in Newfoundland, Canada: A five-year cohort. *Ann Neurol* 1995; 38:518–519.

3. Saliba RM, Annegers JF, Waller DK, Tyson JE, Mizrahi EM. Incidence of neonatal seizures in Harris County, Texas, 1992–1994. *Am J Epidemiol* 1999; 150:763–769.

4. Bergman I, Painter MJ, Hirsch RP, Crumrine PK, David R. Outcome in neonates with convulsions treated in an intensive care unit. *Ann Neurol* 1983; 14:642–647.

5. Scher MS, Aso K, Beggarly M, et al. Electrographic seizures in preterm and full-term neonates: clinical correlates, associated brain lesions, and risk for neurologic sequelae. *Pediatrics* 1993; 91:128–134.

6. Scher MS, Hamid MY, Steppe DA, Beggarly ME, Painter MJ. Ictal and interictal electrographic seizure durations in preterm and term neonates. *Epilepsia* 1993; 34:284–288.

7. Kellaway P, Hrachovy RA. Status epilepticus in newborns: a perspective on neonatal seizures. In: Delgado-Escueta AV, Wasterlain CG, Treiman DM, Porter RJ, eds. *Advances in Neurology. Vol. 34. Status Epilepticus.* New York: Raven Press, 1983:93–99.

8. Volpe JJ. Neonatal seizures. In: *Neurology of the Newborn.* Philadelphia: WB Saunders, 1995:172–207.

9. Dreyfus-Brisac C, Monod N. Electroclinical studies of status epilepticus and convulsions in the newborn. In: Kellaway P, Petersen I, eds. *Neurological and Electroencephalographic Correlative Studies in Infancy.* New York: Grune & Stratton, 1964:250–272.

10. Rose AL, Lombroso CT. A study of clinical, pathological, and electroencephalographic features in 137

full-term babies with a long-term follow-up [or is it neonatal seizure states]. *Pediatrics* 1970; 45:404–425.

11. Volpe JJ. Neonatal seizures. *N Engl J Med* 1973; 289:413–416.

12. Mizrahi EM, Kellaway P. Characterization and classification of neonatal seizures. *Neurology* 1987; 37:1837–1844.

13. Mizrahi EM, Kellaway P. *Diagnosis and Management of Neonatal Seizures.* New York: Lippincott-Raven, 1998.

14. Clancy RR. The management of neonatal seizures. In: Stevenson DK, Seins P, eds. *Fetal and Neonatal Brain Injury.* 2nd ed. New York: Oxford University Press, 1997:432–461.

15. Clancy RR, Chung HJ, Temple JP. Neonatal electroencephalography. Vol. 1. In: Sperling MR, Clancy RR, eds. *Atlas of Electroencephalography.* Amsterdam: Elsevier, 1993.

16. Laroia N, Guillet R, Burchfiel J, McBride MC. EEG background as predictor of electrographic seizures in high-risk neonates. *Epilepsia* 1998; 39:545–551.

17. Mizrahi EM. Pediatric electroencephalographic video monitoring. *J Clin Neurophysiol* 1999; 16:100–110.

18. Leppert M, Anderson VE, Quattlebaum TG, et al. Benign familial neonatal convulsions linked to genetic markers on chromosome 20. *Nature* 1989; 337:647–648.

19. Ronen GM, Rosales TO, Connolly M, et al. Seizure characteristics in chromosome 20 benign familial neonatal convulsions. *Neurology* 1993; 43:1355–1360.

20. Lerche H, Biervert C, Alekov AK, et al. A reduced K$^+$ current due to a novel mutation in KCNQ2 causes neonatal convulsions. *Ann Neurol* 1999; 46:305–312.

21. Salbert BA, Pellock JM, Wolf B. Characterization of seizures associated with biotinidase deficiency. *Neurology* 1993; 43:1351–1355.

22. Haagerup A, Andersen JB, Blichfeldt S, Christensen MF. Biotinidase deficiency: two cases of very early presentation. *Dev Med Child Neurol* 1997; 39:832–835.

23. Takahashi Y, Suzuki Y, Kumazaki K, et al. Epilepsy in peroxisomal diseases. *Epilepsia* 1997; 38:182–188.

24. Nabbout R, Soufflet C, Plouin P, Dulac O. Pyridoxine dependent epilepsy: a suggestive electroclinical pattern. *Arch Dis Child Fetal Neonatal Ed* 1999; 81:F125–F129.

25. Sue CM, Hirano M, DiMauro S, De Vivo DC. Neonatal presentations of mitochondrial metabolic disorders. *Semin Perinatol* 1999; 23:113–124.

26. Evans DJ, Levene MI. Hypoxic-ischemic injury. In: Rennie JM, Roberton NRC. *Textbook of Neonatology.* New York: Churchill Livingstone, 1999; 1231–1251.

27. Committee on Obstetric Practice and American Academy of Pediatrics: Committee on Fetus and Newborn. ACOG committee opinion. Use and abuse of the Apgar score. Number 174–July 1996. American College of Obstetricians and Gynecologists. *Int J Gynaecol Obstet* 1996; 54:303–305.

28. Perlman JM. Intrapartum hypoxic-ischemic cerebral injury and subsequent cerebral palsy: medicolegal issues. *Pediatrics* 1997; 99:851–859.

29. Vannucci RC. Hypoxia-ischemia: clinical aspects. In: Fanaroff A, Martin RJ, eds. *Neonatal-Perinatal Medicine.* 6th ed. St. Louis: Mosby, 1997:877–891.

30. Baley JE, Toltzis P. Viral infections. In: Fanaroff A, Martin RJ, eds. *Neonatal-Perinatal Medicine.* 6th ed. St. Louis: Mosby, 1997:769–811.

31. Hickey S, McCracken G Jr. Postnatal bacterial infections. In: Fanaroff A, Martin RJ, eds. *Neonatal-Perinatal Medicine.* 6th ed. St. Louis: Mosby, 1997:769–811.

32. Barkovich JA. *Pediatric Neuroimaging.* 2nd ed. New York: Raven Press, 1995:668.

33. Morrison SC, Fletcher BD. Diagnostic imaging. In: Fanaroff A, Martin RJ, eds. *Neonatal-Perinatal Medicine.* 6th ed. St. Louis: Mosby, 1997:639–671.

34. Leth H, Toft PB, Herning M, Petersen B, Lou HC. Neonatal seizures associated with cerebral lesions shown by magnetic resonance imaging. *Arch Dis Child Fetal Neonatal Ed* 1997; 77:F105–F110.

34a. Kalhan S, Saker F. Metabolic and endocrine disorders. In: Fanaroff AA, Martin RJ, eds. *Neonatal-Perinatal Medicine: Diseases of the Fetus and Infant.* St. Louis: Mosby, 1997:1439–1563.

34b. Koo WW, Tsang RC. Calcium and magnesium homeostasis. In: Avery GB, Fletcher MA, MacDonald MB. *Neonatal Pathophysiology and Management of the Newborn.* Philadelphia, Lippincott, 1994:585–604.

34c. Fenichel GM. *Neonatal Neurology.* 3rd ed. New York: Churchill-Livingstone, 1990.

35. Deshmukh A, Wittert W, Schnitzler E, Mangurten HH. Lorazepam in the treatment of refractory neonatal seizures. *Am J Dis Child* 1986; 140:1042–1044.

36. André M, Vert P, Wasterlain CG. To treat or not to treat: a survey of current medical practice toward neonatal seizures. In: CG Wasterlain CG, Vert P, eds. *Neonatal Seizures.* New York: Raven Press, 1990:303–307.

37. Painter MJ, Alvin J. Choice of anticonvulsants in the treatment of neonatal seizures. In: CG Wasterlain CG, Vert P, eds. *Neonatal Seizures.* New York: Raven Press, 1990:243–256.

38. Maytal J, Novak GP, King KC. Lorazepam in the treatment of refractory neonatal seizures. *J Child Neurol* 1991; 6:319–323.

39. Massingale TW, Buttross S. Survey of treatment practices for neonatal seizures. *J Perinatol* 1993; 13:107–110.

40. Jalling B. Plasma concentrations of phenobarbital in the treatment of seizures in the newborn. *Acta Paediatr Scand* 1975; 64:14.

41. Painter MJ, Pippenger C, MacDonald H, Pitlick W. Phenobarbital and diphenylhydantoin levels in neonates with seizures. *J Pediatr* 1978; 92:315–319.

42. Painter MJ, Pippenger C, Wasterlain C, et al. Phenobarbital and phenytoin in neonatal seizures. *Neurology* 1981; 31:1107–1112.

43. Lockman LA, Kriel R, Zaske D. Phenobarbital dosage for control of neonatal seizures. *Neurology* 1979; 29:1445–1449.

44. Gal P, Toback J, Boer HR, Erkan NV, Wells TJ. Efficacy of phenobarbital monotherapy in treatment of neonatal

seizures-relationship to blood levels. *Neurology* 1982; 32:1401–1404.

45. Painter MJ, Gaus LM. Neonatal seizures: diagnosis and treatment. *J Child Neurol* 1991; 6:101–108.

46. Painter MJ, Minnigh MB, Gaus L, et al. Neonatal phenobarbital and phenytoin binding profiles. *J Clin Pharmacol* 1994; 34:312–317.

47. Painter MJ, Scher MS, Stein AD, et al. Phenobarbital compared with phenytoin for the treatment of neonatal seizures. *N Engl J Med* 1999; 341:485–489.

48. Hellström-Westas L, Svenningse NW, Westgren U, et al. Lidocaine for treatment of severe seizures in newborn infants. II. Blood concentrations of lidocaine and metabolites during intravenous infusion. *Acta Paediatr Scand* 1992; 81:35–39.

48a. Barr PA, Buettiker VE, Antony JH. Efficacy of lamotrigine in refractory neonatal seizures. *Pediatr Neurol* 1999; 20:161–163.

49. André M, Boutray MJ, Dubruc O, et al. Clonazepam pharmacokinetics and therapeutic efficacy in neonatal seizures. *Eur J Clin Pharmacol* 1986; 305:585–589.

50. Norell E, Gamstorp I. Neonatal seizures: effect of lidocaine. *Acta Paediatr Scand* 1970; 206 (Suppl):97–98.

51. Hellström-Westas L, Westgren U, Rosen I, Svenningsen NW. Lidocaine for treatment of severe seizures in newborn infants. I. Clinical effects and cerebral electrical activity monitoring. *Acta Paediatr Scand* 1988; 77:79–84.

52. Radvany-Bouvet MF, Torricelli A, Rey E, et al. Effects of lidocaine on seizures in the neonatal period. Some electroclinical aspects. In: CG Wasterlain CG, Vert P, eds. *Neonatal Seizures.* New York: Raven Press, 1990:275–283.

53. Jacqz AE, Daoud P, Burtin P, Desplanques L, Beaufils F. Placebo-controlled trial of midazolam sedation in mechanically ventilated newborn babies. *Lancet* 1994; 344:646–650.

54. Sheth RD, Buckley DJ, Gutierrez AR, et al. Midazolam in the treatment of refractory neonatal seizures. *Clin Neuropharmacol* 1996; 19:165–170.

55. Glasgow AM, Boeckx RL, Miller MK, et al. Hyperosmolality in small infants due to propylene glycol. *Pediatrics* 1983; 72:353–355.

56. Nathenson G, Cohen MI, McNamara H. The effect of Na benzoate on serum bilirubin of the Gunn rat. *J Pediatr* 1975; 86:799–803.

57. Malacrida R, Fritz ME, Suter PM, Crevoisier C. Pharmacokinetics of midazolam administered by continuous intravenous infusion to intensive care patients. *Crit Care Med* 1992; 20:1123–1126.

58. McDermott CA, Kowalczyk AL, Schnitzler ER, et al. Pharmacokinetics of lorazepam in critically ill neonates with seizures. *J Pediatr* 1992; 120:479–483.

59. Koren G, Warwick B, Rajchgot R, et al. Intravenous paraldehyde for seizure control in newborn infants. *Neurology* 1986; 36:108–111.

60. Giacoia GP, Gessner PK, Zaleska MM, et al. Pharmacokinetics of paraldehyde disposition in the neonate. *J Pediatr* 1984; 104:291–296.

61. Mackintosh DA, Baird-Lampert J, Buchanan N. Is carbamazepine an alternative maintenance therapy for neonatal seizures. *Dev Pharmacol Ther* 1987; 10:100–106.

62. Bain.

63. Sapin JI, Riviello JJ Jr, Grover WD. Efficacy of primidone for seizure control in neonates and young infants. *Pediatr Neurol* 1988; 4:292–295.

64. Powell C, Painter MJ, Pippenger CE. Primidone therapy in refractory neonatal seizures. *J Pediatr* 1984; 105:651–654.

65. Gal P, Otis K, Gilman J, Weaver R. Valproic acid efficacy, toxicity and pharmacokinetics in neonates with intractable seizures. *Neurology* 1988; 38:467–471.

66. Baxter PS, Gardner-Medwin D, Barwick DD, et al. Vigabatrin monotherapy in resistant neonatal seizures. *Seizure* 1995; 4:57–59.

67. Aicardi J, Sabril IS, Investigator and Peer Review Groups, Mumford JP, Dumas C, Wood S. Vigabatrin as initial therapy for infantile spasms: a European retrospective survey. *Epilepsia* 1996; 37:638–642.

68. Wheless JW. Pediatric use of intravenous and intramuscular phenytoin: lessons learned. *J Child Neurol* 1998; 13(Suppl 1):S11–S14; S30–2.

69. Allen et al., 1995.

70. Morton LD, Pellock JM, Gilman JT, et al. Fosphenytoin pharmacokinetics and safety in pediatric patients. *Ann Neurol* 1997; 42:504. Abstract.

71. Morton LD, Pellock JM, Marin BL, et al. Fosphenytoin safety and pharmacokinetics in children, abstract. *Epilepsia* 1997; 38(Suppl 8):194.

72. Mizrahi EM. Neonatal seizures. In: Shinnar S, Amir N, Branski D, eds. *Childhood Seizures. Pediatric and Adolescent Medicine.* Vol. 6. Basel: Karger, 1995:18–31.

73. Moshé SL. Epileptogenesis and the immature brain. *Epilepsia* 1987; 28(Suppl 1):S3–S15.

74. Wasterlain CG. Recurrent seizures in the developing brain are harmful. *Epilepsia* 1997; 38:728–734.

75. Camfield, PR. Recurrent seizures in the developing brain are not harmful. *Epilepsia* 1997; 38:735–737.

76. Holmes GL. Epilepsy in the developing brain: lessons from the laboratory and clinic. *Epilepsia* 1997; 38:12–30.

77. Mizrahi EM. Consensus and controversy in the clinical management of neonatal seizures. In: Volpe JJ, ed. *Clinics in Perinatology.* Vol. 16, No. 2: Neonatal Neurology. Philadelphia: WB Saunders, 1989:485–500.

78. Hrachovy RA, Mizrahi EM, Kellaway P. Electroencephalography of the newborn. In: Daly D, Pedley TA, eds. *Current Practice of Clinical Electroencephalography.* 2nd ed. New York: Raven Press, 1990:201–242.

79. Mizrahi EM. Clinical diagnosis and management of neonatal seizures. *Int Pediatr* 1994; 9:94–101.

80. Mizrahi EM, Kellaway P. Learning to recognize neonatal seizures (20 minutes). University of Texas Health Science Center Medical Television, 1992.

81. Mizrahi EM, Kellaway P. Neonatal seizures: Review of assessment skills. Part one (10 minutes). University of Texas Health Science Center Medical Television, 1992.

82. Mizrahi EM, Kellaway P. Neonatal seizures: review of assessment skills. Part two (10 minutes). University of Texas Health Science Center Medical Television, 1992.

83. Diaz J, Schain RJ. Phenobarbital: effects of long-term administration on behavior and brain of artificially reared rats. *Science* 1978; 199:90.

84. Diaz J, Schain RJ, Bailey BG. Phenobarbital-induced brain growth retardation in artificially reared rat pups. *Biol Neonate* 1977; 32:77–82.

85. Bergey GK, Swaiman KF, Schrier BK, et al. Adverse effects of phenobarbital on morphological and biochemical development of fetal mouse spinal cord neurons in culture. *Ann Neurol* 1981; 9:584–589.

86. Neale EA, Sher PK, Graubard BI, et al. Differential toxicity of chronic exposure to phenytoin, phenobarbital, or carbamazepine in cerebral cortical cell cultures. *Pediatr Neurol* 1985; 1:143–150.

87. Goldberg RN, Moscoso P, Bauer CR, et al. Use of barbiturate therapy in severe perinatal asphyxia: a randomized controlled trial. *J Pediatr* 1986; 109:851.

88. Gal P, Sharpless MK, Boer HR. Outcome in neonates with seizures: are chronic anticonvulsants necessary? *Ann Neurol* 1984; 15:610–611.

89. Donn SM, Grasela TH, Goldstein GW. Safety of a higher loading dose of phenobarbital in the term newborn. *Pediatrics* 1985; 75:1061–64.

90. Bourgeois BFD, Dodson WE. Phenytoin elimination in newborns. *Neurology* 1983; 33:173–78.

91. Dodson WE. Antiepileptic drug utilization in pediatric patients. *Epilepsia* 1984; 25:S132–S139.

92. Boer HR, Gal P. Neonatal seizures: a survey of current practice. *Clin Pediatr* 1982; 21:453–457.

93. Gal P, Toback J, Erkan NV, Boer HR. The influence of asphyxia on phenobarbital dosing requirements in neonates. *Dev Pharmacol Ther* 1984; 7:145.

94. Brod SA, Ment LR, Ehrenkranz RA, Bridgers S. Predictors of success for drug discontinuation following neonatal seizures. *Pediatr Neurol* 1988; 4:13–17.

95. Fenichel GM. Paroxysmal disorders. In: *Clinical Pediatric Neurology*. 3rd ed. Philadelphia: WB Sanders, 1997:1–43.

96. Ellison PH, Largent JA, Bahr JP. A scoring system to predict outcome following neonatal seizures. *J Pediatr* 1981; 99:455–459.

97. Rowe JC, Holmes GL, Hafford J, et al. Prognostic value of the electroencephalogram in term and preterm infants following neonatal seizures. *Electroencephalogr Clin Neurophysiol* 1985; 60:183–196.

98. André M, Matisse N, Vert P, Debruille C. Neonatal seizures: recent aspects. *Neuropediatrics* 1988; 19:201–207.

99. Clancy RR, Legido A. Postnatal epilepsy after EEG-confirmed neonatal seizures. *Epilepsia* 1991; 32:69–76.

100. Ortibus EL, Sum JM, Hahn JS. Predictive value of EEG for outcome and epilepsy following neonatal seizures. *Electroencephalogr Clin Neurophysiol* 1996; 98:175–185.

101. Bye AME, Cunningham CA, Chee KY, Flanagan D. Outcome of neonates with electrographically identified seizures, or at risk of seizures. *Pediatr Neurol* 1997; 16:225–231.

CHAPTER 12

Febrile Seizures

N. Paul Rosman, M.D.

Children are likely to have convulsions if their fever is high and if they are constipated, if they are wakeful, frightened, cry and change color, turning pale, livid, or red. This most commonly happens in children under the age of 7 years. As they grow up and reach adult years, they are no longer likely to be attacked by convulsions in the course of a fever, unless one of the most severe and worst signs appear as well, as happens in inflammation of the brain — Hippocrates (1)

CHARACTERISTICS OF FEBRILE SEIZURES

Febrile seizures are the most common form of childhood seizures. They were defined by a 1980 consensus panel of the National Institutes of Health (NIH) as "an event in infancy or childhood, usually occurring between 3 months and 5 years of age, associated with fever but without evidence of intracranial infection or defined cause. Seizures with fever in children who have suffered a previous non-febrile seizure are excluded" (2,3). In 1993 the International League Against Epilepsy (ILAE) modified this definition to "an epileptic seizure occurring in childhood after age 1 month, associated with a febrile illness not caused by an infection of the CNS, without previous neonatal seizures or a previous unprovoked seizure, and not meeting criteria for other acute symptomatic seizures" (4). While there has been no firm consensus on the level of body temperature elevation needed to define a seizure as "febrile," most would probably agree that a temperature of at least 38.5 °C is required, although the temperature elevation may not be evident until after the seizure (5). Febrile seizures have a frequency of 2 percent to 5 percent in children in the United States and Western Europe (6–8) and as high as 8 percent to 10 percent in Japan (9) and 14 percent in Guam (10). They are termed *simple* if they are generalized *and* last less than 10 or 15 minutes *and* do not recur within 24 hours; such seizures comprise as many as 85 percent of all febrile seizures (11). When febrile seizures are longer than 10 or 15 minutes (12) *or* focal in nature *or* if they recur

within a day, they are called *complex* (13). The frequency of prolonged and/or focal febrile seizures has varied from 4 percent to 35 percent in different series (14). Approximately three-quarters of all prolonged febrile seizures are the first febrile seizure experienced by the child (14). When an initial febrile seizure is prolonged, a febrile seizure recurrence is more likely to be prolonged (12,15). Although febrile status epilepticus accounts for only 5 percent of febrile seizures, it accounts for approximately 25 percent of all status epilepticus in children (16).

The diagnosis of febrile seizure is clinical. Of the disorders that can be *misdiagnosed* as a febrile seizure, a shaking rigor (shivering) in a febrile child is the most frequent; less often, in the presence of fever, breathholding spells, syncope, reflex anoxic seizures or a febrile delirium can serve to confuse (13). Most febrile seizures occur in children between the ages of 6 months and 3 years, with a median age of 18 to 22 months (6). The first febrile seizure occurs after age 4 years in only 15 percent of children (14), and only occasionally do they occur after age 5 (6,17,18). As to gender, febrile seizures occur more often in boys than in girls (13,19).

Three-quarters of children with febrile seizures have temperatures of 39 °C or higher at the time of the seizure, and one-quarter have temperatures higher than 40 °C (14). Of note, a child who has had a febrile seizure not uncommonly will later tolerate an even higher fever without developing a seizure (20). Although it is often contended that a febrile seizure is more likely to occur when temperature rises rapidly, there are no clinical data to support this (21). Febrile seizures usually occur early in the course of a febrile illness, in the majority within the first 24 hours (14), with a few hours of premonitory symptoms of illness occurring in most cases (18). Sometimes, however, a febrile seizure is the first evidence of illness; in one series this occurred in 30 percent of cases (22), in another in only 7 percent (23). Of the causative illnesses, viral infections are more frequent than bacterial infections. Some viral infections, such as roseola (from human herpesvirus 6), appear to be particularly provocative (24,25). When gastroenteritis is the underlying illness, it has a significant inverse (i.e., protective) association with febrile seizures (26).

There is an increased incidence of febrile seizures in relatives of children with febrile seizures, with frequencies in first-degree relatives varying from 7 percent to 31 percent (13). Most studies suggest a dominant mode of inheritance with reduced penetrance and variable expression or a polygenic mode of inheritance (14). Two recent family studies of febrile convulsions with apparent autosomal dominant inheritance found linkage to chromosome 8q in one of the families (27) but to chromosome 19p in the other (28).

The recently described syndrome of generalized epilepsy with febrile seizures plus has been localized to chromosome 2q; within these families many individuals have typical febrile convulsions, whereas others have febrile seizures continuing beyond age 6 years; some have afebrile tonic-clonic seizures, less often absence, myoclonic, and atonic seizures; and rarely, members have myoclonic-astatic epilepsy or complex partial seizures. The syndrome is transmitted as an autosomal dominant with variable penetrance (28a,28b).

If a child has a febrile seizure, the risk that a sibling will also have a febrile seizure is one in five unless both parents have also had febrile seizures, in which case the risk for the sibling is one in three (6). Whether afebrile seizures are more common in families of children with febrile seizures is still not settled (14).

EVALUATING THE CHILD WITH A FEBRILE SEIZURE

History

The history should focus on three main areas:

1. What is the illness that triggered the febrile seizure, and more important, is there anything to suggest meningitis? Because bacterial meningitis is a very serious illness, particularly in young children, it is essential that one not neglect the possibility that the febrile seizure was signaling the presence of an underlying meningitis.
2. Was the febrile seizure simple or complex? Was the child developmentally and neurologically

normal or abnormal beforehand? Is there a family history of epilepsy in the child's parents or siblings? These clinical features are important because each of them increases the likelihood that the child will develop later unprovoked afebrile seizures, including those that recur (epilepsy). With focal febrile seizures or abnormal neurologic findings, the likelihood of underlying meningitis is increased.
3. Could something other than (or in addition to) fever have caused the seizure? Examples include drugs, toxins, discontinuance of anticonvulsants (previously prescribed), head trauma, hypoglycemia, and a phakomatosis.

Examination

The most crucial part of the examination is the evaluation of symptoms and signs that may indicate an underlying central nervous system (CNS) infection. Bacterial meningitis in children is almost always accompanied by evidence of acutely increased intracranial pressure. This can include alteration in mental status, vomiting, impaired abduction in one or both eyes, downward deviation of the eyes ("setting sun" sign), and changes in vital signs (increased blood pressure, decreased or increased pulse rate, decreased respirations). In the infant in whom the anterior fontanelle is still open, it may be full and fail to pulsate. Signs of accompanying illness, such as otitis media or gastroenteritis, should be sought, along with evidence of trauma and skin lesions (brown, white, or red) that can suggest a phakomatosis. An identification bracelet may indicate that the child has an established seizure disorder. The neurologic examination of the child with a febrile seizure often shows transient abnormalities that in this circumstance lack localizing value (13).

Investigations

Many laboratory studies have been shown to be *un*helpful in the management of the child with a febrile seizure, including a complete blood count, blood sugar, serum electrolytes, serum calcium, blood urea nitrogen, urinalysis, skull x-rays, and cranial computed tomography (CT) scan (13). Such studies should not be done routinely in the evaluation of a child with a first simple febrile seizure (8). An electroencephalogram (EEG) usually is not indicated, but a lumbar puncture may be essential.

Is Lumbar Puncture Necessary to Exclude Bacterial Meningitis?

Seizures have been reported in from 18 percent to 80 percent of cases of acute bacterial meningitis (29), and in 13 percent to 16 percent of children with meningitis, seizures are the presenting sign of disease (8). In approximately 30 percent to 35 percent of the latter children, however, meningeal signs and symptoms may be lacking (8). In a review of 42 cases of acute bacterial meningitis in children and adults, 60 percent of the seizures began within the first 2 days of the illness (29). Most febrile seizures associated with meningitis are complex (30,31), but even complex febrile seizures are almost never the *sole* manifestation of meningitis (31–33). Nonetheless, every child with a first febrile seizure that is complex probably should have a lumbar puncture. Also, every child younger than 1 year of age with a febrile seizure should have a lumbar puncture because the clinical signs and symptoms of meningitis may be minimal or absent at this age. Between 12 and 18 months, a lumbar puncture should be strongly considered because the clinical signs and symptoms of meningitis may be subtle. In a child older than 18 months, a lumbar puncture should be done when meningeal signs and symptoms are present or whenever the history or examination suggests the presence of an intracranial infection. A lumbar puncture should be strongly considered in infants and children with febrile seizures who have received antibiotic treatment because such treatment can mask evidence of meningitis (8,34).

The Electroencephalogram in Febrile Seizures

The EEG is of limited value in the management of febrile seizures. It is probably most helpful in those children in whom it is uncertain whether a febrile seizure has occurred. EEGs done on the same day as the seizure have been abnormal in as many as 88 percent of cases, usually with bilateral posterior slow-wave activity. This same type of abnormality is present in about one-third of children between 3 and 7 days after a febrile seizure and usually disappears by 7 to 10 days (13,35). The presence of an EEG abnormality that later disappears thus serves to confirm the clinical impression of seizure. EEG abnormalities accompanying febrile seizures can be seen ictally, postictally, and in serial tracings over several years, but none is convincingly associated with the later appearance of epilepsy (35).

ACUTE MANAGEMENT OF FEBRILE STATUS EPILEPTICUS

The majority of febrile seizures will have ended by the time the child is seen by a physician. Occasionally, however, seizure activity has continued and must be treated aggressively because febrile status epilepticus has the potential to cause substantial neurologic morbidity and even death. Supportive measures are a top priority. The child should be placed in a semiprone position, an adequate airway ensured, and oxygen given. Endotracheal intubation and assisted ventilation are needed on occasion. An intravenous line should be inserted to obtain blood specimens, maintain hydration, and facilitate administration of medications. A solution containing 5% dextrose in 0.25% normal saline is then infused at a rate of 1000 mL/m^2/per day. A nasogastric tube should be inserted to empty the gastric contents. The child must be protected against injury from hard objects and from pillows and blankets that could compromise air entry. Clothing should be loosened and excess clothing (coats, jackets, sweaters) removed. Fever is treated by sponging with tepid water, wrapping the child in a cooling blanket, and giving antipyretics such as acetaminophen or ibuprofen. Vital signs should be monitored frequently.

The most useful anticonvulsants for a febrile child who is still seizing are diazepam, lorazepam, or phenobarbital. Diazepam (Valium) is given intravenously in a dose of 0.2 to 0.5 mg/kg (maximum rate: 1 to 2 mg/min), with the total dosage not greater than 2 to 4 mg for the infant or 5 to 10 mg for the older child. The same dose can be repeated every 10 to 30 minutes, for a total of three doses, if necessary. Lorazepam (Ativan), a benzodiazepine structurally similar to diazepam but with a longer duration of action, is given intravenously in a dose of 0.05 to 0.10 mg/kg (maximum rate: 1 mg/min), with a maximum total dose of 4 mg. If needed, an additional 0.05 mg/kg can be given 10 minutes later. Phenobarbital is given intravenously in a dose of 15 to 20 mg/kg (rate: 30 to 100 mg/min). If necessary, half of the initial dose can be repeated in an hour (36,37).

FACTORS THAT FAVOR DEVELOPMENT OF A FIRST FEBRILE SEIZURE

A number of factors have been associated with a significantly increased risk of a first febrile seizure (Table 12-1). These include patient age between 6 months and 3 years (6), degree of temperature elevation (38), febrile seizures in first- or second-degree relatives

Table 12-1. Risk Factors for a First Febrile Seizure

- Patient age (6 months–3 years)
- Degree of temperature elevation
- Febrile seizures in first- or second-degree relatives
- Family history of afebrile seizures
- Neonatal discharge at 28 days or later
- Slow development in the child
- Attendance at day care
- Maternal smoking and drinking during pregnancy

(39,40), a family history of afebrile seizures (40), neonatal discharge at 28 days or later (39), slow development in the child (39), attendance at day care (39), and maternal smoking (38,40,41) and drinking (41) during pregnancy.

RECURRENCES OF FEBRILE SEIZURES

Depending on the number of risk factors present, the frequency with which febrile seizures recur varies from 12 percent to 90 percent (32). On average, one-third of children who have had a febrile seizure have at least one recurrence. The most consistent risk factors are the child's age at the time of the first febrile seizure and a family history of febrile seizures (Table 12-2). Recurrences are more frequent when the first febrile seizure occurs at a young age (6,15,32,42,43); if the first febrile seizure occurs before the age of 1 year, 50 percent recur, while only 20 percent recur if the first febrile seizure occurs after age 3 years (6). Recurrences are also more frequent when there is a family history of febrile seizures (15,18,32,39,42,44,45). Additionally, febrile seizures are more likely to recur when the fever triggering the first febrile seizure has been relatively brief (46) and when the fever has been relatively low grade (15,46). Berg and coworkers found the risk of febrile seizure recurrence at 1 year to be 44 percent when the causative fever had lasted less than 1 hour, 23 percent for fever lasting 1 to 24 hours, and 13 percent for fever lasting more than 24 hours (46). They also found that with each degree of increase in temperature from 101 °F to 105 °F or greater, the risk of recurrence at 1 year declined, from 35 percent (101 degrees) to 30 percent (102 °F), 26 percent (103 °F), 20 percent (104 °F) and 13 percent (105 °F and higher) (46). Offringa and colleagues found that children who seized with a temperature of less than 40 °C had twice the risk of recurrence than children who seized with higher temperatures (15). In one study of 180 children with an initial febrile seizure, each degree increase in temperature (Celsius) during subsequent fevers almost doubled the febrile seizure recurrence risk (47).

Table 12-2. Risk Factors for Febrile Seizure Recurrence

- First febrile seizure before 1 year
- Family history of febrile seizures
- Febrile seizures following low-grade fevers
- Febrile seizures following brief fevers
- Epilepsy in first-degree relatives*
- Complex febrile seizures*
- Neurodevelopmental abnormalities in the child*
- Attendance at day care

*Not all studies agree.

Many studies have shown an increase in febrile seizure recurrence risk when there is a family history of epilepsy in first-degree relatives (15,18,32,42,44), but there have been exceptions (48). When the initial febrile seizure is complex, some studies have found an increased febrile seizure recurrence risk (42,43), some have found this only when the child has had multiple febrile seizures initially (32), and others have found recurrence risk to be no greater when the initial febrile seizure is complex than when it is simple (48,49). There is also disagreement about febrile seizure recurrence risk in children who are developmentally or neurologically abnormal, with some studies demonstrating an increased recurrence risk (18,32) and others not (49). Attendance at a day nursery appears to be another risk factor for febrile seizure recurrence (42). EEG findings do not help predict febrile seizure recurrences (13). One-half of febrile seizure recurrences are within 6 months, three-quarters within 1 year, and 90 percent within 2 years (50).

FEBRILE SEIZURES AND RISK OF LATER EPILEPSY

There unquestionably is a relationship between early febrile seizures and later development of epilepsy (Table 12-3). All studies agree that children with febrile seizures are at increased risk for later unprovoked afebrile seizures, including those that recur (epilepsy). Of children who develop epilepsy, 15 percent have preceding febrile seizures (51). Millichap reviewed reports of spontaneous afebrile seizures among 5,576 children with febrile convulsions recorded in 35 publications between 1929 and 1964 from various parts of the world. Of 2,343 patients followed up by 14 investigators for periods up to 29 years, 29 percent had at least one spontaneous afebrile seizure; of 4,459 patients followed up by 31 authors, 20 percent developed epilepsy (the lowest incidence was 2.6 percent, the highest 100 percent) (17). When single afebrile seizures and epilepsy are examined separately, two of three children with febrile seizures who develop a first afebrile seizure proceed to epilepsy (18). More recent studies have found the risk of unprovoked seizures after febrile convulsions to be from 2 percent to 4 percent, depending on the duration of follow-up, with a 7 percent risk when such

Table 12-3. Risk Factors for Later Epilepsy in Febrile Seizures

- Complex febrile seizures
- Neurodevelopmental abnormalities in the child
- Afebrile seizures in first-degree relatives
- Recurrent febrile seizures, especially if complex
- Febrile seizures following brief fevers
- Febrile seizure onset in first year
- Abnormal neonatal history
- Family history of mental retardation

patients are followed to age 25 years (52). Of 54,000 offspring born to women who had registered in the U.S. National Collaborative Perinatal Project (NCPP) and whose children were followed to age 7 years, follow-up data were available in 1,706 children with a history of at least one febrile seizure. Three major risk factors were found to increase the risk of later epilepsy in these children: (1) a complex first febrile seizure, (2) an abnormal neurologic state before the first febrile seizure, (3) afebrile seizures in the child's parents or siblings or both (although others have not found the last to be a risk factor for later afebrile seizures) (53). In the absence of any of these major risk factors, the frequency of later epilepsy was 1 percent, twice that found in the population without febrile seizures. With one major risk factor, the risk for later epilepsy was 2 percent. With two or more major risk factors, the risk for later epilepsy was 10 percent (50).

In the Rochester, Minnesota, epidemiology project, with follow-up to age 25 years, children with simple febrile seizures had a 2.5 percent risk of developing unprovoked seizures. With febrile seizures with a single complex feature, the risk of later unprovoked seizures was 6 percent to 8 percent. When febrile seizures had two complex features, the risk of later unprovoked seizures was 17 percent to 22 percent; and when febrile seizures had all three complex features, later unprovoked seizures occurred in 49 percent of patients. When a first febrile seizure occurred at under a year of age, later afebrile seizures were more likely, especially when the febrile seizure was complex. Complex febrile seizures were found to be strongly associated with later partial unprovoked seizures, while later unprovoked generalized seizures were significantly associated with the number of febrile seizures (52). In a prospective inquiry in 1,005 patients seen for evaluation in an epilepsy clinic, 133 (13.2%) had a history of febrile convulsions. Temporal lobe epilepsy (TLE) was more often preceded by febrile convulsions than extratemporal epilepsy or generalized epilepsy. Patients with generalized epilepsy were more likely than those with TLE to have had simple febrile convulsions, while those with partial epilepsy, particularly of temporal lobe origin, were much more likely to have had complex febrile convulsions, especially convulsions that were prolonged (54).

Although complex febrile seizures carry a higher risk of later epilepsy than simple febrile seizures, most children with febrile seizures who go on to epilepsy have had simple febrile seizures (50) (undoubtedly because simple febrile seizures are much more frequent than complex seizures). Most workers have found the risk for later unprovoked seizures and epilepsy to increase when febrile seizures recur, both when the recurrences are simple and particularly when they are complex (18,55). Others, however, have found febrile

seizure recurrences to be associated with an increased risk of later epilepsy only if the recurrences are complex (56) or if the children are already at increased risk because of preexisting neurologic disorders (57). Also, the risk of later afebrile seizures has been found to be increased in children with a brief duration of fever before their initial febrile seizure (55), in those with an abnormal neonatal history, or in children with a family history of mental retardation (53). Febrile seizures beginning in the first year, especially in the first 6 months, are more likely to be followed by epilepsy than ones that began later (57).

Wallace's comprehensive review of febrile seizures followed by later afebrile seizures found the latter to develop within one year in 40 percent to 70 percent of cases, within three years in 67 percent to 77 percent, and within four years in 85 percent (18).

SHOULD FEBRILE SEIZURES BE PREVENTED?

Opinion is divided on whether febrile seizures should be prevented (58–60). Although a substantial number of febrile seizures recur, most do not. Thus, one might argue that if a child has had only a single febrile seizure, no preventive treatment is needed, particularly if the child is at relatively low risk for febrile seizure recurrence (older than one year of age, normal neurologic development, no family history of febrile or afebrile seizures). Even stronger arguments can be advanced in support of febrile seizure prophylaxis, however, for there are many reasons why this is desirable (58). Seizures are upsetting to both children and their parents. Indeed, many parents witnessing a child's first seizure think their child is dying or is already dead (13,61). After having seen a febrile seizure in their child, most parents continue to be anxious, even after speaking with physicians, viewing slide or tape programs, and reading educational materials, with family disruption in three-fourths (62). Medical costs for the child with a febrile seizure can be considerable, and seizures are potentially dangerous. Although death is rare following a febrile seizure (63), a seizing child may fall, strike his head, and suffer a brain contusion, which could cause later epilepsy. If a seizure is complicated by respiratory compromise, hypoxic brain injury and, again, later epilepsy might result.

Although it is generally agreed that motor handicaps are not residua of febrile seizures (64), there is less agreement about possible adverse effects of febrile seizures on later mental development. Wallace has summarized studies showing adverse effects of febrile seizures on intellectual outcome (18) and has found children with repeated febrile seizures who show a significant decrease in IQ that is not explained by effects of treatment (65). On the other hand, neither of two major prospective studies of childhood febrile seizures, the National Collaborative Perinatal Project in the United States (with 431 children with febrile seizures followed to age 7 years) (66) and the Child Health and Education Study in the United Kingdom (with 398 children with febrile seizures followed to age 10 years) (67) found any relationship between febrile seizures, including those that recurred, and later cognitive decline.

FEBRILE SEIZURES, MESIAL TEMPORAL SCLEROSIS, AND LATER EPILEPSY

The relationship between frequency of febrile seizures, particularly complex seizures, and later development of afebrile seizures, including epilepsy, can be viewed in two ways. It could mean simply that a child predetermined to develop later epilepsy is also predetermined to have frequent febrile seizures. Alternatively, it could mean that frequent febrile seizures can cause brain injury and, in that way, later epilepsy. Support for the latter view is seen in retrospective clinical studies from epilepsy surgery centers where many patients undergoing surgery for intractable TLE have been found to have mesial temporal sclerosis (MTS) and a history of prolonged, focal, and often febrile seizures in infancy (68). This was found in the magnetic resonance imaging (MRI) study by Cendes and coworkers of 43 patients with incompletely controlled TLE, which demonstrated a correlation between more severe degrees of MTS (hippocampus, entorhinal cortex, and amygdala) and prolonged febrile convulsions in early childhood (69). Yet the importance of febrile seizures in the causation of MTS and later TLE remains controversial (70) because most population-based studies and prospective studies of febrile seizures have failed to show such a cause-and-effect association (71). An exception is the very recent MRI study of Van Landingham and coworkers, which provided convincing evidence that prolonged and focal febrile seizures can occasionally cause hippocampal injury that evolves to hippocampal atrophy (68). Preexisting hippocampal abnormalities were present in some of those cases and could have predisposed those children to focal and prolonged febrile seizures and rendered their hippocampi more susceptible to seizure-induced damage, including MTS. Fernandez and associates performed MRI studies on 23 members of two families, of whom 13 had febrile seizures and 10 had not. They found hippocampal malformations in 6 of the 10 patients with no febrile seizures and in 11 of the 13 who had febrile seizures; the remaining 2 patients with febrile seizures had hippocampal sclerosis (and later TLE) (72). Hippocampal malformations therefore may (1) predispose children to both early febrile seizures and later epilepsy, (2) facilitate febrile convulsions that in turn can cause hippocampal sclerosis, with later epilepsy, or (3) render the hippocampi more vulnerable to damaging effects of fever. The last possibility is supported by the elegant experimental studies of Germano and coworkers, who induced neuronal migration disorders (NMD) in offspring of pregnant rats and later exposed those offspring to hyperthermia. In the rats with NMD, seizure thresholds were lower and hippocampal damage (independent of seizure activity) was greater than in controls (73). Therefore, clinically, among the reasons one may want to treat children with febrile seizures to prevent recurrence is the possibility that such treatment might reduce the likelihood of later epilepsy.

Treatment options in febrile seizure prophylaxis include (1) *daily medication* and (2) *intermittent medication* that is given only at times of fever (Table 12-4). If both approaches are of equal efficacy, intermittent treatment (necessitating medication for only a relatively few days a year when the child is febrile) is clearly preferable. Nonetheless, there are a number of circumstances in which daily medication (which also requires monitoring of anticonvulsant blood levels) should be considered: (1) if intermittent treatment proves to be ineffective, (2) if parents repeatedly fail to take their child's temperature when the child is ill, (3) if a child typically experiences sudden elevations in body temperature without premonitory signs of illness (providing inadequate time to give medication before a febrile seizure occurs), and (4) if

Table 12-4. Treatment Options in Febrile Seizure Management

Continuous Prophylaxis (daily oral medication)		Intermittent Prophylaxis (medication only with fever)		
Ineffective	Often effective	Ineffective	Highly effective	Potentially effective
Phenytoin	Phenobarbital	Antipyrexis	Diazepam (rectal)	Nitrazepam (oral)
Carbamazepine	Primidone		Diazepam (oral)	Clobazam (oral)
	Valproic acid			

medicine given intermittently has unacceptable side effects. Children with febrile seizures for whom a daily anticonvulsant might be considered are those with a substantially increased risk of later epilepsy. These include (1) children with complex febrile seizures, an abnormal neurologic examination, or a family history of epilepsy; (2) those with febrile seizures beginning at less than a year of age; and (3) those with frequent febrile seizures, especially if complex. A daily anticonvulsant should also be considered for children with highly anxious parents who cannot be relied on to give medication whenever their child becomes febrile.

If the decision is to treat, since three-quarters of febrile seizures recur within one year, and 90 percent within two years, treatment (whether daily or intermittent) should be continued for at least two years or for one year after the last febrile seizure, which ever is longer.

Daily Medication

Oral phenytoin or oral carbamazepine taken daily have been ineffective in preventing febrile seizures (13,18). By contrast, three other medications, taken orally daily, have usually prevented febrile seizure recurrence: phenobarbital, primidone, and sodium valproate.

Phenobarbital

Daily phenobarbital has been the most frequently used drug for febrile seizure prophylaxis for more than 25 years, and in most studies it has been effective (18,22,74). In six prospective, randomized studies with concurrent controls and blood level monitoring, phenobarbital in a dose of 4 to 5 mg/kg/day was shown to decrease significantly the recurrence rate of febrile convulsions (14). In most phenobarbital studies, the febrile seizure recurrence rate has been reduced to 4 percent to 13 percent, compared with an average recurrence rate in controls of 20 percent to 30 percent (14). More recently, however, the place of phenobarbital in febrile seizure prophylaxis has been questioned (75–77). Concern has centered on the frequency of behavioral side effects (irritability, inattention, overactivity, aggression, drowsiness, sleep disturbances) (13,78), consistently poor drug compliance (no better than 65%) (74,77), and possible cognitive decline (79). A group of 217 children with febrile seizures were randomly assigned to treatment with either daily phenobarbital or placebo, treated for 2 years and followed up for 2.5 years. In the phenobarbital group, there was a significant fall in IQ of 7 points by 2 years, with a 4-point fall still present at 2.5 years; furthermore, phenobarbital failed to produce a significant reduction in febrile seizure recurrence (77). Additional evidence indicating lack of efficacy of daily phenobarbital is seen in the pooled results from six British febrile seizure trials, analyzed by intention-to-treat, which showed phenobarbital to provide no significant benefit (75,76).

Primidone

Primidone has been found to prevent febrile seizure recurrence as effectively as phenobarbital and sodium valproate (80). When compared with phenobarbital (to which it is partially metabolized), primidone was effective in 88 percent of patients, compared with an 80 percent efficacy with phenobarbital. Side effects were frequent, however, occurring in 53 percent of the children receiving primidone and in 77 percent of those receiving phenobarbital (81).

Sodium Valproate

Most studies have found sodium valproate to be at least as effective as phenobarbital and primidone in preventing febrile seizure recurrence (14,18,80,82). In a study in Wales, Wallace and Aldridge Smith found febrile seizure recurrences in 13 percent of children treated with sodium valproate, in 13 percent of those treated with phenobarbital, and in 34 percent of controls (83). In Spain, Herranz and coworkers found febrile seizure recurrences in 20 percent of their patients treated with phenobarbital, in 12 percent of those given primidone, and in only 8 percent of those who received sodium valproate (81). In a study in France, 69 children were placed on daily treatment with phenobarbital, sodium valproate, or placebo after a first generalized febrile seizure and followed up for an average of 21 months. Fourteen children had febrile seizure recurrences, with a relapse rate of 19 percent in the phenobarbital group, 5 percent in the sodium valproate group, and 35 percent in the controls (84). Although sodium valproate is much less likely than phenobarbital or primidone to cause behavioral side effects (13,79), complications do occur, as seen in 45 percent of the patients of Herranz and coworkers (81), with gastrointestinal symptoms the side effect most frequently seen. Other side effects found with sodium valproate are weight gain, hair loss, pancreatitis, and potentially fatal acute liver failure (13). Furthermore, as with phenobarbital, pooled results from four British febrile seizure trials of valproate, analyzed by intention-to-treat, showed no treatment benefit (75,76). Although daily anticonvulsant may therefore be appropriate in some children with febrile seizures, there are many reasons not to treat with daily medication.

Intermittent Prophylaxis

Fevers are frequent early in life, and parents are skillful in anticipating the onset of a febrile illness. Dianese found that 86 percent of mothers were able to recognize that their child was ill at least 6 hours before a fever occurred (85). Banco and Veltri found that mothers who said their children were febrile were correct 52 percent of the time and were correct 90 percent of the time with children 2 years of age or younger (86).

Antipyrexis

Unfortunately, children with febrile seizures who are given antipyretics for their fevers are not protected against febrile seizure recurrence. Camfield and coworkers carried out a randomized double-blind study comparing febrile seizure recurrences in children who at times of fever were given either daily oral phenobarbital and antipyretics or antipyretics and daily oral placebo. The febrile seizure recurrence rate was 5 percent for the children who were given phenobarbital and antipyretics, while it was 25 percent for those receiving placebo and antipyretics (19). More recently, acetaminophen has been given to children with fevers to try to prevent febrile seizure recurrence. Whether given in moderate dose (10 mg/kg four times a day) (87) or in a relatively high dose (15–20 mg/kg every four hours) (88), acetaminophen failed to reduce febrile seizure recurrences.

Oral Phenobarbital

Phenobarbital given at times of fever to children with a history of febrile seizures has failed to prevent febrile seizure recurrence (22). This failure can be explained by the slow rate of absorption of oral phenobarbital—90 minutes before a therapeutic blood level is reached following an oral dose of 15 mg/kg (89).

Rectal Diazepam

Rectal diazepam, given only at times of fever, is effective in preventing febrile seizure recurrence (90). Side effects are infrequent and rarely serious, with mild sedation and ataxia the most common (13). Plasma levels of 150 to 300 ng/mL appear to be protective (91). Rectal diazepam can be given either as a liquid or in suppository form; it is cumbersome to administer as a liquid; although easier to manage, diazepam suppositories are not available in the United States. Where available, diazepam suppositories, given only at times of fever, have been as effective as daily oral phenobarbital in preventing febrile seizure recurrence (18). Knudsen in Denmark studied 289 consecutive children hospitalized with a first febrile seizure, randomized into two groups, one given prophylaxis (rectal diazepam solution at times of fever), the other not. He found the 18-month febrile seizure recurrence rate to be reduced from 39 percent to 12 percent in the diazepam group (23).

In another study in Denmark, Thorn followed up 586 children with a first febrile seizure for 2 years; 153 children received no febrile seizure prophylaxis, 226 children were given daily oral phenobarbital, and 207 children were given diazepam suppositories when febrile. Febrile seizures recurred in 41 percent of the placebo group, in 20 percent of the phenobarbital group, and in 12 percent of the diazepam group (92).

In Japan, Shiraiand and coworkers treated 133 children with two or more previous febrile convulsions with rectal diazepam suppositories at the first sign of fever, with a second dose if the child was still febrile 8 hours later. Follow-up was from 6 to 43 months. The children had a total of 787 fevers, for 722 of which diazepam was given. There were 58 febrile seizure recurrences, but in 17 of these diazepam was not given and in 39 it was given after the seizure had occurred; in only two instances did febrile seizures recur following timely administration of rectal diazepam (93).

A rectal diazepam gel (Diastat) has recently been released in the United States. This preparation has been very effective in aborting acute repetitive seizures (ARS) when given by caretakers to children or adults at ARS onset (94). Diastat may prove to be similarly effective in preventing febrile seizure recurrence.

Oral Diazepam

Like the rectal preparation, oral diazepam is effective in reducing febrile seizure recurrences (90). Peak serum diazepam levels in children are achieved rapidly when it is taken by mouth (with levels of greater than 150 ng/mL reached in 3 to 30 minutes; mean: 5 minutes), more rapidly than when diazepam is given by rectal suppository (95). Side effects of oral diazepam are infrequent but may include drowsiness, dizziness and, less often, hypersalivation, drooling, and tracheobronchial hypersecretion. Serious toxic effects (hematopoietic, hepatic, renal) are rare and have followed chronic oral use (13).

In two uncontrolled studies, oral diazepam taken at the onset of illness appeared to be very effective in preventing febrile seizure recurrence (85,96). Ninety children with febrile seizures were prescribed oral diazepam at the first sign of illness until the second day after recovery. Forty-eight children took the diazepam and only 4 percent had febrile seizure recurrences; of the 42 who did not take the diazepam, febrile seizures recurred in 48 percent (85). Forty children with two or more previous febrile seizures were prescribed oral diazepam to be taken with fevers; if the child was still febrile eight hours later, the diazepam dose was repeated. There were 112 fevers in the 40 children, during 89 of which diazepam was given; 13 febrile seizures occurred but none in a child given diazepam (96).

In a study done in India, 120 children hospitalized with a first febrile seizure were given antipyretics (and antibiotics, if indicated) and randomized to one of four treatment groups: (1) daily oral phenobarbital; (2) oral phenobarbital only with fevers; (3) oral diazepam only with fevers; (4) no anticonvulsant. Follow-up was for 5 to 6 years. The percentages of children with febrile seizure recurrences in the four groups were (1) 30 percent, (2) 17 percent, (3) 0 percent, (4) 20 percent, with significant treatment efficacy found only with the oral diazepam group (97).

In France Autret and coworkers have reported a double-blind, randomized trial of oral diazepam for the prevention of febrile seizure recurrence. A group of 185 children with a first febrile seizure were to receive oral diazepam or placebo every 12 hours at times of fevers. The rates of febrile seizure recurrence did not differ between the two groups (diazepam — 16 percent; placebo — 19.5 percent) but only 1 of 15 diazepam children and only seven of 18 children in the placebo group had received their treatment correctly. Thus, no conclusion could be drawn about the efficacy of intermittent diazepam treatment (98).

In the United States we have reported a 5.5-year, double-blind, randomized clinical trial of intermittent oral diazepam in the prevention of febrile seizure recurrence (99). In our study, in contrast to that of Autret (98), there was a sufficient diazepam experience to ascertain its efficacy. All enrolled children were given oral diazepam (0.33 mg/kg every 8 hours) or placebo at times of fever (at least 38.1 °C). Simultaneously, they took a small amount of riboflavin (which was later excreted in the urine, causing the urine to fluoresce when exposed to an ultraviolet light and by that means confirming drug compliance). A group of 406 children were enrolled in the clinical trial. During a mean follow-up of 1.9 years (by which time 90% of febrile seizures recur), an intention-to-treat analysis showed a reduction of 44 percent in the risk of febrile seizures per person-year with diazepam. There was a considerable dilution effect in the intention-to-treat analysis because of randomized children who had no fevers and/or who never received study medication. An analysis of febrile seizure recurrence restricted to children who had seizures while actually receiving the study medication showed an 84 percent risk reduction with diazepam. Moderate side effects (usually ataxia, lethargy, or irritability) occurred with 111 of 661 fevers (16.8 percent) in children who took diazepam and always reversed after a reduction in drug dosage. There were no severe side effects.

More recently, in Finland, Uhari and colleagues in a two-year, placebo-controlled, double-blind trial of acetaminophen and low-dose diazepam found neither to be effective in preventing febrile seizure recurrence (87). The diazepam dose given by mouth (after an initial dose by rectal solution) was only 0.2 mg/kg three times a day [i.e., only 60 percent of the dose given in our study (99)]; furthermore, there was no information provided about compliance with the treatment protocol (87).

In addition, in Colombia Nuñez-Lopez and colleagues reported a 1-year, open, randomized prospective controlled clinical trial of 87 children assigned to one of three treatment groups: (1) daily phenobarbital, 5 mg/kg; (2) diazepam, sublingual or rectal, 0.5 mg/kg every 12 hours at times of fever; (3) acetaminophen, 10 mg/kg every 6 hours at times of fever. Percentages of children in the three groups who had febrile seizure recurrences were (1) 32 percent, (2) 7 percent, (3) 40 percent, demonstrating efficacy of intermittent diazepam in febrile seizure prevention. Twenty percent of the children treated with phenobarbital developed hyperactivity; 12.5 percent of those who received diazepam had transient lethargy and ataxia (100).

Other Oral Benzodiazepines

Uncontrolled studies of two other benzodiazepines taken orally at times of fever have suggested possible efficacy in febrile seizure prevention. In a study in Canada, nitrazepam was prescribed for 55 children with a history of febrile seizures and a high risk of recurrence. The nitrazepam, at 0.25 to 0.5 mg/kg/day in three divided doses, was to be taken for fevers of 38 °C or higher and continued until the child was afebrile for 12 hours. Of the 55 children, only 31 received the nitrazepam as directed; febrile seizures recurred in 19 percent of these 31 children. Twenty-four children did not receive the nitrazepam at all or were given it incorrectly, and there were febrile seizures recurrences in 46 percent of these 24 (101). In Italy, Tondi and colleagues prescribed clobazam for 69 children with a history of one or more simple febrile seizures to be taken in two daily doses whenever the child developed a fever of 38 °C or higher. Of the 39 children who complied, only one had a febrile seizure recurrence (3%), while in the 30 who did not comply, febrile seizures recurred in eight (27%) (102).

DOES PREVENTION OF FEBRILE SEIZURES REDUCE THE RISK OF LATER EPILEPSY?

Because the frequency of febrile seizure recurrences can be substantially reduced by medication, this is an important question. The answer is not yet known. Two studies have suggested that preventing febrile seizures may not lower the risk of later afebrile seizures, but neither study lends itself to a definitive conclusion. Wolf and Forsythe randomized 400 U.S. children with febrile seizures into one of three groups: daily phenobarbital, phenobarbital taken only with fevers, and no phenobarbital. After 6 years, 14 children had developed afebrile seizures; 7 had been on daily phenobarbital, 6 on intermittent phenobarbital, and 1 on no phenobarbital. For all 7 children with afebrile seizures in the daily phenobarbital group, the phenobarbital had been stopped before the afebrile seizure occurred (53). Knudsen followed up 289 Danish children with a first febrile seizure, with half the children given rectal diazepam with fevers and the other half given no prophylaxis. After 2 years, 5 children had developed two or more afebrile seizures: 3 of the 5 had received diazepam, 2 had not (23). Twelve-year follow-up of the same group of children again showed no difference between the diazepam and control groups in the occurrence of later epilepsy, but the occurrence rate was remarkably low in both groups: 0.7 percent for diazepam, 0.8 percent for no prophylaxis (103).

On the other hand, Farwell and coworkers have reported 2.5 years of follow-up in 217 U.S. children with febrile seizures treated with either daily phenobarbital or daily placebo. Two years after the index febrile seizure, afebrile seizures had occurred in 4 percent of the phenobarbital group and in 7 percent of the placebo group (77).

SUMMARY AND CONCLUSIONS

Febrile seizures are common events, affecting at least 2 percent to 5 percent of children, most often between the ages of 6 months and 3 years. They occur more often in boys. Most are "simple" — generalized, shorter than 10 or 15 minutes, and without recurrence within 24 hours. When focal, or prolonged, or recurrent within a day, they are called "complex." The evaluation of such children, including the need for lumbar puncture, and the acute management of febrile status epilepticus demand prompt action.

One-third of febrile seizures recur, with recurrences more frequent when febrile seizures begin in the first year, when there is a family history of febrile seizures, and when the fever triggering the first febrile seizure has been low-grade or brief. Children with febrile seizures are at increased risk for later epilepsy, particularly when febrile seizures are complex, when the child shows neurodevelopmental abnormalities, and when there is a family history of afebrile seizures. Additional risk factors for later epilepsy are febrile seizures that recur, particularly if complex, seizures that begin in the first year, and seizures that follow brief fevers. Epilepsy is also more likely when there is an abnormal neonatal history and a family history of mental retardation.

Most febrile seizures are benign with a good outcome. For that reason one may elect not to treat such children to prevent recurrence. There are equally strong and perhaps stronger arguments that favor treatment, however, including prevention of major parental anxiety and family disruption, reduction of medical costs consequent to recurring seizures, and the possibility of lowering the risk of accompanying neurologic morbidity. Daily medication with oral phenobarbital, primidone, or valproic acid is often effective in febrile seizure prophylaxis, but intermittent medication, taken only at times of fever, is preferable because treatment efficacy is higher and side effects are fewer. When a child becomes febrile, antipyretics alone do not prevent febrile seizures from recurring, but oral or rectal diazepam is highly effective in lowering the recurrence risk. Prolonged and focal febrile seizures can sometimes cause brain injury (MTS), with later development of epilepsy. Whether preventing febrile seizures can lower the risk of later epilepsy is not yet known.

REFERENCES

1. Lloyd GER. *Hippocratic Writings.* Harmondsworth, England: Penguin Books, 1978:185.

2. National Institutes of Health. Febrile seizures: Long-term management of children with fever-associated seizures. Summary of an NIH consensus statement. *Br Med J* 1980; 281:277–279.

3. Consensus statement on febrile seizures In: Nelson KB, Ellenberg JH, eds. *Febrile Seizures.* New York: Raven Press, 1981:301–306.

4. Commission on Epidemiology and Prognosis, International League Against Epilepsy. Guidelines for epidemiologic studies on epilepsy: *Epilepsia* 1993; 34:592–596.

5. Section discussion on consequences of febrile seizures In: Nelson KB, Ellenberg JH, eds. *Febrile Seizures.* New York: Raven Press, 1981:35–42.

6. Hirtz DG. Generalized tonic-clonic and febrile seizures. *Pediatr Clin N Am* 1989; 36:375–382.

7. Berg AT. Febrile seizures and epilepsy: The contributions of epidemiology. *Pediatr Perinat Epidemiol* 1992; 6:145–152.

8. Provisional Committee on Quality Improvement, Subcommittee on Diagnosis and Treatment of Febrile Seizures. American Academy of Pediatrics Practice Parameter: the neurodiagnostic evaluation of the child with a first simple febrile seizure. *Pediatrics* 1996; 97:769–775.

9. Tsuboi T. Epidemiology of febrile and afebrile convulsions in children in Japan. *Neurology* 1984; 34:175–181.

10. Lessell S, Torres JM, Kurland LT. Seizure disorders in a Guamanian village. *Arch Neurol* 1962; 7:37–44.

11. Nelson KB, Hirtz DG. Febrile seizures. In: Swaiman KF, ed. *Pediatric Neurology: Principles and Practice.* 2nd ed. St. Louis: Mosby, 1994:565–569.

12. Berg AT, Shinnar S. Complex febrile seizures. *Epilepsia* 1996; 37:126–133.

13. Rosman NP. Febrile seizures. *Emerg Med Clin North Am* 1987; 5:719–737.

14. Aicardi J. Febrile convulsions. In: Aicardi J, ed. *Epilepsy in Children*. 2nd ed. New York: Raven Press, 1994:253–275.

15. Offringa M, Bossuyt PMM, Lubsen J, et al. Risk factors for seizure recurrence in children with febrile seizures: A pooled analysis of individual patient data from five studies. *J Pediatr* 1994; 124:574–584.

16. Shinnar S, Pellock JM, Moshe SL, et al. In whom does status epilepticus occur: Age-related differences in children. *Epilepsia* 1997; 38:907–914.

17. Millichap JG. *Febrile Convulsions*. New York: Macmillan, 1968:1–222.

18. Wallace SJ. *The Child with Febrile Seizures*. Boston: John Wright 1988:1–182.

19. Camfield PR, Camfield CS, Shapiro SH, et al. The first febrile seizure — antipyretic instruction plus either phenobarbital or placebo to prevent recurrence. *J Pediatr* 1980; 97:16–21.

20. Lennox-Buchthal MA. *Febrile Convulsions — A Reappraisal*. Amsterdam: Elsevier, 1973:1–138.

21. Berg AT. Are febrile seizures provoked by a rapid rise in temperature? *Am J Dis Child* 1993; 147:1101–1103.

22. Wolf SM, Carr A, Davis DC, et al. The value of phenobarbital in the child who has had a single febrile seizure: a controlled prospective study. *Pediatrics* 1977; 59:378–385.

23. Knudsen FU. Effective short-term diazepam prophylaxis in febrile convulsions. *J Pediatr* 1985; 106:487–490.

24. Kondo K, Nagafuji H, Hata A, et al. Association of human herpesvirus 6 infection of the central nervous system with recurrence of febrile convulsions. *J Infect Dis* 1993; 167:1197–1200.

25. Suga S, Yoshikawa T, Asano Y, et al. Clinical and virological analyses of 21 infants with exanthem subitum (roseola infantum) and central nervous system complications. *Ann Neurol* 1993; 33:597–603.

26. Berg AT, Shinnar S, Shapiro ED, et al. Risk factors for a first febrile seizure: A matched case-control study. *Epilepsia* 1995; 36:334–341.

27. Wallace RH, Berkovic SF, Howell RA, et al. Suggestion of a major gene for familial febrile convulsions mapping to 8q13-21. *J Med Genet* 1996; 33:308–312.

28. Johnson EW, Dubovsky J, Rich SS, et al. Evidence for a novel gene for familial febrile convulsions, FEB2, linked to chromosome 19p in an extended family from the midwest. *Hum Mol Genet* 1998; 7:63–67.

28a. Scheffer IE, Berkovic SF. Generalized epilepsy with febrile seizures plus: a genetic disorder with heterogeneous clinical phenotypes. *Brain* 1997; 120:479–490.

28b. Singh R, Scheffer IE, Crossland K, Berkovic SF. Generalized epilepsy with febrile seizures plus: a common childhood-onset genetic epilepsy syndrome. *Ann Neurol* 1999; 45:75–81.

29. Rosman NP, Peterson DB, Kaye EM, et al. Seizures in bacterial meningitis: prevalence, patterns, pathogenesis and prognosis. *Pediatr Neurol* 1985; 1:278–285.

30. Akpede GO, Sykes RM. Convulsions with fever as a presenting feature of bacterial meningitis among preschool children in developing countries. *Dev Med Child Neur* 1992; 34:524–529.

31. Green SM, Rothrock SG, Clem KJ, et al. Can seizures be the sole manifestation of meningitis in febrile children? *Pediatrics* 1993; 92:527–534.

32. Offringa M. Seizures associated with fever: current management controversies. *Semin Pediatr Neurol* 1994; 1:90–101.

33. Offringa M, Beishuizen A, Derksen-Lubsen G, et al. Seizures and fever: can we rule out meningitis on clinical grounds alone? *Clin Pediatr* 1992; 31:514–522.

34. American Academy of Neurology, Practice Handbook. *Practice Parameters: lumbar puncture. Report of the Quality Standards Subcommittee*. 2/22/93, 149–155.

35. Stores G. When does an EEG contribute to the management of febrile seizures? *Arch Dis Child* 1991; 66: 554–557.

36. Rosman NP. Evaluation and management of febrile seizures. *Curr Opin Pediatr* 1989; 1:318–323.

37. Oppenheimer EY, Rosman NP. Recurring seizures (status epilepticus). In: Reece RM, ed. *Manual of Emergency Pediatrics*. 4th ed. Philadelphia: WB Saunders, 1992, pp. 105–111.

38. Berg AT, Shinnar S, Shapiro ED, et al. Risk factors for a first febrile seizure: a matched case-control study. *Epilepsia* 1995; 36:334–341.

39. Bethune P, Gordon K, Dooley J, et al. Which child will have a febrile seizure? *Am J Dis Child* 1993; 147:35–39.

40. Nelson KB, Ellenberg JH. Prenatal and perinatal antecedents of febrile seizures. *Ann Neurol* 1990; 27:127–131.

41. Cassano PA, Keopsell TD, Farwell JR: Risk of febrile seizures in childhood in relation to prenatal maternal cigarette smoking and alcohol intake. *Am J Epidemiol* 1990; 132:462–473.

42. Knudsen FU: Recurrence risk after first febrile seizure and effect of short term diazepam prophylaxis. *Arch Dis Child* 1985; 60:1045–1049.

43. Al-Eissa YA. Febrile seizures: rate and risk factors of recurrence. *J Child Neurol* 1995; 10:315–319.

44. Offringa M, Derksen-Lubsen G, Bossuyt PM, et al. Seizure recurrence after a first febrile seizure: a multivariate approach. *Dev Med Child Neurol* 1992; 34:15–24.

45. van Esch A, Steyerberg EW, Berger MY, et al. Family history and recurrence of febrile seizures. *Arch Dis Child* 1994; 70:395–399.

46. Berg AT, Shinnar S, Hauser WA, et al. A prospective study of recurrent febrile seizures. *N Engl J Med* 1992; 327:1122–1127.

47. Tarkka R, Rantala H, Uhari M, et al. Risk of recurrence and outcome after the first febrile seizure. *Pediatr Neurol* 1998; 18:218–220.

48. Annegers JF, Blakley SA, Hauser WA, et al. Recurrence of febrile convulsions in a population-based cohort. *Epilepsy Res* 1990; 3:209–216.

49. Berg AT, Shinnar S, Darefsky AS, et al. Predictors of recurrent febrile seizures. A prospective cohort study. *Arch Pediatr Adolesc Med* 1997; 151:371–378.

50. Nelson KB and Ellenberg JH. Prognosis in children with febrile seizures. *Pediatrics* 1978; 61:720–727.

51. Camfield P, Camfield C, Gordon K, Dooley J: What types of epilepsy are preceded by febrile seizures? A population-based study of children. *Dev Med Child Neurol* 1994; 36:887–892.

52. Annegers JF, Hauser WA, Shirts SB, et al. Factors prognostic of unprovoked seizures after febrile convulsions. *N Engl J Med* 1987; 316:493–498.

53. Wolf SM, Forsythe A. Epilepsy and mental retardation following febrile seizures in childhood. *Acta Pediatr Scand* 1989; 78:291–295.

54. Hamati-Haddad A, Abou-Khalil B. Epilepsy diagnosis and localization in patients with antecedent childhood febrile convulsions. *Neurology* 1998; 50:917–922.

55. Berg AT, Shinnar S. Unprovoked seizures in children with febrile seizures: short-term outcome. *Neurology* 1996; 47:562–568.

56. Annegers JF, Hauser WA, Elveback LR, et al. The risk of epilepsy following febrile convulsions. *Neurology* 1979; 29:297–303.

57. Nelson KB, Ellenberg JH. Predictors of epilepsy in children who have experienced febrile seizures. *N Engl J Med* 1976; 295:1029–1033.

58. Rosman NP. The case for treating febrile seizures. *Contemp Pediatr* 1992; 9(6):12–34.

59. Freeman JM. The best medicine for febrile seizures. *N Engl J Med* 1992; 327:1161–1163.

60. Freeman JM. Just say no! Drugs and febrile seizures. *Pediatrics* 1990; 86:624.

61. Balslev T. Parental reactions to a child's first febrile convulsion. *Acta Pediatr Scand* 1991; 80:466–469.

62. Camfield CS, Camfield PR. Febrile seizures: an Rx for parent fears and anxieties. *Contemp Pediatr* 1993; 10:26–44.

63. Hauser WA. The natural history of febrile seizures. In: Nelson KB, Ellenberg JH, eds. *Febrile Seizures*. New York, Raven Press, 1981:5–17.

64. Nelson KB, Ellenberg JH. Febrile seizures. In: Dreifuss FE, ed. *Pediatric Epileptology*. Boston: John Wright, 1983:173–198.

65. Smith JA, Wallace SJ. Febrile convulsions: intellectual progress in relation to anticonvulsant therapy and to recurrence of fits. *Arch Dis Child* 1982; 57:104–107.

66. Ellenberg JH, Nelson KB. Febrile seizures and later intellectual performance. *Arch Neurol* 1978; 35:17–21.

67. Verity CM, Greenwood R, Golding J. Long-term intellectual and behavioral outcomes of children with febrile convulsions. *N Engl J Med* 1998:338:1723–1728.

68. Van Landingham KE, Heinz ER, Cavazos JE, et al. Magnetic resonance imaging evidence of hippocampal injury after prolonged focal febrile convulsions. *Ann Neurol* 1998; 43:413–426.

69. Cendes F, Andermann F, Dubeau F, et al. Early childhood prolonged febrile convulsions, atrophy and sclerosis of mesial structures, and temporal lobe epilepsy: An MRI volumetric study. *Neurology* 1993; 43:1083–1087.

70. Sloviter RS, Pedley TA: Subtle hippocampal malformation. Importance in febrile seizures and development of epilepsy. *Neurology* 1998; 50:846–849.

71. Shinnar S. Prolonged febrile seizures and mesial temporal sclerosis. *Ann Neurol* 1998; 43:411–412.

72. Fernandez G, Effenberger O, Vinz B, et al. Hippocampal malformation as a cause of familial febrile convulsions and subsequent hippocampal sclerosis. *Neurology* 1998; 50:909–917.

73. Germano IM, Zhang YF, Sperber EF, et al. Neuronal migration disorders increase susceptibility to hyperthermia-induced seizures in developing rats. *Epilepsia* 1996; 37:902–910.

74. Wolf SM. Prevention of recurrent febrile seizures with continuous drug therapy: efficacy and problems of phenobarbital or phenytoin therapy. In: Nelson KB, Ellenberg JH, eds. *Febrile Seizures*. New York, Raven Press, 1981:127–134.

75. Newton RW, McKinlay I. Subsequent management of children with febrile convulsions. *Dev Med Child Neurol* 1988; 30:402–406.

76. Newton RW. Randomized controlled trials of phenobarbitone and valproate in febrile convulsions. *Arch Dis Child* 1988; 63:1189–1191.

77. Farwell JR, Lee YJ, Hirtz DG, et al. Phenobarbital for febrile seizures — effects on intelligence and on seizure recurrence. *N Engl J Med* 1992; 326:144.

78. Trimble MR, Cull CA. Antiepileptic drugs, cognitive function, and behavior in children. *Cleve Clin J Med* 1989; 56 (Suppl, Part 1):140–146.

79. American Academy of Pediatrics Committee on Drugs. Behavioral and cognitive effects of anticonvulsant therapy. *Pediatrics* 1995; 96:538–540.

80. Minagawa K, Miura H. Phenobarbital, primidone and sodium valproate in the prophylaxis of febrile convulsions. *Brain Dev* 1981; 3:385–393.

81. Herranz JL, Armijo JA, Arteaga R. Effectiveness and toxicity of phenobarbital, primidone, and sodium valproate in the prevention of febrile convulsions, controlled by plasma levels. *Epilepsia* 1984; 25:89–95.

82. Ngwane E, Bower B. Continuous sodium valproate or phenobarbitone in the prevention of 'simple' febrile convulsions. *Arch Dis Child* 1980; 55:171–174.

83. Wallace SJ, Aldridge Smith J. Successful prophylaxis against febrile convulsions with valproic acid or phenobarbitone. *Br Med J* 1980; 280:353–354.

84. Mamelle N, Mamelle JC, Plasse JC, et al. Prevention of recurrent febrile convulsions — A randomized therapeutic assay: sodium valproate, phenobarbital and placebo. *Neuropediatrics* 1984; 15:37–42.

85. Dianese G. Prophylactic diazepam in febrile convulsions. *Arch Dis Child* 1979; 54:244–245.

86. Banco L, Veltri D. Ability of mothers to subjectively assess the presence of fever in their children. *Am J Dis Child* 1984; 138:976–978.

87. Uhari M, Rantala H, Vainionpää L, et al. Effect of acetaminophen and of low intermittent doses of diazepam

on prevention of recurrences of febrile seizures. *J Pediatr* 1995; 126:991–995.

88. Schnaiderman D, Lahat E, Sheefer T, et al. Antipyretic effectiveness of acetaminophen in febrile seizures: ongoing prophylaxis versus sporadic usage. *Eur J Pediatr* 1993; 152:747–749.

89. Pearce JL, Sharman JR, Forster RM. Phenobarbital in the acute management of febrile convulsions. *Pediatrics* 1977; 60:569–572.

90. Knudsen FU. Intermittent diazepam prophylaxis in febrile convulsions. Pros and cons. *Acta Neurol Scand* 1991; 83 (Suppl 135):1–24.

91. Agurell S, Berlin A, Ferngren H, et al. Plasma levels of diazepam after parenteral and rectal administration in children. *Epilepsia* 1975; 16:277–283.

92. Thorn I. Prevention of recurrent febrile seizures: intermittent prophylaxis with diazepam compared with continuous treatment with phenobarbital. In: Nelson KB and Ellenberg JH, eds. *Febrile Seizures*. New York, Raven Press, 1981:119–126.

93. Shirai H, Miura H, Sunaoshi W. A clinical study on the effectiveness of intermittent therapy with rectal diazepam suppositories for the prevention of recurrent febrile convulsions: a further study. *J Japan Epil Soc* 1988; 6:1–10.

94. Dreifuss FE, Rosman NP, Cloyd JC, et al. A comparison of rectal diazepam gel and placebo for acute repetitive seizures. *N Engl J Med* 1998; 338:1869–1875.

95. Minagawa K, Mizuno S, Shirai H, et al. A pharmacokinetic study on the effectiveness of intermittent oral diazepam in the prevention of recurrent febrile convulsions. *No To Hattatsu* 1985; 17:162–167.

96. Hohjo M, Miura H, Minagawa K, et al. A clinical study on the effectiveness of intermittent therapy with oral diazepam syrups for the prevention of recurrent febrile convulsions: a preliminary report. *Brain Dev* 1986; 8:559–560.

97. Ramakrishnan K, Thomas K. Long term prophylaxis of febrile seizures. *Indian J Pediatr* 1986; 53:397–400.

98. Autret E, Billard C, Bertrand P, et al. Double-blind, randomized trial of diazepam versus placebo for prevention of recurrence of febrile seizures. *J Pediatr* 1990; 117:490–494.

99. Rosman NP, Colton T, Labazzo J, et al. A controlled trial of diazepam administered during febrile illnesses to prevent recurrence of febrile seizures. *N Engl J Med* 1993; 329:79–84.

100. Nuñez-Lopez LC, Espinosa-Garcia E, Hernandez-Arbelaez E, et al. Efficacy of diazepam to prevent recurrences in children with a first febrile convulsion. *Acta Neuropediatr* 1995; 1:187–195.

101. Vanasse M, Masson P, Geoffroy G, et al. Intermittent treatment of febrile convulsions with nitrazepam. *J Can Neurol Sci* 1984; 11:377–379.

102. Tondi M, Carboni F, Deriu A, et al. Intermittent therapy with clobazam for simple febrile convulsions. *Dev Med Child Neurol* 1987; 29:830–831.

103. Knudsen FU, Paerregaard A, Andersen R, et al. Long term outcome of prophylaxis for febrile convulsions. *Arch Dis Child* 1996; 74:13–18.

CHAPTER 13

Severe Encephalopathic Epilepsy in Infants: West Syndrome

Shunsuke Ohtahara, M.D., and Yasuko Yamatogi, M.D.

Infantile spasms is a unique disorder that is peculiar to infancy and early childhood. The seizures have been described in the literature as massive spasms, flexion spasms, jackknife seizures, infantile myoclonic seizures, and the like, and they have been recognized as an epileptic phenomenon since they were first described by William West in 1841 (1). Approximately 100 years later, Gibbs and Gibbs (2) described the interictal electroencephalogram (EEG) pattern, hypsarrhythmia, which was noted to occur in a large number of patients with infantile spasms. Most patients with infantile spasms have some degree of mental and developmental retardation. The triad of infantile spasms, retardation, and hypsarrhythmia has become known as West syndrome. In 1958 the first therapeutic breakthrough was reported by Sorel and Dusaucy-Bauloye (3), who observed improvement in EEGs and amelioration of spasms in patients treated with adrenocorticotropic hormone (ACTH).

A considerable amount of literature pertaining to this disorder has accumulated over the past several decades. However, classifications and clinical descriptions of the seizures, based largely on routine bedside observations, have been highly variable, and this lack of uniformity has led to considerable confusion and controversy. Our understanding of the clinical manifestations of this disorder was greatly increased by the development of long-term polygraphic-video monitoring techniques in the 1970s (4). These techniques also provided objective means of evaluating the acute effects of therapy on seizure frequency and the EEG.

In this chapter, we briefly describe the clinical and EEG features of infantile spasms and review some of the more controversial and as yet unresolved issues, including therapy and pathophysiology.

EPIDEMIOLOGY

The incidence of this disorder in the United States has been estimated at 1 in 4,000 to 6,000 live births (5). Spasm onset is usually within the first 4 to 8 months of life. There is no clear evidence of a preponderance of one sex over the other, and a familial occurrence is rare (6,7).

CLINICAL MANIFESTATIONS

The motor spasm typically consists of a brief, bilaterally symmetrical contraction of the muscles of the neck, trunk, and extremities. The exact character of the seizure depends on whether the flexor or extensor muscles are predominantly affected and on the distribution of the muscle groups involved (4,8). The position of the body (e.g., supine versus sitting) usually influences the type of spasm. The intensity of the spasm may vary from a massive contraction of all flexor muscles, resulting in a jackknife at the waist, to a minimal contraction of muscles such as the abdominal recti.

Three main types of motor spasms have been identified: flexor, extensor, and mixed flexor-extensor. In our polygraphic-video monitoring experience, mixed spasms occur most commonly (approximately 42%), flexor spasms were the next most common (approximately 34%), and extensor spasms occurred least commonly (approximately 25%). Asymmetrical infantile spasms were rare (less than 1%). Periods of attenuated responsiveness, which have been termed *arrest phenomena,* may occur following a motor spasm or may occur independently. Most infants with this disorder have more than one type of spasm.

Approximately 60 percent of spasms are associated with eye deviation, either alone or followed by rhythmic nystagmoid movements. Pauses in respiration also occur in about 60 percent of spasms, while changes in heart rate occur rarely (less than 1%). Although many infants cry following a spasm, crying does not occur as an ictal phenomenon.

There is little variation in the number of spasms recorded from the same patient in consecutive 24-hour monitoring periods; however, there is a marked variation in spasm frequency when patients are monitored at two-week intervals (9). The number of spasms recorded during 24-hour periods has ranged from as few as three to as many as 763 in different patients.

Approximately the same number of spasms occur during the day as at night; however, infantile spasms rarely occur when the infant is actually asleep (less than 3%). Instead, they frequently occur immediately upon, or soon after, arousal. The spasms are not precipitated by feeding or photic stimulation but may occasionally be elicited by tactile stimulation or unexpected loud noises, although this is uncommon.

Although infantile spasms may occur in an isolated fashion, about 80 percent occur in clusters. During long-term polygraphic-video monitoring, the number of spasms per cluster varied from two to 138. Succession rates of up to 15 spasms per minute have been recorded, and the intensity of the motor spasms within a cluster usually waxes and then wanes.

ELECTROENCEPHALOGRAPHIC FEATURES

Interictal Patterns

A variety of interictal EEG patterns may be associated with this disorder (6). These include diffuse slowing of the background activity, focal slowing, focal or multifocal spikes and sharp waves, and generalized slow-spike-and-slow-wave activity. In a small number of infants, the background activity may appear normal; however, the interictal pattern most commonly associated with infantile spasms is hypsarrhythmia. Gibbs and Gibbs (2) originally defined hypsarrhythmia as

...random high voltage slow waves and spikes. These spikes vary from moment to moment, both in duration and in location. At times they appear to be focal, and a few seconds later they seem to originate from multiple foci. Occasionally the spike discharge becomes generalized, but it never appears as a rhythmically repetitive and highly organized pattern that could be confused with a discharge of the petit mal or petit mal variant type. The abnormality is almost continuous, and in most cases it shows as clearly in the waking as in the sleeping record.

This prototypic pattern is usually seen in the early stages of the disorder and most often in younger infants (less than 1 year of age). However, long-term monitoring of these patients has shown that variations of this pattern (modified hypsarrhythmia) are more common. These variations include hypsarrhythmia with a consistent focus of abnormal discharge, hypsarrhythmia with increased interhemispheric synchronization, hypsarrhythmia comprising primarily high-voltage, slow-wave activity with very little spike or sharp-wave activity, asymmetrical or unilateral hypsarrhythmia, and hypsarrhythmia with episodes of generalized, regional, or localized voltage attenuation, which, in its maximal expression, is referred to as the "suppression-burst variant" (10). Recognition of the suppression-burst variant is important because of its prognostic significance. Patients whose EEGs show this pattern invariably have poor long-term outcomes, regardless of therapy.

In addition to demonstrating these basic variations, long-term monitoring has shown that hypsarrhythmia is a highly dynamic pattern, with transient alterations in the pattern occurring throughout the day. The hypsarrhythmic activity tends to be most pronounced and to persist to the latest age in slow-wave sleep and is least evident or completely absent during rapid eye movement (REM) sleep, when the background activity may appear normal (11). Transient disappearance or reduction of the hypsarrhythmic activity is usually seen on arousal from sleep; this normalization may last from a few seconds to many minutes. In addition, there is usually a reduction or disappearance of the hypsarrhythmic pattern during a cluster of spasms, with the pattern returning immediately following cessation of the spasms (10).

Ictal Patterns

A variety of ictal EEG patterns have been identified (8). These include generalized slow-wave transients, sharp-and-slow-wave transients, and attenuation episodes, occurring alone or with superimposed faster frequencies. These patterns occur singly or in various combinations. The most common ictal EEG change associated with infantile spasms is a generalized slow-wave transient, followed by an abrupt attenuation of background activity in all regions. The duration of the ictal EEG event may range from less than 1 second to more than 1 minute, with the longer episodes being associated with arrest phenomena. There is no close correlation between the character of the ictal EEG event and the type of spasm.

DIFFERENTIAL DIAGNOSIS

The diagnosis of infantile spasms is often delayed for weeks or months because parents, and even physicians, do not recognize the motor phenomena as seizures. Colic, Moro reflexes, and startle responses are diagnoses frequently made by pediatricians. Parents also may confuse infantile spasms with hypnagogic jerks occurring during sleep, transient flexor-extensor posturing of trunk and extremities of nonepileptic origin, and other types of myoclonic activity.

Infants with *benign myoclonic epilepsy* may have repetitive jerks, but the seizures are much briefer than spasms, and the EEG during the seizures reveals 3-Hz spike-and-wave or polyspike-and-wave activity. The background EEG activity is usually normal. These myoclonic seizures are treated with standard anticonvulsants (e.g., ethosuximide), and the long-term prognosis in these patients is favorable. Another type of myoclonic movement that has been reported to be confused with infantile spasms is so-called *benign myoclonus of early infancy* (12). Infants with this disorder reportedly have tonic and myoclonic movements involving either the axial or limb musculature, which, like infantile spasms, may occur in clusters. The age at onset of this disorder (3 to 8.5 months) coincides with the age at onset of infantile spasms. In none of the reported cases did these movements persist beyond the age of two years. Unlike infantile spasm patients, infants with benign myoclonus of early infancy have normal development, normal neurologic examinations, and normal EEGs. The motor movements are not accompanied by EEG changes, thus suggesting a nonepileptiform basis for the events. Differentiation of infantile spasms from nonepileptic events and other types of myoclonic activity usually requires that an EEG, including a sleep recording, be obtained. In instances in which the routine EEG fails to shed light on the diagnosis of the patient's seizures, polygraphic-video monitoring studies should be performed to capture the questionable episodes and thus provide a definitive diagnosis.

RELATED SYNDROMES

Ohtahara (13) proposed that the syndrome of infantile spasms and suppression-burst activity in the EEG, when seen in the neonatal period, represents a disorder different from that seen in older infants and termed this disorder *early infantile epileptic encephalopathy*. This syndrome is associated with a wide variety of central nervous system (CNS) insults, particularly brain malformations (see Chapter 14). Other investigators do not consider early infantile epileptic encephalopathy to be a separate entity but rather an early variant of infantile spasms.

A similar syndrome, neonatal myoclonic encephalopathy, has also been described (14). In this syndrome, with onset within the first few weeks of life, patients are reported to have erratic fragmentary myoclonus associated with other types of seizures. The EEG shows a suppression-burst pattern. This syndrome has been associated with brain malformations and inborn errors of metabolism, for example, nonketotic hyperglycinemia and proprionic acidemia. Familial cases are stated to be frequent, and all infants have severe neurologic deficits.

Whether early infantile epileptic encephalopathy and neonatal myoclonic encephalopathy are truly two different syndromes is not known. Furthermore, it is not clear whether these two syndromes should be differentiated from other cases of infantile spasms associated with the suppression-burst pattern. Further investigation in this area is needed. As stated previously, when patients with infantile spasms show the suppression-burst variant of hypsarrhythmia, the prognosis for long-term outcome is poor, regardless of whether the pattern developed in the neonatal period or in later months of life.

PATIENT CLASSIFICATION

In the past, the classification of infantile spasm patients was variable and inconsistent (6). Currently, patients are best classified on the basis of past medical history, developmental history, neurologic examination, and computed tomographic (CT) and magnetic resonance imaging (MRI) findings. Based on these criteria, patients can be divided into two main groups: cryptogenic or symptomatic. We classify a patient as cryptogenic if there is no abnormality on neurologic examination, no known associated etiological factor, normal development before onset of the spasms, and normal CT and MRI scans before institution of therapy. Using these criteria, approximately 10 percent to 15 percent of patients may be classified as cryptogenic (15–18), with the remaining patients classified as symptomatic. The use of functional imaging technologies [e.g., positron emission tomography (PET) or functional MRI (fMRI)] probably will reduce the percentage of patients classified as cryptogenic. Classifying a patient as cryptogenic or symptomatic is crucial when considering long-term outcome (see next section).

ASSOCIATED ETIOLOGICAL AND CLINICAL FACTORS

In approximately 40 percent of patients, no associated etiological factor can be clearly identified. In the other 60 percent, various pre-, peri-, and postnatal factors have been implicated. Prenatal factors include cerebral dysgenesis (e.g., lissencephaly), intrauterine infection, hypoxia-ischemia, prematurity, and genetic disorders (e.g., tuberous sclerosis). Perinatal factors include traumatic delivery and hypoxia-ischemia, and postnatal factors include inborn errors of metabolism (e.g., nonketotic hyperglycinemia), head injury, CNS infection, hypoxia-ischemia, and intracranial hemorrhage.

Approximately 85 percent to 90 percent of patients with infantile spasms show some degree of mental and developmental retardation. Approximately 50 percent have major neurologic deficits, and another 40 percent have minor ones (6,19). In a study we conducted on 54 patients with infantile spasms, CT scans revealed the following: normal, 31 percent; generalized atrophy, 15 percent; predominantly focal atrophy, 35 percent; and congenital anomalies, 19 percent (20). Similar findings have been reported by others (21,22).

Diffuse and focal abnormalities, similar to those identified with CT, may also be seen with MRI. In addition, MRI reportedly also reveals evidence of delayed myelination (23–25). PET reportedly detects changes in up to 97 percent of infantile spasm patients (26). In this study of 139 patients multifocal abnormalities were seen most commonly (62%), followed by unifocal abnormalities (47%), and rarely diffuse changes (3%).

Serial PET studies have shown that focal cortical areas of hypometabolism do not necessarily persist over time, suggesting that cortical hypometabolism in some infantile spasms patients does not represent a structural lesion, but only a functional change (25,27,28). The value of PET in the routine evaluation of infantile spasms patients is still being assessed, and its restricted availability limits its usefulness. Other more readily accessible functional imaging studies (e.g., fMRI) may provide similar information.

IMMUNIZATION

During the last several decades, there has been a major disagreement as to whether immunization is an etiological factor for infantile spasms. This is an important issue, not only from a medical standpoint but also from a legal point of view, as evidenced by the large number of lawsuits against manufacturers of vaccines. Of the various vaccines that have been reported to be associated with infantile spasms, the one most frequently implicated is the diphtheria-pertussis-tetanus (DPT) vaccine. The pertussis agent has generated the most concern, and a number of publications have reported its apparent relationship to the development of infantile spasms (29–35). The major problem in determining whether there is a causal relationship between DPT immunization and infantile spasms is that the vaccine is given at the same age as the usual onset of infantile spasms. Therefore, if a large population were studied, an association between infantile spasms and DPT immunization would be expected on the basis of coincidence alone. Few studies have approached this problem in a manner amenable to statistical analysis; however, those that have done so have demonstrated that the apparent association between DPT immunization and infantile spasms is coincidental and that no causal relationship exists (36–39).

COUPLING OF INFANTILE SPASMS WITH OTHER SEIZURES

The coexistence of partial seizures with infantile spasms has been recognized for many years (6,19,30,40–42). Partial seizures may appear before the onset of infantile spasms, concurrently with spasms, or after spasms have ceased, either spontaneously or following treatment. Recently, there has been increased interest in the observation that in some infantile spasm patients focal electrical seizure discharges (FS) may be tightly coupled with infantile spasms. Our group first described this association in 1984 (10), and since that time several additional reports of this phenomenon in small groups of patients have appeared (43–48). Although this is an interesting phenomenon, its significance remains questionable. These observations have been used by some investigators to support the hypothesis that infantile spasms occur as a result of an interaction between a primary cortical generator and subcortical structures (45,49) (see subsequent section). To further investigate the significance of coupling of FS and infantile spasms, we analyzed the video-EEG studies performed on 96 consecutive patients newly diagnosed with infantile spasms and hypsarrhythmic EEGs (50). Ten patients demonstrated FS; however, in only five patients was there an apparent coupling of FS with infantile spasms. More importantly, in only three patients (3% of the entire population) was the observed coupling statistically significant. Three different couplings were documented. FS could precede a cluster of spasms, could occur during a cluster of spasms, or could follow a cluster of spasms. FS always arose independently from various sites in a given patient, and in some patients coupling of infantile spasms and FS always occurred on arousal from sleep.

Our conclusion from this study is that coupling of FS and infantile spasms at the time of diagnosis of infantile spasms occurs only rarely. We believe there are several possible explanations for this coupling phenomenon. In some instances, apparent coupling of FS and infantile spasms may best be explained by random coincidence. A second possibility is that FS may facilitate or induce the appearance of infantile spasms (or vice versa), as has been the major explanation suggested by others. Finally, the coupling of infantile spasms and FS may result from the effect of some "critical factor" that simultaneously affects the seizure thresholds of the neuronal systems involved in the generation of both seizure types. This final hypothesis assumes that in the presence of the "critical factor," the seizure thresholds for FS and infantile spasms are concurrently altered, resulting in the simultaneous or near simultaneous occurrence of both seizure types. In some of our patients the "critical factor" appeared to be the arousal mechanism, a known potent activator of infantile spasms and other seizures.

Tonic seizures may also be coupled with infantile spasms. These two seizures may be difficult to differentiate because the clinical and EEG features are very similar. The major distinguishing features between the two are that tonic seizures usually are more prolonged and lack the intense initial phasic component seen with infantile spasms. An interesting observation is that tonic seizures may rarely immediately precede a cluster of infantile spasms. A review of video-EEG monitoring studies of 57 consecutive infantile spasm patients revealed coupling of tonic seizures with infantile spasms in three (5%) cases (personal observations). Because of the similarities between tonic seizures and infantile spasms, these two seizures are possibly generated by a similar mechanism and arise from the same region of the brain, possibly the brain stem.

SPONTANEOUS REMISSION

The phenomenon of spontaneous remission of infantile spasms is poorly understood. Published data concerning the duration of this disorder have been infrequent and imprecise. In 1973 Jeavons and coworkers (51) reported that 28 percent of patients were free of spasms by age 1, 49 percent before age 2, 65 percent before age 3, and 74 percent by age 4. Unfortunately, some of their patients had been treated with steroids, and EEG findings were not presented. To further investigate spontaneous remission in this disorder, we retrospectively studied 44 patients who had not been treated with hormonal drugs (52). Our results indicate that spontaneous remission of infantile spasms and disappearance of the hypsarrhythmic EEG pattern can begin within one month of the onset of this disorder and that 25 percent of patients experience spontaneous remission within one year of spasm onset.

Spontaneous remission in two consecutively identified infantile spasms patients being evaluated for possible admission to a trial of ACTH therapy are

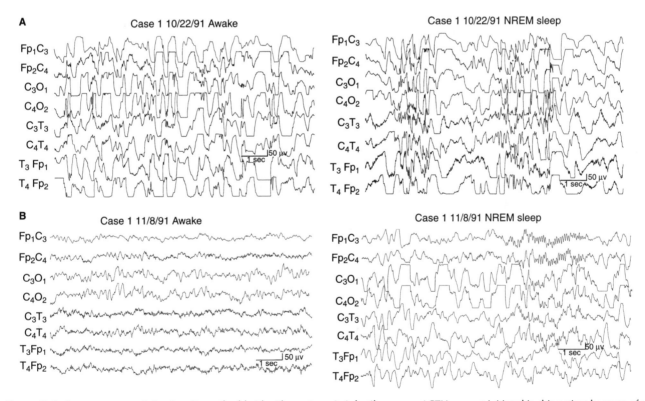

Figure 13-1. Spontaneous remission in a 7-month-old girl with cryptogenic infantile spasms. ACTH was not initiated in this patient because of a concurrent infection. Representative samples of the awake and NREM-sleep EEG selected from 18-channel 24-hour polygraphic-video monitoring records. **A.** Recording at the time of initial diagnosis shows hypsarrhythmia. Infantile spasms were recorded. **B.** Repeat study three weeks later showing normal activity awake and during NREM sleep. Awake sample shown was taken with the patient's eyes open (eyes-closed recording revealed a well-defined occipital dominant rhythm of 5–5.5 Hz). No infantile spasms were recorded during the 24-hour monitoring study.

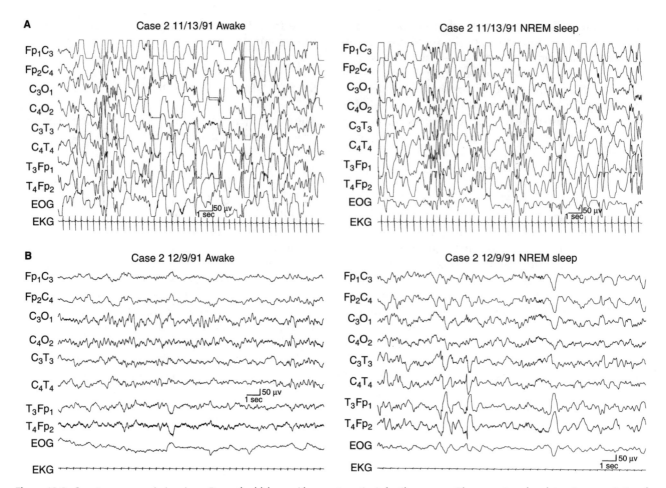

Figure 13-2. Spontaneous remission in a 5-month-old boy with symptomatic infantile spasms. The parents refused to give permission for treatment. Representative samples of the awake and NREM-sleep EEG selected from 18-channel 24-hour polygraphic/video monitoring records. **A.** Recording at the time of initial diagnosis shows hypsarrhythmia. Infantile spasms were recorded. **B.** Repeat study three weeks later, showing normal background activity for age. NREM-sleep sample shows right temporal spikes. Left temporal spikes (not shown) were also present in the sleep tracing. No infantile spasms were recorded during the 24-hour monitoring study.

illustrated in Figures 13-1 and 13-2. This phenomenon must always be remembered when interpreting results of any therapeutic trial in this disorder and must also be considered in discussing possible pathophysiological mechanisms underlying infantile spasms.

PATHOPHYSIOLOGY

The pathophysiological mechanism underlying infantile spasms is not known. Considerable evidence implicates the brain stem as the area in which infantile spasms and the hypsarrhythmic EEG pattern originate (11,53–55). We previously described a pathophysiological model of infantile spasms, based on our long-term polygraphic-video monitoring experience (11,56), which suggested that dysfunction of certain monoaminergic or cholinergic regions of the brain stem involved in the control of sleep cycling

may be responsible for the generation of the spasms and the EEG changes seen in this disorder (56). Various other investigators have also suggested that dysfunction of monoaminergic neurotransmitter systems may be responsible for the generation of infantile spasms (57–61). This model did not exclude the possibility that these critical brain stem region(s) might be affected by distant sites because the brain stem sleep system receives input from many other areas (56). Several years later, Chugani and coworkers (49) expanded our hypothesis. Primarily on the basis of PET scan studies, these authors suggested that the brain stem dysfunction causing infantile spasms was produced by abnormal functional interaction between the brain stem (raphe nuclei) and a "focal or diffuse cortical abnormality." According to this hypothesis, the cortical abnormality exerts a "noxious" influence over the brain stem from where the discharges spread caudally and rostrally to produce spasms and the hypsarrhythmic EEG pattern. The association of partial seizures with infantile spasms (previously described) was further evidence used to support the hypothesis that a primary cortical generator interacts with subcortical structures, resulting in infantile spasms. Other pathophysiological mechanisms underlying this disorder have also been proposed. First, it has been suggested that infantile spasms result from a failure or delay of normal developmental processes (62). This theory is based largely on the assumption that ACTH and corticosteroids accelerate certain normal developmental processes in immature animals (63–67). Another major hypothesis is that infantile spasms are the results of a defect in the immunological system (56,68,69). Supportive evidence for this hypothesis includes the presence of antibodies to extracts of normal brain tissue in the sera of infantile spasm patients (70,71), the presence of increased numbers of activated B cells and T cells in the peripheral blood of infantile spasms patients (72), and an increased frequency of the HLA-DRw52 antigen in infantile spasms patients compared with controls (73). Finally, it has been suggested that corticotropin-releasing hormone, a reported potent convulsant in the rodent, with age-specific potency during infancy, may play a mechanistic role in infantile spasms (74).

TREATMENT

No aspect of this disorder has created as much confusion and controversy as the area of therapy. During the past four decades, numerous studies on the treatment of infantile spasms have been published; however, the results of these studies are so diverse that no consensus exists, and no true "standard of care" has been established. In this section, we briefly review the prevailing attitudes and opinions on the treatment of this disorder and make recommendations for the most appropriate therapy based on the best available data (see Chapter 40). Areas in which further investigation is needed are also noted.

Hormonal Therapy

Acute Effects

Since 1958, when Sorel and Dusaucy-Bauloye (3) reported that treatment of infantile spasms patients with ACTH resulted in cessation or amelioration of spasms and disappearance of the hypsarrhythmic EEG pattern, many reports have appeared on the treatment of this disorder with ACTH and corticosteroids. To date, most of these studies have been plagued with methodological shortcomings that hamper interpretation and comparison of results. Some of the problems encountered are the following:

1. The natural history of the disorder is not completely understood — particularly the phenomenon of spontaneous remission (see above).
2. Few well-controlled prospective single- or double-blind studies have been performed.
3. There have been marked variations in dosages of medications used and durations of treatment.
4. Until recently, objective means of determining the acute effects of hormonal treatment were not used. Instead, previous studies relied on parental observation to determine spasm frequency, which, as we have learned from our monitoring experience, is unreliable. As shown in Figure 13-3, parents often underestimate spasm frequency to such an extent that they might report that no spasms occurred in a child who, in fact, is experiencing many spasms per day. In 8 of 24 patients, parents reported complete cessation of spasms during ACTH or prednisone therapy; however, in three of these patients, the presence of spasms was documented by long-term polygraphic-video monitoring. Conversely, parents may report that spasms did occur in a child who, in reality, does not have spasms.
5. In most studies, response to therapy has been defined in a graded fashion. Our long-term monitoring of patients with infantile spasms treated with ACTH and prednisone indicates that the

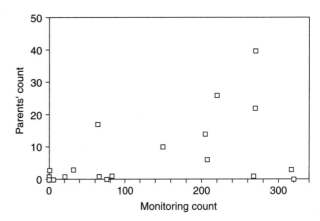

Figure 13-3. Spasm frequency after institution of ACTH or prednisone therapy: comparison of parents' estimates with results of 24-hour polygraphic-video monitoring. The coefficient of determination (r^2) between the parents' and video monitoring counts was 0.26. The 24-hour monitoring studies were performed two to four weeks after institution of ACTH or prednisone therapy. Patients who failed to respond to ACTH were treated with prednisone, and vice versa. Sixteen patients eventually responded to hormonal therapy.

response to therapy is an all-or-none phenomenon — complete control or no control.

Because of these problems, several divergent opinions have evolved regarding hormonal therapy. Some individuals consider ACTH and corticosteroids to be equipotential, whereas others consider ACTH to be superior (6,75–80). Furthermore, two therapeutic approaches have evolved for treating infantile spasms with ACTH. Some investigators recommend using large doses of ACTH (40–160 U/day) and long durations of therapy (3–12 months) (42,77,80–86), whereas others advocate low doses of ACTH (5–40 U/day) for relatively brief periods (1–6 weeks) (79,87–89). Some proponents of high-dose, long-duration therapy report better control of seizures and greater EEG improvement with such therapy compared with low-dose, short-duration therapy. The most dramatic results were reported by Snead and coworkers (77,86) in two noncontrolled, nonblinded, nonrandomized studies of high-dose, long-duration ACTH therapy in which seizure frequency was determined by parents' observations. The most remarkable finding of these two studies is that the EEGs were reported to have reverted to normal following ACTH therapy in 29 of 30 patients in one study (77) and in 14 of 15 patients in a subsequent study (86). A similar response rate to high-dose ACTH has also been reported by Baram and colleagues (80) in a recently completed study comparing high-dose ACTH to prednisone.

We began our investigations in this very complex area by performing controlled studies of the relative efficacies of low-dose ACTH and prednisone. Serial 24-hour polygraphic-video monitoring studies were performed to determine objectively the acute response to therapy (15–17). The results of these studies were as follows:

1. Response to therapy is all or none.
2. There is no major difference in therapeutic efficacy between low-dose ACTH (20–30 U/day) and prednisone (2 mg/kg/day) in stopping the spasms and improving the EEG.
3. Only a short course (2 weeks) of hormonal therapy is required for most patients to obtain a response.
4. After a response to hormonal therapy is documented, the therapy can be discontinued immediately and the response maintained.
5. ACTH failures may respond to prednisone and vice versa.
6. Approximately 60 percent of infantile spasm patients respond to either low-dose ACTH or corticosteroid therapy.
7. Approximately one third of the patients experience a relapse — a figure comparable to that

previously reported by Lacy and Penry (6). If a relapse occurs, a second course of therapy is usually effective.
8. Cause and treatment lag are not useful predictors of response. Patients with long treatment lags respond just as well as those with short treatment lags, and symptomatic patients respond just as well as cryptogenic patients.
9. Disappearance of the hypsarrhythmic EEG pattern may occur in patients who continue to have spasms. This is an important point because many physicians rely heavily on the EEG to determine whether an acute response to therapy has occurred.

After completion of the studies of low-dose ACTH versus prednisone, we performed a single-blind study of high-dose ACTH versus low-dose ACTH in newly diagnosed infantile spasm patients (90). Patients receiving high-dose ACTH were treated as follows: $150 \ U/m^2/day$ for 3 weeks, then $80 \ U/m^2/day$ for 2 weeks, then $80 \ U/m^2$ every other day for 3 weeks, then $50 \ U/m^2/day$ for 1 week, with the dose tapered to none during a final 3-week period. Patients assigned to low-dose ACTH therapy received 20–30 U/day for 2–6 weeks. The results of this study were as follows:

1. There was no significant difference in response rates between the patients assigned to high-dose or low-dose ACTH therapy. Fifty-eight percent of patients receiving low-dose ACTH responded compared with 50 percent of those treated with high-dose ACTH.
2. There was no significant difference in the number of normal EEG findings in patients who responded to either low-dose or high-dose ACTH therapy.
3. There was no significant difference in the relapse rate between the two groups.
4. The side-effect profiles of low-dose ACTH and high-dose ACTH were similar, with the exception of hypertension, which occurred more frequently in the high-dose group.

The various EEG patterns evident at the time of spasm cessation after hormonal therapy are outlined in Table 13-1.

Long-Term Outcome

Unique to hormonal treatment of infantile spasms has been the belief that ACTH or corticosteroids not only improve the EEG and control the spasms but also improve the outlook for mental and motor development. Approximately 9 percent to

Table 13-1. EEG Findings at Time of Documented Cessation of Spasms (N = 53)

EEG Findings	Number of Patients
Hypsarrhythmia	0
Normal	5
Normal background activity	17
Sharp- or spike-and-slow-wave foci	16
in temporal region only	8
in temporal and other regions	8
Focal slow activity only in temporal region	2
Intermittent rhythmic bifrontal sharp-and-slow-wave activity	2
Unilateral suppression of background activity	3
High-voltage fast activity	4
Abnormally slow and disorganized background activity	31
Alpha-rhythm present	11
Sharp- or spike-and-slow-wave foci	27
in temporal region only	8
in temporal and other regions	16
in other regions only	2
Intermittent rhythmic bifrontal sharp-and-slow-wave activity	6
Intermittent rhythmic bifrontal delta activity	10
Intermittent rhythmic bioccipital delta activity	4
Unilateral suppression of background activity	4
No foci	1

13 percent of patients with infantile spasms have been reported to develop normally when lower doses and shorter durations of hormonal treatment were used (51,75,91–95). However, some investigators have found that outcomes in treated and untreated patients were similar (51,75,96), and still others have reported an improved prognosis for long-term mental and motor development when higher doses and longer durations of ACTH therapy were used (22,42). Many authors also imply that long-term outcome is adversely affected when the treatment lag is prolonged (6,22,42). However, like the studies that evaluated the acute effects of hormonal therapy in infantile spasm patients, the designs of most studies concerned with long-term outcome do not permit definitive conclusions. Past reports of long-term prognosis have typically been retrospective or have not used such diagnostic tests as CT and MRI scans to aid in classifying patients as symptomatic or cryptogenic.

Our own study of the long-term outcome in 64 patients followed prospectively and treated with low doses of ACTH (20–30 U/day for 2–6 weeks) and prednisone (2 mg/kg/day for 2–6 weeks) (18) revealed the following:

1. The overall prognosis was poor, with only 5 percent of the total patient population having normal outcomes.
2. Severe or very severe impairment was observed in 67 percent of the patients.
3. There was no significant difference between responders and nonresponders with respect to long-term outcome.
4. There was no significant difference between patients who responded to ACTH and those who responded to prednisone with respect to long-term outcome.
5. There was no significant difference in outcome between patients initially treated within five weeks of the diagnosis of infantile spasms and those whose treatment began more than five weeks after the diagnosis. Early treatment (within five weeks of diagnosis), even in the cryptogenic group, did not ensure a normal long-term outcome.
6. The only factor that appeared to affect long-term outcome was whether the patient was classified as cryptogenic or symptomatic. This has also been noted by other investigators (42,49,78,97). In our study, cryptogenic patients had a significantly better outcome than symptomatic patients: 38 percent of the cryptogenic patients were normal or only mildly impaired, in contrast to 5 percent of the symptomatic patients.
7. We were unable to predict which cryptogenic patients would have normal outcomes and which would not.

At the current time, there are no controlled, prospective studies comparing the effects of high-dose ACTH versus low-dose ACTH on long-term outcome.

Recommended Treatment Regimen

On the basis of the best evidence currently available, the following treatment regimen is recommended for all patients with infantile spasms, regardless of treatment lag, age, or patient classification (cryptogenic vs. symptomatic). A baseline EEG should be obtained before institution of therapy. CT and MRI scans should also be performed to aid in classifying the patient as cryptogenic or symptomatic. Either ACTH or prednisone may be given initially. If ACTH is chosen, the drug should be started at a dose of 20 U/day and continued for two weeks; if there is no response at that time, the dose should be increased to 30 U/day. This dose should be continued for four weeks and then tapered to zero over one week. If prednisone is chosen, the drug should be administered at 2 mg/kg/day for two weeks; if there is no response, that dose should be continued for an additional four weeks and then tapered to zero over one week. Response to either ACTH or prednisone is defined as cessation of infantile spasms and improvement in the EEG. If a patient fails to respond to a course of ACTH, prednisone should be tried after a one-week washout period, and vice versa. If a relapse occurs after hormonal therapy has been discontinued, the effective drug should be restarted at the dose that produced the initial response and continued for two to six weeks depending on response. Serum electrolyte studies should be performed weekly throughout the entire course of ACTH or prednisone therapy, and the patient's blood pressure should be monitored closely.

Side Effects of Hormonal Therapy

The side effects of ACTH or corticosteroid therapy, some of which may preclude treatment or require its termination, include hypertension, suppression of the immune system, ocular opacities, electrolyte imbalances, gastrointestinal disturbances, cardiomegaly, and transient brain shrinkage. The most common and significant side effect from a clinical standpoint is hypertension, which has been reported in 10 percent to 25 percent of infantile spasm patients treated with ACTH or corticosteroids (6,15–17,88,90).

Anticonvulsant, Pyridoxine, and Other Therapies

Some of the various other agents that have been used to treat infantile spasms are listed in Table 13-2. Of these,

Table 13-2. Other Therapy for Infantile Spasms

1. Anticonvulsants
   - Benzodiazepines
     Nitrazepam
     Clonazepam
     Clobazam
   - Lamotrigine
   - Tiagabine
   - Topiramate
   - Valproate
   - Vigabatrin
2. Immunoglobulins
3. Pyridoxine
4. Other
   - Thyroid-releasing hormone
   - Antiserotonergic drugs
   - Antiadrenergic drugs
   - Ketogenic diet

valproate at a dose of 15–100 mg/kg/day (98–102), the benzodiazepines, particularly nitrazepam, at a dose of 0.3–1.0 mg/kg/day (6,103–107), and vigabatrin are reportedly the most effective. Currently, vigabatrin is generating the most enthusiasm (see Chapter 38). The effective dose of vigabatrin appears to be between 60 and 150 mg/kg/day, and reported response rates have ranged from 43 percent to 69 percent, with the best responses in patients with tuberous sclerosis (108–112). Pyridoxine has also been reported to be effective in treating small numbers of patients with infantile spasms (113–118). However, studies reporting use of these drugs have the same methodological shortcomings as those concerned with hormonal therapy. The function of these agents in treating infantile spasms cannot be determined until appropriately designed and objectively evaluated studies are performed.

Surgical Treatment

Over the decades, several anecdotal reports have appeared reporting the beneficial effects of the surgical removal of anatomical lesions from the brains of infantile spasm patients. These lesions include choroid plexus papilloma (119), temporal lobe astrocytoma (120), anaplastic ependymoma (121), and porencephalic cyst (122,123). In recent years, there has been a greater emphasis on the surgical treatment of infantile spasms, even in those patients without apparent lesions on traditional neuroimaging. The largest surgical series to date has been reported by Chugani and coworkers (124). In their series of 23 patients, 17 of whom reportedly had infantile spasms at the time of surgery, 15 underwent focal cortical resection and 8 underwent hemispherectomy. At an average follow-up of 28 months, 15 patients were reported to be seizure-free. There are several problems in interpreting the results of these surgical studies.

1. Not all of the patients identified in these reports actually had infantile spasms at the time of surgery. Many of the patients had a prior history of infantile spasms but at the time of surgery were actually experiencing other seizure types (e.g., partial seizures).
2. The time required for cessation of infantile spasms following surgical treatment is usually not provided. In most instances, it is not possible to determine whether spasms stopped immediately following surgery or weeks to months later. This point is extremely important when one considers the phenomenon of spontaneous remission.
3. In most cases, video-EEG monitoring was not used to document the presence of spasms

immediately before surgery or the cessation of spasms following surgery.

The problem in determining the effect of surgical treatment on spasm frequency can be further demonstrated by comparing studies of the long-term outcome in a group of surgically treated infantile spasm patients with a group of patients who failed to respond to hormonal therapy but were not treated surgically. Of the 17 patients reportedly experiencing infantile spasms at the time of surgery in Chugani's series (124), 10 (59%) were reportedly seizure-free at follow-up. In a study of 26 patients who failed to respond to hormonal therapy but were not treated surgically (18), 12 (46%) were seizure-free at follow-up. Therefore, it is difficult to determine whether cessation of spasms in all of the surgically treated patients was secondary to the surgical procedure itself or to some other factor (i.e., spontaneous remission). Of equal importance is the question whether surgical treatment of infantile spasm patients affects long-term development. Although some authors report that infantile spasm patients treated surgically show some improvement in developmental skills following surgery (124), the degree of improvement is difficult to assess because of the limited developmental information provided and the lack of control subjects. Although surgical treatment may abolish seizures in some infantile spasm patients, further controlled, prospective studies are needed to determine which patients may benefit from surgery and whether long-term development is significantly improved following surgical intervention.

OTHER SEIZURE TYPES

Other types of seizures have been reported to occur in 35 percent to 60 percent of patients who stopped having infantile spasms (6,51,88,91). The most common types of seizures that subsequently develop are tonic, simple partial, and generalized tonic-clonic. In our prospective study of long-term outcome (18), other types of seizures occurred in 53 percent of patients. An important observation is that none of the cryptogenic patients who responded to hormonal therapy developed other types of seizures.

Approximately one-third to one-half of cases of infantile spasms reportedly develop the Lennox-Gastaut syndrome (125,126). However, the time at which the transition from infantile spasms to the Lennox-Gastaut syndrome occurs is very difficult to determine in most patients because by clinical observation alone it may be impossible to differentiate the seizures associated with these syndromes. In some patients, the clinical and EEG features of both syndromes may coexist, suggesting that these two disorders actually represent a continuum.

MORTALITY RATE

The mortality rate reported in previous studies of infantile spasms ranges from 11 percent to 23 percent (6). However, we documented a mortality rate of only 5 percent in our study of long-term outcome (18), a finding probably reflecting the availability of better medical care today.

REFERENCES

1. West WJ. On a peculiar form of infantile convulsions. *Lancet* 1841; 1:724–725.
2. Gibbs FA, Gibbs EL. *Atlas of Electroencephalography.* Vol. 2. *Epilepsy.* Cambridge: Addison-Wesley, 1952.
3. Sorel L, Dusaucy-Bauloye A. A propos de 21 cas d'hypsarythmie de Gibbs. Son traitement spectaculaire par l'A. C. T. H. *Acta Neurol Psychiatr Belg* 1958; 58:130–141.
4. Frost JD Jr, Hrachovy RA, Kellaway P, Zion T. Quantitative analysis and characterization of infantile spasms. *Epilepsia* 1978; 19:273–282.
5. van den Berg BJ, Yerushalmy J. Studies on convulsive disorders in young children. I. Incidence of febrile and nonfebrile convulsions by age and other factors. *Pediatr Res* 1969; 3:298–304.
6. Lacy JR, Penry JK. *Infantile Spasms.* New York: Raven Press, 1976.
7. Dulac O, Feingold J, Plouin P, et al. Genetic predisposition to West syndrome. *Epilepsia* 1993; 34:732–737.
8. Kellaway P, Hrachovy RA, Frost JD Jr, Zion T. Precise characterization and quantification of infantile spasms. *Ann Neurol* 1979; 6:214–218.
9. Hrachovy RA, Frost JD Jr. Intensive monitoring of infantile spasms. In: Schmidt D, Morselli PL, eds. *Intractable Epilepsy: Experimental and Clinical Aspects.* New York: Raven Press, 1986:87–97.
10. Hrachovy RA, Frost JD Jr, Kellaway P. Hypsarrhythmia: variations on the theme. *Epilepsia* 1984; 25:317–325.
11. Hrachovy RA, Frost JD Jr, Kellaway P. Sleep characteristics in infantile spasms. *Neurology* 1981; 31:688–694.
12. Lombroso CT, Fejerman N. Benign myoclonus of early infancy. *Ann Neurol* 1977; 1:138–143.
13. Ohtahara S. Clinico-electrical delineation of epileptic encephalopathies in childhood. *Asian Med J* 1978; 21:499–509.
14. Aicardi J. Early myoclonic encephalopathy. In: Roger J, Dravet C, Bureau M, Dreifuss FE, Wolf P, eds. *Epileptic Syndromes in Infancy, Childhood and Adolescence.* London: John Libbey, 1985:12–22.
15. Hrachovy RA, Frost JD Jr, Kellaway P, Zion T. A controlled study of prednisone therapy in infantile spasms. *Epilepsia* 1979; 20:403–407.

16. Hrachovy RA, Frost JD Jr, Kellaway P, Zion T. A controlled study of ACTH therapy in infantile spasms. *Epilepsia* 1980; 21:631–636.

17. Hrachovy RA, Frost JD Jr, Kellaway P, Zion TE. Double-blind study of ACTH vs prednisone therapy in infantile spasms. *J Pediatr* 1983; 103:641–645.

18. Glaze DG, Hrachovy RA, Frost JD Jr, Kellaway P, Zion TE. Prospective study of outcome of infants with infantile spasms treated during controlled studies of ACTH and prednisone. *J Pediatr* 1988; 112:389–396.

19. Kellaway P. Neurologic status of patients with hypsarrhythmia. In: Gibbs FA, ed. *Molecules and Mental Health*. Philadelphia: Lippincott, 1959:134–149.

20. Glaze DG, Hrachovy RA, Frost JD Jr, Zion TE, Bryan RN. Computed tomography in infantile spasms: effects of hormonal therapy. *Pediatr Neurol* 1986; 2:23–27.

21. Gastaut H, Gastaut JL, Regis H, et al. Computerized tomography in the study of West's syndrome. *Dev Med Child Neurol* 1978; 20:21–27.

22. Singer WD, Haller JS, Sullivan LR, et al. The value of neuroradiology in infantile spasms. *J Pediatr* 1982; 100:47–50.

23. Schropp C, Staudt M, Staudt F, et al. Delayed myelination in children with West syndrome: an MRI-study. *Neuropediatrics* 1994; 25:116–120.

24. Kasai K, Watanabe K, Negoro T, et al. Delayed myelination in West syndrome. *Psychiatr Clin Neurosci* 1995; 49:S265–S266.

25. Natsume J, Watanabe K, Maeda N, et al. Cortical hypometabolism and delayed myelination in West syndrome. *Epilepsia* 1996; 37:1180–1184.

26. Chugani H, Conti J. Classification of infantile spasms in 139 cases: the role of positron emission tomography. *Epilepsia* 1994; 35(Supp 8):19.

27. Maeda N, Watanabe K, Negoro T, et al. Transient focal cortical hypometabolism in idiopathic West syndrome. *Pediatr Neurol* 1993; 9:430–434.

28. Maeda N, Watanabe K, Negoro T, et al. Evolutional change of cortical hypometabolism in West's syndrome. *Lancet* 1994; 343:1620–1623.

29. Baird HW, Borofsky LG. Infantile myoclonic seizures. *J Pediatr* 1957; 50:332–339.

30. Jeavons PM, Bower BD. *Infantile Spasms: A Review of the Literature and a Study of 112 Cases*. London: Spastics Society and Heinemann, 1964. Clinics in Developmental Medicine, No. 15.

31. Kulenkampff M, Schwartzman JS, Wilson J. Neurological complications of pertussis inoculation. *Arch Dis Child* 1974; 49:46–49.

32. Miller DL, Ross EM, Alderslade R, Bellman MH, Rawson NSB. Pertussis immunization and serious acute neurologic illness in children. *Br Med J (Clin Res)* 1981; 282:1595–1599.

33. Millichap JG, Bickford RG, Klass DW, Backus RE. Infantile spasms, hypsarrhythmia, and mental retardation. A study of etiologic factors in 61 patients. *Epilepsia* 1962; 3:188–197.

34. Strom J. Further experience of reactions, especially of a cerebral nature, in conjunction with triple vaccination: a study based on vaccinations in Sweden 1959–65. *Br Med J* 1967; 4:320–323.

35. Wilson J. Neurological complications of DPT inoculation in infancy. *Arch Dis Child* 1973; 48:829–830.

36. Bellman MH, Ross EM, Miller DL. Infantile spasms and pertussis immunization. *Lancet* 1983; 1:1031–1034.

37. Cody CL, Baraff LJ, Cherry JD, Marcy SM, Manclark CR. Nature and rates of adverse reactions associated with DPT and DT immunizations in infants and children. *Pediatrics* 1981; 68:650–660.

38. Fukuyama Y, Tomori N, Sugitate M. Critical evaluation of the role of immunization as an etiological factor of infantile spasms. *Neuropaediatrie* 1977; 8:224–237.

39. Melchior JC. Infantile spasms and early immunization against whooping cough. Danish survey from 1970 to 1975. *Arch Dis Child* 1977; 52:134–137.

40. Druckman R, Chao D. Massive spasms in infancy and childhood. *Epilepsia* 1955; 4:61–72.

41. Fukuyama Y. Studies on the etiology and pathogenesis of flexor spasms. *Adv Neurol Sci* (Tokyo) 1960; 4:861–867.

42. Lombroso CT. A prospective study of infantile spasms. *Epilepsia* 1983; 24:135–158.

43. Bour F, Chiron C, Dulac O, Plouin P. Caractéres électrocliniques des crises dans le syndrome d'Aicardi. *EEG Neurophysiol Clin* 1986; 16:341–353.

44. Carrazana EJ, Barlow JK, Holmes GL. Infantile spasms provoked by partial seizures. *J Epilepsy* 1990; 3:97–100.

45. Carrazana EJ, Lombroso CT, Mikati M, Helmers S, Holmes GL. Facilitation of infantile spasms by partial seizures. *Epilepsia* 1993; 34:97–109.

46. Donat JF, Wright FS. Simultaneous infantile spasms and partial seizures. *J Child Neurol* 1991; 6:246–250.

47. Plouin P, Jalin C, Dulac O, Chiron C. Enregistrement ambulatoire de l'EEG pendant 24 heures dans les spasmes infantiles épileptiques. *Rev EEG Neurophysiol Clin* 1987; 17:309–318.

48. Yamamoto N, Watanabe K, Negoro I, et al. Partial seizures evolving to infantile spasms. *Epilepsia* 1988; 29:34–40.

49. Chugani HT, Shewmon DA, Sankar R, Chen BJ, Phelps ME. Infantile spasms: II. Lenticular nuclei and brain stem activation on positron emission tomography. *Ann Neurol* 1992; 31:212–219.

50. Hrachovy RA, Frost JD Jr, Glaze DG. Coupling of focal electrical seizure discharges with infantile spasms: Incidence during long-term monitoring in newly diagnosed patients. *J Clin Neurophysiol* 1994; 11:461–464.

51. Jeavons PM, Bower BD, Dimitrakoudi M. Long-term prognosis of 150 cases of "West syndrome." *Epilepsia* 1973; 14:153–164.

52. Hrachovy RA, Glaze DG, Frost JD Jr. A retrospective study of spontaneous remission and long-term outcome in patients with infantile spasms. *Epilepsia* 1991; 32:212–214.

53. Morimatsu Y, Murofushi K, Handa T, Shinohara T, Shiraki H. Pathology in severe physical and mental disabilities in children—with special reference to four cases of nodding spasms. *Adv Neurol Sci* (Tokyo) 1972; 16:465–470.

54. Satoh J, Mizutani T, Morimatsu Y, et al. Neuropathology of infantile spasms. *Brain Dev* 1984; 6:196.

55. Chugani HT, Mazziotta JC, Engel J Jr, Phelps ME. Positron emission tomography with ^{18}F-2-fluorodeoxyglucose in infantile spasms. *Ann Neurol* 1984; 16:376–377.

56. Hrachovy RA, Frost JD Jr. Infantile spasms: a disorder of the developing nervous system. In: Kellaway P, Noebels JL, eds. *Problems and Concepts in Developmental Neurophysiology*. Baltimore: Johns Hopkins University Press, 1989:131–147.

57. Coleman M. Infantile spasms associated with 5-hydroxytryptophan administration in patients with Down's syndrome. *Neurology* 1971; 21:911–919.

58. Klawans HL Jr, Goetz C, Weiner WJ. 5-hydroxytryptophan-induced myoclonus in guinea pigs and the possible role of serotonin in infantile myoclonus. *Neurology* 1973; 23:1234–1240.

59. Nausieda PA, Carvey PM, Braun A. Long-term suppression of central serotonergic activity by corticosteroids: a possible model of steroid-responsive myoclonic disorder. *Neurology* 1982; 32:772–775.

60. Ross DL, Anderson G, Shaywitz B. Changes in monoamine metabolites in CSF during ACTH treatment of infantile spasms. *Neurology* 1983; 33(Suppl 2):75.

61. Silverstein F, Johnston MV. Cerebrospinal fluid monoamine metabolites in patients with infantile spasms. *Neurology* 1984; 34:102–104.

62. Riikonen R. Infantile spasms: some new theoretical aspects. *Epilepsia* 1983; 24:159–168.

63. Palo J, Savolainen H. The effect of high doses of synthetic ACTH on rat brain. *Brain Res* 1974; 70:313–320.

64. Ardeleanu A, Sterescu N. RNA and DNA synthesis in developing rat brain: Hormonal influences. *Psychoneuroendocrinology* 1978; 3:93–101.

65. Huttenlocher PR, Amemiya IM. Effects of adrenocortical steroids and of adrenocorticotrophic hormone on (Na^+-K^+)-ATPase in immature cerebral cortex. *Pediatr Res* 1978; 12:104–107.

66. Doupe AJ, Patterson PH. Glucocorticoids and the developing nervous system. In: Ganton D, Pfaff D, eds. *Current Topics in Neuroendocrinology: Adrenal Actions on Brain*. Berlin: Springer-Verlag, 1982:23–43.

67. Pranzatelli MR. On the molecular mechanism of adrenocorticotrophic hormone in the CNS: Neurotransmitters and receptors. *Exp Neurol* 1994; 125:142–161.

68. Mandel P, Schneider J. Sur le mode d'action de l'A. C. T. H. dans l'E. M. I. H. In: Gastaut H, Roger J, Soulayrol R, Pinsard N, eds. *L'encéphalopathie myoclonique infantile avec hypsarythmie*. Paris: Masson & Cie, 1964:177–189.

69. Martin F. Physiopathogénie. In: Gastaut H, Roger J, Soulayrol R, Pinsard N, eds. *L'encéphalopathie myoclonique infantile avec hypsarythmie*. Paris: Masson & Cie, 1964:169–76.

70. Reinskov T. Demonstration of precipitating antibody to extract of brain tissue in patients with hypsarrhythmia. *Acta Paediatr Scand* 1963; (Suppl):140–73.

71. Mota NGS, Rezkallah-Iwasso MT, Peracoli MTS, Montelli TCB. Demonstration of antibody and cellular immune response to brain extract in West and Lennox-Gastaut syndromes. *Arq Neuropsiquiatr* 1984; 42:126–131.

72. Hrachovy RA, Frost JD Jr, Shearer WT, et al. Immunological evaluation of patients with infantile spasms. *Ann Neurol* 1985; 18:414.

73. Hrachovy RA, Frost JD Jr, Pollack M, Glaze DG. Serologic HLA typing in infantile spasms. *Epilepsia* 1988; 29:817–819.

74. Baram TZ. Pathophysiology of massive infantile spasms (MIS): Perspective on the role of the brain adrenal axis. *Ann Neurol* 1993; 33:231–237.

75. Kurokawa T, Goya N, Fukuyama Y, et al. West syndrome and Lennox-Gastaut syndrome: A survey of natural history. *Pediatrics* 1980; 65:81–88.

76. Low NL. Infantile spasms with mental retardation. II. Treatment with cortisone and adrenocorticotropin. *Pediatrics* 1958; 22:1165–1169.

77. Snead OC III, Benton JW, Myers CJ. ACTH and prednisone in childhood seizure disorders. *Neurology* 1983; 33:966–970.

78. Snyder CH. Infantile spasms. Favorable response to steroid therapy. *JAMA* 1967; 201:198–200.

79. Willoughby JA, Thurston DL, Holowach J. Infantile myoclonic seizures: An evaluation of ACTH and corticosteroid therapy. *J Pediatr* 1966; 69:1136–1138.

80. Baram T, Mitchell WG, Tournay A, et al. High-dose corticotropin (ACTH) versus prednisone for infantile spasms: a prospective, randomized, blinded study. *Pediatrics* 1996; 97:375–379.

81. Chevrie J, Aicardi J. Le pronostic psychique des spasmes infantiles traites par l'ACTH ou les corticoides. Analyse statistique de 78 cas suivis plus d'un an. *J Neurol Sci* 1971; 12:351–368.

82. Hagberg B. The nosology of epilepsy in infancy and childhood. In: Birkmayer W, ed. *Epileptic Seizures—Behaviour—Pain*. Bern: Huber, 1976:51–64.

83. Lagenstein I, Willig RP, Iffland E. Behandlung frühkindlicher Anfälle mit ACTH und Dexamethason unter standardisierten Bedingungen. I. Klinische Ergebnisse. *Monatsschr Kinderheilkd* 1978; 126:492–499.

84. Lerman P, Kivity S. The efficacy of corticotropin in primary infantile spasms. *J Pediatr* 1982; 101:294–296.

85. Singer WD, Rabe EF, Haller JS. The effect of ACTH therapy upon infantile spasms. *J Pediatr* 1980; 96:485–489.

86. Snead OC III, Benton JW Jr, Hosey LC, et al. Treatment of infantile spasms with high-dose ACTH: efficacy and plasma levels of ACTH and cortisol. *Neurology* 1989; 39:1027–1031.

87. Jeavons PM, Bower BD. The natural history of infantile spasms. *Arch Dis Child* 1961; 36:17–21.

88. Riikonen R. A long-term follow-up study of 214 children with the syndrome of infantile spasms. *Neuropediatrics* 1982; 13:14–23.

89. Trojaborg W, Plum P. Treatment of "hypsarrhythmia" with ACTH. *Acta Paediatr Scand* 1960; 49:572–582.

90. Hrachovy RA, Frost JD Jr, Glaze DG. High dose/long duration vs. low dose/short duration corticotropin therapy n infantile spasms: a single blind study. *J Pediatr* 1994; 124:803–806.

91. Jeavons PM, Harper JR, Bower BD. Long-term prognosis of infantile spasms: a follow-up report on 112 cases. *Dev Med Child Neurol* 1970; 12:413–421.

92. Matsumoto A, Watanabe K, Negoro T, et al. Long-term prognosis after infantile spasms: a statistical study of prognostic factors in 200 cases. *Dev Med Child Neurol* 1981; 23:51–65.

93. Pache HD, Trögen H. Das West-syndrom und seine behandlung mit ACTH. *Munch Med Wochenschr* 1967; 109:2408–2413.

94. Wiszczor-Adamczyk B, Koslacz-Folga A. Results of treatment and clinico-electroencephalographic evolution of infantile spasms. *Pol Med J* 1969; 8:193–199.

95. Wiszczor-Adamczyk B, Slenzak J. Neurological and psychological evaluation of children with infantile spasms in the light of observation during many years. *Pediatr Pol* 1972; 47:601–605.

96. Friedman E, Pampiglione C. Prognostic implications of electroencephalographic findings of hypsarrhythmia in first year of life. *Br Med J* 1971; 4:323–325.

97. Chevrie JJ, Aicardi J, Thieffry S. Traitement hormonal de 58 cas de spasmes infantiles. Resultats et pronostic psychique a long terme. *Arch Fr Pediatr* 1968; 25:263–276.

98. Bachman D. Use of valproic acid in treatment of infantile spasms. *Arch Neurol* 1982; 39:49–52.

99. Dyken PR, DuRant RH, Minden DB, King DW. Short-term effects of valproate on infantile spasms. *Pediatr Neurol* 1985; 1:34–37.

100. Siemes H, Spohr HL, Michael TH, Nau H. Therapy of infantile spasms with valproate: results of a prospective study. *Epilepsia* 1988; 29:553–560.

101. Prats JM, Garaizar C, Rua MJ, García-Nieto ML, Madoz P. Infantile spasms treated with high doses of sodium valproate. Initial response and follow-up. *Dev Med Child Neurol* 1991; 33:617–625.

102. Pavone L, Incorpora G, La Rosa M, Li Volti S, Mollica F. Treatment of infantile spasms with sodium dipropylacetic acid. *Dev Med Child Neurol* 1981; 23:454–461.

103. Dreifuss F, Farwell J, Holmes G, et al. Infantile spasms: comparative trial of nitrazepam and corticotropin. *Arch Neurol* 1986; 43:1107–1110.

104. Fukushima T, Akihama Y, Shibuki K, Sato A. The treatment of infantile spasms with nitrazepam. *No To Shinkei* 1968; 20:1297–1301.

105. Hagberg B. The chlordiazepoxide HC1 (Librium) analogue, nitrazepam (Mogadon), in the treatment of epilepsy in children. *Dev Med Child Neurol* 1968; 10:302–308.

106. Jan JE, Riegl JA, Crichton JU, Dunn HG. Nitrazepam in the treatment of epilepsy in childhood. *Can Med Assoc J* 1971; 104:571–575.

107. Markham CH. The treatment of myoclonic seizures of infancy and childhood with LA-I. *Pediatrics* 1964; 34:511–518.

108. Livingston JH, Beaumont D, Arzimanoglou A, Aicardi J. Vigabatrin in the treatment of epilepsy in infants. *Br J Clin Pharmacol* 1989; 27:109–112.

109. Chiron C, Dulac O, Luna D, et al. Vigabatrin in infantile spasms. *Lancet* 1990; 335:363–364.

110. Chiron C, Dulac O, et al. Therapeutic trial of vigabatrin in refractory infantile spasms. *J Child Neurol* 1991; 6:S52–S59.

111. Vles JSH, van der Heyden AMHG, Glijjs A, Troost J. Vigabatrin in the treatment of infantile spasms. *Neuropediatrics* 1993; 28:230–231.

112. Aicardi J. Vigabatrin treatment for infantile spasms. *Acta Neuropediatr* 1996; 2:9–11.

113. Bankier A, Turner M, Hopkins IJ. Pyridoxine dependent seizures — a wide clinical spectrum. *Arch Dis Child* 1983; 58:415–418.

114. Blennow G, Starck L. High dose B$_6$ treatment in infantile spasms. *Neuropediatrics* 1986; 17:7–10.

115. French JH, Grueter BB, Druckman R, O'Brien D. Pyridoxine and infantile myoclonic seizures. *Neurology* 1965; 15:101–113.

116. Ohtsuka Y, Matsuda M, Kohno C, et al. Pyridoxal phosphate in the treatment of West syndrome. In: Akimoto H, Kazamatsuri H, Seino M, Ward AA Jr, eds. *The XIIIth Epilepsy International Symposium*. New York: Raven Press, 1982:311–313. Advances in Epileptology.

117. Ohtsuka Y, Matsuda M, Ogino T, et al. Treatment of the West syndrome with high-dose pyridoxal phosphate. *Brain Dev* 1987; 9:415–417.

118. Pietz J, Benninger C, Shaffer H, et al. Treatment of infantile spasms with high-dosage vitamin B6. *Epilepsia* 1993; 34:757–763.

119. Branch CE, Dyken PR. Choroid plexus papilloma and infantile spasms. *Ann Neurol* 1979; 5:302–304.

120. Mimaki T, Ono J, Yabuuchi H. Temporal lobe astrocytoma with infantile spasms. *Ann Neurol* 1983; 14:695–696.

121. Ruggieri V, Caraballo R, Fejerman N. Intracranial tumors and West syndrome. *Pediatr Neurol* 1989; 5:327–329.

122. Palm DG, Brandt M, Korinthenberg R. West syndrome and Lennox-Gastaut syndrome in children with porencephalic cysts: Long-term follow-up after neurosurgical treatment. In: Niedermeyer E, Degen R, eds. *The Lennox-Gastaut Syndrome*. New York: Alan R. Liss, 1988:491–526.

123. Uthman BM, Reid SA, Wilder BJ, Andriola MR, Beydoun AA. Outcome for West syndrome following surgical treatment. *Epilepsia* 1991; 32:668–671.

124. Chugani HT, Shewmon A, Shields D, et al. Surgery for intractable infantile spasms: neuroimaging perspectives. *Epilepsia* 1993; 34:764–771.

125. Ohtahara S. Seizure disorders in infancy and childhood. *Brain Dev* 1984; 6:509–519.

126. Weinman HM. Lennox-Gastaut syndrome and its relationship to infantile spasms (West syndrome). In: E. Niedermeyer, R. Degen, eds. *The Lennox-Gastaut syndrome*. New York: Alan R. Liss, 1988:301–316.

CHAPTER 14

Severe Encephalopathic Epilepsy in Early Infancy

Shunsuke Ohtahara, M.D., and Yasuko Yamatogi, M.D.

From the neonatal to the early infantile periods, seizures are relatively rarely observable, compared with other periods of childhood because of the structural and biochemical immaturity of the brain, which may regulate the seizure susceptibility or threshold. Only a few epileptic syndromes begin to occur in these periods, and most of them are severe epilepsies (1). Peculiar representatives are early myoclonic encephalopathy (EME) (2) and early-infantile epileptic encephalopathy with suppression-bursts or Ohtahara syndrome (OS) (3). Both syndromes are classified into symptomatic generalized epilepsies with nonspecific etiology (1) and could be inclusively called "early infantile epileptic syndromes with suppression-burst" (4) because of shared common characteristics: very early onset with frequent minor seizures and suppression-burst (S-B) pattern on the electroencephalogram (EEG).

EARLY-INFANTILE EPILEPTIC ENCEPHALOPATHY WITH SUPPRESSION-BURSTS, OHTAHARA SYNDROME

Ohtahara syndrome (OS) was first described by Ohtahara and coworkers in 1976 (5) as the earliest form of an age-dependent epileptic encephalopathy and is characterized by frequent tonic spasms of early onset within a first few months of life and S-B pattern in EEG.

The age-dependent epileptic encephalopathies include OS, West syndrome, and Lennox-Gastaut syndrome. Although each of these syndromes is an independent clinicoelectrical entity with its own specific features, they have the following common characteristics (5–7):

1. Age preference in a certain period of life
2. Peculiar types of frequent, minor generalized seizures
3. Severe and continuous massive epileptic EEG abnormality
4. Heterogeneous cause
5. Frequent association with mental defect
6. Therapy resistance and grave prognoses

Furthermore, transition is often observed with age among patients with these syndromes. A considerable number of OS cases evolve into West syndrome and from West to Lennox-Gastaut syndrome in their clinical course (8–11). Because of these common characteristics and mutual transition with age, the inclusive term *age-dependent epileptic encephalopathy* has been applied to this group of syndromes (6,7,12).

As the clinicoelectrical feature specific to each syndrome is based on many causes commonly observed in the three syndromes, the age factor should be considered as the common denominator responsible for the manifestation of their individual characteristics. These syndromes, therefore, may be the age-specific epileptic reaction to various nonspecific exogenous brain insults acting at the specific developmental stage.

Several dozens of cases of OS have been reported (13–17), but its incidence is rare compared with those of West and Lennox-Gastaut syndromes. No obvious sex difference has been observed.

Clinical Manifestations

The onset of seizures is very early and is confined to within the first 2 or 3 months after birth, mainly within 1 month. The main seizure type is tonic spasms with or without clustering. The duration of each tonic spasm is up to 10 seconds. One series, that is, a cluster, consists of 10 to 40 spasms, at intervals of 5 to 15 seconds. These epileptic spasms occur not only in waking states but also in sleeping states, in most cases. Daily seizure frequency is very high, ranging from 100 to 300 isolated spasms or 10 to 20 series in those with clustering spasms. In addition to tonic spasms, partial seizures such as erratic focal motor seizures and hemiconvulsions are observed in about one-third of the cases.

EEG Findings

The most characteristic feature is the S-B pattern that is persistently observed regardless of the circadian cycle (Figure 14-1). The S-B pattern is characterized by high voltage bursts alternating with nearly flat patterns at an approximately regular rate. Bursts of 1 to 3 seconds' duration comprise 150 to 350 microvolt high-voltage slow waves intermixed with multifocal spikes. Duration of the suppression phase is 3 to 4 seconds. The burst-burst interval, measured from onset to onset of the bursts, ranges from 5 to 10 seconds. Presumably reflecting the underlying organic brain lesion, some asymmetry in S-B occurs in about two-thirds of cases, but no remarkable asynchrony is found except in the case of Aicardi syndrome (18).

The ictal EEG of tonic spasms shows principally a desynchronization with or without evident, sometimes remarkable, initial rapid activity. A low-voltage fast activity is also often observed. Tonic spasms appear concomitant with bursts. Partial seizures usually start from some fixed foci and are followed by tonic spasms in series or sometimes follows them.

Other Investigations

Brain imaging such as CT and MRI reveal structural abnormalities, notably asymmetric lesions at even the early stage of presentation in most cases. Progressive brain atrophy is often suspected with seizure persistence, particularly in infancy. With evoked potentials, peak latencies of central components are often prolonged in auditory brain stem responses (ABRs) and visual evoked potentials (VEPs) (3). No abnormalities are found in routine laboratory examinations of blood, urine, cerebrospinal fluid, bone marrow, and liver functions, in metabolic studies including amino acid analysis, lysosomal enzyme assay, pyruvate and lactate, and organic acid; or in immunological and virological examinations.

Cause

Although the causes of OS are heterogeneous, obvious brain lesions including brain malformations are often found. Porencephaly, Aicardi syndrome (3,18), olivary-dentate dysplasia (17,19), hemimegalencephaly (16), linear sebaceous naevus (20), Leigh encephalopathy (21), and subacute diffuse encephalopathy (3) have all been associated with the syndrome. In a few cases no cause has been identified, and these are labelled cryptogenic (3,15).

Treatment and Prognoses

Seizures are intractable. Natural or synthetic adrenocorticotropic hormone (ACTH) therapy is partially effective in only a few cases. Successful resection of focal cortical dysplasia is reported (22). Although seizures are possibly suppressed by school age in about half of the cases, developmental and life prognoses are poor. All those surviving are severely handicapped, both mentally and physically. Mortality is high, especially in the early stage of the disease.

EARLY MYOCLONIC ENCEPHALOPATHY

Early myoclonic encephalopathy is a rare epileptic syndrome of very early onset with frequent myoclonias and partial seizures and S-B in EEG. It was first described by Aicardi and Goutieres in 1978 (23).

Clinical Manifestations

The onset of seizures is in the first three months of life, mostly during the neonatal period. No sex difference is observed in its incidence.

The cardinal seizures are myoclonias, which are mostly fragmentary. Frequent erratic partial seizures, massive myoclonias, and tonic spasms are also seen. Among these types of seizures, fragmentary myoclonias are the essential symptom in EME and the initial seizure type in most cases (2). Such myoclonias are characterized by only a slight twitching of the distal ends of the extremities, eyelids, and corners of the mouth, and are sometimes too subtle to detect without careful observation. The frequency of these myoclonias varies greatly from several times a day to several dozen times a minute. The ictal EEG usually shows no consistent change with myoclonia, although some myoclonias coincidentally occur with bursts (24–27). This suggests that myoclonias in EME are mainly of a nonepileptic type.

Throughout the course of the syndrome, the main seizure types are partial seizures; those include complex partial seizures with eye-deviation or autonomic symptoms such as apnea and facial flushing, clonic seizures at various parts of the body, and asymmetric tonic posturing with or without generalization. Partial seizures following erratic myoclonias are particularly

Awake

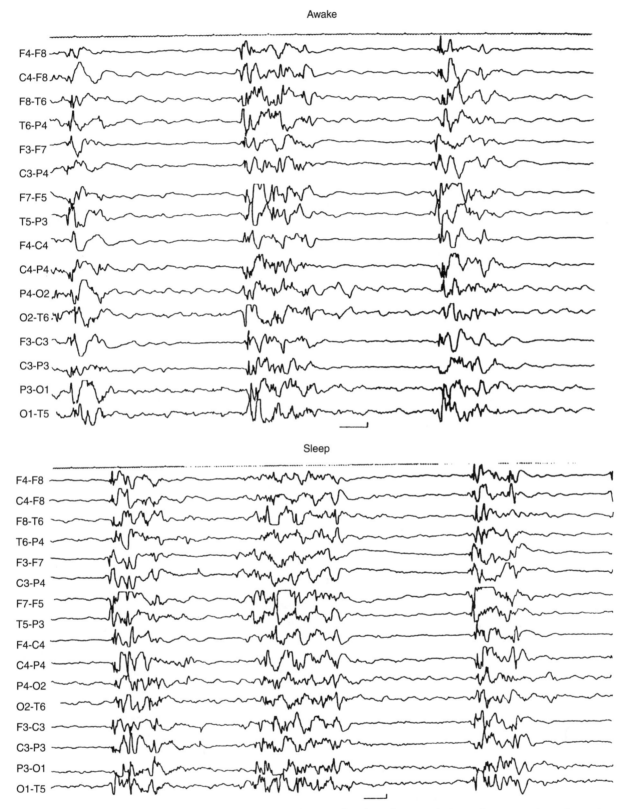

Sleep

Figure 14-1. Interictal EEG (Ohtahara syndrome). Two-month-old boy. High voltage bursts and almost flat suppressions alternately repeat continuously and consistently throughout the waking (upper) and sleeping (lower) states. The horizontal calibration mark; 1 sec, the vertical one; 50 microvolts.

characteristic of this syndrome (25,26). Partial seizures have a tendency to cluster in the early stage. They are seen during both waking and sleeping states. The frequency of partial seizures is remarkably high, ranging from 7 to 8 times to 30 to 100 times a day but decreases with age.

Massive myoclonias and tonic spasms are not necessarily observed in all cases. Tonic spasms are often observed. Cases are considered West syndrome when tonic spasms appear at 3 to 4 months of age. The period of West syndrome is, however, transient, and the EME state recurs and persists for a long period thereafter. Tonic spasms are usually seen during both waking and sleeping states and appear either in series or in isolation. Tonic spasms in series sometime appear following a partial seizure, but a partial seizure may appear just after tonic spasms in other infants.

EEG Findings

Interictal EEG of EME is also characteristically a S-B pattern with bursts lasting 1 to 5 seconds and nearly flat periods of 3 to 10 seconds. This pattern becomes more distinct during sleep, and more pronounced as sleep deepens (24,26) (Figure 14-2).

The S-B pattern tends to be replaced by atypical hypsarrhythmia or by multifocal paroxysms after 3 to 5 months of age. In most cases, however, the appearance of atypical hypsarrhythmia is transient, lasting up to 2 years 6 months of age at the latest (24), after which S-B pattern returns and persists for a long period (24–27). In addition to the S-B pattern, multifocal spikes persist throughout the clinical course. The location of spike foci varies in every case and is not consistent in a given patient.

With the ictal EEG of partial seizures, various patterns of focal onset, such as fast activity, alpha or theta patterns, rhythmic sharp waves, and irregular spike-waves are observed, usually from two or more sites with migration in each individual case (2,24–27). Ictal EEG of tonic spasms shows desynchronization, which appears concomitant with bursts. Myoclonic seizures also occur during bursts (4,27).

Other Investigations

Neuroimaging is often normal at the onset, but progressive cortical and periventricular atrophies are observed in some cases (2,26). Abnormalities are often detected from 3 to 10 months of age, that is, 3 to 8 months after the onset. Diffuse cortical atrophy is noted in all, with associated ventricular dilatation in some cases, but focal abnormalities are exceptional. Abnormalities in evoked potentials affect are detected ABR, and VEP, often in somatosentory evoked potentials (SSEPs), and sometimes in photo-evoked eyelid microvibration (MV) (24).

Etiology

The most striking feature of this disorder is the high incidence of familial cases as found in 4 of 12 families in the series of Aicardi and coworkers (2) and 2 of 8 families in the series of Dalla Bernardina and coworkers (25,26). This suggests the etiologic participation of some kinds of genetic and congenital metabolic errors in many cases. Non-ketotic hyperglycinemia (24,28–30), propionic acidemia, methylmalonic acidemia and D-glyceric acidemia (30), sulphite and xanthine oxidase deficiency (2), Menkes disease (32), and Zellweger syndrome (31) have been reported to be associated with EME. In many cases; however, the cause remains unknown.

Treatment and Prognoses

None of the conventional antiepileptic drugs, ACTH, corticosteroids, or pyridoxine have been effective. Both partial seizures and myoclonias, however, decrease gradually with age. Early myoclonic encephalopathy has an extremely poor prognosis including a high mortality, with death usually occurring before two years of age. Survivors have persistent partial seizures and progressive psychomotor deterioration to a vegetative state (2,24).

DEVELOPMENTAL ASPECTS

Compared to EME, the remarkable characterstic of OS is its age-dependent evolutional change; that is the development from OS to West syndrome in middle infancy, particularly during 3 to 6 months of age, in many cases, and further from West to Lennox-Gastaut syndrome in early childhood, at 1 to 3 years of age, in some cases (11).

The EEG also evolves from the S-B pattern to hypsarrhythmia in many cases at around 3 to 6 months of age, and further from hypsarrhythmia to diffuse slow spike-waves in some cases at around 1 year of age (11).

Concerning the changing process of S-B pattern in OS, its transition to hypsarrhythmia starts with a gradual increase in the amplitude of the suppression phase. Disappearance of the S-B pattern in waking precedes that in sleep, and S-B remains in the sleeping EEG even after the waking EEG has already transformed to hypsarrhythmia. In the course of evolution from hypsarrhythmia to diffuse slow spike-waves, the change in the waking EEG is followed by that in the sleeping EEG. Thus, the evolution from a S-B pattern to hypsarrhythmia and further to diffuse slow spike-waves proceeds in a close relation with the waking and sleeping cycle (8,11). The timing of transition among

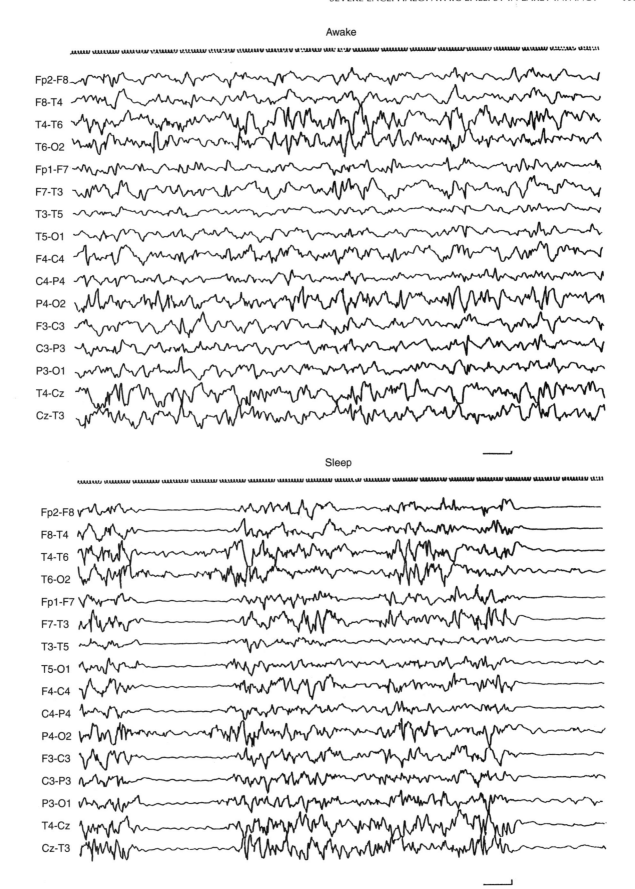

Figure 14-2. Interictal EEG (early myoclonic encephalopathy). Six-month-old girl. Multifocal spikes are noted frequently in the disorganized background activity in the waking record (upper), but suppression-burst pattern is apparent in the sleeping record (lower).

the three clinical syndromes and EEG patterns is specific; evolving syndromes and EEG patterns appear at characteristic ages.

EME, however, manifests no fundamental change in the clinicoelectrical feature throughout its course, except for the EEG change from suppression-burst or burst-suppression pattern to a disorganized pattern with frequent multifocal spikes that occur within a few months of life (2,27) and transient manifestation of West syndrome and hypsarrhythmia in some cases (24).

DIFFERENTIAL DIAGNOSIS

Differential Diagnosis of OS from West Syndrome

The age of onset of the two syndromes is different: OS appears the neonatal to early infantile periods and West syndrome in middle infancy. Although the main seizure type is tonic spasms in both syndromes, tonic spasms in OS appear not only while awake but also during sleep, and not only in clusters. Partial seizures also occur in some OS cases but are rare in West syndrome. Most cases with OS have severe cortical pathology, often displaying asymmetric lesions in neuroimaging.

The EEG discriminates the S-B pattern in OS from hypsarrhythmia in West syndrome. The S-B pattern differs from the periodic type of hypsarrhythmia in which periodicity becomes evident only during sleep.

Seizures are more intractable in OS, and ACTH therapy is usually not effective. Furthermore, children with OS have a less favourable prognoses than those with West syndrome.

Differential Diagnosis Between EME and OS

As EME and OS have common clinical and electrical characteristics, such as early onset within a few months of life and the S-B pattern on EEG, differentiation can be difficult. The main seizure type is tonic spasms, and myoclonias are rarely seen in OS. In contrast, myoclonias, especially erratic myoclonias, and frequent partial seizures predominate in EME (24).

Electroencephalographically, the S-B pattern is a common feature of both syndromes, but its relation to the circadian cycle and age of its appearance and disappearance differ considerably. The S-B pattern in OS is characterized by consistent appearance during both waking and sleeping states, whereas in EME, it is enhanced by sleep and often not manifest in the waking state. Concerning the duration of appearance, the S-B pattern appears at the beginning of the disease and disappears within the first six months of life in OS, while in EME, it becomes distinct at 1 to 5 months of age in some cases and characteristically persists for a long period (24–27).

The evolution of the EEG abnormalities during the clinical course is a characteristic feature of OS: from the S-B pattern to hypsarrhythmia in many cases and further from hypsarrhythmia to diffuse slow spike-waves in some cases (3,11). In EME, the S-B pattern persists for a long time, although appears atypical hypsarrhythmia transienly in some cases. Therefore, the age-related evolutional pattern differs considerably between OS and EME (24).

Regarding epileptic syndromes, OS shows a characteristic evolution as the earliest form of an age-dependent epileptic encephalopathy, while EME has no specific evolution with age.

Etiologically, OS is usually based on evident organic brain lesions including brain malformations. Neuroimaging demonstrates abnormal findings even at the early stage. No familial cases have been reported in OS. In contrast, the frequent incidence of familial cases suggests some undetermined inborn metabolic disorder as the cause in many cases of EME.

The differences between OS and EME, indicate that they are independent clinicoelectrical entities. This is in agreement with Schlumberger and coworkers who found definite clinical and symptomatological differences and no overlap between the two syndromes (4).

REFERENCES

1. Commission on Classification and Terminology of the International League Against Epilepsy. Proposal for revised classification of epilepsies and epileptic syndromes. *Epilepsia* 1989; 30:389–99.

2. Aicardi J. Early myoclonic encephalopathy (neonatal myoclonic encephalopathy). In: Roger J, Bureau M, Dravet C, et al. eds. *Epileptic Syndromes in Infancy, Childhood and Adolescence*, 2nd ed. London: John Libbey, 1992: 13–23.

3. Ohtahara S, Ohtsuka Y, Yamatogi Y, et al. Early-infantile epileptic encephalopathy with suppression-bursts. In: Roger J, Bureau M, Dravet C, et al. eds. *Epileptic Syndromes in Infancy, Childhood and Adolescence*, 2nd ed. London: John Libbey, 1992: 25–34.

4. Schlumberger E, Dulac O, Plouin P. Early infantile epileptic syndrome(s) with suppression-burst: nosological considerations. In: Roger J, Bureau M, Dravet C, et al. eds. *Epileptic Syndromes in Infancy, Childhood and Adolescence*, 2nd ed. London: John Libbey, 1992:35–42.

5. Ohtahara S, Ishida T, Oka E, et al. On the specific age dependent epileptic syndrome: the early-infantile epileptic encephalopathy with suppression-bursts. *No To Hattatsu* 1976; 8:270–280.

6. Ohtahara S. A study on the age-dependent epileptic encephalopathy. *No To Hattatsu* 1977; 9:2–21.

7. Ohtahara S. Clinico-electrical delineation of epileptic encephalopathies in childhood. *Asian Med J* 1978; 21:499–509.

8. Ohtahara S, Yamatogi Y. Evolution of seizures and EEG abnormalities in childhood onset epilepsy. In: Wada JA, Ellingson RJ, eds. *Clinical Neurophysiology of Epilepsy, Handbook of Electroencephalography and Clinical Neurophysiology, Revised Series*, Vol. 4. Amsterdam: Elsevier, 1990:457–477.

9. Ohtsuka Y, Ogino T, Murakami N, et al. Developmental aspects of epilepsy with special reference to age-dependent epileptic encephalopathy. *Jpn J Psychiatry Neurol* 1986; 40:307–313.

10. Yamatogi Y, Ohtahara S. Age-dependent epileptic encephalopathy: a longitudinal study. *Folia Psychiatr Neurol Jpn* 1981; 35:321–331.

11. Ohtahara S, Ohtsuka Y, Yamatogi Y, et al. The early-infantile epileptic encephalopathy with suppression-bursts: developmental aspects. *Brain Dev* 1987; 9:371–376.

12. Donat JF. The age-dependent epileptic encephalopathies. *J Child Neurol* 1992; 7:7–21.

13. Martin H-J, Deroubaix-Tella P, Thelliez Ph. Encephalopathie epileptique neonatale a bouffees periodiques. *Rev EEG Neurophysiol* 1981; 11:397–403.

14. Konno K, Miura Y, Suzuki H, et al. A study on clinical features of the early infantile epileptic encephalopathy with suppression burst of Ohtahara syndrome. *No To Hattatsu* 1982; 14:395–404.

15. Clark M, Gill J, Noronka M, et al. Early infantile epileptic encephalopathy with suppression burst: Ohtahara syndrome. *Dev Med Child Neurol* 1987; 29:508–519.

16. Bermejo AM, Martin VL, Arcas J, et al. Early infantile epileptic encephalopathy: a case associated with hemimegalencephaly. *Brain Dev* 1992; 14:425–428.

17. Robain O, Dulac O. Early infantile epileptic encephalopathy with suppression bursts and olivary-dentate dysplasia. *Neuropediatrics* 1992; 23:162–164.

18. Ohtsuka Y, Oka E, Terasaki T, et al. Aicardi syndrome: a longitudinal clinical and electroencephalographic study. *Epilepsia* 1993; 34:627–634.

19. Harding BN, Boyd SG. Intractable seizures from infancy can be associated with dentato-olivary dysplasia. *J Neurol Sci* 1991; 104:157–165.

20. Hirata Y, Ishikawa A, Somiya K. A case of linear nevus sebaceous syndrome associated with early-infantile epi-leptic encephalopathy with suppression burst (EIEE). *No To Hattatsu* 1985; 17:577–582.

21. Tatsuno M, Hayashi M, Iwamoto H, et al. Leigh's encephalopathy with wide lesions and early infantile epileptic encephalopathy with burst-suppression: an autopsy case. *No To Hattatsu* 1984; 16:68–75.

22. Pedespan JM, Loiseau H, Vital A, et al. Surgical treatment of an early epileptic encephalopathy with suppression-bursts and focal cortical dysplasia. *Epilepsia* 1995; 36:27–40.

23. Aicardi J, Goutières F. Encéphalopathie myoclonique neonatale. *Rev EEG Neurophysiol* 1978; 8:99–101

24. Murakami N, Ohtsuka Y, Ohtahara S. Early infantile epileptic syndromes with suppression-bursts: early myoclonic encephalopathy vs. Ohtahara syndrome. *Jpn J Psychiatry Neurol* 1993; 47:197–200.

25. Dalla Bernardina B, Dulac O, Bureau M, et al. Encéphalopathie myoclonique précoce avec épilepsie. *Rev EEG Neurophysiol* 1982; 12:8–14.

26. Dalla Bernardina B, Dulac O, Fejerman N, et al. Early myoclonic epileptic encephalopathy (EMEE). *Eur J Pediatr* 1983; 140:248–252.

27. Otani K, Abe J, Futagi Y, et al. Clinical and electro-encephalographical follow-up study of early myoclonic encepahlopathy. *Brain Dev* 1989; 11:332–337.

28. Dalla Bernardina B, Aicardi J, Goutieres F, et al. Glycine encephalopathy. *Neuropädiatrie* 1979; 10:209–225.

29. Terasaki T, Yamatogi Y, Ohtahara S, et al. A long-term follow-up study on a case with glycine encephalopathy. *No To Hattatsu* 1988; 20:15–22.

30. Lombroso CT. Early myoclonic encephalopathy, early infantile epileptic encephalopathy, and benign and severe infantile myoclonic epilepsies: a critical review and personal contributions. *J Clin Neurophysiol* 1990; 7:380–408.

31. Spreafico R, Angelini L, Binelli S, et al. Burst-suppression and impairment of neocortical ontogenesis: electroclinical and neuropathologic findings in two infants with early myoclonic encephalopathy. *Epilepsia* 1993; 34:800–808.

32. Aicardi J. *Epilepsy in Children*. 2nd ed. New York: Raven Press, 1995:40–42.

CHAPTER 15

Encephalopathic Epilepsy after Infancy

Tracy A. Glauser, M.D., and Diego A. Morita, M.D.

Among the numerous epileptic syndromes occurring during childhood, a subset are characterized by severe treatment-resistant seizures usually associated with progressive loss of higher intellectual functions and characteristic electroencephalogram (EEG) abnormalities. These age-dependent epileptic syndromes are often called encephalopathic epilepsies or epileptic encephalopathies, a descriptive terminology that does not shed light on their underlying pathophysiologies or specific etiologies. It has been proposed that these syndromes are age-specific epileptic reactions to nonspecific and diverse exogenous insults (1).

This subgroup of pediatric epilepsy syndromes includes early infantile epileptic encephalopathy with suppression-burst (EIEE, Ohtahara syndrome) and infantile spasms (West syndrome), both of which are discussed in detail elsewhere in this book (see Chapters 13 and 14). The emphasis of this chapter is on other encephalopathic epilepsies, specifically childhood epileptic encephalopathy with diffuse slow spike waves (Lennox-Gastaut syndrome, or LGS), acquired epileptic aphasia (Landau-Kleffner syndrome, or LKS), and electrical status epilepticus during sleep (ESES), which is also called continuous spike and wave during sleep (CSWS).

LENNOX-GASTAUT SYNDROME

History

The clinical manifestations of the Lennox-Gaustat syndrome have been recognized for more than two centuries. In 1772 Tissot described a mentally retarded boy who had multiple daily brief motor seizures with drop attacks (2). Over 100 years later, Jackson in 1886 reported a young child who had been having stiffening spells (with subsequent falling and facial injury) occurring 20 to 50 times a day since the age of two years (2). In the early twentieth century, Hunt reported more than 10 patients suffering abrupt loss of postural tone resulting in falls with subsequent significant facial and knee injuries (2).

With the advent of the EEG, neurologists began to look at clinical-electrographic correlates (both ictal and interictal) in patients with epilepsy. In 1935 the 3-Hz spike and wave discharge associated with "petit mal" seizures was first described by Gibbs, Davis, and Lennox (3). Subsequently, in 1939, Gibbs, Gibbs, and Lennox identified similar yet slower patterns (approximately 2 per second) and proposed to call it a "petit mal variant" to distinguish it from the classic 3-Hz spike and wave (4).

In 1945 William Lennox assembled the clinical manifestations and the EEG manifestations into the first semblance of the electroclinical syndrome (5) that we now call childhood epileptic encephalopathy with diffuse slow spike waves or the Lennox-Gastaut syndrome. Lennox's triad consisted of the slow spike and wave interictal EEG pattern, mental retardation, and three types of seizures considered characteristic: myoclonic jerks, atypical absence, and "drop attacks" (also known as akinetic seizures or astatic seizures) (2,5–7).

This constellation of symptoms initially was not given a formal syndrome name. Renewed interest in this syndrome began in 1964, when Sorel and Doose each described about 20 cases (8,9). Three meetings held in Marseille (the 13th, 14th, and 16th Symposia of Marseille in 1964, 1966, and 1968, respectively) examined the syndrome in depth (2). After the first meeting ended with very "divergent" views on the subject, multiple investigators sought to better define the electroclinical manifestations of this syndrome (2). Dravet, in her doctoral thesis in 1965 and two subsequent papers in 1966, reported the results of these intensive studies (10–12). The 1966 Marseille meeting culminated in the proposal to name the syndrome the "Lennox-Gastaut" syndrome, acknowledging the significant contributions of both the U.S. and French groups to the understanding of the syndrome (2). The 1968 meeting in Marseille reinforced the existence of this syndrome in every country of the participants and solidified its position in the pantheon of epileptic syndromes (2).

The importance of recognizing patients with the LGS increased in the early 1990s, when this population was identified as a target group to participate in trials of investigational antiepileptic drugs (AEDs). The factors contributing to the targeting of this group for study with investigational AEDs include their high daily seizure frequency, the lack of very effective therapy, and the desire to examine safety and efficacy issues for investigational AEDs in pediatric populations before general release.

Diagnostic Criteria

The definition of LGS by the International League Against Epilepsy (ILAE) classification is: "LGS manifests itself in children aged 1–8 years, but appears mainly in preschool-age children. The most common seizure types are tonic-axial, atonic, and absence seizures, but other types such as myoclonic, generalized tonic-clonic seizures (GTCS), or partial seizures are frequently associated with this syndrome. Seizure frequency is high, and status epilepticus is frequent (stuporous states with myoclonias, tonic and atonic seizures). The EEG usually has abnormal background activity, slow spike-waves <3 Hz and, often, multifocal abnormalities, During sleep, bursts of fast rhythms (10 Hz) appear. In general, there is mental retardation. Seizures are difficult to control, and the development is unfavorable. In 60 percent of cases, the syndrome occurs in children suffering from a previous encephalopathy, but is primary in other cases" (13). A triad of basic elements needed to make a diagnosis of LGS is usually stated based on this definition coupled with clinical experience and research:

- multiple types of seizures including tonic seizures, atypical absences, and atonic seizures;
- an EEG pattern consisting of interictal diffuse slow spike-wave discharges occurring at a 1.5 to 2 Hz frequency; and
- diffuse cognitive dysfunction and/or mental retardation (2,13–18).

There remains abundant discussion among epileptologists about the minimal necessary and sufficient criteria to diagnose a patient with LGS. Some investigators do not consider cognitive dysfunction

and/or mental retardation indispensable for diagnosis, especially at onset if the seizures and EEG pattern are typical (15,19–21). Other authors use a stricter EEG criteria requiring that the diagnostic EEG pattern include bursts of generalized fast spikes (10 Hz) during non–rapid eye movement sleep (NREMS) (22).

Ohtahara proposed a more comprehensive set of diagnostic criteria consisting of indispensable, supportive, and suggestive criteria (19). The indispensable criteria are the combination of tonic seizures, atypical absences, atonic seizures, myoclonic seizures, and astatic seizures with an interictal EEG pattern of diffuse slow spike-wave. Mental retardation, bursts of generalized fast spikes (10 Hz) during NREMS, onset in early childhood, and treatment-resistant seizures are among the supportive features (19).

Differential Diagnosis

Because of the nonspecific nature of multiple seizure types and cognitive dysfunction, multiple other pediatric epilepsy syndromes may be confused with the LGS. A useful approach to understanding and differentiating these syndromes is to first consider LGS and similar epilepsy syndromes as part of a continuum and then try to identify characteristics that separate the syndromes. Two scenarios have been proposed. In both scenarios, one end of the spectrum is fixed at LGS. In one scenario, the other end of the continuum is placed in the broad term *myoclonic epilepsies* (16), while another scenario places the end at myoclonic astatic epilepsy (23). In both scenarios, the epilepsy syndromes encountered moving from one end of the spectrum to the other are in the same order: LGS, the "myoclonic variant" of LGS, myoclonic astatic epilepsy, and then the lumped "myoclonic epilepsies" (e.g., benign myoclonic epilepsy of infancy, severe myoclonic epilepsy of infancy, and progressive myoclonic epilepsy) (17).

Compared with classic LGS, the "myoclonic variant" of LGS has less frequent and less severe mental retardation, rarer tonic seizures but an "unusually marked myoclonic component," and frequently faster (>2.5 Hz) spike wave complexes on EEG (16,24).

Myoclonic astatic epilepsy (Doose syndrome) and LGS have in common myoclonic seizures, atonic seizures, and atypical absences. However, there are major differences: myoclonic astatic epilepsy is predominately idiopathic, is genetically determined, usually has a favorable outcome, and does not follow West syndrome, whereas LGS is mainly symptomatic, is not genetically determined, usually has an unfavorable outcome, and can follow West syndrome (18,23). Kaminska and coworkers differentiate LGS and myoclonic astatic epilepsy using a sophisticated statistical approach called multiple correspondence analysis to study different clinical and EEG parameters. They recognized a group of children with LGS characterized by later onset of epilepsy, atypical absences, tonic and partial seizures, no myoclonus or vibratory tonic seizures, mental retardation, and an EEG pattern with slow spike-wave that were, as a group, different than the group with myoclonic astatic epilepsy features (23).

Compared with patients with LGS, patients with myoclonic epilepsies (in the broadest sense) have myoclonic seizures as the clearly predominant seizure type, only occasionally have tonic seizures, only occasionally have slow spike-wave on EEG, almost always have fast (>2.5 Hz) spike wave complexes on EEG, and have variable frequency and levels of mental retardation (16,17).

Classification

Lennox-Gastaut syndrome can be classified according to its suspected etiology as either idiopathic or symptomatic. Patients may be considered to have idiopathic LGS if there is normal psychomotor development before the onset of symptoms, if there are no underlying disorders or definite presumptive causes, and if there are no neurologic or neuroradiologic abnormalities (19). In contrast, patients have symptomatic LGS if there is an identifiable cause for the syndrome.

Population-based studies found that 22 percent to 30 percent of patients have idiopathic LGS, while 70 percent to 78 percent have symptomatic LGS (19,20,25,26). Examples of underlying pathologies responsible for symptomatic LGS include encephalitis/meningitis, tuberous sclerosis, brain malformations (e.g., cortical dysplasias), birth injury, hypoxic-ischemic injury, frontal lobe lesions, and trauma (18,19,24). Infantile spasms precede the development of LGS in 9 percent to 39 percent of cases (14,21,24).

Some investigators add cryptogenic as a different etiological category, in which there is no identified cause when a cause is suspected and the epilepsy is presumed to be symptomatic. In an epidemiological study in Atlanta, 44 percent of all LGS patients were classified in the cryptogenic group (21).

Reports of a family history of epilepsy and febrile seizures for patients with LGS range from 2.5 percent to 47.8 percent (noted in a series of 23 patients with cryptogenic LGS) (26,27).

Pathophysiology

The pathophysiology of LGS is not known (14), and there are no animal models (18). A variety of possible pathophysiologies have been proposed including developmental, immunologic, or metabolic. One hypothesis is that there is excessive permeability in the excitatory interhemispheric pathways in the frontal areas at the time the anterior parts of the brain mature. This maturation commonly occurs around the age of onset of LGS and would allow for synchronization of both frontal lobes (18).

Immunogenetic mechanisms are hypothesized to play a role in triggering or maintaining some cases of LGS. A strong association between LGS and the HLA class I antigen B7 (28) was found in one study, but another group found no statistical difference in the presence of HLA class I antigens including the antigen B7 (29). This latter study found an increased frequency of HLA class II antigen DR5 and a decrease DR4 antigen (29). No clear-cut or homogeneous metabolic pattern was noted in two positron emission tomography (PET) studies done in 10 and 15 children with LGS (30,31).

Epidemiology

Overall, LGS accounts for 1 percent to 4 percent of all cases of childhood epilepsy but 10 percent of cases that start in the first 5 years of life (20,21,32–37). Epidemiological studies in the Western or industrialized world (Israel, Spain, Estonia, Italy, and the United States) demonstrated that the proportion of LGS seems relatively consistent across various populations (21,33–36). The annual incidence of LGS in childhood is 2 per 100,000 children (38,39). The prevalence of LGS ranges from 0.1 to 0.28 per 1,000 in Europe and the United States (21,39–41).

The prevalence and percentage of LGS in mentally retarded children was reported as 0.06 per 1,000 and 7 percent, respectively (37). The proportion of LGS in institutionalized patients with mental retardation is as high as 16.3 percent (42).

Males are affected more often than females. Most studies do not report this gender difference to be statistically significant, but in an epidemiological study in Atlanta, Georgia, the difference between males and females was significant ($p = 0.005$) (21,26,27,38). The relative risk of occurrence of LGS is significantly higher in boys (prevalence rate 0.1 per 100 for boys, 0.02 per 1,000 for girls; rate ratios 5.31; 95% confidence intervals, 1.16–49.35) (40). There are no racial differences in the occurrence of LGS (21).

The mean age at epilepsy onset is 26 to 28 months (range 1 day–14 years) (20,27). The peak age at epilepsy onset is older in the symptomatic LGS group, but the difference in age of onset between the group with a history of West syndrome compared with the group without such a history was not significant. The average age at diagnosis of LGS in Japan was 6 years (range 2–15 years) (20). Compared with other patients with less severe epilepsies, patients with LGS have a younger age of onset of epilepsy (38).

Electroclinical Features

Interictal Manifestations

Before onset, 20 percent to 30 percent of children with LGS are free from neurologic and neuropsychological deficits. These problems inevitably appear during the evolution of LGS. Factors associated with mental retardation are symptomatic LGS, a previous history of West syndrome, onset of symptoms before 12 to 24 months of age, and higher seizure frequency (18,25,26,43).

The average IQ in a series of 72 patients with LGS followed up for more than 10 years was significantly lower in the symptomatic group compared with the cryptogenic group (20). At the time of the first examination, the IQ showed a variable degree of mental retardation in 66 percent of the cryptogenic group and in 76 percent of the symptomatic group. At the last examination, mental retardation was found in 95 percent of the cryptogenic group and in 100 percent of the symptomatic group (20). A significant correlation exists between age of onset of seizures and mental deterioration. In one study almost 98 percent of the patients who had the onset of seizures before age 2 years and 63 percent of those with onset after the age of 2 years had definite cognitive impairment (43).

Psychiatric symptoms in young children consist of mood instability and personality disturbances, while slowing or arrest of psychomotor development and educational progress characterize the neuropsychological symptoms. Character problems predominate in older children, and acute psychotic episodes or chronic forms of psychosis with aggressiveness, irritability, or social isolation may occur (26). Prolonged reaction time and information processing are the most impaired of the cognitive functions (18). Kaminska found that the main characteristics of mental deterioration were apathy, memory disorders, impaired visuomotor speed, and perseverance (23).

The interictal EEG is characterized by a slow background that can be constant or transient. Permanent slowing of the background is associated with poor cognitive prognosis (26). The hallmark of the awake interictal EEG is the diffuse slow spike-wave. This pattern consist of bursts of irregular, generalized spikes or sharp waves followed by a sinusoidal 35 to 400 milliseconds slow wave (18) with an amplitude that ranges from 200 to 800 µV (43), which can be symmetrical or asymmetrical. The amplitude is very often higher in the anterior region and in the frontal or frontocentral areas, but in some cases the activity may dominate in the posterior regions of the head (43). The frequency of the slow spike-wave activity is commonly found between 1.5 and 2.5 Hz (43) (Figure 15-1).

Slow spike-waves are usually not activated by photic stimulation. In one series of 83 patients with LGS,

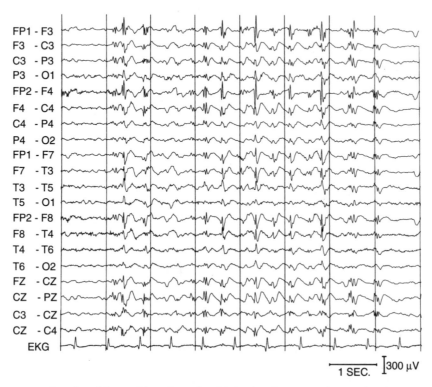

Figure 15-1. Slow spike-wave pattern in a 24-year-old awake male with Lennox-Gastaut syndrome. The slow posterior background rhythm has frequent periods of 2–2.5 Hz discharges maximal in the bifrontocentral areas occurring in trains up to 8 seconds without any clinical accompaniment.

activation of slow spike-waves with photic stimulation occurred in two patients (3 tracings), and decrease in slow spike-wave activity was noted in 9 percent of the tracings (43). Hyperventilation rarely induces slow spike-waves (18), although in many patients mental retardation prevents an adequate cooperation (43). During NREMS, discharges are more generalized, occur more frequently, and consist of polyspikes and slow waves. In rapid eye movement sleep (REMS) there is a decrease in spike waves (18). There is a reduction in the total duration of REMS during periods of frequent seizures (18).

Ictal Manifestations

Several types of seizures occur in LGS including tonic, atonic, myoclonic, and atypical absences, often associated with other less common types.

Tonic Seizures

Tonic seizures are said to be the most characteristic type of seizure and occur in 17 percent to 95 percent of children with LGS (16,24). Tonic seizures are more frequent during NREMS; therefore, researchers who have systematically obtained sleep tracings reported higher prevalences. These seizures can occur during wakefulness or sleep, but if they occur only during sleep they may go unnoticed (26).

Tonic seizures may be (1) axial tonic, involving the head and the trunk with head and neck flexion, contraction of masticatory muscles, and eventual vocalizations; (2) axorhizomelic tonic, in which there is tonic involvement of the proximal upper limbs with elevation of the shoulders and abduction of the arm; or (3) global tonic with contraction of the distal part of the extremities, sometimes leading to a sudden fall and other times mimicking infantile spasms (18,22,26).

Tonic seizures can be asymmetric, and some patients may show gestural automatisms after the tonic phase. Duration is from a few seconds to a minute, and, if prolonged, they can end in a vibratory component. In some seizures, the activity may be limited to upward deviation of the eyes (sursum vergens) and a slowing of respiration (18,26), and these may be mistaken for physiologic phenomena.

The EEG is characterized by a diffuse, rapid (10–13 Hz), low-amplitude activity, mainly in the anterior and vertex areas ("recruiting rhythm") that progressively decreases in frequency and increases in amplitude (Figure 15-2). When the seizure is limited to brief upward deviation of the eyes, the EEG activity may be accentuated in the posterior regions (22). A brief

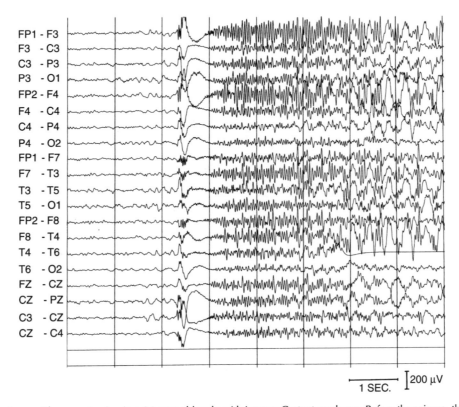

Figure 15-2. Tonic seizure with arm extension in a 24-year old male with Lennox-Gastaut syndrome. Before the seizure, the patient is watching television and then has a sudden body jerk, leans forward with arms extended and fixed at shoulder level. The EEG shows a diffuse burst of high-voltage polyspike and slow wave activity followed by 1 second of relative attenuation and then paroxysmal fast activity maximal in the bifrontocentral regions of the head.

generalized discharge of slow spike-waves or flattening of the recording may precede this pattern. Diffuse slow waves and slow spike-waves may follow it. These fast discharges are common during NREMS. Unlike tonic-clonic seizures, no postictal flattening occurs. Clinical manifestations appear 0.5 to 1 seconds after the onset of EEG manifestations and last several seconds longer than the discharge (18,26). Yaqub also reported synchronous 3-Hz spike-waves associated with tonic seizures (22).

Atypical Absences
The reported frequency ranges from 17 percent to 100 percent (16,22). In most studies, the frequency of the different types of seizures reported is based on parental counting of seizures, reviews from charts, or not specifically stated. Unfortunately, parental ability to recognize and identify atypical absences correctly is poor. In one study using video-EEG monitoring in a cohort of children with LGS, parental recognition was 27 percent for atypical absences, while the sensitivity was as high as 80 percent for myoclonic seizures and 100 percent for tonic, atonic, tonic-clonic, clonic, and complex partial seizures (44).

Atypical absences may be difficult to diagnose because the onset may be gradual (18,22,26) and there may be an incomplete loss of consciousness that allows the patient to continue activities to some degree. They may be associated with eyelid myoclonias, not as rhythmic as in typical absences, but often associated with perioral myoclonias or progressive flexion of the head secondary to a loss of tone (26). Automatisms may be observed (18). The seizure end may be gradual in some cases or abrupt in others (18,22,26).

The EEG is characterized by diffuse, slow (2–2.5 Hz) and irregular spike-waves, which may be difficult to differentiate from interictal bursts (18). Discharges of rapid rhythms sometimes may be seen preceded by flattening of the record for 1 to 2 seconds followed by a progressive development of irregular fast rhythm in the anterior and central regions, ending with brief spike-waves (22,26).

Atonic Seizures, Massive Myoclonic Seizures, and Myoclonic-Atonic Seizures
Atonic seizures, massive myoclonic seizures, and myoclonic-atonic seizures can be difficult to differentiate by clinical observation alone, and there are considerable discrepancies in how these terms are used. The reported frequency ranges from 10 percent to 56 percent (16,18,20,21,25,27). They produce sudden fall, producing injuries ("drop attacks," "Sturzanfälle"), sometimes limited to the head, resulting in the head falling on the chest ("head drop," "head nod," "nictatio capitis") (2,26,45). Ikeno found that pure atonic seizures are exceptional

and that most so-called atonic seizures had a tonic or myoclonic component (45). The EEG is characterized by slow spike-waves, polyspike-waves, or rapid diffuse rhythms (26). Simultaneous video-EEG recording and polygraphy is necessary for precise diagnosis. However, in 95 percent of affected patients, all three types of seizures occur in the same patient (26).

Other Types of Seizures
Generalized tonic-clonic seizures are reported in 15 percent of patients with LGS, while complex partial seizures occur in 5 percent (18). Status epilepticus of different types (absence status epilepticus, tonic status epilepticus, nonconvulsive status epilepticus) can occur (16,18) and is characterized by a long duration and resistance to treatment. The EEG during absence status epilepticus reveals continuous spike-wave discharges, usually at a lower frequency than at baseline, and rapid rhythms during tonic status epilepticus (26).

Donat and Wright reported in patients with LGS, infantile spasms–like seizures with clinical characteristics and ictal EEG changes similar to those typically seen in West syndrome. These seizures consisted of brief myoclonic jerks and brief stiffening or flexion of the upper body at the waist. The interictal EEG showed generalized slow spike-wave discharges (1–2.5 Hz) with occasional multifocal spike-waves. The ictal changes consisted of generalized decrement in cerebral activity, identical to the pattern that can be observed with infantile spasms (46).

Prognosis

The long-term prognosis is variable, but overall it is unfavorable. Four studies (presented here chronologically by publication date) have followed cohorts of children with LGS over time and illustrate this unevenness:

1. Beaumanoir found that 47 percent of the patients with LGS still had typical characteristics after 10 years of follow-up (41).
2. Roger followed 338 patients with LGS until adulthood. In 46.9 percent of patients, the clinical characteristics and EEG findings persisted into adulthood. In 15.5 percent of patients, mainly symptomatic cases, the syndrome disappeared but a severe, multifocal epilepsy persisted. About 17 percent of patients in which LGS followed another type of epilepsy seemed to have been cured (47).
3. Ohtahara reported persistent seizures in 76.4 percent of patients and mental retardation present in 91 percent of patients with LGS in a long-term follow-up study (48).

4. Yagi examined a cohort of 102 patients with LGS followed up for an average of 16 years; 11.8 percent of them worked normally, 35.3 percent worked part-time or at a sheltered workshop, and the remaining 52.9 percent were under home care or institutionalized (49). The characteristic clinical symptoms and EEG pattern remained in one-third of the patients at the end of the study. In the remaining patients, seizures decreased in type and frequency with treatment (49).

A worse prognosis is associated with symptomatic LGS, particularly those with a prior history of West syndrome (25), early onset of seizures (25), higher frequency of seizures (18), or constant slow EEG background activity (26). In one report, tonic seizures became more difficult to control over time and persisted (97.8% of the patients), while myoclonic and atypical absences appeared easier to control, persisting in 22.5 percent and 39.3 percent of the patients, respectively (50). The characteristic diffuse slow spike-wave pattern of LGS gradually disappears with age and is replaced by focal epileptic discharges, especially multiple independent spikes. This may reflect that subcortical epileptic discharges are suppressed and focal cortical discharges gain preponderance with brain maturation (25).

Mortality has been reported to range from 3 percent (mean follow-up of 8.5 years) to 7 percent (mean follow-up of 9.7 years) (26).

Treatment

Overview

The goals of treatment for patients with LGS are the same as for all epilepsy patients: the best quality of life with the fewest seizures (hopefully none), the fewest treatment side effects, and the least number of medications.

The various treatment options for patients with LGS can be divided into three major groups (Table 15-1):

- First-line treatments based on clinical experience or conventional wisdom;
- Suspected effective treatments based on open-label uncontrolled studies; and
- Effective treatments based on double-blind placebo-controlled studies.

In the first and second groups, the efficacy and safety of individual treatment options have not been formally tested. Only options in the third group have been rigorously and scientifically evaluated and found to be effective and safe for specific seizure types in LGS patients. Each treatment group can be subdivided

Table 15-1. Treatments for Children with Lennox-Gastaut Syndrome

First-line treatments based on clinical experience or conventional wisdom
Valproic acid
Benzodiazepines
Pyridoxine
Suspected effective treatments based on open-label uncontrolled studies
Adrenocorticotropic hormone–corticosteroids
Intravenous immunoglobulin
Vigabatrin
Zonisamide
Ketogenic diet
Corpus callosotomy
Vagus nerve stimulation
Effective treatments based on double-blind, placebo-controlled studies
Felbamate
Lamotrigine
Topiramate

into medical, dietary, and surgical therapies. Unfortunately, no treatment by itself in any of the three groups gives satisfactory relief for all or even a majority of patients with LGS. Combination of treatment modalities is frequently needed (51).

First-Line Treatments Based on Clinical Experience or Conventional Wisdom

Medications
Over the past two decades, valproic acid has been considered as a first-line treatment option for children with LGS (24,52,53). From a practical viewpoint, by the time a clinician makes a diagnosis of LGS, the patient has already been diagnosed with epilepsy and treatment has been initiated. Because these children have multiple types of generalized seizures and at times coexisting partial seizures, clinicians may initially select a broad-spectrum AED such as valproic acid. Valproic acid has been reported to be more effective in cryptogenic LGS than in symptomatic LGS (54).

Benzodiazepines, specifically clonazepam, nitrazepam, and clobazam, are also first-line AED therapy options (24,53,55). All are considered effective against seizures associated with LGS, but side effects and the development of tolerance limit their usefulness over time (24). Side effects of clonazepam include hyperactivity, sedation, drooling, and incoordination, which can significantly affect the quality of life for patients with LGS (24). The efficacy and tolerability profile of nitrazepam is similar to that of clonazepam (24). Clobazam is considered the least sedating benzodiazepine with the longest time to the development of tolerance (55). Some recommendations to slow the development of tolerance include dosing on an every-other-day schedule or alternate two different benzodiazepines on an alternate-day basis (56,57). Unfortunately, not all benzodiazepines are beneficial: intravenous diazepam and lorazepam have been reported to induce tonic status epilepticus in some patients (58,59). Based on clinical experience, some authors believe a combination of valproic acid and a benzodiazepine may be better than either drug alone, but no data exist to confirm this impression (24).

Although carbamazepine, phenobarbital, phenytoin, and ethosuximide may be first-line therapy for a variety of seizure types or other epilepsy syndromes, none is considered first-line therapy for LGS. Carbamazepine may exacerbate atypical absence seizures despite reducing generalized tonic-clonic seizures (60,61). Phenobarbital may be effective against a variety of seizures but can exacerbate hyperactivity and aggressiveness or produce sedation and drowsiness (which may exacerbate tonic seizures) (24,54). Phenytoin can be effective for tonic seizures and tonic status epilepticus but not for atypical absence seizures (62). In contrast, ethosuximide may be useful in atypical absence seizures but is ineffective in other seizure types (51).

Because patients with pyridoxine (vitamin B6) dependency may have seizures and a slow spike and wave pattern on EEG, some clinician investigators have suggested trials of vitamin B6 in all children with treatment-resistant epilepsy who are younger than 5 years old (53). One study examined the efficacy of high-dose vitamin B6 in five patients with LGS and found mixed results; three of the five patients with LGS had no response, whereas the others had a more noticeable response (63). Given the lack of serious side effects and the ease of performing a therapeutic vitamin B6 trial, it is reasonable and appropriate to conduct a vitamin B6 trial early in treatment of a child with LGS (64). Doses and duration of vitamin B6 therapy vary widely. In the aforementioned clinical trial, vitamin B6 was given for the first five days 50 to 100 mg/day intramuscularly and then after 5 days 200 to 300 mg/day orally (63). Some clinicians (mainly in Japan) administer high doses of pyridoxal phosphate (30–40 mg/kg/day) (53). Wheless prescribes 100 mg of vitamin B6 three times daily for 2 weeks, discontinuing vitamin B6 if there is no response to therapy after 2 weeks (53).

Dietary Treatment
At this time the ketogenic diet is not a first-line therapy for the seizures associated with LGS.

Surgical Treatment
At this time neither corpus callosotomy nor the vagus nerve stimulator are first-line therapies for the seizures associated with LGS.

Suspected Effective Treatments Based on Open-Label Uncontrolled Studies

Medications
Medications suspected to have some effectiveness against seizures associated with LGS based on open-label uncontrolled trials include (in alphabetical order): adrenocorticotropic hormone (ACTH) (65,66), corticosteroids (26,53,67), intravenous immunoglobulin (IVIG) (68,69), vigabatrin (70), and zonisamide (ZNS) (71).

Both ACTH and corticosteroid therapy are proposed to be effective against the seizures associated with LGS. Roger proposes that prolonged corticosteroid therapy initiated at the onset of cryptogenic LGS can yield "excellent" results (26). Despite this effectiveness, there are multiple potentially significant side effects associated with therapy, and relapse frequently occurs when the drugs are withdrawn (24,53,64–67).

The efficacy of adjunctive high-dose IVIG in patients with LGS has been investigated in at least seven open-label trials (68,69,72–74). The results of these trials were very encouraging because 30 percent to 92 percent of LGS patients receiving IVIG experienced at least 50% seizure reduction during treatment (68). Dosing schedules varied between studies. Later well-controlled trials (detailed below) did not confirm the effectiveness of IVIG against seizures associated with LGS (75,76).

Six studies involving 78 patients treated with vigabatrin showed that 15 percent of these patients became completely seizure-free and 44 percent of the patients had at least 50 percent reduction in their seizure frequency (70,77–81). The best results were noted in an open-label, dose-ranging, adjunctive therapy study of vigabatrin in 20 children with LGS who had failed first-line monotherapy with valproic acid. Seventeen children (85%) experienced at least 50% reduction in their seizure frequency, and eight children (40%) were seizure-free at doses ranging from 1 to 3 grams/day at study end (70). The authors concluded that vigabatrin–valproic acid duotherapy was effective and well tolerated in children with LGS (70).

The most common adverse effects of vigabatrin are generally CNS-related and include hyperactivity, agitation, weight gain, drowsiness, insomnia, facial edema, ataxia, stupor, and somnolence (79,82–84). However, vigabatrin may exacerbate myoclonic seizures and even absence seizures in some patients, and visual field constriction has been identified in children (78,79,82,85,86). Both of these side effects significantly limit consideration of vigabatrin as long-term therapy for patients with LGS (83).

The effectiveness of ZNS in LGS has been investigated in three small studies. Although Sakamoto reported that ZNS was "effective" in 39 percent of patients with LGS, the definition of effectiveness was not clear (71). In 1991 Yamatogi reported 50 percent

(10 of 20) of Lennox-Gastaut patients treated with ZNS had at least 50% reduction in seizure frequency (87). In a recent report by Iinuma, 26 percent (10 of 39) of patients with LGS treated with ZNS responded with a 50 percent or greater reduction in seizure frequency. (Data on file, Dianippon Pharmaceutical, Japan).

There have been no formal published open-label studies investigating the effectiveness and safety of gabapentin, tiagabine, levetiracetam, or oxcarbazepine in the treatment of seizures associated with LGS. Single reports have suggested that L-tryptophan (transient improvement), amantadine, and DN-1417, a thyrotropin-releasing hormone analogue may reduce seizure frequency in patients with LGS (88–90).

Dietary Treatment

A number of studies have shown the ketogenic diet to be useful for patients with LGS (64,65,91,92). Response to the diet usually is evident within 1 month of starting the diet (53). In a recent study, the atonic or myoclonic seizures in 17 consecutively treated patients with LGS at The Johns Hopkins Hospital decreased "by more than 50% immediately" (93). The benefits of the diet can include fewer seizures along with less drowsiness, better behavior, and fewer concomitant AEDs (53).

Surgical Treatment

Surgical procedures that have been reported to be beneficial for patients with LGS include corpus callosotomy, vagus nerve stimulation (VNS), and, rarely, focal resection (53). Corpus callosotomy is effective in reducing drop attacks but typically does not appear to be helpful for other seizure types (24,94–96). A recent study from Taiwan reported that anterior corpus callosotomy was effective for "all kinds of medically intractable seizures, especially generalized" in a cohort of 74 patients (80% had LGS) (97). In general, callosotomy is considered palliative rather than curative, and seizure freedom is rare although it can occur (54,97).

In six studies (three published reports and three abstracts), VNS appears effective for patients with LGS (98–103). The three published studies reported a total of 13 of 18 (72%) patients with LGS experienced at least 50% reduction in seizure frequency with follow-up as long as 5 years (98–100). In the largest cohort of LGS patients treated with VNS ($n = 46$), Frost reported in abstract form that the mean reduction in seizure frequency at 1 month ($n = 46$), 3 months ($n = 29$), and 6 months ($n = 15$) was 38 percent, 41 percent, and 71 percent, respectively (101). Two other studies (reported in abstract form) have concluded that VNS is effective as adjunctive therapy for patients with LGS (102,103).

In rare cases, resection of a localized lesion (e.g., vascular lesion or tumor) can improve seizure control in patients with LGS (24,104).

Effective Treatments Based on Double-Blind Placebo-Controlled Studies

Medications

The gold standard for evaluation of the safety and efficacy of an anticonvulsant medication is the randomized, double-blind, placebo-controlled clinical trial. Five drugs have undergone this rigorous testing to determine safety and efficacy in patients with LGS: cinromide, IVIG, felbamate, lamotrigine, and topiramate. The latter three AEDs successfully demonstrated efficacy against seizures in patients with LGS, whereas the former two did not. Despite the lack of proven efficacy for cinromide and immunoglobulins in double-blind studies, both therapies had open-label trials suggesting efficacy in patients with LGS, reinforcing the need for randomized double-blind controlled trials to definitively establish the efficacy of any proposed therapy.

Cinromide. In 1980 cinromide was reported to be effective for seizures associated with LGS in an open-label uncontrolled trial (105). These results prompted a subsequent double-blind, placebo-controlled adjunctive therapy trial of cinromide in patients with LGS (106). Overall, 73 patients enrolled, but "sufficient data for analysis" were available only for 56 patients (26 receiving cinromide, 30 receiving placebo). There was no difference between cinromide adjunctive therapy and placebo adjunctive therapy in terms of seizure reduction or global evaluations (106). The development of cinromide was halted in 1981 (106).

Immunoglobulins. Two blinded placebo-controlled studies have been published examining the efficacy of IVIG in children with LGS (75,76). The first study enrolled 10 children, aged 4 to 14 years, in an add-on, placebo-controlled, single-blind study design. Only 2 children showed a response to IVIG (42% and 100% decrease in seizure frequency), while the remaining 8 children were "unaffected" (75). Sixty-one patients with various forms of refractory epilepsy (including LGS and West syndrome) participated in a randomized, double-blind, placebo-controlled, dose-ranging (three different doses) trial of IVIG. Despite 52.5 percent of the IVIG group having a greater than 50% reduction in seizure frequency compared with the 27.8 percent in the placebo group, this difference did not reach statistical significance (76).

Felbamate. Felbamate (FBM) was found to be safe and effective in patients with LGS in a randomized, double-blind, placebo-controlled adjunctive therapy trial (107). Seventy-three patients with LGS aged 4 to 36 years enrolled. The FBM dose in the double-blind portion was 45 mg/kg/day (maximum 3600 mg/day). The

FBM treatment group experienced a 34 percent reduction in atonic seizures compared with 9 percent in the placebo group ($p = 0.01$). Total seizure frequency dropped 19 percent in the FBM group compared with a 4 percent increase in the placebo group ($p = 0.002$). The percentage of patients experiencing at least 50 percent reduction in atonic seizures was 57 percent for the FBM group compared with 9 percent in the placebo group ($p < 0.001$). The percentage of patients experiencing at least 50% reduction in total seizure frequency was 50 percent for the FBM group compared with 11 percent in the placebo group ($p < 0.001$) (Table 15-2). FBM was significantly better than placebo in improving global evaluation scores. The types and frequency of side effects were similar in the two treatment groups (107). A 12-month follow-up in patients who completed the controlled part of the study confirmed long-term efficacy (108).

Unfortunately, FBM is associated with dangerous idiosyncratic reactions involving the blood and liver. The most common severe FBM-associated idiosyncratic reaction is aplastic anemia, which has been seen to date in 34 patients receiving FBM (109). The incidence of FBM-associated aplastic anemia is approximately 127 cases per million treated with FBM (approximately 1 in 4,000 to 8,000 FBM-treated patients) versus 2 to 2.5 per million people in the general population (83,109,110). Another report estimates the risk of aplastic anemia in patients receiving FBM to be 1:3,000, with a death rate of 1 in 10,000 FBM-treated patients (83,111). In perspective, this estimated risk is approximately 20 times greater than that for carbamazepine-associated aplastic anemia (109). Risk factors for FBM-associated aplastic anemia are Caucasian, adult, female, history of autoimmune disorder, history of prior AED toxicity or allergy, prior cytopenia, and treatment with FBM for less than 1 year (109,112).

The second most common severe FBM-associated idiosyncratic reaction is hepatotoxicity. Reported in 18 patients receiving FBM, its estimated incidence is between 64 and 164 per million (approximately 1 in 18,500–25,000 FBM-treated patients) (109). This suggests that the frequency of FBM-associated hepatotoxicity and VPA-associated hepatotoxicity are approximately the same (109). There is no evidence that laboratory monitoring of blood counts and liver function during FBM therapy anticipates these severe idiosyncratic reactions (109). A suggested management strategy is to employ careful clinical monitoring, perform routine laboratory testing, and discontinue the drug if no substantial clinical benefit is observed after 3 to 6 months of therapy.

Although effective, there are significant risks associated with felbamate use. In general, it is regarded as a good third-line or fourth-line drug for LGS.

Lamotrigine. The efficacy of lamotrigine (LTG) against seizures associated with LGS has been examined in multiple open-label studies and two controlled trials. In five open-label trials of LTG in patients with LGS, 58 percent (31 of 53) experienced at least 50 percent reduction in seizure frequency (113–117). A double-blind, placebo-controlled, crossover study of LTG as adjunctive therapy in 30 patients with treatment-resistant generalized epilepsy was reported in 1998. Twenty study patients had LGS. Seven of the 20 children with LGS responded to LTG therapy with a greater than 50 percent reduction in seizure frequency. Two patients became seizure-free (118).

Lamotrigine was found to be safe and effective in patients with LGS in a randomized, double-blind, placebo-controlled, adjunctive therapy trial (119). A total of 169 patients enrolled and were randomized to either LTG ($n = 79$) or placebo ($n = 90$) adjunctive therapy. Patients on the LTG treatment arm had a greater median percent reduction from baseline in weekly seizure counts (for drop attacks, tonic-clonic seizures, and all major seizures—defined as drop attacks plus tonic clonic) compared with patients on the placebo treatment arm. The responder rate (percentage of patients experiencing at least 50% reduction in seizures) for major seizures (drop attacks and tonic-clonic seizures) was greater in the LTG group (33%) than in the placebo group (16%, $p = 0.01$). For drop attacks, 37 percent of LTG-treated patients responded

Table 15-2. Responder Rates (at least 50% reduction in seizure frequency) for Three Antiepileptic Medications Tested in Double-Blind, Placebo-Controlled Trials in Lennox-Gastaut Syndrome

Seizure Type	Felbamate vs. Placebo	Lamotrigine vs. Placebo	Topiramate vs. Placebo
Total seizures	50% vs. 11%*		
All major seizures (drop attacks plus tonic-clonic)		33% vs.16%*	33% vs. 8%*
Drop attack or atonic seizures	57% vs. 9%*	37* vs. 22%*	28% vs. 14%
Tonic-clonic seizures	60% vs. 23%*	43% vs. 20%*	

*$p < 0.05$

compared with 22 percent of the placebo-treated patients ($p = 0.04$). Finally, for tonic-clonic seizures, 43 percent of the LTG-treated patients responded compared with 20 percent of patients receiving placebo ($p = 0.007$) (119) (Table 15-2).

Unfortunately, LTG can be associated with idiosyncratic reactions predominantly involving the skin. The most common skin manifestation is a rash affecting 10 percent to 12 percent of LTG patients (83,120,121). The rash rapidly resolves following LTG withdrawal; sometimes the rash may even resolve without changing LTG dosage (122). However, this dermatologic reaction can progress in some patients to erythema multiforme, Stevens-Johnson syndrome, or even toxic epidermal necrolysis (83,120,122). Stevens-Johnson syndrome and toxic epidermal necrolysis are related severe mucocutaneous disorders with mortality rates of 5 percent and 30 percent, respectively (120). The risk of a potentially life-threatening rash (based on clinical trials and postmarketing reports) in adults is 0.3 percent and approximately 1 percent in children 16 years old and younger (122).

Risk factors for LTG-associated severe dermatologic reactions include younger age (children more than adults), comedication with valproic acid, a rapid rate of LTG titration, and a high LTG starting dose (83,120,122). Careful attention should be given to initial LTG starting dose, titration rate, and comedications. The prompt evaluation of any rash is prudent.

Despite the risk of idiosyncratic reactions, LTG is a very valuable medication for patients with LGS and should be considered for use as soon as the diagnosis of LGS is made. Proper attention to concomitant medications, a low starting dose, and a very slow titration can minimize the risk of dermatologic idiosyncratic reactions.

Topiramate. Topiramate (TPM) was found to be safe and effective as adjunctive therapy for patients with LGS in a multicenter, double-blind, placebo-controlled trial (123). Ninety-eight patients with LGS (aged >1 year to <30 years) were randomized to either TPM adjunctive therapy (target dose 6 mg/kg/day) or placebo adjunctive therapy. The median percentage reduction from baseline in average monthly seizure rate for drop attacks was 14.8 percent for the TPM group and −5.1 percent (an increase) for the placebo group ($p = 0.041$). Using parental global evaluations, TPM-treated patients demonstrated greater improvement in seizure severity than did placebo-treated patients ($p = 0.037$). The responder rate for major seizures (drop attacks and tonic-clonic seizures) was greater in the topiramate group (15 of 46, or 33%) than in the control group (4 of 50, or 8%; $p = 0.002$). The responder rate for drop attacks in the TPM group was higher than in the placebo group (28%

versus 14%) but did not reach statistical significance (123) (Table 15-2).

In the long-term, open-label extension portion of the above trial, 97 patients were followed up and had their TPM dose adjusted as clinically indicated (124). The mean TPM dose in those patients who had completed 6 months of therapy was 10 mg/kg/day. For those patients who had completed 6 months of TPM therapy, drop attacks were reduced at least 50 percent in 55 percent of patients; 15 percent of patients were free of drop attacks for at least 6 months at the last visit. The median percent reduction in drop attacks was 56 percent. The median percent reduction in overall seizure frequency was 44 percent, with 45 percent of the patients having at least 50 percent reduction in all seizure types and 2 percent being seizure-free for the previous 6 months. Long-term TPM therapy was well tolerated. The most common adverse events were somnolence, injury, and anorexia. Behavioral problems during the last 6 months of TPM long-term therapy were reported in only 5 percent of the patients. During long-term therapy, TPM is effective and well tolerated in controlling drop attacks and seizures associated with LGS (124).

Comparison Among FBM, LTG, and TPM. Since the FBM, LTG, and TPM double-blind, placebo-controlled, adjunctive therapy trials for patients with LGS showed efficacy and safety, attention turns to the issue of which medication is ''better.'' Because no comparative trial of anticonvulsant medications has been performed in patients with LGS, the best method of resolving the issue is a meta-analysis of these three trials.

A clinically useful measure of treatment effect of a study medication is the ''number needed to treat'' (NNT) (125). This calculated number represents the number of patients a clinician must treat with a study medication to expect to find one with the desired outcome. In clinical trials of AEDs involving patients with treatment-resistant epilepsy, the desired outcome is usually at least 50 percent reduction in seizure frequency. A patient who achieves this reduction is called a ''responder.'' If the percentage of responders in the active treatment arm is called A and the percentage of responders in the placebo treatment arm is called P, the NNT is calculated by $1/(A-P)$. This represents the inverse of the absolute risk reduction (125). The 95 percent confidence interval (CI) can then be calculated. (G. Pledger, personal communication)

To date, only trials involving adults with treatment-resistant partial seizures have been considered in other meta-analysis studies of AEDs (126). It is possible to calculate the NNT using the FBM, LTG, and TPM double-blind, placebo-controlled, adjunctive therapy trials described previously. In each study, drop attacks (atonic/tonic seizures) were used as the seizure outcome variable because they are the most debilitating type of seizure. Felbamate's NNT was calculated as 2.1 (95% CI 1.4, 3.8), lamotrigine's 6.4 (95% CI 3.4, 54.8), and topiramate's 7.2 (95% CI 3.3, 1000). Because the confidence intervals overlap, these differences are not statistically significant.

Dietary Treatment

The efficacy of the ketogenic diet for patients with LGS is currently being examined in an ongoing double-blind controlled trial (J. Freeman, personal communication).

Surgical Treatment

There are no double-blind trials examining the efficacy of surgical intervention in patients with LGS completed or under way at this time.

Additional Considerations

The severity of the seizures, frequent injuries, developmental delays, and behavioral problems take a large toll on even the strongest parents and family structures. Attention needs to be paid to the psychosocial needs of the family (especially siblings). The proper educational setting is also important to help the patients with LGS reach their maximal potential. Because of the high rate of injuries associated with atonic/tonic seizures, some patients with LGS may need to wear a protective helmet. Helmets need to have a faceguard to maximize protection of the patient's forehead, nose, and teeth. Unfortunately, some patients will not tolerate a helmet with a faceguard, and even if tolerated helmets are often uncomfortable and rarely "cosmetically acceptable" (24).

ACQUIRED EPILEPTIC APHASIA (LANDAU-KLEFFNER SYNDROME)

History

Landau and Kleffner first described the syndrome of acquired epileptic aphasia (Landau-Kleffner syndrome, LKS) in six children in 1957 (127). These children exhibited "normal acquisition of speech" followed by aphasia, seizures, and EEG abnormalities (127). Approximately 200 cases have been reported since 1957 (128,129).

Diagnostic Criteria

The definition of LKS by the International League Against Epilepsy (ILAE) classification is: "The Landau-Kleffner syndrome is a childhood disorder in which an acquired aphasia, multifocal spike, and spike and wave discharges are associated. Epileptic seizures and behavioral and psychomotor disturbances occur in two-thirds of the patients. There is verbal auditory agnosia and rapid reduction in spontaneous speech. The seizures, usually GTCS or partial motor, are rare, and remit before the age of 15 years, as do the EEG abnormalities" (13).

Uniformly accepted diagnostic criteria are lacking. The most commonly accepted criteria for making this diagnosis are the occurrence of an acquired aphasia in a previously normal child and multifocal epileptiform discharges on EEG predominantly in the temporal-parietal-occipital areas and activated by sleep (128,130). Behavioral and psychomotor disorders may be seen in children with LKS. Clinical seizures may occur but are not a prerequisite for making the diagnosis (128).

Epidemiology

The prevalence and incidence of LKS is not known (128). Males are affected more than females (24).

Clinical Manifestations

Symptoms, especially aphasia, are usually recognized in patients between the ages of 3 and 9 years (70% before 6 years of age) (131–133). The majority of patients have normal language development before development of symptoms; a minority (13%) may have "preexisting difficulties in language acquisition" (128). The aphasia commonly begins as a verbal auditory agnosia with a reduction in spontaneous verbal expression (134). These symptoms may lead to the patient's being diagnosed as autistic or deaf (24,133). The language difficulties can evolve in a progressive or stepwise fashion (12% of cases) (128). Seven percent of patients experience relapse (128).

While the patient is awake, the EEG usually has normal background activity with bilateral, asymmetric, high-amplitude focal epileptiform discharges in either the temporal (>50% of cases) or parieto-occipital (33% of cases) regions (24,128,133). Although well-localized, the spikes vary in space and time (128). Hyperventilation and photic stimulation do not activate any additional abnormalities (128). The spikes do not necessarily occur in the dominant hemisphere and may not be temporally related to the aphasia. Although the interictal multifocal EEG abnormalities imply local bihemispheric dysfunction, it is not certain whether these foci precede or follow the pathophysiologic processes responsible for the aphasia (128).

Sleep, especially slow sleep, activates the EEG; the spikes appear with a bihemispheric, bisynchronous distribution; and "short bursts of diffuse slow spikes and wave may arise" (128,133). This has led investigators to make comparisons between LKS and LGS and ESES (128).

The actual frequency of seizures is not known; best estimates are that approximately 70 percent to 80 percent of patients with LKS experience one or more seizures (24,128). Seizures can range from nocturnal simple partial seizures to generalized tonic-clonic seizures or atypical absence seizures (24,131). Tonic seizures are not seen in patients with LKS (131). Seizure frequency is often low but can be very high in some patients (135). Only 20 percent of patients older than 10 years experience seizures, and a few patients have been reported with seizures after 15 years of age (24,128). Family history of epilepsy ranges from 5 percent (children with LKS without seizures) to 12 percent (children with LKS with seizures) (128).

Behavioral and psychomotor disturbances are reported to occur in approximately three-fourths of children with LKS (128,133). The most common symptoms are hyperkinesia and rage outbursts (128,133). Some patients may exhibit anxiety, avoid interpersonal contact, or have very bizarre behavior (24). There are few detailed characterizations of these behavioral and psychomotor abnormalities in LKS children.

Etiology

The etiology of LKS is not known (24). One proposed etiology was subacute bitemporal encephalitis, although no definitive data exist to support this hypothesis (132). Neuroimaging studies, including computed tomography (CT) and magnetic resonance imaging (MRI), show no evidence of structural lesions (136). Several PET studies suggests that temporal lobe structures are important in the pathophysiology of LKS (136,137). There is a single report that depicts LKS in a child with neurocysticercosis (138). Pascual-Castroviejo reported a series of four children with LKS and associated cerebral vasculitis (139).

Treatment

There are no reports of controlled clinical trials using standard AEDs for children with LKS. In general, conventional AEDs usually are ineffective (24). Corticosteroid therapy appears to be the most successful treatment in uncontrolled anecdotal reports but has potential for significant side effects (24,131,140). Aicardi recommends prolonged therapy (at least 3 months) with large doses (prednisolone 2–3 mg/kg/day) (24). Multiple subpial transection has been useful in selected cases. In a recent report, 11 of 14 children with LKS had "significant postoperative improvement on measures of receptive or expressive vocabulary" (141). The ketogenic diet was recently reported to be effective in three

children with LKS (142). Felbamate therapy resulted in a "dramatic, rapid, and prolonged improvement in seizure control, language skills and EEG" in one patient with LKS (135).

Outcome

Outcome is not affected by the frequency or type of seizures (128). As described previously, the prognosis for seizure control is good. In contrast, language recovery is variable (143,144). One report of long-term follow-up in nine patients (including the six patients initially used to describe the condition), 10 to 28 years after the onset of the aphasia, revealed that four patients had recovered fully, one had mild language dysfunction, and four had moderate language disability (143). For many patients "speech functions return before adulthood" but only 40 percent to 50 percent of patients with LKS lead a normal social and professional life (128). Indicators for a good prognosis are onset of symptoms after age 6 years and early speech therapy (128,130).

ELECTRICAL STATUS EPILEPTICUS DURING SLEEP (ESES)

History

Electrical status epilepticus during sleep, which is characterized by continuous spike-wave discharges during slow sleep, partial or generalized seizures, and neuropsychological disturbances, was first described in 1971 by Patry and collaborators as a "subclinical 'electrical status epilepticus' induced by sleep in children" (145). Some years later, Tassinari, one of the collaborators in the original description, called this entity "electrical status epilepticus during sleep (ESES)" (146). Some investigators use the term *continuous spike-wave discharges during sleep* (CSWS) (147), emphasizing the principal electrophysiologic criteria for its diagnosis.

Epidemiology

The epidemiology of ESES has not been well characterized. Its incidence is not known, but it is consider to be rare (148). One study found "a preponderance of males" (149). A family history of epilepsy is rare (128).

EEG Manifestations

During wakefulness, paroxysmal abnormalities can be found, varying between 1.9 percent and 24.4 percent of the total recording time (145). They are characterized by either isolated or bursts of generalized spike-wave discharges, with a frequency of 2 to 3 Hz, predominantly over the anterior regions of the head. Some investigators reported occasional focal epileptiform abnormalities in awake and drowsy states (147).

The characteristic pattern appears with the onset of sleep, with an increase of the spike-wave discharges persisting throughout the whole sleep and subsiding upon awakening. The frequency of spike-waves tends to be slower (1.5–2 Hz) than during wakefulness (145). Patry and collaborators placed special emphasis in that the "spike-wave index" should be more than 85 percent (145). In other words, the total duration of the spike-wave recording should be more than 85 percent of the total slow sleep tracing. During REM sleep, both the spike-wave index and the spike-wave frequency are similar to those observed during wakefulness. The paroxysmal pattern disappears upon awakening as suddenly as it appears at the onset of sleep (145). Patry considered that the continuous spike-waves during sleep had to be present in at least three recordings over a period of at least 1 month (145). Other researchers used two recordings over a period of at least 1 month as a diagnostic criterion (150), while others did not mention the number of recordings used (147).

These EEG abnormalities are long-lasting, persisting for years. In Tassinari's series of 29 patients, the average age of ESES diagnosis was 8 years, 1 month (range 3 years, 1 month–15 years, 1 month), and the average age of ESES disappearance was 11 years, 1 month (149).

Seizures

Seizures are partial or generalized, are commonly nocturnal, and may precede the recognition of the characteristic EEG pattern (148). Atypical absences can also be observed, and their appearance is usually preceded by that of partial onset seizures (147).

Based on the clinical semiology of the seizures, three groups have been described. One group of patients were having only motor seizures throughout their evolution. The seizures, usually nocturnal, tended to disappear in adolescence. The second group initially had unilateral partial motor seizures or generalized tonic-clonic seizures, mainly during sleep, and typical absences appearing at the onset of ESES. Their seizures remitted between the ages of 10 and 16 years. The third group had rare unilateral seizures or generalized tonic-clonic seizures that became associated with atypical absences at the time of ESES (149,151).

Tonic seizures have not been observed in ESES (148,149). In his series of 29 children, Tassinari found that the average age of seizure onset was 4 years, 7 months (range 8 months–12 years), with the average age of disappearance 12 years (range 4 years, 1 month–17 years, 8 months) (149).

Neuropsychological Development

Most patients have a normal neuropsychological development before the onset of ESES. Those children with abnormal development experience a worsening in their cognitive function during the stage of ESES.

Neuropsychological disturbances are characterized by decrease in IQ, reduction in language function, abnormal perception of space and body image, reduced attention span, hyperactivity, and aggressiveness (149,152). There is a global improvement in cognitive performance and behavior after ESES disappears (148,149), although in a significant number of patients there is a residual neuropsychological dysfunction.

Treatment

Several AEDs have been used with variable influence on seizures, including valproic acid, carbamazepine, phenytoin, ethosuximide, various benzodiazepines, and barbiturates (148,149). The treatment of the electrographic abnormality is less favorable. Clobazam, lorazepam, nitrazepam, and ACTH were tried with temporary suppression of the paroxysmal tracing (149). A recent report details successful use of TPM in two patients with ESES (153).

REFERENCES

1. Ohtahara S, Ohtsuka Y, Yamatogi Y, et al. Prenatal etiologies of West syndrome. *Epilepsia* 1993; 34:716–722.
2. Gastaut H. The Lennox-Gastaut syndrome: comments on the syndrome's terminology and nosological position amongst the secondary generalized epilepsies of childhood. *Electroencephalogr Clin Neurophysiol* 1982; 35 (Suppl):71–84.
3. Gibbs F, Davis H, Lennox W. Electroencephalogram in epilepsy and in conditions of impaired consciousness. *Arch Neurol Psychiat* 1935; 34:1133–1148.
4. Gibbs F, Gibbs E, Lennox W. Influence of blood sugar level on wave and spike formation in petit mal epilepsy. *Arch Neurol Psychiat* 1939; 41:1111–1114.
5. Lennox W. The petit mal epilepsies: their treatment with tridione. *JAMA* 1945; 129:1069–1074.
6. Lennox WG, Davis JP. Clinical correlates of the fast and the slow spike-wave electroencephalogram. *Pediatrics* 1950; 5:626–644.
7. Lennox W. *Epilepsy and Related Disorders*. Vol. 1. Boston: Little, Brown, 1960:156–169.
8. Doose H. Das akinetische petit mal. *Ach Psychiatr Nervenkr* 1964; 205:625–654.
9. Sorel L. L'epilepsie myokinetique grave de la premiere enfance avec pointe-onde lente (petit mal variant) et son traitement. *Rev Neurol* 1964; 110:215–233.
10. Dravet C. *Encephalopathie Epileptique de l''Enfant avec Pointe-onde Lente Diffuse*. These, Marseille, 1965.
11. Bernard R, Pinsard N, Draver C, et al. Aspets diagnostiquest et evolutifs d'ume encephalopathie epileptique de l'enfant avec pointe-ondes lents diffuses. *Pediatrie* 1966; 21:712–730.

12. Gastaut H, Roger J, Soulayrol R, et al. Childhood epileptic encephalopathy with diffuse slow spike-waves (otherwise known as "petit mal variant") or Lennox syndrome. *Epilepsia* 1966; 7:139–179.

13. Commission on Classification and Terminology of the International League Against Epilepsy. Proposal for revised classification of epilepsies and epileptic syndromes. *Epilepsia* 1989; 30:389–399.

14. Beaumanoir A, Dravet C. The Lennox-Gastaut syndrome. In: Roger J, Bureau M, Dravet C, Dreifuss F, Perret A, Wolf P, eds. *Epileptic Syndromes in Infancy, Childhood and Adolescence.* London: John Libbey, 1992:115–132.

15. Farrell K. Classifying epileptic syndromes: problems and a neurobiologic solution. *Neurology* 1993; 43:S8–S11.

16. Aicardi J. Epileptic syndromes in childhood. *Epilepsia* 1988; 29:S1–S5.

17. Livingston JH. The Lennox-Gastaut syndrome. *Dev Med Child Neurol* 1988; 30:536–540.

18. Dulac O, N'Guyen T. The Lennox-Gastaut syndrome. *Epilepsia* 1993; 34:S7–S17.

19. Ohtahara S. Lennox-Gastaut syndrome. Considerations in its concept and categorization. *Jpn J Psychiatry Neurol* 1988; 42:535–542.

20. Oguni H, Hayashi K, Osawa M. Long-term prognosis of Lennox-Gastaut syndrome. *Epilepsia* 1996; 37:44–47.

21. Trevathan E, Murphy CC, Yeargin-Allsopp M. Prevalence and descriptive epidemiology of Lennox-Gastaut syndrome among Atlanta children. *Epilepsia* 1997; 38:1283–1288.

22. Yaqub BA. Electroclinical seizures in Lennox-Gastaut syndrome. *Epilepsia* 1993; 34:120–127.

23. Kaminska A, Ickowicz A, Plouin P, et al. Delineation of cryptogenic Lennox-Gastaut syndrome and myoclonic astatic epilepsy using multiple correspondence analysis. *Epilepsy Res* 1999; 36:15–29.

24. Aicardi J. Epilepsy in children. In: Procopis PG, Rapin I, eds. *The International Review of Child Neurology.* New York: Raven Press, 1994:44–66.

25. Ohtsuka Y, Amano R, Mizukawa M, Ohtahara S. Long-term prognosis of the Lennox-Gastaut syndrome. *Jpn J Psychiatry Neurol* 1990; 44:257–264.

26. Roger J, Dravet C, Bureau M. The Lennox-Gastaut syndrome. *Cleve Clin J Med* 1989; 56:S172–S180.

27. Chevrie JJ, Aicardi J. Childhood epileptic encephalopathy with slow spike-wave. A statistical study of 80 cases. *Epilepsia* 1972; 13:259–271.

28. Smeraldi E, Scorza Smeraldi R, Cazzullo CL, et al. Immunogenetics of the Lennox-Gastaut syndrome: frequency of HL-A antigens and haplotypes in patients and first-degree relatives. *Epilepsia* 1975; 16:699–703.

29. van Engelen BG, de Waal LP, Weemaes CM, Renier WO. Serologic HLA typing in cryptogenic Lennox-Gastaut syndrome. *Epilepsy Res* 1994; 17:43–47.

30. Theodore WH, Rose D, Patronas N, et al. Cerebral glucose metabolism in the Lennox-Gastaut syndrome. *Ann Neurol* 1987; 21:14–21.

31. Chugani HT, Mazziotta JC, Engel J Jr, Phelps ME. The Lennox-Gastaut syndrome: metabolic subtypes determined by 2-deoxy-2[18F]fluoro-*D*-glucose positron emission tomography. *Ann Neurol* 1987; 21:4–13.

32. Hauser WA. The prevalence and incidence of convulsive disorders in children. *Epilepsia* 1994; 35(Suppl 2):S1–S6.

33. Kramer U, Nevo Y, Neufeld MY, et al. Epidemiology of epilepsy in childhood: a cohort of 440 consecutive patients. *Pediatr Neurol* 1998; 18:46–50.

34. Prats JM, Garaizar C. Etiology of epilepsy in adolescents. *Rev Neurol* 1999; 28:32–5.

35. Beilmann A, Talvik T. Is the International League Against Epilepsy classification of epileptic syndromes applicable to children in Estonia? [In Process Citation]. *Europ J Paediatr Neurol* 1999; 3:265–272.

36. Cavazzuti GB. Epidemiology of different types of epilepsy in school age children of Modena, Italy. *Epilepsia* 1980; 21:57–62.

37. Steffenburg U, Hedstrom A, Lindroth A, et al. Intractable epilepsy in a population-based series of mentally retarded children. *Epilepsia* 1998; 39:767–75.

38. Heiskala H. Community-based study of Lennox-Gastaut syndrome. *Epilepsia* 1997; 38:526–531.

39. Rantala H, Putkonen T. Occurrence, outcome, and prognostic factors of infantile spasms and Lennox-Gastaut syndrome. *Epilepsia* 1999; 40:286–289.

40. Beilmann A, Napa A, Soot A, Talvik I, Talvik T. Prevalence of childhood epilepsy in Estonia. *Epilepsia* 1999; 40:1011–1019.

41. Beaumanoir A. The Lennox-Gastaut syndrome: a personal study. *Electroencephalogr Clin Neurophysiol* 1982; 35(Suppl):85–99.

42. Mariani E, Ferini-Strambi L, Sala M, Erminio C, Smirne S. Epilepsy in institutionalized patients with encephalopathy: clinical aspects and nosological considerations. *Am J Ment Retard* 1993; 98(Suppl):27–33.

43. Markand ON. Slow spike-wave activity in EEG and associated clinical features: often called 'Lennox' or 'Lennox-Gastaut' syndrome. *Neurology* 1977; 27:746–757.

44. Bare MA, Glauser TA, Strawsburg RH. Need for electroencephalogram video confirmation of atypical absence seizures in children with Lennox-Gastaut syndrome. *J Child Neurol* 1998; 13:498–500.

45. Ikeno T, Shigematsu H, Miyakoshi M, et al. An analytic study of epileptic falls. *Epilepsia* 1985; 26:612–621.

46. Donat JF, Wright FS. Seizures in series: similarities between seizures of the West and Lennox-Gastaut syndromes. *Epilepsia* 1991; 32:504–509.

47. Roger J, Remy C, Bureau M, et al. Lennox-Gastaut syndrome in the adult. *Rev Neurol* 1987; 143:401–405.

48. Ohtahara S, Ohtsuka Y, Kobayashi K. Lennox-Gastaut syndrome: a new vista. *Psychiatry Clin Neurosci* 1995; 49:S179–S183.

49. Yagi K. Evolution of Lennox-Gastaut syndrome: a long-term longitudinal study. *Epilepsia* 1996; 37:48–51.

50. Ohtsuka Y, Ohmori I, Oka E. Long-term follow-up of childhood epilepsy associated with tuberous sclerosis. *Epilepsia* 1998; 39:1158–1163.

51. Mattson RH. Efficacy and adverse effects of established and new antiepileptic drugs. *Epilepsia* 1995; 36 (Suppl):S13–S26.

52. Jeavons P, Clark J, Maheshwari M. Treatment of generalized epilepsies of childhood and adolescence with sodium valproate ('Epilim'). *Dev Med Child Neurol* 1977; 19:9–25.

53. Wheless JW, Constantinou JEC. Lennox-Gastaut syndrome. *Pediatr Neurol* 1997; 17:203–211.

54. Farrell K. Secondary generalized epilepsy and Lennox-Gastaut syndrome. In: Wyllie E, ed. *The Treatment of Epilepsy: Principles and Practice*. Philadelphia: Lea & Febiger, 1993:604–613.

55. Gastaut H, Lowe M. Antiepileptic properties of clobazam, a 1-5 benzodiazepine, in man. *Epilepsia* 1979; 20:437–446.

56. Snead OC, Saito M. Encephalopathic epilepsy after infancy. In: Dodson WE, Pellock JM, eds. *Pediatric Epilepsy: Diagnosis and Therapy*. New York: Demos Publications, 1993:147–156.

57. Sher P. Alternate day clonazepam treatment of intractable seizures. *Arch Neurol* 1985; 42:787–788.

58. Bittencourt PR, Richens A. Anticonvulsant-induced status epilepticus in Lennox-Gastaut syndrome. *Epilepsia* 1981; 22:129–134.

59. DiMario FJ, Jr., Clancy RR. Paradoxical precipitation of tonic seizures by lorazepam in a child with atypical absence seizures. *Pediatr Neurol* 1988; 4:249–251.

60. Snead O. Exacerbation of seizures in children by carbamazepine. *N Engl J Med* 1985; 323:916–921.

61. Horn CS, Ater SB, Hurst DL. Carbamazepine-exacerbated epilepsy in children and adolescents. *Pediatr Neurol* 1986; 2:340–345.

62. Erba G, Browne T. Atypical absence, myoclonic, atonic and tonic seizures and the "Lennox-Gastaut syndrome." In: Browne T, Feldman R, eds. *Epilepsy, Diagnosis and Management*. Boston: Little, Brown, 1983:75–94.

63. Zouhar A, Slapal R. Administration of high doses of B6 in age-related epileptic encephalopathies. *Cesk Neurol Neurochir* 1989; 52:28–31.

64. Bourgeois BFD. Antiepileptic drugs in pediatric practice. *Epilepsia* 1995; 36:S34–S45.

65. Brett E. The Lennox-Gastaut syndrome: therapeutic aspects. In: Niedermeyer E, Degen R, eds. *The Lennox-Gastaut Syndrome*. New York: Alan Liss, 1988:317–339.

66. Yamatogi Y, Ohtsuka Y, Ishida T, et al. Treatment of the Lennox syndrome with ACTH: a clinical and electroencephalographic study. *Brain Dev* 1979; 1:267–276.

67. Snead O, Benton J, Myers C. ACTH and prednisone in childhood seizure disorders. *Neurology* 1983; 33:966–970.

68. Duse M, Notarangelo LD, Tiberti S, et al. Intravenous immune globulin in the treatment of intractable childhood epilepsy. *Clin Exp Immunol* 1996; 104(Suppl 1): 71–76.

69. van Engelen BG, Renier WO, Weemaes CM, et al. High-dose intravenous immunoglobulin treatment in cryptogenic West and Lennox-Gastaut syndrome; an add-on study. *Eur J Pediatr* 1994; 153:762–769.

70. Feucht M, Brantner-Inthaler S. Gamma-vinyl-GABA (vigabatrin) in the therapy of Lennox-Gastaut syndrome: an open study. *Epilepsia* 1994; 35:993–998.

71. Sakamoto K, Kurokawa T, Tomita S, et al. Effects of zonisamide on children with epilepsy. *Curr Ther Res* 1988; 43(3):378–383.

72. van Rijckevorsel-Harmant K, Delire M, Rucquoy-Ponsar M. Treatment of idiopathic West and Lennox-Gastaut syndromes by intravenous administration of human polyvalent immunoglobulins. *Eur Arch Psychiatry Neurol Sci* 1986; 236:119–122.

73. Gross-Tsur V, Shalev RS, Kazir E, Engelhard D, Amir N. Intravenous high-dose gammaglobulins for intractable childhood epilepsy. *Acta Neurol Scand* 1993; 88:204–209.

74. Ariizumi M, Baba K, Shiihara H. High dose gamma-globulin for intractable childhood epilepsy. *Lancet* 1983; 2:162–163.

75. Illum N, Taudorf K, Heilmann C, et al. Intravenous immunoglobulin: a single-blind trial in children with Lennox-Gastaut syndrome. *Neuropediatrics* 1990; 21:87–90.

76. van Rijckevorsel-Harmant K, Delire M, Schmitz-Moorman W, Wieser HG. Treatment of refractory epilepsy with intravenous immunoglobulins. Results of the first double-blind/dose finding clinical study. *Int J Clin Lab Res* 1994; 24:162–166.

77. Livingston J, Beaumont D, Arzimanoglou A. Vigabatrin in the treatment of epilepsy in children. *Br J Clin Pharmacol* 1989; 27:109S–112S.

78. Gibbs J, Appleton R, Rosenbloom L. Vigabatrin in intractable childhood epilepsy: a retrospective study. *Pediatr Neurol* 1992; 8:338–340.

79. Luna D, Dulac O, Pajot N. Vigabatrin in the treatment of childhood epilepsies. A single-blind placebo-controlled study. *Epilepsia* 1989; 30:430–437.

80. Fois A, Buoni S, Bartolo RD. Vigabatrin treatment in children. *Childs Nerv Syst* 1994; 10:244–248.

81. Maldonado C, Castello J, Fuentes E. Vigabatrin in the management of Lennox-Gastaut Syndrome. *Epilepsia* 1995; 36:S102.

82. Dulac O, Chiron C, Luna D, et al. Vigabatrin in childhood epilepsy. *J Child Neurol* 1991; Suppl 2:S30–S37.

83. Pellock JM. New antiepileptic drugs in pediatric epilepsy syndromes. *Pediatrics* 1999; 104:1106–1116.

84. Shields WD, Sankar R. Vigabatrin. *Semin Pediatr Neurol* 1997; 4:43–50.

85. Appleton RE. Vigabatrin in the management of generalized seizures in children. *Seizure* 1995; 4:45–48.

86. Sankar R, Wasterlain CG. Is the devil we know the lesser of two evils? Vigabatrin and visual fields. *Neurology* 1999; 52:1537–1538.

87. Yamatogi Y, Ohtahara S. Current topics of treatment. In: Ohtahara S, Roger J, eds. *Proceedings of the International Symposium, New Trends in Pediatric Epileptology.* Okayama, 1991:136–148.

88. Prusinski A, Stepien-Barcikowska A. A trial of using tryptophane in the treatment of Lennox-Gastaut Syndrome. *Neurochir Polska* 1984; 18:287–289.

89. Slapal R, Zouhar A. Therapeutic effect of dopaminergic substances in drug-resistant Lennox-Gastaut syndrome. *Cesk Neurol Neurochir* 1989; 52:32–35.

90. Inanaga K, Kumashiro H, Fukuyama Y, Ohtahara S, Shirouzu M. Clinical study of oral administration of DN-1417, a TRH analog, in patients with intractable epilepsy. *Epilepsia* 1989; 30:438–445.

91. Ros Perez P, Zamarron Cuesta I, Aparicio Meix M, Sastre Gallego A. Evaluation of the effectiveness of the ketogenic diet with medium-chain triglycerides, in the treatment of refractory epilepsy in children. Apropos of a series of cases. *An Esp Pediatr* 1989; 30:155–158.

92. Wheless J. The ketogenic diet: Fa(c)t or fiction. Editorial. *J Child Neurol* 1995; 10:419–423.

93. Freeman JM, Vining EP. Seizures decrease rapidly after fasting: preliminary studies of the ketogenic diet. *Arch Pediatr Adolesc Med* 1999; 153:946–949.

94. Wheless J. Evaluation of children for epilepsy surgery. *Pediatr Ann* 1991; 20:41–49.

95. Baumgartner J, Clifton G, Wheless J. Corpus callostomy. *Tech Neurosurg* 1995; 1:45–51.

96. Chevrie J-J, Aicardi J. Lennox-Gastaut syndrome. In: Luders H, ed. *Epilepsy Surgery.* New York: Raven Press, 1991:197–202.

97. Kwan SY, Wong TT, Chang KP, et al. Seizure outcome after corpus callosotomy: the Taiwan experience. *Childs Nerv Syst* 2000; 16:87–92.

98. Hornig GW, Murphy JV, Schallert G, Tilton C. Left vagus nerve stimulatin in children with refractory epilepsy: an update. *South Med J* 1997; 90:484–488.

99. Ben-Menachem E, Hellstrom K, Waldton C, Augustinsson LE. Evaluation of refractory epilepsy treated with vagus nerve stimulation for up to 5 years. *Neurology* 1999; 52:1265–1267.

100. Lundgren J, Amark P, Blennow G, Stromblad LG, Wallstedt L. Vagus nerve stimulation in 16 children with refractory epilepsy. *Epilepsia* 1998; 39:809–813.

101. Frost M, Gates J, Conry J, et al. Vagus nerve stimulation (VNS) in Lennox-Gastaut syndrome (LGS). *Epilepsia* 1999; 40:95.

102. Hosain S, Harden C, Nikolov B, Fraser R, Labar D. Vagus nerve stimulation in children with symptomatic generalized epilepsy. *Epilepsia* 1999; 40:125.

103. Tatum W, Ferriera J, Benbadis S, Vale F. Vagus nerve stimulation and antiepileptic drug reduction. *Epilepsia* 1999; 40:223.

104. Angelini L, Broggi G, Riva D, Lazzaro Solero C. A case of Lennox-Gastaut syndrome successfully treated by removal of a parietotemporal astrocytoma. *Epilepsia* 1979; 20:665–669.

105. Lockman L, Rothner A, Erenberg G, et al. Cinromide in the treatment of seizures in the Lennox-Gastaut syndrome. *Epilepsia* 1980; 22:241.

106. Anonymous. Double-blind, placebo-controlled evaluation of cinromide in patients with the Lennox-Gastaut syndrome. The Group for the Evaluation of Cinromide in the Lennox-Gastaut Syndrome. *Epilepsia* 1989; 30:422–429.

107. Ritter FJ. Efficacy of felbamate in childhood epileptic encephalopathy (Lennox-Gastaut syndrome). *N Engl J Med* 1993; 328:29–33.

108. Jensen PK. Felbamate in the treatment of Lennox-Gastaut syndrome. *Epilepsia* 1994; 35(Suppl 5):S54–S57.

109. Pellock JM. Felbamate. *Epilepsia* 1999; 40:S57–S62.

110. Patton W, Duffull S. Idiosyncratic drug-induced haematological abnormalities. Incidence, pathogenesis, management and avoidance. *Drug Safety* 1994; 11:445–462.

111. Bourgeois BF. Felbamate. *Semin Pediatric Neurol* 1997; 4:3–8.

112. Pellock JM, Brodie MJ. Felbamate: 1997 update. *Epilepsia* 1997; 38:1261–1264.

113. Donaldson JA, Glauser TA, Olberding LS. Lamotrigine adjunctive therapy in childhood epileptic encephalopathy (the Lennox Gastaut syndrome). *Epilepsia* 1997; 38:68–73.

114. Timmings PL, Richens A. Lamotrigine as an add-on drug in the management of Lennox-Gastaut syndrome. *Eur Neurol* 1992; 32:305–307.

115. Schlumberger E, Chavez F, Palacios L, et al. Lamotrigine in treatment of 120 children with epilepsy. *Epilepsia* 1994; 35:359–367.

116. Uvebrant P, Bauziene R. Intractable epilepsy in children. The efficacy of lamotrigine treatment, including non-seizure related benefits. *Neuropediatrics* 1994; 25:284–289.

117. Buchanan N. Lamotrigine: clinical experience in 93 patients with epilepsy. *Acta Neurol Scand* 1995; 92:28–32.

118. Eriksson AS, Nergardh A, Hoppu K. The efficacy of lamotrigine in children and adolescents with refractory generalized epilepsy: a randomized, double-blind, crossover study. *Epilepsia* 1998; 39:495–501.

119. Motte J, Trevathan E, Arvidsson JF, et al. Lamotrigine for generalized seizures associated with the Lennox-Gastaut syndrome. *N Engl J Med* 1997; 337:1807–1812.

120. Pellock JM. Overview of lamotrigine and the new antiepileptic drugs: the challenge. *J Child Neurol* 1997; 12:S48–52.

121. Schlienger RG, Shapiro LE, Shear NH. Lamotrigine-induced severe cutaneous adverse reactions. *Epilepsia* 1998; 39:S22–S26.

122. Matsuo F. Lamotrigine. *Epilepsia* 1999; 40:S30–S36.

123. Sachdeo RC, Glauser TA, Ritter F, et al. A double-blind, randomized trial of topiramate in Lennox-Gastaut syndrome. *Neurology* 1999; 52:1882–1887.

124. Glauser TA, Levisohn PM, Ritter F, Sachdeo RC. Topiramate in Lennox-Gastaut syndrome: open-label treatment of patients completing a randomized controlled trial. Topiramate YL Study Group. *Epilepsia* 2000; 41:S86–S90.

125. Cook RJ, Sackett DL. The number needed to treat: a clinically useful measure of treatment effect [published erratum appears in *Br Med J* 1995 Apr 22; 310(6986):1056]. *Br Med J* 1995; 310:452–454.

126. Marson AG, Kadir ZA, Chadwick DW. New antiepileptic drugs: a systematic review of their efficacy and tolerability. *Br Med J* 1996; 313:1169–1174.

127. Landau W, Kleffner F. Syndrome of acquired aphasia with convulsive disorder in children. *Neurology* 1957; 7:523–530.

128. Beaumanoir A. The Landau-Kleffner syndrome. In: Roger J, Bureau M, Dravet C, Dreifuss FE, Perret A, Wolf P, eds. *Epileptic Syndromes in Infancy, Childhood and Adolescence*. London: John Libbey, 1992:231–243.

129. Kaga M. Language disorders in Landau-Kleffner syndrome. *J Child Neurol* 1999; 14:118–122.

130. Hirsch E, Marescaux C, Maquet P, et al. Landau-Kleffner syndrome: a clinical and EEG study of five cases. *Epilepsia* 1990; 31:756–767.

131. Deonna TW. Acquired epileptiform aphasia in children (Landau-Kleffner syndrome). *J Clin Neurophysiol* 1991; 8:288–298.

132. Gordon N. Acquired aphasia in childhood: the Landau-Kleffner syndrome. *Dev Med Child Neurol* 1990; 32:267–274.

133. Roger J, Genton P, Bureau M, Dravet C. Less common epileptic syndromes. In: Wyllie E, ed. *The Treatment of Epilepsy: Principles and Practice*. Philadelphia: Lea & Febiger, 1993:624–635.

134. Rapin I, Mattis S, Rowan AJ, Golden GG. Verbal auditory agnosia in children. *Dev Med Child Neurol* 1977; 19:197–207.

135. Glauser TA, Olberding LS, Titanic MK, Piccirillo DM. Felbamate in the treatment of acquired epileptic aphasia. *Epilepsy Res* 1995; 20:85–89.

136. da Silva EA, Chugani DC, Muzik O, Chugani HT. Landau-Kleffner syndrome: metabolic abnormalities in temporal lobe are a common feature. *J Child Neurol* 1997; 12:489–495.

137. Maquet P, Hirsch E, Dive D, et al. Cerebral glucose utilization during sleep in Landau-Kleffner syndrome: a PET study. *Epilepsia* 1990; 31:778–783.

138. Otero E, Cordova S, Diaz F, Garcia-Teruel I, Del Brutto OH. Acquired epileptic aphasia (the Landau-Kleffner syndrome) due to neurocysticercosis. *Epilepsia* 1989; 30:569–572.

139. Pascual-Castroviejo I, Lopez Martin V, Martinez Bermejo A, Perez Higueras A. Is cerebral arteritis the cause of the Landau-Kleffner syndrome? Four cases in childhood with angiographic study. *Can J Neurol Sci* 1992; 19:46–52.

140. Marescaux C, Hirsch E, Finck S, et al. Landau-Kleffner syndrome: a pharmacologic study of five cases. *Epilepsia* 1990; 31:768–777.

141. Grote CL, Van Slyke P, Hoeppner JA. Language outcome following multiple subpial transection for Landau-Kleffner syndrome. *Brain* 1999; 122:561–566.

142. Bergqvist AG, Chee CM, Lutchka LM, Brooks-Kayal AR. Treatment of acquired epileptic aphasia with the ketogenic diet. *J Child Neurol* 1999; 14:696–701.

143. Mantovani J, Landau W. Acquired aphasia with convulsive disorder; course and prognosis. *Neurology* 1980; 30:524–529.

144. Deonna T, Peter C, Ziegler AL. Adult follow-up of the acquired aphasia-epilepsy syndrome in childhood. Report of 7 cases. *Neuropediatrics* 1989; 20:132–138.

145. Patry G, Lyagoubi S, Tassinari CA. Subclinical 'electrical status epilepticus' induced by sleep in children. A clinical and electroencephalographic study of six cases. *Arch Neurol* 1971; 24:242–252.

146. Tassinari CA, Bureau M, Dravet C, Roger J, Daniele-Natale O. Electrical status epilepticus during sleep in children (ESES). In: Sterman MB, Shouse MN, Passouant P, eds. *Sleep and Epilepsy*. London, New York: Academic Press, 1982:465–479.

147. Morikawa T, Seino M, Osawa T, Yagi K. Five children with continuous spike-wave discharges during sleep. In: Roger J, Dravet C, Bureau M, Dreifuss FE, Wolf P, eds. *Epileptic Syndromes in Infancy, Childhood and Adolescence*. London: John Libbey, 1985:205–212.

148. Jayakar PB, Seshia SS. Electrical status epilepticus during slow-wave sleep: a review. *J Clin Neurophysiol* 1991; 8:299–311.

149. Tassinari CA, Bureau M, Dravet C, Dalla Bernardina B, Roger J. Epilepsy with continuous spikes and waves during slow sleep—otherwise described as ESES (epilepsy with electrical status epilepticus during slow sleep). In: Roger J, Bureau M, Dravet C, Dreifuss FE, Perret A, Wolf P, eds. *Epileptic Syndromes in Infancy, Childhood and Adolescence*. London: John Libbey, 1992:245–256.

150. Veggiotti P, Beccaria F, Guerrini R, Capovilla G, Lanzi G. Continuous spike-and-wave activity during slow-wave sleep: syndrome or EEG pattern? *Epilepsia* 1999; 40:1593–1601.

151. Tassinari CA, Bureau M, Dravet C, Dalla Bernardina B, Roger J. Epilepsy with continuous spikes and waves during slow sleep—otherwise described as ESES (epilepsy with electrical status epilepticus during slow sleep). In: Roger J, Dravet C, Bureau M, Dreifuss FE, Wolf P, eds. *Epileptic Syndromes in Infancy, Childhood and Adolescence*. London: John Libbey, 1985:194–204.

152. Boel M, Casaer P. Continuous spikes and waves during slow sleep: a 30 months follow-up study of neuropsychological recovery and EEG findings. *Neuropediatrics* 1989; 20:176–180.

153. Symann S, Rucquoy M, Misson J, et al. New hope for CSWS/ESES treatment: topiramate? In: Evrard P, Richelme C, Tardieu M, eds. *3rd EPNS Congress*. Bologna: Monduzzi Editore S.p.A., 199:155–159.

CHAPTER 16

Absence Seizures

Phillip L. Pearl, M.D., and Gregory L. Holmes, M.D.

The absence seizure is characterized by sudden discontinuation of activity with loss of awareness, responsiveness, and memory, and an equally abrupt recovery. The first description of such an event was by Poupart in 1705 (1). The use of "petit mal" to describe all nonconvulsive seizures, proposed by Esquirol in 1815, has contributed to confusion that persists today. "Petit mal" was used to more or less imply the severity of a seizure before the EEG description of 3 Hz spike-and-wave by Gibbs, Davis, and Lennox in 1935 (2). Clarification and delineation of absence seizure types remained elusive until the past 25 years, when systematic neurophysiological studies using video-EEG monitoring techniques aided the description of the protean manifestations and clinical syndromes associated with absence seizures.

CLASSIFICATION

The revised classification of epileptic seizures by the International League Against Epilepsy (ILAE) categorizes absence seizures as generalized seizures, indicating bihemispheric initial involvement clinically and electroencephalographically (3). Absence seizures are divided into typical and atypical (Table 16-1), the features of which are discussed later. Many children with absence seizures can be further categorized as having a characteristic epileptic syndrome. The various syndromes featuring absence seizures include both idiopathic and symptomatic generalized epilepsies (Table 16-2), and these are described later in this chapter.

EPIDEMIOLOGY

Absence seizures are relatively uncommon, comprising 2 percent to 11 percent of seizure types in all ages (4–9). The prevalence is highest in the first decade (10,11). The incidence is 9.6 per 100,000 in the age group 0 to 15 years (10). Sato and coworkers (12), in a study of 83 patients with absence seizures, reported the age of onset was most commonly in the 5- to 9-year-old group (versus 4 or less, or 10 or more), while Wirrel (13) and colleagues found an average age of onset of 5.7 years in 72 children.

A population-based case control study found that only a history of febrile seizures was a significant risk factor for the development of absence seizures ($p < 0.01$) (14). None of the other factors studied were significant, including those that were previously

Table 16-1. Classification of Absence Seizures

I. Typical absence seizures
  A. Simple — impairment of consciousness only
  B. Complex
    1. With mild clonic components
    2. With changes in tone
    3. With automatisms
    4. With autonomic components
II. Atypical absence seizures
III. Absence status

Table 16-2. Classification of Absence Syndromes

I. Generalized idiopathic epilepsies
  A. Childhood absence (pyknolepsy)
  B. Juvenile absence
  C. Juvenile myoclonic epilepsy (impulsive petit mal of Janz)
II. Generalized symptomatic epilepsies
  A. Lennox-Gastaut syndrome
  B. Epilepsy with myoclonic-astatic seizures
  C. Epilepsy with myoclonic absences

suggested such as twin pregnancy, breech presentation, being first-born, and perinatal asphyxia.

CHARACTERIZATION OF ABSENCE SEIZURES

The terms *typical absence seizure* (TAS) and *atypical absence seizure* (AAS) were used by the International Classification of Epileptic Seizures to describe and categorize the various absence types (3). As shown in Table 16-1, the simple typical absence seizure consists of the sudden onset of impaired consciousness, usually associated with a blank facial appearance without other motor or behavioral phenomena. This subtype is actually relatively rare and comprises only 9 percent of 374 absence seizures videorecorded from 48 patients by Penry and associates (15). The complex typical absence seizure, alternatively, is accompanied by other motor, behavioral, or autonomic phenomena.

Clonic components may be quite subtle and most frequently consist of eye blinking. Clonic activity may range from nystagmus (16) to rapid jerking of the arms. Changes in tone may include a tonic postural contraction, leading to flexion or extension of the trunk (17). Decreases in tone leading to head nodding or dropping objects may also occur, although they rarely cause a fall.

In a study of 476 typical absence seizures monitored by simultaneous video-EEG radiotelemetry, automatisms were the most common clinical accompaniment, occurring in 44 percent of 27 patients (18). Automatisms are semipurposeful behaviors of which the patient is unaware and subsequently cannot recall. They may be either perseverative, reflecting continuation of preictal activities, or de novo. Simple behaviors, such as rubbing the face or hands, licking the lips, chewing, grimacing, scratching, or fumbling with clothes tend to be de novo automatisms. Complex activity such as dealing cards, playing pattycake, or handling a toy are generally perseverative. If it occurs, speech is usually perseverative and often slowed and dysarthric, but it may be totally normal and include both expressive and receptive abilities (19).

Autonomic phenomena associated with absence seizures include pupil dilatation, pallor, flushing, sweating, salivation, piloerection, and even urinary incontinence (17,20). Neither the autonomic changes or automatisms allow one to distinguish absence seizures from other seizure types.

Atypical absence seizures have traditionally been characterized as having less abrupt onset or cessation, more pronounced changes in tone, and longer duration than typical absence (3). They usually begin before 5 years of age and are associated with other generalized seizure types and mental retardation. The ictal EEG is more heterogeneous, showing 1.5 to 2.5 Hz slow spike-and-wave or multiple spike-and-wave discharges that may be irregular or asymmetrical (4,5). The interictal EEG is usually abnormal, with slowing and multifocal epileptiform features (21).

Using the aforementioned ictal EEG criteria to operationally differentiate atypical from typical absence seizures, Holmes and coworkers (18) compared 426 typical and 500 atypical absence seizures in 54 children. The average duration of the AAS, 10.24 seconds, was significantly longer than that of the TAS, 8.69 seconds ($p < 0.01$). A change in facial expression or appearance of a blank stare was the most common initial clinical manifestation in either type. A pause or slowing of motor activity was also frequently noted as the initial finding in either seizure type. Either diminished postural tone or tonic or myoclonic activity was significantly more likely to be the initial clinical feature in AAS than in TAS. A blank stare or change in facial expression was the sole clinical finding in only 16 percent of TAS and 28 percent of AAS. Automatisms, eye blinking, and lip smacking occurred more commonly in TAS. A change in postural tone, either an increase or a decrease, was more commonly seen in AAS. Automatisms were more common in TAS than in AAS and are usually perseverative, such as often playing with a toy or game. De novo automatisms were associated with longer spells and most commonly consisted of rubbing the face or hands in TAS and smiling in AAS.

In the study by Holmes and coworkers (18), the authors found that both TAS and AAS started abruptly without an aura, lasted from a few seconds to half a minute, and ended abruptly. Both were frequently associated with eye blinking, lip smacking, decrease in tone, and automatisms. Although statistically significant differences can be identified between TAS and AAS, there is considerable overlap between the two seizure types, and they more likely represent a clinical continuum. This overlap pertains to the EEG as well as the proposed pathophysiology.

PATIENT CHARACTERISTICS

Most patients with typical absence seizures have normal neurologic examinations. In two large studies, abnormalities were found in 23 percent of patients by Sato and associates (12) and 16 percent by Dalby (7). Neurologic abnormalities tend to be mild and nonprogressive.

Intelligence scores are more variable, largely attributable to the diverse patient populations. In patients with typical 3-Hz spike-and-wave discharges, Dalby (7) found 17 percent of patients had IQs below 90, whereas Sato and coworkers (12) found 52 percent had IQs below 90. Holmes (18) found 22 percent of 27 patients with typical absence seizures to be mentally retarded, whereas 93 percent of 27 patients with atypical absence were retarded.

Table 16-3. Differential Diagnosis of Typical Absence Seizures

Clinical Data	Absence	Complex Partial	Daydreaming
Frequency/day	Multiple	Rarely over 1–2	Multiple; situation-dependent
Duration	Frequently <10 sec	Average duration over 1 min, 10 sec	Seconds to minutes; rarely more rarely less
Aura	Never	Frequently	No
Eye blinking	Common	Occasionally	No
Automatisms	Common	Frequently	No
Postictal impairment	None	Frequently	No
Seizures activated by:			
HV	Very frequently	Occasionally	No
Photic	Frequently	Rarely	No
EEG			
Ictal	Generalized spike and wave	Usually unilateral or bilateral temporal frontal discharges	Normal
Interictal	Usually normal	Variable; may be spikes or sharp waves in frontal or temporal lobes	Normal

Source: With permission from publisher and author, Holmes GL. *Diagnosis and Management of Seizures in Children.* Philadelphia: W.B. Saunders Company, 1987:177.

Between 40 percent and 60 percent of patients with typical absence seizures have generalized tonic-clonic seizures (7,10,12,22–25). The time from the first absence to the first generalized tonic-clonic seizure may range from 1 to 16 years (mean 6.6 years) (25). Nearly all patients with atypical absence seizures have generalized tonic-clonic seizures, and many also have myoclonic, tonic, and atonic seizures. Partial seizures are unusual in patients with absences (18).

DIFFERENTIAL DIAGNOSIS

The primary diagnostic considerations to be differentiated from absence seizures are complex partial seizures and daydreaming (Table 16-3). Complex partial seizures are more common than absence seizures and are also manifested by an alteration in consciousness with staring, automatisms, changes in tone, and autonomic symptoms (26). The complex partial seizure tends to be longer and less frequent, but clinically there may be no absolute distinguishing factor. The presence of an aura or postictal impairment is strongly suggestive of a complex partial seizure. When positive, the EEG is the best confirmation of either seizure type.

Daydreaming is associated with boredom, can be "broken" with stimulation, and is not associated with motor activity. Absence seizures, however, may sometimes be terminated with stimulation and tend to increase during periods of relaxation and tiredness. Tics and pseudoseizures may need to be considered as well. A normal EEG that includes several trials of 3 to 5 minutes of hyperventilation, however, virtually rules out absence seizures. Repeated studies or prolonged monitoring occasionally are necessary when diagnostic confusion persists (27).

ELECTROENCEPHALOGRAPHY

The EEG signature of a typical absence seizure is the sudden onset of 3-Hz generalized symmetrical spike- or multiple spike-and-slow wave complexes (Figure 16-1). The voltage of the discharges is often maximal in the frontocentral regions. The frequency tends to be faster, about 4 Hz, at the onset and slows to 2 Hz toward the end of discharges longer than 10 seconds. The ictal discharges during an atypical absence seizure are more variable. They occur at frequencies between 1.5 and 2.5 Hz or may be faster than 2.5 Hz but are irregular or asymmetrical in voltage.

The interictal EEG background is generally normal in TAS and abnormal in AAS. Utilizing the aforementioned ictal EEG criteria to classify absence seizures, Holmes and colleagues (18) found that only 44 percent of 27 patients with TAS had normal EEG backgrounds. Diffuse slowing was seen in 22 percent, paroxysmal spikes or sharp waves in 37 percent, and posterior rhythmic delta (less than 4 Hz) slowing in 15 percent. Conversely, only 11 percent of 27 patients with AAS had a normal interictal EEG. Diffuse slowing and focal or multifocal spikes or sharp waves were seen in 85 percent.

The discharges are more numerous during all sleep states except REM (28–30). The bursts have a modified appearance in sleep, as they are briefer, irregular, and slow to 1.5 to 2.5 Hz. Hyperventilation, photic stimulation, and hypoglycemia activate typical absence

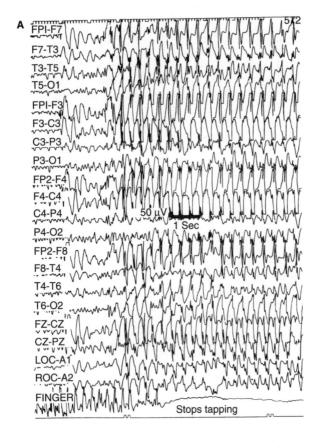

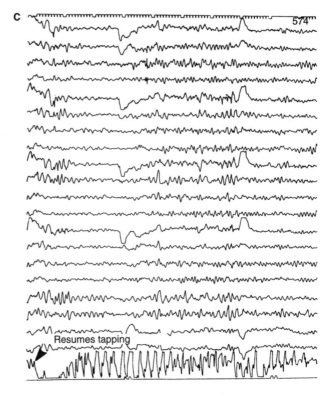

Figure 16-1. (*Continued*)

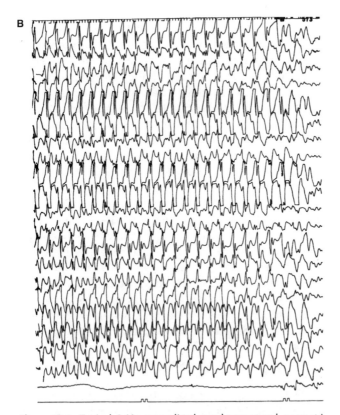

Figure 16-1. Typical 3-Hz generalized synchronous and symmetrical spike-and-wave EEG discharge during hyperventilation in an 8-year-old girl with pyknolepsy. Note the drop out of finger tapping 2 seconds into the paroxysm and return on cessation of the discharge.

seizures, but hyperventilation is the most effective procedure (7,31).

Clinical effects are generally perceived accompanying discharges lasting longer than 3 seconds. Detailed neuropsychological investigations have demonstrated functional impairment from a spike-and-wave burst of any duration. Auditory reaction times were delayed 56 percent of the time when a stimulus was presented at the onset of the EEG paroxysm (32). They were abnormal in 80 percent when the stimulus was delayed 0.5 second. Responsiveness may improve as the paroxysm continues (33).

ETIOLOGY

Both acquired and inherited factors are implicated in the etiology of absence seizures, reflecting the heterogeneity of the patient population. Genetic factors predominate in children who match the syndromes of idiopathic generalized epilepsy. Alternatively, acquired disorders are frequently found in retarded children with abnormal neurologic findings, abnormal interictal EEGs, and atypical absence seizures. Typical absence seizures, both clinically and electrographically, have been rarely seen in patients with mesial frontal lesions, with diencephalic lesions, and after withdrawal from sedatives (34–37). Nonconvulsive status epilepticus of frontal lobe origin can mimic absence status epilepticus once it has progressed to a full-blown phase (38).

The lack of structural pathology and the age-specific window observed in most patients with typical absence seizures implicate a hereditary etiology. Metrakos and Metrakos (39) showed that absence seizures and generalized spike-and-wave EEG discharges are both inherited traits. Generalized spike-and-wave activity was seen in 37 percent of siblings of patients with generalized spike-and-wave on EEG and absence or generalized tonic-clonic seizures compared with 9 percent of controls. Only 25 percent of the family members with the EEG trait actually had seizures. They theorized that the inheritance of generalized spike-and-wave discharges is autosomal dominant with age-dependent penetrance, regardless of whether seizures occur. Doose and associates (40) suggested a multigenic inheritance, with both independent and interactive genetic factors.

An exciting discovery in epileptology has been the mapping of chromosome locus 6p21.3 to juvenile myoclonic epilepsy (41). Using both epileptic and asymptomatic "EEG-affected" family members of 68 probands with juvenile myoclonus epilepsy (JME), DNA linkage analysis revealed that the JME gene is tightly linked to the properdin factor B (Bf)-HLA loci in chromosome 6 in some families. Some family members had different seizure types than their JME probands, including absence or tonic-clonic seizures alone or in combination, and even febrile seizures. In addition, other families with JME do not map to 6p21.3.

The genetic diversity of JME and the other inherited epilepsies awaits exploration and may be the result of different genetic loci or different alleles at the same locus. The even larger query of "genetic susceptibility" to epilepsy after acquired insults is among the next frontiers of molecular epileptology (see Chapter 5).

PATHOPHYSIOLOGY

The observation that 3-Hz spike-and-wave discharges in absence seizures appear simultaneously and synchronously in all electrode locations led early investigators to speculate that the pathophysiological mechanisms must involve "deep" structures with widespread connections between the two hemispheres (43–45). The term *centrencephalon* was coined to describe this unknown structure. Although this term was useful in emphasizing the fundamental differences between partial seizures and generalized seizures, it has outlived its usefulness. Work over the last decade has led to a better understanding of the basic mechanism of this disorder.

A number of studies have recently suggested that the basic underlying mechanism in generalized absence epilepsies involves thalamocortical circuitry and the generation of abnormal oscillatory rhythms in this neuronal network (46–49). Studies using both in vivo and in vitro models have now demonstrated the neuronal circuit responsible for the generation of the oscillatory thalamocortical burst-firing observed during absence

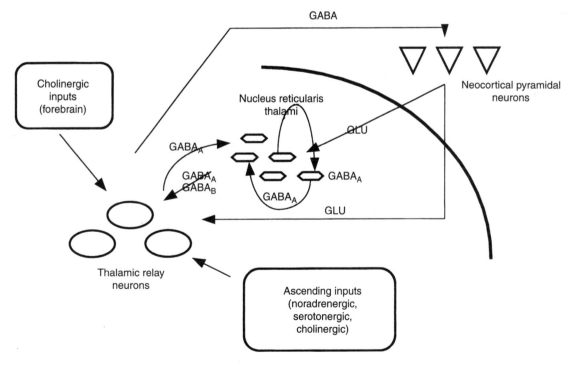

Figure 16-2. Thalamocortical circuit and neuronal networks implicated in the genesis of absence seizures. For discussion, see text.

seizures. The key role of the thalamus is corroborated by a selective increase in blood flow during absence seizures using positron emission tomography (PET) imaging technology (50).

This circuit includes cortical pyramidal neurons, thalamic relay neurons, and the nucleus reticularis thalami (NRT) (49,51). The principal synaptic connections of the thalamocortical circuit include glutamatergic fibers between neocortical pyramidal cells and the NRT, and GABAergic fibers from NRT neurons that activate $GABA_A$ and $GABA_B$ receptors on thalamic relay neurons. In addition, recurrent collateral GABAergic fibers from the NRT activate $GABA_A$ receptors on adjacent NRT neurons. As can be seen in Figure 16-2, the NRT is in a position to influence the flow of information between the thalamus and cerebral cortex (52). The NRT cells have rhythmic burst firing (oscillatory firing) during periods of sleep and continuous single spike firing (tonic firing) during wakefulness.

The cellular events that underlie the ability of NRT neurons to shift between an oscillatory and tonic firing mode are the low-threshold Ca^{++} spikes that are present in thalamocortical and NRT neurons (52). Low-threshold, transient Ca^{++} channels (T-channels) are a key membrane property involved in burst firing excitation and are associated with the change from oscillatory to burst firing in thalamocortical cells (47,48,53,54). Mild depolarization of these neurons is sufficient to activate these channels and to allow the influx of

extracellular Ca^{++}. Further depolarization produced by Ca^{++} inflow exceeds the threshold for firing a burst of action potentials. After T-channels are activated, they become inactivated rather quickly; hence the name *transient*. Deinactivation of T-channels requires a relatively lengthy hyperpolarization. $GABA_B$ receptor–mediated hyperpolarization is able to deinactivate T-channels.

There is considerable evidence that the pathophysiological basis of absence seizures is the generation of excessive abnormal oscillatory rhythms (55). These abnormal oscillatory rhythms could be caused by abnormalities of the T-channels or enhanced $GABA_B$ function (43,56). In some animal models of absence seizures T-channel activation in the NRT is significantly different than in control animals (57). These aberrant T-channels may be one basis for absence seizures. In other models, there has been an increase in $GABA_B$ receptors in thalamic and neocortical neuronal populations compared with controls (55). As would be predicted from the thalamocortical circuits involved in absence seizures, in animal models of absences $GABA_B$ agonists produce an increase in seizure frequency, while $GABA_B$ antagonists reduce seizure frequency (58–60).

As demonstrated in Figure 16-2, recurrent collateral GABAergic fibers from the NRT neurons activate $GABA_A$ receptors on adjacent NRT neurons. Activating $GABA_A$ receptors in the NRT therefore results in inhibition of output to the thalamic relay neurons and serves to reduce hyperpolarization and delay deinactivation of the T-channels. In animals studies, injection of the $GABA_A$ agonists bilaterally into the NRT reduces absence seizure frequency. This occurs because the GABA output to the thalamic relay neurons is reduced. Because of the decreased $GABA_B$ activation, there would be a reduced likelihood that the Ca^{++} deinactivation would occur. This would result in decreased oscillatory firing. However, direct $GABA_A$ and $GABA_B$ activation of thalamic relay neurons would be expected to have detrimental effects, increasing depolarization and deinactivation of the T-channels.

As would be expected from these animal findings are the clinical observations that three drugs that are effective in the treatment of absence seizures—valproate acid, ethosuximide, and trimethodione—all suppress T-currents. In addition, there is some clinical evidence that vigabatrin, which increases endogenous GABA levels and thereby increases the activation of $GABA_B$ receptors, worsens absence seizures in patients. However, clonazepam, which preferentially activates $GABA_A$ receptors in the NRT, can be a highly effective antiabsence drug (61). Hosford and Wang (62) evaluated the effects of a number of new antiepileptic drugs (AEDs) on seizure frequency in the lethargic (lh/lh) model of absence seizures. Previous studies had demonstrated the efficacy of ethosuximide,

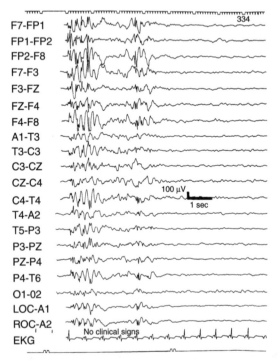

Figure 16-3. EEG of an 11-year-old girl with juvenile myoclonic epilepsy, showing brief paroxysms of multiple-spike-and-wave discharges. There were no associated clinical signs.

clonazepam, and valproate in this model. The authors found that lamotrigine significantly reduced seizure frequency, while vigabatrin and tiagabine increased seizure frequency and duration. Gabapentin and topiramate had no significant effects on seizure frequency.

Other neurotransmitter systems (i.e., serotonergic, noradrenergic, and cholinergic) can influence the thalamocortical circuits and therefore influence absence seizure frequency. However, the GABA system appears to be the most important system in the pathogenesis of absence seizures.

ABSENCE SYNDROMES

Most physicians use the term *petit mal* to describe a syndrome of simple absence seizures in school-age children who are otherwise neurologically and intellectually normal. The ILAE classification of epileptic syndromes recognizes three syndromes of the idiopathic generalized epilepsies that prominently feature absence seizures (63,64). These are childhood absence epilepsy (pyknolepsy), juvenile absence epilepsy, and juvenile myoclonic epilepsy (impulsive petit mal).

Pyknolepsy describes typical absence seizures (i.e., both simple and complex) in children between the ages of 3 to 5 years and puberty who are otherwise normal. There is a strong genetic predisposition, and girls are more frequently affected. The absences are very frequent, occurring at least several times daily, and tend to cluster. The EEG reveals a bilateral, synchronous symmetrical 3-Hz spike-and-wave discharge with normal interictal background activity. The absences may remit during adolescence, but generalized tonic-clonic seizures often develop.

Juvenile absence epilepsy begins around puberty and differs from pyknolepsy in that the seizures are more sporadic and retropulsive movements are less common. This syndrome blurs with juvenile myoclonic epilepsy, as generalized tonic-clonic seizures and myoclonic seizures are often seen on awakening. Sex distribution is equal, and on EEG the spike-waves are often slightly faster than 3 Hz.

Impulsive petit mal, or juvenile myoclonic epilepsy of Janz (JME), is a syndrome that appears between 12 and 18 years of age with early morning mild to moderate myoclonic jerks of the neck, shoulders, and arms. These may be quite subtle, as the patient may only realize in retrospect that he feels shaky or nervous for an hour or two after awakening. The irregular upper body jerks may cause the patient to drop or even toss items. Generalized tonic-clonic seizures occur in almost all patients (65) and are often the reason for seeking medical advice. The myoclonic jerks may actually culminate in a generalized tonic-clonic seizure. The seizures are aggravated by lack of sleep or premature awakening,

fatigue, stress, alcohol, or recreational drugs (65,66). Between 15 percent and 40 percent of these patients have absence seizures as well (67–69). Studies are difficult to compare, as some include patients that appear to be in overlap groups that do not quite fit the JME classification, for example, adolescent females with photically sensitive myoclonic jerks and an occasional generalized tonic-clonic seizure. The interictal EEG shows fast (3.5 to 6 Hz), often irregular, spike-and-wave and multiple-spike-and-wave complexes (see Figure 16-3). Rapid, 10- to 16-Hz spikes, followed by irregular slow waves, often occur during the myoclonic seizures. Photic stimulation and sleep deprivation are particularly good activation procedures.

A particular diagnostic difficulty is predicting whether a patient with absences will develop the JME syndrome. The distinction is more than academic because JME persists for life and AED withdrawal is not recommended. In JME, absences may begin 1 to 9 years before the onset of myoclonic jerks and tonic-clonic seizures (69). Recent comparative studies of absence seizures have identified characteristic EEG differences between these syndromes (69,70). The ictal EEG discharge tends to be briefer in JME (mean 6.6 ± 4.2 sec) than in childhood absence (12.4 ± 2.1 sec) or juvenile absence epilepsy (16.3 ± 7.1 sec). Frequent multiple spikes of variable frequency and amplitude, and fragmented interictal spike-and-wave discharges, occur in JME.

Absence seizures may also be prominent in the generalized symptomatic epilepsies. These syndromes include the Lennox-Gastaut syndrome, epilepsy with myoclonic-astatic seizures, and epilepsy with myoclonic absences. These absence seizures tend to be atypical and carry a much less favorable prognosis.

Lennox-Gastaut syndrome usually appears in preschool-age children, although it may manifest between ages 1 and 8 years. It typically comprises tonic, atonic, and absence seizures but also myoclonic, generalized tonic-clonic, or partial seizures. The EEG shows slow spike-and-wave less than 3 Hz, with an abnormal background and often multifocal abnormalities. A diverse group of etiologies, from structural to metabolic, may be identified in 60 percent of cases. The seizures are usually refractory, and developmental outcome is poor.

Epilepsy with myoclonic-astatic seizures is a syndrome with onset between the ages of 7 months and 6 years, usually between 2 and 5 years. The developmental background is usually normal, and there is a hereditary predisposition. Boys are affected twice as often unless onset is within the first year. The seizures are myoclonic, astatic, myoclonic-astatic, absence, and tonic-clonic. Status epilepticus is frequent. The EEG is initially normal except for 4- to 7-Hz theta rhythms, but it develops irregular fast spike-

or multiple spike-and-wave complexes. The prognosis is variable.

The syndrome of epilepsy with myoclonic absences (71) is characterized by absence seizures accompanied by severe bilateral rhythmical clonic, and sometimes tonic, activity. Age of onset averages 7 years, and boys are more often affected. The ictal EEG discharges are similar to those of pyknolepsy. Seizures are frequent and less responsive to medication than those of pyknolepsy. Mental deterioration and evolution to Lennox-Gastaut syndrome may occur.

MANAGEMENT

The extent of diagnostic evaluation required in patients with absence seizures is variable and depends somewhat on which epileptic syndrome might best "fit" the patient. A patient who meets the criteria for one of the idiopathic generalized syndromes by clinical and electroencephalographic criteria requires no further studies. Not every patient, however, fits these descriptions. The presence of typical absence seizures with consistent EEG ictal and interictal features and normal intelligence and neurologic examinations is reassuring that further tests are not necessary. Atypical features or history of developmental delay warrant an imaging study, generally MRI, and possibly more specific tests such as lumbar puncture, metabolic studies, and tissue examinations.

Antiepileptic drug therapy is recommended for all children with adequate documentation of absence seizures. Although they are not life-threatening, they may lead to poor school performance, ridicule, and accidents. As even a 1-second generalized spike-and-wave discharge sometimes affects cognitive function (32), it is prudent to try to control the seizures as well as possible with minimal drug toxicity.

Injury prevention counseling should not be underestimated. Accidental injury is common in patients with absence epilepsy and indeed usually occurs after anticonvulsant medication is already started (72). Specific recommendations, including mandatory use of bicycle helmets and avoidance of unsupervised swimming or climbing without protection, are common-sense precautions for any child. JME is particularly associated with a higher accident risk, and driving restrictions, although state-regulated, are applicable while seizures are active.

The primary drugs of choice are ethosuximide, valproic acid, and clonazepam. All three agents are effective, and a previously untreated patient receiving any one of these medications has a better than 70 percent chance of significant reduction or total elimination of seizures (72–79). A single agent should be chosen and, after appropriate laboratory studies, initiated at a low dose and gradually increased. AED levels may

be helpful, but dose changes in either direction should follow clinical indications. Upon dosage modifications, drug levels should be obtained only after sufficient time has elapsed to reach steady-state serum concentrations. The efficacy of ethosuximide and clonazepam may be noted with 48 hours, but valproic acid may take 3 to 4 weeks for full effect (79,80).

Many clinicians begin therapy with ethosuximide, primarily because of the rare but severe hepatotoxicity and pancreatitis associated with valproic acid (38,81–83). Valproic acid is equally effective (84–87) and generally considered the drug of choice in the patient who has both absence seizures and generalized tonic-clonic seizures (16,57). Clonazepam is usually reserved for refractory cases because of the high incidence of drowsiness and behavioral side effects (73,74) (see Chapters 27, 31, and 32).

The combination of ethosuximide and valproic acid may be more effective than either drug alone (87,88), although drug interactions do occur, requiring monitoring of clinical toxicity and serum drug levels (89). The combination of valproic acid and clonazepam has been associated with precipitation of absence status (90) but this is rare.

There have been few studies evaluating the new AEDs in the absence epilepsies. Lamotrigine appears to be a promising drug in the treatment of absence seizures, with a number of studies demonstrating its efficacy (91–94). Lamotrigine has demonstrated some efficacy in the treatment of myoclonic absence seizures (95). In a small, open-label extension study Biton found that four of five patients with absence seizures had a 50 percent or greater reduction in seizure frequency with topiramate (96). Based on animal studies and limited clinical experience, it does not appear that vigabatrin is effective in the treatment of absence seizures (97). Felbamate may sometimes be useful in the treatment of absence seizures, although the drug is rarely used for this indication because of the associated aplastic anemia (98). Gabapentin also does not appear to be effective in the treatment of absences (99,100). Although trimethadione is rarely used because of its side-effect profile and significant teratogenic potential, it is an effective compound to be considered only in truly refractory absence seizures (101).

The cellular mechanisms of action of the antiabsence drugs remain unclear. Valproate increases GABA levels through several possible pathways, but the relevance of this mechanism to its clinical effect has not been demonstrated (102). Valproate has been shown to limit sustained high-frequency repetitive firing of action potentials at therapeutic levels using mouse neurons in cell culture (103). Clonazepam, along with other benzodiazepines and phenobarbital, augments postsynaptic GABA responses (103). The antiabsence action of ethosuximide is not known. Recent studies have demonstrated that dimethadione, the active metabolite of trimethadione, blocks the low threshold, transient (T-type) calcium current in thalamic neurons, an effect shared by ethosuximide but not phenytoin, carbamazepine, or valproate (101).

As discussed in the section on pathophysiology, the *lh/lh* genetic mouse model has contributed extensively to the investigation of the cellular and molecular mechanisms underlying absence seizures. The model has correctly predicted the therapeutic effects of ethosuximide, clonazepam, and valproate, in contrast to phenobarbital, phenytoin, and carbamazepine, against absence seizures. This same model demonstrated antiabsence efficacy of lamotrigine, proabsence effects of vigabatrin and tiagabine, and lack of effects by gabapentin and topiramate (62).

Duration of Therapy

The duration of therapy is variable, although a general rule is to taper patients off therapy after 2 seizure-free years in those with childhood absence epilepsy. The EEG is very helpful in this situation, as even a 1-second generalized spike-and-wave discharge can result in subtle functional impairment (32). A brief discharge in sleep, however, would not preclude drug withdrawal. Hyperventilation should be performed during the EEG for 3 to 5 minutes, and the presence of discharges indicates a high recurrence risk.

An important caveat is that knowledge of the patient's syndrome may significantly alter this plan. JME is a case in point. Between 80 percent and 90 percent of JME patients are controlled with valproate, alone or in combination with other antiepileptic medications (104). Valproate is effective against the gamut of generalized seizure components of JME — myoclonic, tonic-clonic, and absence seizures. Relapses are nearly always associated with drug noncompliance or precipitating events in the patient's life, be it stress, anxiety, sleep deprivation, alcohol consumption, or menses. The disorder is life-long, however, and antiepileptic therapy generally should be continued indefinitely or relapses are likely to occur.

Withdrawal seizures may occur with ethosuximide and valproic acid but are more likely to be precipitated by rapid reduction of clonazepam (78). Clonazepam should not be tapered faster than 0.25 mg per week (105). Withdrawal seizures may be delayed weeks after stopping valproic acid.

Treatment of Absence Status Epilepticus

Absence status epilepticus is a unique form of nonconvulsive status epilepticus manifested by sustained impairment of consciousness associated with generalized, irregular, approximately 3-Hz spike-and-wave EEG discharges. Most patients are dull and confused but partially responsive and able to carry out tasks of daily living (106). They often exhibit facial twitching, eye blinking, staring, and automatisms (34,107–109). Absence status often presents as periods of stupor in adolescents with a history of childhood absences after a relatively seizure-free interval. The EEG may also show multispike-and-wave discharges or prolonged generalized bursts of spike activity or irregular slow spike-and-wave discharges (106). Treatment is usually with intravenous diazepam (109), although intravenous acetazolamide (500 mg, or 250 mg for children weighing less than 35 kg) has been advocated (110). Intravenous valproate is likely to be useful for treatment of absence status (see Chapter 31).

PROGNOSIS

The average age of cessation of absence seizures is 10.5 years (11); however, some children continue to have absence seizures beyond puberty. Typical absence seizures generally have a favorable prognosis, with remission rates of approximately 80 percent (6,111–113). A recent analysis of 52 patients with childhood absence by Loiseau and coworkers (65) demonstrated complete control in 95 percent of patients with absence seizures only and in 77 percent of patients with absence plus generalized tonic-clonic seizures. In contrast, of 62 patients with juvenile absence epilepsy, control was achieved in 77 percent of patients with absence seizures only and in 37 percent of patients with absence plus generalized tonic-clonic seizures (66).

Patients with pyknolepsy have a favorable response to medication and good prognosis for remission when taken off medication. Sato and colleagues (21) identified favorable prognostic signs for "outgrowing" both absence seizures and other seizure types as a negative family history of epilepsy, normal EEG background activity, and normal intelligence. Yet a recent long-term follow-up study of 72 patients having mean seizure onset at 5.7 years (range, 1–14 years) and studied at a mean age of 20.4 years (range, 12–31 years) determined only a 65 percent remission rate, and furthermore that 15 percent of the total cohort developed JME. Adverse prognostic factors were cognitive difficulties at diagnosis, history of absence status, presence of generalized tonic-clonic or myoclonic seizures during AED treatment, abnormal EEG background, and family history of generalized seizures in first-degree relatives (13). Also troubling is the observation of psychosocial difficulties, in the areas of academic-personal and behavioral categories, in a recent report on 56 young adults having a history of typical childhood absence epilepsy. Remission occurred in 32 (57 percent) of the patients, and the least favorable outcomes correlated with persistence of seizures (115).

Juvenile absence epilepsy may persist in adulthood, and JME, as already outlined, does not usually remit spontaneously. Patients with the symptomatic generalized epilepsies have an even dimmer outlook. In the Lennox-Gastaut syndrome, seizures tend to be frequent and refractory, and status epilepticus is common. The course and prognosis of epilepsy with myoclonic-astatic seizures and with myoclonic absences are variable but less favorable than that of pyknolepsy. Onset of generalized tonic-clonic seizures before absence seizures carries a poorer prognosis than the reverse order (21). Other poor prognostic factors are onset before 4 years of age, impaired intelligence, abnormal neurologic examination, other seizure types, and abnormal interictal EEG background activity.

REFERENCES

1. Temkin O. *The Falling Sickness. A History of Epilepsy from the Greeks to the Beginnings of Modern Neurology.* 2nd ed. Baltimore: Johns Hopkins University Press, 1971.

2. Ajmone-Marsan D, Lewis WR. Pathologic findings in patients with "centrencephalic" electroencephalographic patterns. *Neurology* 1960; 10:922–930.

3. Commission on Classification and Terminology of the International League Against Epilepsy. Proposal for revised clinical and electroencephalographic classification of epileptic seizures. *Epilepsia* 1981; 22:489–501.

4. Blom S, Heijbel J, Bergfors PG. Incidence of epilepsy in children: a follow-up study three years after the first seizure. *Epilepsia* 1978; 19:343–350.

5. Blume WT, David RB, Gomez MR. Generalized sharp and slow wave complexes. Associated clinical features and long-term follow-up. *Brain* 1973; 96:289–306.

6. Cavazzuti GB. Epidemiology of different types of epilepsy in school age children of Modena, Italy. *Epilepsia* 1980; 21:57–62.

7. Dalby MA. Epilepsy and 3 per second spike and wave rhythms. A clinical electroencephalographic and prognostic analysis of 346 patients. *Acta Neurol Scand* 1969; 45(Suppl. 40):1–83.

8. Livingston S, Torres I, Pauli LL, et al. Petit mal epilepsy. Results of a prolonged follow-up study of 117 patients. *JAMA* 1965; 194:227–232.

9. Okuma T, Kumashiro J. Natural history and prognosis of epilepsy: report of a multiinstitutional study in Japan. *Epilepsia* 1981; 22:35–53.

10. Hauser WA, Kurland LT. The epidemiology of epilepsy in Rochester, Minnesota, 1935 through 1967. *Epilepsia* 1975; 16:1–66.

11. Blume WT. Abnormal EEG: Epileptiform potentials. In: Blume WT, ed. *Atlas of Pediatric EEG.* New York: Raven Press, 1982:139–148.

12. Sato S, Dreifuss FE, Penry JK, et al. Long-term followup of absence seizures. *Neurology* 1983; 33:1590–1595.

13. Wirrel EC, Camfield CS, Camfield PR, Gordon KE, Dooley JM. Long-term prognosis of childhood absence epilepsy: remission or progression to juvenile myoclonic epilepsy. *Neurology* 1996; 47:912–918.

14. Rocca WA, Sharbrough FW, Hauser WA, Annegers JF, Schoenberg BS. Risk factors for absence seizures: a population-based case-control study in Rochester, MN. *Neurology* 1987; 37:1309–1314.

15. Penry JK, Porter RJ, Dreifuss FE. Simultaneous recording of absence seizures with videotape and electroencephalography. A study of 374 seizures in 48 patients. *Brain* 1975; 98:427–440.

16. Watanabe K, Negoro T, Matsumoto A, et al. Epileptic nystagmus associated with typical absence seizures. *Epilepsia* 1984; 25:22–24.

17. Sato S. Generalized seizures: Absence. In: Dreifuss FE, ed. *Pediatric Epileptology.* Littleton, MA: John Wright, 1983:65–91.

18. Holmes GL, McKeever M, Adamson M. Absence seizures in children: clinical and electrographic features. *Ann Neurol* 1987; 21:268–273.

19. McKeever M, Holmes GL, Russman BS. Speech abnormalities in seizures: a comparison of absence and partial complex seizures. *Brain Lang* 1983; 19:25–32.

20. Mirsky AF, Van Buren JM. On the nature of the "absence" in centrencephalic epilepsy: a study of some behavioral, electroencephalographic, and autonomic factors. *Electroencephalogr Clin Neurophysiol* 1965; 18:334–348.

21. Sato S, Dreifuss FE, Penry JK. Prognostic factors in absence seizures. *Neurology* 1976; 26:788–796.

22. Charlton MH, Yahr MD. Long-term follow-up of patients with petit mal. *Arch Neurol* 1967; 16:595–598.

23. Gibberd FB. The clinical features of petit mal. *Acta Neurol Scand* 1966; 42:176–190.

24. Gibberd FB. Prognosis of petit mal. *Brain* 1966; 89:531–538.

25. Loiseau P, Pestre M, Dartigues JF, et al. Long-term prognosis in two forms of childhood epilepsy: typical absence seizures and epilepsy with rolandic (centrotemporal) EEG foci. *Ann Neurol* 1983; 13:642–648.

26. So ES, King DW, Murvin AJ. Misdiagnosis of complex absence seizures. *Arch Neurol* 1984; 41:640–641.

27. Duchowny MS, Resnick TJ, Deray MJ, Alvarez LA. Video EEG diagnosis of repetitive behavior in early childhood and its relationship to seizures. *Ped Neurol* 1988; 4:162–164.

28. Niedermeyer E. Sleep electroencephalograms in petit mal. *Arch Neurol* 1965; 12:625–630.

29. Ross JJ, Johnson LC, Walter RD. Spike and wave discharges during stages of sleep. *Arch Neurol* 1966; 14:399–407.

30. Sato S, Dreifuss FE, Penry JK. The effect of sleep on spike-wave discharges in absence seizures. *Neurology* 1973; 23:1335–1345.

31. Adams DJ, Lüders H. Hyperventilation and six-hour EEG recording in evaluation of absence seizures. *Neurology* 1981; 31:1175–1177.

32. Porter RJ, Penry JK, Dreifuss FE. Responsiveness at the onset of spike-wave bursts. *Electroencephalogr Clin Neurophysiol* 1973; 34:239–245.

33. Browne TR, Penry JK, Porter RJ, et al. Responsiveness before, during, and after spike-wave paroxysms. *Neurology* 1974; 24:659–665.

34. Andermann F, Roble JP. Absence status: a reappraisal following review of thirty-eight patients. *Epilepsia* 1972; 31:177–187.

35. Farwell JR, Stuntz JT. Frontoparietal astrocytoma causing absence seizures and bilaterally synchronous epileptiform discharges. *Epilepsia* 1984; 25:695–698.

36. Madsden JA, Bray PF. The coincidence of diffuse electroencephalographic spike-wave paroxysms and brain tumors. *Neurology* 1966; 16:546–555.

37. Stevens JR. Focal abnormality in petit mal epilepsy. *Neurology* 1970; 20:1069–1076.

38. Kudo T, Sato K, Yagi K, Seino M. Can absence status epilepticus be of frontal lobe origin? *Acta Neurol Scand* 1995; 92:472–477.

39. Metrakos K, Metrakos JD. Genetics of convulsive disorders. II. Genetic and electroencephalographic studies in centrencephalic epilepsy. *Neurology* 1961; 11:474–483.

40. Doose H, Gerken H, Horstmann F, et al. Genetic factors in spike-wave absences. *Epilepsia* 1973; 14:57–75.

41. Delgado-Escueta AV, Greenberg DA, Treiman L, et al. Mapping the gene for JME. *Epilepsia* 1989; 30(S4):S8–S18.

42. Gloor P, Testa G. Generalized penicillin epilepsy in the cat: effect of intracarotid and intravertebral pentylenetetrazole and amobarbital injections. *Electroencephalogr Clin Neurophysiol* 1974; 36:499–515.

43. Gloor P. Generalized spike and wave discharges: a consideration of cortical and subcortical mechanisms of their genesis and synchronization. In: Petsche H, Brazier MAB, eds. *Synchronization of EEG Activities in Epilepsies*. New York and Vienna: Springer Verlag, 1972:382–402.

44. Gloor P. Generalized corticoreticular epilepsies. Some considerations on the pathophysiology of generalized bilaterally synchronous spike and wave discharges. *Epilepsia* 1968; 9:249–263.

45. Gloor P. Neurophysiological bases of generalized seizures termed "centrencephalic." In: Gastaut H, Jasper H, Bancaud J, et al., eds. *The Physiopathogenesis of the Epilepsies*. Springfield, IL: Charles C Thomas, 1969:209–246.

46. Coulter DA and Zhang Y. Thalamocortical rhythm generation in vitro: physiological mechanisms, pharmacological control, and relevance to generalized absence epilepsy. In: Malafosse A, Genton P, E Hirsch E, et al., eds. *Idiopathic Generalized Epilepsies: Clinical, Experimental, and Genetic Aspects*. London: John Libbey, 1994:123–131.

47. Crunelli V, Leresche N. A role for GABA$_B$ receptors in excitation and inhibition of thalamocortical cells. *TINS* 1991; 14:16–21.

48. Huguenard JR, Prince DA. Intrathalamic rhythmicity studied *in vitro*: nominal T current modulation causes robust anti-oscillatory effects. *J Neurosci* 1994; 14:5485–5502.

49. Steriade M, McCormick DA, Sejnowski TJ. Thalamocortical oscillations in the sleeping and aroused brain. *Science* 1993; 262:679–685.

50. Prevett MC, Duncan JS, Jones T, Fish DR, Brooks EB. Demonstration of thalamic activation during typical absence seizures using H$_2$(15)O and PET. *Neurology* 1995; 45:1396–1402.

51. Steriade M, Llinas RR. The functional states of the thalamus and the associated neuronal interplay. *Physiol Rev* 1988; 68:649–742.

52. Snead III OC. Basic mechanisms of generalized absence seizures. *Ann Neurol* 1995; 37:146–152.

53. Coulter DA, Huguenard JR, Prince DA. Specific petit mal anticonvulsants reduce calcium currents in thalamic neurons. *Neurosci Lett* 1989; 98:74–78.

54. Coulter DA, Huguenard JR, Prince DA. Characterization of ethosuximide reduction of low-threshold calcium current in thalamic neurons. *Ann Neurol* 1989; 25:582–593.

55. Hosford DA, Wang Y. Utility of the lethargic *(lh/lh)* mouse model of absence seizures in predicting the effects of lamotrigine, vigabatrin, tiagabine, gabapentin, and topiramate against human absence seizures. *Epilepsia* 1997; 38:408–414.

56. Liu Z, Vernes M, Depaulis A, Marescaux C. Involvement of intrathalamic GABA$_B$ neurotransmission in the control of absence seizures in the rat. *Neuroscience* 1992; 48:87–93.

57. Tsakiridou E, Bertollini L, de Curtis M, Avanzini G, Pape H-C. Selective increase in T-type calcium conductance of reticular thalamic neurons in a rat model of absence epilepsy. *J Neurosci* 1995; 15:3110–3117.

58. Hosford DA, Clark S, Cao Z, et al. The role of GABA-B receptor activation in absence seizures of lethargic *(lh/lh)* mice. *Science* 1992; 257:398–401.

59. Marescaux C, Vergnes M, Bernasconi R. GABA$_B$ receptor antagonists: potential new anti-absence drugs. *J Neural Transm* 1992; 35:179–188.

60. Marescaux C, Vergnes M, Depaulis A. Genetic absence epilepsy in rats from Strasbourg—a review. *J Neural Transm* 1992; 35(Suppl.):37–69.

61. Huguenard JR, Prince DA. Clonazepam suppresses GABA$_B$-mediated inhibition in thalamic relay neurons through effects in nucleus reticularis. *J Neurophysiol* 1994; 71:2576–2581.

62. Hosford DA, Wang Y. Utility of the lethargic *(lh/lh)* mouse model of absence seizures in predicting the effects of lamotrigine, vigabatrin, tiagabine, gabapentin, and topiramate against human absence seizures. *Epilepsia* 1997; 38:408–414.

63. Commission on Classification and Terminology of the International League Against Epilepsy. Proposal for classification of epilepsies and epileptic syndromes. *Epilepsia* 1985; 26:268–278.

64. Commission on Classification and Terminology of the International League Against Epilepsy. Proposal for

classification of epilepsies and epileptic syndromes. *Epilepsia* 1989; 30:389–399.

65. Asconape J, Penry JK. Some clinical and EEG aspects of benign juvenile myoclonic epilepsy. *Epilepsia* 1984; 25:108–114.

66. Dreifuss FE. JME: Characteristics of a primary generalized epilepsy. *Epilepsia* 1989; 30(Suppl 4):S1–S7.

67. Delgado-Escueta AV, Enrile-Bascal FE. Juvenile myoclonic epilepsy of Janz. *Neurology* 1984; 34:285–294.

68. Janz D. *Die Epilepsien*. Stuttgart: Thieme, 1969.

69. Panayiotopoulos CP, Obeid T, Waheed G. (1989): Absences in JME: a clinical and video-electroencephalographic study. *Ann Neurol* 25: 391–397.

70. Panayiotopoulos CP, Obeid T, Waheed G. Differentiation of typical absence seizures in epileptic syndromes. *Brain* 1989; 112:1039–1056.

71. Tassinari CA, Bureau M. Epilepsy with myoclonic absence. In: Roger J, Dravet C, Bureau M, Dreifuss FE, Wolf P, eds. *Epileptic Syndromes in Infancy, Childhood and Adolescence*. London: John Libbey, 1985:121–129.

72. Wirrel EC, Camfield PR, Camfield CS, Dooley JM, Gordon KE. Accidental injury is a serious risk in children with typical absence epilepsy. *Arch Neurol* 1996; 53:929–932.

73. Browne TR. Clonazepam: a review of a new anticonvulsant drug. *Arch Neurol* 1976; 33:326–332.

74. Browne TR. Clonazepam. *N Engl J Med* 1978; 299: 812–816.

75. Browne TR, Dreifuss FE, Dyken PR, et al. Ethosuximide in the treatment of absence (petit mal) seizures. *Neurology* 1975; 25:515–524.

76. Bruni J, Wilder BJ, Baumann AW, et al. Clinical efficacy and long-term effects of valproic acid therapy on spike-and-wave discharges. *Neurology* 1980; 30:42–46.

77. Holmes GL. Absence seizures. In: *Diagnosis and Management of Seizures in Children*. Philadelphia: WB Saunders, 1987:173–186.

78. Lund M, Trolle E. Clonazepam in the treatment of epilepsy. *Acta Neurol Scand* 1973; 49(Suppl 53):82–90.

79. Sherard ES, Steiman GS, Couri D. Treatment of childhood epilepsy with valproic acid: results of the first 100 patients in a 6-month trial. *Neurology* 1980; 30:31–35.

80. Dreifuss FE. Treatment of the nonconvulsive epilepsies. *Epilepsia* 1983; 24(Suppl 1): S45–S54.

81. Committee on Drugs. Valproic acid: benefits and risks. *Pediatrics* 1982; 70:316–319.

82. Dreifuss FE. How to use valproate. In: Morselli PL, Pippenger CE, Penry JK, eds. *Antiepileptic Drug Therapy in Pediatrics*. New York: Raven Press, 1983:219–227.

83. Schmidt D. Adverse effects of valproate. *Epilepsia* 1984; 25(Suppl 1):S44–S49.

84. Callaghan N, O'Hare J, O'Driscoll D, et al. Comparative study of ethosuximide and sodium valproate in the treatment of typical absence seizures (petit mal). *Dev Med Child Neurol* 1982; 24:830–836.

85. Santavuori P. Absence seizures: Valproate or ethosuximide? *Acta Neurol Scand* 1983; 68(Suppl 97):41–48.

86. Sato S, White BG, Penry JK, et al. Valproic acid versus ethosuximide in the treatment of absence seizures. *Neurology* 1982; 32:157–163.

87. Suzuki M, Maruyama H, Ishibashi Y, et al. A double-blind comparative trial of sodium dipropylacetate and ethosuximide in epilepsy in children with special emphasis on pure petit mal seizures. *Med Prog* 1972; 82:470–488.

88. Rowan AJ, Meijer JW, deBeer-Pawlikowski NKB, et al. Sodium valproate: serial monitoring of EEG and serum levels. *Neurology* 1979; 29: 1450–1459.

89. Mattson RH, Cramer JA. Valproic acid and ethosuximide interaction. *Ann Neurol* 1980; 7:583–584.

90. Jeavons PM. Non-dose-related side effects of valproate. *Epilepsia* 1984; 25(Suppl 1): S50–S55.

91. Besag FMC, Wallace SJ, Dulac O, et al. Lamotrigine for the treatment of epilepsy in childhood. *J Pediatr* 1995; 127:991–997.

92. Frank LM, Enlow T, Holmes GL, et al. Lamictal (lamotrigine) monotherapy for typical absence seizures in children. *Epilepsia* 1999; 40:973–979.

93. Fitton A, Goa KL. Lamotrigine. An update on its pharmacology and therapeutic use in epilepsy. *Drugs* 1995; 50:691–713.

94. Schlumberger E, Chavez F, Palacios L, et al. Lamotrigine in treatment of 120 children with epilepsy. *Epilepsia* 1994; 35:359–367.

95. Manonmani V, Wallace SJ. Epilepsy with myoclonic absences. *Arch Dis Child* 1994; 870:288–290.

96. Biton V. Preliminary open-label experience with topiramate in primary generalized seizures. *Epilepsia* 1997; 38(Suppl 10):S42–S44.

97. Michelucci R, Tassnari CA. Response to vigabatrin in relation to seizure type. *Br J Clin Pharmacol* 1989; 27(Suppl 1):119S–124S.

98. Theodore WH, Jensen PK, Kwan RMF. Felbamate. Clinical use. In: Levy RH, Mattson SN, Meldrum BS, eds. *Antiepileptic Drugs*. 4th ed. New York: Raven Press, 1995:817–822.

99. Chadwick D, Leiderman DB, Sauermann W, Alexander J, Garofalo E. Gabapentin in generalized seizures. *Epilepsy Res* 1996; 25:191–197.

100. Trudeau V, Myers S, LaMoreaux L, et al. Gabapentin in generalized seizures. *Epilepsy Res* 1996; 25:191–197.

101. Pellock JM, Coulter DA. Oxazolidinedione: Trimethodione. In: Levy RH, Mattson RH, Meldrum BS, eds. *Antiepileptic Drugs*. 4th ed. New York: Raven Press, 1995:689–694.

102. Fariello R, Smith MC. Valproate: mechanisms of action. In: Levy R, Mattson R, Meldrum B, Penry JK, Dreifuss FE, eds. *Antiepileptic Drugs*. 3rd ed. New York: Raven Press, 1989:567–575.

103. MacDonald RL, McLean MJ. Mechanisms of anticonvulsant drug action. *Electroencephalogr Clin Neurophysiol* 1987; 39 (Suppl):200–208.

104. Penry JK, Dean JC, Riela AR. JME: Long-term response to therapy. *Epilepsia* 1989; 30 (Suppl 4):S19–S23.

105. Schmidt D. How to use benzodiazepines. In: Morselli PL, Pippenger CE, Penry JK, eds. *Antiepileptic Drug Therapy in Pediatrics*. New York: Raven Press, 1983:271–280.

106. Porter RJ, Penry JK. Petit mal status. In: Delgado-Escueta AV, Wasterlain CG, Treiman DM, et al., eds. *Advances in Neurology: Status Epilepticus*. New York: Raven Press, Vol. 34, 1983:61–67.

107. Belafsky MA, Carwille S, Miller P, et al. Prolonged epileptic twilight states: continuous recordings with nasopharyngeal electrodes and videotape analysis. *Neurology* 1978; 28:239–245.

108. Geier S. Prolonged psychic absence seizures: a study of the absence status. *Epilepsia* 1978; 19:431–445.

109. Moe PG. Spike-wave stupor. *Am J Dis Child* 1971; 121:307–313.

110. Browne TR. Status epilepticus. In: Browne TR, Feldman RG, eds. *Epilepsy: Diagnosis and Management*. Boston: Little, Brown, 1983:341–354.

111. Annegers JF, Hauser WA, Elveback LR. Remission of seizures and relapse in patients with epilepsy. *Epilepsia* 1979; 20:729–737.

112. Sofijanov NG. Clinical evolution and prognosis of childhood epilepsies. *Epilepsia* 1982; 23:61–69.

113. Turnbull DM, Rawling MD, Weightman D, et al. A comparison of phenytoin and valproate in previously untreated adult epileptic patients. *J Neurol Neurosurg Psychiatry* 1982; 45:55–59.

114. Loiseau P, Duche B, Pedespan JM. Absence epilepsies. *Epilepsia* 1995; 36:1182–1186.

115. Wilder BJ, Ramsay RE, Murphy JV, et al. Comparison of valproic acid and phenytoin in newly diagnosed tonic-clonic seizures. *Neurology* 1983; 33:1474–1476.

CHAPTER 17

Progressive Myoclonus Epilepsies

Samuel F. Berkovic, M.D., F.R.A.C.P.

The syndrome of progressive myoclonus epilepsy (PME) consists of myoclonic seizures, tonic-clonic seizures, and progressive neurologic dysfunction, particularly ataxia and dementia. Onset may be at any age but is usually in late childhood or adolescence. Myoclonus in PME is typically fragmentary and multifocal and often is precipitated by posture, action, or external stimuli such as light, sound, or touch. It is particularly apparent in facial and distal limb musculature. Bilateral massive myoclonic jerks, which tend to involve proximal limb muscles, may also occur.

In its fully developed form with florid, unremitting myoclonic seizures and progressive neurologic deterioration, diagnosis of the PME syndrome can hardly be missed. Diagnosis may be more difficult in the early stages, and confusion with more benign epilepsies is common. There are a large number of causes of the PME syndrome; most are due to specific genetic disorders, which can now be accurately diagnosed in life. Spectacular advances in the molecular genetics of these disorders have occurred in the last few years (Table 17-1). Diagnosis of the specific type of PME is challenging, as most individual clinicians have limited experience with these rare disorders. The main causes of PME are described in subsequent sections. Description of the rarer forms can be found elsewhere (1–3).

UNVERRICHT-LUNDBORG DISEASE

Unverricht-Lundborg disease is the prototypic cause of PME (4,5). No storage material is present, but there is neuronal loss and gliosis, particularly affecting the cerebellum, medial thalamus, and spinal cord (6).

Clinical Features

Clinical onset is with myoclonus or tonic-clonic seizures between the ages of 8 and 13 years (mean 10, range

Table 17-1. Molecular Genetics of Major Progressive Myoclonus Epilepsies

Specific Disorder	Linkage	Gene
Unverricht-Lundborg disease	21q22	Cystatin B
Myoclonus epilepsy ragged-red fiber syndrome	mt DNA	t-RNA^{Lys}
Lafora disease	6q24	Tyrosine phosphatase
Late-infantile ceroid lipofuscinosis	11p15	Lysosomal peptidase
Finnish late-infantile variant ceroid lipofuscinoses	13q	Novel membrane protein
Late-infantile variant ceroid lipofuscinoses	15q	?
Juvenile ceroid lipofuscinosis	16p	Hydrophobic protein of unknown function
Adult ceroid lipofuscinosis	?	?
Sialidosis type I	6p21	Neuraminidase
Sialidosis type II	20q13	"Protective" protein

6–16). The myoclonus usually is quite severe and may be precipitated by movement, stress, and sensory stimuli. Repetitive morning myoclonus is also typical, frequently building up and culminating in a major tonic-clonic seizure (7,8). Seizures may be difficult to control, but progression in terms of ataxia and dementia is mild and late. The clinical course is variable, and there may be considerable intrafamily variation in the severity of the seizures. Some patients are relatively mildly affected and survive to old age. Others have a more fulminant course, with death within a few years of onset; this outcome seems to be rare now and may have been due to unrecognized deleterious effects of phenytoin (9,10).

The electroencephalogram (EEG) background may show some diffuse theta that increases over years as well as some frontal beta activity. Epileptic activity comprises 3–5 Hz spike wave or multiple spike-wave activity with the maximum field being anterior. Sporadic focal spikes, particularly in the occipital region may be seen but are usually not prominent. Photosensitivity typically is marked. The spike-wave activity is diminished during non–rapid eye movement (non-REM) sleep (8,11).

Genetics

Unverricht-Lundborg disease is an autosomal recessive condition (12) initially recognized as a geographic cluster in Finland and eastern Sweden ("Baltic myoclonus"). An erroneous but frequently held view is that this disorder is confined to the Baltic region. Clusters of a phenotypically identical disorder, the so-called "Mediterranean myoclonus," occur in southern Europe and North Africa; (13). It is also found sporadically worldwide in caucasians, blacks, and Japanese (10,14,15).

The disorder was linked to the long arm of chromosome 21 (16). Subsequently, using a positional cloning approach, the gene for cystatin B was identified as the culprit (17). Cystatin B is an intracellular protease inhibitor. Mutations in cystatin B that cause a marked reduction in functional activity cause the disease, but the mechanism of this remains to be unraveled. A variety of mutations are observed, but the most frequent one is an expansion of a dodecamer repeat near the promoter region of the gene. The clinical prediction that cases seen outside the Baltic region have the same condition was confirmed by showing mutations in cystatin B in families from diverse racial backgrounds (18–20).

Diagnosis

Unverricht-Lundborg disease is recognized clinically by its characteristic age of onset and clinical pattern, with an absence of other clinical or pathologic features. Presently, there is no routine diagnostic laboratory test. Vacuoles have recently been reported in skin biopsies, but the diagnostic usefulness of this finding is uncertain (21). Molecular analysis of the cystatin B gene is likely to become the confirmatory diagnostic method in the near future, as screening for the expanded dodecamer repeat can be simply performed .

MYOCLONUS EPILEPSY WITH RAGGED RED FIBERS

The syndrome of myoclonus epilepsy with ragged red fibers (MERRF) has emerged as a one of the most common causes of PME. It may be familial or sporadic, and its clinical features and severity are extremely variable.

Clinical Features

Myoclonus epilepsy with ragged red fibers was first described in cases with a florid clinical myopathy and myoclonus epilepsy (22,23). It is now clear that the clinical spectrum of MERRF is extremely broad. It should be suspected in a wide variety of situations, even when clinical and pathologic evidence of myopathy are absent (24). Symptoms may begin at any age, and there may be marked intrafamily variation in the age of onset and clinical severity (24,25). The clinical features include myoclonus, tonic-clonic seizures, dementia, and ataxia, with less common findings of myopathy, neuropathy, deafness, and optic atrophy. Some cases show striking axial lipomas. Occasional patients or families have focal neurologic events, and there is an overlap with the syndrome of mitochondrial encephalomyopathy, lactic acidosis, and strokelike episodes (MELAS) in which strokelike episodes, frequently preceded by migrainous headaches with vomiting, are characteristic.

The EEG shows slowly progressive background slowing paralleling degree of clinical deterioration. There are generalized spike-and-wave discharges at 2–5 Hz or multiple spike-and-wave discharges. Sporadic occipital spikes and sharp waves may be seen. Prominent photosensitivity may occur. Non-REM sleep is disorganized, and spike-and-wave discharges are diminished (11,26).

Genetics

All familial cases of MERRF are transmitted through the maternal line and are examples of mitochondrial inheritance (25). The peculiarities of mitochondrial inheritance provide an explanation for the wide phenotypic variability in patients with MERRF and the extraordinary intrafamily variation.

A single base substitution at nucleotide pair 8344 of mitochondrial DNA, causing an A-to-G substitution in the tRNA^{Lys} gene occurs in many familial cases of MERRF (27). The fact that this mutation affects tRNA rather than a gene for a respiratory enzyme probably explains the heterogeneous results for respiratory enzyme assays reported in MERRF. This tRNA^{Lys} mutation has been confirmed in numerous laboratories around the world and appears to underlie most but not all familial cases and some sporadic examples of MERRF. Other rare identified molecular causes of MERRF are mutations at nucleotides 8356 and 8363 in the same tRNA^{Lys} (28,29) and mutations in tRNA^{Ser} (30), but in some cases no molecular defect has been found.

Diagnosis

Diagnosis can usually be suspected clinically but may be difficult to confirm with laboratory markers. The clinical clues to the diagnosis include deafness, optic atrophy, myopathy, lipomas, intrafamily variation in age of onset and severity, and a pattern of inheritance compatible with maternal transmission. Serum lactate, ragged red fibers, and respiratory enzyme activities in muscle can all be normal in patients known to be affected (e.g., family members of proven cases). Magnetic resonance spectroscopy of muscle may show elevated levels of inorganic phosphate and a decrease of the phosphocreatine to inorganic phosphate concentration ratio (31). When present, molecular defects in mitochondrial DNA can be detected in peripheral blood or muscle (32,33).

LAFORA DISEASE

Lafora disease is characterized by the presence of Lafora bodies, which are polyglucosan inclusions found in neurons and in a variety of other sites, including the heart, skeletal muscle, liver, and sweat gland duct cells (34,35).

Clinical Features

Onset of Lafora disease is between the ages of 10 and 18 years, with a mean age of onset of 14 years. Clinical features are myoclonus, tonic-clonic seizures, and relentless cognitive decline. Focal seizures, particularly that arise from the occipital regions, occur in approximately half the patients. Recognition of Lafora disease in its fully developed form is not difficult. At the onset, however, the disorder may resemble a typical benign adolescent generalized epilepsy with no evidence of cognitive decline. It also may present as a dementing illness with relatively infrequent seizures, or it may mimic a nonspecific secondary generalized epilepsy because myoclonus is not obvious (36,37). The prognosis of Lafora disease is dismal, with death occurring 2 to 10 years after onset and the mean age of death being 20 years.

The clinical picture, including the relatively narrow age range of onset and relentlessly progressive course to death within 2 to 10 years of onset, is constant in all reports with the exception of a few cases. These cases, sometimes erroneously labeled "type Lundborg," had symptoms beginning in late adolescence or early adult life with a milder protracted course. They may represent a genetic subtype of Lafora disease separate from the classic form (38,39).

At onset the EEG background is well organized, and there are multiple spike-and-wave discharges that are increased by intermittent photic stimulation. Erratic myoclonus is seen without EEG correlation. Spike-and-wave discharges are not accentuated during sleep. Over the next few months to years, the background deteriorates, the physiologic elements of sleep become disrupted, and only REM sleep can be identified. Multifocal, particularly posterior, epileptiform abnormalities appear in addition to the generalized bursts, and in the terminal phase of the illness the EEG is quite disorganized (40).

Genetics

Lafora disease is an autosomal recessive condition. The largest series have been reported from southern Europe (40), but it is found worldwide, apparently without a marked racial or ethnic predilection.

A locus for Lafora disease was identified on chromosome 6q23-25 (41), and the genetic defect on 6q was recently found to be in a gene for a tyrosine phosphatase (42). The mechanism by which tyrosine phosphatase defects cause accumulation of polyglucosans remains to be elucidated. Some families do not link to the 6q locus, so other undiscovered genetic defects may also cause the disease.

Diagnosis

The age of onset, eventual inexorable dementia, and frequent occurrence of focal occipital seizures are clinical clues to the diagnosis (36). Lafora bodies can be demonstrated in many tissues, but diagnosis is most simply made by examination of eccrine sweat gland ducts by a simple skin biopsy (35).

NEURONAL CEROID LIPOFUSCINOSES

The neuronal ceroid lipofuscinoses (NCL) are characterized by the accumulation of abnormal amounts of lipopigment in lysosomes. Five types — late infantile (Jansky-Bielschowsky, CLN2), late infantile variants (CLN5, CLN6), juvenile (Spielmeyer-Vogt-Sjögren, CLN3), and adult NCL (Kufs, CLN4) — may cause the PME syndrome. The infantile form (CLN1) presents differently, with regression, hypotonia, and impaired vision, and it is not considered here. The childhood forms are sometimes collectively referred to as Batten's disease.

Clinical Features

The late infantile form has an onset between 2.5 and 4 years. Seizures usually are the first manifestation, with myoclonic seizures, tonic-clonic seizures, atonic seizures, and atypical absences. Ataxia and psychomotor regression are seen within a few months of onset, with visual failure generally developing late.

Examination of the optic fundi reveals attenuated retinal vessels and macular degeneration. The seizures are usually intractable, dementia is relentless, and there is progressive spasticity, with death approximately 5 years after onset (37). The EEG shows background slowing and disorganization with generalized epileptiform discharges. Photosensitivity is marked, and single flashes may provoke giant posterior evoked responses. Visual evoked potentials (VEPs) are abnormally broad and of high amplitude and sensory evoked potentials (SEPs) are enlarged. The electroretinogram (ERG) becomes progressively attenuated (37,43).

The late infantile variant form, described in Finland, differs in that onset is later, between 5 and 7 years; psychomotor regression and visual failure occur earlier; myoclonic and tonic-clonic seizures generally appear at approximately age 8 years; and progression is somewhat slower (44). Electrophysiologic findings are similar to those of the late-infantile form except that the marked response to photic stimulation develops at approximately age 7–8 years and disappears by age 10–11 years, and the visual evoked response (VER), which initially is large, progressively attenuates (44).

Juvenile NCL begins between the ages of 4 and 10 years. The majority of patients present with visual failure and have gradual development of dementia and extrapyramidal features, with seizures being a relatively minor manifestation. Other patients present with myoclonus and tonic-clonic seizures with visual, cognitive, and motor signs developing later. This is sometimes called the early juvenile variant. Funduscopy reveals optic atrophy, macular degeneration, and attenuated vessels. Inheritance is autosomal recessive. The course is variable, with death approximately 8 years after onset (37,45). The EEG shows background slowing and generalized epileptiform discharges that often are of the slow-spike-and-wave type. Sleep activates the epileptic abnormality, but photic stimulation does not. VEPs are of low amplitude and sometimes cannot be elicited. The ERG is flat (37,43).

The adult form is considerably rarer. It can present as a PME syndrome around the age of 30, although other patients present with a picture of dementia and extrapyramidal or cerebellar disturbance. Visual auras may occur before some seizures. Blindness is notably absent, and the optic fundi are normal. The clinical course from onset to death is approximately 12 years (46). The EEG shows generalized fast spike-and-wave discharges with marked photosensitivity. Single flashes may evoke paroxysmal discharges. The background activity may be normal in the early stages, and ERGs are normal (11,46).

Genetics

The various forms are genetically distinct and occur worldwide but with peculiar patterns of geographic clustering. In Finland there are large numbers of infantile and juvenile cases, whereas in Newfoundland late-infantile and juvenile cases occur with increased frequency (47,48). All forms are autosomal recessive disorders. Kufs' disease, however, also occurs in families with dominant inheritance (49).

The storage material(s) in the NCLs has been extremely difficult to characterize and for many years was thought to be lipid. Subunit c of mitochondrial ATP synthase, a very hydrophobic protein, subsequently was identified as the major storage protein in an ovine model (50) and in human late-infantile, juvenile, and adult cases (50,51).

Considerable progress in the molecular genetics of this complex group of disorders has recently occurred. Juvenile NCL (CLN3) was linked to chromosome 16 (52), and the responsible gene was found to be a large hydrophobic protein whose function is as yet uncertain (53). The Finnish late-infantile variant (CLN5) links to chromosome 13q (54), and a novel putative transmembrane protein has recently been identified as the cause (55). The common late-infantile form (CLN2) was very difficult to map, but recently the locus for the classic form was found at 11p15 (56), and mutations in a lysosomal peptidase were found (57). Another variant late-infantile form (CLN6) was found to link to 15q21-23, but the gene has not yet been found (56). Loci for the adult forms are not presently known.

Diagnosis

Diagnosis may often be suspected clinically, particularly if there are visual changes. The electrophysiologic findings previously described previously may be helpful. Vacuolated lymphocytes may occur in the juvenile form. Neuroradiologic studies show cerebral atrophy and particularly cerebellar atrophy. Definitive diagnosis presently requires the demonstration of characteristic inclusions by electron microscopy. These can be found most simply in eccrine secretory cells. The inclusions take various forms, with curvilinear profiles being characteristic of a late-infantile NCL, fingerprint profiles being usual in the juvenile and adult forms, and granular osmiophilic deposits occurring in the infantile form. Considerable expertise may be required in the pathologic interpretation of the electron micrographs (58).

SIALIDOSES

The sialidoses are the least common of the major forms of PME. They are autosomal recessive disorders associated with deficiencies of a-N-acetyl-neuraminidase.

Clinical Features

In sialidosis type I ("cherry-red spot-myoclonus syndrome"), there is onset in adolescence with myoclonus, gradual visual failure, tonic-clonic seizures, ataxia, and a characteristic cherry-red spot in the fundus. The myoclonus is usually very severe. Lens opacities and a mild peripheral neuropathy with burning feet may occur. Dementia is absent (37,59).

Juvenile sialidosis type II presents as a PME with features similar to those of sialidosis type I except that onset is sometimes a little later. There may be additional features of coarse facies, corneal clouding, dysostosis multiplex, hearing loss, and low intellect, which may be present from early life (59,60).

The EEG background shows low-voltage fast activity, but some slowing can be seen in demented patients. Generalized spike-and-wave bursts are absent or infrequent; rather massive myoclonus is associated with trains of 10- to 20-Hz small vertex positive spikes preceding the electromyogram (EMG) artifact. Non-REM sleep is disorganized, and although myoclonus diminishes, the vertex spikes persist and become very frequent in deep sleep (37).

Genetics

Sialidosis type I is caused by a primary deficiency in a neuraminidase. Many of the published cases were of Italian origin (59). The locus of the sialidosis type I gene is on chromosome 6p21.3 (61).

Sialidosis type II comprises a complex group of phenotypes. The juvenile form presents as a PME and occurs predominantly in Japan. In addition to the neuraminidase deficiency, a partial deficiency of β-galactosidase is also found in most if not all cases (58,59). The combination of neuraminidase and β-galactosidase deficiency (galactosialidosis) is due to a lack of protein that is required to protect galactosidase from degradation and is essential for the catalytic action of neuraminidase (62,63). This protein, subsequently shown to be identical to cathepsin A, is coded for on chromosome 20 (64).

Diagnosis

Sialidoses should be identified clinically because of the characteristic optic fundus. Periodic acid-Schiff–positive inclusions may be seen in lymphocytes, bone marrow cells, neurons, and Kupfer cells. Diagnosis is confirmed by grossly elevated urinary sialyloligosaccharides and by a deficiency of cryolabile a-N-acetylneuraminidase in leukocytes or cultured fibroblasts (59).

DIFFERENTIAL DIAGNOSIS

Distinguishing PME from Other Epilepsies and Myoclonic Syndromes

It usually is not difficult to diagnose the syndrome of PME some years after onset with the distinctive diagnostic triad of myoclonic seizures, tonic-clonic seizures, and progressive neurologic decline. At the beginning of the illness, however, the clinical and EEG features may be similar to those of benign idiopathic generalized epilepsies, particularly mimicking juvenile myoclonic epilepsy. Initial response to therapy may be relatively favorable. However, seizures may become more frequent with the passage of time, and progressive neurologic decline occurs. Failure to respond to therapy and progressive neurologic signs should lead to consideration of the presence of a PME. Conversely, the clinical picture of patients with idiopathic generalized epilepsies may mimic that of PME if they are inappropriately treated and intoxicated with antiepileptic drugs leading to ataxia, impaired cognitive function, and poorly controlled seizures.

Myoclonus in PMEs is usually quite severe, but in some patients it may be relatively obscure, with convulsive seizures and intellectual decline dominating the clinical picture, leading to a misdiagnosis of a nonspecific symptomatic (secondary) generalized epilepsy or Lennox-Gastaut syndrome. In such cases, a careful search for myoclonus should lead to consideration of the PME syndrome.

Neurophysiologic assessment may also provide clues to the presence of a PME. The EEG background rhythm may be relatively well preserved in the early phases, but generalized slow activity appears as the condition progresses. This is particularly so in those forms of PME associated with relentless dementia, such as Lafora disease and NCL. Generalized epileptiform abnormalities are seen during the resting record, usually in the form of fast spike-and-wave, multiple spike-and-wave, or multiple spike discharges. Photosensitivity is common and may be marked. Focal, particularly posterior, epileptiform abnormalities are common in Lafora disease but also may occur in other forms (11). Somatosensory evoked potentials (SEPs) frequently show giant responses (65).

PMEs should be distinguished from degenerative disorders in which seizures and/or myoclonus can occur but do not form part of the clinical core or usual initial presentation of the disorder. The causes of such progressive encephalopathies with seizures are numerous and include GM_2 gangliosidosis, nonketotic hyperglycinemia, Niemann-Pick type C, juvenile Huntington's disease, Alzheimer's disease, and so forth. The distinction between this diverse group of disorders and the PMEs, while not absolute, is clinically useful and provides a practical framework on which to begin specific differential diagnosis. For example, typical Alzheimer's disease may have myoclonus as a relatively late feature and would not be confused with a PME. Rare early-onset cases may, however, present as a PME in early adult life (66). Myoclonus is also prominent in certain static encephalopathies, of which postanoxic myoclonus (Lance-Adams syndrome) is the best known. The absence of progression and the usual clear history of the causative encephalopathy enable clear distinction from PME.

The PME syndrome should also be distinguished from the *progressive myoclonic ataxias*. This term was introduced to denote a group of patients, usually adults, with progressive ataxia and myoclonus but with few if any tonic-clonic seizures and little or no evidence of dementia (14). Previously, some authors used the term *Ramsay Hunt syndrome* for these patients, although others used this term for quite different clinical groups, which led to considerable confusion in the literature. The causes of progressive myoclonic ataxia partially overlap with those of PME but also include spinocerebellar degeneration, celiac disease, and Whipple's disease. While it is now possible to specifically diagnose most patients with the PME syndrome in life (see next section), a larger proportion of carefully studied cases with progressive myoclonic ataxia remain without a known specific cause (14,67).

Recently, Japanese authors have highlighted a condition of benign myoclonic epilepsy of adulthood. In this autosomal dominant disorder, onset is usually between 20 and 40 years, with myoclonus and rare tonic-clonic seizures. Generalized epileptiform EEG abnormalities and giant SEPs are present, but there is little or no evidence of progression (68,69). This condition may be the same as or similar to that previously described in the German literature as myoclonus epilepsy of Hartung type (38).

Finally, the condition of benign familial myoclonus should be distinguished. In this autosomal dominant disorder, nonepileptic myoclonus begins in the first three decades of life but is not associated with major seizures, epileptiform EEG abnormalities, or neurologic deterioration (70)

Diagnosing the Specific Type of PME

Once the clinician is convinced that a patient has the PME syndrome, the critical question is to determine which specific disorder is present. This is essential for proper clinical and genetic counseling of the family (see "Treatment" section).

It is now possible to provide a specific diagnosis in life for the majority of patients with PME using clinical methods and minimally invasive investigations. An approach to this problem has been described previously. The clinician should first consider the five major disorders causing PME. Once these conditions are excluded, the rarer disorders should be considered (1,3).

Clinical Features

Although patients with the PME syndrome superficially may appear to have similar clinical features, knowledge of the specific clinical patterns of the common causes of PME often allows the differential diagnosis to be narrowed. Age at onset of symptoms provides some guidance in making the diagnosis, although MERRF may begin at any age. Certain seizure patterns are helpful; very prominent myoclonus suggests Unverricht-Lundborg disease, MERRF, or sialidosis. Partial seizures, particularly of occipital origin, can occur in a variety of the disorders but are often noted in Lafora disease. Characteristic fundal changes are almost invariable in sialidosis and are frequent in the NCLs. Dementia is a constant feature of Lafora disease and NCLs, whereas it is characteristically absent or mild in Unverricht-Lundborg disease and sialidosis type I. The presence of deafness, lipomas, optic atrophy, myopathy, or neuropathy are clinical pointers to MERRF. Neuropathy may also occur in sialidosis. Dysmorphic features are usual in sialidosis type II and may occur in MERRF.

Family History

A detailed family history, including examination of relatives, is essential. Recessive inheritance is usual, and the finding of parental consanguinity or early clinical signs in asymptomatic siblings would support this pattern. Maternal transmission is characteristic of MERRF. In MERRF and the autosomal dominant disorders, older relatives may be found to have mild, incomplete forms of the condition (71).

Neurophysiology

Findings that may be useful in specific diagnosis include vertex spikes as the main epileptiform abnormality in sialidosis, activation of epileptiform abnormalities in non-REM sleep in the sialidoses and the late-infantile and juvenile forms of NCL, photosensitivity to single flashes in late-infantile and adult NCL, and absent ERG in late-infantile and juvenile NCL (11).

Laboratory Findings

Hematologic examination may reveal lymphocyte vacuolation in sialidosis and in certain cases of NCL. Routine biochemical tests are not helpful, with the exception elevated lactate levels in blood and cerebrospinal fluid in some cases of MERRF.

Pathologic Studies

A tissue diagnosis is essential for a number of these disorders. Skin biopsy with or without skeletal-muscle biopsy is the initial procedure. Lafora disease can be reliably diagnosed by examining eccrine sweat-gland duct cells with stains for polysaccharides (35). The diagnosis of NCL may be suggested by an acid phosphatase stain, but electron microscopy of the skin biopsy specimen is essential for the definitive identification of inclusions. These inclusions are detectable in many cell types in the late-infantile form of the disease, but diagnostic inclusions may be limited to eccrine secretory cells in the juvenile and adult varieties (58). False-negative skin biopsies in Lafora disease and in late-infantile and juvenile NCL are due to failure to examine the appropriate cell type properly. In suspected Lafora disease sweat gland ducts must be included in the biopsy and properly examined. Where doubt remains, skin biopsy should be repeated because of the serious prognostic implications of the diagnosis of Lafora disease. The reliability of diagnosis of Kufs' disease from skin biopsy is not yet clear.

Study of muscle biopsy specimens with modified Gomori's trichome and oxidative enzyme reactions may demonstrate ragged-red fibers in MERRF. Abnormal mitochondria may be identified in muscle or skin using electron microscopy. Normal light and electron microscopic studies of muscle do not rule out the diagnosis of MERRF, and a second biopsy may be indicated in clinically suspicious cases.

Molecular Biological Studies

Molecular biological studies will play an increasing role in the diagnosis of the PMEs. A test for the common mitochondrial DNA mutation in MERRF is available in many centers. Molecular diagnosis for Unverricht-Lundborg disease should be available in the near future.

TREATMENT

Treatment of these disorders may be distressingly difficult. Accurate diagnosis is the first step, as informed genetic counseling must be given. It is very important to distinguish MERRF, which may show maternal inheritance, from autosomal recessive disorders, such as Unverricht-Lundborg disease, Lafora disease, sialidoses, and the NCLs, and from rare dominant families with Kufs' disease. Genetic counseling may now be extended to prenatal diagnosis in some cases. Specific diagnosis also allows an accurate prognosis to be given, including a realistic appraisal of the educational and vocational goals of the patient.

Valproate and/or clonazepam should be used for symptomatic control of myoclonus. Phenytoin has a clear deleterious effect in Unverricht-Lundborg disease (9,10), and neither should it be used in the other PMEs. Small doses of barbiturates may be helpful, but sedation should be avoided. Piracetam may be useful in certain cases (72,73). Care must be taken not to intoxicate the patient with drugs, although there is some evidence that carefully monitored polytherapy may be more effective in some patients than the usual practice of aiming for monotherapy (74). Zonisamide was found to be remarkably effective in two patients (75).

Programs of physical therapy may be of benefit, and attempts should be made to search for strategies that allow movement without precipitating myoclonus in individual patients. Alcohol may provide symptomatic benefit in some patients, but must be used judiciously (76).

Strategies for replacing enzymes in the storage disorders and augmenting mitochondrial function in the mitochondrial disorders are being developed, but presently they remain in the experimental phase, and results to date have been disappointing.

REFERENCES

1. Berkovic SF, Andermann F, Carpenter S, Wolfe LS. Progressive myoclonus epilepsies: specific causes and diagnosis. *N Engl J Med* 1986; 315:296–305.
2. Roger J. Progressive myoclonic epilepsy in childhood and adolescence. In: Roger J, Bureau M, Dravet C, Dreifuss FE, Perret A, Wolf P, eds. *Epileptic Syndromes in Infancy, Childhood and Adolescence.* 2nd ed. London: John Libbey, 1992:381–400.
3. Berkovic SF. Progressive myoclonus epilepsies. In: Engel J Jr, Pedley TA, eds. *Epilepsy: A Comprehensive Textbook.* Philadelphia: Lippincott-Raven, 1997:2455–2468.
4. Unverricht H. *Die Myoclonie.* Leipzig: Franz Deuticke, 1891:1–128.
5. Koskiniemi M. Baltic myoclonus. In: Fahn S, Marsden CD, Van Woert MH, eds. *Myoclonus.* New York: Raven Press, 1986:57–64. Advances in Neurology, Vol. 43.
6. Haltia M, Kristensson K, Sourander P. Neuropathological studies in three Scandinavian cases of progressive myoclonus epilepsy. *Acta Neurol Scand* 1969; 45:63–77.
7. Koskiniemi M, Donner M, Majuri H, Haltia M, Norio R. Progressive myoclonus epilepsy: a clinical and histopathological study. *Acta Neurol Scand* 1974; 50:307–332.
8. Koskiniemi M, Toivakka E, Donner M. Progressive myoclonus epilepsy: electroencephalographic findings. *Acta Neurol Scand* 1974; 50:333–359.

9. Iivanainen M, Himberg JJ. Valproate and clonazepam in the treatment of severe progressive myoclonus epilepsy. *Arch Neurol* 1982; 39:236–28.

10. Eldridge R, Iivanainen M, Stern R, Koerber T, Wilder BJ. "Baltic" myoclonus epilepsy: hereditary disorder of childhood made worse by phenytoin. *Lancet* 1983; 2:838–842.

11. Berkovic SF, So NK, Andermann F. Progressive myoclonus epilepsies: clinical and neurophysiological diagnosis. *J Clin Neurophysiol* 1991; 8:261–274.

12. Norio R, Koskiniemi M. Progressive myoclonus epilepsy: genetic and nosological aspects with special reference to 107 Finnish patients. *Clin Genet* 1979; 15:382–398.

13. Genton P, Michelucci R, Tassinari CA, Roger J. The Ramsay Hunt syndrome revisited: Mediterranean myoclonus versus mitochondrial encephalomyopathy with ragged-red fibers and Baltic myoclonus. *Acta Neurol Scand* 1990; 81:8–15.

14. Marseille Consensus Group. Classification of progressive myoclonus epilepsies and related disorders. *Ann Neurol* 1990; 28:113–116.

15. Cochius J, Figlewicz DA, Kalvianen et al. Unverricht-Lundborg disease: absence of non-allelic genetic heterogeneity. *Ann Neurol* 1993; 34:739–741.

16. Lehesjoki AE, Koskiniemi M, Sistonen P, et al. Localization of a gene for progressive myoclonus epilepsy to chromosome 21q22. *Proc Natl Acad Sci USA* 1991; 88:3696–3699.

17. Pennacchio LA, Lehesjoki AE, Stone NE, et al. Mutations in the gene encoding cystatin B in progressive myoclonus epilepsy (EPM1). *Science* 1996; 271:1731–1734.

18. Lafreniere RG, Rochefort DL, Chretien N, et al. Unstable insertion in the 5′ flanking region of the cystatin B gene is the most common mutation in progressive myoclonus epilepsy type 1, EPM1. *Nat Genet* 1997; 15:298–302.

19. Virtaneva K, D'Amato E, Miao J, et al. Unstable minisatellite expansion causing recessively inherited myoclonus epilepsy type, EPM1. *Nat Genet* 1997; 15:393–396.

20. Lalioti MD, Scott HS, Buresi C, et al. Dodecamer repeat expansion in cystatin B gene in progressive myoclonus epilepsy. *Nature* 1997; 386:847–851.

21. Cochius J, Carpenter S, Andermann E, et al. Sweat gland vacuoles in Unverricht-Lundborg disease: a clue to diagnosis. *Neurology* 1994; 44:2372–2375.

22. Tsairis P, Engel WK, Kark P. Familial myoclonic epilepsy syndrome associated with skeletal muscle mitochondrial abnormalities. *Neurology* 1973; 23:408.

23. Fukuhara N, Tokiguchi S, Shirakawa K, Tsubaki T. Myoclonus epilepsy associated with ragged-red fibres (mitochondrial abnormalities): disease entity or a syndrome? *J Neurol Sci* 1980; 47:117–133.

24. Berkovic SF, Carpenter S, Evans A, et al. Myoclonus epilepsy and ragged-red fibers (MERRF) 1. A clinical, pathological, biochemical, magnetic resonance spectroscopic and positron emission tomographic study. *Brain* 1989; 112:1231–1260.

25. Rosing HS, Hopkins LC, Wallace DC, Epstein CM, Weidenheim K. Maternally inherited mitochondrial myopathy and myoclonic epilepsy. *Ann Neurol* 1985; 17:228–237.

26. So N, Berkovic SF, Andermann F, et al. Myoclonus epilepsy and ragged-red fibers (MERRF) 2. Electrophysiological studies and comparison with the other progressive myoclonus epilepsies. *Brain* 1989; 112:1261–1276.

27. Shoffner JM, Lott MT, Lezza AMS, et al. Myoclonic epilepsy and ragged-red fiber disease (MERRF) is associated with a mitochondrial DNA tRNA^{Lys} mutation. *Cell* 1990; 61:931–937.

28. Silvestri G, Moraes CT, Shanske S, Oh SJ, DiMauro S. A new mtDNA mutation in the tRNA^{Lys} gene associated with myoclonic epilepsy and ragged red fibers (MERRF). *Am J Hum Genet* 1992; 51:1213–1217.

29. Ozawa M, Nishino I, Horai S, Nonaka I, Goto Y. Myoclonus epilepsy associated with ragged-red fibers—a G-to-A mutation at nucleotide pair 8363 in mitochondrial tRNALys in two families. *Muscle Nerve* 1997; 20:271–278.

30. Jaksch M, Klopstock T, Kurlemann G, et al. Progressive myoclonus epilepsy and mitochondrial myopathy associated with mutations in the tRNA$^{Ser(UCN)}$ gene. *Ann Neurol* 1998; 44:635–640.

31. Matthews PM, Berkovic SF, Shoubridge EA, et al. In vivo magnetic resonance spectroscopy of brain and muscle in a type of mitochondrial encephalomyopathy (MERRF). *Ann Neurol* 1991; 29:435–438.

32. Hammans SR, Sweeney MG, Brockington M, Morgan-Hughes JA, Harding AE. Mitochondrial encephalopathies: molecular genetic diagnosis from blood samples. *Lancet* 1991; 337:1311–1313.

33. Zeviani M, Amati P, Bresolin N, et al. Rapid detection of the A → G (8344) mutation of mtDNA in Italian families with myoclonus-epilepsy and ragged red fibers (MERRF). *Am J Hum Genet* 1991; 48:203–211.

34. Lafora GR, Glueck B. Beitrag zur Histopathologie der myoklonischen Epilepsie. *Z Gesamte Neurol Psychiatr* 1911; 6:1–14.

35. Carpenter S, Karpati G. Sweat gland duct cells in Lafora disease: diagnosis by skin biopsy. *Neurology* 1981; 31:1564–1568.

36. Roger J, Pellissier JF, Bureau M, et al. Le diagnostic precoce de la maladie de Lafora: importance des manifestations paroxystiques visuelles et interet de la biopsie cutanee. *Rev Neurol (Paris)* 1983; 139:115–124.

37. Rapin I. Myoclonus in neuronal storage and Lafora diseases. In: Fahn S, Marsden CD, Van Woert MH, eds. *Myoclonus*. New York: Raven Press, 1986:65–85. Advances in Neurology, Vol. 43.

38. Diebold K. Vier Erbtypen oder Krankheitsformen der progressiven Myoklonusepilepsien. *Arch Psychiatr Nervenkr* 1972; 215:362–375.

39. Footitt DR, Quinn N, Kocen R, Oz B, Scaravilli F. Familial Lafora body disease of late onset: report of four cases in one family and a review of the literature. *J Neurol* 1997; 244:40–44.

40. Tassinari CA, Bureau-Paillas M, Dalla Bernardina B, et al. La maladie de Lafora. *Rev Electroencephalogr Neurophysiol Clin* 1978; 8:107–122.

41. Serratosa JM, Delgado-Escueta AV, Posada I, et al. The gene for progressive myoclonus epilepsy of the Lafora type maps to chromosome 6q. *Hum Mol Genet* 1995; 4:1657–1664.

42. Minassian BA, Lee JR, Herbrick JA, et al. Mutations in a gene encoding a novel protein tyrosine phosphatase cause progressive myoclonus epilepsy. *Nat Genet* 1998; 20:171–174.

43. Pampiglione G, Harden A. So-called neuronal ceroid lipofuscinosis: neurophysiological studies in 60 children. *J Neurol Neurosurg Psychiatry* 1977; 40:323–330.

44. Santavuori P, Rapola J, Sainio K, Raitta Ch. A variant of Jansky-Bielschowsky disease. *Neuropediatrics* 1982; 13:135–141.

45. Lake BD, Cavanagh NPC. Early-juvenile Batten's disease: a recognisable subgroup distinct from other forms of Batten's disease. *J Neurol Sci* 1978; 36:265–271.

46. Berkovic SF, Carpenter S, Andermann F, Andermann E, Wolfe LS. Kufs' disease: a critical reappraisal. *Brain* 1988; 111:27–62.

47. Rapola J, Santavuori P, Savilahti E. Suction biopsy of rectal mucosa in the diagnosis of infantile and juvenile types of neuronal ceroid lipofuscinoses. *Hum Pathol* 1984; 15:352–360.

48. Andermann E, Jacob JC, Andermann F, et al. The Newfoundland aggregate of neuronal ceroid-lipofuscinosis. *Am J Med Genet* 1988 (Suppl); 5:111–116.

49. Boehme DH, Cottrell JC, Leonberg SC, Zeman W. A dominant form of neuronal ceroid-lipofuscinosis. *Brain* 1971; 94:745–760.

50. Palmer DN, Fearnley IM, Medd IM, et al. Lysosomal storage of the DCCD reactive proteolipid subunit of mitochondrial ATP synthase in human and ovine ceroid lipofuscinosis. *Adv Exp Med Biol* 1990; 266:211–222.

51. Hall NA, Lake BD, Dewji NN, Patrick AD. Lysosomal storage of subunit c of mitochondrial ATP synthase in Batten's disease (ceroid-lipofuscinosis). *Biochem J* 1991; 275:269–272.

52. Gardiner M, Sandford A, Deadman M, et al. Batten disease (Spielmeyer-Vogt disease, juvenile onset neuronal ceroid lipofuscinosis) gene (CLN3) maps to human chromosome 16. *Genomics* 1990; 8:387–390.

53. Lerner TJ, Boustany RMN, Anderson JW, et al. Isolation of a novel gene underlying Batten disease, CLN3. *Cell* 1995; 6:949–957.

54. Savukoski M, Kestilä M, Williams R, et al. Defined chromosomal assignment of CLN5 demonstrates that at least four genetic loci are involved in the pathogenesis of human ceroid lipofuscinosis. *Am J Hum Genet* 1994; 55:695–701.

55. Savukoski M, et al. CLN5, a novel gene encoding a putative transmembrane protein mutated in Finnish variant late infantile neuronal ceroid lipofuscinosis. *Nat Genet* 1998; 19:286–288.

56. Sharp JD, Wheeler RB, Lake BD, et al. Loci for classical and a variant late infantile neuronal ceroid lipofuscinosis map to chromosomes 11p15 and 15q21-23. *Hum Mol Genet* 1997; 4:591–596.

57. Sleat DE, Donnelly RJ, Lackland H, et al. Associations of mutations in a lysosomal protein with classical late-infantile neuronal ceroid lipofuscinosis. *Science* 1997; 277:1802–1805.

58. Carpenter S, Karpati G. Andermann F, Jacob JC, Andermann E. The ultrastructural characteristics of the abnormal cytosomes in Batten-Kufs' disease. *Brain* 1977; 100:137–156.

59. Lowden JA, O'Brien JS. Sialidosis: a review of human neuraminidase deficiency. *Am J Hum Genet* 1979; 31:1–18.

60. Matsuo T, Egawa I, Okada S, et al. Sialidosis type 2 in Japan: clinical study in two siblings' cases and review of literature. *J Neurol Sci* 1983; 58:45–55.

61. Pshezhetsky AV, Richard C, Michaud L, et al. Cloning expression and chromosomal mapping of human sialidase and characterization of mutations in sialidosis. *Nat Genet* 1997; 15:316–320.

62. D'Azzo A, Hoogeveen A, Reuser AJJ, Robinson D, Galjaard H. Molecular defect in combined β-galactosidase and neuraminidase deficiency in man. *Proc Natl Acad Sci USA* 1982; 79:4535–4539.

63. Palmer DN, Martinus RD, Cooper SM, et al. Ovine ceroid lipofuscinosis: the major lipopigment protein and the lipid-binding subunit of mitochondrial ATP synthase have the same NH_2-terminal sequence. *J Biol Chem* 1989; 264:5736–5740.

64. Zhou'X-Y, van der Spoel A, Rottier R, et al. Molecular and biochemical analysis of protective protein/cathepsin A mutations; correlation with clinical severity in galactosialidosis. *Hum Mol Genet* 1996; 5:1977–1988.

65. Shibasaki H, Yamashita Y, Neshige R, Tobimatsu S, Fukui R. Pathogenesis of giant somatosensory evoked potentials in progressive myoclonic epilesy. *Brain* 1985; 108:225–240.

66. Melanson M, Nalbantoglou J, Berkovic SF, et al. Progressive myoclonus epilepsy in young adults with neuropathologic features of Alzheimer's disease. *Neurology* 1997; 49:1732–1733.

67. Marsden CD, Harding AE, Obeso JA, Lu CS. Progressive myoclonic ataxia (the Ramsay Hunt syndrome). *Arch Neurol* 1990; 47:1121–1125.

68. Kuwano A, Takakubo F, Morimoto Y, et al. Benign adult familial myoclonus epilepsy (BAFME): an autosomal dominant form not linked to the dentatorubral pallidoluysian atrophy (DRPLA) gene. *J Med Genet* 1996; 33:80–81.

69. Okino S. Familial benign myoclonus epilepsy of adult onset—a previouly unrecognized myoclonic disorder. *J Neurol Sci* 1997; 135:113–118.

70. Daube JR, Peters HA, Madison WIS. Hereditary essential myoclonus. *Arch Neurol* 1966; 15:587–594.

71. Berkovic SF, Cochius J, Andermann E, Andermann F. Progressive myoclonus epilepsies: clinical and genetic aspects. *Epilepsia* 1993; 34(Suppl 3):S19–S30.

72. Obeso JA, Artieda J, Luquin MR, et al. Antimyoclonic action of piracetam. *Clin Neuropharmacol* 1986; 9:58–64.

73. Koskiniemi M, Van Vleymen B, Hakamies L, Lamusoo S, Taalas J. Piracetam relieves symptoms in progresssive myoclonus epilepsy; a multicentre randomised, double blind, crossover study comparing efficacy and safety of three dosages of oral piracetam with placebo. *J Neurol Neurosurg Psychiatry* 1998; 64:344–348.

74. Obeso JA, Artieda J, Rothwell JC, et al. The treatment of severe action myoclonus. *Brain* 1989; 112:765–77.

75. Henry TR, Leppik IE, Gumnit RJ, Jacobs M. Progressive myoclonus epilepsy treated with zonisamide. *Neurology* 1988; 38:928–931.

76. Genton P, Guerrin R. Antimyoclonic effects of alcohol in progressive myoclonus epilepsy. *Neurology* 1990; 40:1412–1416.

CHAPTER 18

Localization-Related Epilepsies: Simple Partial Seizures, Complex Partial Seizures, Benign Focal Epilepsy of Childhood, and Epilepsia Partialis Continua

G. Arunkumar, M.D., Prakash Kotagal, M.D., and A. David Rothner, M.D.

The International Classification of Epilepsies and Epileptic syndromes (1) divides epilepsy first on the basis of whether the seizures are partial (localization-related epilepsies) or generalized (generalized epilepsies) and second by etiology (idiopathic, symptomatic or cryptogenic epilepsy). Idiopathic epilepsies are defined by age-related onset, clinical and electroencephalographic characteristics, and a presumed genetic etiology. Symptomatic epilepsies comprise syndromes based on anatomic localization and are considered to be the consequence of a known or suspected disorder of the central nervous system. Cryptogenic epilepsies are presumed to be symptomatic, but the etiology is not known. Localization-related epilepsies include the following types of seizures:

1. Simple partial seizures
2. Complex partial seizures
   a. With impairment of consciousness at onset
   b. Simple partial onset followed by impairment of consciousness.
3. Partial seizures evolving to generalized tonic-clonic (GTC) convulsions
   a. Simple partial evolving into GTC
   b. Complex partial evolving into GTC including those with simple partial onset

DEFINITIONS

A simple partial seizure is one that arises from a localized area within one hemisphere without impairment of consciousness. A complex partial seizure is a partial onset seizure that is characterized by impaired consciousness, unresponsiveness, and automatic behavior often followed by postictal confusion. Impaired consciousness is defined as the inability to respond normally to exogenous stimuli by virtue of altered awareness or responsiveness (2). *Awareness* refers to the patient's contact with events during the period in question and its recall (2), whereas *responsiveness* is the ability of the patient to carry out simple commands or willed movements.

ETIOLOGY

By definition, partial seizures imply the presence of a focal abnormality in one cerebral hemisphere. A definite etiological factor can be identified by magnetic resonance imaging (MRI) in approximately 75 percent to 90 percent of patients with partial seizures (3–5). These include birth asphyxia, intrauterine infections (toxoplasmosis, cytomegalovirus, rubella, and syphilis), congenital anomalies head trauma, meningitis, viral encephalitis, parasitic infections (cysticercosis and echinococcosis), neoplasms, arteriovenous malformations, cerebral embolization from congenital heart disease, or disorders affecting the intracranial vessels as in fibromuscular dysplasia and moyamoya disease. Head injury and viral encephalitis have a predilection for the temporal lobe (6–7). Approximately 30 percent of patients who undergo surgical treatment for intractable partial seizures have a foreign tissue lesion detected on pathological examination (8). Mesial temporal sclerosis (MTS) has been established as a causative factor in 50 percent to 60 percent of adolescents and adults with temporal lobe epilepsy (TLE) (9–11). Hippocampal pathology shows neuronal loss and gliosis in the Sommer sector, end folium, and dentate gyrus in 50 percent of cases (12). However, other etiologies predominate in children below the age of 12 years. Duchowny and coworkers found in their surgical series of 16 patients with TLE, only 2 had MTS, 7 had abnormalities of neuroblast migration, and 3 had ganglioglioma (13). The common tumors associated with intractable partial epilepsy include low-grade gliomas, gangliogliomas, and dysembryoplastic neuroepitheliomas (DNT) (14,15). Neuronal migration disorders have been increasingly recognized as a cause of epilepsy. Focal cortical dysplasia (16–18), lissencephaly (19), band heterotopia (20), nodular heterotopia (21), the bilateral perisylvian syndrome (22–23), and schizencephaly (24) often present with seizures. In a study correlating pathology and MRI findings in children with intractable partial seizures, Kuzniecky and coworkers (25) described the presence of cortical lesions in 23 percent of patients. Tuberous sclerosis, Sturge-Weber syndrome, neurofibromatosis, epidermal nevus syndrome, and hypomelanosis of Ito are neurocutaneous disorders associated with early-onset seizures (26). Coexistence of certain tumors such as ganglioglioma and DNT with cortical dysplasia, most frequently observed in the pediatric population, may suggest a hamartomatous nature of the neoplasms (27–28). The association of hippocampal sclerosis with cortical dysplasia remote from the mesial structures is well established in patients with TLE (29–30).

SEIZURE PHENOMENA

The symptomatology of partial seizures depends greatly on the location of the seizure focus within the cerebral cortex. Although a given symptom may occur with seizures arising from different locations, the combined information from seizure symptomatology and electroencephalogram (EEG) findings enables one to determine the location of seizure focus. Simple partial seizures with motor manifestations may result from ictal onset within or propagation to the precentral and postcentral gyri of the contralateral hemisphere

or the supplementary motor area (31). The ictal symptomatology of epileptic seizures in general is a reflection of activation of symptomatogenic zones. This activation is usually the result of spreading of the epileptiform discharges from the epileptogenic zone to adjacent cortex, which when activated produces the ictal semiology. Auras consist exclusively of subjective warning symptoms and usually occur at the beginning of a seizure; depending on methodology and selection of patients, auras have been reported anywhere from 20 percent to 90 percent of those with partial-onset seizures (32–34). Complex partial seizures (CPS) arise from the temporal lobes in the majority of cases. However, in 15 percent to 20 percent of CPS an extratemporal focus in the mesial frontal, opercular insular region, cingulate gyrus, orbitofrontal cortex is seen (35). Postictal dysfunction has localizing value but does not reliably identify the site of ictal onset. The International Classification of Epileptic Seizures provides a useful approach to understanding the symptomatology of partial seizures (2).

Simple Partial Seizures with Motor Signs

Simple partial seizures with motor signs are the most common form of simple partial seizures because of the prominent representation of the motor cortex and high epileptogenicity of the frontal cortex. These symptoms are contralateral (at least at onset) and usually consist of positive (irritative) symptoms, less often negative (inhibitory) symptoms, or a combination of the two.

Focal Motor Seizures With and Without March

Motor seizures can be clonic or tonic, involving any portion of the body, depending on the site of origin of the ictal discharge. Focal motor seizures may remain strictly focal or they may spread to contiguous cortical areas producing a sequential involvement of body parts in an epileptic march. This pattern is often referred to as a Jacksonian march. Postictally, a temporary weakness, Todd's paralysis, may be seen, especially if the seizure is severe or prolonged (7). Focal clonic seizures can occur with ictal discharges in any cortical region. The name *epilepsia partialis continua* (EPC) is given to continuous focal motor seizure activity.

Versive Seizures

Seizures beginning in or spreading to area 8, the frontal eye field, and the supplementary motor area or mesial part of premotor area 6 produce contralateral conjugate deviation of the eyes and turning of the head. When this movement is unquestionably forced and involuntary, the seizures are termed versive seizures and lateralize seizure onset to the contralateral hemisphere (36). Forced and sustained head and eye version continuing through generalization or occurring within 10 seconds before generalization was the best lateralizing sign, identifying a contralateral seizure focus in more than 90 percent of seizures (37).

Supplementary Sensorimotor Area Seizures

The supplementary sensorimotor area (SSMA) may be activated during seizures arising in patients with an epileptogenic zone in the posterior mesial or superior frontal area of one hemisphere. Seizures are frequent, brief, and usually out of sleep with abrupt bilateral asymmetric tonic posturing of the extremities. The posturing predominantly affects the proximal musculature with stiffening and gross flailing movements (15,16,38,39). Speech arrest and vocalization are common, but consciousness is often preserved. Ictal contraversive head and eye version may serve as a lateralizing feature if they precede secondary generalization. SSMA seizures may be confused with psychogenic seizures and parasomnias such as night terrors or confusional arousals.

Aphasic Seizures

Ictal language disturbances during epileptic seizures include speech arrest, aphasia, or vocalization. Seizures that begin with aphasic speech arrest, without altered consciousness, are generally considered to originate in the dominant posterolateral temporal region (42,43). Lüders and coworkers (44) demonstrated the presence of a basal temporal language area (BTLA) by electrical stimulation with subdural electrodes (44,45). Speech arrest has been demonstrated in seizures originating in the dominant BTLA (46,47). Seizures arising in the frontal operculum of the dominant hemisphere can give rise to epileptic aphasia (48). Vocalizations, sounds of no speech quality, may be seen with simple partial seizures affecting the suprasylvian area of the frontal lobe as well as complex partial seizures. They have no lateralizing value (49).

Simple Partial Seizures with Somatosensory or Special Sensory Signs

Sensory or motor phenomena are often the initial symptom of seizures starting in or near the postcentral area. Sensory phenomena include tingling, numbness, or paresthesias contralateral to the epileptogenic focus. The sensory phenomena may march to adjacent sensory or motor areas. The frequency of motor phenomena is due to intimate connections between the sensory and motor areas (6), as shown by motor phenomena observed in 25 percent of cases during electrical stimulation of the postcentral gyrus. Sensory symptoms that are ipsilateral or bilateral in distribution and

identical to those occurring only contralaterally are believed to originate in the second sensory area at the base of the motor strip in the frontoparietal operculum (50). Benign focal epilepsy of childhood (BFEC) often manifests with focal motor seizures with preserved consciousness or as partial-onset, secondarily generalized tonic-clonic seizures. They usually involve the face, oropharyngeal muscles, or arm on one side, and less commonly the leg. Sometimes they are associated with sensory phenomena such as tingling or numbness. BFEC and EPC (a form of focal motor status epilepticus) are discussed separately in this chapter.

Visual seizures are simple partial seizures involving the visual cortex in the region of the calcarine fissure. They usually consist of flashes of light or colors in the contralateral hemifield. Visual seizures should be distinguished from migraine, which usually produces negative phenomena such as scotomas or hemianopsia. More elaborate visual phenomena (i.e., formed visual hallucinations) are seen with seizures starting in the posterior temporal regions. Seizures starting from the occipital cortex may spread to the temporal lobes producing complex partial seizures (51).

Auditory seizures are seen with onset from the auditory cortex in the superior temporal gyrus. They usually manifest with sounds such as humming, buzzing, roaring, or whistling. More elaborate hallucinations (music, voices, etc.) result from involvement of the auditory association areas (6).

Olfactory and gustatory seizures present with an aura of an unpleasant odor or a bad taste in the mouth. They are usually observed with seizures arising from the anterior temporal lobe or insular region.

Vertiginous phenomena are sometimes reported by patients as the aura preceding their complex partial seizures. This may be a light-headed feeling or actual vertigo. Vertiginous phenomena are encountered with CPS of posterior temporal lobe onset (52–53).

Simple Partial Seizures with Autonomic Symptoms or Signs

Autonomic symptoms in the form of flushing, pallor, sweating, pupillary dilation, nausea, vomiting, borborygmi, piloerection, or epigastric sensations are often seen in CPS, especially those starting in the anterior temporal lobe, opercular-insular region, and orbitofrontal cortex (53–55). Ictal gastrointestinal symptoms that are limited to visceral sensations are more common in children; they include painful cramping, periumbilical pain, bloating, nausea, vomiting, and diarrhea. Pallor and cold sweating may accompany the abdominal symptoms in children and may be misdiagnosed as psychogenic pain (56). Sinus tachycardia, the most frequent cardiac concomitant of seizures, has been reported in several case studies (57–58). Sinus bradycardia, sinus arrest, atrioventricular block, and prolonged asystole occur much less frequently. Sudden unexplained death has been postulated to be a result of autonomically mediated fatal cardiac arrhythmia or sudden "neurogenic" pulmonary edema associated with seizures (59–61).

Simple Partial Seizures with Psychic Symptoms

Simple partial seizures with psychic symptoms refer to alterations of higher cerebral function — dysphasia, dysmnesia (déjà vu or ja mais vu), affective (fear, anger), cognition (distortion of time sense, dreamy states), illusions (micropsia or macropsia), or hallucinations (voices, music, or scenes). They are usually followed by a complex partial phase; only rarely do they occur in isolation.

As mentioned previously, simple partial seizures may evolve to secondarily generalized tonic-clonic seizures directly or after a complex partial phase. Likewise, CPS may give rise to secondarily generalized tonic-clonic seizures (2). The ictal discharge may spread from the focus to contiguous areas or to distant regions by way of specific pathways or callosal fibers connecting homologous areas of the cortex in the opposite hemisphere.

Complex Partial Seizures

Approximately 50 percent of patients with CPS report a warning symptom or aura. An aura is, by definition, a simple partial seizure. It may take different forms depending on the location of the seizure focus, as described previously. CPS of mesial temporal onset are most commonly preceded by a rising epigastric sensation. Young children sometimes run to the mother and cling to her fearfully (62). The aura is more clearly expressed as the child gets older. The aura is followed by the complex partial phase with partial or complete loss of consciousness, unresponsiveness often with a vacant stare, behavioral arrest, and some stiffening of the body. Duchowny and coworkers (63) noted that CPS in infants under 2 years of age frequently consisted of behavioral arrest with forced lateralized deviation of the head and eyes and tonic upper extremity extensor stiffening. Automatisms defined as more or less coordinated, involuntary movements occurring during a period of altered awareness are frequently seen in CPS. These invariably take place during the ictus, less commonly in the postictal period. They may consist of stereotyped movements of the mouth and lips, oroalimentary automatisms such as lip smacking or swallowing, fumbling or grasping movements of the hands, blinking, grimacing, bicycling movements of the legs, walking or running about, laughing, crying, or complex motor activity. Automatisms tend to

be simpler in the younger children, whereas highly organized behavioral sequences and complex gestural automatisms are observed in the older children and adults (63–65). The motor phenomena in preschool children may consist of symmetric tonic or clonic movements of the limbs and atonic phenomenon such as head nodding resembling infantile spasms or hypermotor turning movements and postures similar to frontal lobe seizures in adults. Unilateral dystonic posturing has been reported in CPS of temporal and frontal lobe onset and has good lateralizing value (66,67). CPS usually last 60 to 90 seconds and are followed by a postictal period lasting several minutes or hours (68). The child is often lethargic during the postictal period and may complain of headache. Postictal dysphasia may also be seen. The patient is usually confused postictally and may engage in automatic behavior. Attempts to restrain the patient may result in aggressive behavior, which is usually nondirected (69). One-third to one-half of patients with CPS may go on to have a secondarily generalized tonic-clonic seizure. Version may occur during such a seizure and is of lateralizing significance (36).

Occasionally, patients may develop complex partial status epilepticus that may present as a prolonged confusional state, similar to absence status. This may last several hours or even days. The patient appears to be in a daze, is slow to respond, frequently is unable to talk, and often is restless and disoriented. The diagnosis is established by the finding of a continuous focal ictal pattern on the EEG (70).

Frontal Lobe Seizures

Frontal lobe seizures represent the largest subgroup of extratemporal epilepsy, accounting for 30 percent of partial epilepsy (71,72). The most recent epilepsy classification scheme (43) suggests seven different types of frontal lobe seizures related to specific regions of seizure origin (Table 18-1). In practice, large epileptogenic zones, high speed and pattern of seizure propagation, and extensive overlap among different types make it impossible to accurately subclassify CPS of frontal lobe origin into distinct anatomic subregions based on clinical characteristics. Frontal lobe CPS (73–76) are uncommon, but their unique clinical features allow identification possible in most cases (Table 18-2). These seizures often have a bizarre clinical presentation, have minimal or absent interictal and ictal EEG abnormalities, and sometimes are mistaken for psychogenic seizures.

Autosomal Dominant Nocturnal Frontal Lobe Epilepsy

Autosomal dominant nocturnal frontal lobe epilepsy (ADNFLE) was first described as a distinct clinical

Table 18-1. Summary of International League Against Epilepsy (ILAE) Classification of Frontal Lobe Epilepsies

Region	Clinical Features According to ILAE Classification
Primary motor cortex	Contralateral tonic or clonic movements according to somatotopy, speech arrest and swallowing with frequent secondary generalization
SMA	Simple focal tonic seizures with vocalization, speech arrest, fencing postures, and complex focal motor activity
Cingulate	Complex focal motor activity with initial automatisms, sexual features, vegetative signs, changes in mood and affect, and urinary incontinence
Frontopolar	Early loss of consciousness, "pseudo absence," adversive and subsequent contraversive movements of head and eyes, axial clonic jerks, falls, autonomic signs with frequent generalization
Orbitofrontal	Complex focal motor seizures with initial automatisms or olfactory hallucinations, autonomic signs, and urinary incontinence
Dorsolateral (premotor)	Simple focal tonic with versive movements and aphasia and complex focal motor activity with initial automatisms
Opercular	Mastication, salivation, swallowing and speech arrest with epigastric aura, fear, and autonomic phenemena. Partial clonic facial seizures may be ipsilateral, and gustatory hallucination is common

Table 18-2. Features of Frontal Lobe Complex Partial Seizures

- Frequent, brief seizures occurring in clusters
- Nonspecific aura
- Abrupt onset and end with little or no postictal confusion
- Nocturnal preponderance
- Complex motor and sexual automatisms
- Prominent vocalization from simple humming, screaming, or expletives
- Bizarre hysterical appearance
- Complex partial status epilepticus

syndrome in six families in 1994 (77). The gene for this partial seizure syndrome was initially assigned to chromosome 20q13.2 (78) (see Chapter 5). The seizures begin in childhood (mean age 11.7 years, range 2 months–52 years) and usually persist through adult life. Individuals frequently have an aura followed by a gasp, grunt, or vocalization, and thrashing hyperkinetic activity or tonic stiffening with or without superimposed clonic activity (79). Seizures typically occur in clusters during sleep, and awareness is usually retained. Patients are of normal intellect with normal neurologic examination and neuroimaging tests. Interictal EEG is usually normal. When not obscured by movement artifact, ictal EEG may show bifrontal epileptiform discharges. Seizures are often misdiagnosed as parasomnias, paroxysmal nocturnal dystonia (which may in actuality be ADNFLE), familial dyskinesia, or a psychiatric disorder. The seizures frequently respond to carbamazepine monotherapy.

Benign Focal Epilepsy of Childhood (BFEC)

Benign focal epilepsy of childhood (BFEC), which includes benign epilepsy with central temporal spikes (BECTS, rolandic epilepsy), is the most common focal epilepsy in childhood, accounting for 13 percent to 23 percent of all childhood epilepsies (80–82) (Table 18-3). It has its onset between 3 and 13 years, with a peak at 7 to 8 years, and resolves by age 16. A nocturnal seizure, usually occurring after falling asleep or before awakening, in a neurologically and cognitively normal child is quite typical, and the diagnosis may be suspected on clinical grounds. However, in 15 percent of patients they occur in both sleep and wakeful state, and in 20 percent to 30 percent, they occur only in the waking state (83,84). Secondarily generalized tonic-clonic seizures at night are the most common type, followed by simple partial seizures (85–89). During the partial seizures (1) unilateral paresthesias of the tongue, lips, gum, and cheek; (2) unilateral clonic or tonic activity involving the face, lips, and tongue; and (3) speech arrest, salivation, and vocalization with preserved consciousness are seen. Children under the age of

Table 18-3. Benign Focal Epilepsy of Childhood (BFEC)

Clinical Criteria

- Onset between 18 months and 13 years, peak age 8–9 years
- Genetic predisposition
- Infrequent partial seizures, most specific type facial motor seizures, and the most common presentation, nocturnal generalized tonic-clonic seizures
- Normal neurologic examination, intelligence, and neuroimaging
- Remission in the second decade of life
- No long-term behavioral or cognitive impairment
- Good response to medication

EEG Criteria

- Normal background activity and sleep organization
- Characteristic interictal focal sharp waves, activated by sleep
- Tendency of discharges to shift and be multifocal
- Possible coexistence of generalized spike-and-wave discharges
- Remission of typical discharges, as a rule, before adolescence

5 years are more likely to have a hemiconvulsion or a GTC seizure (90,91). Postictal Todd's paresis has been reported in 7 percent to 16 percent of cases (92).

The diagnosis of BFEC is confirmed by finding a characteristic EEG pattern consisting of a high-voltage, usually diphasic spikes or sharp waves with a prominent negative polarity, often blunt sharp wave, preceded by a well-defined prepositivity (93). The after-following slow wave is less than the height of the sharp component. Marked activation of the spikes in drowsiness and sleep is characteristic, and 30 percent of cases show spikes only during sleep (94). They may occur singly or in clusters at the midtemporal and central (rolandic) region. The focus is maximum at the electrode position C6 between the central C4 and midtemporal T4 electrodes where the rolandic fissure meets the sylvian fissure. Rolandic spikes typically have a horizontal dipole (Figure 18-1, A and B) with maximum negativity over the midtemporal-central region and positivity over the superior frontal area (95,96). These discharges may also occur in multiple regions, particularly bifrontal and bioccipital locations in the same patient, often shifting in location on serial EEGs. Approximately 60 percent of patients show a unilateral spike focus, whereas in 40 percent it is bilateral and may be synchronous or asynchronous (84). There is no relationship between the discharge rate and seizure frequency. Lüders and coworkers found that only 8 percent of children who have BFEDCs on their EEGs actually manifest seizures (93). The seizure frequency is low; approximately a quarter of patients have only a single seizure, and one-half of patients have fewer than five seizures (97). Status epilepticus is extremely rare in BFEC (98,99).

In the presence of a typical clinical history, normal neurologic examination, and characteristic EEG findings, an MRI scan is not necessary. However, in the presence of an atypical clinical or EEG features or abnormal neurologic examination, an MRI scan is recommended to look for a structural abnormality. No treatment is recommended in patients with infrequent, nocturnal, partial seizures if the child and family are comfortable with this approach. If seizures are frequent, or if the seizures are sufficiently disturbing to the child or the family, treatment with carbamazepine or phenytoin is usually successful. A larger fraction of the dose may be given at bedtime, and treatment should be continued for at least 2 years after the last seizure. It is important to educate the parents regarding the benign nature of this syndrome and its good prognosis.

Benign Epilepsy of Childhood with Occipital Paroxysms

Benign epilepsy of childhood with occipital paroxysms (BEOP) was first described by Gastaut (100,101) as a benign form of partial epilepsy in childhood, characterized by ictal visual symptoms and interictal occipital rhythmic spikes appearing only after eye closure. The age of onset is from 15 months to 17 years, with a peak between 5 and 7 years (102,103). The seizures are characterized by visual symptomatology followed by psychomotor or sensorimotor phenomenon and or migraine-type headache, nausea, and vomiting (104–107).

The visual symptoms consist of amaurosis, elementary and complex visual hallucinations, or visual illusion including micropsia, metamorphopsia, or palinopsia. Gastaut and Zifkin divided the cases into three forms: a complete syndrome including seizures with ictal visual symptoms and interictal occipital paroxysmal activity and two incomplete syndromes in which either the ictal visual symptoms or the interictal EEG abnormalities were absent. Only about half the patients had the complete syndrome. The EEG is characterized by high-amplitude diphasic occipital spikes, appearing rhythmically at a frequency of 1 to 3 Hz in bursts or trains. An important feature is the prompt suppression of the spikes with eye opening and reappearance within 1 to 20 seconds after eye closure. Intermittent photic stimulation and sleep have no significant effect on the occipital epileptiform activity. BEOP carries a good prognosis, although it is not as benign as BFEC. Gastaut found that complete seizure control was achieved in 60 percent of patients (101). Panayiotopoulos reported remission in 16 of 18 children with BEOP (103).

Landau-Kleffner Syndrome

Landau-Kleffner syndrome (LKS), or acquired epileptic aphasia, is characterized by language regression following normal acquisition of language skills, accompanied by epileptiform abnormalities in the central-temporal or parietooccipital regions primarily during sleep, with or without clinical seizures. The disorder makes its appearance between 2 and 5 years of age. The onset may be subacute or stuttering, and the initial language abnormality consists of a loss of verbal understanding in an otherwise normal child who has already developed age-appropriate language. Speech output is soon reduced, and paraphasias and phonological errors appear. Behavioral abnormalities similar to autism can occur, and ultimately the child may become completely mute. Seizures may vary in type but most commonly are associated with eye blinking or brief eye deviation, head dropping, and minor automatisms with occasional secondary generalization. CPS with psychomotor automatisms are rare. Status epilepticus occurs in approximately 15 percent of children with LKS. The seizures bear a variable relationship to the language deficit, and, indeed, 20 percent to 30 percent of patients do not

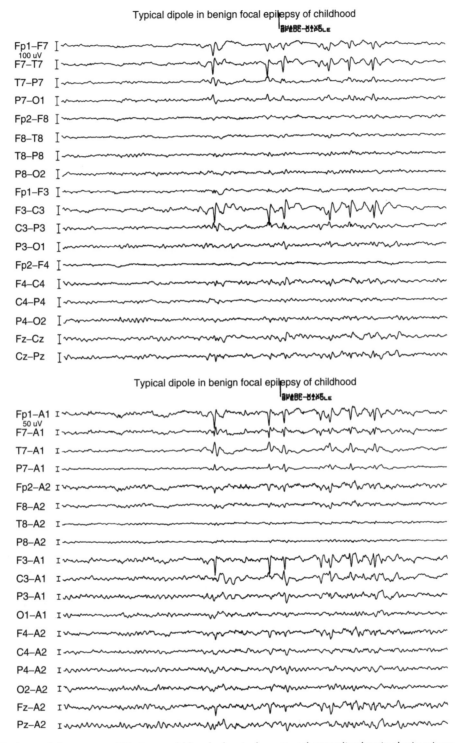

Figure 18-1. Rolandic focus of sharp waves. This 8-year-old boy had a single nocturnal generalized tonic-clonic seizure. **A.** shows runs of left centrotemporal sharp waves. **B.** is a referential montage using ear reference electrode showing upward deflection (negativity) at T7 and C3 and downward deflections (positivity) at FP1, F7, and F3 electrodes, indicating a dipole.

have behavioral seizures (108). EEG findings during wakefulness may be normal. The typical EEG consists of repetitive high-amplitude spikes and sharp waves, predominantly bitemporal and activated by sleep, especially slow-wave sleep. A continuous 1.5 to 5 Hz spike-and-wave discharges during slow-wave sleep

is an important component of the LKS, but it is not essential to make the diagnosis. Neuroimaging studies with CT and MRI scans are usually normal. Several studies using positron emission tomography (PET) and single photon emission computed tomography (SPECT) have shown temporal lobe abnormalities in glucose metabolism and brain perfusion (109–112). Treatment of LKS can be quite frustrating. Valproate with or without benzodiazepine (113) has had partial effects on clinical and EEG symptoms of LKG. If epileptiform EEG abnormalities and cognitive dysfunction persists, treatment with steroids (114,115), intravenous (IV) immunoglobulin (116,117), or, in select LKG patients, subpial cortical transections (118) should be seriously considered. Although prognosis for seizure control is good (119), permanent neuropsychological consequences are common, with normal clinical status and speech recovery in less than 50 percent of patients (120,121).

Epilepsia Partialis Continua

Epilepsia partialis continua (EPC) is characterized by regular or irregular muscular twitches affecting a limited part of the body, occurring for a minimum of 1 hour, and recurring at intervals of no more than 10 seconds (122). Epilepsia partialis continua was first described in 1895 by Koshewnikow, who hypothesized that the seizures arose from an area of localized encephalitis (123). Later in a series of 52 patients, Omorokow came to the same conclusion based on numerous cortical biopsies (124). Useful reviews of the syndrome appear in papers by Juul-Jensen (125), Bancaud (126), and Thomas (122). EPC often has a changing pattern from hour to hour or day to day, changing in rhythm, amplitude, and extent of involvement in a limb. It usually affects distal limb muscles and face but may also involve the trunk, diaphragm, neck, and throat muscles. Asynchrony of muscle twitching is often present, suggesting the presence of multiple foci within a larger epileptogenic zone (122).

Bancaud pointed out the existence of two types of EPC. The first type is seen in both adults and children. It usually is due to a focal discrete epileptogenic lesion such as a cavernous angioma, astrocytoma, or infarct. It has been reported in Sjögren's syndrome (127) and following metrizamide myelography (128) and nonketotic hyperglycemia in adults (129) and children (130). It has also been observed in the MELAS (mitochondrial encephalopathy with lactic acidosis and stroke-like episodes) syndrome (131). Focal cortical dysplasia should be suspected when EPC occurs in children without another obvious cause. Normal magnetic resonance studies do not exclude neuronal migration disorders (132). PET and SPECT reveal the metabolic effects of EPC in the setting of normal MRI scans (133). Penicillin, azlocillin, and cefotaxime have been incriminated in some cases of EPC (134). The EEG shows normal background activity and the presence of spikes, sharp waves, or rhythmic slow waves in the rolandic region (122,125). In some patients a definite relationship can be seen between the sharp waves and muscular jerks, while others may have a variable or unclear relationship. There is controversy in the literature regarding the role of cortical and subcortical mechanisms in its pathogenesis. Some patients have been found to have destructive lesions of the subcortical white matter, striatum, and thalamus in addition to the cortex (135). Many of the cases that showed subcortical lesions associated with EPC increased focal cortical excitability (136–138) by partially undercutting and deafferenting the overlying cortex. Several investigators have postulated that there is a unilateral enhancement of the somatosensory evoked potential (139–140). Using the jerk-locked averaging technique, Kuroiwa and coworkers found time-locked sharp waves preceding the muscle jerks, enhanced transcortical long-loop reflexes, and increased cerebral blood flow in the region of the focus (141). Cowan and coworkers postulated that stimulus-sensitive myoclonus sometimes seen in such patients is the result of an abnormal discharge in the precentral motor cortex (seen on scalp EEG as a spike), which may be triggered by peripheral sensory afferents (142). Occasionally, the EEG does not show any abnormalities in a patient with EPC. This may happen if the seizure focus is too small to be picked up by scalp EEG or if it lies within the infolded cortex of a gyrus or in the region of the interhemispheric fissure (143,144). Spikes may also be obscured by EMG and movement artifacts. The use of closely spaced scalp electrodes and proper montages is helpful in such instances (143). Sleep recordings may activate spikes and help reduce artifacts. However, corticography shows spike discharges even when scalp EEG fails to reveal them (122).

The second form of EPC begins exclusively in childhood and is referred to as Rasmussen's syndrome (RS). It is characterized by intractable focal motor seizures, declining cognitive function, progressive hemiparesis, visual field abnormality, and contralateral focal, predominantly perisylvian cortical atrophy. The onset of the disease occurs at 10 years or younger in 85 percent of patients (145). EPC occurs in one-half of patients at some point in their course (146). The etiology is not known, but an autoimmune process is important in the pathogenesis of RS, and it is believed that the glutamate receptor subunit, Glu R3 may be an important autoantigen (147–149). Neuropathology characteristically shows perivascular lymphocytic cuffing and proliferation of microglial nodules in the cortex of the affected hemisphere (150–152). The EEG may show background slowing, disruption of sleep architecture, and frequent epileptiform discharges over the affected hemisphere; with progression of the disease, the spikes may become bilaterally synchronous and appear in the contralateral hemisphere (153–155). CT and MRI scans may show diffuse atrophy of the involved hemisphere (156). Proton MR-spectroscopy may reveal decreased N-acetylaspartate (NAA) concentration in patients with RS (157). This finding correlates well with brain atrophy and neuronal loss.

Rasmussen's syndrome is notoriously difficult to treat and does not show the same dramatic response to IV medications as do other forms of status (122). IV immunoglobulin, high-dose steroids, or both may produce some reduction of seizure frequency in the short term in a few cases (158), but surgical removal of the affected hemisphere is the standard therapy (159). In the Johns Hopkins experience, 88 percent of children who underwent hemispherectomy became seizure-free or have occasional, nondisabling seizures (159–161). Early hemispherectomy, although increasing the hemiparesis, reduces the overall burden of the illness because of a marked decrease in both frequency and severity of seizures. Because hemiplegia is inevitable with or without surgery, early surgery may allow the child to return to a more normal life by preventing the cognitive decline that is the result of constant seizures.

DIFFERENTIAL DIAGNOSIS

Pseudoseizures are in the differential diagnosis of any seizure, especially if presenting with bizarre and unusual patterns or prolonged generalized seizures with intact memory for the event. There usually is no postictal confusion. Pseudoseizures often can be terminated abruptly with suggestion (162–163). The frequency of pseudoseizures may be unrelated to antiepileptic drug (AED) levels. Video-EEG monitoring reveals no seizure pattern during the episode. Psychogenic unresponsiveness, that is, unresponsiveness during the presence of a preserved alpha background rhythm, is also very helpful. Pseudoseizures occasionally coexist with true seizures, and the monitoring must document all the seizure types reported by the family. Migrainous phenomena (164) may be difficult to distinguish from CPS, especially if they are associated with visual hallucinations or confusion. Migraine and partial seizures may coexist, or at times migraine may be followed by a partial seizure. The prodrome of the migraine attack usually develops more slowly than the epileptic aura. The frequent occurrence of vomiting and family history make this diagnosis more likely. The recording of a typical episode in the laboratory with EEG and video monitoring is helpful. EPC is sometimes mistaken for segmental myoclonus or paroxysmal choreoathetosis.

Radiological Findings

Magnetic resonance imaging is the imaging modality of choice in a child with partial or localization-related epilepsy because of its inherent advantages in soft tissue contrast, spatial resolution, multiplanar capabilities, and lack of bone artifact. Kuzniecky and coworkers (165) correlated the MRI imaging results with pathology in 44 children with intractable epilepsy and showed a potential epileptogenic abnormality in 86 percent of patients (165). CT scanning is inferior in detecting lesions that may be seen only on MRI, with the exception of revealing intracranial calcification in Sturge-Weber syndrome, congenital brain infections such as toxoplasmosis, or cytomegalovirus. MRI reliably demonstrates hippocampal atrophy in 70 percent to 90 percent of patients with mesial TLE (166,167). Accurate assessment of hippocampal size by volumetric studies has been shown to correlate with severity of neuronal loss in the hippocampus (168) and seizure outcome following resection (169). MRI has led to increased recognition, better characterization, and improved understanding of neuronal migration disorder (NMD). The generalized NMDs include lissencephaly, pachygyria, band or laminar heterotopia, and subependymal heterotopias. Focal forms of NMDs include focal cortical dysplasia, polymicrogyria, focal subependymal heterotopias, and schizencephaly (170, 171). The identification of a focal NMD and complete removal of the lesion is followed by good seizure control in 77 percent of the patients (172). MRI is very sensitive in detection of tumors, vascular malformations such as cavernous hemangiomas, arteriovenous malformations and subependymal nodules, and cortical tubers in tuberous sclerosis. PET scans may show an area of hypometabolism interictally and a focus of hypermetabolism on ictal scans (173,174). Unilateral temporal lobe hypometabolism is present in 70 percent to 80 percent of patients with TLE (175) and corresponds pathologically and anatomically to the depth electrode localization of the epileptic zone (176). Focal cortical dysplasia (FCD) is difficult to visualize in very young children because of incomplete myelination. Interictal PET is useful in demonstrating areas of hypometabolism corresponding to FCD in infants and children with catastrophic epilepsy. In the early stages of Rasmussen's encephalitis, the MRI may be normal, but the PET scan may show focal or diffuse hemispheric hypometabolism. Flumazenil PET reveals a reduction in benzodiazepine receptor binding in the epileptic focus of partial epilepsy (177). Carfentanil PET studies of TLE have revealed increased mu-opiate receptor binding in the neocortex of the epileptogenic temporal lobe, correlating directly with a decrease of glucose metabolism seen on FDG-PET (178). SPECT has been used in patients with refractory seizures considered for epilepsy surgery. Interictal SPECT demonstrates hypoperfusion in 40 percent to 70 percent of patients with focal epilepsy (179). Ictal SPECT scan with hexamethylpropyleneamineoxime (HMPAO) has been reported to have a localization accuracy of 70 percent to 100 percent in TLE (180) and in up to 90 percent of patients with frontal lobe epilepsy (181,182).

Interictal EEG

The interictal EEG may be normal in 30 percent to 40 percent of patients with clinically documented partial seizures. A normal EEG, however, does not rule out the diagnosis of epilepsy. The chance of finding an abnormality is increased by performing repeated or prolonged EEGs, sleep recordings, additional closely spaced electrodes, appropriate montages, and hyperventilation. With these techniques, the yield may be increased up to 90 percent (183–185). A unilateral temporal lobe focus is found in most cases of CPS. Bitemporal sharp wave foci are seen in 25 percent to 33 percent of patients (186). An extratemporal focus is seen in 15 percent to 20 percent of patients, usually in the frontal lobe (13). Focal intermittent rhythmic slowing may be seen intermittently in approximately half the patients with focal seizures (183,186) and has the same significance as focal spikes. One may also find focal slowing that is nonrhythmic with suppression of the normal background rhythms in 75 percent of patients (183). It is important to exclude nonepileptiform sharp transients such as small sharp spikes, psychomotor variant or 14- and 6-Hz spikes. Additionally, benign focal epileptiform discharges of childhood may occur in asymptomatic children (187). These usually are found in the central or midtemporal location, have a characteristic stereotyped waveform, and are markedly activated during sleep.

Ictal EEG

According to Gastaut (188), the ictal EEG is abnormal in more than 95 percent of cases. In 75 percent of patients, the interictal spikes or sharp waves show an abrupt cessation or decrease just before ictal onset. This is then followed by rhythmic activity that shows a progressive build-up of amplitude and frequency (most often in the 13–30 Hz range but may be in the theta or delta range). This may be well localized to the area of the focus or it may be more widespread over that hemisphere (183). Postictally, one may find slowing or flattening, which, if focal, may be helpful in lateralization (189). Sometimes it is difficult to localize or lateralize the seizure onset from scalp recordings. Invasive recordings with subdural or depth electrodes may be indicated in such cases (190–195).

Medical Treatment

Table 18-4 lists the principal AEDs used in partial seizures, their half-lives, therapeutic range, dosage, and side effects (196). Carbamazepine, phenytoin, primidone, and phenobarbital are equally effective in controlling CPS, differing mainly in their propensity to produce side effects.

Carbamazepine (Tegretol) is a drug of first choice in children and adults (197,198). It is safe (199), can be titrated to high enough levels, and is well tolerated. It has few side effects and favorable effects on cognitive performance (200). It is effective in both partial and generalized seizures (197). Beginning at 10 to 20 mg/kg/day in two or three divided doses, it can be increased every 5 to 7 days by an additional 10 mg/kg/day. The therapeutic range is between 6 and 12 µg/ml. It is best to use it alone in maximally tolerated doses until seizures are controlled or toxicity occurs.

Table 18-4. Antiepileptic Drugs: Pharmacokinetics and Dosage

Medication	Half-life (hours)	Metabolism	Protein Binding (%)	Adult Dose (mg/day)	Pediatric Dose (mg/kg/day)
Carbamazepine	12[a]	Hepatic	60–70	600–1600	5–20
Phenytoin	24[b]	Hepatic	85–90	200–500	4–7
Valproate	10	Hepatic	70–90	1000–3000	10–15
Phenobarbital	96	Hepatic	45–50	90–180	2–6
Primidone[c]	12	Hepatic	<30	300–1500	10–20
Ethosuximide	36	Hepatic	<10	750–1500	15–40
Fosphenytoin	8–17 min	Hepatic	85–90	See below[d]	See below[d]
Felbamate	14–23	Hepatic and renal	30	1200–3600	15–45
Gabapentin	6–8	Renal	Negligible	900–4800	10–30
Lamotrigine	24[c]	Hepatic	55	200–700	5–15
Topiramate	18–24	Renal	<15	200–800	1–9
Vigabatrin	5–7	Renal	Negligible	2000–4000	50–150
Tiagabine	7	Hepatic	95	52	0.25–1.5

[a]Carbamazepine induces its own metabolism.

[b]Phenytoin has nonlinear kinetics.

[c]Primidone's primary metabolites, phenobarbital and phenylethylmalonomide, are pharmacologically active; values given for the parent compound.

[d]Loading dose in status epilepticus: 15–20 mg/kg intravenously at 150 mg/minute in adults or 2–3 mg/kg/minute in children weighing <50 kg; maintenance dose: 4–7 mg/kg intramuscularly or intravenously at 150 mg/min in adults or 2–3 mg/kg/min in children <50 kg twice daily.

[e]Lamotrigine's half-life is affected by other antiepileptic drugs.

Two extended-release formulations of carbamazepine, Carbatrol and Tegretol-XR, allow convenient twice-a-day dosing, predictable bioavailability, and lower risk of cognitive impairment (see Chapter 30).

Phenytoin (Dilantin) is one of the first-line drugs for partial and generalized tonic-clonic seizures. The dose is 5 to 10 mg/kg/day, and the therapeutic range is 10 to 20 µg/ml. Phenytoin has zero-order kinetics, so that a small increase in dose may produce marked elevations in plasma levels into the toxic range, particularly at plasma levels over 18 µg/ml. It can be given parenterally, which makes it useful in status epilepticus (see Chapter 20). Phenytoin suspension is absorbed erratically and should be avoided when possible (see Chapter 29).

Fosphenytoin is a water-soluble prodrug that is metabolized completely and rapidly to phenytoin in approximately 15 minutes and may be infused three times more rapidly than IV phenytoin with the same pharmacologic effects. It is significantly better tolerated at the infusion site and represents a true advance in the treatment of acute seizures in children of all ages. Clinical studies with IV and IM fosphenytoin have shown that the efficacy, safety, and pharmacokinetics of this drug are similar in young and older children (see Chapters 15, 24, and 29).

Phenobarbital is also effective in partial seizures but has significant effects on behavior and cognition and may exacerbate hyperactivity in children (201). The dose for children under 5 years is 3 to 5 mg/kg/day and 2 to 3 mg/kg for children above the age of 5, given in one or two divided doses.

Primidone (Mysoline) is also effective in controlling partial seizures in 84 percent of patients (202). The starting dose is 10 to 20 mg/kg/day in two or three divided doses. Primidone is metabolized to phenobarbital and phenylethylmalonamide (PEMA). Primidone and its two metabolites have independent anticonvulsant activity. Approximately 25 percent of the primidone dose is converted to phenobarbital. Efficacy appears to correlate better with phenobarbital serum levels rather than the primidone level. Phenytoin and carbamazepine induce the conversion of primidone to phenobarbital, whereas valproate, acetazolamide, and isoniazid have an inhibitory effect on the conversion of primidone to phenobarbital. Long-term side effects of primidone are similar to those of phenobarbital (see Chapter 28).

Valproate has been used for partial seizures given alone or in combination with carbamazepine (203). The starting dose is 15 to 20 mg/kg/day in two to four divided doses and increased to over 60 mg/kg/day depending on response and serum blood levels. Valproate is highly protein bound, but the binding is concentration-dependent and nonlinear. The free fraction increases at plasma concentrations greater than 75 µg/ml because the protein binding sites are saturated resulting in side effects. Valproate increases the concentration of carbamazepine epoxide by blocking epoxide hydrolase. In rare cases, it may produce pancreatitis (204) and fatal hepatic failure (205). The risk of fatal hepatic failure is 1 in 600 for the highest risk group (age < 2 years, on polytherapy), decreasing to 1 in 45,000 for patients in the low-risk group (over age 2 years, on monotherapy) (205). Valproate should not be used as the initial treatment for partial seizures in very young children.

If a patient has been seizure-free for more than 2 to 3 years on AEDs, the possibility of tapering them should be discussed with patient and family. An EEG done at this time if free of epileptiform discharges is a favorable sign that anticonvulsants may be tapered. Although some authors initially suggested waiting 4 years after being seizure-free (206), others (207,208) believe that a 2 to 3 year seizure-free interval is adequate. The drugs should be tapered slowly over a period of 6 to 12 months (209). Should the patient have a seizure during withdrawal, it is advisable to wait for additional seizures before resuming medications to avoid treating a withdrawal seizure (210) (see Chapter 21).

Newer Antiepileptic Drugs

Felbamate which was introduced in 1993, is effective in the treatment of refractory partial and generalized seizures in children and adults (211). Common side effects include anorexia, vomiting, weight loss, headache, insomnia, and somnolence (212–214). Felbamate increases the blood concentrations of phenytoin, valproate, and the epoxide metabolite of carbamazepine. In children, the recommended dose ranges from 15 to above 45 mg/kg. Unfortunately, a significant number of patients developed fatal aplastic anemia and severe hepatitis, a presumed idiosyncratic reaction (215), and felbamate usage sharply declined. The estimated incidence of fatal aplastic anemia is 1 in 3,600 to 5,000 exposed patients (214). The risk of fatal hepatic failure is approximately 1 in 24,000 to 34,000 (214). Because of these serious side effects, the use of felbamate is now restricted to children with intractable seizures such as Lennox-Gastaut syndrome in whom alternative medications are ineffective (see Chapter 35).

Gabapentin is approved by the U.S. Food and Drug Administration (FDA) as adjunctive therapy for partial and secondarily generalized seizures in adults and children 12 years of age or older. It has demonstrated efficacy as adjunctive therapy in 5 controlled studies and 18 uncontrolled studies of patients with medically refractory partial seizures (216,217). Gabapentin has shown similar efficacy in children with refractory and benign focal epilepsy (218). Gabapentin has a very short half-life, but it is not metabolized, does not bind to plasma proteins, and does not appear to possess enzyme-inducing or enzyme-inhibiting properties. Its absorption is dose-dependent, not dose proportional; the fraction absorbed falls as higher doses are administered (219). There is no significant interaction with other AEDs or oral contraceptives. Common reported side effects include somnolence, dizziness, fatigue, and ataxia. Other reported side effects include aggression, hyperactivity, and weight gain (220–223). The usual pediatric dose of gabapentin varies from 10 to over 90 mg/kg/day (see Chapter 33).

Lamotrigine appears to be effective in partial and generalized seizures (224,225). It has linear kinetics, is approximately 55 percent bound to plasma proteins, and has a half-life of 24 to 36 hours, but it is greatly influenced by concomitant conventional AEDs. In patients taking enzyme-inducing AEDs (phenytoin, carbamazepine, or barbiturates), its half-life is reduced by approximately 50 percent. When lamotrigine is given concomitantly with valproate, the half-life is significantly prolonged. Frequently reported side effects include dizziness, diplopia, ataxia, nausea, vomiting, somnolence, laryngitis, and adverse reaction–aggravated seizure increase. Overall, maculopapular skin rash occurs in 10 percent of patients. Potentially life-threatening skin rash appears to be greatest in children receiving valproate and with rapid escalation of lamotrigine dose (226). For children receiving enzyme-inducing AEDs, initial recommended dosage is 2 mg/kg daily for the first 2 weeks, followed by 5 mg/kg in weeks 3 and 4, until a maintenance dose of 5 to 15 mg/kg is attained. If the child is receiving valproate, the initial recommended dosage is 0.2 mg/kg, increasing to 0.5 mg/kg after the first 2 weeks, and then gradually increased in 2-week intervals to a maintenance dose between 1 and 5 mg/kg/day (227) (see Chapter 34).

Vigabatrin is an irreversible inhibitor of GABA transaminase, which increases brain concentrations of GABA, an inhibitory neurotransmitter. It is effective in the treatment of refractory partial seizures and infantile spasms (228–232). Between 45 percent and 80 percent of patients demonstrate a greater than 50 percent reduction in seizures (233–238), with 8 to 10 percent of children becoming seizure-free. Vigabatrin is neither protein bound nor metabolized by the microsomal oxidase enzyme system. Initially reported neuropathological findings have not been verified in humans (239–241). The principal adverse effects reported in add-on trials were somnolence, fatigue, irritability, depression, ataxia, weight gain, psychosis, and hyperactivity in children (230,235–238,242). Rare side effects include cataracts, macular degeneration, central

scotomas (243), and visual field constriction (244). Vigabatrin is not approved by the FDA in the United States. The recommended starting dose is 40 to 50 mg/kg/day, increasing to 80 to 100 mg/kg/ day given as a twice-daily dose (see Chapter 38).

Topiramate is indicated for refractory partial seizures and Lennox-Gastaut syndrome (245–248). It is rapidly absorbed, has linear pharmacokinetics, is not significantly metabolized, and is predominantly excreted by the kidneys; protein binding is low. Topiramate plasma clearance is higher and half-life shorter in children compared with adults. Seizure reduction in a refractory partial-onset pediatric epilepsy population of at least 50 percent have been reported in U.S. multicenter, double-blind, placebo-controlled, add-on trials (249,250). Psychomotor slowing, concentration difficulty, speech and language problems, somnolence, dizziness, and ataxia have been the most common adverse effects (251,252). There is a 1.5 percent incidence of renal stones, and paresthesias may occasionally occur (see Chapter 36).

Tiagabine is indicated as adjunctive therapy for partial seizures. It blocks GABA reuptake into presynaptic neurons (253). It may be effective in intractable complex partial seizures (254–257). It is 95 percent bound to plasma proteins, has a short half live of 7 to 9 hours, and is metabolized in the liver (258,259). Although tiagabine has no effect on other AEDs, hepatic enzyme-inducing AEDs increase tiagabine clearance, shortening its half-life to 4 to 7 hours (260). In adolescents 12 to 18 years old, tiagabine should be initiated at 4 mg daily. The total daily dose may be increased by 4 mg at weekly intervals until clinical response is achieved. Doses higher than 32 mg/day have been tolerated with better efficacy. Preliminary reports suggest a dose-dependent effect, with 25 percent of patients achieving a 50 percent reduction in seizure frequency. Adverse effects include ataxia, dizziness, tremor, and cognitive changes (261,262) (see Chapter 37).

Three newer AEDs, oxcarbazepine, zonisamide, and levetiracetam, are discussed in Chapters 30, 39, and 40, respectively.

ROLE OF EPILEPSY SURGERY

As mentioned previously, partial-onset seizures arise from a localized focus in one hemisphere. Surgical resection to remove the epileptic focus should be considered under the following circumstances:

1. *Medically intractable seizures.* When seizures are poorly controlled despite high-dose monotherapy with at least three of the major AEDs (263,264), as well as one or two combinations of drugs, one should

consider evaluating the patient with intensive video-EEG monitoring. This can help establish the exact seizure type, which is important in selection of appropriate medications. A child should be referred for surgical evaluation if the seizures remain uncontrolled despite adequate trial of appropriate major AEDs with documentation of therapeutic serum levels or unacceptable side effects. Inability to control seizures with AEDs after 2 years is sufficient reason to consider epilepsy surgery in adults, but this time concept is not applicable to many young children with catastrophic epilepsy. Several issues must be considered when judging intractability in pediatric epilepsy. These factors include nature of the underlying seizure disorder, frequency of seizures, negative effects of seizures and AEDs on cognitive development, and plasticity of the developing brain.

2. When seizures interfere in a significant way with the patient's lifestyle. This criterion is relative because a child who has frequent seizures only at night is less handicapped than an otherwise normal adult with one seizure a month who is not able to drive or hold a job.

All patients should have a psychological evaluation to determine what effect controlling the seizures will have on their lifestyle. For some patients, whose identity is closely linked to their long-standing epilepsy, becoming seizure-free can have disastrous consequences (265).

The patient should be physically and psychologically capable of participating in the evaluation process, which can be prolonged and stressful. We do not automatically exclude mentally retarded or behaviorally handicapped individuals unless their condition precludes any testing whatsoever (see Chapter 47).

We believe that the age of a patient is not in itself a contraindication to epilepsy surgery, provided the other criteria are met. Studies on the outcome of partial seizures show that except for BFEC, the likelihood of spontaneous remission, especially in CPS, is quite small (266,267). The 2 or 3 years it takes to document medical intractability gives the clinician an opportunity to satisfy himself that he is dealing with a stable epileptic syndrome. Waiting additional years only prolongs the intellectual, social, and psychological disability of a child already impaired by the seizures and side effects of AEDs. In fact, they may have a better psychosocial outcome than patients operated on later in life (268,269). A surgical series from the Cleveland Clinic reported 75 percent of 12 infants seizure-free or with rare seizures. These patients had severe intractable epilepsy before the age of 2 years and underwent frontal, temporal, or temporoparietal-occipital resections or functional

hemispherectomy before the age of 2.5 years. Etiologies included focal cortical dysplasia, Sturge-Weber syndrome, hemimegalencephaly, and gangliioglioma (270). Vigevano and DiRocco demonstrated the effectiveness of hemispherectomy with seizure-free and good developmental outcome in five patients with hemimegalencephaly at age 4 months to 3 years with intractable seizures (271). Hoffman and coworkers reported seizure-free outcome after complete hemispherectomy for five of seven infants younger than 1 year of age with Sturge-Weber syndrome and attributed good cognitive and motor development to early surgical intervention (272). Duchowny reported that temporal lobectomy in the first decade of life is a safe and effective procedure for children with intractable TLE (273). In several series of temporal lobectomy in children, seizure outcome was comparable to that of adult patients (274–280). Palmini and coworkers reported a favorable surgical outcome in 26 of 53 patients exclusively with extratemporal cortical dysplasia (281). Teixeira and coworkers reported 65 percent seizure-free or greatly improved outcome in 20 patients presenting only with extratemporal dysplastic lesions (282). In general, results are better in patients with temporal focal cortical dysplasia (283–285).

In addition to lateralizing and localizing information obtained from scalp or invasive recordings, imaging studies, functional imaging (PET or SPECT scans), neuropsychological, and WADA testing to determine language and memory dominance are performed before epilepsy surgery. The goal of epilepsy surgery is to improve seizure control without compromising language, memory, or sensorimotor function.

Results of cortical resection for temporal lobectomy are quite uniform in studies from various centers across the world. Mortality is low (<1 percent), and 60 percent to 80 percent of patients become seizure free (286,287). Results in those with extratemporal foci are less favorable, with only a third of patients becoming seizure-free while another one-third report a significant reduction in seizure frequency (286,288–289).

PROGNOSIS

Contrary to previous reports that stated that up to one-third of patients with CPS became seizure-free (290), our experience and that of others indicates that although some patients do become seizure-free on medication, spontaneous remission, that is, seizure-free off medications, is rare (266). Pazzaglia and coworkers reported that good seizure control was achieved in 31 percent of patients with simple partial seizures, 37 percent of those with complex partial seizures, and 61 percent of those with secondarily generalized epilepsy (291). Loiseau and coworkers found that seizure control could be predicted after 1 year of treatment (292). Therefore, it should be possible to document intractability within a couple of years after seizure onset. Such patients should undergo prolonged EEG-video monitoring. If found to be suitable candidates, epilepsy surgery should be performed sooner rather than later to minimize compromise of psychosocial and intellectual function.

REFERENCES

1. Dreifuss FE. Proposal for classification of epilepsies and epileptic syndromes. *Epilepsia* 1985; 26:268–278.

2. Dreifuss FE. Proposal for a revised clinical and electrographic classification of Epileptic seizures. *Epilepsia* 1981; 22:489–501.

3. Jackson GD. New techniques in magnetic resonance and epilepsy. *Epilepsia* 1994; 35:S2–S13.

4. Li LM, Fish DR, Sisodiya SM, et al. High-resolution resonance imaging in adults with partial or secondarily generalized epilepsy attending a tertiary referral unit. *J Neurol Neurosurg Psychiatry* 1995; 59:384–387.

5. Kuzniecky R, Murro A, King D, Morawetz R, Smith J. Magnetic resonance imaging in childhood intractable partial epilepsies: pathologic correlations. *Neurology* 1993; 43:681–687.

6. Scarpa P, Carassini B. Partial epilepsy in childhood: clinical and EEG study of 261 cases. *Epilepsia* 1982; 23:333–341.

7. Ounsted C, Lindsay J, Norman R. Biological factors in temporal lobe epilepsy. *Clin Dev Med* 1966; 22.

8. Babb TL, Brown WJ. Pathological findings in epilepsy. In: Engel J Jr, ed. *Surgical Treatment of the Epilepsies.* New York: Raven Press; 1987:511–540.

9. Falconar MA, Taylor DC. TLE: clinical features, pathology, diagnosis and treatment. In: Price JH, ed. *Modern Trends in Psychological Medicine.* London: Butterworths, 1970:346–373.

10. Brown WJ. Structural substrate of seizure foci in the temporal lobe. In: Brazier MAB, ed. *Epilepsy: Its Phenomena in Man.* New York: Academic Press, 1973:339–374.

11. Brown WJ, Babb TL. Central pathological considerations of complex partial seizures. In: Hopkins A, ed. *Epilepsy.* London: Chapman and Hall, 1987.

12. Falconer MA, Taylor DC. Surgical treatment of drug resistant epilepsy due to mesial temporal sclerosis. *Arch Neurol* 1968; 19:353–361.

13. Duchowny M, Levin B, Jayakar P, et al. Temporal lobectomy in early childhood. *Epilepsia* 1992; 33:298–303.

14. Mercuri S, Russo A, Palma L. Hemispheric supratentorial astrocytomas in children: long term results in 29 cases. *J Neurosurgery* 1981; 55:170–173.

15. Gol A. Cerebral astrocytomas in childhood. *J Neurosurgery* 1962; 19:577–582.

16. Taylor DC, Falconer MA, Bruton CJ, Corsellis JAN. FD of the cerebral cortex in epilepsy. *J Neurol Neurosurg Psychiatry* 1971; 34:369–387.

17. Palmini A, Andermann F, Oliver A, Tampieri D, Rabitallia Y. Neuronal migration disorder and intractable partial epilepsy. Results of surgical treatment. *Ann Neurol* 1991; 30:750–757.

18. Guerrini R, Dravet C, Raybaud C, et al. Epilepsy and focal abnormalities detected by MRI: electroclinicomorphological relations and follow up. *Dev Med Child Neurol* 1992; 34.

19. Dieker H, Edwards RH, Zukhein G, et al. The lissencephaly syndrome. *Birth Defects* 1969; 5:53–64.

20. Palmini A, Andermann F, Aicardi J, et al. Diffuse cortical dysplasia, 'the double cortex' syndrome: the clinical and epileptic syndrome in 10 patients. *Neurology* 1991; 41:1656–1662.

21. Barkovitch AJ, Kjos B. Grey matter heterotopias: MR characteristics and correlation with developmental and neurologic manifestations. *Radiology* 1992; 182:493–499.

22. Kuzniecky R, Andermann F, Guerrini R, and the CBPS Collaborative Study. Congenital perisylvian syndrome: a study of 31 patients. *Lancet* 1993; 341:608–612.

23. Kuzniecky R, Andermann F, Tampieri D, et al. Bilateral central microgyria: epilepsy, pseudobulbar palsy and mental retardation: a recognizable neuronal migration disorder. *Ann Neurol* 1989; 25:547–554.

24. Liblan CR, Tampieri D, Robitaille Y, Feindel W, Andermann F. Surgical treatment of intractable epilepsy associated with schizencephaly. *Neurosurgery* 1991; 29:421–429.

25. Kuzniecky R, Murro A, King D, et al. MRI in childhood intractable partial epilepsy: pathological correlations. *Neurology* 1993; 43:681–687.

26. Kotagal P, Rothner AD. Epilepsy in the setting of neurocutaneous syndrome. *Epilepsia* 1993; 34 (Suppl 3):S71–S78.

27. Prayson R, Estes M, Morris H. Coexistence of neoplasia and cortical dysplasia in patients presenting with seizures: *Epilepsia* 1993; 34:609–615.

28. Prayson RA, Estes ME. Dysembryoplastic neuroepithelial tumor. *Am J Clin Pathol* 1992; 97:398–401.

29. Raymond AA, Fish DR, Stevens JM, et al. Association of hippocampal sclerosis with cortical dysgenesis in patients with epilepsy. *Neurology* 1994; 44:1841–1845.

30. Rush E, Morrell MJ. Cortical dysplasia with mesial temporal sclerosis: evidence for kindling in humans. *Epilepsia* 1993; 34(Suppl 6):15. Abstract.

31. Penfield W, Jasper H. *Epilepsy and the Functional Anatomy of the Brain.* Boston: Little, Brown, 1954.

32. Quesney LF, Constain M, Fish DR, Rasmussen T. The clinical differentiation of seizures arising in the parasagittal and anterolateral dorsal frontal convexities. *Arch Neurol* 1990; 47:677–684.

33. Quesney LF. Clinical and EEG features of complex partial seizures of temporal lobe origin. *Epilepsia* 1986 (Suppl 2); 27:S27–S45.

34. Kotagal P, Lüders H, Williams G, et al. Temporal lobe complex partial seizures: analysis of symptom clusters and sequences. *Epilepsy Res* 1995; 20:49–67.

35. Jovanovic UJ. *Psychomotor Epilepsy: A Polydimensional Study*. Springfield, Ill: Charles C Thomas, 1974.

36. Wyllie E, Lüders H, Morris HH, Dinner DS. The lateralizing significance of versive head and eye movements during epileptic seizures. *Neurology* 1986; 36:606–611.

37. Kernan JC, Devinsky O, Luciano DJ, Vasquez B, Perrine K. Lateralizing significance of head and eye deviation in secondary generalized tonic clonic seizures. *Neurology* 1993; 43:1308–1310.

38. Morris HH, Dinner DS, Lüders H, Wyllie E, Kramer RE. Supplementary motor seizures: clinical and electroencephalographic findings. *Neurology* 1988; 38:1075–1082.

39. Kanner A, Morris HH, Dinner DS, et al. Supplementary motor seizures mimicking pseudoseizures: how to distinguish one from the other. *Neurology* 1988; 38(Supp 1):347.

40. Wyllie E, Bass NE. Supplementary sensory motor area seizures in children and adolescents. *Adv Neurol* 1996; 70:301–308.

41. Bass NE, Wyllie E, Commair Y, et al. Supplementary sensorimotor area seizures in children and adolescents. *J Pediatr* 1995; 126:537–544.

42. Commission on Classification and Terminology of the ILAE. Proposal for classification of epilepsies and epileptic syndromes. *Epilepsia* 1985; 26:268–278.

43. Commission on Classification and Terminology of the ILAE. Proposal for classification of epilepsies and epileptic syndromes. *Epilepsia* 1989; 30:389–399.

44. Lüders H, Lesser RP. Hahn J, et al. Basal temporal language area demonstrated by electrical stimulation. *Neurology* 1986; 36:505–510.

45. Lüders H, Lesser RP, Hahn J, et al. Basal temporal language area. *Brain* 1991; 114:743–754.

46. Suzuki I, Shimizu H, Ishijima B, et al. Aphasic seizures caused by focal epilepsy in the left fusiform gyrus. *Neurology* 1992; 42:2207–2210.

47. Abou-Khalil B, Wilch L, Blumenkopf B, Newman K, Whatsell JR. Global aphasia with seizure onset in the dominant basal temporal region. *Epilepsia* 1994; 35:1097–1084.

48. Sakai K, Hidari M, Fukai M, et al. A chance SPECT study of ictal aphasia during simple partial seizures. *Epilepsia* 1997; 38:374–376.

49. Gabr M, Lüders H, Dinner DS, Morris H, Wyllie E. Speech manifestations in lateralization of temporal lobe seizures. *Ann Neurol* 1980; 25:82–87.

50. Penfield W, Jasper H. *Epilepsy and the Functional Anatomy of the Human Brain*. Boston: Little, Brown, 1954:517–518.

51. Williamson PD, et al. Complex partial seizures with occipital lobe onset. *Epilepsia* 1981; 22:247–255.

52. Smith BH. Vestibular disturbances in epilepsy. *Neurology* 1960; 10:465.

53. King DW, Ajmone-Marsan C. Clinical features and ictal patterns in epileptic patients with EEG temporal lobe foci. *Ann Neurol* 1977; 2:138–147.

54. Tharp BR. Orbital frontal seizures: a unique electroencephalographic and clinical syndrome. *Epilepsia* 1972; 627–642.

55. Kramer RE, Lüders H, Goldstick LP, et al. Ictus emeticus: an electroclinical analysis. *Neurology* 1988; 48:1048–1052.

56. Singhi PD, Kaur S. Abdominal epilepsy misdiagnosed as psychogenic pain. *Postgrad Med J* 1988; 64:281–282.

57. Marshall DW, Westmoreland BF, Sharbrough FW. Ictal tachycardia during temporal lobe seizures. *Mayo Clin Proc* 1983; 58:443–446.

58. Devinsky O, Price BH, Cohen SI. Cardiac manifestations of complex partial seizures. *Am J Med* 1986; 80:195–202.

59. Neuspiel DR, Kuller LH. Sudden and unexpected natural death in childhood and adolescence. *JAMA* 1985; 254:1321–1325.

60. Leestma JE, Kelkar MB, Teas SS, et al. Sudden unexpected death associated with seizures: analysis of 66 cases. *Epilepsia* 1984; 25:84–88.

61. Terrence CF, Rao GR, Perper JA. Neurogenic pulmonary edema in unexpected death of epileptic patients. *Ann Neurol* 1981; 9:458–64.

62. Blume WT. Temporal lobe seizures in childhood. Medical aspects. In: Blaw ME, Rapin I, Kinsbourne M, eds. *Topics in Child Neurology*. New York, Spectrum, 1977:105–125.

63. Duchowny MS. Complex partial seizures of infancy. *Arch Neurol* 1987; 44:911–914.

64. Brockhaus A, Elger CE. Complex partial seizures of temporal lobe origin in children of different age groups. *Epilepsia* 1995; 36:1173–1181.

65. Bye AME, Foo S. Complex partial seizures in young children. *Epilepsia* 35 1994:482–488.

66. Kotagal P, Lüders H, Morris HH, et al. Dystonic posturing in complex partial seizures of temporal lobe onset: a new lateralizing sign. *Neurology* 1989; 39:196–201.

67. Varelas M, Wada JA. Lateralizing significance of unilateral upper limb dystonic posturing in temporal/frontal lobe seizures. *Neurology* 1988; 38(Suppl 1):107.

68. Delgado-Escueta AV, Mattson R, King L, et al. The nature of aggression during epileptic seizures. *N Engl J Med* 1981; 305:711–716.

69. Delgado-Escueta AV, Bascal FE, Treiman DM. Complex partial seizures on closed-circuit television and EEG. A study of 691 attacks in 79 patients. *Ann Neurol* 1982; 11:292–600.

70. Mayeux R and Lüders H. Complex partial status epilepticus. A case report and proposal for diagnostic criteria. *Neurology* 1978; 28:957.

71. Wieser HG, Hajek M. Frontal lobe epilepsy: compartmentalization, presurgical evaluation, and operative results. In: Jasper HH, Riggio S, Goldman-Rakic PS, eds. *Epilepsy and the Functional Anatomy of the Frontal Lobe*. New York: Raven Press, 1995:297–319.

72. Manford M, Hart YM, Sander JW, Shorvon SD. National General Practice Study of Epilepsy (NGPSE):

partial seizure patterns in a general population. *Neurology* 1992: 42:1911–1917.

73. Williamson PD, Spencer DD, Spencer SS, Novelly R, Mattson RH. Complex partial seizures of frontal lobe origin. *Ann Neurol* 1985; 18:497–504.

74. Williamson PD. Frontal lobe epilepsy: some clinical characteristics. In: Jasper HH, Riggio S, Goldman-Rakic PS, eds. *Epilepsy and the Functional Anatomy of the Frontal Lobe.* New York: Raven Press, 1995:297–319.

75. Salanova V, Morris HH, Van Ness P, et al. Frontal lobe seizures: electroclinical syndromes. *Epilepsia* 1995; 36:16–24.

76. Manford M, Fish DR, Shorvon SD. An analysis of clinical seizure patterns and their localizing value in frontal and temporal lobe epilepsies. *Brain* 1996; 119:17–40.

77. Scheffer I, Bhatia K, Lopes-Cendes I, et al. Autosomal dominant frontal epilepsy misdiagnosed as sleep disorder. *Lancet* 1994; 343:515–517.

78. Phillips H, Scheffer I, Berkovic S, et al. Localization of a gene for autosomal dominant nocturnal frontal lobe epilepsy to chromosome 20q13.2. *Nat Genet* 1995; 10:117–118.

79. Scheffer I, Bhatia K, Lopes-Cendes I, et al. Autosomal dominant frontal epilepsy. A distinctive clinical disorder. *Brain* 1995; 118:61–73.

80. Heijbel J, Blom S, Bergfors PG. Benign epilepsy of children with centrotemporal EEG foci. A study of incidence rate in outpatient care. *Epilepsia* 1975; 16:657–64.

81. Cavazzuti GB, Capella L, Nalin A. Longitudinal study of epileptiform EEG patterns in normal children. *Epilepsia* 1980; 21:43–45.

82. Lerman P, Kivity S. Benign focal epilepsy of childhood. A follow-up study of 100 recovered patients. *Arch Neurol* 1975; 32:261–264.

83. Beaussart M. Benign epilepsy of children with rolandic (centro-temporal) paroxysmal foci: a clinical entity. Study of 221 cases. *Epilepsia* 1972; 13:795–811.

84. Lerman P. Benign partial epilepsy with centrotemporal spikes. In: Roger J, Dravet C, Bureau M, et al., eds. *Epileptic Syndromes in Infancy, Childhood and Adolescence.* London: John Libbey, 1985:150–158.

85. Faure J, Loiseau P. Une correlation clinique particuliere des pointes-ondes rolandique sans signification focale. *Rev Neurol* 1959; 102:399–406.

86. Heijbel J, Blom S, Rasmuson M. Benign focal epilepsy of childhood with centro-temporal foci: a genetic study. *Epilepsia* 1975; 16:285–293.

87. Bray P, Wiser WC. Evidence for a genetic etiology of temporal central abnormalities in focal epilepsy. *N Engl J Med* 1964; 271:926–933.

88. Gibbs FA, Gibbs EL. *Atlas of Electroencephalography: Vol. 2. Epilepsy.* Cambridge: Addison-Wesley, 1952.

89. Loiseau P, Pestre M, Dartigues JF, et al. Long-term prognosis in two forms of childhood epilepsy: typical absence seizures and epilepsy with rolandic (centrotemporal) EEG foci. *Ann Neurol* 1983; 13:642–648.

90. Kajitani T, Nakamura M, Ueoka K, Kobuchi S. Three pairs of monozygotic twins with rolandic discharges. In: Wada JA, Penry JK, eds. *Advances in Epileptology: The Xth Epilepsy International Symposium.* New York: Raven Press, 1980:171–175.

91. Nishiura N, Miyazaki T. Clinico-electroencephalographical study of focal epilepsy with special reference to 'benign epilepsy of children with centro-temporal EEG foci' and its age dependency. *Folia Psychiatr Neurol Jpn* 1976; 30:253–261.

92. Wirrel EC, Camfield PR, Gordon KE, Dooley JM, Camfield CS. Benign rolandic epilepsy: atypical features are very common. *J Child Neurol* 1995; 10:455–458.

93. Lüders H, Lesser RP, Dinner DS, Morris HH. Benign focal epilepsy of childhood. In: Lüders H, Lesser RP, eds. *Electroclinical Syndromes (Clinical Medicine and Nervous System Series).* New York: Springer-Verlag, 1987:303–346.

94. Blom S, Heijbel J. Benign epilepsy of children with centro-temporal EEG foci. Discharge rate during sleep. *Epilepsia* 1975; 16:133–140.

95. Gregory DL, Wong PK. Topographic analysis of the centrotemporal discharges in benign rolandic epilepsy of childhood. *Epilepsia* 1984; 25:705–711.

96. Gregory DL, Wong PK. Clinical relevance of a dipole field in rolandic spikes. *Epilepsia* 1992; 33:36–44.

97. Loiseau P, Beaussart M. The seizures of benign childhood epilepsy with rolandic paroxysmal discharges. *Epilepsia* 1973; 14:381–389.

98. Fejerman N, Di Blasi AM. Status epilepticus of benign partial epilepsies in children: report of two cases. *Epilepsia* 1987; 28:351–355.

99. Colamaria V, Sgro V, Caraballo R, et al. Status epilepticus in benign rolandic epilepsy manifesting as anterior opercular syndrome. *Epilepsia* 1991; 32:329–334.

100. Gastaut H. A new type of epilepsy: benign partial epilepsy of childhood with occipital spike-waves. *Clin Electroencephalogr* 1982; 13:13–22.

101. Gastaut H. Benign epilepsy of childhood with occipital paroxysms. In: Roger J, Dravet C, Bureau M, Dreifuss FE, Wolf P, eds. *Epileptic Syndromes in Infancy, Childhood and Adolescence.* London: John Libbey, 1985:150–158.

102. Lerman P, Kivity S. Benign focal epilepsy of childhood. A follow up of 100 recovered patients. *Arch Neurol* 1975; 32:261–264.

103. Panayiotopoulos CP. Benign childhood epilepsy with occipital paroxysms: a 15-year prospective study. *Ann Neurol* 1989; 26:51–56.

104. Gastaut H. A new type of epilepsy: benign partial epilepsy of childhood with occipital spike-waves. In: Akimoto H, Kazamatsuri H, Seino M, Ward A, eds. *Advances in Epileptology: XIII Epilepsy International Symposium.* New York: Raven Press, 1982:19–24.

105. Beaumanoir A. Infantile epilepsy with occipital focus and good prognosis. *Eur Neurol* 1983; 22:43–52.

106. Newton R, Aicardi J. Clinical findings in children with occipital spike-wave complexes suppressed by eye-opening. *Neurology* 1983; 33:1526–1529.

107. Niedermeyer E, Riggio S, Santiago M. Benign occipital lobe epilepsy. *J Epilepsy* 1988; 1:3–11.

108. Beaumanoir A. The Landau-Kleffner syndrome. In: Roger J, Dravet C, Bureau M, Dreifuss FE, Wolf P, eds. *Epileptic Syndromes in Infancy, Childhood and Adolescence*. London: John Libbey; 1985:181–191.

109. Guerreiro MM, Camargo EE, Kato M, et al. Brain single photon emission computed tomography imaging in Landau-Kleffner syndrome. *Epilepsia* 1996; 37:60–67.

110. Maquet P, Hirsch E, Dive D, et al. Cerebral glucose utilization during sleep in Landau-Kleffner syndrome: a PET study. *Epilepsia* 1990; 31:778–783.

111. O'Tuama LA, Urion DK, Janicek MJ, et al. Regional cerebral perfusion in Landau-Kleffner syndrome and related childhood aphasias. *J Nucl Med* 1992; 33:1758–1765.

112. Dasilva EA, Chugani DC, Muzik O, Chugani HT. Landau-Kleffner syndrome: metabolic abnormalities in temporal lobe are a common feature. *J Child Neurol* 1997; 12:489–495.

113. Marescaux C, Hirsch E, Finck S, et al. Landau-Kleffner syndrome. A pharmacological study of five cases. *Epilepsia* 1990; 31:768–777.

114. Lerman P, Lerman-Sagie T, Kivity S. Effect of early corticosteroid therapy for Landau-Kleffner syndrome. *Dev Med Child Neurol* 1991; 33:257–260.

115. Deonna T, Roulet E. Epilepsy and language disorder in children. In: Fukuyama Y, Kamoshita S, Ohtsuka C, Suzuki Y, eds. *Modern Perspectives of Child Neurology*. The Japanese Society of Child Neurology; 1991:259–266.

116. Fayad MN, Choeiri R, Mikati M. Landau-Kleffner syndrome: consistent response to repeated intravenous gamma-globulin doses: a case report. *Epilepsia* 1997; 38:489–494.

117. Lagae LG, Silberstein J, Cullis PL, Casaer PJ. Successful use of intravenous immunoglobulin in Landau-Kleffner syndrome. *Pediatr Neurol* 1998; 18:165–168.

118. Morrel F, Whisler WW, Smith MC, et al. Landau-Kleffner syndrome: treatment with subpial intracortical transection. *Brain* 1995; 118:1529–1546.

119. Bureau M. Outstanding cases of CSWS and LKS analysis of the data sheets provided by the participants. In: Beaumanoir A, Bureau M, Deonna T, Mira L, Tassinari CA, eds. *Continuous Spikes and Waves During Slow Sleep Electrical Status Epilepticus During Slow Sleep*. London: John Libbey; 1995:213–216.

120. Mantovani JF, Landau WM. Acquired aphasia with convulsive disorder: course and Prognosis. *Neurology* 1980; 30:524–529.

121. Soprano AM, Garcia EF, Caraballo R, Fejerman N. Acquired epileptic aphasia: neuropsychological follow-up of 12 patients. *Pediatr Neurol* 1995; 11:230–235.

122. Thomas JE, Reagan TJ, Klass DW. Epilepsia partialis continua. A review of 32 cases. *Arch Neurol* 1977; 34:266–275.

123. Koshewnikow AY. Eine besondere form von corticaler epilepsie. *Neurol Centralbl* 1895; 14:47.

124. Omorokow L. Die Kojewnikoffske epilepsie in Siberien. *Z Ges Neurol Psych* 1927; 107:487–496.

125. Juul-Jensen, Denny-Brown D. Epilepsia partialis continua. A clinical, electroencephalographic and neuropathological study of 9 cases. *Arch Neurol* 1966; 15:563–578.

126. Bancaud J, et al. Syndrome de Kojewnikov et acces somato-moteurs (etude clinique, EEG, EMG, SEEG). *Encephale* 1970; 59:391–438.

127. Bansal SK, Sawhney MS, Chopra JS. Epilepsia partialis continua in Sjögren's syndrome. *Epilepsia* 1987; 28:362–363.

128. Shiozawa Z, Sasaki H, Ozaki Y, Nakanishi T, Yun PH. Epilepsia partialis continua following metrizamide cisternography. *Ann Neurol* 1981; 10:400–401.

129. Singh BM, Gupta DR, Strobos RJ. Nonketotic hyperglycemia and epilepsia partialis continua. *Arch Neurol* 1973; 187–190.

130. Sabharwal RK, Gupta M, Sharma D, Puri V. Juvenile diabetes manifesting as EPC. *J Assoc Physicians India* 1989; 37:603–604.

131. Chevrie JJ, Aicardi J, Goutieres F. Epilepsy in childhood mitochondrial myopathies. In: *Advances in Epileptology. The XVI Epilepsy International Symposium*. New York, Raven Press, 1986.

132. Desbiens R, Berkovic SF, Dubeau F, et al. Life threatening focal status epilepticus due to occult cortical dysplasia. *Arch Neurol* 1993; 50:695–700.

133. Katz A, Bose A, Lind SJ, Spencer SS. SPECT in patients with EPC. *Neurology* 1990; 40:1848–1850.

134. Wroe SJ, Ellershaw JE, Whittaker JA, Rulens A. Focal motor status epilepticus following treatment with azlocillin and cefataxime. *Med Toxicol* 1987; 2:233–234.

135. Kristiansen K, Kaada BR, Henriksen GF. Epilepsia partialis continua. *Epilepsia* 1971; 12:263–267.

136. Juul-Jensen P, Denny-Brown D. EPC. *Arch Neurol* 1966; 15:563–578.

137. Kristiansen K, Kaada BR, Henriksen GF. EPC. *Epilepsia* 1971; 12:263–267.

138. Boetz M, Bossard L. EPC with well-delimited subcortical frontal tumor. *Epilepsia* 1974; 15:39–43.

139. Chauvel P, Liegeois-Chauvel C, Marquis P, Bancaud J. Distinction between the myoclonus-related potential and the epileptic spike in EPC. *Electroencephalogr Clin Neurophysiol* 1986; 64:304–307.

140. Wiser HG, Graf HP, Bernoulli C, Siegfried J. Quantitative analysis of intracerebral recordings in EPC. *Electroencephalogr Clin Neurophysiol* 1978; 44:14–22.

141. Kuroiwa Y, Tohgi H, Takashahi A, Kanaya H. Epilepsia partialis continua: active cortical spike discharges and high cerebral blood flow in the motor cortex and enhanced transcortical long loop reflex. *J Neurol* 1985; 232:162–166.

142. Cowan JMA, Rothwell JC, Wise RJS, Marsden CD. Electrophysiological and positron emission studies in patients with cortical myoclonus, epilepsia partialis continua and motor epilepsy. *J Neurol Neurosurg Psychiatry* 1986; 49:796–807.

143. Morris HH, Lüders H. Electrodes. In: Gotman J, Ives JR, Gloor P, eds. *Long-Term Monitoring in Epilepsy.* Amsterdam, Elsevier Biomedical Press, 1985:326.

144. Goldensohn ES, Zablow L, Stein B. Interrelationships of form and latency of spike discharge from small areas of human cortex. *Electroencephalogr Clin Neurophysiol* 1970; 29:321–322.

145. Rasmussen T, Andermann F. Update on the syndrome of "chronic encephalitis" and epilepsy. *Cleve Clin J Med* 1989; 56(Suppl):181–184.

146. Oguni H, Andermann F, Rasmussen TB. The natural history of the syndrome of chronic encephalitis and epilepsy: a study of the MNI series of 48 cases. In: Andermann F, ed. *Chronic Encephalitis and Epilepsy: Rasmussen Syndrome.* Boston: Butterworth-Heinemann, 1991:7–25.

147. Rogers SW, Andrews PI, Gahring LC, et al. Autoantibody to glutamate receptor Glu R3 in Rasmussen's encephalitis. *Science* 1994; 265:648–651.

148. Pardo CA, Arroyo S, Ringing EPG, Freeman JM. Neuronal injury in Rasmussen's chronic encephalitis is mediated by cytotoxic T-cells. *Epilepsia* 1994; 35(Suppl 8):89.

149. Andrews PI, Dichter MA, Berkovic SF, McNamara JO. Plasmapheresis in Rasmussen's encephalitis. *Neurology* 1996; 46:242–246.

150. Aguilar MJ, Rasmussen T. Role of encephalitis in the pathogenesis of epilepsy. *Arch Neurol* 1960; 2:663–676.

151. Verhagen WIM, Renier, Ter Laak H, Jaspar HHJ, Gabreels FJM. Anomalies of the cerebral cortex in a case of epilepsia partialis continua. *Epilepsia* 1988; 29:57–62.

152. Robitaille Y. Neuropathological aspects of chronic encephalitis. In: Andermann F, ed. *Chronic Encephalitis and Epilepsy: Rasmussen Syndrome.* Boston: Butterworth-Heinemann, 1991:79–110.

153. Andrews PI, McNamara JO, Lewis DV. Clinical and electroencephalographic correlates in Rasmussen's encephalitis. *Epilepsia* 1997; 38:189–194.

154. Vining EPG, Freeman JM, Brandt J, Carson BS. Progressive unilateral encephalopathy of childhood (RS): a reappraisal. *Epilepsia* 1993; 34:639–650.

155. So NK, Gloor P. Electroencephalographic and electrocorticographic findings in chronic encephalitis of the Rasmussen type. In: Andermann F, ed. *Chronic Encephalitis and Epilepsy: Rasmussen Syndrome.* Boston: Butterworth-Heinemann, 1991:37–46.

156. Tien RD, Ashdown BC, Lewis DV, Atkins MR, Burger PC. Rasmussen's encephalitis: neuroimaging findings in 4 patients. *AJR* 1992; 158:1329–1332.

157. Matthews PM, Andermann F, Arnold DL. A proton magnetic resonance spectroscopic study of focal epilepsy in humans. *Neurology* 1990; 40:985–989.

158. Hart YM, Cortez M, Andermann F, et al. Medical treatment of Rasmussen's syndrome (chronic encephalitis and epilepsy): effect of high dose steroids or immunoglobulins in 19 patients. *Neurology* 1994; 44:1030–1036.

159. Vining PG, Freeman JM, Pillas DJ, et al. Why would you remove half a brain? The outcome of 58 children after hemispherectomy—The Johns Hopkins Experience: 1968 to 1996.

160. Villemure JG, Andermann F, Rasmussen T. Hemispherectomy for the treatment of epilepsy due to chronic encephalitis. In: Andermann F, ed. *Chronic Encephalitis and Epilepsy: Rasmussen Syndrome.* Boston: Butterworth-Heinemann, 1991:235–41.

161. Vining PG, Carson B, Brandt J. Hemispherectomy for Rasmussen syndrome: report of 24 cases. *Epilepsia* 1995; 36:S241. Abstract.

162. Theodore WH, Porter RJ, Penry JK. Complex partial seizures: clinical characteristics and differential diagnosis. *Neurology* 1983; 33:1115–1221.

163. Wyllie E, Friedman D, Rothner AD, et al. Psychogenic seizures in children and adolescents: outcome after diagnosis by ictal video and electroencephalographic recording. *Pediatrics* 1990; 85(Suppl 4):480–484.

164. Rothner AD. The migraine syndrome in children and adolescents. *Pediatr Neurol* 1986; 2:121–126.

165. Kuzniecky R, Murro A, King D, et al. Magnetic resonance imaging in in childhood intractable partial epilepsies: pathologic correlation. *Neurology* 1993; 43:681–687.

166. Berkovic SF, Andermann F, Olivier A, et al. Hippocampal sclerosis in temporal lobe epilepsy demonstrated by magnetic resonance imaging. *Ann Neurol* 1991; 29:175–182.

167. Jackson GD, Berkovic SF, Duncan JS, Connelly A. Optimizing the diagnosis of hippocampal sclerosis using MRI. *Am J Nucl Radiol* 1993; 14(3):753–762.

168. Cascino GD, Jack CR, Parsi JE, et al. Magnetic resonance imaging based volume studies in temporal lobe epilepsy: pathological correlation. *Ann Neurol* 1991; 30:31–36.

169. Jack C, Sharbrough FW, Cascino GD, Hirschorn KA, O'Brein PC. Magnetic resonance image-based hippocampal volumetry: correlation with outcome after temporal lobectomy. *Ann Neurol* 1992; 31:138–146.

170. Kuzniecky R, Cascino G, Palmini A, et al. Structural neuroimaging. In: Engel JE, ed. *Surgical Treatment of Epilepsies.* New York, Raven Press, 1993:197.

171. Palmini A, Andermann F, Olivier A, et al. Focal neuronal migrational disorder and intractable partial epilepsy: a study of 30 patients. *Ann Neurol* 1991; 30:741–749.

172. Palmini A, Andermann F, Olivier A, et al. Neuronal migration disorders. A contribution of modern neuroimaging to the etiological diagnosis of epilepsy. *Can J Neurol Sci* 1991; 18:580–587.

173. So NK, Gloor P. Electroencephalographic and electrocorticographic findings in chronic encephalitis of the Rasmussen type. In: Andermann F, ed. *Chronic Encephalitis and Epilepsy: Rasmussen Syndrome.* Boston:Butterworth-Heinemann, 1991:37–46.

174. Tien RD, Ashdown BC, Lewis DV, Atkins MR, Burger PC. Rasmussen's encephalitis: neuroimaging findings in 4 patients. *AJR* 1992; 158:1329–1332.

175. Theodore WH. Neuroimaging in the evaluation of patients for focal resection. In: Wyllie E, ed.

The Treatment of Epilepsy: Principles and Practice. Philadelphia: Lea & Febiger, 1993:1039–1050.

176. Henry TR, Chugani HT, Abou-Khalil BW, et al. Positron emission tomography. In: Engel J Jr, ed. *Surgical Treatment of Epilepsies.* 2nd ed. New York: Raven Press, 1993:211–243.

177. Savic I, Persson A, Roland P, et al. In vivo demonstration of BZ receptor binding in human epileptic foci. *Lancet* 1988; 2:863–866.

178. Frost JJ, Mayberg HS, Fisher RS, et al. Mu-opiate receptors measured by positron emission tomography are increased in temporal lobe epilepsy. *Ann Neurol* 1988; 23:231–237.

179. Adams C, Hwang P, Gilday DL, et al. Comparison of SPECT, EEG, CT, MRI and pathology in partial epilepsy. *Pediatr Neurol* 1992; 8:97–103.

180. Markhand ON, Shen W, Park HM, et al. Single photon imaging computed tomography (SPECT) for localization of epileptogenic focus in patients with intractable complex partial seizures. *Epilepsy Res* 1992 (Suppl 5):121–126.

181. Harvey A, Hopkins I, Bowe J, et al. Frontal lobe epilepsy: clinical seizure characteristics and localization with ictal 99m Tc-HMPAO SPECT. *Neurology* 1993; 43:1966–1980.

182. Marks DA, Katz A, Hoffer P, et al. Localization of extratemporal epileptic foci during ictal single-photon emission computed tomography. *Ann Neurol* 1992; 31:250–255.

183. Geiger LR, Harner RN. EEG seizure patterns at the time of focal seizure onset. *Arch Neurol* 1978; 35:276–286.

184. Gibbs FA, Gibbs EL. Atlas of electroencephalography. In: *Epilepsy.* Vol III. Reading, MA: Addison-Wesley, 1960.

185. Klass DW, Fischer-Williams M. Activation and provocation methods in clinical neurophysiology. I. Sensory stimulation. Sleep and sleep deprivation. In: Remond A, ed. *Handbook of Electroencephalography and Clinical Neurophysiology.* Amsterdam: Elsevier, 1975.

186. Harner RN. The significance of focal hypersynchrony in clinical EEG. *Electroencephalogr Clin Neurophysiol* 1971; 31:293.

187. Eeg-Olofson O, Peterson I, Seliden U. The development of the electroencephalogram in normal children from the age of 1 through 15 years: paroxysmal activity. *Neuropediatrie* 1971; 2:375–404.

188. Gastaut H, Broughton R. *Epileptic Seizures.* Springfield, Ill: Charles C Thomas, 1972.

189. Gastaut H, Vigoroux M. Electroclinical correlation in 500 cases of psychomotor seizures. In: Baldwin E, and Bailey P, eds. *Temporal Lobe Epilepsy.* Springfield, Ill: Charles C Thomas, 1958:118–128.

190. Wyllie E, Lüders H, Morris HH, et al. Subdural electrodes in the evaluation for epilepsy surgery in children and adults. *Neuropediatrics* 1988; 19:80–86.

191. Lüders H, Lesser RP, Dinner DS, et al. Commentary: chronic intracranial recording and stimulation with subdural electrodes. In: Engel J, ed. *Surgical Treatment of the Epilepsies.* New York, Raven Press, 1987:297–321.

192. Munari C, Bancaud J. The role of stereo-electroencephalography in the evaluation of partial epileptic seizures. In: Porter RJ, Morselli PL, eds. *Epilepsies.* London, Butterworths, 1985:267–306.

193. Engel J, Rausch R, Lieb JP, Kuhl DE, Crandall PH. Correlation of criteria used for localizing epileptic foci considered for surgical therapy of epilepsy. *Ann Neurol* 1981; 9:215–224.

194. Spencer SS, Spencer DD, Williamson PD, Mattson R. The localizing value of depth electroencephalography in 32 patients with refractory epilepsy. *Ann Neurol* 1982; 12:248–253.

195. Oliver A, Gloor P, Andermann F, Ives J. Occipito-temporal epilepsy studied with stereotaxically implanted depth electrodes and successfully treated by temporal resection. *Ann Neurol* 1982; 11:428–432.

196. Lesser RP, Pippenger CE. Choosing an antiepileptic drug. The case for individualized treatment. *Postgrad Med* 1985; 77:225–237.

197. Troupin AS. Carbamazepine reexamined. In: Pedley TA and Meldrum BS, eds. *Recent Advances in Epilepsy.* Vol. I. Edinburgh: Churchill Livingstone, 1983:47–56.

198. Wallace SJ. Carbamazepine in childhood seizures. *Dev Med Child Neurol* 1978: 20:223–226.

199. Porter RJ, Penry JK. Efficacy and choice of antiepileptic drugs. In: Meinardi H, Rowan AJ, eds. *Advances in Epileptology.* Amsterdam: Swets & Zeitlinger 1978:220–230.

200. Thompson PJ, Trimble MR. Anticonvulsant drugs and cognitive functions. *Epilepsia* 1982; 23:531–544.

201. Reynolds EH, Trimble MR. Adverse neuropsychiatric effects of anticonvulsant drugs. *Drugs* 1985; 29:570–581.

202. Tassinari CA, Roger J. Prognosis and therapy of complex partial seizures with barbiturates, hydantoins and other drugs. In: Penry JK and Daly DD, eds. *Advances in Neurology.* Vol XI. New York: Raven Press, 1975:201–219.

203. Gupta AK, Jeavons PN. Complex partial seizures, EEG foci and response to carbamazepine and sodium valproate. *J Neurol Neurosurg Psychiatry* 1985; 48:1010–1014.

204. Wyllie E, Wyllie R, Cruse RP, Erenberg G, Rothner AD. Pancreatitis associated with valproic acid therapy. *Am J Dis Child* 1984; 138:912–914.

205. Alton E. Bryant III, Dreifuss FE. Valproic acid hepatic fatalities III: US experience since 1984. *Neurology* 1996; 46:465–469.

206. Holowach-Thurston J, Thurston DL, Hixon BB, Keller AJ. Prognosis in childhood epilepsy. Additional follow-up of 148 children after withdrawal of anticonvulsant therapy. *N Engl J Med* 1982; 306:831–836.

207. Janz D, Sommer-Burkhardt EM. Discontinuation of antiepileptic drugs in patients with epilepsy who have been seizure free for more than two years. In: Janz D, ed. *Epileptology.* Stuttgart: Thieme, 1976:228–234.

208. Shinnar S, et al. Discontinuing antiepileptic medication in children with epilepsy after two years without seizures: a prospective study. *N Engl J Med* 1985; 313:976–980.

209. Chadwick D. The discontinuation of antiepileptic therapy. In: Pedley TA and Meldrum BS, eds. *Recent Advances in Epileptology*. Edinburgh: Churchill Livingstone, 1985:111–124.

210. Spencer SS, Spencer DD, Williamson PD, Mattson RH. Ictal effects of anticonvulsant medication withdrawal in epileptic patients. *Epilepsia* 1981; 22:297–307.

211. Felbamate study group in Lennox-Gastaut syndrome. Efficacy of felbamate in childhood epileptic encephalopathy (LGS). *N Engl J Med* 1993; 328:29–33.

212. Bourgeois MD, Leppik IE, Sackellares JC, et al. Felbamate: a double blind control trial in patients undergoing presurgical evaluation of partial seizures. *Neurology* 1993; 43:693–696.

213. Pellock JM, Boggs JG. Felbamate: a unique anticonvulsant. *Drugs Today* 1995; 31:9–17.

214. Brodie MJ, Pellock JM. Taming the brain storms: felbamate updated. *Lancet* 1995; 346:918–919.

215. Dodson WE. Felbamate in the treatment of Lennox-Gastaut syndrome: results of a 12 month, open-label study following a randomized clinical trial. *Epilepsia* 1993; 34(Suppl 7):S18–S24.

216. US Gabapentin Study Group No. 5. Gabapentin as add-on therapy in refractory partial epilepsy: a double-blind placebo-controlled, parallel-group study. *Neurology* 1993; 43:2292–2298.

217. Abou-Khalil B, Shellenberger MK, Anhut H. Two open-label, multicenter studies of the safety and efficacy of gabapentin in patients with refractory epilepsy. *Epilepsia* 1992:33(Suppl 3):77. Abstract.

218. Hes MS, Trudeau VL, Kilgore MB, et al. A double-blind, placebo controlled randomised multicenter trial of gabapentin in pediatric patients with BECTS. *Epilepsia* 1995; 36(Suppl 4):S125.

219. Vollmer KO, Archut H, Thomann P, Wagner F, Jahnchen D. Pharmacokinetic model and absolute bioavailability of the new anticonvulsant gabapentin. *Advances in Epileptology*. Vol. 17. New York: Raven Press, 1989:209–211.

220. Litzinger MJ, Wiscombe N, Hanny A, Yau J, Green D. Increased seizures and aggression seen in persons with mental retardation and epilepsy treated with Neurontin. *Epilepsia* 1995; 36(Suppl 4):71.

221. Asconape J, Collins T. Weight gain associated with the use of gabapentin. *Epilepsia* 1995; 36(Suppl 4):S74.

222. Cugley AL, Swartz BE. Gabapentin associated mood changes. *Epilepsia* 1995; 36(Suppl 4):S74.

223. Shantz D, Towbin JA, Spitz MC. Changes in mood and affect in patients on gabapentin. *Epilepsia* 1995; 36(Suppl 4):S75.

224. Brodie MJ, Richens A, Yuen AWC. Double-blind comparison of lamotrigine and carbamazepine in newly diagnosed epilepsy. *Lancet* 1995; 345:476–479.

225. Steiner TJ, Silveira C, Yuen AWC, et al. Comparison of lamotrigine (Lamictal) and phenytoin monotherapy in newly diagnosed epilepsy. *Epilepsia* 1994; 35(Suppl 7):61.

226. Besag FMC, Wallace SJ, Dulac O, et al. Lamotrigine for the treatment of epilepsy in childhood. *J Pediatr* 1995; 127:991–997.

227. Pellock JM. Utilization of new antiepileptic drugs in children. *Epilepsia* 1996; 37(Suppl 1):S66–S73, 1996.

228. Gibbs JM, Appleton RE, Rosenbloom L. Vigabatrin in intractable childhood epilepsy: a retrospective study. *Pediatr Neurol* 1992; 8:338–340.

229. Bernardina BD, Fontana E, Vigevano F, et al. Efficacy and tolerability of vigabatrin in children with refractory partial seizures: a single-blind dose-increasing study. *Epilepsia* 1995; 36:687–691.

230. Uldall P, Alving J, Gram L, et al. Vigabatrin in childhood epilepsy: a 5-year follow-up study. *Neuropediatrics* 1995; 26:253–256.

231. Aicardi J, Sabril IS, Investigator and Peer Review Groups, et al. Vigabatrin as initial therapy for infantile spasms: a European retrospective survey. *Epilepsia* 1996; 37:638–642.

232. Nabbout RC, Chiron C, Mumford J, Dumas C, Dulac O. Vigabatrin in partial seizures in children. *J Child Neurol* 1997; 12:172–177.

233. Luna D, Dulac O, Pajot N, Beaumont D. Vigabatrin in the treatment of childhood epilepsies: a single-blind placebo-controlled study. *Epilepsia* 1989; 30:430–437.

234. Uldall P, Alving J, Gram L. Vigabatrin in pediatric epilepsy — an open long term study. *J Child Neurol* 1991; 6(Suppl 2):S38–S44.

235. Gibbs J, Appleton RE, Rosenbloom L. Vigabatrin in intractable childhood epilepsy: a retrospective study. *Pediatr Neurol* 1992; 8:338–340.

236. Fois A, Buoni S, Di Bartolo RM, et al. Vigabatrin treatment in children. *Childs Nerv Syst* 1994; 10:244–248.

237. Wong V. Open label trial with vigabatrin in children with intractable epilepsy. *Brain Dev* 1995; 17:249–252.

238. Dulac O, Chiron C, Luna D, et al. Vigabatrin in childhood epilepsy. *J Child Neurol* 1991; 6(Suppl 2):S30–S37.

239. Cannon DJ, Butler WH, Mumford JP, et al. Neuropathological findings in patients receiving long-term vigabatrin therapy for chronic intractable epilepsy. *J Child Neurol* 1991; 6:2S17–2S24.

240. Ben-Menachem E, Nordborg C, Hedstrom A, Augustinsson LF, Silvenius H. Case report of surgical brain sample after 2 1/2 years of vigabatrin therapy. *Epilepsia* 1988; 29:699.

241. Paljarvi L, Vapalahti M, Sivenius J, Riekkinen P. Neuropathological examination in 5 patients with vigabatrin treatment. *Neurology* 1990; 40(Suppl 1):157.

242. Martinez AC, Baines JPO, Marques MB, et al. Vigabatrin associated reversible acute psychosis in a child. *Ann Pharmacother* 1995; 29:1115–1117.

243. Krauss GL, Johnson MA, Miller NR, et al. Vigabatrin associated retinal cone system dysfunction: electroretinogram and ophthalmologic findings. *Neurology* 1998; 50:614–618.

244. Eke T, Talbot JF, Lawden MC. Severe persistent visual field constriction associated with vigabatrin. *Br Med J* 1997; 314:180–181.

245. Glauser TA. Topiramate. *Semin Pediatr Neurol* 1997; 4:34–42.

246. Elterman R, Glauser TA, Riter FJ, Reife R, Wu SC. Topiramate as adjuvant therapy in pediatric patients with partial-onset seizures. *Epilepsia* 1997; 38(Suppl 8):98. Abstract.

247. Glauser TA, Sachdeo RC, Ritter FJ, Reife R, Lim P. A double blind trial of topiramate in Lennox-Gastaut syndrome (LGS). *Epilepsia* 1997; 38(Suppl 3):131. Abstract.

248. Glauser TA, Sachdeo RC, Ritter FJ, Reife R, Lim P. Topiramate in Lennox-Gastaut syndrome: a double blind trial. *Neurology* 1997; 48:1729. Abstract.

249. Elterman R, Glauser TA, Ritter FJ, Reife R, Wu SC. Efficacy and safety of topiramate in partial seizures in children. *Neurology* 1997; 48:1729. Abstract.

250. Glauser TA, Elterman R, Wyllie E. Long-term topiramate therapy in children with partial-onset seizures. *Neurology* 1998; 50(Suppl 4):A312. Abstract.

251. Ben-Menachem E, Henriksen O, Dam M, et al. Double-blind, placebo controlled trial of topiramate as add-on therapy in patients with refractory partial seizures. *Epilepsia* 1996; 37:539–543.

252. Reife RA, Lim P, Pledger G. Topiramate: side effect profile double blind studies. *Epilepsia* 1995; 36(Suppl 4):34. Abstract.

253. Suzdak PD, Jansen JA. A review of the preclinical pharmacology of tiagabine: a potent and selective anticonvulsant GABA uptake inhibitor. *Epilepsia* 1995; 36:612–626.

254. Chadwick D, Richens A, Duncan J, et al. Tiagabine HCl: safety and efficacy as adjunctive treatment for complex partial seizures. *Epilepsia* 1991; 32(Suppl 3):20.

255. Richens A, Chadwick DW, Duncan JS, et al. Adjunctive treatment of partial seizures with tiagabine: a placebo-controlled trial. *Epilepsy Res* 1995; 21:37–42.

256. Sachdeo RC, Leroy RF, Krauss GL, et al. Tiagabine therapy for complex partial seizures: a dose-frequency study. *Arch Neurol* 1997; 54:595–601.

257. Uthman BM, Rowan AJ, Ahmann PA, et al. Tiagabine for complex partial seizures. *Arch Neurol* 1998; 55:56–62.

258. Perucca E, Bialer M. The clinical pharmacokinetics of the new antiepileptic drugs: focus on topiramate, zonisamide and tiagabine. *Clin Pharmacokinet* 1996; 31:29–46.

259. Lau AH, et al. Pharmacokinetics and safety of tiagabine in subjects with various degrees of hepatic function. *Epilepsia* 1997; 38:445–451.

260. Brodie MJ. Tiagabine pharmacology in profile. *Epilepsia* 1995; 36(Suppl 6):S7–S9.

261. Dodrill CB, Arnett JL, Sommerville KW, Shu V. Cognitive and quality of life effects of differing dosages of tiagabine in epilepsy. *Neurology* 1997; 48:1025–1031.

262. Kalviainen R, Aikia M, Saukkonen AM, et al. Cognitive effects of tiagabine. *Epilepsia* 1994; 35(Suppl 4):74.

263. Mattson RH, Cramer JA, Collins JF, et al. Comparison of carbamazepine, phenobarbital, phenytoin and primidone for partial and secondarily generalized tonic-clonic seizures. *N Engl J Med* 1985; 313:145–151.

264. Schmidt D. Two antiepileptic drugs for intractable epilepsy with complex partial seizures. *J Neurol Neurosurg Psychiatry* 1982; 45:1119–1124.

265. Ferguson SM, Rayport M. The adjustment to living without epilepsy. *J Nerv Ment Dis* 1965; 140:26–37.

266. Kotagal P, Rothner AD, Erenberg G, Cruse RP, Wyllie E. Complex partial seizures of childhood-onset: a five-year follow-up study. *Arch Neurol* 1987; 44:1177–1180.

267. Iemolo F, Farnarier G, Serbanescu T, Menendez P. Etude longitudinale des epilepsies survenant dans l'adolescence. *Rev EEG Neurophysiol* 1981; 11:502–508.

268. Taylor DC. Mental state and temporal lobe epilepsy. A correlative account of 100 patients treated surgically. *Epilepsia* 1972; 13:727–765.

269. Ogunmekan AO, Hwang PA, and Hoffman HJ. Sturge-Weber-Dimitri disease: role of hemispherectomy in prognosis. *Can J Neurol Sci* 1989; 16:78–80.

270. Wyllie E, Comair Y, Kotagal P, Raja S, Ruggieri P. Epilepsy surgery in infants. *Epilepsia* 1996; 37:625–637.

271. Vigevano F, DiRocco C. Effectiveness of hemispherectomy in hemimegalencephaly with intractable seizures. *Neuropediatrics* 1990; 21:222–223.

272. Hoffman HH, Hendrick EB, Dennis M, Armstrong D. Hemispherectomy for Sturge-Weber syndrome. *Child Brain* 1979; 5:233–248.

273. Duchowny M, Levin B, Jayakar P, Resnick TJ. Temporal lobectomy in early childhood. *Epilepsia* 1992; 33:298–303.

274. Pieper T, Tuxhorn I, et al. Surgical outcome after temporal lobectomy in children with temporal lobe epilepsy. *Epilepsia* 1996; 37(Suppl 4):72.

275. Hopkins IJ, Klug GL. Temporal lobectomy for the treatment of intractable complex partial seizures temporal lobe origin in early childhood. *Dev Med Child Neurol* 1991; 33:26–31.

276. Erba G, Winston K, et al. Temporal lobectomy for complex partial seizures that began in childhood. *Surg Neurol* 1992; 38:424–432.

277. Meyer FB, Marsh RW, Laws ER, Sharbrough FW. Temporal lobectomy in children with epilepsy. *J Neurosurg* 1986; 64:371–376.

278. Rapport RL, Ojemann GA, Wyler AR, Ward AA. Surgical management of epilepsy. *West J Med* 1977; 127:185–189.

279. Whittle IR, Ellis HJ, Simpson DS. The surgical treatment of intractable childhood and adolescent epilepsy. *Aust NZ J Surg* 1981; 51:190–196.

280. Stepien L, Bacia T, Bidzinski, Wislawski J. Late results of operation in temporal lobe epilepsy in adults and children. *Neurosurg Rev* 1981; 4:61–69.

281. Palmini A, Costa Da Costa J, Andermann F, et al. Surgical results in epilepsy patients with localized cortical dysplastic lesions. In: Tuxhorn I, Holthausen H, eds. *Pediatric Epilepsy Syndromes and Their Surgical Treatment*. London: John Libbey, 1997:371–376.

282. Teixeira W, Holthausen H, Tuxhorn I, et al. Factors influencing surgical outcome in patients with severe

epilepsy and focal cortical dysplasia. Proceedings of the 6th International Bethel-Cleveland Clinic Epilepsy Symposium, Bielefeld, March 1995.

283. Taylor DC, Falconer MA, Bruton CJ, Corsellis JAN, et al. Focal dysplasia of the cerebral cortex in epilepsy. *J Neurol Neurosurg Psychiatry* 1971; 34:369–387.

284. Raymond AA, Fish DR, Sisodiya SM, et al. Abnormalities of gyration, heterotopias, tuberous sclerosis, focal cortical dysplasia, microdysgenesis, dysembrioplastic neuroepithelial tumor and dysgenesis of the archicortex in epilepsy: clinical, EEG and neuroimaging features in 100 adult patients. *Brain* 1995; 118:629–660.

285. Kuzniecky R, Garcia J, Faught E, Marawetz R, et al. Cortical dysplasia in temporal lobe epilepsy: magnetic resonance imaging correlations. *Ann Neurol* 1991; 29:293–298.

286. Wyllie E, Lüders H, Morris HH, Lesser RP, et al. Clinical outcome after complete or partial cortical resection for intractable epilepsy. *Neurology* 1987; 37:1634–1641.

287. Wyllie E, Rothner AD, Lüders H. Partial seizures in children. *Pediatr Clin North Am* 1989; 36:343–364.

288. Lüders H, Dinner DS, Morris HH, Wyllie E, Godoy J. EEG evaluation for epilepsy surgery in children. *Cleve Clin J Med* 1989; 56:S53–S61.

289. Gaser GH. Treatment of intractable temporal lobe epilepsy(complex partial seizures) by temporal lobectomy. *Ann Neurol* 1980; 8:455–459.

290. Lindsay J, Ounsted C, Richards P. Long-term outcome in children with temporal lobe epilepsy: I. Social outcome and childhood factors. *Dev Med Child Neurol* 1979; 21:285–298.

291. Pazzaglia P, D'Alesaandro R, Lozito A, Lugaresi E. Classification of partial epilepsies according to the symptomatology of seizures: Practical value and prognostic implications. *Epilepsia* 1982; 23:343–350.

292. Loiseau P, Dartigues JF, Pestre M. Prognosis of partial epileptic seizures in the adolescent. *Epilepsia* 1983; 24:472–481.

CHAPTER 19

Selected Disorders Associated with Epilepsy

Edwin C. Myer, M.D., and Lawrence D. Morton, M.D.

Certain diseases and clinical syndromes should be suspected by their presentation with particular types of epilepsy. A typical example is the onset of infantile spasms in an infant who has a hypsarrhythmic electroencephalogram (EEG). The clinical evaluation in any infant with this type of generalized seizure should include an ultraviolet light (Woods lamp) examination of the skin for hypomelanotic macules (1,2). The diagnosis is, of course, confirmed by neurologic evaluation and brain imaging with either computed tomography (CT) or magnetic resonance imaging (MRI). Thus, a variety of uncommon diseases in which epilepsy is a prominent symptom can be suspected by recognizing distinctive forms of epilepsy. This chapter discusses important examples of childhood disorders in which epilepsy plays a major role.

RETT SYNDROME

Rett syndrome is a unique disorder of unknown etiology occurring in girls due to a mutation on the X chromosome affecting methyl-CpG-binding protein 2 (3,4). Abnormalities of cerebrospinal fluid (CSF) biogenic amines have also been demonstrated, suggesting neurotransmitter dysfunction (4,5). After an apparently questionably normal early development (6), Rett syndrome patients lose acquired skills. This deterioration involves loss of acquired purposeful motor and hand skills and loss of communication and cognitive functions between 6 and 30 months. Of particular significance is the loss of acquired speech. Deceleration of head growth, stereotypic hand-wringing movements, and gait apraxia occur between 1 and 5 years (7). Apnea, hyperpnea, and breathholding spells occur. Seizures usually appear at 3 to 4 years of age. Aberrant behavior manifesting as irritability, sleeplessness, screaming spells, and self-abusiveness is common. Subsequently,

hypertonicity and spasticity can occur and progressive scoliosis develops.

The progression of the syndrome has been divided into four stages (8,9). Stage I is the period of apparently normal development lasting 6 to 18 months. Stage II, the regression period with stereotypy and autistic features, lasts 1 to 4 years. Stage III begins at approximately 3 years of age when seizures and ataxia occur. The deterioration may stop and the patient appears stationary. Stage IV is associated with severe disability and scoliosis. These stages can overlap. The ultimate prognosis is dependent on the degree of immobility and scoliosis and on the level of subsequent care (10).

Seizures occur in 70 percent to 80 percent of Rett syndrome patients. These may be generalized tonic, tonic-clonic, atypical absence, complex partial, myoclonic, or atonic seizures (8). Multiple seizure types occur in 30 to 40 percent of patients and may be intractable (9). The seizures usually appear at the age of 3 or 4 years. After 10 years of age it is uncommon for seizures to begin. Seizure types may appear refractory; however, some patients spontaneously improve on reaching adulthood (8,10,11). EEG may be helpful in the diagnosis of Rett syndrome in stages I and II by ruling out Angelman's syndrome, in which seizures occur before 2 years of age (12).

EEG changes similarly stratify into stages but do not correlate with the clinical course. During stage I the EEG may be normal or minimally slow. In stage II a rapid EEG deterioration occurs with slowing, loss of both occipital rhythms, and loss of normal sleep characteristics during quiet sleep [non–rapid eye movement (REM)]. Focal epileptiform activity, first during sleep and then in wakefulness with subsequent multifocal discharges then occurs. Stage III is represented by further deterioration with generalized slow spike-wave activity and multifocal discharges during sleep and wakefulness. The EEG remains markedly abnormal during stage IV.

The evolution of EEG changes is distinctive and can aid in the diagnosis of Rett syndrome (13). Multifocal central spikes and spike waves of short duration enhanced by sleep and predating seizure activity is a fairly consistent finding (14–16). These parasagittal spikes are present during the early stages of non-REM sleep and in the early morning hours and can help in differentiating the diagnosis of Rett syndrome from primary autism, in which the EEG usually is normal (17). In some of the episodes, apnea may not be seizure activity (18).

NEUROCUTANEOUS DISORDERS

Tuberous Sclerosis

Tuberous sclerosis complex is a congenital neurocutaneous disease of autosomal-dominant inheritance and variable expressivity (2). Two different mutations have been described that cause the tuberous sclerosis complex. The foci have been mapped to chromosomes 9q34.3 and 16p13.3, respectively (19,20). Hamartomas or benign growths may effect almost any organ but notably the skin, central nervous system (CNS), retina, heart, and kidney. The incidence of tuberous sclerosis varies in different studies from 1 in 10,000 to 1 in 170,000 but with increased evaluation appears to be more prevalent and is not a rare disease (21).

Tuberous sclerosis most often presents with seizures. In all, 80 percent to 90 percent of tuberous sclerosis patients develop seizures at some point in their lifetime. Generalized seizures are the most frequent, with infantile spasms occurring in 68 percent of selected patients. Complex partial seizures also occur frequently. Infantile spasms and myoclonic seizures are common in infants. Tonic, atonic, and atypical absences are also seen, especially in patients who have slow spike-wave EEG patterns and thus conform to the Lennox-Gastaut syndrome. Tonic-clonic seizures usually occur after 1 year of age, replacing other seizure types (22).

Various EEG abnormalities have been documented, depending on the clinical seizure type. Infantile spasms are associated with a hypsarrhythmic pattern, which may progress to multifocal EEG abnormalities including, most frequently, sharp-and-slow-wave discharges and spike-and-wave discharges. In general, the EEG abnormalities relate to the age of onset of the seizures (23,24).

The neurologic examination is frequently nonfocal; however, focal or diffuse signs occur with increasing size of subependymal or cortical lesions. These include hydrocephalus, movement disorders, visual disturbances, mental retardation, and rare focal motor deficits. The prognosis depends on the number and location of intracerebral lesions. The number and location of these lesions correlates with an early onset of difficult-to-control seizures and mental retardation. Approximately 37 percent of patients with tuberous sclerosis have average intelligence; 50 percent to 60 percent are mentally retarded. Seizure-free children usually have normal intelligence. Involvement of other organ systems, especially the heart and kidneys, may effect longevity. Aberrant behavior frequently becomes the most difficult management issue in these children as they become older.

Patients with infantile spasms and myoclonic seizures need to be treated immediately. The treatment of choice for each patient depends on their seizure type, age, and comorbidity (21,25,26) (see Chapters 31, 34, 38, and 40). Surgical treatment for focal abnormalities or tubers primarily correlated by EEG evidence of partial seizures has been quite successful (26) (see chapter on surgical treatment).

Neurofibromatosis (von Recklinghausen's Disease)

Neurofibromatosis is inherited as an autosomal-dominant disorder. Two forms have been characterized, NF1 and NF2. NF1 is the most common and the classic form; it has an incidence of 1 in 4,000 births. Central or acoustic neurofibromatosis, NF2, causes acoustic neuromas, not cutaneous or bony abnormalities. NF1 has been mapped to 17q11.2 and NF2 to the long arm of chromosome 22 (27,28).

Classic neurofibromatosis is characterized by pigmentary abnormalities and neurofibromas (27,29). Skin lesions include cafT au lait spots (6 or more >0.5 cm in prepubertal children and >1.5 cm in postpubertal children) and intertriginous freckles. Lisch nodules in the iris are present in a minority of affected young children but increase with age. Neurologic features include seizures in 3 percent to 5 percent (30), occasional mental retardation, learning disorders, and a heightened risk of developing glial CNS tumors, with visual path glioma being most common in NF1. Although cortical heterotopias are found in rare cases, most often the pathogenesis of epilepsy and learning problems is unclear. Other features include growth disturbances, osseous aplasia or hyperplasia, macrocephaly, scoliosis, precocious puberty, and cerebrovascular lesions causing stroke. There is an increased risk of malignancies, which can limit longevity.

The treatment of seizures associated with neurofibromatosis is dependent on seizure type and whether a specific intracranial mass lesion is present. Most patients are treated with chronic antiepileptic drug (AED) therapy, with very few having spontaneous remission of their epilepsy.

Sturge-Weber Syndrome

Sturge-Weber syndrome is characterized by a port wine stain unilaterally over the upper face, superior eyelid, or supraorbital region. Buphthalmos is common, resulting in glaucoma, and intracranial calcification occurs in 90 percent of cases. Partial or secondary generalized seizures occur in almost all patients with increasing frequency with age. EEG reveals decreased amplitude and frequency over the affected hemisphere with diffuse multiple and independent spikes (31). Surgical removal of the affected lobe or hemisphere should be considered when seizures are refractory (see Chapter 48).

Hypomelanosis of Ito

Hypomelanosis of Ito is characterized by macular cutaneous hypopigmentation in patterns of whorls, streaks, and patches, as well as generalized abnormalities.The associated CNS abnormalities produce a clinical picture characterized by delayed development and frequently refractory seizures, including infantile spasms. Cortical atrophy is seen on imaging studies. The EEG abnormality shows no consistent pattern (32).

Incontinentia Pigmenti

The skin lesion of incontinentia pigmenti, which is seen mostly in girls, has three stages. Initially, one sees macular papular vesicular and even bullous lesions occurring in the first 2 weeks of life and located primarily over the limbs or trunk. This stage is followed by a keratotic verrucous lesion over the limbs followed by hypopigmentation or skin atrophy. Subsequent pigmentation then occurs. The CNS is commonly involved, with generalized and focal seizures in 9 percent to 13 percent of patients. Retardation, spasticity, and microcephaly occur in 5 percent to 16 percent. Ocular abnormalities occur in one-third of the patients (33).

METABOLIC DISORDERS

Various diseases with underlying inborn metabolic abnormalities may cause epilepsy characterized by a particular EEG abnormality (34). Early identification and appropriate treatment of these specific disorders frequently lead to the best treatment of seizures and optimal developmental outcome. AEDs, however, are sometimes necessary despite identification and treatment.

Urea cycle disorders occur in 1 in 30,000 births. Seizure activity may be the presenting symptom associated with hyperammonemia, which can be precipitated or worsened by valproate therapy in unrecognized ornithine transcarbamylase deficiency (35). Deficiencies of ornithine transcarbamylase and arginosuccinic acid lyase have resulted in abnormal EEG activity characterized mainly by multiple spikes, spike waves, or slow-and-sharp-wave activity. The EEG normalizes with successful treatment of the metabolic disorder (36). Citrullinemia also has presented with seizure activity and an EEG with multifocal spikes (37). However, there is a lag in EEG normalization after treatment (peritoneal dialysis) in this condition. Neurologic deficits persist in reported cases (38).

Phenylketonuria when untreated may be associated with infantile spasms and a hypsarrhythmic EEG. In treated phenylketonuria there is an increased prevalence of EEG abnormalities manifesting as generalized slowing with or without spikes (39). With advancing age, the EEG abnormalities increase but lack any relationship to IQ or dietary treatment (40).

Menkes' kinky hair disease, a sex-linked disorder with its gene located on the long arm of the X chromosome, causes a marked reduction of serum copper and serum ceruloplasmin levels. The clinical findings consist of mental retardation, poorly pigmented fragile hair, hypotonia, and generalized seizure activity, frequently infantile spasms (41).

Other inborn errors of metabolism may be associated with generalized seizure activity. These include maple syrup urine disease, galactosemia, hyperglycinemia, and hyperammonemia, to mention only a few.

Although *porphyria* does not become symptomatic until after puberty, it occasionally affects older adolescents. Seizures commonly occur in 15 percent of patients with porphyria, usually during an acute attack. Seizures may be partial or generalized. Therapy of chronic seizures in these patients must avoid drugs that increase porphyria precursors and induce attacks. This includes all commonly used AEDs (42), although gabapentin is safe and effective.

Skin rashes and striking neurologic symptoms with seizures are prominent signs of biotinidase deficiency. Hypotonia, developmental delay, and seizures are presenting features in the neonatal form. In the late-onset type, 1 week to 2 years onset, the most common presenting feature is seizures. The most common seizure type is myoclonus, although generalized tonic-clonic and focal clonic seizures have been described (43). Ataxia and hypotonia are present, as are rash and alopecia. Hearing loss may occur. Treatment is oral biotin with rapid response within 24 hours (43,44).

INFECTIONS

Infants with prenatal intracranial infections are liable to have generalized postnatal seizures. A common infection is cytomegalovirus (45). In particular, infants with neonatal herpes simplex encephalitis may have specific EEG patterns consisting of periodic or quasi-periodic patterns. Thus, a periodic pattern in a young infant with partial motor seizures and lymphocytic cerebrospinal fluid (CSF) pleocytosis is highly suggestive of herpes virus encephalitis (46), cytomegalovirus, or toxoplasmosis (47).

Human immunodeficiency virus (HIV) has emerged as a major prenatal infection with significant neurologic morbidity. Approximately 90 percent of prepubertal cases reflect intrauterine or intrapartum infection. The predominant clinical finding is a triad of impaired brain growth, progressive motor dysfunction, and plateau or loss of developmental milestones (48,49). In children, CNS effects usually result from direct HIV-1 infection, not from tumors or opportunistic infections, in contrast to adults (48). Seizures occur at only a slightly higher incidence in the pediatric HIV-1 population (50) compared with the uninfected population. The presence of a seizure leads to a workup, including neuroimaging, to look for coexisting focal pathology (51).

Subacute sclerosing panencephalitis was first reported in 1993 as an inclusion body encephalitis. Measles virus is the causal agent and persists in the CNS. Virus persistence appears to be a result of a defect in replication. The progression of the illness has been broken into four stages, with stage I including mild behavioral and intellectual changes and stage IV including flexor posture, mutism, and autonomic instability. Seizures typically develop in stage II. Myoclonus is the best known and typically is periodic and stereotypic. The EEG demonstrates periodic complexes of high-amplitude delta waves occurring every 4 to 12 seconds and are synchronous with the myoclonic jerks (52). Other seizure types include akinetic, atypical absence, generalized tonic-clonic, and focal clonic (53). The prognosis is grave even with treatment, with a median survival of 1 year.

CHROMOSOMAL ABNORMALITIES AND CONGENITAL BRAIN ABNORMALITIES

Chromosomal abnormalities, including trisomy 13 and 21, may result in infants and children with seizure activity. Approximately 20 percent of patients with fragile X syndrome have seizures (generalized or partial) with spikes similar to rolandic spikes, which are noted during sleep tracings (54,55). Five percent to 6 percent of children with Down syndrome (trisomy 21) have seizures (56). Infantile spasms may occur but are fairly responsive to therapy.

Congenital malformations with neurologic deficits can cause infantile spasms and hypsarrhythmic patterns as well as other seizure types. The Aicardi syndrome, an X-linked dominant syndrome limited to females, is marked by agenesis of the corpus callosum, mental retardation, vertebral anomalies, and chorioretinal lacunae. In patients with seizures, 97 percent have had infantile spasms, with many having other seizure types (57). Septico-optic dysplasia with absence of septum pellucidum, optic nerve hypoplasia, and hypothalamic-pituitary dysfunction can also present with infantile spasms (58). Various brain gyral malformations such as lissencephaly, agyria-pachygyria, and others may cause infantile spasms or other seizure types (59–61).

Angelman's Syndrome (Happy Puppet Syndrome)

Angelman's syndrome occurs in children with a history of nonprogressive delayed development from infancy. Jerky limb movements, stiff ataxic-like gait, paroxysms of inappropriate laughter, and lack of speech are characteristic. Distinctive facial features with a prominent lower jaw, wide mouth, frequent tongue thrusting, and a thin upper lip are consistent. A chromosomal abnormality of maternal origin 15q11-13 has been detected in patients with Angelman's syndrome (62).

Seizure activity is a frequent presenting symptom and is present in 86 percent of patients (63). Seizures commence at an early age, appearing by age 11 months at the earliest but often by 2 years of age. Myoclonic, atypical absence, generalized tonic-clonic, and unilateral clonic seizures are the typical clinical patterns, whereas infantile spasms are rare (64–66). This is an earlier age of onset for seizures than is seen in Rett syndrome, in which seizures usually begin at 3 to 4 years of age (12). Seizures are usually preceded by an abnormal EEG. The EEG demonstrates large- amplitude generalized spike-wave activity not unsimilar to the EEG pattern in Lennox-Gastaut syndrome, but unlike this syndrome, seizures in Angelman's syndrome are not severe. The large rhythmic activity persists in sleep. The spike-wave activity tends to be accentuated with eye closure. Thus, this facilitation of the EEG pattern with eye closure and the general pattern present from 1 year of age is suggestive of Angelman's syndrome (67). This EEG pattern appears to persist and is not modified by AEDs. Brain imaging shows variable results, with brain atrophy in perhaps 50 percent of patients. Correlation exists between epilepsy phenotypes and genotypes (68).

Prader-Willi Syndrome

Prader-Willi syndrome consists of short stature, small hands and feet, obesity, and mental retardation preceded in infancy by hypotonia and feeding difficulty. Males have hypoplastic, flat scrotums with inguinal or abdominal testes. Seizures occur in 15 percent to 20 percent (69,70). Although most cases are sporadic, concordance in monozygotic twins has been reported (71).

The disorder results from the specific deletion of 15q11q13 of paternal origin (72). The same region is deleted in Angelman's syndrome but the different syndromes result from genetic imprinting (73).

Miller-Dieker Syndrome

Miller-Dieker syndrome includes microcephaly and lissencephaly, epilepsy, profound mental retardation, and occasional anomalies of the heart and genitalia (74,75). Characteristic features include flat midface, prominent forehead, protuberant upper lip, and small jaw. It results from a deletion of the terminal end of the long arm of chromosome 17p13.3. Smaller deletions in chromosome 17 have also resulted in lissencephaly but lack the typical facies (76,77).

Acquired Epileptic Aphasia (Landau-Kleffner Syndrome)

Landau-Kleffner syndrome is typified by the loss of receptive and expressive language in association with paroxysmal EEG changes and in some cases seizures (78). Partial seizures in the dominant hemisphere both acutely and postictally may be associated with transient aphasia. However, in this disorder children who have developed normal language then experience a progressive deterioration of language (79). Diffuse or focal spike-waves with temporal preponderance are present, as are temporal metabolic abnormalities. Seizure activity may occur at a much later stage. The aphasia rarely improves with seizure control (80,81). These children occasionally may have autistic-like features. Recognition of the progressive nature of the language dysfunction may result in earlier intervention (82). Autistic-like features also may be seen in children with epilepsy–generalized tonic-clonic, absence, and partial complex seizures, either primary or secondary (83).

MITOCHONDRIAL ENCEPHALOMYOPATHIES

The mitochondrial encephalomyopathies consist of a heterogeneous group of multisystem disorders. Seizures are a common finding in this class of disease. Seizures are a defining symptom in myoclonic epilepsy with ragged red fibers (MERRF) and are a common feature in mitochondrial encephalomyopathy, lactic acidosis, and strokelike episodes (MELAS). Seizures are uncommon in Kearns-Sayre syndrome.

MERRF

Ataxia, intention and action myoclonus, and progressive mental deterioration have been reported in MERFF. Associated with these features, muscle biopsy has demonstrated aggregates of mitochondria in skeletal muscle known as ragged red fibers. Generalized tonic-clonic seizures, which are photosensitive, are a feature and may be a presenting symptom. Spike-wave complexes occurring spontaneously and coinciding with myoclonic activity occur (84).

Mitochondrial myopathies associated with myoclonic epilepsy have been described occurring in families. Recent mitochondrial abnormalities occurring in Rett syndrome have been reported (6). In most reported mitochondrial myopathies, EEGs typically show abnormal spike-wave activity. Seizure control is difficult in severe cases (85).

MELAS

MELAS has among its defining features strokelike episodes typically before age 40; encephalopathy characterized by dementia, seizures, or both; and evidence of a mitochondrial myopathy with ragged red fibers and/or lactic acidosis. Patients with MELAS frequently have seizures. In one group, seizures were the initial clinical symptom in 28 percent. They were sometimes associated with a strokelike episode. Seizure were both generalized and partial (86). Partial seizures were most typically motor. Seizures typically respond to conventional antiseizure agents.

ALPERS' DISEASE (POLIODYSTROPHY)

Progressive infantile poliodystrophy designates a pattern of symptoms including seizures and overall deterioration called Alpers' disease. The early cases in the literature were heterogeneous, and confusion about diagnosis and nomenclature has been a hallmark of this group of diseases (87,88). Two distinct groups of patients have emerged. One group has microcephaly with shrunken "walnut" brains, a progressive degeneration (89). The second group indicates a more uniform spectrum of clinical and pathologic phenotypes that are due to several inborn errors that affect energy metabolism, the Krebs cycle, respiratory chain, and mitochondrial function (90–94). Some of these patients have insidious but progressive liver disease (88,95) while others are without hepatic failure (96). In recent years, when some of these patients have died with liver failure, valproic acid hepatotoxicity has been blamed (88).

Usually thought to be normal at birth, the children develop a progressive illness manifest by developmental delay, failure to thrive, focal myoclonus, seizures with a propensity for status epilepticus, hypotonia, visual disturbances (blindness is common), eventual paralysis, spasticity, and liver failure (94,97–99). In addition, many of these patients develop multifocal myoclonic twitching or epilepsia partialis continua of the Kojewnikow variety (100–102). Variable features include deafness, chorea, and ataxia. They often worsen rapidly during an intercurrent illness.

At autopsy, there is atrophy of the hemispheres and the cerebellum. The cortex has diffuse foci of degeneration with neuronal necrosis, astrocytosis, and spongiosis with perivascular and pericellular edema. Other affected structures include the basal ganglia, thalamus, brain stem nuclei, dentate nucleus, cerebellar cortex, and lumbar spinal ganglia. The predominant hepatic lesions are microvesicular fatty infiltration and cirrhosis sometimes with a micronodular pattern (99).

Distinctive EEG features include slow (≤ 1 Hz), high-amplitude (200–1,000 μV) background mixed with lower amplitude polyspikes, often with focal prominence in the occipital area. The polyspikes on the EEG persist despite intravenous doses of barbiturates that suppress clinical seizures. Evoked potentials have been variably abnormal. Flash visual evoked potentials (VEPs) have ranged from normal to absent and often are asymmetric. Brain stem auditory evoked potentials (BAEPs) in some cases have been absent (100).

Several enzyme deficiencies have been reported as a biochemical basis for this disorder. These include abnormalities of the pyruvate dehydrogenase (PDH) complex, pyruvate carboxylase, coenzyme Q, and complexes I and IV, in the second part of the citric acid cycle (after the oxoglutarate dehydrogenase complex) in nicotinamide-adenine dinucleotide (reduced form) (NADH) oxidation, in cytochrome aa$_3$, and in pyruvate carboxylase activity (94). Additional defects in cerebral energy metabolism are likely to be discovered. The types of enzyme defects described thus far have been associated with elevated concentrations of lactic acid in CSF.

COCKAYNE'S SYNDROME

Cockayne's syndrome is characterized by paucity of growth with developmental delay, loss of subcutaneous fat, cold cyanosed extremities, increased pigmented nevi, and decreased scalp hair. With increasing cachexia the patient's distinctive facies, enophthalmos, and absent fat are prominent features. Mental retardation and microcephaly with ventriculomegaly and questionable normal-pressure hydrocephalus is present. Hypertonicity with various movement disorders and myoclonic jerks is present. Optic atrophy and retinal pigmentary changes occur. It is inherited as an autosomal recessive trait caused by several different mutations on chromosomes 5, 10, 13, and 19. Seizure activity usually has an early onset but can occur initially in adults. Status epilepticus resulting in death has been reported (103,104).

COLLAGEN VASCULAR DISEASES

Fourteen percent to 17 percent of patients with systemic lupus erythematosus (SLE) develop seizures unrelated to renal disease, cardiac disease, or drugs. These generalized or partial seizures usually occur early in the disease. As a true vasculitis is uncommon, the precise cause is not defined, although disordered immunoregulation involving antineuronal antibodies has been suggested. Cerebral microinfarcts and subarachnoid hemorrhage have been demonstrated. When seizures are associated with psychiatric symptoms, a generalized vasculitis is probably present. Infective causes need to be ruled out in the immunosuppressed patient. In polyarteritis nodosa, seizure activity occurs in 40 percent to 50 percent of older children. Seizures typically appear early in the course and are difficult to control (42). Phenytoin, ethosuximide, and carbamazepine can cause symptoms similar to those of SLE (105).

CONCLUSIONS

Many disease states may present with generalized or partial seizures in infancy and childhood. On occasion, the type of seizure and EEG pattern can be helpful in making the specific diagnosis. In particular, the cause, if demonstrable, may help in treatment and genetic counseling. The absence of seizure activity and a normal EEG can be equally useful in arriving at a diagnosis in girls with autism and self-mutilation resembling Rett syndrome. The early abnormal EEG in girls with similar clinical features without concomitant seizures is helpful in diagnosing Angelman's syndrome.

Infantile spasms can occur in multiple diseases, and treatable etiologies such as metabolic disorders and infections need to be aggressively evaluated and treated as well as the epilepsy. Seizures, after all, represent a symptom of CNS dysfunction. Associated symptoms should encourage the treating physician to further evaluate these children when they present with evidence of more widespread disorders as reviewed herein.

REFERENCES

1. Oppenheimer EY, Roosman NP, Dooling EC. The late appearance of hypopigmented maculae in tuberous sclerosis. *Am J Dis Child* 1985; 139:408–409.

2. Gomez MR. Tuberous sclerosis. In: Gomez MR, ed. *Neurocutaneous Diseases*. London: Butterworth, 1987:33–37.

3. Amir RE, Van den Veyver IB, Wan M, et al. Rett syndrome is caused by mutations in X-linked MECP2, enclosing methyl-CpG-binding protein 2. *Nat Genet* 1999; 23:185–188.

4. Van den Veyver IB, Zoghbi HY. Methyl-CpG-binding protein 2 mutations in Rett syndrome. *Curr Opin Genet Dev* 2000; 10:275–279.

5. Zoghbi HY, Milstien S, Beebler IJ, et al. Cerebrospinal fluid biogenic amines and biopterin in Rett syndrome. *Ann Neurol* 1989; 25:56–60.

6. Naidu S. Rett syndrome: a disorder affecting early brain growth. *Ann Neurol* 1997; 42:3–10.

7. The Rett Syndrome Diagnostic Work Group. Diagnostic criteria for Rett syndrome. *Ann Neurol* 1988; 23:425–428.

8. Hagbert BA. Rett syndrome: clinical peculiarities, diagnostic approach, and possible causes. *Pediatr Neurol* 1989; 5:75–83.

9. Trevalhan E, Naidu S. The clinical recognition and differential diagnosis of Rett syndrome. *J Child Neurol* 1988; 3(Suppl):S6–S16.

10. Naidu S, Murphy M, Moser HW, et al. Rett syndrome—natural history in 70 cases. *Am J Med Genet* 1986; 24(Suppl):61–72.

11. Coleman M, Brubaker J, Hunter K, Smith G. Rett syndrome: a survey of North American patients. *J Ment Defic Res* 1988; 32:117–124.

12. Laan LA, Brouwer OF, Begeer CH, Zwinderman AH, Gert van Dijk J. The diagnostic value of EEG in Angelman and Rett syndrome at a young age. *Electroencephalogr Clin Neurophysiol* 1998; 106:404–408.

13. Glaze DG, Frost JD, Zoghbi H, Percy AK. Rett syndrome: correlation of electroencephalographic characteristics with clinical staging. *Arch Neurol* 1987; 44:1053–1056.

14. Garofalo EA, Drury I, Goldstein GW. EEG abnormalities aid diagnosis of Rett syndrome. *Pediatr Neurol* 1988; 4:350–353.

15. Hagne I, Witt-Engerstrom I, Hagberg B. EEG development in Rett syndrome—a study of 30 cases. *Electroencephalogr Clin Neurophysiol* 1989; 72:1–6.

16. Robb SA, Harden A, Boyd SG. Rett syndrome: an EEG study in 52 girls. *Neuropediatrics* 1989; 20:192–195.

17. Aldrich MS, Garofalo EA, Drury I. Epileptiform abnormalities during sleep in Rett syndrome. *Electroencephalogr Clin Neurophysiol* 1990; 75:365–370.

18. Glaze DG, Schultz RJ, Frost JD. Rett syndrome: characterization of seizures versus non-seizures. *Electroencephalogr Clin Neurophysiol* 1998; 106:79–83.

19. Fryer AE, Chalmers AH, Connor JM, et al. Evidence that the gene for tuberous sclerosis is on chromosome 9. *Lancet* 1987; 1:659–661.

20. European Chromosome 16 Tuberous Sclerosis Consortium. Identification and characterization of tuberous sclerosis gene on chromosome 16. *Cell* 1993; 75:1305–1315.

21. Gomez MR. Tuberous sclerosis. In: Gomez MR, ed. *Neurocutaneous Diseases*. London: Butterworth, 1887:21–49.

22. Franz DN. Diagnosis and management of tuberous sclerosis complex. *Semin Ped Neurol* 1998; 5:253–268.

23. Riikonen R, Simell O. Tuberous sclerosis and infantile spasms. *Dev Med Child Neurol* 1990; 32:203–209.

24. Ohtsuka Y, Ohmori I, Oka E. Long-term follow-up of childhood epilepsy associated with tuberous sclerosis. *Epilepsia* 1998; 39:1158–1163.

25. Shields WD, Sankar R. Vigabatrin. *Semin Pediatr Neurol* 1997; 4:43–50.

26. Baumgartner JE, Wheless JW, Kulkarni S, et al. On the surgical treatment of refractory epilepsy in tuberous sclerosis complex. *Pediatr Neurosurg* 1997; 27:311–318.

27. Listernick R, Charrow J. Neurofibromatosis type 1 in childhood. *J Pediatr* 1990; 116:845–853.

28. Wertelecki W, Rouleau GA, Superneau DW, et al. Neurofibromatosis 2: clinical and DNA linkage studies of a large kindred. *N Engl J Med* 1988; 319:278–283.

29. Riccardi V. Neurofibromatosis. In: Gomez MR, ed. *Neurocutaneous Diseases*. London: Butterworth, 1987.

30. Kulkantrakorn K, Geller TJ. Seizures in neurofibromatosis 1. *Pediatr Neurol* 1998; 19:347–350.

31. Maria BL, Neufeld JA, Rosainz LC, et al. High prevalence of bihemispheric structural and functional defects in Sturge-Weber syndrome. *J Child Neurol* 1998; 13:595–605.

32. Glover MT, Brett EM, Atherton DJ. Hypomelanosis of Ito: spectrum of the disease. *J Pediatr* 1989; 115:75–80.

33. Rossman P. Incontinentia pigmenti. In: Gomez MR, ed. *Neurocutaneous Diseases*. London: Butterworth, 1987:293–300.

34. Verma NP, Hart ZH, Kooi KA. Electrographic findings in urea-cycle disorders. *Electroencephalogr Clin Neurophysiol* 1984; 57:105–112.

35. Burton BK. Inborn errors of metabolism: a guide to diagnosis. *Pediatrics* 1998; 102:E69.

36. Oechsner M, Steen C, Sturenburg HJ, Kohlschutter A. Hyperammonaemic encephalopathy after initiation of valproate therapy in unrecognized ornithine transcarbamylase deficiency. *J Neurol Neurosurg Psychiatry* 1998; 64:680–682.

37. Engel RC, Buist NRM. The EEGs of infants with citrullinemia. *Dev Med Child Neurol* 1985; 27:199–206.

38. Origuchi Y, Ushijima T, Sakaguchi M, et al. Citrullinemia presenting as uncontrollable epilepsy. *Brain Dev* 1984; 6:328–331.

39. Korinthenberg R, Ullrich K, Fullenkemper F. Evoked potentials and electroencephalography in adolescents with phenylketonuria. *Neuropediatrics* 1988; 19:175–178.

40. Pietz J, Benninger CH, Schmidt H, et al. Long-term development of intelligence (IQ) and EEG in 34 children with phenylketonuria treated early. *Eur J Pediatr* 1988; 147:361–367.

41. Menkes JH. Kinky hair disease: twenty-five years later. *Brain Dev* 1988; 10:77–79.

42. Zadra M, Grandi R, Erli LC, Mirabile D, Brambilla A. Treatment of seizures in acute intermittent porphyria: safety and efficacy of gabapentin. *Seizure* 1998; 7:415–416.

43. Salbert BA, Pellock JM, Wolf B. Characterization of seizures associated with biotinidase deficiency. *Neurology* 1993; 43:1351–1355.

44. Wolf B, Heard GS, Weissbecker KA, et al. Biotinidase deficiency: initial clinical features and rapid diagnosis. *Ann Neurol* 1985; 18:614–617.

45. Bale JF, Blackman JA, Sato Y. Outcome in children with symptomatic congenital cytomegalovirus infection. *J Child Neurol* 1990; 5:131–136.

46. Mizrahi EM, Thorp BR. A characteristic EEG pattern in neonatal herpes simplex encephalitis. *Neurology* 1982; 32:1215–1220.

47. Wright R, Johnson D, Neumann M, et al. Congenital lymphocytic choriomeningitis virus syndrome: a disease that mimics congenital toxoplasmosis or cytomegalovirus infection. *Pediatrics* 1997; 100:E9.

48. Brouwers P, Belman AL, Epstein LG. Central nervous system involvement: manifestations, evaluation, and pathogenesis. In: Pizzo PA and Wilfert CM, eds. *Pediatric AIDS.* Baltimore: Williams & Wilkins, 1994: 433–455.

49. Belman AL. Acquired immune deficiency in the child's central nervous system. *Pediatr Clin North Am* 1992; 39:691–714.

50. Mintz M, Epstein LG, Koenigsberger MR. Neurologic manifestations of acquired immunodeficiency syndrome (AIDS) in children. *International Pediatrics* 1989; 4:161–171.

51. Wong MC, Suite AND, Labar DR. Seizures in human immunodeficiency virus infection. *Arch Neurol* 1990; 47:640–642.

52. Rish WAS, Haddard FS. The variable natural history of subacute sclerosing panencephalitis: a study of 118 cases from the Middle East. *Arch Neurol* 1979; 36:610–614.

53. Markland CN, Panszi JG. The elective encephalogram in subacute sclerosing panencephalitis. *Arch Neurol* 1975; 32:719–726.

54. Musumeci SA, Colognola RM, Ferri R, et al. Fragile X syndrome: a particular epileptogenic EEG pattern. *Epilepsia* 1988; 29:41–47.

55. Kluger G, Bohm I, Laub MC, Waldenmaier C. Epilepsy and fragile X mutations. *Pediatr Neurol* 1996; 15:358–360.

56. Stafstrom CE, Patxot OF, Gilmore HE, Wisniewski KE. Seizures in children with Down syndrome: etiology, characteristics and outcome. *Dev Med Child Neurol* 1991; 33:191–220.

57. Chevrie J, Aicardi J. The Aicardi syndrome. In: Pedley T and Meldram J, eds. *Recent Advances in Epilepsy.* 3rd ed. Edinburgh: Churchill-Livingstone, 1986:189–210.

58. Kuriyama M, Shigematsu Y, Konishi K, et al. Septo-optic dysplasia with infantile spasms. *Pediatr Neurol* 1988; 4:62–66.

59. Dobyns WB, Truwit CL. Lissencephaly and other malformations of cortical development: 1995 update. *Neuropediatrics* 1995; 26:132–147.

60. Paladin F, Chiron C, Dulac O, et al. Electroencephalographic aspects of hemimegalencephaly. *Dev Med Child Neurol* 1989; 31:377–383.

61. Gastaut H, Pinsard N, Raybaud C, et al. Lissencephaly (agyria-pachygyria) clinical findings and serial EEG studies. *Dev Med Child Neurol* 1987; 29:167–180.

62. Robb SA, Pohl KR, Baraitser M, Wilson J, Brett EM. The happy "puppet" syndrome of Angelman: review of the clinical features. *Arch Dis Child* 1989; 64:83–86.

63. Laan LA, Renier WO, Arts WF, et al. Evolution of epilepsy and EEG findings in Angelman syndrome. *Epilepsia* 1997; 38:195–199.

64. Geurrini R. DeLorey TM, Bonanni P, et al. Cortical myoclonus in Angelman syndrome. *Ann Neurol* 1996; 40:39–48.

65. Matsumoto A, Kumagai T, Miura K, et al. Epilepsy in Angelman syndrome associated with chromosome 15q deletion. *Epilepsia* 1992; 33:1083–1090.

66. Viani F, Romeo A, Viri M, et al. Seizure and EEG patterns in Angelman's syndrome. *J Child Neurol* 1995; 10:467–471.

67. Rubin DI, Patterson MC, Westmoreland BF, Klass DW. Angelman's syndrome: clinical and electrographic findings. *Electroencephalogr Clin Neurophysiol* 1997; 102:299–302.

68. Minassian BA, DeLorey TM, Olsen RW, et al. Angelman syndrome: correlations between epilepsy phenotypes and genotypes. *Ann Neurol* 1998; 43:485–493.

69. Williams MS, Rooney BL, Williams J, Josephson K, Pauli R. Investigation of thermoregulatory characteristics in patients with Prader-Willi syndrome. *Am J Med Genet* 1994; 49:302–307.

70. Hall BD, Smith DW. Prader-Willi syndrome. *J Pediatr* 1972; 81:286–293.

71. Brissenden JE, Levy EP. Prader-Willi syndrome in infant monozygotic twins. *Am J Dis Child* 1973; 126:110–112.

72. Ledbetter DH, Riccardi VM, Airhart SD, et al. Deletions of chromosome 15 as a cause of the Prader-Willi syndrome. *N Engl J Med* 1981; 304:325–329.

73. Knoll JH, Nicholls RD, Magenis RE, et al. Angelman and Prader-Willi syndromes share a common chromosome 15 deletion but differ in parental origin of the deletion. *Am J Med Genet* 1989; 32:285–290.

74. Izmeth MG, Parameshwar E. The Miller-Dieker syndrome: a case report and review of the literature. *J Ment Defic Res* 1989; 33:267–270.

75. Schnizel A. Microdeletion syndromes, balanced translocations, and gene mapping. *J Med Genet* 1988; 25:454–462.

76. Dobyns WB, Reiner O, Carrozzo R, Ledbetter DH. Lissencephaly: a human brain malformation associated with deletion of the LIS1 gene located at chromosome 17p13. *JAMA* 1993; 270:2838–2842.

77. Fogli A, Guerrini R, Moro F, et al. Intracellular levels of LIS1 protein correlate with clinical and neuroradiological findings in patients with classical lissencephaly. *Ann Neurol* 1999; 45:154–161.

78. Landau WM, Kleffner FR. Syndrome of acquired aphasia with convulsive disorder in children. *Neurology* 1957; 7:523–530.

79. Msall M, Shapiro B, Balfour PB, et al. Acquired epileptic aphasia. *Clin Pediatr* 1986; 25:248.

80. Da Silva EA, Chugani DC, Muzik O, Chugani HT. Landau-Kleffner syndrome: metabolic abnormalities in temporal lobe are a common feature. *J Child Neurol* 1997; 12:489–495.

81. Nakano S, Okuno T, Mikawa H. Landau-Kleffner syndrome EEG topographic study. *Brain Dev* 1989; 11:43–50.

82. Nass R, Gross A, Devinsky O. Autism and autistic epileptiform regression with occipital spikes. *Dev Med Child Neurol* 1998; 40:453–458.

83. Olsson I, Steffenberg S, Gellberg C. Epilepsy in autism and autistic-like conditions. *Arch Neurol* 1988; 45:666–668.

84. Garcia-Silva MR, Aicardi J, Goutieres F, Chevrie JJ. The syndrome of myoclonic epilepsy with ragged-red fibres. Report of a case and review of the literature. *Neuropediatrics* 1987; 18:200–204.

85. Rosing HS, Hopkins LC, Wallace DC, et al. Maternally inherited mitochondrial myopathy and myoclonic epilepsy. *Ann Neurol* 1985; 17:228–237.

86. Hirano M, Pavlakis SG. Mitochondrial myopathy, encephalopathy, lactic acidosis and stroke-like episodes (MELAS): current concepts. *J Child Neurol* 1994; 9:4–13.

87. Alpers BJ. Progressive cerebral degeneration of infancy. *J Nerv Ment Dis* 1960; 130:442–448.

88. Harding BN. Progressive neuronal degeneration of childhood with liver disease (Alpers-Huttenlocher syndrome): a personal review. *J Child Neurol* 1990; 5:273–287.

89. Laurence KM, Cavanaugh JB. Progressive degeneration of the cerebral cortex in infancy. *Brain* 1968; 91:261–280.

90. Prick MJ, Gabreels FJ, Renier WO, et al. Pyruvate dehydrogenase deficiency restricted to brain. *Neurology* 1981; 31:398–404.

91. Prick MJ, Gabreels FJ, Renier WO, et al. Progressive infantile poliodystrophy. Association with disturbed pyruvate oxidation in muscle and liver. *Arch Neurol* 1981; 38:767–772.

92. Prick MJ, Gabreels FJ, Renier WO, et al. Progressive infantile poliodystrophy (Alpers' disease) with a defect in citric acid cycle activity in liver and fibroblasts. *Neuropediatrics* 1982; 13:108–111.

93. Harding BN, Alsanjari N, Smith SJ. Progressive neuronal degeneration of childhood with liver disease (Alpers' disease) presenting in young adults. *J Neurol Neurosurg Psychiatry* 1995; 58:320–325.

94. Gabreels FJ, Prick MJ, Trijbels JM, et al. Defects in citric acid cycle and the electron transport chain in progressive poliodystrophy. *Acta Neurol Scand* 1984; 70:145–154.

95. Huttenlocher PR, Solitare GB, Adams G. Infantile diffuse cerebral degeneration with hepatic cirrhosis. *Arch Neurol* 1976; 33:186–192

96. Burgeois M, Goutieres F, Chretien D, et al. Deficiency in complex II of the respiratory chain, presenting as a leukodystrophy in two sisters with Leigh syndrome. *Brain Dev* 1992; 14:404–408.

97. Naviaux RK, Nyhan WL, Barshop BA, et al. Mitochondrial DNA polymerase gamma deficiency and mtDNA depletion in a child with Alpers' syndrome. *Ann Neurol* 1999; 45:54–58.

98. Egger J, Harding BN, Boyd SG, Wilson J, Erdohazi M. Progressive neuronal degeneration of childhood (PNDC) with liver disease. *Clin Pediatr* 1987; 26:167–173.

99. Harding BN, Egger J, Portmann B, Erdohazi M. Progressive neuronal degeneration of childhood with liver disease. A pathological study. *Brain* 1986; 109:181–206.

100. Boyd SG, Harden A, Egger J, Pampliglione G. Progressive neuronal degeneration of childhood with liver disease ("Alpers' disease"): characteristic neurophysiological features. *Neuropediatrics* 1986; 17:75–80.

101. Bickenese A, Dodson WE, May W, Hickey WF. Hepatocerebral degeneration (Alpers' disease) presenting as valproate toxicity. *Ann Neurol* 1990; 28:438–439.

102. Bickenese AR, May W, Hickey WF, Dodson WE. Early childhood hepatocerebral degeneration misdiagnosed as valproate hepatotoxicity. *Ann Neurol* 1992; 32:767–775.

103. Zimmerman R. Cockayne's syndrome. In: Gomez MR, ed. *Neurocutaneous Diseases*. London: Butterworth, 1987:128–135.

104. Ozdirim E. Topcu M, Ozon A, Cila A. Cockayne syndrome: review of 25 cases. *Pediatr Neurol* 1996; 15:312–316.

105. Hess E. Drug-related lupus. *N Engl J Med* 1988; 318:1460–1462. Editorial.

CHAPTER 20

Status Epilepticus

David J. Leszczyszyn, M.D., Ph.D., and John M. Pellock, M.D.

Status epilepticus (SE) is a true neurologic emergency (1). Both convulsive and nonconvulsive SE affect people of all ages, being more common and carrying greater morbidity and mortality in infants and the elderly (2–5). Recent large population studies have revealed an incidence 2 to 2.5 times greater than previously recognized (6). In addition, hospital-based studies have disclosed that SE is underrecognized and is the cause of coma in a significant number of patients who demonstrate no overt seizure activity (7,8). Prompt recognition and management certainly lead to the best chance for successful outcome. Because of the potentially significant morbidity and mortality, there are strong arguments to redefine the duration of seizures equating with SE to encourage earlier intervention in this important public health issue (9). Additionally, several recent advances in treatment have occurred, including improved prehospital care for acute seizures, new anticonvulsant formulations, and improved emergency room and intensive care management. These approaches and a deeper understanding of the pathophysiology and prognosis of SE are discussed.

DEFINITION AND CLASSIFICATION

Although the malady had been recognized for centuries, in 1824 Calmeil first used the term *etat de mal* (status epilepticus) to describe the state in which grand mal (generalized tonic-clonic) seizures occurred in rapid succession without recovery between convulsions (10). The International League Against Epilepsy and the World Health Organization currently define SE as a "condition characterized by an epileptic seizure that is so frequently repeated or so prolonged as to create a fixed and lasting condition" (11). The lack of recovery for a fixed period, possible frequent repetition, prolongation, and possible propagation of further seizures are inherent in the definition.

Status epilepticus is defined functionally as a seizure lasting more than 30 minutes or recurrent seizures lasting more than 30 minutes from which the patient does not regain consciousness (ILAE, 1981). The classification of individual episodes of SE should be based on observation of clinical events combined with electrographic information when possible (Table 20-1). Clinical care requires intervention for seizures lasting longer than 5 minutes, recognizing that any type of seizure can develop into SE (Table 20-2). The current definition of 30 minutes is not, as described earlier, universally accepted, and several clinical studies have been published using durations of 10 or 20 minutes. DeLorenzo recently confirmed a nearly 10-fold greater mortality for seizures lasting 30 minutes or greater compared with those lasting 10 to 29 minutes (12). More information is needed to clarify and allow acceptance of a standard operational definition for SE.

This chapter deals primarily with convulsive tonic-clonic SE that is primarily or secondarily generalized using the 30-minute operational definition. This is the most commonly recognized form of SE in children. Partial seizures that evolve to SE most commonly are secondarily generalized convulsive seizures and may occur at any age but probably account for the overwhelming majority of adult cases. Status epilepticus also encompasses several nonconvulsive entities, including complex partial, simple partial, and absence seizures. Complex partial SE usually is characterized by an epileptic twilight state in which there is a cyclical variation between periods of partial responsiveness and episodes of motionless staring and complete unresponsiveness accompanied, at times, by automatic behavior (7,13,14). Simple partial SE is characterized by focal seizures that may persist or be repetitive for at least 30 minutes without impairment of consciousness.

Table 20-1. Proposed Classification of Status Epilepticus

Partial
Convulsive
- Tonic — Hemiclonic status epilepticus, hemiconvulsion-hemiplegia-epilepsy,
- Clonic — hemi-grand mal status epilepticus, grand mal

Nonconvulsive
- Simple — Focal motor status, focal sensory, epilepsia partialis continua, adversive status epilepticus
- Complex partial — Epileptic fugue state, prolonged epileptic stupor, prolonged epileptic confessional state, temporal lobe status epilepticus, psychomotor status epilepticus, continuous epileptic twilight state

Generalized
Convulsive
- Tonic-clonic — Grand mal, epilepticus convulsivus
- Tonic
- Clonic
- Myoclonic — Myoclonic status epilepticus

Nonconvulsive
- Absence — Spike-and-wave stupor, spike-and-slow-wave or 3/s spike-and-wave SE, petit mal. epileptic fugue, epilepsia minora continua, epileptic twilight state, minor SE

Undetermined
- Subtle — Epileptic coma
- Neonatal — Erratic status epilepticus

Table 20-2. Status Epilepticus Precipitating Events

Antiepileptic drug alterations
Withdrawal
Noncompliance
Drug interactions
Toxicity
Infections
   Central nervous system
   Systemic
Toxins
   Alcohol
   Drugs
   Poisons
   Convulsive agents
Structural
   Trauma
   Ischemic stroke
   Hemorrhagic stroke
   Acute hydrocephalus
Hormonal change
Electrolyte imbalance
Diagnostic procedures and medications
Emotional stress
Progressive-degenerative disease
Sleep deprivation
Primary apnea
Cardiac arrhythmias
Fever

When this condition lasts for hours or days, it is termed *epilepsia partialis continua*. Absence, or petit mal, status has also been referred to as spike-wave stupor. This type of nonconvulsive SE may be extremely difficult to differentiate from complex partial SE without the aid of an electroencephalogram (EEG) evaluation. Classically, in absence status there is a continuous alteration of consciousness without cyclical variations seen with complex partial SE. The EEG recording exhibits prolonged, sometimes continuous, generalized synchronous 3-hertz (Hz) spike and wave complexes rather than focal ictal discharges that characterize partial SE (7,15). The child presenting with a prolonged confused state, fluctuating level of consciousness, or prolonged unconsciousness needs both clinical and EEG evaluations in addition to other studies.

Myoclonic, generalized clonic, and generalized tonic SE are seen primarily in children. Such children usually are those with encephalopathic epilepsies (3,7,16), and their consciousness seems to be preserved throughout the attacks. The EEG pattern is bilaterally symmetric with polyspike discharges coinciding with the myoclonic jerks. The term *myoclonic SE*

should not be used when children with severe encephalopathy exhibit repetitive myoclonic jerks not accompanied by ictal discharges on EEG. These patients have subtle, generalized, convulsive SE as defined by Treiman (7). About one-half of the cases of generalized clonic SE occur in normal children and are associated with prolonged febrile seizures; the other half are distributed among those with acute and chronic encephalopathies (17). Generalized tonic SE appears most frequently in children, particularly those with the Lennox-Gastaut syndrome. Prolonged generalized tonic convulsions have been precipitated by benzodiazepine administration.

EPIDEMIOLOGY

Status epilepticus is usually a manifestation of symptomatic epilepsy with preexisting neurologic dysfunction or a manifestation of acute disease primarily or secondarily affecting the central nervous system (CNS). In infants and young children, it is uncommon for SE to occur in the unstressed patient with idiopathic epilepsy. A child who has prolonged resistant seizures should receive a full diagnostic evaluation for all etiologies of seizures, along with a search for those precipitating events listed in Table 20-2. Interestingly, there also is evidence for a genetic predisposition for SE (18). The major causes vary with age, such as febrile SE in children 1 to 2 years of age and remote symptomatic etiologies in the 5 to 10 year range (19). Acute symptomatic etiologies most commonly lead to prolonged SE lasting over 1 hour (20,21). Similarly, recurrent SE is more frequent in children with remote symptomatic etiologies or progressive degenerative disease (19,22).

A recent prospective population-based study of SE revealed the incidence of SE to be 41 patients per year per 100,000 population, resulting in a total of 50 episodes of SE per year per 100,000. It is projected that between 102,000 and 152,000 events occur in the United States annually, an incidence 2 to 2 1/2 times greater than that previously proposed by Hauser (6,23). Approximately one-third of the cases present as the initial seizure of epilepsy, one-third occur in patients with previously established epilepsy, and one-third occur as the result of an acute isolated brain insult. Among those previously diagnosed as having epilepsy, estimates of SE occurrence range from 0.5 percent to 6.6 percent. Hauser reported that up to 70 percent of children who have epilepsy that begins before the age of 1 year experience an episode of SE. Also, within 5 years of the initial diagnosis of epilepsy, 20 percent of all patients experience an episode of SE. A greater incidence of SE was reported by Shinnar from a cohort of patients with childhood-onset epilepsy. One-third of the patients experienced SE over a 30-year period, 50 percent presenting as the first seizure and an additional 22 percent occurring within 12 months of onset of epilepsy. In this group, SE occurred in 44 percent of those with remote symptomatic epilepsy and 20 percent of those with idiopathic or cryptogenic epilepsy (24).

Although adults with SE as their first unprovoked seizure are likely to develop subsequent epilepsy (23), a prospective study of children with SE found that only 30 percent of those initially presenting with SE later developed epilepsy (20). Hesdorffer has presented more recent data indicating a greater likelihood of epilepsy following SE in a group of 95 people, one-third of whom were children. Over the ensuing 10-year period following a symptomatic bout of SE, there was a 41 percent risk of an unprovoked seizure (25).

Among children, SE is most common in infants and young toddlers, with more than 50 percent of cases of SE occurring under the age of 3 years (26). In the Richmond, Virginia, study, total SE events and incidence per 100,000 individuals per year showed a bimodal distribution with the highest values during the first year of life and after 60 years of age (6,17,27). Infants younger than 1 year of age represent a subgroup of children with the highest incidence of SE whether events, total incidents, or recurrence is counted. The recurrence rate of SE in the Richmond study was 10.8 percent (6), but 38 percent of patients younger than 4

years old had repeat episodes, findings supported by the Finnish study (24). In another cohort of pediatric epilepsy patients followed up by Berg and coworkers for 5 years, only 4.3 percent had their first episode of SE, while 19.6 percent of those who presented with status had one or more episodes of SE (28).

Extrapolating these figures worldwide, more than one million cases of SE occur annually. Because SE is a neurologic emergency that requires immediate, effective treatment to prevent residual neurologic complications or death, SE poses a substantial health risk. Mortality rates as high as 30 percent have been reported in overall studies. Children have a far lower mortality rate than do adults with the exception of those in the first year of life (29). Age, etiology, and duration directly correlate with mortality (4,6,30). Multiple studies confirm the lower mortality rate in most children following adequate emergency treatment (20,26,31–33)

PATHOPHYSIOLOGY

The pathophysiology of SE has been reviewed recently and is discussed in other chapters of this book. The mechanisms by which chronic seizures evolve to SE remain unclear (3). There seems to be a loss of inhibitory mechanisms, and neuronal metabolism is not able to keep up with the demand of continuing ictal activity. The pathophysiologic changes that accompany SE can be divided into neuronal (cerebral) and systemic effects. Continuing seizures lead to both biochemical changes within the brain and systemic derangements that further complicate these cerebral changes.

Prolonged convulsive seizures can lead to excitotoxic brain injury. Glutamate, the primary excitatory amino acid neurotransmitter, binds to several neuronal receptors, including the N-methyl-D-aspartate (NMDA) receptor, which is activated by depolarization. The resulting calcium influx causes further depolarization and perpetuates seizures. Glutamate also activates receptors that open channels that conduct sodium and calcium into the cell. Further neuronal damage results through this excessive excitatory neurotransmission. Although gamma-aminobutyric acid (GABA) is the most prevalent inhibitory neurotransmitter in the brain, excessive GABA may in fact increase activity on both $GABA_A$ and $GABA_B$ receptors. Activation of the presynaptic $GABA_B$ receptors can provide feedback inhibition of $GABA_A$ receptors and paradoxically exacerbate seizures. Other neurotransmitters that may be important in the initiation and maintenance of SE include acetylcholine, adenosine, and nitric oxide (34).

Neuronal injury and cell death from SE are most prominent in areas that are rich in NMDA glutamate receptors, including the limbic region. The increase in intracellular calcium concentration is critical to cell death. Calcium activates proteases and lipases that degrade intracellular elements, leading to mitochondrial dysfunction and cellular necrosis. Laminar necrosis and neuronal damage after prolonged seizures are similar to that following cerebral hypoxia. Although young animals may be less likely to develop brain damage from SE (35,36), studies using alternative models demonstrate hippocampal cellular injury even in immature rodents (37). It is believed that the glutamate-initiated calcium-dependent cascade is similar to the mechanism of NMDA receptor–mediated cell death during cerebral ischemia. Absence SE associated with excessive inhibitory influences generated by $GABA_B$-mediated hyperpolarization and activation of folinic T-type calcium channels does not cause cerebral injury (34). Furthermore, recent evidence suggests that acute and long-term changes in gene expression may occur following prolonged seizures and may directly contribute to hyperexcitability (38).

Systemic metabolic abnormalities increase the risk of brain damage in convulsive SE. These include alterations of blood pressure, heart rate, acidosis, hypoxia, changes in respiratory function, body temperature, leukocytosis, rhabdomyolysis, and heightened demands on cerebral oxygen and glucose utilization (39). Circulating catecholamine concentrations increase during the initial 30 minutes of SE, resulting in a hypersympathetic state. Tachycardia sometimes associated with severe cardiac dysrhythmias occurs and rarely may be fatal (40). Furthermore, cardiac output diminishes and total peripheral resistance increases along with mean arterial blood pressure, perhaps because of the sympathetic overload. Hyperpyrexia may become significant during the course of SE even without prior febrile illness in both children and adults and may contribute to neuronal injury (41).

Hypoventilation leads to hypoxia and respiratory acidosis. In addition, serum pH and glucose levels are frequently abnormal as lactic acidosis develops following increased anaerobic metabolism. A leukemoid reaction of peripheral blood frequently occurs in the absence of infection. Rhabdomyolysis, which is not uncommonly seen, may compromise renal function. Recovery from this complicated derangement of metabolism is time-dependent. More prolonged seizures produce further neuronal injury and death.

PROGNOSIS

The morbidity and mortality of SE are direct consequences of its basic pathophysiology and the efficiency of treatment. Previously, overall mortality figures for SE were quoted as 10 percent to 30 percent (30,42,43).

The mortality rate for the Richmond, Virginia, population was 22 percent overall. Based on this study, which includes all age groups, there are approximately 126,000 to 195,000 SE events with 22,000 to 42,000 deaths per year in the United States. However, the mortality rate in children was only 3 percent, and most of the pediatric deaths occurred between the ages of 1 and 4 years (Table 20-3). The pediatric and aged populations had an increased number of recurrences of SE following a single episode. In general, children had chronic neurologic disabilities but rarely went on to die. Among those patients who died, death rarely occurred during the acute episode of SE. Rather, most patients succumbed 15 to 30 days later. Children with chronic epilepsy and low anticonvulsant drug levels have the lowest mortality rate overall.

The morbidity of SE in children was examined in the same database from Virginia. Before their SE event, 81 percent of children with no prior history of seizures were neurologically normal in contrast to only 31 percent of children with seizure histories. Of the neurologically normal children with no prior seizures, more than 25 percent deteriorated after their first SE event in comparison with less than 15 percent of neurologically normal children with a seizure history. Children who were neurologically abnormal without prior seizure deteriorated further in 6.7 percent compared with 11.3 percent of the abnormal children with a seizure history. Morbidity was determined at the time of hospital discharge, and in some children the abnormalities certainly improve as minor degrees of ataxia, incoordination, or motor deficits can be attributed to the acute therapies or clinical changes after prolonged seizures and may not persist. Determining whether language deficits and school performance difficulties were transient or more permanent was much more difficult. In the prospective study, 11 percent to 15 percent had a significant morbidity after an episode of SE (Table 20-3). These findings suggest a neurologic morbidity substantially lower than the "greater than 50 percent" rate previously reported in children having SE (42), but the morbidity and mortality of very sick infants is higher than in older children (29).

Hesdorffer and colleagues in Rochester, Minnesota, have recently demonstrated a 41 percent 10-year risk

Table 20-3. Childhood Status Epilepticus Prognosis

Patient Series	Aicardi and Chevrie (42)	Pellock (31)	Maytal (20)	DeLorenzo et al. (6)
Patients	239	97	193	229
Status epilepticus duration	60	30	30	30
Symptomatic (%)	75	72	77	73
Morbidity (%)	>50	23	9.1	11–15
Mortality (%)	11	8	3.6	3

of having an unprovoked seizure following an acute seizure with SE. This 95-person cohort included 17 individuals under 1 year in age and 17 from 1 to 19 years. This risk was increased 18.8-fold for SE as a result of anoxic encephalopathy, 7.1-fold for structural causes, and 3.6-fold for metabolic causes when compared with a population of patients who experienced a less prolonged acute symptomatic seizure (25).

Electrographic and biochemical markers for increased morbidity and mortality in SE exist. The duration of the individual seizure, especially if it evolves to nonconvulsive SE (NCSE), has been directly correlated with death or poor outcome as defined by inability to return to prehospital level of function (44). Serum and cerebrospinal fluid (CSF) levels of neuron-specific enolase (NSE) rise above normal after both brief and prolonged seizures. Serum levels following SE are significantly higher and are at their highest in patients following NCSE where levels above 37 ng/mL correlate with poor outcome (45). CSF lactate is certainly elevated following SE, and levels three times greater than the accepted normal have been associated with poor outcome, while those elevated twofold or less had better outcomes. CSF lactate dehydrogenase (LDH) and creatinine kinase do not appear to be valid indicators of prognosis in SE (46). CSF pleocytosis also does not appear to be a valid indicator of prognosis in SE. In all ages it is typically related to the acute illness or injury precipitating the seizure. Greater than 6 WBC/mm^3 or any polymorphonuclear lymphocytes (PMNs) in the adults or greater than 8 WBC/mm^3 (and greater than 4 PMNs/mm^3) in children should prompt a search for an etiology other than the seizure itself (47,48).

Radiographic findings following SE, typically reversible focal magnetic resonance imaging (MRI) T2-weighted abnormalities, have been recognized for years (49). It is currently assumed that these findings are benign. However, there is a growing collection of case reports suggesting that there is brain injury despite radiographic normalization as evidenced by persistent EEG abnormalities and proton MR spectroscopy abnormalities (50,51). There is also strong evidence that structural brain injury in the form of ischemic stroke has a synergistic effect with SE, leading to increased mortality (52).

THERAPY

Extrapolating the statistical figures worldwide, more than one million cases of SE occur annually. As a true neurologic emergency, it requires mobilization of significant personal and medical resources and certainly qualifies as a substantial public health concern. With mortality rates as high as 30 percent reported in all-age

inclusive studies, immediate effective treatment is necessary to prevent residual neurologic complications or death. Age, etiology, and duration directly correlate with mortality (4,6). The highest mortality is seen in the elderly; fortunately, children have a far lower mortality rate than do adults (4,20,23,30). Some of this improved prognosis is probably a result of fewer coexisting medical conditions. That said, multiple studies confirm a lower mortality rate in children following adequate emergency treatment (20,26,31–33).

Because SE frequently occurs away from a medical center, appropriate first-aid recommendations are discussed for completeness. The Epilepsy Foundation of America (EFA) recommends that you:

- Look for medical identification.
- Protect the person from nearby hazards.
- Loosen ties or shirt collars.
- Protect the head from injury.
- Turn the person on his side to keep the airway clear.
- Reassure when consciousness returns.
- If a single seizure lasted more than 5 minutes, ask if hospital evaluation is wanted.
- If multiple seizures, or if one seizure lasts longer than 5 minutes, call an ambulance.
- If the person is pregnant, injured, or diabetic, call for aid at once.

The EFA also recommends that you:

- Do not put any hard implement in the mouth.
- Do not try to hold the tongue. It cannot be swallowed.
- Do not try to give liquids during or just after the seizure.
- Do not use artificial respiration unless breathing is absent after muscle jerks subside or water has been inhaled.
- Do not restrain the person (53).

The person should be transferred to a medical center as soon as possible if their seizure continues beyond 5 minutes or if it begins again after ceasing.

The neurologic emergency of SE requires maintenance of respiration, general medical support, and specific treatment of seizures while the etiology is sought (1,54,55). The most typical and frequent mistake made in the treatment of SE is that inadequate doses of drugs are given initially, and physicians wait for more seizures to occur before administering the necessary total dose (54,56). The ideal antiepileptic drug (AED) for the treatment of SE should have the following properties: rapid onset of action, broad spectrum of activity, ease of administration including intravenous

(IV) and intramuscular (IM) preparations, minimal redistribution from the CNS, and wide therapeutic safety margin. Because of these desired properties, and particularly because it is longer acting, lorazepam (LZP) has become more popular in many centers as the initial agent thus replacing diazepam (DZP). Recent studies in both children and adults also support the use of midazolam (MDZ). Its rapid absorption from varied sites of administration and rapid onset of anticonvulsant activity make MDZ a very attractive agent for use in multiple settings. If, however, SE continues after the initial dosing of a benzodiazepine and persists after a primary AED such as phenytoin (PHT) (as fosphenytoin, FOS) or phenobarbital (PB) is given, a second dose of the same AED should be administered before switching to alternative medications. SE refractory to these established agents carries a more grave prognosis (55). Numerous studies suggest that additional bolus administration followed by titrated IV infusions of DZP, MDZ, pentobarbital, or the anesthetic agents, lidocaine or propofol, may break these seizures. The role of IV valproic acid (VPA) in the treatment of SE is currently being explored.

The primary goal of treatment is to stop the convulsive discharges in the brain. Table 20-4 lists the steps of the emergency management of SE (54,57). The child presenting in SE must have cardiorespiratory function assessed immediately by vital sign determination, auscultation, airway inspection, arterial blood gas determination, and suction if necessary. Although spontaneously breathing on presentation, children may already be hypoxic with respiratory or metabolic acidosis from apnea, aspiration, or central respiratory depression (1). The need for ventilator support depends not only on respiratory status at the time of presentation but also on the conditions before arrival and the ability to maintain adequate oxygenation throughout ongoing seizures and during the IV administration of drugs, all of which cause some amount of respiratory depression. Elective intubation and respiratory support are urged in the neurologically depressed patient. In most patients, placement of an oral airway and/or nasal cannula oxygen is insufficient as respiratory drive is depressed. Significant hypoxia is a principal factor determining morbidity and mortality (6). Rapid assessment of vital signs and general neurologic examination give clues to the etiology of SE. Blood drawn to determine blood gases, glucose, calcium, electrolytes, complete blood count, AED levels, culture, and virologic and toxicologic studies help with the overall determination of etiology. Similarly, urine for drug and metabolic screens should be collected. The roles of CSF NSE and lactate, as well as serum NSE, in the prognostication of outcomes in SE were discussed previously.

Intravenous fluids should be administered judiciously, with appropriate corrections for fever, suction, and chemical abnormality. Fluid restriction is rarely necessary. Immediately following placement of the IV line, 25% glucose (2–4 mL/kg) should be given by bolus. In the case in which IV access cannot be established, the intraosseous route has been shown efficient for both fluid and medication administration (58). Because of the high incidence of febrile SE resulting from CNS infection in infants, a lumbar puncture should be done early in the course of management but not necessarily during the initial phase of stabilization. It is rarely necessary to wait for imaging studies to be performed in this group. If lumbar puncture is deferred for any reason, appropriate antimicrobial coverage for possible meningitis or encephalitis should be considered. Electrocardiographic (ECG) and EEG monitoring is desirable when available (55).

EEG monitoring is extremely useful in both the initial and the subsequent management of SE (57,59–61). The classification of SE, clues to etiology, and prognosis may be suggested from EEG and its response to therapy. This includes patients with completely hysterical attacks and those presenting with overdose of drugs or focal pathology. Definition of seizures as being mainly partial versus primarily or secondarily generalized is easily recognized; in nonconvulsive cases the EEG easily establishes the diagnosis as complex partial or absence. The use of EEG is mandatory in the presence of neuromuscular blockade or whenever recurrence of seizures cannot be documented on a clinical basis (1,57).

An electroclinical dissociation may exist after large doses of AEDs have been given so that the clinical manifestations are absent while electrographic seizures continue. The recognition of EEG patterns, such as paroxysmal lateralized epileptiform discharges (PLEDs), periodic epileptiform discharges (PEDS), and evidence of continued post-SE ictal discharges without clinical correlation while the patient remains in coma require ongoing therapy and may be helpful in establishing the etiologic diagnosis and prognosis (8). One recent study of 50 patients with SE reported poor outcomes, including death or persistent vegetative states in 44 percent of those whose records demonstrated PEDS compared with 19 percent without PEDS (62). ECG changes seen in adults during and after SE range from evidence of ischemia to tachyarryhmias. These changes must be promptly and appropriately treated (39,63). These relatively new findings suggest that EEG be more aggressively used in the evaluation and treatment of SE. Practical limitations must be realized, however, because many treatment sites do not have EEG readily available. Nevertheless, urgent use of this monitoring must be considered when patients do not

Table 20-4. The Steps of Status Epilepticus Emergency Management

1. Ensure adequate brain oxygenation and cardiorespiratory function
2. Terminate clinical and electrical seizure activity as rapidly as possible
3. Prevent seizure recurrence
4. Identify precipitating factors such as hypoglycemia, electrolyte imbalance, lowered drug levels, infection, and fever
5. Correct metabolic imbalance
6. Prevent systemic complications
7. Further evaluate and treat the cause of status epilepticus

regain consciousness or when seizures are continuous or recurrent.

DRUG THERAPY OF STATUS EPILEPTICUS

There are multiple regimens for treating SE successfully. Benzodiazepines and FOS (PHT equivalent) as initial therapy are preferred by our group at the Medical College of Virginia of Virginia Commonwealth University (MCV/VCU), but others may wish to continue alternative agents if the patient is known to be on maintenance therapy or has already received smaller doses of PHT or PB (64,65). LZP, DZP, FOS, and PB are accepted agents for initial and continued therapy of SE. The large SE treatment study done in adults and sponsored by the U.S. Veterans Administration suggests that there is no significant difference between three IV drug regimens: (1) DZP, 0.15 mg/kg, and PHT, 18 mg/kg; (2) LZP, 0.1 mg/kg; or (3) PB, 15 mg/kg, for initial management of generalized convulsive SE when results were measured at 20 minutes (66). Each was superior to PHT, 18 mg/kg, used alone. It is important to note that the rate of PHT administration probably biased the study. The much more rapid speed at which FOS can be administered may significantly change these results. The choice of an initial agent may depend on individual patient characteristics, prior AED therapy, and physician preference. Recommended doses of

commonly used drugs for the treatment of convulsive SE are listed in Table 20-5. Protocols presently used by our group at MCV/VCU for the management of SE in children, adolescents, and adults are given in Tables 20-6 and 20-7 (64).

Benzodiazepines

As a group the benzodiazepines are the most potent and efficacious drugs in the treatment of SE (67). Lasting control of SE is achieved in approximately 80 percent of patients treated with either LZP, DZP, or clonazepam (66). Because the IV preparation of clonazepam is not available in the United States, lorazepam and diazepam are most frequently used. A recent prospective, randomized study determined that IM MDZ is as effective as DZP in stopping seizures and is faster than DZP because it avoids the requirement of starting an IV line (68). Nasal and buccal administration of benzodiazepines have demonstrated efficacy in aborting acute seizures, but no prospective studies support these routes in treating SE (69,70).

Lorazepam

Lorazepam is a potent benzodiazepine with rapid onset and more prolonged duration of anticonvulsant action compared with DZP. With a half-life of approximately 10 to 15 hours in adults and children, LZP continues to have an effective brain level for 8 to 24 hours. A favorable lipid partition coefficient allows LZP to remain in the brain longer than DZP, which redistributes more rapidly. The recommended IV bolus LZP dose is 0.1 mg/kg up to a total of 5 to 8 mg. Tachyphylaxis develops, making repeated doses less effective (71,72). LZP is also less useful in patients receiving chronic benzodiazepine therapy.

The efficacy of LZP equals that of DZP in neonates, children, and adults (71a–78). Adverse effects include hypoventilation, ataxia, vomiting, amnesia, lethargy, respiratory depression, and hypotension. These symptoms are exacerbated when barbiturates, paraldehyde,

Table 20-5. Recommended Initial IV Doses for Status Epilepticus

Patient Age	LZP (0.1 mg/kg)	DZP (0.3 mg/kg)	MDZ (0.15–0.3 mg/kg)	FOS or PE (20 mg/kg)	PB (20 mg/kg)
<6 mo	0.3–1.0	1–2	0.5–2	60–200	60–200
6–12 mo	0.5–1.2	2–4	1–4	100–250	100–250
1–5 yr	0.8–2.5	3–10	1.5–10	160–250	160–250
5–12 yr	1.5–6.0	5–15	2.5–15	300–1200	300–1200
13 yr +	3.0–6.0	10–20	5–20	500–1500+	500–1500+

LZP = lorazepam; DZP = diazepam; MDZ = midazolam; FOS or PE = fosphenytoin or phenytoin equivalent; PB = phenobarbital.

Table 20-6. Medical College of Virginia Hospital's Status Epilepticus (SE) Protocol for Children*

Step	Time from Start of Intervention	Procedure
1	0–5 min	Determination of SE. As soon as the diagnosis is made, institute monitoring of temperature, blood pressure, pulse, respirations, ECG, and EEG. Insert oral airway and administer O_2 if necessary. Insert an IV catheter and draw venous blood levels of anticonvulsants, glucose, electrolytes, calcium, BUN, and CBC. Draw arterial blood for antipyretics (acetaminophen). Perform frequent suctioning.
2	6–9 min	Place an IV line with normal saline. Administer a bolus of 2 mL/kg 50% glucose.
3	10–30 min	Initial treatment consists of an infusion by IV lorazepam given at a rate of 1–2 mg/min (0.1 mg/kg) to a maximal dose of 8 mg. This is followed by IV fosphenytoin (FOS) infused at 150 mg/min [or phenytoin (PHT) infused at a rate not to exceed 1 mg/kg/min or 50 mg/min]. Monitor ECG and blood pressure. May repeat FOS (PHT) 10 mg/kg before proceeding to next step.
4	31–59 min	If seizures persist, administer a bolus infusion of phenobarbital at a rate not to exceed 50 mg/min until seizures stop or to a loading dose of 20 mg/kg.
5	60 min	If control is not achieved, other options include: Diazepam (50 mg) is diluted in a solution of 250 ml 0.9% NaCl or D5W and run as a continuous infusion at 1 ml/kg/h (2 mg/kg/h) to achieve blood levels of 0.2–8.0 mg/ml. The IV solution is changed every 6 h as advised by certain authors and short-length tubing is used. Pentobarbital with an initial IV loading dose of 5 mg/kg with additional amounts given to produce a "burst suppression" pattern on EEG. Maintenance of pentobarbital anesthesia is continued for approximately 4 h by an infusion of 1–3 mg/kg/h. The patient is then checked for the reappearance of seizure activity by decreasing the infusion rate. If clinical seizures and/or generalized discharges persist on EEG, the procedure is repeated; if not, the pentobarbital is tapered over 12–24 h.
6	61–80 min	If seizures are still not controlled, call Anesthesia Department to begin general anesthesia with halothane and neuromuscular blockade.

ECG = electrocardiogram, EEG = electroencephalogram, IV = intravenous, BUN = blood urea nitrogen, CBC = complete blood count, D5W = 5% dextrose in water

*Continuous monitoring of EEG is recommended in an obtunded patient to ensure that SE has not recurred. In the management of intractable status, a neurologist who has expertise in SE should be consulted, and advice from a regional epilepsy center should be sought. Lumbar puncture should be performed as soon as possible, especially in a febrile child or infant <1 year old. For infants with a history of neonatal seizures, infantile spasms, or early-onset seizures, pyridoxine 100 mg IV should be administered while EEG monitoring is being performed to diagnose and treat the rare patient with seizures and a vitamin B_6 deficiency.

or other depressant drugs are administered before LZP. Following rectal administration, LZP has a more delayed onset of action than DZP (77). Sedation that follows IV administration of LZP is longer lasting than that following DZP. Significant sedation is a disadvantage of both drugs when continued observation of level of consciousness is necessary.

Diazepam

Diazepam enters the brain within seconds following IV administration and successfully stops convulsive and nonconvulsive seizures in the majority of adults and children (67). Its primary disadvantages are similar to those of LZP. In addition, because of rapid redistribution, seizures frequently reoccur after 15 to 20 minutes after IV administration, requiring that a second longer-acting drug be given or a second dose of DZP be administered. Respiratory support should be available when DZP is used to treat SE. Recommended dose estimates by age are given in Table 20-4 based on 10 to 15 mg/m², or 0.3 mg/kg. An initial estimate of dose may be made by taking the patient's age and

giving 1 mg per year plus 1 mg (1). DZP may be given by intraosseous or rectal route or by a continuous IV infusion (79). In addition to respiratory depression, laryngospasm may develop during the administration of diazepam.

As LZP is supplanting DZP in many hospital emergency situations, DZP has taken on another important role — that of prehospital treatment by family or other caregivers for prolonged or acute repetitive seizures. A new viscous solution of 5 mg/mL DZP was developed specifically for rectal administration. Its safety and efficacy have been established in two U.S. trials, and considerably fewer of the DZP gel-treated patients required subsequent emergency medical attention for continued seizures following the treatment of their episode (80,81). This leads to a reduced cost of care and in the future may decrease the prolongation of some seizures to SE (82).

Midazolam

Midazolam has been used successfully as a first-line treatment for convulsive SE and for refractory

Table 20-7. Medical College of Virginia Hospital's Status Epilepticus (SE) Protocol for Adults*

Step	Time from Start of Intervention	Procedure
1	0–5 min	Determination of SE. As soon as the diagnosis is made, institute monitoring of temperature, blood pressure, pulse, respirations, ECG, and EEG. Insert oral airway and administer O_2 if necessary. Insert an IV catheter and draw venous blood levels of anticonvulsants, glucose, electrolytes, Ca, Mg, BUN, and CBC. Draw arterial blood for ABG analysis. If necessary, nasotracheal suctioning is performed.
2	6–9 min	Place an IV line with normal saline containing vitamin B complex. Administer a bolus of 50 ml 50% glucose.
3	10–30 min	Infuse IV lorazepam given at a rate of 2 mg/min (0.1 mg/kg) to a maximal dose of 8 mg or alternatively administer IV diazepam given at a rate not to exceed 2 mg/min until seizures stop or to a total of 20 mg. This is followed by IV fosphenytoin (FOS) [phenytoin (PHT)], 20 mg/kg, at a rate no faster than 50 mg/min. Monitor ECG and blood pressure.
4	31–59 min	If seizures persist, perform elective endotracheal intubation before starting a bolus infusion of phenobarbital at a rate not to exceed 100 mg/min until seizures stop or to a loading dose of 20 mg/kg.
5	60 min	If control is not achieved, other options include: Pentobarbital with an initial IV loading dose of 5–10 mg/kg with additional amounts given to produce a "burst suppression" pattern on EEG. Maintenance of pentobarbital anesthesia is continued for approximately 4 h by an infusion of 1–3 mg/kg/h. The patient is then checked for the reappearance of seizure activity by decreasing the infusion rate. If clinical seizures and/or generalized discharges persist on EEG, the procedure is repeated; if not, the pentobarbital is tapered over 12–24 h. Diazepam (50–100 mg) is diluted in a solution of 500 ml 0.9% NaCl or D5W and run as a continuous infusion to achieve blood levels of 0.2–8.0 mg/ml. The IV solution is changed every 6 h as advised by certain authors and short-length tubing is used.
6	61–80 min	If seizures are still not controlled, call Anesthesia Department to begin general anesthesia and neuromuscular blockade.

ECG = electrocardiogram, EEG = electroencephalogram, IV = intravenous, BUN = blood urea nitrogen, CBC = complete blood count, ABG = arterial blood gas, D5W = 5% dextrose in water
*Continuous monitoring of EEG is recommended in an obtunded patient to ensure that SE has not recurred. In the management of intractable status, a neurologist who has expertise in SE should be consulted, and advice from a regional epilepsy center should be sought.

convulsive SE. Clinical evidence supports that IM MDZ is more effective than IM DZP and as effective as IV DZP in abolishing interictal spikes on EEG recordings. At doses from 0.15 to 0.3 mg/kg it effectively terminated convulsive seizure activity (83). More than 100 children with SE are described in the literature as being successfully treated primarily with MDZ, without drug-related cardiac side effects or urgent intubation for ventilatory support (84–86). The dosing of MDZ for SE in children is not established. Suggested values are found in Table 20-5. Although LZP, DZP, and now MDZ are usually considered as the initial drugs of choice, they sometimes are useful as the second or third agent when seizures continue. Respiratory support should be available when any of the benzodiazepines are used because of the cumulative blunting of the respiratory drive centers. Additional intensive monitoring should also be performed to guard against hypotension.

Midazolam undergoes rapid hepatic breakdown, leaving no active metabolites. The elimination half-life of MDZ in children aged 6 months to 10 years ranges from 1.17 to 4 hours, in contrast to longer values in adults (1.8–6.4 hours) and elderly men (5–6 hours) (87). Recall that the active desmethyl metabolite of DZP has a physiologic half-life of 46 to 78 hours. When MDZ is administered as a continuous IV drip, dosing needs to be adjusted upward to achieve continued anticonvulsant or sedative action because of marked tachyphylaxis.

Phenobarbital

Phenobarbital remains the initial drug of choice in some institutions for the treatment of childhood SE (88,89). Its time to onset of action is longer than that of LZP and DZP, with peak brain levels being reached in 20 to 60 minutes. Slow IV bolus infusion of 20 to 25 mg/kg is suggested initially. Repeated 10 to 20 mg/kg doses may be necessary to be successful (1,89). Principal side effects are hypotension and respiratory and sensorial depression. PB should be administered by IV infusion no faster than 100 mg/min. In the VA Cooperative Study PB was just as efficacious in treating SE as LZP and LZP plus PHT, and a better first drug (regimen) than PHT alone (66).

Fosphenytoin (Phenytoin Prodrug Equivalent)

Fosphenytoin has replaced injectable PHT at our institution because of its safety advantages. This prodrug is nearly 100 percent bioavailable and, unlike its product (PHT), is freely soluble in aqueous solutions (90). Given IV, FOS is rapidly converted to PHT by phosphatases in the bloodstream. PHT then enters the brain, reaching peak brain levels at 15 minutes (91,92). FOS is an excellent agent for the treatment of convulsive SE, both partial and generalized, but it is ineffective in the treatment of absence status (1). A marked advantage is that it does not depress respiration like other drugs in this situation (1). The dose is prescribed as milligrams of PHT equivalents (PE). In young children, initial IV FOS dose should be 15 to 25 mg PE/kg (93). In adolescents and adults, a dose of 18 mg PE/kg provides initial serum PHT levels greater than 25 µg/mL and is effective in maintaining serum levels of 10 µg/mL for 24 hours (94). Cardiac conduction disturbances have not been seen, while hypotension is rare with infusion rates up to 150 mg PE/min (95). According to data from animal and human studies, most systemic adverse effects are due to the derived PHT, so the most common CNS effects include nystagmus, headache, ataxia, and somnolence. Intramuscular administration of FOS at doses from 10 to 20 mg PE/kg may allow for treatment in the field or when no IV access is present, potentially allowing for more rapid seizure control. Therapeutic blood levels can be attained in 20 to 30 minutes following IM injection (96).

Although FOS has many advantages over PHT (IM route, safe when IV site infiltrates, faster rates of administration, and lack of solvent, cardiosuppressive effects), it is not available in all facilities and frequently is not available outside the United States. FOS is significantly more expensive that PHT, but pharmacokinetics studies in patients can demonstrate its overall advantage.

Phenytoin

Phenytoin is an excellent agent for the treatment of convulsive SE, both partial and generalized, but it is not indicated in the treatment of absence status (1). After IV administration PHT reaches peak brain levels at 15 minutes (91,92). A marked advantage of PHT is that it does not cause significant respiratory depression (1). As demonstrated by the VA study, it is best administered in combination with a benzodiazepine to ensure a rapid anticonvulsant effect, followed by the long-lasting efficacy of PHT (66). ECG should be monitored during administration because of hypotension and cardiac conduction disturbances, primarily in adults or children with preexisting cardiac disease (1). The rate of infusion should be less than 50 mg/min in adults or 25 mg/min in children. IV injection should be directly into the vein or IV line close to venous access because precipitation is likely to occur in most IV solutions. IM administration of PHT is discouraged because of crystallization, muscle destruction, and unpredictable absorption (97).

Pentobarbital

Pentobarbital is used at many institutions for refractory SE. Following a loading dose of 20 mg/kg, 1 to 2 mg/kg/h is given IV to keep the serum level at 20 to 40 µg/mL to produce electrographic suppression or burst-suppression pattern. Pentobarbital's half-life is approximately 20 hours. Most authorities stop pentobarbital coma at 24 to 48 hours to determine whether SE subsides (98). Cardiac output and blood pressure are compromised at levels above 40 g/mL. Unfortunately, refractory SE requiring coma with pentobarbital or other anesthetic agents to produce EEG suppression is associated with a higher rate of morbidity and mortality (56).

Other Agents

When SE is resistant to benzodiazepines, PB, and PHT, paraldehyde was previously used (1). Paraldehyde IV solution is no longer commercially available in the United States, but rectal solution is sometimes still used. For rectal administration a 2:1 paraldehyde oil (vegetable or peanut) mixture is administered at 0.3 mL/kg per dose with doses repeated every 2 to 4 hours (99). IV lidocaine may alternatively be used for the treatment of SE. There are no large, double-blind, placebo-controlled studies of the efficacy of lidocaine, but numerous case reports and case series suggest an initial bolus of 1 to 3 mg/kg followed by slow infusion of 4 to 10 mg/kg/hour (91,100). The principal side effect is cardiovascular dysfunction. Paradoxical convulsions may occur as levels of lidocaine elevate.

In addition to lidocaine, other anesthetic agents have been used for seizure and EEG suppression (1). The foremost of these is propofol, and its use in the treatment of refractory SE has recently been reviewed (101). Based on case reports and two small, open, uncontrolled studies, propofol is no better than other second-line agents for ultimate control of prolonged seizures, but compared with high-dose barbiturate therapy, the time to attain seizure control appears markedly reduced (102). This promising property of propofol is, however, offset in the pediatric population by two drawbacks. The metabolism of this drug is exceedingly rapid, and escalating doses are required to maintain adequate blood levels, without which breakthrough seizures and SE are common. Several cases of severe metabolic acidosis and rhabdomyolysis also have been reported (103).

Intravenous VPA may be given to patients with epilepsy when it is not possible to maintain concentrations by the oral route. Although there have been no multicenter, controlled trials of IV valproate in SE, two small studies reported improvement in patients with DZP-resistant SE (104). Another small open study demonstrated control of seizures within 20 minutes in more than 80 percent of patients (105). Doses in these studies of seizures and SE were usually an IV bolus of 15 mg/kg followed by continuous or intermittent infusions at rates of 0.5 to 1.0 mg/kg/h. We presently recommend administering the available VPA for IV use diluted 1:1 at a rate of 6 mg/kg/min for rapid replacement or when seizures are refractory to other therapies (106). Steady-state concentrations above 50 mg/L have been reported after administration of IV VPA 15 mg/kg followed 1 to 3 hours later by either IV VPA or sustained-release oral divalproex sodium 7.0 mg/kg every 8 hours or 4 mg/kg every 6 hours. When VPA concentrations need to be maintained above 100 mg/L, the drug may need to be infused every 4 hours (107).

Discussions concerning the optimal or first-choice drug therapy of SE examine morbidity and mortality, along with the practical issues of drug administration and adverse effects. As Holmes (54) recently concluded, no one drug of choice may be acceptable to all clinicians. Certainly LZP, DZP, MDZ, PHT, and PB are all useful agents for both the initial and continued therapy of SE (89,108,109). Thus one's choice of the initial and subsequent medications for the treatment of SE may depend on the individual patient characteristics, prior AED therapy, and physician preference. Most important, a protocol should be established so that prompt and appropriate emergency treatment can be given in an efficient manner (110). The use of IV VPA in SE is currently being defined, as are the roles of alternate forms of administering benzodiazepines.

MEDICAL COMPLICATIONS OF STATUS EPILEPTICUS

The treatment of SE requires close monitoring of physiologic variables and excellent nursing to prevent secondary complications (3,7,59). Besides the underlying or precipitating disease states associated with SE, subsequent medical complications are quite common. Pulmonary care, proper positioning, and careful observation of seizures, noting the possible changes in seizure pattern, are mandatory. Frequent surveillance and normalization of glucose and electrolytes, particularly in neonates and small infants, is mandatory. Optimal oxygenation and expectant observation and treatment for hyperthermia and other medical complications lead directly to a lessening of morbidity and mortality. Cardiovascular, respiratory, and renal effects may be severe. Medical complications of SE, which may occur in both infants and older children, are listed in Table 20-8.

When hyperthermia is resistant to rectally administered antipyretics and cooling blankets, muscular blockade may be necessary. EEG monitoring is a necessity when this is performed. A rise in blood pressure consistently accompanies seizures but rarely requires antihypertensive medication unless the child is at risk for malignant hypertension. Unfortunately, treatment may result in hypotension and reduce cerebral perfusion pressure. Very infrequently does cerebral edema or increased intracranial pressure become problematic during most cases of SE not associated with an intracranial mass. The use of osmotic diuretics and steroids are therefore rarely indicated in the routine treatment of SE.

Table 20-8. Medical Complications of Status Epilepticus

Tachycardia
Bradycardia
Cardiac arrhythmia
Cardiac arrest
Conduction disturbance
Congestive heart failure
Hypertension
Hypotension
Altered respiratory pattern
Pulmonary edema
Pneumonia
Oliguria
Uremia
Renal tubular necrosis
Lower nephron nephrosis
Rhabdomyolysis
Increased creatine phosphokinase
Myoglobinuria
Apnea
Anoxia
Hypoxia
CO_2 narcosis
Intravascular coagulation
Metabolic and respiratory acidosis
Cerebral edema
Excessive perspiration
Dehydration
Endocrine failure
Altered pituitary function
Elevated prolactin
Elevated vasopressin
Hyperglycemia
Hypoglycemia
Increased plasma cortisol
Autonomic dysfunction
Fever

NONCONVULSIVE STATUS EPILEPTICUS

Convulsive generalized tonic-clonic SE may evolve into nonconvulsive or subtle SE either without treatment as part of its natural history or because of partially successful drug treatment. The incidence of posttreatment subtle SE has been placed as high as 48 percent in patients requiring intensive care management (8). The mortality in such cases has been difficult to isolate from the associated acute medical illnesses but ranges from 33 percent to 52 percent, rising well above that for the SE population as a whole. Multifactorial analysis does suggest, however, that the morbidity and mortality in this group is most closely correlated with the delay in time to diagnosis (duration of seizure) and serum levels of NSE. (44,45). Treatment of subtle SE is identical to that of refractory SE, and the central theme to improving outcome is early recognition and intensive EEG monitoring.

In addition to postconvulsive subtle seizures, NCSE also presents as prolonged complex partial, absence, myoclonic, or atonic seizures. These confusional or fugue states are a separate entity from the previously described subtle SE. Childhood conditions with periods of frequently occurring seizures that meet the definition of SE include the syndromes of West (infantile spasms/hypsarrhythmia), Lennox-Gastaut, Landau-Kleffner, childhood absence (pyknolepsy), continuous spike-wave during sleep, and continuous occipital spike-wave during sleep (89). Furthermore, neonatal seizures with their various subtle and sometimes variable symptomatology may sometimes represent SE. Specific etiologies should always be considered in these cases.

EEG monitoring reveals continuous or noncontinuous generalized, symmetric or diffuse and irregular 1.5- to 4-Hz multispike-and-wave complexes in absence status, as opposed to the partial discharges seen in SE because of complex partial seizures (59). Clinically, a child in absence status usually demonstrates partial responsiveness with confusion, disorientation, speech arrest, amnesia, and sometimes automatisms (111). Total unresponsiveness with stereotyped automatisms is usually lacking in absence status (111). Complex partial SE is more likely to be fluctuating, sometimes with nearly cyclical impairment of consciousness, including total unresponsiveness and more complex stereotyped automatisms, with wandering eye movements or eye deviations (112,113).

The therapy of complex partial SE is similar therapy for convulsive SE. For absence status, IV LZP or DZP is excellent. This medication should then be followed quickly by IV VPA or oral, nasogastric, or rectal doses ethosuximide or clonazepam. Rarely, combined administration of VPA and clonazepam may produce absence status. Some children with Lennox-Gastaut syndrome have seizures exacerbated by benzodiazepines (89). Case reports demonstrate the response of refractory partial SE to clobazam (114) and refractory absence SE to propofol or IV VPA (115,116). Respiratory support is less problematic in NCSE than in convulsive forms; however, some patients have difficulties handling secretions in their "twilight state" or spike-wave stupor.

CONCLUSIONS

Similar to other seizure types, SE represents a symptom of CNS dysfunction. However, it signifies severe malfunction. The etiology of SE must be sought out because the highest percentage of SE is symptomatic, particularly in young children. Judicious use of routine laboratory tests coupled with neuroradiologic studies and lumbar puncture should be employed in almost every patient. Those patients who remain in prolonged coma may harbor a disease such as intracranial hemorrhage, meningitis, or encephalitis, and in general have a poorer prognosis, as do all patients with prolonged or uncontrollable SE. Recent studies dispute the prior morbidity and mortality figures for SE at approximately two-thirds. A better prognosis seems possible if seizures are controlled more rapidly while optimal support is given. Promptly recognizing medical complications and treating concomitant diseases further improve outcome in all children.

REFERENCES

1. Pellock JM. Status epilepticus. In: Pellock JM, Myer EC, eds. *Neurologic Emergencies in Infancy and Childhood*. Philadelphia: Harper & Row, 1984.

2. Dodson WE, DeLorenzo RJ, Pedley TA, et al. for the Epilepsy Foundation of America's Working Group on Status Epilepticus. Treatment of convulsive status epilepticus. *JAMA* 1993; 270:854.

3. Pellock JM. Status epilepticus in children: update and review. *J Child Neurol* 1994; 9(Suppl 2):S27–S35.

4. Towne AR, Pellock JM, Ko D, et al. Determinants of mortality in status epilepticus. *Epilepsia* 1994; 35:27.

5. Pellock JM, DeLorenzo RJ. Status epilepticus. In RJ Porter, D Chadwick, eds. *The Epilepsies 2*. Boston: Butterworth-Heinemann, 1997:267.

6. DeLorenzo RJ, Hauser WA, Towne AR, et al. A prospective, population-based epidemiologic study of status epilepticus in Richmond, Virginia. *Neurology* 1996; 46:1029–1035.

7. Treiman DM. Status epilepticus. In: Laidlaw J, Richems A, Chadwick D, eds. *A Textbook of Epilepsy*. Edinburgh: Churchill-Livingstone, 1993:205.

8. DeLorenzo RJ, Waterhouse EJ, Towne AR, et al. Persistent nonconvulsive status epilepticus after the

control of convulsive status epilepticus. *Epilepsia* 1998; 39:833–840.

9. Lowenstein DH, Bleck T, Macdonald RL. It's time to revise the definition of status epilepticus. *Epilepsia* 1999; 40:120–122.

10. Calmeil LE. *De l'epilepsie etudiee sous le raport de son seige et de son influence sur la production de l'alienation mentale.* Master's Thesis. Paris: Didat, 1924.

11. Gastaut H. Classification of status epilepticus. In: Delgado-Escueta AV, Porter RJ, Wasterlain CG, eds. *Status Epilepticus: Mechanisms of Brain Damage and Treatment.* New York: Raven Press, 1982.

12. DeLorenzo RJ, Garnett L, Towne AR, et al. Comparison of status epilepticus with prolonged seizure episodes lasting from 10 to 29 minutes. *Epilepsia* 1999; 40:164–169.

13. Scher MA, Ask K, Beggarly Me, et al. Electrographic seizures in preterm and full term neonates: clinical correlates, associated brain lesions, and risk for neurologic sequelae. *Pediatrics* 1993; 91:128.

14. Delgado-Escueta AV, Treiman DM. Focal status epilepticus: modern concepts. In: Lüders H, Lesser RP, eds. *Epilepsy Electroclinical Syndromes.* London: Springer. 1987:347.

15. Porter RJ, Penry JK. In: Delgado-Escueta AV, Wasterlain CG, et al., eds. *Status Epilepticus.* New York: Raven Press, 1983:61.

16. Lockman LA. Treatment of status epilepticus in children. *Neurology* 1990; 40(Suppl):43–46.

17. DeLorenzo RJ, Towne AR, Pellock JM, et al. Status epilepticus in children, adults, and the elderly. *Epilepsia* 1992; 33(Suppl 4):S15.

18. Corey LA, Pellock JM, Boggs JG, et al. Evidence for a genetic predisposition for status epilepticus. *Neurology* 1998; 50:558–560.

19. Shinnar S, Pellock JM, Moshe SL, et al. In whom does status epilepticus occur. Epilepsia 1997; 38:907–914.

20. Maytal J, Shinnar S, Moshe SL, Alvarez LA. Low-morbidity and mortality of status epilepticus in children. *Pediatrics* 1989; 83:323–331.

21. Driscoll SM, Jack RE, Teasley JE, et al. Mortality in childhood status epilepticus. *Ann Neurol* 1988; 24:318.

22. Driscoll SM, Pellock JM, Towne A, et al. Recurrent status epilepticus in children. *Neurology* 1990; 40:14(Suppl 1):297.

23. Hauser WA, Rich SS, Annegers JF, et al. Seizure recurrence after a first unprovoked seizure: an extended follow-up. *Neurology* 1990; 40:1163.

24. Sillanpaa M, Jalava M, Shinnar S. Status epilepticus in a population-based cohort with childhood-onset epilepsy in Finland. *Epilepsia* 1998; 39(Suppl 6):219–220.

25. Hesdorffer D, Logroscino G, Cascino G, et al. Risk of unprovoked seizure after acute symptomatic seizure: effect of status epilepticus. *Ann Neurol* 1998; 44;908–912.

26. Shinnar S, Pellock JM, Berg AT, et al. An inception cohort of children with febrile status epilepticus: cohort characteristics and early outcomes [abstract]. *Epilepsia* 1995; 36(Suppl 4):31.

27. DeLorenzo RJ, Pellock JM, Towne AR, et al. Pathophysiology of status epilepticus. *J Clin Neurol* 1995; 12:316

28. Berg AT, Shinnar S, Levy SR, et al. Status epilepticus in children with newly diagnosed epilepsy. *Ann Neurol* 1999; 45:618–623.

29. Morton LD, Watemberg NM, Driscoll-Bannister S, et al. Long-term outcome of status epilepticus in the first year of life [abstract]. *Epilepsia* 1998; 39(Suppl 6):220.

30. Hauser WA. Status epilepticus: epidemiologic considerations. *Neurology* 1990; 40 (Suppl):9–13.

31. Pellock JM. Status epilepticus. In: Dodson WE, Pellock JM, eds. *Pediatric Epilepsy: Diagnosis and Therapy.* New York: Demos.1993:197.

32. Dunn W. Status epilepticus in children: etiology, clinical features, and outcome. *J Child Neurol* 1988; 3:167.

33. Phillips SA, Shanahan RJ. Etiology and mortality of status epilepticus in children. *Arch Neurol* 1989; 46:74–76.

34. Fountain N, Lothman EW. Pathophysiology of status epilepticus. *J Clin Neurophysiol* 1995; 12:326–342.

35. Moshe SL. Epileptogenesis and the immature brain. *Epilepsia* 1987; 28(Suppl):53–55.

36. Moshe SL. Brain injury with prolonged seizures in children and adults. *J Child Neurol* 1998; 13(Suppl 1):S3–S6.

37. Thompson K, Wasterlain C. The model of status epilepticus that produces neuronal necrosis in the immature brain. *Neurology* 1994; 44:A272.

38. Rice AC, DeLorenzo RJ. Kindling induces long-term changes in gene expression. In: Cocoran, Moshe SL, eds. *Kindling 5.* New York: Plenum, 1998:267–284.

39. Simon RP, Pellock JM, DeLorenzo RJ. Acute morbidity and mortality of status epilepticus. In: Engel J, Pedley TA, eds. *Epilepsy: A Comprehensive Textbook.* 1997:741–753.

40. Boggs JG, Painter JA, DeLorenzo RJ. Analysis of electrocardiographic changes in status epilepticus. *Epilepsy Res* 1993; 14:87–94.

41. Liu Z, Gatt A, Mikati M, et al. Effect of temperature on kainic acid-induced seizures. *Brain Res* 1993; 631:51–58.

42. Aicardi JF, Chevrie JJ. Convulsive status epilepticus in infants and children: a study of 239 cases. *Epilepsia* 1987; 11:187.

43. Whitty CWM. Status epilepticus. In: Tryer JH, ed. *The Treatment of Epilepsy.* Philadelphia: Lippincott, 1980.

44. Young GB, Jordan KG, Dolg GS. An assessment of nonconvulsive seizures in the intensive care unit using continuous EEG monitoring: an investigation of variables associated with mortality. *Neurology* 1996; 47:89–89.

45. DeGiorgio CM, Heck CN, Rabinowicz AL, et al. Serum neuron-specific enolase in the major subtypes of status epilepticus. *Neurology* 1999; 52:746–749.

46. Calabrese VP, Gruemer HD, James K, et al. Cerebrospinal fluid lactate levels and prognosis in status epilepticus. *Epilepsia* 1991; 32:816–821.

47. Barry E, Hauser WA. Pleocytosis after status epilepticus. *Arch Neurol* 1994; 51:190–193.

48. Rider LG, Thapa PB, Del Beccaro MA, et al. Cerebrospinal fluid analysis in children with seizures. *Ped Emerg Care* 1995; 11:226–229.

49. Chan S, Chin SS, Kartha K, et al. Reversible signal abnormalities in the hippocampus and neocortex after prolonged seizures. *Am J Neuroradiol* 1996; 17:1725–1731.

50. Juhasz C, Scheidl E, Szirmai I. Reversible focal MRI abnormalities due to status epilepticus. An EEG, single photon emission computed tomography, transcranial Doppler follow-up study. *Electroencephalogr Clin Neurophysiol* 1998; 107:402–407.

51. Fazekas F, Kapeller P, Schmidt R, et al. Magnetic resonance imaging and spectroscopy findings after focal status epilepticus. *Epilepsia* 1995; 36:946–949.

52. Waterhouse EJ, Vaughan JK, Barnes TY, et al. Synergistic effect of status epilepticus and ischemic brain injury on mortality. *Epilepsy Res* 1998; 29:175–183.

53. *Seizure Recognition and First Aid*. Epilepsy Foundation of America, 1989.

54. Pellock JM. Recent advances concerning status epilepticus. *Pediatrics* 1990; 5:188–195.

55. Van Ness PC. Pentobarbital and EEG burst suppression in treatment of status epilepticus refractory to benzodiazepines and phenytoin. *Epilepsia* 1990; 31:61–67.

56. Delgado-Escueta AV, Porter RJ, Wasterlain CG, eds. *Status Epilepticus: Mechanisms of Brain Damage and Treatment*. New York: Raven Press, 1982.

57. Pellock JM, Myer EC, eds. *Neurologic Emergencies in Infancy and Childhood*. 2nd ed. New York: Butterworth, 1992.

58. Orlowski JP, Porembha DT, Gallagher BB, et al. Comparison study of intraosseous, central intravenous and peripheral intravenous infusions of emergency drugs. *Am J Dis Child* 1990; 144:112–117.

59. Leppik WA. Status epilepticus: the next decade. *Neurology* 1990; 40(Suppl):4–9.

60. Jaitly R, Sgro JA, Towne AR, et al. Prognostic value of EEG monitoring after status epilepticus: a prospective adult study. *J Clin Neurophysiol* 1997; 14:326–334.

61. Alehan FK, Morton LD, Pellock JM. Electroencephalogram in the pediatric emergency department: is it useful? *Neurology* 1999; 52(Suppl 2):A45.

62. Nei M, Lee JM, Shanker VL, et al. The EEG and prognosis in status epilepticus. *Epilepsia* 1999; 40:157–163.

63. Boggs JG, Marmarou A, Agnew JP, et al. Hemodynamic monitoring prior to and at the time of death in status epilepticus. *Epilepsy Res* 1998; 31:199–209.

64. Pellock JM, DeLorenzo RJ. Status epilepticus. In: Porter RJ, Chadwick D, eds. *The Epilepsies 2*. Boston: Butterworth-Heinemann, 1997:267.

65. Holmes GL. Drug of choice for status epilepticus. I. *Epilepsy* 1990; 3:1.

66. Treiman DM, Meyers PD, Walton NY, et al. A comparison of our treatments for generalized convulsive status epilepticus. Veterans Affairs Status Epilepticus Cooperative Study Group. *N Engl J Med* 1998; 339:792–798.

67. Treiman DM. The role of benzodiazepines in the management of status epilepticus. *Neurology* 1990; 40(Suppl):32–42.

68. Chamberlain J, Alterieri M, Futterman C, et al. A prospective, randomized study comparing intramuscular midazolam with intravenous diazepam for treatment of seizures in children. *Pediatr Emerg Care* 1997; 13:92–94.

69. Wallace S. Nasal benzodiazepines for management of acute childhood seizures? *Lancet* 1997; 25:222.

70. Scott RC, Besag FMC, Neville BGR. Buccal midazolam and rectal diazepam for treatment of prolonged seizures in childhood and adolescence: a randomized trial. *Lancet* 1999; 353:623–626.

71. Homan RW, Unwin DH. Benzodiazepines: lorazepam. In: Levy RH, Dreifuss FE, Mattson RH, et al., eds. *Antiepileptic Drugs*. 3rd ed. New York: Raven Press, 1989:849–854.

71a. Crawford TO, Mitchell WG, Snodgrass SR. Lorazepam in childhood status epilepticus and serial seizures: effectiveness and tachyphylaxis. *Neurology* 1987; 37:190–195.

72. Deshnukh A, Wittert W, Schnitzler E, Margutten HH. Lorazepam in the treatment of refractory neonatal seizures. *Am J Dis Child* 1986; 140:1042–1044.

73. Graing DW, McBride MC. Lorazepam versus diazepam for the treatment of status epilepticus. *Pediatr Neurol* 1988; 4:358–361.

74. Lacey DJ, Singer WD, Horwitz SJ, Gilmore H. Lorazepam therapy of status epilepticus in children and adolescents. *J Pediatr* 1986; 198:771–774.

75. Levy RJ, KraII RL. Treatment of status epilepticus with lorazepam. *Arch Neurol* 1984; 41:605–611.

76. Relling MV, Mulhern RK, Dodge RK, et al. Lorazepam pharmacodynamics and pharmacokinetics in children. *J Pediatr* 1989; 114:641–646.

77. Graves NM, Kriel RL. Rectal administration of antiepileptic drugs in children. *Pediatr Neurol* 1987; 3:321–326.

78. Enrile-Bacsal F, Delgado-Escueta AV. IV diazepam drip in tonic-clonic status epilepticus. In: Delgado-Escueta AV, Porter RJ, Wasterlain CG, eds. *Status Epilepticus: Mechanisms of Brain Damage and Treatment*. New York: Raven Press, 1982.

79. Dreifuss F, Rosman N, Cloyd J, et al. A comparison of rectal diazepam gel and placebo for acute repetitive seizures. *N Engl J Med* 1998; 338:1869–1875.

80. Cereghino JJ, Mitchell W, Murphy J, et al. Treating repetitive seizures with a rectal diazepam formulation: a randomized study. The North American Diastat Study Group. *Neurology* 1998; 51:1274–1282.

81. Pellock JM. Management of acute seizure episodes. *Epilepsia* 1998; 39(Suppl 1):S28–S35.

82. Egli M, Albani C. Relief of status epilepticus after IM administration of the new short-acting benzodiazepine midazolam (Dormicum). In: Program and abstracts of

the 12th World Congress of Neurology. Princeton, NJ: Excerpta Medica; 1981; 44. Abstract 137.

83. Bebin M, Bleck TP. New anticonvulsant drugs. Focus on flunarizine, fosphenytoin, midazolam, and stiripentol. *Drugs* 1994; 48:153–171.

84. Pellock JM. Emergency room management of status epilepticus with midazolam. *Ann Emerg Med* 1999 (in press).

85. Pellock JM. Use of midazolam for refractory status epilepticus in pediatric patients. *J Child Neurol* 1998; 13:581–587.

86. Greenblatt D, Abernathy D, Locniskar A, et al. Effect of age, gender, and obesity on midazolam kinetics. *Anesthesiology* 1984; 61:27–35.

87. Lombroso CT. The treatment of status epilepticus. *Pediatrics* 1974; 53:536–542.

88. Lockman LA. Treatment of status epilepticus in children. *Neurology* 1990; 40(Suppl):43–46.

89. Shaner DM, McCurdy SA, Herring MO, Gabor AJ. Treatment of status epilepticus: a prospective comparison of diazepam and phenytoin versus phenobarbital and optional phenytoin. *Neurology* 1988; 38:202–207.

90. Quon C, Stampfi, H. In-vitro hydrolysis of ACC-9653 (phosphate ester prodrug of phenytoin) by human, dog, rat blood and tissues. *Pharm Res* 1987; 3(Suppl):1349. Abstract.

91. Wilder BJ, Ramsay RE, Hillmore U, et al. Efficacy of intravenous phenytoin in the treatment of status epilepticus: kinetics of central nervous system penetration. *Ann Neurol* 1977; 1:511–518.

92. Ramsey RE, Hammond EJ, Perchalski RJ, et al. Brain uptake of phenytoin, phenobarbital and clonazepam. *Arch Neurol* 1979; 36:535–539.

93. Pellock JM. Seizure disorders. In: Kelley VC, ed. *Practice of Pediatrics*. Hagerstown, MD: Harper & Row, 1987:150.

94. Cranford RE, Leppick IE, Patrick B, et al. Intravenous phenytoin: clinical and pharmacokinetic aspects. *Neurology* 1979; 29:1474–1479.

95. Eldon M, Loewen G, Voightman R, et al. Pharmacokinetics and tolerance of fosphenytoin and phenytoin administration intravenously to healthy subjects. *Can J Neurol Sci* 1993; 20:5180.

96. Knapp LE, Kugler AR. Clinical experience with fosphenytoin in adults: pharmacokinetics, safety, and efficacy. *J Child Neurol* 1998; 13(Suppl 1):S15–S18.

97. Wilensky AJ, Lowden JA. Inadequate serum levels after intramuscular administration of diphenylhydantoin. *Neurology* 1973; 23:318–321.

98. Raskin MC, Younger C, Penowish P. Pentobarbital treatment of refractory status epilepticus. *Neurology* 1987; 37:500–503.

99. Shields WD. Status epilepticus. *Pediatr Clin North Am* 1989; 36:383–393.

100. Walker I, Slovis C. Lidocaine in the treatment of status epilepticus. *Acad Emerg Med* 1997; 4:918–922.

101. Brown LA, Levin GM. Role of propofol in refractory status epilepticus. *Ann Pharmacother* 1998; 32:1053–1059.

102. Stecker MM, Kramer TH, Raps EC, et al. Treatment of refractory status epilepticus with propofol: clinical and pharmacokinetic findings. *Epilepsia* 1998; 39:18–26.

103. Hanna JP, Ramundo ML. Rhabdomyolysis and hypoxia associated with prolonged propofol infusion in children. *Neurology* 1998; 50:301–303.

104. Price DJ. Intravenous valproate: experience in neurosurgery. *Royal Soc Med Int Cong Symp Ser* 1989; 152:197–203.

105. Marlow N, Cooke RWI. Intravenous sodium valproate in the neonatal intensive care unit. *Royal Soc Med Int Cong Symp Ser* 1989:152:208–210.

106. Wheless J, Venkataraman V. Safety of high intravenous valproate doses in epilepsy patients. *J Epilepsy* 1999; 11:319–324.

107. Cavanaugh JH, Hussein Z, Lamm J, et al. Effect of multiple oral dose divalproex sodium after intravenous loading dose administration in healthy volunteers. *Drug Invest* 1994; 7:1–7.

108. Gabor AJ. Lorazepam versus phenobarbital: candidates for drug of choice for treatment of status epilepticus. *J Epilepsy* 1990; 3:3–6.

109. Mitchell WG, Crawford TO. Lorazepam is the treatment of choice for status epilepticus. *J Epilepsy* 1990; 3:7–10.

110. Dodson WE, DeLorenzo RJ Pedley TA, et al. for the epilepsy Foundation of America's Working Group on Status Epilepticus. Treatment of convulsive status epilepticus. *JAMA* 1993; 270:854.

111. Porter RJ, Penry JK. Petit mal status. In: Delgado-Escueta AV, Wasterlain CG, Treiman DM, et al., eds. *Status Epilepticus*. New York: Raven Press, 1987; 61–67. Advances in Neurology, vol. 34.

112. McBride MC, Dooling EC, Oppenheimer IN. Complex partial status epilepticus in young children. *Ann Neurol* 1981; 9:526–530.

113. Treiman DM, Delgado-Escueta AV Complex partial status epilepticus. In: Delgado-Escueta AV, Wasterlain CG, Treiman DM, et al., eds. *Status Epilepticus*. New York: Raven Press, 1987:69–68. Advances in Neurology, vol. 34.

114. Corman C, Guberman A, Benavente O. Clobazam in partial status epilepticus. *Seizure* 1998; 7:243247.

115. Crouteau D, Shevell M, Rosenblatt B, et al. Treatment of absence status in the Lennox-Gastaut syndrome with propofol. *Neurology* 1998; 51:315–316.

116. Alehan FK, Morton LD, Pellock JM. Treatment of absence status with intravenous valproate. *Neurology* 1999; 52:889–890.

CHAPTER 21

Treatment Decisions in Childhood Seizures

Shlomo Shinnar M.D., Ph.D., and Christine O'Dell, R.N., M.S.N.

Not long ago almost all children with a seizure of any type, febrile or afebrile, were placed on long-term therapy with antiepileptic drugs (AEDs). This was based on several assumptions. First, that almost all children with an isolated seizure would go on to have more seizures (1,2). Second, that seizures, even brief ones, could cause brain damage and lead to progressively intractable epilepsy (1–3). Third, that AEDs were not only effective but also safe and that treatment was associated with only minimal morbidity. Finally, that seizures "beget" seizures and that early AED therapy not only prevented seizures but also somehow altered the natural history of the disorder and prevented the development of "chronic" epilepsy (3–6). We now know that these assumptions are not true. Recent research has provided information that has altered the way physicians think about seizures, their consequences, and the drugs used to treat them. The decision whether and for how long to treat a child with AEDs must be weighed against the possible risks of that treatment and must take into account the large body of data that has accumulated; namely, that many children with a single seizure do not go on to experience further seizures (7–16), that many children with epilepsy ultimately go on to become seizure-free (17–20), that most seizures are brief and even prolonged seizures rarely cause brain damage unless they are associated with an acute neurologic insult (21–24), and that AEDs may cause untoward effects (25–27).

The decision of whether to initiate treatment in a child with one or more seizures must balance the risks and benefits of treatment in each case. Similarly, the patient who is seizure-free on medications for some time must weigh the risks of possible seizure recurrence if medications are withdrawn against the risks of continuing long-term AED therapy. This chapter reviews the data relevant to these decisions. The data on the probability of seizure recurrence following a

first unprovoked seizure are presented. Next, the issue of withdrawing AEDs in children with epilepsy who are seizure-free for 2 or more years is considered. This is followed by a review of the risks of not treating (i.e., the risks of subsequent seizures) and of the morbidity of therapy. Finally, recommendations for a therapeutic approach to children with seizures are outlined.

RECURRENCE RISK FOLLOWING A FIRST UNPROVOKED SEIZURE

An understanding of the natural history of children who present with an initial unprovoked seizure is necessary to develop a rational approach to their management. Many studies have attempted to address this issue over the past two decades (7–16). For purposes of this discussion, a first unprovoked seizure is defined as a seizure or flurry of seizures occurring within 24 hours in a patient over 1 month of age with no prior history of unprovoked seizures (28).

The reported overall recurrence risk following a first unprovoked seizure in children varies from 27 percent to 71 percent (7–16). Studies that identified the children at the time of first seizure and carefully excluded those with prior seizures report recurrence risks of 27 percent to 44 percent (7–11). Studies that recruited subjects later, either retrospectively or from electroencephalogram (EEG) laboratories, but excluded those with prior seizures report higher recurrence risks of 48 percent to 52 percent (14,15). Finally, studies that included children who already had recurrent seizures at the time of identification report the highest recurrence risks — 61 percent to 71 percent (12,13). Once methodological issues and differences in the distribution of risk factors among different studies are taken into account, the results are fairly consistent (9). The majority of recurrences occur early, with approximately 50 percent of

Table 21-1. Risk Factors for Recurrence: Multivariable Analysis Using Cox Proportional Hazards Model

Risk Factor	Proportionate Hazards Model		
	Rate Ratio	95% CI	p value
Overall Group (N = 407)			
Abnormal EEG	2.1	1.6, 3.0	<0.001
Remote symptomatic etiology	1.7	1.2, 2.4	0.006
Prior febrile seizures	1.6	1.1, 2.3	0.019
Todd's paresis	1.7	1.0, 2.9	0.038
Seizure while asleep	1.5	1.1, 2.1	0.008
Cryptogenic Cases (N = 342)			
Abnormal EEG	2.5	1.7, 3.6	<0.0001
Seizure while asleep	1.7	1.2, 2.5	<0.003
Remote Symptomatic Cases (N = 65)			
Prior febrile seizures	2.3	1.2, 4.5	<0.02
Age ≤3 years	2.4	1.2, 4.9	<0.02

Reprinted with permission from Shinnar S, Berg AT, Moshe SL, et al. The risk of recurrence following a first unprovoked afebrile seizure in childhood: an extended follow-up. *Pediatrics* 1996; 216:216–225.

recurrences occurring within 6 months and over 80 percent within 2 years of the initial seizure (7–16). Late recurrences are unusual (8).

Similar predictors of recurrent seizures were found in the majority of the studies despite variations in methodology and subject selection (7–16). Factors that are associated with a differential risk of recurrence include the etiology of the seizure, the EEG, whether the first seizure occurred in wakefulness or in sleep, and seizure type. Factors that are not associated with a change in the recurrence risk include age of onset and duration of the initial seizure. The report of a family history of seizures in a first-degree relative is of unclear significance, with conflicting results in the various studies. Risk factors for seizure recurrence from our large prospective study (8) are shown in Table 21-1.

Etiology

The recent International League Against Epilepsy (ILAE) guidelines for epidemiologic research (28) classify seizures as acute symptomatic, remote symptomatic, cryptogenic, or idiopathic. *Acute symptomatic seizures* are associated with an acute insult such as head trauma or meningitis. *Remote symptomatic seizures* are those without an immediate cause but with an identifiable prior brain injury such as major head trauma (loss of consciousness longer than 30 minutes, depressed skull fracture, or intracranial hemorrhage), meningitis or encephalitis, stroke, or the presence of a static encephalopathy such as mental retardation or cerebral palsy, which are known to be associated with an increased risk of seizures. *Cryptogenic seizures* are those occurring in otherwise normal individuals with no clear cause. Factors such as sleep deprivation

are considered trigger factors but do not change the classification of the seizure because they would only be associated with seizures in susceptible individuals. Until recently cryptogenic seizures were also called *idiopathic seizures*. In the new classification, the term *idiopathic* is reserved for seizures that occur in the context of the presumed genetic epilepsies such as benign rolandic and childhood absence (28–30), but many authors still refer to cryptogenic seizures as idiopathic.

Children with a remote symptomatic first seizure have a higher risk of recurrence. In one large prospective study with mean follow-up of 6.3 years, 44 of 65 children (68%) with a remote symptomatic first seizure recurred compared with 127 of 347 children (37%) with a cryptogenic/idiopathic first seizure (p < 0.001) (8). Comparable findings are reported in other studies (9–11,14,15).

Electroencephalogram

The EEG is an important predictor of recurrence, particularly in cryptogenic cases (8–11,14). Epileptiform abnormalities are more important than nonepileptiform abnormalities, but any EEG abnormality increases the recurrence risk in cryptogenic cases (8). In our study, the risk of seizure recurrence by 5 years for children with a cryptogenic first seizure was 27 percent for those with a normal EEG, 44 percent for those with nonepileptiform abnormalities, and 62 percent for those with epileptiform abnormalities (7,8). In our data (8,31), any clearly abnormal EEG patterns, including generalized spike-and-wave, focal spikes, and focal or generalized slowing, increased the risk of recurrence, whereas Camfield and coworkers (14) report that only epileptiform abnormalities substantially increase the risk of recurrence. Hauser and colleagues (10) state that only generalized spike-and-wave patterns are predictive of recurrence, but they studied mostly adolescents and adults, They therefore would not have included many children with centrotemporal spikes (benign rolandic epilepsy), which is the most common focal spike pattern found in studies focusing on children with a first seizure (8,14,31). The EEG appears to be the most important predictor of recurrence in children with a cryptogenic first seizure, (8,9).

Sleep State at Time of First Seizure

Whether the initial seizure occurs while the child is awake or asleep affects the recurrence risk, particularly in cryptogenic cases (8). In our series, the 5-year recurrence risk was 53 percent for children whose initial seizure occurred during sleep compared with 36 percent for those whose initial seizure occurred while awake (p < 0.001) (8). On multivariable analysis, etiology, EEG, and sleep state were the only significant predictors of outcome. The group of children with a cryptogenic first seizure occurring while awake and a normal EEG had a 5-year recurrence risk of only 21 percent. If seizures did recur, they usually recurred in the same sleep state as the initial seizure.

Seizure Classification

Some although not all studies indicate that the risk of recurrence following a partial seizure is higher than that following a generalized seizure (9). However, partial seizures are more common in children with a remote symptomatic first seizure and in children with a cryptogenic first seizure who have an abnormal EEG (7). Once the effects of etiology and the EEG are controlled for, partial seizures are not associated with an increased risk of recurrence (7,8,10). In the meta-analysis no clear association between seizure type and recurrence risk could be found (9).

Family History

At the present time, there are insufficient data to determine whether a positive family history of epilepsy is a risk factor for recurrence. Although one study, primarily of adults, found a substantially increased risk of recurrence in those with a positive family history of epilepsy (10), others have failed to find a major effect (8,14). In our study, family history was only important in children with a cryptogenic first seizure who also had an abnormal EEG. This type of patient constitutes a small fraction of the population (7). These mixed results suggest that the additional risk of a positive family history, if present, turns out to be small or limited to specific subgroups.

Duration of First Seizure and Status Epilepticus

The duration of the first seizure does not affect the risk of recurrence (8–10). This is true whether one analyzes it as a continuous variable or separates the children into those who had status epilepticus and those who had a briefer seizure (8). Most cases of status epilepticus occur as the initial seizure. In our series of 407 children, 48 (12%) had status epilepticus as their first seizure, but only 7 of 171 children (4%) with recurrent seizures recurred with status epilepticus. Although the occurrence of status epilepticus as the first seizure did not alter recurrence risks, a recurrence was more likely to be prolonged. Five of 24 children (21%) with recurrent seizures whose initial seizure was status epilepticus had an episode of status epilepticus as their second seizure compared with 2 of 147 children (1%) with recurrent seizures whose first seizure was brief ($p < 0.001$). None of these children experienced any sequelae (8). Remission rates were not different in those who presented with an episode of status epilepticus (32).

Age at First Seizure

The majority of studies, both in children and in adults, have not found age at first seizure to alter the risk of recurrence (7–11,14–16). This was true whether age was analyzed as a continuous variable or broken up into several age ranges. The only exception is the National Collaborative Perinatal Project, which found an increased risk of recurrence in children under age 2 years with focal motor seizures (13). At the present time, the preponderance of available data indicate that the age at time of first seizure does not affect the risk of recurrence following a first unprovoked seizure.

Treatment Following a First Seizure

In observational studies such as those discussed previously, whether children were treated after their first seizure did not alter the recurrence risk (8,10); however, these studies were not randomized treatment trials. The physicians presumably treated those children they thought to have a high risk of recurrence. Following an initial seizure, patients often are started on a small dose of medication, and compliance may be lax. In randomized clinical trials comparing AED therapy with placebo following a first unprovoked seizure in children and adults AEDs reduce the risk of a second seizure by half (16,33). However, with longer follow-up, there was no difference between the two groups in terms of the probability of achieving remission (6,34).

Conclusions

Knowing these predictors and the recurrence risks, the child with a first unprovoked seizure presents an interesting dilemma. The likelihood that it will be an isolated event must be weighed against whether it is the first of many attacks. A thorough evaluation of the patient, including a detailed history and appropriate laboratory studies such as an EEG, is indicated regardless of whether AED therapy is started. Factors such as the seizure type, family history of seizures, and the possible etiology of the seizure must be ascertained. Of particular importance is a careful history of prior events that may have been seizures. Many children who first come to medical attention because of a convulsive episode are found to have had prior nonconvulsive episodes of absence or complex partial seizures that were not recognized as such by the family. These children clearly fall into the category of newly diagnosed epilepsy and not first seizure.

The majority of children with a first unprovoked seizure do not have additional unprovoked seizures.

Children with an cryptogenic first seizure and a normal EEG have a particularly favorable prognosis. There are small subgroups of children with multiple risk factors who do have a high risk of recurrence; however, although AED therapy reduces the likelihood of further seizures, there is no evidence that it alters the long-term prognosis. In particular, the data from randomized clinical trials and large epidemiologic studies indicate that delaying therapy neither alters the response rate to AEDs nor adversely affects the probability of attaining remission (3,5,6,19,34). The decision to treat or not after a first seizure must be based on the relative risks and benefits of therapy compared with the risks of further seizures. This risk-benefit assessment is discussed at the end of this chapter. The authors rarely treat children with a first unprovoked seizure.

WITHDRAWING AEDS IN CHILDREN WITH EPILEPSY WHO HAVE BEEN SEIZURE-FREE FOR TWO OR MORE YEARS

The available data indicate that children who are seizure-free on medication for 2 or more years have a very high likelihood of remaining in remission on medication (35). In selected populations, withdrawal may be feasible after an even shorter seizure-free interval (35–38). How long should a child be maintained on medication before attempting to withdraw it? This decision is influenced by a variety of factors, including the probability of remaining seizure-free after withdrawal, the potential risk of injury from a seizure recurrence, and the potential adverse effects of continued AED therapy.

The majority of children who are seizure-free on medications for at least 2 years remain seizure-free when medications are withdrawn. A large number of well-designed studies involving more than 700 children have been done over the past 20 years (35,39–50). The overall results have been consistent. Between 60 percent and 75 percent of children with epilepsy who have been seizure-free for more than 2 years (35,39,40,45–49) or 4 years (40–44) on medications remain seizure-free when AEDs are withdrawn. Furthermore, the majority of recurrences occur shortly after medication withdrawal; almost half the relapses occur within 6 months of medication withdrawal, and 60 percent to 80 percent occur within 1 year (35,49,50). These studies are supported by a follow-up study of patients for 15 to 23 years after medication withdrawal (43). Although late recurrences do occur, they are rare (43,49). In a recent randomized study, the increased risk of relapse following AED withdrawal only occurred in the first 2 years after withdrawal. The rate of late recurrences was the same in those who continued to receive AED therapy and those whose AEDs were discontinued (44).

The important question is can one identify risk factors such as etiology, age of onset, type of seizure, EEG features, and specific epilepsy syndromes that allow one to identify subgroups of children with an even better prognosis and subgroups with a much less favorable prognosis for maintaining seizure remission off medication? There is much less agreement in this area. A discussion of the potential risk factors that have been investigated and their possible significance is presented in the following sections.

Etiology and Neurologic Status

In general, children with epilepsy associated with a prior neurologic insult have a lower chance of becoming seizure-free in the first place than do children with cryptogenic epilepsy (17,18,20). In children with remote symptomatic epilepsy who are seizure-free on medication, most studies indicate a higher risk of recurrence after discontinuation of medication than in children with cryptogenic epilepsy (41–43,45,46,49). In a recent meta-analysis of this literature, the relative risk of relapse in those with remote symptomatic seizures was 1.55 (95 percent, CI, 1.21 to 1.98) (50). However, almost half of these children remained seizure-free after withdrawal of medication (41,49,50). Furthermore, even within this group one can identify subgroups with favorable and unfavorable risk factors (49).

Age of Onset and Age at Withdrawal

Age of onset above 12 years of age is associated with a higher risk of relapse following discontinuation of medications (35,38,41,45–47,49,50). In our data, this was the single most important risk factor for recurrence (Relative Risk 4.24, 95 percent, CI 2.54 to 7.08). A meta-analysis (50) also found adolescent-onset seizures to be associated with a higher risk of recurrence than childhood-onset (Relative Risk 1.79, 95 percent, CI 1.46 to 2.19). Whether a very young age of onset (under 2 years) may be a poor prognostic factor is controversial (41). In our data, a young age of onset was associated with a less favorable prognosis only in those with remote symptomatic seizures and was associated with more severe neurologic abnormalities (49). Because most childhood epilepsy is readily controlled with AED therapy, the age at withdrawal of AEDs correlates highly with age of onset; however, the age at AED withdrawal does not appear to be important once age of onset is taken into account. In particular, there is no evidence that discontinuation of AEDs during the pubertal period is associated with a heightened risk of recurrence (35,39,40,49).

Duration of Epilepsy and Number of Seizures

These two variables are closely interrelated. A long duration of epilepsy may increase the risk of recurrence, although the magnitude of the effect is small (35,38,42,43). One study reported that having more than 30 generalized tonic-clonic seizures was associated with a high risk of recurrence after discontinuation of therapy (41). In a community-based practice, most children are easily controlled within a short time after therapy is initiated so that these factors are rarely important.

Seizure Type

Studies on the effect of seizure type on the risk of recurrence after medication withdrawal in children have produced inconsistent results. Children with multiple seizure types have a poorer prognosis (42,43). The data regarding partial seizures are conflicting (35,39–50). At this time it is not clear that any specific seizure type is associated with an increased risk of recurrence following discontinuation of medication.

Electroencephalogram

In several studies (35,36,39–41,49,50), the EEG before discontinuation of medication was one of the most important predictors of relapse in children with cryptogenic epilepsy; however, the specific EEG abnormalities of significance varied across studies. Two other studies found no correlation between the EEG and outcome (42,46). A meta-analysis found that an abnormal

EEG before AED withdrawal was associated with a relative risk of relapse of 1.45 (95% CI 1.18 to 1.79) (50). The preponderance of evidence indicates that an abnormal EEG is associated with an increased recurrence risk in children with cryptogenic-idiopathic epilepsy.

The EEG obtained at the time of initial diagnostic evaluation may also have predictive value. Certain characteristic EEG patterns associated with specific epileptic syndromes, such as benign rolandic epilepsy or juvenile myoclonic epilepsy, provide additional prognostic information (20,29,30,49). Changes in the EEG over time also may have prognostic value (36,39).

Epilepsy Syndromes

Epilepsy syndromes are known to be associated with a differential prognosis for remission (20,29,30). Regrettably, there is little information on the effect of specific epilepsy syndromes on the risk of relapse following AED withdrawal. The majority of studies of AED withdrawal have not provided information by epilepsy syndrome. The results from our investigation (49) are shown in Table 21-2. Overall, patients with both idiopathic and cryptogenic epilepsy syndromes have similar prognosis; however, specific syndromes are associated with a differential risk of relapse. Patients with benign rolandic epilepsy have a particularly favorable prognosis even if their EEGs remain abnormal, whereas all four of our patients with juvenile myoclonic epilepsy relapsed. Clearly, future studies need to focus more on the role of the specific epilepsy syndrome in guiding therapy both in terms of both initiating and discontinuing therapy and the selection of appropriate treatment.

Table 21-2. Epileptic Syndromes in Cohort of Children Being Withdrawn from Antiepileptic Drug Therapy After a Seizure-Free Interval: Cryptogenic and Idiopathic Cases

Epileptic Syndrome	N	Recurred (%)	p value
Idiopathic epilepsy syndromes	79	22 (28)	
Primary generalized epilepsy	61	21 (34)	
Childhood absence	26	5 (19)	
Juvenile absence	9	3 (33)	
Juvenile myoclonic epilepsy	4	4 (100)	0.006
Other primary generalized	22	9 (41)	
Idiopathic partial epilepsy	18	1 (4)	
Benign rolandic epilepsy	14	0 (0)	<0.001
Benign occipital epilepsy	4	1 (25)	
Cryptogenic epilepsy syndromes	86	26 (30)	
Cryptogenic partial epilepsy	50	16 (32)	
Temporal lobe epilepsy	7	3 (43)	
Other partial epilepsy	43	13 (30)	
Unclassified cryptogenic epilepsy	36	10 (28)	
Total Cryptogenic/Idiopathic Cases	165	48 (29)	

*Adapted from Shinnar S, Berg AT, Moshe SL, et al. Discontinuing antiepileptic drugs in children with epilepsy: a prospective study. *Ann Neurol* 1994; 35:534–545.

Type of Medication

The majority of studies have not found that the specific AED used affects recurrence rates. One well-designed randomized study in adults (48) suggests that the risk of recurrence may be higher in those treated with valproate than in those treated with other medications. The significance of this finding remains unclear. It may be related to the ability of valproate to normalize generalized spike-wave abnormalities, thus making the subject appear to be at lower risk than is actually the case. At the present time, there is insufficient evidence to justify basing the decision to continue or withdraw AEDs on the particular AED that the patient is taking.

The serum drug level does not seem to have much impact on recurrence risk. Children who have not had seizures for several years often have "subtherapeutic" levels, and few have toxic levels. Available studies show little or no correlation between drug level before discontinuation and seizure recurrence and outcome (39,41).

Duration of Seizure-Free Interval

The chances of remaining seizure-free after medication withdrawal are similar whether a 2-year (35,39,40,45–49) or 4-year seizure-free interval (35,40–44) is used. One study that evaluated seizure-free intervals of one or more years did find that a longer seizure-free period was associated with a slightly lower recurrence risk (40). Note that among children who are 2 years seizure-free but remain on medication, approximately 3 percent to 5 percent experience another seizure in the third or fourth year of treatment (17). More recent studies that have used a seizure-free interval of 1 year or less have reported higher recurrence risks (35–38). The risk of relapse after a 1-year remission compared with a longer seizure-free interval is also higher in patients who continue on AEDs (17).

Remission Following Relapse

The majority of patients who relapse after medication withdrawal reattain remission after AEDs are restarted, although not necessarily immediately (35,51,52). The prognosis for long-term remission appears to be primarily a function of the underlying epilepsy syndrome. A recent randomized study of medication withdrawal found that the prognosis for seizure control after recurrence in patients with previously well-controlled seizures was no different in those who were withdrawn from AED therapy and relapsed than those who relapsed while continuing to receive AED therapy (51).

RISKS OF NOT TREATING OR DISCONTINUING ANTIEPILEPTIC DRUGS

Seizure recurrence is the major risk associated with not treating the child with one or two seizures or discontinuing AED therapy. Although a seizure is a dramatic and frightening event, the main impact of a brief seizure is psychosocial. There is no convincing evidence that a brief seizure causes brain damage (3,6,53). Serious injury from a brief seizure is a rare event usually related to loss of consciousness and the resultant fall (52). In general, the physical and emotional consequences of a seizure in a child, who usually is in a supervised environment and is not yet driving, are less serious than those in an adult who faces loss of driving privileges and possible adverse effects on his employment (7,49,53–55).

In the past there was concern that delaying treatment would result in a worse long-term prognosis (2,4). This was based on Gower's statement that "the tendency of the disease is toward self-perpetuation; each attack facilitates the occurrence of the next by increasing the instability of the nerve elements" (1). Proponents of this view, most notably Reynolds, have argued that treatment after the first seizure is necessary to prevent the development of "chronic" epilepsy (4,12). Similar concerns have been raised about early discontinuation of AED therapy. Current epidemiologic data and data from controlled clinical trials indicate that this is not the case (3,5,6,19,34,56). Prognosis is primarily a function of the underlying epilepsy syndrome, and although treatment with AEDs does reduce the risk of subsequent seizures, it does not alter the long-term prognosis (34). Several comprehensive reviews of this issue have been published recently (3,6).

In children, even status epilepticus, which is defined as a seizure or a series of seizures lasting more than 30 minutes without regaining consciousness between seizures (21–24,28), is rarely associated with brain damage attributable to the status per se (21–24). In mature animals, generalized convulsive status epilepticus produces biochemical and neuropathologic changes (24). However, although immature animals are more susceptible to the development of status epilepticus with relatively mild insults, they are much less likely to experience brain damage as a result of prolonged seizures than adult animals (24). Adult rats that had experienced status epilepticus as infants do not show a lower seizure threshold or an increased susceptibility to seizures induced by kindling compared with rats who did not experience seizures as pups (57).

Education is the key to empowering the parents and child regardless of which therapeutic option is chosen. Parents must be reassured that the child will not die during a seizure and that keeping the child safe during the seizure is generally the only action that needs to be taken. Parents must be told that most of the child's activities may be continued, although some may children need closer adult supervision. Specific instructions regarding supervision of activities, such as swimming, should be given to the parents. Counseling of this nature often allays the parents' fear and educates them about safety precautions for the child, thereby reducing the chance for injury from seizures whether the child is treated or not. Educational programs are available for school personnel—teachers, nurses, students, and baby-sitters.

The amount of information and the level of content depends in large part on the medical sophistication of the parents and their ability to attend to the information given them at that particular time. The parents' perception of their child's disorder will be an important factor in their later coping and ultimately will affect their perception of quality of life. The practitioner's prejudices regarding treatment options undoubtedly come into play during these discussions, but the different options should be discussed.

Parents usually are interested in information that will help them manage the illness or specific problems; lengthy explanations usually are not helpful. Remember that when giving information to the parents about prognosis you should provide information about how to manage further seizures if they occur. This includes what should be done during a seizure, when to call the physician, and when the child should be taken to the emergency department. Depending on the age of the child, education is necessary for the patient. Children may fear accidents, loss of friends, taking "drugs," and other less well defined outcomes. The practitioner should address these issues with the patient and parents for a comprehensive approach to treatment.

RISKS OF INITIATING OR CONTINUING TREATMENT WITH ANTIEPILEPTIC DRUGS

Antiepileptic drugs are potent medications whose use is associated with a variety of significant side effects (25–27) (see Chapter 25). The adverse effects of the medications must be balanced against the risk of further seizures. The potential adverse effects of AED therapy and of having a seizure are summarized in Table 21-3. Physicians are familiar with idiosyncratic drug effects and the acute toxicities of the drugs. However, subtle behavioral and cognitive effects often are not recognized in children with epilepsy (26), particularly when they have been receiving medications since their preschool years. Only when medication is stopped does it become apparent that the child's performance was impaired by the drug. For teenage girls, a discussion of the risks of treatment must include

Table 21-3. Potential Adverse Consequences of Antiepileptic Drug Therapy and of Seizures

Antiepileptic Drug Therapy	Seizures
Systemic toxicity	Physical injury
Idiosyncratic	Loss of consciousness
Dose-related	Injury from falls
Chronic toxicity	Drowning
Teratogenicity	Status epilepticus
Higher cortical functions	
Cognitive impairment	
Adverse effects on behavior	
Psychosocial	Psychosocial
Need for daily medication	Restrictions on activity
Labelling as chronic illness	Physical
Adverse effect on psychosocial	Social
development	Social stigma of seizure
Economic/temporal	Fear of further seizures
Cost of medications	
Cost/time of physician visits	
Cost/time of laboratory tests	

consideration of the potential teratogenicity of these compounds (54,58,59) (see Chapter 26). Because the major teratogenic effects take place in early gestation and many pregnancies in this group are unplanned, the physician must always consider this issue in advance. For this reason, the author is particularly aggressive in trying to withdraw medications from adolescent females who have been seizure-free for 2 years, even if their other risk factors are not favorable.

A hidden side effect of continued AED therapy is that of being labeled. The person with a single seizure or childhood epilepsy who has not had a seizure in many years and is no longer receiving medications is considered by himself and society to have outgrown his epilepsy. That individual may lead a normal life with few restrictions. In contrast, remaining on chronic medication implies ongoing illness both to the patient and to those around him. Continued use of medication requires ongoing medical care to prescribe and monitor the medication. It also implies certain restrictions in driving licensure and may have an adverse impact on obtaining employment. In addition to the problems associated with having epilepsy, the perception of any chronic illness may adversely affect the normal psychosocial maturation process, particularly in adolescents (60).

A THERAPEUTIC APPROACH

Given the consequences of long-term drug therapy, an attempt should be made to withdraw medications at least once in most children and adolescents with epilepsy who are seizure-free regardless of risk factors. In general, avoid starting medications in the children who has had only one seizure and aggressively pursue withdrawal of medications in children who are seizure-free for 2 or more years. We rarely treat children with a first seizure even if they have risk factors for recurrence. In many cases, treatment may not be necessary even in children with more than one seizure if the seizures are brief and infrequent and the child's underlying syndrome has a favorable prognosis (61).

Whatever the decision, it should be made jointly by the medical care providers and the family after careful discussion that includes not only an assessment of the risks and benefits of treatment but also a review of measures to be taken in the event of a recurrence. Patient and family education is a key factor whether one decides to treat with AEDs or not because both seizures and AEDs are associated with some risks. Even children with good prognostic factors may experience another recurrence. Conversely, children with poor risk factors may nevertheless maintain remission when medications have been discontinued. It is far easier to take these risks while the patient is still in the supervised environment of the home and school. Education assists the family in making an informed decision, helps them to fully participate in the plan of care, and prepares them to deal with psychosocial consequences of the diagnosis. Informed decision making by the physician in consultation with the family maximizes the chances of good long-term outcomes in these children.

The approach presented in this chapter emphasizes that both seizures and available therapies carry some risk and that optimal patient care requires careful balancing of these risks and benefits. Although presented in the context of whether to treat at all, the same approach is useful when seizures persist for deciding whether to add a second drug, try investigational drugs, consider epilepsy surgery for a child who is medically refractory, or offer the ketogenic diet. As more information and newer therapies become available, the risk-benefit ratio may well change. To provide the best care available, the physician must be aware of the available options and individualize them to the needs of the specific patient.

ACKNOWLEDGMENT

Supported in part by grant R01 NS26151 from the National Institute of Neurological Disorders and Stroke, Bethesda, MD, USA.

REFERENCES

1. Gowers WR. *Epilepsy and Other Chronic Convulsive Disorders.* London: J & A Churchill, 1881.

2. Livingston S. *Comprehensive Management of Epilepsy in Infancy, Childhood and Adolescence.* Springfield, Ill: Charles C Thomas, 1972.

3. Berg AT, Shinnar S. Do seizures beget seizures? An assessment of the clinical evidence in humans. *J Clin Neurophysiol* 1997; 14:102–110.

4. Reynolds EH. Do anticonvulsants alter the natural course of epilepsy? Treatment should be started as early as possible. *Br Med J* 1995; 310:176–177.

5. Moshe SL, Shinnar S. Early intervention. In: Engel J Jr, ed. *Surgical Treatment of the Epilepsies.* 2nd ed. New York: Raven Press, 1993:123–132.

6. Shinnar S, Berg AT. Does antiepileptic drug therapy prevent the development of "chronic" epilepsy? *Epilepsia* 1996; 37:701–708.

7. Shinnar S, Berg AT, Moshe SL, et al. The risk of recurrence following a first unprovoked seizure in childhood: A prospective study. *Pediatrics* 1990; 85:1076–1085.

8. Shinnar S, Berg AT, Moshe SL, et al. The risk of seizure recurrence following a first unprovoked afebrile seizure in childhood: an extended follow-up. *Pediatrics* 1996; 98:216–225.

9. Berg A, Shinnar S. The risk of seizure recurrence following a first unprovoked seizure: a quantitative review. *Neurology* 1991; 41:965–972.

10. Hauser WA, Anderson VE, Loewenson RB, McRoberts SM. Seizure recurrence after a first unprovoked seizure. *N Engl J Med* 1982; 307:522–528.

11. Hauser WA, Rich SS, Annegers JF, Anderson VE. Seizure recurrence after a 1st unprovoked seizure: an extended follow-up. *Neurology* 1990; 40:1163–1170.

12. Elwes RDC, Chesterman P, Reynolds EH. Prognosis after a first untreated tonic-clonic seizure. *Lancet* 1985; 2:752–753.

13. Hirtz DG, Ellenberg JH, Nelson KB. The risk of recurrence of nonfebrile seizures in children. *Neurology* 1984; 34:637–641.

14. Camfield PR, Camfield CS, Dooley JM, et al. Epilepsy after a first unprovoked seizure in childhood. *Neurology* 1985; 35:1657–1660.

15. Annegers JF, Shirts SB, Hauser WA, Kurland LT. Risk of recurrence after an initial unprovoked seizure. *Epilepsia* 1986; 27:43–50.

16. First Seizure Trial Group. Randomized clinical trial on the efficacy of antiepileptic drugs in reducing the risk of relapse after a first unprovoked tonic-clonic seizure. *Neurology* 1993; 43:478–483.

17. Annegers JF, Hauser WA, Elveback LR. Remission of seizures and relapse in patients with epilepsy. *Epilepsia* 1979; 20:729–737.

18. Silanpää M, Jalava M, Kaleva O, Shinnar S. Long-term prognosis of seizures with onset in childhood. *N Engl J Med* 1998; 338:1715–1755.

19. Sander JWAS. Some aspects of prognosis in the epilepsies: A review. *Epilepsia* 1993; 34:1007–1016.

20. Berg AT, Hauser WA, Shinnar S. The prognosis of childhood-onset epilepsy. In: Shinnar S, Amir N, Branski D (eds.). *Childhood seizures.* Basel: S Karger, 1995:93–99.

21. Maytal J, Shinnar S, Moshe SL, Alvarez LA. The low morbidity and mortality of status epilepticus in children. *Pediatrics* 1989; 83:323–331.

22. DeLorenzo RJ, Hauser WA, Towne AR et al. A prospective population-based epidemiological study of status epilepticus in Richmond, Virginia. *Neurology* 1996; 46:1029–1035.

23. Dodson WE, DeLorenzo RJ, Pedley TA, et al. The treatment of convulsive status epilepticus: recommendations of the Epilepsy Foundation of America's working group on status epilepticus. *JAMA* 1993; 270:854–859.

24. Shinnar S, Babb TL. Long term sequelae of status epilepticus. In: Engel J Jr, Pedley TA, eds. *Epilepsy: A Comprehensive Text*. Philadelphia: Lippincot-Raven, 1997:755–763.

25. Reynolds EH. Chronic antiepileptic toxicity: A review. *Epilepsia* 1975; 16:319–352.

26. Vining EPG, Mellits ED, Dorsen MM, et al. Psychologic and behavioral effects of antiepileptic drugs in children: a double-blind comparison between phenobarbital and valproic acid. *Pediatrics* 1987; 80:165–174.

27. Committee on Drugs, American Academy of Pediatrics. Behavioral and cognitive effects of anticonvulsant therapy. *Pediatrics* 1995; 96:538–540.

28. Commission on Epidemiology and Prognosis, International League Against Epilepsy. Guidelines for epidemiologic studies on epilepsy. *Epilepsia* 1993; 34:592–596.

29. Commission on Classification and Terminology of the International League Against Epilepsy. Proposal for revised classification of epilepsies and epileptic syndromes. *Epilepsia* 1989; 30:389–399.

30. Roger J, Dravet C, Bureau M, Dreifuss FE, Wolf P. eds. *Epileptic Syndromes in Infancy, Childhood and Adolescence*. 2nd ed. London: John Libbey Eurotext, 1992.

31. Shinnar S, Kang H, Berg AT, et al. EEG abnormalities in children with a first unprovoked seizure. *Epilepsia* 1994; 35:471–476.

32. Shinnar S, Berg AT, Moshe SL. The effect of status epilepticus on the long term outcome of a cohort of children prospectively followed from the time of their first idiopathic unprovoked seizure. *Dev Med Child Neurol* 1995; 37(Suppl 72):116.

33. Camfield P, Camfield C, Dooley J, et al. A randomized study of carbamazepine versus no medication following a first unprovoked seizure in childhood. *Neurology* 1989; 39:851–852.

34. Musicco M, Beghi E, Solari A, Viani F, for the First Seizure Trial Group (FIRST Group). Treatment of first tonic-clonic seizure does not improve the prognosis of epilepsy. *Neurology* 1997; 49:991–998.

35. Berg AT, Shinnar S, Chadwick D. Discontinuing antiepileptic drugs. In: Engel J Jr, Pedley TA, eds. *Epilepsy: A Comprehensive Textbook*. Philadelphia: Lippincott-Raven. 1997; 1275–1284.

36. Braathen G, Melander H. Early discontinuation of treatment in children with uncomplicated epilepsy: a prospective study with a model for prediction of outcome. *Epilepsia* 1997; 38:561–569.

37. Arts WFM. The Dutch study of epilepsy in childhood: early discontinuation. *Epilepsia* 1995; 36(Suppl 3):S29.

38. Dooley J, Gordon K, Camfield P, Camfield C, Smith E. Discontinuation of anticonvulsant therapy in children free of seizures for 1 year: a prospective study. *Neurology* 1996; 46:969–974.

39. Shinnar S, Vining EPG, Mellits ED, et al. Discontinuing antiepileptic medication in children with epilepsy after two years without seizures: a prospective study. *N Engl J Med* 1985; 313:976–980.

40. Todt H. The late prognosis of epilepsy in childhood: results of a prospective followup study. *Epilepsia* 1984; 25:137–144.

41. Emerson R, D'Souza BJ, Vining EP, et al. Stopping medication in children with epilepsy: predictors of outcome. *N Engl J Med* 1981; 304:1125–1129.

42. Holowach J, Thurston DL, O'Leary J. Prognosis in childhood epilepsy: followup study of 148 cases in which therapy had been suspended after prolonged anticonvulsant control. *N Engl J Med* 1972; 286:169–174.

43. Holowach-Thurston JH, Thurston DL, Hixon BB, et al. Prognosis in childhood epilepsy: additional followup of 148 children 15 to 23 years after withdrawal of anticonvulsant therapy. *N Engl J Med* 1982; 306:831–836.

44. Medical Research Council Antiepileptic Drug Withdrawal Study Group. Randomised study of antiepileptic drug withdrawal in patients with remission. *Lancet* 1991; 337:1175–1180.

45. Arts WFM, Visser LH, Loonen MCB, et al. Follow-up of 146 children with epilepsy after withdrawal of antiepileptic therapy. *Epilepsia* 1988; 29:244–250.

46. Bouma PAD, Peters ACB, Arts RJHM, et al. Discontinuation of antiepileptic therapy: a prospective trial in children. *J Neurol Neurosurg Psychiatry* 1987; 50:1579–1583.

47. Juul Jensen P. Frequency of recurrence after discontinuance of anticonvulsant therapy in patients with epileptic seizures: a new followup study after 5 years. *Epilepsia* 1968; 9:11–16.

48. Callaghan N, Garrett A, Goggin T. Withdrawal of anticonvulsant drugs in patients free of seizures for two years. *N Engl J Med* 1988; 318:942–946.

49. Shinnar S, Berg AT, Moshe SL, et al. Discontinuing antiepileptic drugs in children with epilepsy: a prospective study. *Ann Neurol* 1994; 35:534–545.

50. Berg AT, Shinnar S. Relapse following discontinuation of antiepileptic drugs: a meta-analysis. *Neurology* 1994; 44:601–608.

51. Chadwick D, Taylor J, Johnson T. Outcomes after seizure recurrence in people with well-controlled epilepsy and the factors that influence it. The MRC Antiepileptic Drug Withdrawal Group. *Epilepsia* 1996; 37:1043–1050.

52. Shinnar S, Berg AT, Moshe SL, et al. What happens to children with epilepsy who experience a seizure recurrence after withdrawal of antiepileptic drugs. *Ann Neurol* 1996; 40:301–302.

53. Freeman JM, Tibbles J, Camfield C, Camfield P. Benign epilepsy of childhood: a speculation and its ramifications. *Pediatrics* 1987; 79:864–868.

54. Shinnar S. Seizures. In: Friedman SB, Fisher MM, Schonberg SK, Alderman EM, eds. *Comprehensive Adolescent*

Health Care. 2nd ed. St. Louis: Quality Medical Publishing, 1997:501–510

55. Jacoby A, Baker G, Chadwick D, Johnson A. The impact of counseling with a practical statistical model on a patient's decision making about treatment with epilepsy: findings from a pilot study. *Epilepsy Res* 1993; 16:207–214.

56. van Donselaar CA, Brouwer OF, Geerts AT, et al. Clinical course of untreated tonic-clonic seizures in childhood: prospective, hospital based study. *Br Med J* 1997; 314:401–404.

57. Okada R, Moshe SL, Albala BJ. Infantile status epilepticus and future seizure susceptibility in the rat. *Dev Brain Res* 1984; 15:177–183.

58. Yerby MS. Teratogenic effects of antiepileptic drugs: what do we advise patients. *Epilepsia* 1997; 38:957–958.

59. Commission on Genetics, Pregnancy and the Child, International League Against Epilepsy. Guidelines for the care of women of childbearing age with epilepsy. *Epilepsia* 1993; 34:588–589.

60. Hoare P. Does illness foster dependency: a study of epileptic and diabetic children. *Dev Med Child Neurol* 1984; 26:20–24.

61. Shinnar S, Berg AT, O'Dell C, et al. Predictors of multiple seizures in a cohort of children prospectively followed from the time of their first unprovoked seizure. *Ann Neurol* 2000; 48:140–147.

CHAPTER 22

Comparative Anticonvulsant Profiles and Proposed Mechanisms of Action of the Established and Newer Antiepileptic Drugs

H. Steve White, Ph.D.

For the vast majority of people who develop epilepsy, initial therapy consists of pharmacologic treatment with one or more of the established anticonvulsant drugs, These medications include phenytoin (PHT), carbamazepine (CBZ), valproate (VPA), barbiturates such as phenobarbital (PB), certain benzodiazepines (BZDs), and ethosuximide (ESM). For some patients, complete seizure control with this group of "established" antiepileptic drugs (AEDs) may never be achieved at doses that are devoid of various types and severities of AED-related adverse effects.

The 1990s have been marked by a number of advances in AED development. Since 1993 several novel AEDs have been commercialized in one or more countries and are in the process of evaluation for worldwide registration. This is an exciting era for practitioners and their patients who have intractable seizure disorders. For the physician, the new AEDs provide novel therapeutic options for their patients. For the patient with intractable epilepsy, the new drugs represent renewed hope for complete seizure control and lessening of their AED-associated side-effect profile. This chapter addresses the preclinical animal models that led to the initial identification of the new AEDs felbamate (FBM), lamotrigine (LTG), gabapentin (GBP), topiramate (TPM), tiagabine (TGB), vigabatrin (VGB), oxcarbazepine (OCBZ), and zonisamide (ZNS) and the proposed molecular mechanisms of action of the new and the established AEDs.

STRATEGIES FOR ANTIEPILEPTIC DRUG DISCOVERY

The process by which new AEDs are discovered has evolved in the 60 years since PHT was identified by Putnam and Merritt (1). In recent years the strategies employed in the search for new AEDs have been based largely on three different approaches: (1) random drug screening and efficacy-based AED discovery; (2) rational drug design wherein structural modifications of an active pharmacophore are synthesized and tested; and (3) mechanistic-based AED development. All three approaches have led to the identification of clinically effective drugs. Despite this progress, there continues to be a significant need for more effective and less toxic AEDs. Regardless of the process by which a chemical entity is brought forth from the medicinal chemistry laboratory, it must first demonstrate some degree of efficacy in an animal model to become a candidate for clinical trials.

IN VIVO TESTING

No single laboratory test, in itself, establishes the presence or absence of anticonvulsant activity or fully predicts the clinical utility of an investigational antiepileptic drug. Therefore, the true test of a drug's efficacy must always await the results of clinical trials. There are many available animal seizure models that have been fully characterized and possess appropriate properties to qualify as a predictive seizure model. The maximal electroshock (MES) test, the subcutaneous pentylenetetrazol (sc PTZ) test, and the electrical kindling model are the three *in vivo* systems that have been most commonly employed in the search for new AEDs (2). Today newer in vivo models are being introduced that incorporate known genetic defects that more closely resemble the human condition.

Table 22-1. Correlation Between Clinical Utility and Efficacy in Experimental Animal Models of the Established and Newer AEDs

Seizure Type	Experimental Model			
	MES (Tonic Extension)	sc PTZ (Clonic Seizures)	Spike-Wave Discharges[b]	Electrical Kindling (Focal Seizures)
Tonic and/or clonic generalized seizures	CBZ, PHT, VPA, PB [FBM, GBP, LTG, OCBZ, TPM, ZNS]			
Myoclonic/generalized absence seizures		ESM, VPA, PB[a] BZD [FBM, GBP, TGB]		
Generalized absence seizures			ESM, VPA, BZD [LTG, TPM]	
Partial seizures				CBZ, PHT, VPA, PB, BZD [FBM, GBP, LTG, OCBZ, TPM, TGB, VGB, ZNS]

[a]PB blocks clonic seizures induced by sc PTZ but is inactive against generalized absence seizures.
[b]Data summarized from GBL, GAERS, and *lh/lh* spike-wave models (references 5–8)
[ ] Newer AEDs.

To gain a full appreciation for a new AED's overall spectrum of activity (i.e., narrow vs. broad-spectrum), all investigational AEDs should be screened in a variety of seizure and epilepsy models.

CORRELATION OF ANIMAL ANTICONVULSANT PROFILE AND CLINICAL UTILITY

The MES test and the kindling model are two highly predictive models that are useful in the characterization of a drug's potential utility against generalized tonic-clonic and partial seizures, respectively (Table 22-1). For a number of years, positive results obtained in the sc PTZ test were considered suggestive of a drug's potential utility against generalized absence seizures. This interpretation was based largely on the observation that drugs that were active in the clinic (i.e., ETS, trimethadione, VPA, the BZDs, and more recently FBM) were able to block clonic seizures induced by sc PTZ, whereas drugs such as PHT and CBZ were ineffective both experimentally and clinically. However, as summarized in Table 22-1, the PTZ test would also suggest that the barbiturates and TGB should also be effective against generalized absence. For the barbiturates (and possibly TGB), this is the direct opposite of what has been reported clinically. For example, phenobarbital worsens human spike-wave discharges (3). On the other hand, PB is useful for the management of myoclonic seizures. In this respect, the sc PTZ test as conducted by most laboratories may have greater utility in the identification of drugs with activity against myoclonic seizures (4).

In recent years, three other animal models have emerged that are reasonably more predictive than the sc PTZ for efficacy against generalized absence seizures. These include spike-wave seizures induced by the chemoconvulsant γ-butyrolacetone (5), the genetic absence epileptic rat of Strasbourg (GAERS) (6), and most recently the lethargic (*lh/lh*) mutant mouse (7,8). Of these three, the *lh/lh* mouse displays spontaneous spike-wave discharges that are blocked by drugs that have been found clinically effective in reducing spike-wave activity (e.g., the BZDs, ETS, VPA, and LTG). Furthermore, all three models accurately predict the potentiation of spike-wave seizures by drugs that elevate GABA concentrations (e.g., VGB and TGB), drugs that directly activate the $GABA_B$ receptor, and the barbiturates. For these reasons, any drug being evaluated for the potential use against absence seizures should be tested in one or more of these three models.

The remainder of this chapter focuses primarily on a description of the anticonvulsant profile and comparative mechanisms of action between the established AEDs and the newer AEDs. Where appropriate, the reader is referred to more comprehensive reviews and primary citations supporting the proposed mechanisms of action.

MECHANISM OF ACTION: GENERAL CONSIDERATIONS

The mechanisms of action of currently marketed anticonvulsant drugs are not fully understood. Ultimately, there are numerous molecular mechanisms

Table 22-2. Comparative Mechanistic Profile Between the Established and New AEDs

AED	Limit SRF[a]/Na$^+$ Channel Block	Enhance GABA-Mediated Neurotransmission	Reduce VSCC	Reduce Glutamate-Mediated Excitation
Established				
Phenytoin	+			
CBZ	+			
VPA	+	+(?)	+(?)	
BZDs		+		
PB		+		
ESM			+	
Newer				
FBM	+	+	+	+
GBP	+[b]	+[c]	+[f]	
LTG	+		+	
OCBZ	+		+	
TPM	+	+	+	+
ZNS	+	+	+	
VGB		+[d]		
TGB		+[e]		

[a]Sustained repetitive firing.
[b]Mechanism not clearly established; binds to unique site; requires prolonged exposure.
[c]Increases brain GABA levels in brains of epileptic patients.
[d]Inhibits GABA metabolism via GABA-T.
[e]Blocks neuronal and glial uptake of synaptically released GABA.
[f]Binds to the $\alpha_2\delta$ auxiliary subunit of voltage-sensitive Ca^{2+} channels.

through which drugs can alter neuronal excitability and thereby limit or control seizure activity. However, three primary mechanisms appear to be targeted by most of the established anticonvulsants (9) (Table 22-2). The mechanisms include the ability to (1) block sustained high-frequency firing through an effect on voltage-sensitive sodium channels that disrupts burst firing, (2) enhance GABA-mediated neurotransmission that elevates seizure threshold, and (3) reduce voltage-dependent low-threshold (T-type) calcium currents in thalamocortical neurons that interrupts the thalamic oscillatory firing patterns associated with absence seizures. Likewise, drugs that reduce glutamatergic-mediated excitation can be expected to reduce burst firing elicited by synaptic stimulation. Although not a target of standard AEDs, this fourth mechanism does appear to be targeted by some of the new AEDs, including FBM and TPM and the investigational remacemide. Many of the older established and newer antiepileptic drugs have been observed to exert a number of different pharmacologic actions that could account for their anticonvulsant action. In those cases in which multiple actions have been defined, it is highly likely that the separate mechanisms offer some degree of synergy.

As shown in Table 22-3, inhibition of voltage-sensitive Na$^+$ and Ca^{2+} channels, augmentation of GABA-mediated inhibition, and inhibition of glutamate-mediated excitatory neurotransmission has both synaptic and nonsynaptic consequences that, hopefully, when translated to an in vivo effect contributes to a drug's anticonvulsant action. Unfortunately, the ability of an AED to modulate the function of any one of these neuronal processes can have profound consequences not only on abnormal firing of epileptic neurons but also on normal neuronal communication. As a result, for most of the AEDs the same action(s) that decrease seizure frequency are likely to contribute to their CNS-related side-effect profile. Some of the drugs display properties that lead to a greater separation between effective and toxic effects. For example, it is widely accepted that to be a therapeutically useful Na$^+$ channel blocker, drugs should possess both voltage- and use-(frequency) dependent actions. These properties confer a certain level of selectivity toward those epileptic neurons that display a paroxysmal depolarization shift and high-frequency sustained repetitive firing (i.e., epileptic neurons within a seizure focus). Thus, at therapeutic concentrations voltage- and use-dependent Na$^+$ channel blockers would be less likely to affect normal neuronal function than a Na$^+$ channel blocker that lacks these properties. One still needs to reconcile the cognitive impairment that has come to be associated with the voltage- and use-dependent Na$^+$ channel blockers phenytoin

Table 22-3. Functional Consequences of Proposed Mechanism of Action of Established and Newer AEDs

Molecular Mechanism of Action	AED	Consequences of Action
Na$^+$ channel blockers	PHT, CBZ, LTG, FBM, OCBZ, TPM, VPA	1. Block action potential propagation 2. Stabilize neuronal membranes 3. Decrease neurotransmitter release 4. Decrease focal firing 5. Decrease seizure spread
Ca^{2+} channel blockers	ESM, VPA, GBP, LTG	1. Decrease neurotransmitter release (N & P types) 2. Decrease slow-depolarization (T-type) 3. Decrease spike-wave discharges
GABA$_A$ receptor allosteric modulators	BZDs, PB, FBM, TPM	1. Increase membrane hyperpolarization 2. Elevate seizure threshold 3. Attenuate (BZDs) spike-wave discharges 4. Aggravate (barbiturates) spike-wave discharges 5. Decrease focal firing
GABA-uptake inhibitors/ GABA-transaminase inhibitors	TGB, VGB	1. Increase synaptic GABA levels 2. Increase membrane hyperpolarization 3. Decrease focal firing 4. Aggravate spike-wave discharges
NMDA-receptor antagonists	FBM	1. Decrease slow excitatory neurotransmission 2. Decrease excitatory amino acid neutrotoxicity 3. Delay epileptogenesis
AMPA/kainate-receptor antagonists	PB, TPM	1. Decrease fast excitatory neurotransmission 2. Attenuate focal firing

and carbamazepine. This can be done in part by acknowledging the fact that these drugs can, at higher concentrations, attenuate Na$^+$ currents at resting membrane potentials and thereby modify normal neuronal communication. Furthermore, inhibiting neuronal voltage-sensitive Na$^+$ channels can produce a subsequent inhibition of depolarization-dependent neurotransmitter release. Given the critical role that the excitatory neurotransmitter glutamate plays in fast excitatory neurotransmission, slight modification of glutamate release in the absence of abnormal neuronal firing may contribute to the cognitive impairment observed in some patients taking these drugs. In this case, drugs that display greater voltage- and use-dependence would necessarily offer certain potential advantages over less selective Na$^+$ channel blockers.

CORRELATION BETWEEN ANTICONVULSANT PROFILE AND MECHANISM OF ACTION

Does a drug's anticonvulsant profile suggest anything about its potential mechanism of action? The short answer to this question is probably not. However, certain trends have emerged over the years that are worthy

of mention. First, activity against MES-induced tonic extension has been suggested to identify drugs that are effective in preventing seizure spread, whereas activity against PTZ-induced clonic seizures is suggestive of a drug's ability to elevate seizure threshold (10). Another common theme among drugs that prevent MES-induced seizures is that a large fraction of the marketed AEDs have been demonstrated to inhibit sustained repetitive firing of neurons through an action at the voltage-sensitive Na$^+$ channel (11). Besides the Na$^+$ channel blockers, two other classes of drugs that are very effective against MES-induced seizures are the N-methyl-D-aspartate (NMDA) and non-NMDA glutamate receptor antagonists. For the NMDA antagonists, this would include both competitive (e.g., CPP, CPPene, and CGS 19755) and noncompetitive (e.g., MK-801) antagonists, glycine-site antagonists (e.g., ACEA 1021 and FBM), and polyamine-site antagonists such as eliprodil and ifenprodil. Drugs active at the non-NMDA receptor and effective against MES-induced tonic extension include topiramate and the noncompetitive antagonist NBQX.

Na$^+$ channel blockers, nonselective NMDA, and non-NMDA antagonists are for the most part inactive against clonic seizures induced by PTZ. Conversely, drugs that enhance GABA-mediated inhibition (e.g., allosteric modulators, uptake inhibitors, and GABA-transaminase inhibitors) are active against PTZ-induced clonus and inactive against MES-induced seizures at nontoxic doses. Likewise, drugs that selectively block T-type voltage-sensitive Ca^{2+} channels (e.g., ESM and trimethadione) are active against PTZ-induced clonus but not MES-induced tonic extension.

Whereas the MES and sc PTZ tests identify a certain mechanistic class of AEDs, the kindled rat model appears to be less discriminating. For example, in the kindled rat, Na^+ channel blockers, $GABA_A$ receptor modulators and non-NMDA glutamate receptor antagonists (e.g., NBQX, etc.) display activity, whereas the NMDA-receptor antagonists and T-type Ca^{2+} channel antagonists do not. The aforementioned correlations between anticonvulsant activity and mechanism of action are based purely on our knowledge of the currently available AEDs and experimental compounds that display highly selective mechanisms of action. As new drugs with other well-characterized mechanisms of action become available for testing, it will be interesting to see whether other classes of drugs [e.g., subunit selective NMDA, AMPA (α-amino-2,3-dihydro-5-methyl-3-oxo-4-isoxazolepropanoic acid], and kainate antagonists; K^+ channel antagonists; other selective Ca^{2+} channel antagonists: N, P, and Q type; selective adenosine agonists, etc.) fall into a rational classification scheme. Finally, given that a number of the currently available AEDs are active in a variety of experimental models, they may be likely to possess multiple mechanisms of action and a broader clinical profile than drugs with a narrow anticonvulsant profile. As is discussed subsequently, this certainly appears to be the case for VPA, FBM, and TPM.

The value of such an oversimplified discussion lies not in trying to assess the mechanism of action of a drug based on its anticonvulsant profile but in providing a logical rationale for assessing efficacy of an investigational AED emerging from a mechanistically driven drug discovery program. Therefore, based on the available data with reasonably selective drugs, one would not attempt to demonstrate efficacy with a Na^+ channel blocker or NMDA antagonist using the PTZ test, nor would one initially evaluate a T-type Ca^{2+} channel blocker or GABA-uptake blocker against MES seizures. It could be argued that all drugs should be screened initially in the kindled rat, given the broad spectrum of drugs that are active in this model. However, because the kindled rat is an extremely labor-intensive model, it would not necessarily be amenable to high-volume screening. One model not discussed thus far that is often employed as a broad-spectrum screen is the audiogenic

mouse model (e.g., the DBA/2J and the Frings genetically susceptible mouse). Given that the audiogenic mouse model is nondiscriminatory with respect to clinical classes of AEDs, it serves as a useful model for "proof of principle" screening (12). Once an active molecule has been identified, its clinical potential can be further established using more syndrome-specific models.

The remainder of this chapter focuses on the most widely accepted mechanism(s) that have been observed at therapeutically relevant concentrations of the established and newer AEDs. As alluded to previously, this is not to imply that a minor, less-established action does not contribute to a drug's anticonvulsant profile. The reader is referred to reviews by Rogawski and Porter (13) , Macdonald and Meldrum (14) , Meldrum (15), and White (11) for more comprehensive discussions of these effects.

ESTABLISHED AEDS

Phenytoin and Carbamazepine

The anticonvulsant profiles of PHT and CBZ observed in animal seizure models correlate well with their clinical efficacy in generalized tonic-clonic and complex partial seizures (Table 22-1). Therefore, both drugs are effective against tonic extension seizures induced by a number of different stimuli including MES and various chemoconvulsants (16,17), and both AEDs are effective against fully expressed kindled seizures (13). Unlike ESM, both drugs are ineffective against clonic seizures induced by PTZ. Studies conducted to date provide compelling evidence that therapeutic concentrations of PHT and CBZ prevent sustained repetitive firing resulting from extended depolarization (Table 22-2). In addition, both drugs prevent posttetanic potentiation (PTP), a process whereby high-frequency stimulation produces a transiently enhanced responsiveness to subsequent stimulation. The ability of PHT and CBZ to effect a block against PTP may explain in part their ability to limit seizure spread.

The voltage-sensitive Na^+ channel is thought to underlie the ability of neurons to fire repetitively. As such, anticonvulsants that inhibit sustained repetitive firing are likely to exert an effect on voltage-sensitive Na^+ channels. PHT and CBZ have been found to exert an inhibitory effect on voltage-gated Na^+ channels (18–20) that is both use- and voltage-dependent (Table 22-2). These two properties account for the unique ability of PHT, CBZ, and other voltage-dependent Na^+ channel blockers to limit high-frequency firing characteristic of epileptic discharges without significantly altering normal patterns of neuronal firing.

Phenytoin and CBZ also produce a shift in the steady-state inactivation curve in mammalian myelinated nerve fibers to more negative voltages (21), thereby effectively reducing the degree of depolarization required to inactivate Na^+ channels. In addition, both drugs delayed the rate of Na^+ channel recovery from inactivation. Whether slight differences between PHT and CBZ in time dependence of the frequency-dependent block account for differences in anticonvulsant efficacy between these drugs has yet to be established. Thus, by stabilizing the Na^+ channel in its inactive form and slowing its rate of recovery from inactivation, both drugs can prevent sustained repetitive firing evoked by prolonged depolarization such as that found in an epileptic focus.

Similarly, voltage-, frequency-, and time-dependent inactivation of Na^+ channels by PHT has also been confirmed in isolated rat hippocampal neurons and *Xenopus* oocytes injected with human brain mRNA (22,23). All of these studies provide strong experimental evidence supporting an interaction of PHT and CBZ with the voltage-dependent Na^+ channel.

Ethosuximide

Unlike PHT and CBZ, ESM is effective against clonic seizures induced by subcutaneously administered PTZ (Table 22-1). It is also active against spike-wave seizures induced by the chemoconvulsant γ-hydroxybutyrate (5) and against spontaneous spike-wave discharges in the *lh/lh* mouse model of absence. ESM is ineffective against tonic extension seizures induced by MES and focal seizures in the kindled rat. In this respect, the in vivo profile of ESM is consistent with its clinical efficacy against generalized absence seizures and lack of efficacy in generalized tonic-clonic or partial seizures (Table 22-1).

The mechanism of ESM was not elucidated until 1989, when it was shown to reduce low-threshold T-type Ca^{2+} currents in thalamic neurons isolated from rats and guinea pigs (25). Reduction of the T-type current was voltage-dependent and was observed at clinically relevant ESM concentrations, suggesting that this mechanism may be the basis for the efficacy of ESM in controlling absence seizures (Table 22-2). This effect of ESM, which is produced at clinically relevant concentrations, is thought to represent the primary mechanism by which it controls absence epilepsy. Activation of T-channels in thalamic relay neurons generates low-threshold Ca^{2+} spikes that are thought to contribute to the abnormal thalamocortical rhythmicity that underlies the 3-Hz spike-and-wave EEG discharge of absence epilepsy. By preventing Ca^{2+}-dependent depolarization of thalamocortical neurons, ESM and dimethadione, the active metabolite of the antiabsence drug trimethadione (26), are thought to block the synchronized firing associated with spike-wave discharges.

Valproic Acid

Of the standard AEDs, VPA appears to have the broadest preclinical and clinical profile (Table 22-1). It is active in a variety of animal seizure models, including electrical seizures in the MES test, chemically induced clonic seizures in the sc PTZ test, electrically kindled seizures, GBL-induced spike-wave, and spontaneous spike-wave discharges in the *lh/lh* mouse (5,7,24). Clinically, VPA is useful in the management of both partial and generalized seizures.

Based on VPA's rather broad preclinical and clinical anticonvulsant profile, it might be anticipated that VPA would possess more than one mechanism of action. Indeed, a number of studies suggest that VPA possesses at least three different mechanisms of action. First, in vitro studies with VPA support an action at the voltage-sensitive Na^+ channel (11). For example, VPA has been found to inhibit Na^+ currents in isolated *Xenopus leavis* myelinated nerves (27) and in neocortical neurons in vitro (28). Furthermore, in rat hippocampal neurons VPA decreased peak Na^+ currents in a voltage-dependent manner and produced a 10-mV leftward shift in the Na^+ inactivation curve (29). Such an action may contribute to its ability to prevent MES-induced tonic extension in animals and generalized tonic-clonic and partial seizures in humans. Second, VPA, like ESM, has been shown to reduce T-type Ca^{2+} currents in primary afferent neurons (30). This effect, albeit modest and observed at high VPA concentrations, may contribute to VPA's clinical efficacy in absence seizures. Third, VPA-mediated elevations of whole brain GABA levels and potentiation of GABA responses are also found at relatively high drug concentrations (13). This effect, coupled with its effect at the voltage-sensitive Na^+ channel, may also contribute to its efficacy against kindled seizures in rats and human partial seizures.

Benzodiazepines and Barbiturates

In animal seizure models, the BZDs and barbiturates are effective at low doses against sc PTZ-induced clonic seizures and in the kindled rat model of partial seizures. The barbiturates at low doses and BZDs at higher doses are also active against MES-induced tonic extension. One important distinction between these two classes of compounds lies in their efficacy against spike-wave seizures in the GBL and *lh/lh* models of absence. In both models, the BZDs are effective in reducing spike-wave discharges, whereas the barbiturates actually worsen spike-wave discharges (5.7).

BZDs and barbiturates limit high-frequency repetitive firing of action potentials only at high drug concentrations. Once released from GABAergic nerve terminals, the inhibitory neurotransmitter GABA binds to both $GABA_A$ and $GABA_B$ receptors. The $GABA_A$ receptor complex is a multimeric macromolecular protein that forms a chloride-selective ion pore. Thus far, multiple binding sites for GABA, anticonvulsant BZDs, barbiturates, neurosteroids, convulsant β-carbolines, and the chemoconvulsant picrotoxin have been identified (31). The $GABA_B$ receptor is coupled via a GTP binding protein to calcium or potassium channels but does not form an ion pore and does not appear to contribute to the anticonvulsant action of either BZDs or barbiturates. The principle anticonvulsant action of the BZDs and barbiturates is thought to be related to their ability to enhance inhibitory neurotransmission by allosterically modulating the $GABA_A$ receptor complex.

GABA receptor current can be enhanced by increasing channel conductance, open and burst frequency, and/or open and burst duration. Studies indicate that the barbiturates act mainly by increasing the mean channel open duration without affecting channel conductances or opening frequency, whereas the binding of a BZD to its allosterically coupled $GABA_A$ binding site increases opening frequency without affecting open or burst duration (32–35). Results from several reconstitution experiments conducted in a variety of laboratories wherein specific GABA receptor subunits were transiently expressed in either *Xenopus* oocytes, Chinese hamster ovary (CHO) cells, or human embryonic kidney cells have suggested a molecular basis for the differential regulation of GABA receptor current by these two classes of drugs. The results from these studies have suggested that the allosteric regulatory site conferring barbiturate sensitivity appears to be contained in the α and β subunits (36,37). Thus, while GABA receptors formed from $\alpha_1\beta_1$ subunits are barbiturate-sensitive, they are BZD-insensitive (36,38). BZD sensitivity is restored when the γ_2 subunit is coexpressed with α_1 and β_1 subunits. Transient coexpression of the γ_2, α_1, and β_1 subunits in human embryonic kidney cells results in fully functional GABA receptors that are sensitive to the BZDs, barbiturates, β-carbolines, and picrotoxin. These effects at the $GABA_A$ synapse are likely to account for the efficacy of the BZDs and barbiturates against kindled seizures in rats and partial seizures in humans.

One important difference between these two classes of GABA modulators is that the barbiturates can directly activate a Cl^- current in the absence of GABA, whereas the BZDs cannot. This difference, coupled with possible anatomic differences in subunit expression, may explain in part why BZDs attenuate spike-wave seizures in both rodents and humans, whereas the barbiturates actually exacerbate spike-wave discharges. For example, clonazepam

and diazepam selectively augment $GABA_A$-mediated inhibition in neurons of the nucleus reticularis thalami (NRT) but not thalamic neurons. Because the inhibitory synapses in the NRT are primarily reciprocal inhibitory circuits, augmentation of inhibition by the BZDs results in decreased output of NRT onto the thalamus. By decreasing the "pacemaker" activity of the thalamic reticular neurons impinging onto the thalamus, the BZDs selectively and effectively prevent spike-wave discharges. In contrast, barbiturates, by increasing the inhibitory drive within the thalamus, enhance the deinactivation of T-currents, which results in a stronger low-threshold burst and increased thalamocortical rhythms. In contrast to the barbiturates, the BZDs do not augment inhibition within the thalamus and thus do not display the same proconvulsant action.

NEWER AEDS

In some circumstances, the mechanisms of action of the newer AEDs overlap with those defined previously for the established AEDs; however, some of the newer compounds display a unique mechanistic profile relative to the older drugs. AED development has increasingly produced novel molecules that enhance inhibitory neurotransmission by acting on GABA receptors, GABA transporters, and GABA metabolism or reduce excitatory neurotransmission mediated by glutamate.

Felbamate

Felbamate (2-phenyl-1,3-propanediol dicarbamate) received FDA approval by the U.S. Food and Drug Administration in mid-1993 and was the first new AED approved in the United States since 1978. Results from preclinical studies conducted by the NINDS Anticonvulsant Drug Development Program demonstrated that FBM possessed a broad anticonvulsant profile in animal seizure models (40,41) (Table 22-1). It is effective against tonic extension seizures induced by MES and the glutamate agonists NMDA and quisqualic acid. Like VPA, FBM is also active against clonic seizures induced by a number of chemoconvulsants. In syndrome-specific animal models of partial seizures, FBM has been found to reduce the seizure severity in corneal kindled rats and PTZ-kindled rats and to raise the seizure threshold in amygdala-kindled rats (42,43). In addition to its anticonvulsant properties, FBM has been demonstrated to possess neuroprotectant properties both in vitro and in vivo (44–47). Consistent with FBM's broad preclinical profile is its rather broad clinical spectrum. Upon entry into the U.S. market, FBM was approved for treatment of partial seizures, primary and secondary generalized tonic-clonic seizures, and Lennox-Gastaut syndrome.

Felbamate also possesses a broad mechanistic profile that provides a basis for understanding its broad preclinical and clinical anticonvulsant profile, as well as its neuroprotectant action (11). FBM reduces sustained repetitive firing in mouse spinal cord neurons in a concentration-dependent manner. This action suggests an interaction with voltage-dependent Na$^+$ channels, an effect that was confirmed in rat striatal neurons (48) (Table 22-2). At low concentrations, FBM also appears to inhibit dihydropyridine-sensitive high-threshold voltage-sensitive Ca^{2+} currents (49), an effect that is consistent with decreased excitability. One mechanism that appears to be unique to FBM is related to its ability to modulate glutamate receptor function through an action at the strychnine-insensitive glycine site of the NMDA receptor. FBM has been shown to displace a competitive antagonist at the strychnine-insensitive glycine binding site of the NMDA receptor in rat brain membranes (50) and postmortem human brains (51). Furthermore, FBM exerts a neuroprotective effect in the rat hippocampal slice that is reversed by glycine (52). Likewise, its anticonvulsant effect is reversed by strychnine-insensitive glycine receptor agonists (53–55). The ability of FBM to block NMDA-evoked currents is unique among both the standard AEDs and the newer ones. Despite its interaction with this receptor complex, FBM does not appear to produce either the behavioral or pathologic impairment of the CNS associated with either competitive or noncompetitive NMDA antagonists (42).

At substantially higher concentrations, FBM has also been reported to enhance GABA-evoked chloride currents and to inhibit NMDA-evoked currents (56). The mechanism by which FBM enhances GABA-evoked currents is not known. For example, FBM in concentrations up to 1 mM does not appear to affect ligand binding to the GABA, BZD, or picrotoxin binding sites on the GABA$_A$ receptor ionophore, nor does it enhance GABA-stimulated ^{36}Cl$^-$ flux into cultured mouse spinal cord neurons (57).

Felbamate remains a mechanistically interesting AED with an apparently broad anticonvulsant profile. However, its clinical utility has been markedly limited by the serious hematologic and hepatic toxicity reported after its commercialization in the United States (58). A thorough understanding of the mechanisms underlying these idiosyncratic adverse effects and the ability to identify patients at risk will likely lead to an increased use of this highly effective drug in therapy-resistant patients.

Gabapentin

The second member of the newer generation AEDs to be marketed in the United States is GBP. GBP, 1-(aminomethyl)cyclohexaneacetic acid, was originally designed and synthesized as a drug to enhance GABA-mediated inhibition by mimicking the steric conformation of the endogenous neurotransmitter GABA (59).

In animal seizure models, GBP is active in a number of anticonvulsant tests (8,60–62). It reduces electrically and chemically induced tonic extension seizures, as well as clonic seizures induced by sc PTZ (Table 22-1), and blocks sound-induced seizures in DBA mice but not absence-like spike-wave seizures. GBP is also effective against fully kindled seizures in the kindled rat. These findings support its clinical efficacy against human partial seizures and secondarily generalized seizures.

Although the chemical structure and steric conformation of GBP were originally designed to enhance GABA-mediated inhibition, GABA mimetic activity was surprisingly absent in early studies. Despite demonstrated efficacy in both animal and human studies and numerous in vitro studies that have described several potential mechanisms of action, the precise mode of action of GBP remains unknown.

Findings from in vitro studies suggest that GBP can increase the concentration of GABA in both the glial and neuronal the compartments (63). More recently, GBP has been shown to increase in vivo occipital lobe GABA levels in patients with epilepsy (64) (Table 22-2). GBP may increase brain GABA turnover by interacting with a number of different metabolic processes. It has been demonstrated to enhance glutamate dehydrogenase and glutamic acid decarboxylase and inhibit branched-chain amino acid aminotransferase and GABA aminotransferase. Although any one of these effects could singly or in concert with each other contribute to the anticonvulsant action of GBP, it is not clear at this point which effects are important (60,63). After prolonged administration, a voltage- and frequency-dependent limitation of Na$^+$-dependent sustained action potential firing in mouse cortical neurons was observed at clinically relevant concentrations of GBP (65). The ability of GBP to limit sodium-dependent sustained action potential firing in cultured mouse spinal cord neurons was voltage- and frequency-dependent. The precise mechanism of this effect is not known; however, it is unlikely that GBP inhibits sodium currents in a manner similar to that of established sodium channel blockers PHT and CBZ. The delayed effect of GBP against sustained repetitive firing is consistent with the substantial time lag between the appearance of peak plasma and brain concentrations and GBP's time to peak anticonvulsant effect observed following intravenous administration (66). This delay in anticonvulsant effect suggests that prolonged synaptic and/or cytosolic exposure to GBP is important and supports an indirect mechanism of action for GBP.

Gabapentin has also been reported to bind to a novel site in rat brain that is not affected by any of the standard AEDs and is not significantly displaced by NMDA or AMPA receptor ligands (60). GBP is displaced stereospecifically by certain L-amino acids, suggesting a relationship between the GBP binding site and system-L transporter membrane. More recently, GBP has been found to bind to the $\alpha_2\delta$ regulatory subunit of the voltage-sensitive Ca^{2+} channel (67). The precise function of this auxiliary subunit is not known, but it has been suggested that GBP may modify monamine neurotransmitter release through its interaction with Ca^{2+} channels (63).

In summary, GBP displays a unique anticonvulsant profile in animal studies and has demonstrated efficacy in human trials. Furthermore, results from a number of in vitro and in vivo studies also suggest that the mechanism of action of GBP is unique among the existing AEDs. Among the many possible hypotheses being tested, the two that appear most closely associated with its anticonvulsant action are its ability to (1) enhance GABA turnover and release and (2) interact with a unique binding site that appears to be coupled to some voltage-sensitive Ca^{2+} channels.

Lamotrigine

Lamotrigine (3,5-diamino-6-[2,3-dichlorphenyo]-1,2,4-triazine) was the third new-generation AED to be marketed in the United States since 1993. LTG was derived from an antifolate drug development program based on the observation that chronic use of phenobarbital, primidone, and phenytoin reduced folate levels (68) and that folates induce seizures in laboratory animals (69). However, despite its structural similarity to other antifolate drugs, LTG displays only weak antifolate activity. Furthermore, results from structure-activity studies suggest that there is little correlation between antifolate activity and anticonvulsant potency (13).

In some respects, the preclinical profile of LTG is very similar to that observed with PHT and CBZ (Table 22-1). For example, LTG is active in the kindled rat and against tonic extension seizures in the MES test but is ineffective against sc PTZ-induced clonus (61,70,71). However, the preclinical profile of LTG differs significantly from that of PHT and CBZ in one important manner. LTG is effective in the *lh/lh* model of absence (9), whereas PHT and CBZ are not only ineffective but also can on occasion actually worsen spike-wave seizures (5,7) (Table 22-1). In this respect, the preclinical profile of LTG supports its clinical utility against partial seizures, generalized tonic-clonic, and generalized absence seizures (72–74).

In in vitro experiments, LTG selectively blocks veratrine-evoked but not potassium-evoked release of endogenous glutamate (75). These findings suggested that LTG, like PHT, acts at voltage-sensitive Na^+ channels to stabilize neuronal membranes (Table 22-2). Evidence favoring this mechanism includes the documented capacity of LTG to inhibit [^{3}H]batrachotoxin binding and veratrine-stimulated [^{14}C]quanidinium transport into synaptosomes (76,77), its capacity to inhibit sustained repetitive firing (76), and its demonstrated concentration-dependent inhibition of Na^+ currents in mouse neuroblastoma cells (18). Effects of all three AEDs on Na^+ currents were voltage-dependent, and all three slowed recovery from inactivation.

As mentioned previously, however, the clinical profile of LTG appears broader than would be expected based on this single mechanism. Given the lack of efficacy of other Na^+ channel blockers against generalized absence seizures, the efficacy of LTG against this seizure type is likely unrelated to this mechanism unless, as suggested by Coulter (39), LTG exerts an effect on a particular isoform of the brain Na^+ channel that is either anatomically involved in the generation of spike-wave discharges or whose expression is selectively altered in the thalamocortical circuitry of absence patients. LTG has been found to decrease voltage-gated Ca^{2+} currents (49). This effect may contribute to a decrease in neurotransmitter release and thereby contribute to its anticonvulsant action (Table 22-3). Additional investigations are required to resolve whether this effect contributes to the broader clinical profile of LTG compared with that of PHT and CBZ.

Oxcarbazepine

Oxcarbazepine (10,11-dihydro-10-oxo-carbamazepine) is structurally related to CBZ (78). The keto substitution at the 10,11 position of the dibenzazepine nucleus does not affect the therapeutic profile of OCBZ but does contribute to better tolerability in humans (79–82). In vivo, OCBZ is rapidly and completely reduced to its active metabolite (10,11-dihydro-10-hydroxy-carbamazepine [HCBZ]), which is thought to be responsible for the anticonvulsant action of OCBZ (83). HCBZ is a racemate that can be separated into two enantiomers, both of which appear to contribute to the anticonvulsant activity of HCBZ (84).

The anticonvulsant profiles of OCBZ and HCBZ are virtually identical to that of CBZ (Table 22-1). For example, they are both active against tonic-extension seizures induced by MES and essentially inactive against clonic seizures induced by PTZ, picrotoxin, and strychnine (84,85). Both compounds possess activity against focal seizures in monkeys with chronic aluminum foci (83). In comparative clinical trials, OCBZ was demonstrated to be as efficacious and better tolerated than CBZ (80–82). Clinically, OCBZ seems to represent a less toxic and equally effective alternative to CBZ, which appears to exert its anticonvulsant effect through a similar mechanism of action. Furthermore, OCBZ appears to be highly effective and safe as a first-line treatment in adults with partial and generalized tonic-clonic seizures (86).

OCBZ, HCBZ, and CBZ all appear to share a similar mechanistic profile (87) (Table 22-2). (See ref. for review). OCBZ and HCBZ, like other drugs that block MES seizures, both block sustained repetitive firing in cultured spinal cord neurons in a voltage- and frequency-dependent manner (88). Additional results from electrophysiologic studies suggest that HCBZ may mediate some of its anticonvulsant effect through an action at high-threshold voltage-gated Ca^{2+} channels (49).

Topiramate

Topiramate [2,3:4,5-*bis*-O-(1-methylethylidene)-β-D-fructopyranose sulfamate] is a chemically novel AED. In animal tests, the anticonvulsant profile of TPM most closely approximates that of PHT, CBZ, and LTG. For example, it is active against MES-induced tonic extension seizures. TPM does not prevent seizures induced by sc PTZ; however, it does elevate the seizure threshold for PTZ-induced seizures (89,90). In the amygdala-kindled rat, TPM reduced both the seizure score and the afterdischarge duration of fully expressed kindled seizures (91) and with pretreatment appears to delay the acquisition of kindling (92). This latter effect suggests an antiepileptic versus purely anticonvulsant effect. In the spontaneously epileptic rat, which displays both tonic extension seizures and absence-like spike-wave discharges, TPM was as effective as PHT in reducing tonic extensions and, like ESM, decreased the duration of spike-wave discharges in a dose- and time-dependent fashion (93) (Table 22-1). These findings support the apparent broad clinical profile that has emerged for TPM. For example, it appears to be effective against a broad range of seizure types, including partial and generalized tonic-clonic seizures (Table 22-1). Anecdotal reports suggest that TPM may be effective against uncomplicated absence seizures, an action supported by findings in the spontaneously epileptic rat (93) but not the *lh/lh* mouse (8).

In studies conducted thus far, TPM has been found to possess multiple potential mechanisms of action (89,94) (Table 22-2). In cultured hippocampal neurons, therapeutic concentrations (3–30 µM) of TPM inhibit sustained repetitive firing in a use- and concentration-dependent manner (95) and reduce voltage-activated Na^+ currents in cultured neocortical neurons (96).

TPM has also been shown to reduce kainate-evoked inward currents and to block kainate-evoked cobalt influx, indicating that TPM has antagonistic effects on the kainate-AMPA subtype of glutamate receptor (97,98). The effect of TPM on kainate-evoked currents appears to be unique to TPM among the new AEDs and is consistent with a decrease in neuronal excitability and may, when coupled with its effects against Na^+ currents, contribute to its effectiveness against partial and generalized convulsive seizures.

Effects at the Na^+ channel and AMPA-kainate receptor do not necessarily support the ability of TPM to block absence-like spike-wave discharges in the spontaneously epileptic rat and anecdotal reports suggesting efficacy against generalized absence epilepsy. TPM has been reported to enhance GABA-evoked chloride single-channel currents in cultured neocortical neurons (99,100). Kinetic analysis of single-channel recordings from excised outside-out patches demonstrated that TPM increased the frequency of channel opening and the burst frequency but was without effect on open-channel duration or burst duration. This effect of TPM on $GABA_A$ channel activity was similar to that observed with BZDs; however, the ability of TPM to enhance $GABA_A$-evoked current was not reversed by the BZD antagonist flumazenil. Although consistent with the ability of TPM to block spike-wave discharges and its apparent efficacy against absence epilepsy, enhancement of GABA-mediated inhibition would not be predicted from previous invitro studies wherein TPM did not displace radiolabeled ligand binding to known binding sites on $GABA_A$ receptors (90).

In other preclinical studies, TPM was shown to inhibit certain carbonic anhydrase isoforms, an activity that may through an alteration of HCO_3^- homeostasis contribute to TPM's mechanism of action (101). Furthermore, TPM has been observed to decrease high voltage–activated Ca^{2+} currents (HVACC) in CA1 pyramidal neurons (102). This effect at both L- and non–L-type Ca^{2+} channels required a short preincubation period.

The results to date suggest that the effects of TPM on Na^+ channels, $GABA_A$ receptors, HVACC, and AMPA-kainate receptors are unique when compared with prototypical modulators of these processes. For example, the effects of TPM on all four of these protein complexes can be highly variable. TPM has been observed to produce both immediate and delayed effects; sometimes its effect is reversible and sometimes it is not; in some preparations, the action of TPM appears to be dependent on the age of neurons in culture. All of these observations, albeit frustrating, are suggestive of a unique interaction with the target protein that may be dependent in part on its molecular structure (i.e., subunit specificity) and/or, as has been suggested, the state of phosphorylation of the protein (94). Clearly, additional studies are required to further elucidate its precise mechanism of action.

Tiagabine

Tiagabine [(R)-N-(4,4-di-(3-methyl-thien-2-yl)but-3-enyl) nipecotic acid hydrochloride] is a selective GABA uptake inhibitor (Table 22-3), which emerged from a mechanistic-based drug discovery program designed to identify lipophilic GABA uptake inhibitors for the treatment of epilepsy (103).

In animals, TGB is effective against several types of chemically induced seizures, including DMCM-induced clonic seizures and sc PTZ-induced tonic (potent inhibitor) and clonic (partial inhibitor) seizures (103) (Table 22-1). TGB reduces both seizure severity and afterdischarge duration in the amygdala-kindled rat, was active against audiogenic seizures in DBA/2 mice, and was only partially effective against photically induced myoclonus in the photosensitive baboon. However, it is active in the MES test only at doses two- to threefold higher than that producing motor impairment. Like VGB, TGB also worsens spike-wave discharges in the GAERS, GBL, and lh/lh models of absence (8).

In vitro studies have shown TGB to be a potent inhibitor of neuronal and glial GABA uptake (103) (Table 22-2). TGB binds selectively and reversibly to the GAT-1 GABA uptake carrier of both glia and neurons but does not stimulate GABA release. It is ineffective at other receptor binding and uptake sites evaluated to date, including the glutamate receptor, Na^+, or Ca^{2+} channels. Inhibition of GABA uptake by TGB leads to increased synaptic concentrations of GABA and a consequent enhancement and prolongation of GABA-mediated inhibitory neurotransmission, an effect that is assumed to be the basis of TGB's anticonvulsant activity against partial seizures and its ability to aggravate spike-wave seizures in rodents and, potentially, humans. Indeed, TGB treatment has been demonstrated to increase extracellular fluid GABA levels in vivo in both animal brains (104) and human brains (105). The mechanism of its proconvulsive action is probably much like that of VGB in that elevated synaptic concentrations of GABA at the level of the thalamus are thought to potentiate $GABA_B$ -mediated slow after-hyperpolarization, which leads to enhanced deinactivation of T-currents and increased amplification of thalamocortical rhythms necessary to support spike-wave discharges.

Vigabatrin

Vigabatrin [4-amino-5-hexenoic acid; (γ-vinyl GABA)] is widely available in Europe and Canada for the treatment of partial seizures and is in late-stage clinical development in the United States. In experimental seizure models, VGB is active in photosensitive baboons, strychnine- and sound-induced seizures, and amygdala kindling. VGB is essentially inactive in the MES test and in DMCM (methyl-6-7-dimethoxy-4-ethyl-β-carboline-3-carboxylate)-induced clonic seizures and worsens spike-wave seizures in the lh/lh mouse and GAERS rat (8,11,13,106) (Table 22-1). Furthermore, direct injection of VGB into the median part of the lateral thalamus of GAERS significantly increased the cumulative duration of spike and wave discharges (107,108). The anticonvulsant activity of VGB in the kindled rat and worsening of spike-wave seizures in the lh/lh mouse and GAERS correlates well with its clinical utility against partial seizures and its potential exacerbation of spike-wave seizures, respectively.

VGB, a close structural analogue of GABA, arose from a synthesis program designed to develop molecules that target GABA α-oxoglutarate transaminase (GABA-T; EC 2.6.1.19), the enzyme responsible for GABA metabolism. VGB binds to GABA-T and permanently inactivates the enzyme, thereby increasing brain GABA levels and enhancing GABAergic neurotransmission (Table 22-2). VGB administration to laboratory animals produces a prolonged, dose-related inhibition of GABA-T and corresponding elevation of whole-brain GABA levels (109,110). An increase in all brain regions examined was observed; however, quantitative differences between brain regions were noted (111). Likewise, in human studies VGB produces a dose-dependent increase in cerebrospinal fluid GABA levels (112–114). In animal studies, there does appear to be a preferential increase in the GABA concentration in the synaptosomal versus nonsynaptosomal pool (115). Thus, VGB treatment leads to an increased amount of presynaptic GABA available for release, which indirectly causes increased GABAergic activity at postsynaptic GABA receptors.

The consequent increased activity of GABA on postsynaptic GABA receptors results in increased inhibition of neurons involved in seizure activity and represents the most likely basis for VGB's clinical activity against partial seizures. The same mechanism that affords efficacy in partial seizures likely contributes to aggravation of generalized absence seizures (8,39,106). For example, increased GABA release in the thalamus causes a greater activation of $GABA_B$ receptors. Enhanced $GABA_B$ receptor activation leads to a prolonged hyperpolarization and subsequent deactivation of T-type Ca^{2+} currents, which contribute to the synchronized burst firing of thalamocortical neurons.

Zonisamide

Zonisamide (1,2-benzisoxazole-3-methanesulfonamide) was discovered as a result of routine biological screening of 1,2-benzisoxazole derivatives. ZNS possesses a broad anticonvulsant profile in animal seizure models (13,116) (Table 22-1). It blocks MES seizures in a number of different species and restricts the spread of focal cortical seizures in cats. In addition, ZNS blocks tonic extension seizures in spontaneous epileptic rats and audiogenic seizures in DBA/2 mice (93). In cats and rats, ZNS also suppresses focal seizure activity induced by cortical freezing and tungstic acid gel, respectively. Moreover, in hippocampal kindled rats, amygdala-kindled rats, and cats, ZNS suppresses subcortically evoked seizures. In geniculate-kindled cats, ZNS decreases photically induced myoclonus. In the spontaneous epileptic rat, ZNS did not affect spike-wave discharges (93). Clinically, ZNS appears to possess efficacy against a number of seizure types, including partial and secondarily generalized seizures, generalized tonic-clonic, generalized tonic, atypical absence, atonic, and myoclonic seizures (116).

The broad anticonvulsant profile of ZNS can likely be accounted for by a similarly broad mechanistic profile (see Table 22-2). For example, it blocks sustained repetitive firing in cultured spinal cord neurons (117) through an effect on voltage-sensitive Na channels (118). In voltage-clamped *Myxicola* giant axons, ZNS, like PHT, CBZ, and LTG, appears to retard recovery from fast and slow Na channel inactivation and produces a hyyerpolarizing shift in the steady-state inactivation curve. ZNS has also been demonstrated to reduce voltage-dependent T-type calcium currents in cultured neurons (119) and neuroblastoma cells (120). ZNS also appears to modulate GABA-mediated inhibition. For example, ZNS has been reported to decrease [^{3}H]flunitrazepam and [^{3}H]muscimol binding to the BZD and GABA$_A$ receptors, respectively. Similarly, [^{3}H]ZNS binding to rat whole brain membranes is reduced by clonazepam and enhanced by GABA (121). In contrast, ZNS did not affect ion currents evoked by iontophoretically applied GABA (117). Obviously, additional experiments are required to resolve this apparent discrepancy.

Effects on voltage-sensitive Na$^+$ channels are likely to contribute to the ability of ZNS to block MES-induced tonic extension in animals and generalized tonic seizures in humans; whereas, effects on low voltage–activated T currents and perhaps GABA receptors are more likely to correlate with its efficacy against generalized absence and myoclonic seizures, respectively.

CONCLUSIONS

In recent years, an improved understanding of the mechanisms associated with epileptiform events and the anticonvulsant activity of AEDs have contributed to the synthesis of new AEDs specifically designed to reduce excitation or enhance inhibition. This mechanistic approach has been successful in identifying two new

drugs that modify GABA-mediated inhibition by either blocking reuptake of synaptically released GABA (i.e., TGB) or inhibiting metabolism of neuronal and glial GABA (i.e., VGB). These two examples clearly support the validity of the mechanistic approach.

Unfortunately, the mechanistic approach has been less successful at the excitatory synapse, despite an extensive understanding of the processes underlying excitatory neurotransmission. For example, the drugs developed thus far to specifically target the NMDA-preferring glutamate receptor have not only lacked efficacy in the limited clinical trials conducted to date but also resulted in intolerable side effects (122). Increased understanding of the molecular biology of not only the NMDA but also the AMPA and kainate receptors may ultimately lead to the development of selective, less toxic, and clinically effective glutamate antagonists.

Many of the new AEDs appear to act through a combination of mechanisms that likely extend beyond effects on Na$^+$ and Ca^{2+} channels and GABA receptors; however, these effects alone are probably not sufficient to account for the apparent efficacy of the newer AEDs in highly refractory seizure patients. Two of the newer drugs (FBM and TPM) appear to possess a unique ability to inhibit glutamate-mediated neurotransmission through an effect on NMDA (FBM) and AMPA-kainate (TPM) receptors. The finding that these drugs limit glutamatergic neurotransmission without producing the typical behavioral disturbances associated with selective glutamate antagonists may suggest that they target a different glutamate receptor subtype. Newly developed molecular biologic techniques will undoubtedly make it possible to address this issue in the near future.

Mechanisms of action beyond those discussed are likely to contribute to the underlying efficacy of the new AEDs. The continued search to thoroughly understand the molecular mode of action of the available drugs will indirectly provide important information concerning the underlying causes of seizure disorders. Ultimately, the results obtained from these and other studies will continue to assist in the rational design of newer, more effective, and less toxic drugs. It is likely that we will eventually identify novel drugs that not only inhibit acute seizures but also interfere with the pathologic processes that underlie the development of drug-resistant epilepsy. Only at that point will we be able to conclude the search for the ideal AED.

REFERENCES

1. Putnam TJ, Merritt HH. Experimental determination of the anticonvulsant properties of some phenyl derivatives. *Science* 1937; 85:525–526.

2. White HS, Wolf HH, Woodhead JH, Kupferberg HJ. The National Institutes of Health Anticonvulsant Drug Development Program: Screening for Efficacy. In: French J, Leppik I, Dichter MA, eds. *Antiepileptic Drug Development*. Philadelphia: Lippincott-Raven, 1998:29–39. Advances in Neurology, Vol. 76.

3. Mattson RH. General principles: selection of antiepileptic drug therapy. In: Levy RH, Mattson RH, Meldrum BS, eds. *Antiepileptic Drugs*. 4th ed. New York: Raven Press, 1995:123–135.

4. Loscher W, Honack D, Fassbender CP, Nolting B. The role of technical, biological and pharmacological factors in the laboratory evaluation of anticonvulsant drugs. 3. Pentylenetetrazole seizure models. *Epilepsy Res* 1991; 8:171–189.

5. Snead OC. Pharmacological models of generalized absence seizures in rodents. *J Neural Transm* 1992; 35:7–19.

6. Marescaux C, Vergnes M. Genetic absence epilepsy in rats from Strasbourg (GAERS). *Ital J Neurol Sci* 1995; 16:113–118.

7. Hosford DA, Clark S, Cao Z, et al. The role of GABAB receptor activation in absence seizures of lethargic (*lh/lh*) mice. *Science* 1992; 257:398–401.

8. Hosford DA, Wang Y. Utility of the lethargic (*lh/lh*) mouse model of absence seizures in predicting the effects of lamotrigine, vigabatrin, tiagabine, gabapentin, and topiramate against human absence seizures. *Epilepsia* 1997; 38:408–414.

9. Macdonald RL, Kelly KM. Antiepileptic drug mechanisms of action. *Epilepsia* 1995; 36(Suppl 2):S2–S12.

10. Swinyard EA, Woodhead JH, White HS, Franklin MR. General principles: experimental selection, quantification, and evaluation of anticonvulsants. In: Levy R, Mattson R, Meldrum B, Penry JK, Dreifuss FE, eds. *Antiepileptic Drugs*. 3rd ed. New York: Raven Press, 1989:85–102.

11. White HS. Mechanisms of antiepileptic drugs. In: Porter R, Chadwick D, eds. *Epilepsies II*. Boston: Butterworth-Heinemann, 1997:1–30.

12. Chapman AA, Croucher MJ, Meldrum BS. Evaluation of anticonvulsant drugs in DBA/2 mice with sound-induced seizures. *Arzneim Forsch/Drug Res* 1984; 34:1261–1264.

13. Rogawski MA, Porter RJ. Antiepileptic drugs: pharmacological mechanisms and clinical efficacy with consideration of promising developmental stage compounds. *Pharmacol Rev* 1990; 42:223–286.

14. Macdonald RL, Meldrum BS. General principles. Principles of antiepileptic drug action. In: Levy RH, Mattson RH, Meldrum BS, eds. *Antiepileptic Drugs*. 4th ed. New York: Raven Press, 1995:61–77.

15. Meldrum B. Action of established and novel anticonvulsant drugs on the basic mechanisms of epilepsy. *Epilepsy Res Suppl* 1996; 11:67–77.

16. Piredda SG, Woodhead JH, Swinyard EA. Effect of stimulus intensity on the profile of anticonvulsant activity of phenytoin, ethosuximide and valproate. *J Pharmacol Exp Ther* 1985; 232:741–745.

17. White HS, Johnson M, Wolf HH, Kupferberg HJ. The early identification of anticonvulsant activity: role of the maximal electroshock and subcutaneous pentylenetetrazol seizure models. *Ital J Neurol Sci* 1995; 16:73–77.

18. Lang DG, Wang CM, Cooper BR. Lamotrigine, phenytoin and carbamazepine interactions on the sodium current present in N4TG1 mouse neuroblastoma cells. *J Pharmacol Exp Ther* 1993; 266:829–835.

19. Willow M, Catterall WA. Inhibition of binding of [^{2}H]batrachotoxinin A20-α-benzoate to sodium channels by the anticonvulsant drugs diphenylhydantoin and carbamazepine. *Mol Pharmacol* 1982; 22:627–635.

20. Willow M, Kuenzel EA, Catterall WA. Inhibition of voltage-sensitive sodium channels in neuroblastoma cells and synaptosomes by the anticonvulsant drugs diphenylhydantoin and carbamazepine. *Mol Pharmacol* 1984; 25:228–234.

21. Schwarz JR, Grigat G. Phenytoin and carbamazepine: potential- and frequency-dependent block of Na currents in mammalian myelinated nerve fibers. *Epilepsia* 1989; 30:286–294.

22. Tomaselli G, Marban E, Yellen G. Sodium channels from human brain RNA expressed in Xenopus oocytes basic electrophysiologic characteristics and their modifications by diphenylhydantoin. *J Clin Invest* 1989; 83:1724–1732.

23. Wakamori M, Kaneda M, Oyama Y, Akaike N. Effects of chlordiazepoxide, chlorpromazine, diazepam, diphenylhydantoin, flunitrazepam and haloperidol on the voltage-dependent sodium current of isolated mammalian brain neurons. *Brain Res* 1989; 494:374–378.

24. White HS, Woodhead JH, Franklin MR, Swinyard EA, Wolf HH. General principles: Experimental selection, quantification, and evaluation of antiepileptic drugs. In: Levy RH, Mattson RH, Meldrum BS, eds. *Antiepileptic Drugs*. 4th ed. New York: Raven Press, 1995:99–110.

25. Coulter DA, Hugenard JR, Prince DA. Characterization of ethosuximide reduction of low threshold calcium current in thalamic neurons. *Ann Neurol* 1989; 25:582–593.

26. Coulter DA, Hugenard JR, Prince DA. Differential effects of petit mal anticonvulsants and convulsants on thalamic neurones: calcium current reduction. *Br J Pharmacol* 1990; 100:800–806.

27. Van Dongen AMJ, Van Erp MG, Voskuyl RA. Valproate reduces excitability by blockage of sodium and potassium conductance. *Epilepsia* 1986; 27:177–182.

28. Zona C, Avoli M. Effects induced by the antiepileptic drug valproic acid upon the ionic currents recorded in rat neocortical neurons in cell culture. *Exp Brain Res* 1990; 81:313–317.

29. Van den Berg RJ, Kok P, Voskuyl RA. Valproate and sodium currents in cultured hippocampal neurons. *Exp Brain Res* 1993; 93:279–287.

30. Kelly KM, Gross RA, Macdonald RL. Valproic acid selectively reduces the low-threshold (T) calcium in rat nodose neurons. *Neurosci Lett* 1990; 116:233–238.

31. Macdonald RL, Olsen RW. GABA$_A$ receptor channels. *Annu Rev Neurosci* 1994; 17:569–602.

32. Rogers CJ, Twyman RE, Macdonald RL. Benzodiazepine and β-carboline regulation of single GABA$_A$ receptor channels of mouse spinal neurones in culture. *J Physiol* 1994; 475:69–82.

33. Study RE, Barker JL. Diazepam and (–)-pentobarbital: fluctuation analysis reveals different mechanisms for potentiation of gamma-aminobutyric acid responses in cultured central neurons. *Proc Natl Acad Sci USa* 1981; 78:7180–7184.

34. Twyman RE, Rogers CJ, Macdonald RL. Differential regulation of gamma-aminobutyric acid receptor channels by diazepam and phenobarbital. *Ann Neurol* 1989; 25:213–220.

35. Vicini S, Mienville JM, Costa E. Actions of benzodiazepine and β-carboline derivatives on gamma-aminobutyric acid-activated Cl-channels recorded from membrane patches of neonatal rat cortical neurons in culture. *J Pharmacol Exp Ther* 1987; 243:1195–1201.

36. Moss SJ, Smart TA, Porter NM, et al. Cloned GABA receptors are maintained in a stable cell line: allosteric and channel properties. *Eur J Pharmacol* 1990; 189:177–188.

37. Verdoorn TA, Draguhn A, Ymer S, Seeburg PH, Sakmann B. Functional properties of recombinant rat GABA$_A$ receptors depend upon subunit composition. *Neuron* 1990; 4:919–928.

38. Pritchett DB, Sontheimer H, Shivers BD, et al. Importance of a novel GABA$_A$ receptor subunit for benzodiazepine pharmacology. *Nature* 1989; 338:582–584.

39. Coulter DA. Antiepileptic drug cellular mechanisms of action: where does lamotrigine fit in? *J Child Neurol* 1997; 12(Suppl 1):S2–S9.

40. Swinyard EA, Sofia RD, Kupferberg HJ. Comparative anticonvulsant activity and neurotoxicity of felbamate and four prototype antiepileptic drugs in mice and rats. *Epilepsia* 1986; 27:27–34.

41. White HS, Wolf HH, Swinyard EA, Skeen GA, Sofia RD. A neuropharmacological evaluation of felbamate as a novel anticonvulsant. *Epilepsia* 1992; 33:564–572.

42. Sofia RD. Felbamate. Mechanisms of action. In: Levy RH, Mattson RH, Meldrum BS, eds. *Antiepileptic Drugs*. 4th ed. New York: Raven Press, 1995:791–797.

43. Wlaz P, Loscher W. Anticonvulsant activity of felbamate in amygdala kindling model of temporal lobe epilepsy in rats. *Epilepsia* 1997; 38:1167–1172.

44. Wallis RA, Panizzon KL, Fairchild MD, Wasterlain CG. Protective effects of felbamate against hypoxia in the rat hippocampal slice. *Stroke* 1992; 23:547–551.

45. Wasterlain CG, Adams LM, Hattori H, Schwartz PH. Felbamate reduces hypoxic-ischemic brain damage in vivo. *Eur J Pharmacol* 1992; 212:275–278.

46. Wasterlain CG, Adams LM, Schwartz PH, et al. Post-hypoxic treatment with felbamate is neuroprotective in a rat model of hypoxia-ischemia. *Neurology* 1994; 43:2303–2310.

47. Chronopoulos A, Stafstrom C, Thurber S, et al. Neuroprotective effect of felbamate after kainic acid-induced status epilepticus. *Epilepsia* 1993; 34:359–366.

48. Pisani A, Stefani A, Siniscalchi A, et al. Electrophysiological actions of felbamate on rat striatal neurones. *Br J Pharmacol* 1995; 116:2053–2061.

49. Stefani A, Spadoni F, Bernardi G. Voltage-activated calcium channels: targets of antiepileptic drug therapy? *Epilepsia* 1997; 38:959–965.

50. McCabe RT, Wasterlain CG, Kucharczyk N, Sofia RD, Vogel JR. Evidence for anticonvulsant and neuroprotectant action of felbamate mediated by strychnine-insensitive glycine receptors. *J Pharmacol Exp Ther* 1993; 264:1248–1252.

51. Wamsley JK, Sofia RD, Faull RLM, et al. Interaction of felbamate with [^{3}H]DCKA-labeled strychnine-insensitive glycine receptors in human postmortem brain. *Exp Neurol* 1994; 129:244–250.

52. Wallis RA, Panizzon KL. Glycine reversal of felbamate hypoxic protection. *NeuroReport* 1993; 4:951–954.

53. White HS, Harmsworth WL, Sofia RD, Wolf HH. Felbamate modulates the strychnine-insensitive glycine receptor. *Epilepsy Res* 1995; 20:41–48.

54. Coffin V, Cohen-Williams M, Barnett A. Selective antagonism of the anticonvulsant effects of felbamate by glycine. *Eur J Pharmacol* 1994; 256:R9–R10.

55. De Sarro G, Ongini E, Bertorelli R, Aguglia U, De Sarro A. Excitatory amino acid neurotransmission through both NMDA and non-NMDA receptors is involved in the anticonvulsant activity of felbamate in DBA/2 mice. *Eur J Pharmacol* 1994; 262:11–19.

56. Rho JM, Donevan DC, Rogawski MA. Mechanism of action of the anticonvulsant felbamate: Opposing effects on NMDA and GABA$_A$ receptors. *Ann Neurol* 1994; 35:229–234.

57. Ticku MK, Kamatchi GL, Sofia RD. Effect of anticonvulsant felbamate on GABA$_A$ receptor system. *Epilepsia* 1991; 32(3):389–391.

58. Pennell PB, Ogaily MS, Macdonald RL. Aplastic anemia in a patient receiving felbamate for partial seizures. *Neurology* 1995; 45:456–460.

59. Schmidt B. Potential antiepileptic drugs: gabapentin. In: Levy RH, Driefuss FE, Mattson RH, Meldrum BS, Penry JK, eds. *Antiepileptic Drugs*. 3rd ed. New York: Raven Press, 1989:925–935.

60. Taylor CP. Gabapentin. Mechanisms of action. In: Levy RH, Mattson RH, Meldrum BS, eds. *Antiepileptic Drugs*. 4th ed. New York: Raven Press, 1995:829–841.

61. Dalby NO, Nielsen EB. Comparison of the preclinical anticonvulsant profiles of tiagabine, lamotrigine, gabapentin and vigabatrin. *Epilepsy Res* 1997; 28:63–72.

62. Bartoszyk GD, Meyerson N, Reimann W, Satzinger G, von Hodenberg A. Gabapentin. In: Meldrum BS, Porter RJ, eds. *Current Problems in Epilepsy: New Anticonvulsant Drugs*. London: John Libbey, 1986:147–164.

63. Taylor CP, Gee NS, Su T-Z, et al. A summary of mechanistic hypotheses of gabapentin pharmacology. *Epilepsy Res* 1998; 29:233–249.

64. Petroff OAC, Rothman DL, Behar KL, Lamoureux D, Mattson RH. Gabapentin increases brain gamma-aminobutyric acid levels in patients with epilepsy. *Ann Neurol* 1995; 38:295–296.

65. Wamil AW, McLean MJ. Limitation by gabapentin of high frequency action potential firing by mouse central neurons in cell culture. *Epilepsy Res* 1994; 17:1–11.

66. Welty DF, Schielke GP, Vartanian MG, Taylor CP. Gabapentin anticonvulsant action in rats: disequilibrium with peak drug concentrations in plasma and brain microdialysate. *Epilepsy Res* 1993; 16:175–181.

67. Gee NS, Brown JP, Dissanayake VUK, et al. The novel anticonvulsant drug gabapentin (Neurontin), binds to the $\alpha 2\delta$ subunit of a calcium channel. *J Biol Chem* 1996; 271:5768–5776.

68. Reynolds EH, Milner G, Matthews DM. Anticonvulsant therapy, megaloblastic haemopoiesis and folic acid metabolism. *Q J Med* 1966; 35:521–537.

69. Hommes OR, Obbens EAMT. The epileptogenic action of sodium folate in the rat. *J Neurol Sci* 1972; 20:269–272.

70. Wheatley PL, Miller AA. Effects of lamotrigine on electrically induced afterdischarge duration in anaesthetised rat, dog and marmoset. *Epilepsia* 1989; 30:34–40.

71. Miller AA, Wheatley P, Sawyer DA, Baxter MG, Roth B. Pharmacological studies on lamotrigine, a novel potential antiepileptic drug, I: anticonvulsant profile in mice and rats. *Epilepsia* 1986; 27:483–489.

72. Leach JP, Brodie MJ. Lamotrigine. Clinical use. In: Levy RH, Mattson RH, Meldrum BS, eds. *Antiepileptic Drugs*. 4th ed. New York: Raven Press, 1995:889–895.

73. Yuen AWC. Lamotrigine: a review of antiepileptic efficacy. *Epilepsia* 1994; 35(Suppl 5):S33–S36.

74. Buchanan N. Lamotrigine in the treatment of absence seizures. *Acta Neurol Scand* 1995; 92:348.

75. Leach MJ, Marden CM, Miller AA. Pharmacological studies on lamotrigine, a novel potential antiepileptic drug, II: neurochemical studies on the mechanism of action. *Epilepsia* 1986; 27:490–497.

76. Cheung H, Kamp D, Harris E. An in vitro investigation of the action of lamotrigine on neuronal voltage-activated sodium channels. *Epilepsy Res* 1992; 13:107–112.

77. Riddall DR, Clackers M, Leach MJ. Correlation of inhibition of veratrine evoked [^{14}C] guanidine uptake with inhibition of veratrine evoked release of glutamate by lamotrigine and its analogues. *Can J Neurol Sci* 1993; 20(Suppl 4):S181.

78. Dam M, Ostergaard LH. Other antiepileptic drugs. Oxcarbazepine. In: Levy RH, Mattson RH, Meldrum BS, eds. *Antiepileptic Drugs*. 4th ed. New York: Raven Press, 1995:987–995.

79. Gram L, Philbert A. Oxcarbazepine. In: Meldrum BS, Porter RJ, eds. *New Anticonvulsant Drugs*. London: John Libbey, 1986:229–235.

80. Houtkooper MA, Lammertsma A, Meyer JMA, et al. Oxcarbazepine (GP 47.680): a possible alternative to carbamazepine? *Epilepsia* 1987; 28:693–698.

81. Reinikainen KJ, Keranen T, Halonen T, Komulainen H, Riekinen PJ. Comparison of oxcarbazepine and carbamazepine: a double-blind study. *Epilepsy Res* 1987; 1:284–289.

82. Dam M, Ekberg R, Loyning Y, Waltimo O, Jakobsen K. A double-blind study comparing oxcarbazepine and carbamazepine in patients with newly diagnosed, previously untreated epilepsy. *Epilepsy Res* 1989; 3:70–76.

83. Jensen PK, Gram L, Schmutz M. Oxcarbazepine. *Epilepsy Res* 1991; 3:135–140.

84. Schmutz M, Ferret T, Heckendorn R, et al. GP 47779, the main human metabolite of oxcarbazepine (Trileptal), and both enantiomers have equal anticonvulsant activity. *Epilepsia* 1993; 34(Suppl 2):122.

85. Baltzer V, Schmutz M. Experimental anticonvulsant properties of GP 47680 and of MHD, its main human metabolite: compounds related to carbamazepine. In: Meinardi H, Rowan AJ, eds. *Advances in Epileptology*. Amsterdam: Swets & Zeitlinger BV, 1978:295–299.

86. Christe W, Kramer G, Vigonius U, et al. A double-blind controlled clinical trial: oxcarbazepine versus sodium valproate in adults with newly diagnosed epilepsy. *Epilepsy Res* 1997; 26:451–460.

87. McLean MJ, Schmutz M, Wamil AW, et al. Oxcarbazepine: mechanisms of action. *Epilepsia* 1994; 35(Suppl 3):S5–S9.

88. Wamil AW, Porter C, Jensen PK, Schmutz M, McLean MJ. Oxcarbazepine and its monohydroxy metabolite limit action potential firing by mouse central neurons in cell culture. *Epilepsia* 1991; 32(Suppl 3):65.

89. White HS, Brown SD, Woodhead JH, Skeen GA, Wolf HH. Topiramate enhances GABA-mediated chloride flux and GABA-evoked chloride currents in murine brain neurons and increases seizure threshold. *Epilepsy Res* 1997; 23:167–179.

90. Shank RP, Gardocki JF, Vaught JL, et al. Topiramate: preclinical evaluation of a structurally novel anticonvulsant. *Epilepsia* 1994; 35(Suppl 2):450–460.

91. Wauquier A, Zhou S. Topiramate: a potent anticonvulsant in the amygdala-kindled rat. *Epilepsy Res* 1996; 24:73–77.

92. Amano K, Hamada K, Yagi K, Seino M. Antiepileptic effects of topiramate on amygdaloid kindling in rats. *Epilepsy Res* 1998; 31:123–128.

93. Nakamura J, Tamura S, Kanda T, et al. Inhibition by topiramate of seizures in spontaneously epileptic rats and DBA/2 mice. *Eur J Pharmacol* 1994; 254:83–89.

94. Shank RP, Gardocki JF, Streeter AJ, Maryanoff BE. An overview of the preclinical aspects of topiramate: pharmacology, pharmacokinetics and mechanism of action. *Neurology* (in press).

95. Coulter DA, Sombati S, DeLorenzo RJ. Selective effects of topiramate on sustained repetitive firing and spontaneous bursting in cultured hippocampal neurons. *Epilepsia* 1993; 34(Suppl 2):123.

96. Zona C, Ciotti MT, Avoli M. Topiramate attenuates voltage-gated sodium currents in rat cerebellar granule cells. *Neurosci Lett* 1997; 231:123–126.

97. Severt L, Coulter DA, Sombati S, DeLorenzo RJ. Topiramate selectively blocks kainate currents in cultured hippocampal neurons. *Epilepsia* 1995; 36(Suppl 4):S38.

98. Skradski S, White HS. The novel antiepileptic drug topiramate blocks kainate-evoked cobalt influx into cultured neurons. *Neurology* (in press).

99. Brown SD, Wolf HH, Swinyard EA, Twyman RE, White HS. The novel anticonvulsant topiramate enhances GABA-mediated chloride flux. *Epilepsia* 1993; 34(Suppl 2):122–123.

100. White HS, Brown D, Skeen GA, Wolf HH, Twyman RE. The anticonvulsant topiramate displays a unique ability to potentiate GABA-evoked chloride currents. *Epilepsia* 1995; 36(Suppl 3):S39–S40.

101. Staley KJ, Soldo BL, Proctor WR. Ionic mechanisms of neuronal excitation by inhibitory GABA$_A$ receptors. *Science* 1995; 269:977–981.

102. Zhang X, Velumian AA, Jones OT, Carlen PL. Topiramate reduces high-voltage activated Ca^{2+} currents in CA1 pyramidal neurons in vitro. *Epilepsia* 1998; 39(Suppl. 6):44.

103. Suzdak PD, Jansen JA. A review of the preclinical pharmacology of tiagabine: a potent and selective anticonvulsant GABA uptake inhibitor. *Epilepsia* 1995; 36:612–626.

104. Fink-Jensen A, Suzdak PD, Swedberg MBD, et al. The GABA uptake inhibitor tiagabine increases extracellular brian levels of GABA in awake rats. *Eur J Pharmacol* 1992; 220:197–201.

105. During M, Mattson R, Scheyer R, et al. The effect of tiagabine HCl on extracellular GABA levels in the human hippocampus. *Epilepsia* 1992; 33(Suppl 3):83.

106. Vergnes M, Marescaux C. Pathophysiological mechanisms underlying genetic absence epilepsy in rats. In: Malafosse A, Genton P, Hirsch E, et al, eds. *Idiopathic Generalized Epilepsies: Clinical Experimental and Genetic Aspects.* London: John Libbey, 1994:151–168.

107. Liu Z, Vergnes M, Depaulis A, Marescaux C. Evidence for a critical role of GABAergic transmission within the thalamus in the genesis and control of absence seizures. *Brain Res* 1991; 545:1–7.

108. Marescaux C, Micheletti G, Vergnes M, Rumbach L, Warter JM. Diazepam antagonizes GABAmimetics in rats with spontaneous petit mal–like epilepsy. *Eur J Pharmacol* 1985; 113:19–24.

109. Jung MJ, Lippert B, Metcalf B, Bohlen P, Schechter PJ. Gamma-vinyl GABA (4-amino-hex-5-enoic acid), a new irreversible inhibitor of GABA-T: effects on brain GABA metabolism in mice. *J Neurochem* 1977; 29:797–802.

110. Schechter PJ, Tranier Y, Jung MJ, Bohlen P. Audiogenic seizure protection by elevated brain GABA concentration in mice: effects of gamma-acetylenic GABA and gamma-vinyl GABA, two irreversible GABA-T inhibitors. *Eur J Pharmacol* 1977; 45:319–328.

111. Chapman AG, Riley K, Evans MC, Meldrum BS. Acute effects of sodium valproate and gamma-vinyl GABA on regional amino acid metabolism in the rat brain: incorporation of 2-[^{14}C]glucose into amino acids. *Neurochem Res* 1982; 7:1089–1105.

112. Ben-Menachem E. Pharmacokinetic effects of vigabatrin on cerebrospinal fluid amino acids in humans. *Epilepsia* 1989; 30(Suppl 3):S12–S14.

113. Grove J, Schechter PJ, Tell G, et al. Increased gamma-aminobutyric acid (GABA), homocarnosine and β-alanine in cerebrospinal fluid of patients treated with gamma-vinyl GABA (4-amino-hex-5-enoic acid). *Life Sci* 1981; 28:2431–2439.

114. Schechter PJ, Hanke NFJ, Grove J, Huebert N, Sjoerdsma A. Biochemical and clinical effects of gamma-vinyl GABA in patients with epilepsy. *Neurology* 1984; 34:182–186.

115. Sarhan S, Seiler N. Metabolic inhibitors and subcellular distribution of GABA. *J Neurosci Res* 1979; 4:399–421.

116. Seino M, Naruto S, Ito T, Miyazaki H. Other antiepileptic drugs. Zonisamide. In: Levy RH, Mattson RH, Meldrum BS, eds. *Antiepileptic Drugs.* 4th ed. New York: Raven Press, 1995:1011–1023.

117. Rock DM, Macdonald RL, Taylor CP. Blockade of sustained repetitive action potentials in cultured spinal cord neurons by zonisamide (AD 810, CI 912), a novel anticonvulsant. *Epilepsy Res* 1989; 3:138–143.

118. Schauf CL. Zonisamide enhances slow sodium inactivation in Myxicola. *Brain Res* 1987; 413:185–188.

119. Suzuki S, Kawakami K, Nishimura S, et al. Zonisamide blocks T-type calcium channel in cultured neurons of rat cerebral cortex. *Epilepsy Res* 1992; 12:21–27.

120. Kito M, Maehara M, Watanabe K. Mechanisms of T-type calcium channel blockade by zonisamide. *Seizure* 1996; 5:115–119.

121. Mimaki T, Suzuki Y, Tagawa T, Tanaka J, Itoh N, Yabuuchi H. [^{3}H]Zonisamide binding in rat brain. *Jpn J Psychiatry Neurol* 1988; 42:640–642.

122. Meldrum BS. Neurotransmission in epilepsy. *Epilepsia* 1995; 36(Suppl 1):S30–S35.

CHAPTER 23

Pharmacokinetic Principles of Antiepileptic Therapy in Children

W. Edwin Dodson, M.D.

Pharmacokinetics is the study of drug concentrations over time for the purpose of understanding the time course of drug actions (1–4). The unique pharmacokinetics of each drug result from both drug-related and host-related factors (Table 23-1). Host-related factors are responsible for most of the variability in the relationship between drug doses and drug concentrations. However, differences in drug formulation can substantially influence the time course of drug action.

FUNDAMENTAL PHARMACOKINETIC CONCEPTS

Pharmacokinetic principles are based on mathematical models. When a model is selected for a specific pharmacokinetic analysis, assumptions must be made to simplify complex physiological processes. Models are named according to the number of compartments that are considered and according to the type of kinetics that are applied: linear versus nonlinear. A one-compartment model assumes that the body is a single compartment; a two-compartment model assumes the body has two compartments, a

central compartment and a peripheral compartment. Although two-compartment models are preferable to one-compartment models, one-compartment models have been used most frequently in pharmacokinetic studies in patients (5).

The physical properties of a drug, such as its size, ionization constant (pK_a), lipid and aqueous solubility, and dissolution rate determine how the drug interacts with physiological processes in the body. These interactions result in kinetic patterns of absorption, distribution, metabolism (biotransformation), and excretion that are characteristic for each drug (6). The drug elimination rate constant (k_{el}) summarizes all of the mechanisms that act to remove a drug from the body. The elimination of antiepileptic drugs (AEDs) is largely due to hepatic biotransformation and renal excretion. Although hepatic biotransformation can produce active metabolites, which contribute to drug action, most of the time drug metabolites do not have antiepileptic activity.

$$k_{el} = k_{renal} + k_{hepatic} + k_{other} \qquad (1)$$

LINEAR DRUG ELIMINATION KINETICS

The mechanisms that eliminate most AEDs are capable of removing much more drug than is usually present. In these circumstances, the elimination mechanisms dispose of a constant fractional amount of the drug per unit of time, independent of the drug concentration. These processes have linear, first-order kinetics. When the elimination of a drug has linear kinetics, the relationship between the drug dose and the drug concentration in serum is linear and intuitively predictable.

Table 23-1. Factors That Determine the Pharmacokinetics of a Drug

Drug-Related Factors	Patient-Related Factors
Size	Pharmacogenetics
Ionization constant	Age
Lipid solubility	Nutritional state
Aqueous Solubility	Disease
Formulation	Comedication
	Route of administration

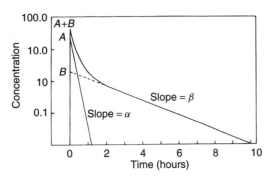

Figure 23-1. Semilogarithmic plot of intravenous concentration versus time curve based on a two-compartment model. Curve A is obtained by subtracting the extrapolated terminal portions of curve $A + B$. For more on exponential curve peeling see Riggs (53) and Greenblatt and Koch-Weser (2,3).

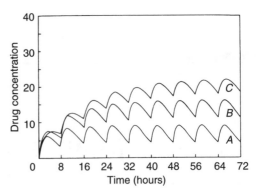

Figure 23-2. Effect of varying half-life on time to reach steady state and on the eventual concentration at steady state. The half-lives of curves A, B, and C are 4, 8, and 12 hours, respectively. Increasing the half-life delays steady state and results in higher concentrations.

Intravenous Dose and Drug Half-life

It is easiest to evaluate drug elimination after intravenous (IV) dosing when drug absorption is not an issue (2,3) (Figure 23-1). Immediately after an IV bolus dose, drug concentrations are very high in serum. At first, the drug level declines very rapidly, but later the rate of decline becomes slower. The initial rapid decline (α phase) is due to the distribution of drug from the central vascular compartment into peripheral tissue compartments. Later, the slower decline (β phase) is determined predominantly by drug elimination. For a two-compartment model, the concentration-time curve after an IV dose is described by the equation:

$$C_t = A \cdot e^{-\alpha t} + B \cdot e^{-\beta t} \qquad (2)$$

The terminal portion of the concentration-time curve is used to determine the half-life ($t_{1/2}$) and the elimination rate constant (k_{el}). The half-life is defined as the time that is required for the amount of drug in the body to decline by one-half. In a single-compartment model, the elimination rate constant is the slope of the declining curve, but in two-compartment models the elimination rate constant is more complex because of the simultaneous effects of drug distribution into the peripheral compartment. In a two-compartment model, the β half-life is calculated from the terminal portion of the concentration-time curve. The half-life is related to the elimination rate constant according to the following relationship: $k_{el} \cdot t_{1/2} = \ln 2$. The elimination rate constant has the dimensions of a fraction per unit of time; the half-life has the dimension of time.

The half-life is important for several reasons. First, it indicates how much time is required for drug levels to stabilize after the dose is changed (Figure 23-2.) Whenever the dose is changed, five half-lives must transpire before a steady state is reached and drug levels stabilize. Second, under steady-state conditions, the drug concentration is directly proportional to the half-life. If the half-life changes, the steady-state concentration changes. Third, the half-life ordinarily dictates how frequently doses should be administered. In most cases, doses should be administered at intervals equal to or less than the half-life to limit the fluctuation in drug levels between doses. For drugs that have a short half-life, retarding absorption by the administration of slow-release formulations also limits the fluctuation in drug levels between doses. This is discussed further with other aspects of drug absorption. Finally, if the half-life changes, the steady-state drug concentration changes.

Volume of Distribution

The apparent volume of distribution (Vd) is the volume that the drug seems to occupy in the body. It is an imaginary volume that does not necessarily conform to anatomical compartments. The volume of distribution is the quotient of the amount of drug in the body divided by the drug concentration. Although the volume of distribution can be calculated several ways, the simplest approach is to extrapolate the terminal phase of the IV concentration-time curve back to time zero and use that concentration (the theoretical concentration at time zero) to calculate Vd (2,3). For example, if there is 100 mg of drug in the body and the drug level at time zero is 10 mg/L, the volume of distribution is 10 L. The relative volume of distribution is the Vd divided by the patient's weight. If the patient with a Vd of 10 L weighed 20 kg, the patient's relative volume of distribution (Vd_{rel}) would be 0.5 L/kg.

The volume of distribution has two important applications. First, it can be used to calculate loading doses. For example, a 100-mg loading dose results in a level of 20 mg/L in a 10-kg child who has a Vd_{rel} of 0.5 L/kg (dose $= Vd_{rel} \cdot$ concentration $\cdot$ weight). Second, it is an important component of clearance.

Clearance

Clearance (Cl) summarizes all of the factors that act to reduce the drug concentration. Clearance is defined as the volume of distribution that is completely rid of drug per unit of time; it has the dimensions of volume per time. Operationally, clearance is the product of the volume of distribution times the elimination rate constant; $Cl = Vd \cdot k_{el}$. Clearance is inversely related to half-life; a long half-life causes a low clearance ($Cl = Vd \cdot \ln 2 / t_{1/2}$). The relative clearance (Cl_{rel}) is the clearance divided by weight.

The relative clearance is the best parameter for comparing drug dose requirements among different groups of patients. It also provides the most reliable basis for determining initial doses because clearance accommodates variations in body water and fat content. However, clearance is rarely used to calculate doses because the values are harder to remember than doses based on weight.

Steady State

A *steady state* exists when the rate of drug input equals the rate of drug output. When drug administration is initiated at a constant dose, the drug progressively accumulates in the body until the clearance equals the dosing rate. Five half-lives are required to nearly reach a steady state.

Although the administration of large, loading doses causes drug levels to increase rapidly, loading doses do not necessarily produce the same concentration that occurs at steady state (Figure 23-3). Steady-state concentrations depend on the maintenance doses, which are administered repeatedly. Thus, a steady state should never be assumed until a constant dose has been administered for a sufficient amount of time.

Under steady-state conditions, the average drug level in serum (C_m^{ss}) is constant and is equal to the dosing rate divided by the clearance.

$$C_m^{ss} = \frac{D}{\tau} \div Cl \tag{3}$$

After replacing clearance with its components, Vd and $t_{1/2}$, it can be seen that the average drug level at steady state is directly related to the dosing rate and to the half-life and inversely related to the volume of distribution.

$$C_m^{ss} = \frac{D}{\tau} \cdot \frac{t_{1/2}}{Vd \cdot \ln 2} \tag{4}$$

Drug Absorption

Drug absorption is described both in terms of the *absorption rate* and in terms of the extent of absorption, or *bioavailability*. The rate of absorption determines when the peak concentration occurs. Slowing the absorption rate postpones and reduces the peak concentration, attenuating the range of the fluctuations in drug concentrations between doses. Bioavailability (*F*) is a measure of the extent of drug absorption that is independent of time. Bioavailability is the quotient of the areas under the concentration-time curves for a non-IV dose divided by an IV dose. For example, the area under the curve after an oral dose divided by the area after the same IV dose is the bioavailability of the orally administered formulation. Bioavailability is expressed as either a fraction or a percent.

Several factors reduce the bioavailability of orally administered drugs. Failure to absorb the drug because of gastrointestinal (GI) disease, lack of tablet dissolution, and drug insolubility are obvious reasons. Bioavailability is also reduced when drugs are metabolized in the GI tract or in the liver before they reach the systemic circulation, so-called first-pass metabolism.

Bioequivalence is a measure that compares both the extent of absorption and the rate of absorption, but it does not require an IV dose. The bioequivalence of various oral formulations of a drug is determined before generic formulations are authorized for marketing. Operationally, the absorption rate or time to peak concentration and the areas under the concentration-time curves for different formulations are compared. According to the U.S. Food and Drug Administration's definition of bioequivalence, different oral formulations of the same drug are bioequivalent if they differ by no more than 20 percent. However, these tolerance limits may be too broad for some patients with epilepsy that is difficult to control.

The route of drug administration influences the absorption rate and thereby affects the onset of drug action. IV administration increases drug levels fastest, making the drug available for entry into tissues almost instantaneously. However, drugs that have limited aqueous solubility such as carbamazepine can not be formulated for IV administration. Intramuscular

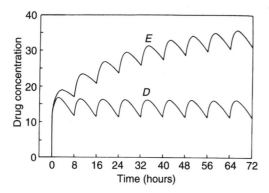

Figure 23-3. Effect of varying half-life after loading doses. Note that independent of the administration of a loading dose, five half-lives are required for levels to stabilize. The half-life for curve D is 8 hours and for curve E is 20 hours.

(IM) administration of some drugs results in slower absorption than oral administration. In the case of lipophilic drugs with relatively poor aqueous solubility such as phenytoin, absorption after IM administration is slow and erratic, although eventually complete. Among the AEDs, phenobarbital is best documented to be rapidly and reliably absorbed after IM administration. Phenobarbital concentrations usually reach peak values in less than 90 minutes in children (7).

Oral administration of AEDs is the cornerstone of the treatment of epilepsy. By and large, drugs with erratic or low bioavailability are not suitable for chronic antiepileptic therapy. Drugs with rapid absorption and short half-lives are manufactured in delayed or slowly absorbed formulations to help sustain drug levels between doses. Examples include valproate (Depakote Sprinkles) and carbamazepine (Tegretol XR and Carbitrol). As a general principle, slowly absorbed formulations are preferable for chronic antiepileptic therapy because they attenuate the fluctuations in drug concentrations between doses. The differing absorption rates of different drug formulations have important implications for generic substitution.

Rectal administration of AEDs is important for patients who take drugs that lack parenteral formulations and for emergency situations when drugs cannot be administered either intravenously or orally. Rectal administration is also helpful when epileptic patients undergo surgery and cannot take their medications by mouth (8). Lipophilic AEDs such as diazepam are rapidly and well absorbed after rectal administration (9). Typically, drugs in solution are absorbed faster and more reliably than drugs in suppositories. Rectal administration also reduces first-pass hepatic metabolism.

Many AEDs have been given rectally, including diazepam, clonazepam, lorazepam, nitrazepam, ethosuximide, valproic acid, carbamazepine, paraldehyde, and phenytoin (8,10,11). Diazepam has an extensive history of rectal administration and has been used to interrupt serial seizures and status epilepticus and to prevent febrile seizures. After rectal administration of diazepam solutions in doses of 0.5 to 1 mg/kg, peak concentrations usually occur in less than 10 minutes (12,13). The absorption kinetics of carbamazepine in suspension is similar after oral and rectal administration, but rectal administration of carbamazepine suspension produces a strong defecatory urge (14).

Drug Elimination

The route of drug elimination plays an important role in determining a drug's pharmacokinetics and its vulnerability to pharmacokinetic interactions. Drugs that are eliminated mainly by hepatic metabolism to inactive metabolites include carbamazepine, ethosuximide, phenytoin, lamotrigine, zonisamide, and

various benzodiazepines. Several AEDs are eliminated by both hepatic biotransformation and renal excretion of unmetabolized drug. These include phenobarbital, felbamate, oxcarbazepine, tiagabine, topiramate, and valproate. All of these are subject to substantial hepatic metabolism, and altered hepatic processing affects serum levels substantially. Vigabatrin and gabapentin are eliminated exclusively by urinary excretion and are impervious to the effects of other drugs on hepatic drug metabolizing capacity.

The vulnerability of an AED to pharmacokinetic interactions depends on how it is eliminated, the extent of induction and/or inhibition of the elimination processes, and the resultant capacity of the drug-eliminating mechanisms relative to the amount of drug available for elimination. Additional factors that influence the propensity for a drug to participate in pharmacokinetic interactions include which enzymes catalyze its metabolism, which enzymes it induces, and which other drugs are shared as substrates by the enzyme. Drugs that are substrates for the same cytochrome P-450 component enzyme tend to interact, usually inhibiting each other's elimination. The effects of various AEDs on hepatic drug metabolizing capacity are summarized in Table 23-2.

Drugs that depend on hepatic biotransformation for elimination are prone to pharmacokinetic interactions. Among those drugs that are likely to participate in pharmacokinetic interactions, phenytoin is arguably the most sensitive because the phenytoin-eliminating enzymes are partially saturated at usual doses and concentrations.

In the 1990s knowledge about the hepatic cytochrome P-450 complex expanded considerably. The components of the P-450 system that are most relevant to the metabolism of AEDs are CYP2C9, CYP2C19, and CYP3A4. Information about these enzymes and their substrates are summarized in Table 23-3. Potent inducers of hepatic drug metabolism increase the activity of these three enzymes plus the activities of epoxide hydrolase and uridine diphosphate glucuronosyl transferase. Uridine diphosphate glucuronosyl transferase catalyzes the

Table 23-2. Effects of Antiepileptic Drugs on Hepatic Drug Metabolizing Enzyme Systems

Potent Inducers	Feeble or No Effect	General Inhibitor
Carbamazepine	Ethosuximide	Felbamate
Phenobarbital	Gabapentin	Valproate
Phenytoin	Lamotrigine	
Primidone	Oxcarbazepine	
	Tiagabine	
	Topiramate	
	Vigabatrin	
	Zonisamide	

Table 23-3. The Three Major Components of Cytochrome P 450 Drug Metabolizing Enzymes That Participate in the Elimination of Antiepileptic Drugs Are Listed Along with Their Substrates. These Relationships Provide the Basis for Numerous Pharmacokinetic Interactions (46–49). Shared Substrates That Produce Inhibition of Drug Metabolism Consistently Are Noted. Other Shared Substrates That Have Only Mild or Inconsistent Inhibitory Effects Are Listed as Other Substrates

CYP2C9	CYP2C19	CYP3A4
Major AED Substrates		
Phenytoin (major)	Phenytoin (minor)	Carbamazepine
		Zonisamide
		Several
		benzodiazepines
Other Substrates		
Amiodarone	Cimetidine	**Inhibited by**
Azapropazone	Diazepam	Fluvoxamine
Cotrimoxazole	Felbamate	Nefazadone
Disulfiram	Fluoxetine	Fluoxetine
Fluconazole	Imipramine	Sertraline
Metronidazole	Omeprazole	Macrolide
		antibiotics:
		erythromycin and
		trioleandomycin
Miconazole		Ketoconazole
Phenylbutazone	**Inhibited by**	Cyclosporin A
Propoxyphene	Felbamate	Miconazole
Stiripental	Fluvoxamine	
Sulfaphenazole	Topiramate	

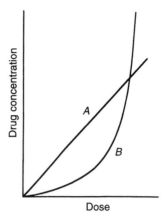

Figure 23-4. Dose versus concentration curves for drugs with linear (A) versus nonlinear (B) elimination kinetics.

formation of glucuronide conjugates and plays a major role in valproate elimination.

Valproic acid has a distinctive pattern of elimination. It is metabolized by β oxidation like a fatty acid, and it is conjugated with glucuronic acid to facilitate urinary excretion. Underdevelopment of the glucuronidation pathway is the major reason infants and young children eliminate valproate slowly.

Valproate and felbamate are inhibitors of hepatic drug metabolism. This has important implications for pediatric polytherapy of epilepsy. The addition of valproate substantially increases lamotrigine and phenobarbital concentrations. Furthermore, in children, valproate approximately doubles the $t_{1/2}$ of tiagabine with average the $t_{1/2}$ increasing from 3.2 to 5.7 hours (15) . Likewise, add-on felbamate increases the concentrations of phenobarbital, phenytoin, and valproate. When either valproate or felbamate is added to phenobarbital, phenytoin, and valproate, the doses of the preexistent drug should be reduced (16).

NONLINEAR KINETICS

Although the pharmacokinetics of most AEDs are linear or first-order, notable exceptions exist. When the mechanisms that result in drug elimination have linear

kinetics, a constant fraction of the drug is absorbed, transported, and eliminated per unit of time. The elimination mechanisms for phenytoin have a low capacity relative to the phenytoin concentrations that are usually present and are partially saturated (17,18). This results in nonlinear elimination kinetics and causes the relationship between the phenytoin dose and concentration to be nonlinear and intuitively unpredictable (Figure 23-4). Other AED pharmacokinetics that are nonlinear include gabapentin absorption and valproate binding. Gabapentin transport into brain is likely to be saturable, too. Nonlinear kinetic patterns are also designated as saturable, concentration-dependent, or dose-dependent.

When drugs are eliminated by processes with nonlinear kinetics, the fractional rate of drug disposition varies with the dose or drug concentration. As drug concentrations increase, the elimination mechanism becomes progressively saturated. This prolongs the half-life that is measured because a smaller percentage of the drug is eliminated per unit of time as the concentration increases. In this situation, the half-life that is observed should be designated as the $t_{50\%}$ to differentiate it from the usual $t_{1/2}$.

When drug elimination has nonlinear kinetics the apparent half-life ($t_{50\%}$) changes with the dose or concentration. The apparent half-life is directly proportional to the initial concentration that is present when the half-life is measured (19) Thus, increasing doses lead to disproportionate increases in drug concentrations. When drug doses are reduced, the opposite occurs; small reductions in dose can cause precipitous declines in drug concentration. Finally, the amount of drug in the body and the concentration of the drug in blood progressively increase if the dosing rate exceeds the capacity for drug elimination.

$$t_{50\%} = \frac{0.5Ci}{V_{\max}} + \frac{K_m(\ln 2)}{V_{\max}} \qquad (5)$$

The Michaelis-Menten equations that describe the kinetics of enzyme reactions can be applied to describe nonlinear drug elimination (6). This is done by measuring drug levels at two or more steady states and then solving for the nonlinear kinetic parameters — the maximal reaction velocity (V_{max}) and the drug concentration at which the reaction rate is one-half of the maximal elimination velocity (K_m). The critical assumption that underlies these calculations is that at steady state the rate of drug dosing equals the rate of drug elimination. Hence, at steady state the dosing rate equals the reaction velocity. Similarly, the drug concentration is analogous to a substrate concentration. To calculate the nonlinear kinetic parameters V_{max} and K_m, you need to know two or more pair of doses and concentrations. Several methods have been described for calculating V_{max} and K_m (20). These are discussed further in Chapter 29.

$$V = \frac{V_{max} \cdot C}{K_m + C} \qquad (6)$$

For drugs with nonlinear kinetics, varying the absorption rate changes the apparent bioavailability. Martis and Levy described the effects of bioavailability (F), absorption rate (k_a), K_m, and V_{max} on the rate of phenytoin concentration change (21).

$$dC/dt = k_a F C_0 e^{-kat} - K_1 C - \left[\frac{V_{max} C}{K_m + C} \right] \qquad (7)$$

In this equation k_a is the first-order absorption rate; C_0 is the drug concentration at zero time; C is the concentration at any time t; F is the bioavailability or fraction of the drug that is ultimately absorbed; and K_1 is the overall apparent first-order rate constant. This equation has been used to evaluate the relationship between absorption rate and apparent bioavailability (22). Based on computer simulations using average values of K_m and V_{max}, the apparent bioavailability declines by 25 percent as the half-time for absorption increases from 0 (IV administration) to 1.2 hours.

DRUG-PROTEIN BINDING

Ordinarily, only total (bound plus unbound) AED levels are measured. However, it is the unbound drug concentration in plasma that is in equilibrium with the unbound drug concentration in brain. The unbound level correlates better with drug action than the total level (23,24). Nevertheless, measuring the total drug concentration in plasma usually works well because total concentrations correlate highly with the unbound concentrations in most patients.

Various AEDs differ in the extent to which they are bound to serum constituents (25,26) (Table 23-4). The binding of ethosuximide, phenobarbital, and

Table 23-4. Binding of Antiepileptic Drugs to Serum Proteins (18,50,51)

Drug	Percent Unbound
Carbamazepine	27–40
Ethosuximide	90–100
Felbamate	78–64
Gabapentin	100
Lamotrigine	35–45
Oxcarbazepine	60
Phenobarbital	50–55
Phenytoin	7–15
Primidone	70–100
Tiagabine	4
Topiramate	83–91
Valproic acid (high)	10–30
Valproic acid (low)	8–10
Vigabatrin	100
Zonisamide	50–60

primidone is so low as to be clinically irrelevant. However, the binding of carbamazepine, phenytoin, and valproate is sufficiently high that significant changes in unbound drug levels occur when binding is altered (25). Conditions that cause hypoalbuminemia, such as renal disease and hepatic disease, and certain drug interactions with acidic compounds, such as fatty acids, aspirin, and valproate, increase the unbound drug concentrations of phenytoin and carbamazepine. Newborns also have reduced drug-protein binding because of hypoalbuminemia (26). When drug-protein binding is disturbed, therapeutic ranges based on total levels of phenytoin and carbamazepine no longer apply.

High concentrations of valproate exceed the binding capacity of plasma constituents, resulting in a nonlinear relationship between the total valproate level and the unbound valproate level (27). When total valproate levels are high, the unbound valproate level increases disproportionately.

ADJUSTING DOSES AND THE APPLICATION OF DRUG LEVEL MEASUREMENTS

The practical worth of any drug is specified by its therapeutic index. The therapeutic index is defined as the dose that produces toxicity divided by the dose that produces the desired therapeutic effect. Most AEDs have a narrow therapeutic index compared with antibiotic drugs such as penicillin. Furthermore, there is great variability in the therapeutic index of AEDs among individual patients because different types of seizures have variable susceptibility to drugs and patients vary in their sensitivity to dose-related neurotoxicity.

Among groups of patients the AEDs seem to have therapeutic indices of 2 to 4. However, the therapeutic index is often much lower in individual patients. Approximately 15 percent of patients are not adequately treated with any of the currently available drugs because intolerable dose-related neurotoxicity occurs at doses and levels that are less than those required to prevent the patient's seizures. In clinical practice this high degree of heterogeneity among patients with epilepsy makes it necessary to adjust the doses of AEDs on an individual, patient-by-patient basis. Published therapeutic ranges provide only loose and often unreliable guidelines to adequate therapy.

GENERIC ANTIEPILEPTIC DRUG FORMULATIONS

Generic substitution of AEDs has the potential to reduce the cost of antiepileptic therapy. Generic formulations are produced by several manufacturers and are distributed by more numerous intermediate suppliers. These factors facilitate low cost through open-market competition but make it difficult to track down the origin of a specific generic formulation.

Despite the need for low-cost antiepileptic therapy, the overriding goal of treating epilepsy with antiepileptic drugs is to administer enough drug to prevent seizures while maintaining drug levels below those which cause dose-related neurotoxicity in the individual patient. In practical terms, fluctuations in antiepileptic drug levels between doses need to be minimized.

As discussed previously, the magnitude of expected fluctuation in levels between doses depends on two factors: first, the drug's elimination rate or half-life, and second, the absorption rate. Because generic AEDs tend to have faster absorption rates than brand-name products, generic substitution sometimes increases the fluctuations in levels between doses, increasing the risk of both subtherapeutic and toxic levels (Figure 23-5). For certain drugs such as phenobarbital, which has a very long half-life, this is a trivial issue and generic substitution is indicated.

The problems that result from switching among formulations with different absorption rates are

most severe for phenytoin because it has nonlinear kinetics. Different phenytoin formulations with different absorption rates have different apparent bioavailability. When a formulation is absorbed rapidly, it produces a higher peak concentration, which in turn causes the apparent half-life to be prolonged. As a result, steady-state concentrations can change significantly when phenytoin formulations are switched. Generic substitution of phenytoin should be prohibited for this reason.

For carbamazepine, which has an intermediate to short half-life (18 hours or less), depending on the patient, the issue of generic substitution is complex. Changing the formulation can modify the extent of fluctuation between doses but does not alter the average concentration at steady state unless there also is a problem with tablet dissolution and bioavailability. For some patients who require only low carbamazepine levels to hold seizures in abeyance, generic substitution works well. For others who have a narrow therapeutic index for carbamazepine, generic substitution is highly problematic. These types of patients are at risk for both toxicity and recurrent seizures if they are switched to a formulation that is more rapidly absorbed. Thus, the patient and the treating physician should be consulted when generic carbamazepine substitution is contemplated.

EFFECT OF AGE ON ANTIEPILEPTIC DRUG PHARMACOKINETICS

Age and prior drug exposure affect the child's capacity for drug elimination (28). For the purposes of categorizing the affects of age on drug elimination, the following groups have been used: newborns (birth–6 weeks), infants (6 weeks–12 months), children (1 year–11 years), adolescents (11 years–15 years), adults (>15 years). These age groupings are somewhat arbitrary because the pharmacokinetic changes that occur are gradual and because of individual variation in growth and maturation. Adolescence is heralded in individual patients by the transition from Tanner stage 1 to stage 2. For each age group, the children who have prior drug exposure need to be considered separately from those who lack prior drug treatment.

Newborns exposed to drugs in utero usually eliminate AEDs at rates that are comparable to those of adults (18). The older AEDs that induce drug-metabolizing pathways in adults also do so prenatally and postnatally. Drugs such as valproate that inhibit hepatic drug elimination do so dramatically in newborns and young children. Valproate has an extremely long half-life in newborns and infants who have not been exposed to other inducing agents. Furthermore,

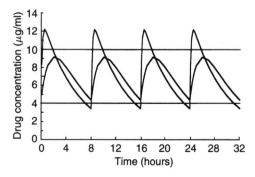

Figure 23-5. Effect of rapid versus slow absorption rate on fluctuations in drug levels between doses. Reproduced with permission from Dodson WE. Aspects of antiepileptic drug treatment in children. *Epilepsia* 1988; 29(Suppl 3):S10–S14.

most newborns who have seizures do not have prior intrauterine drug exposure. Consequently, they tend to eliminate AEDs far more slowly than any other age group. Furthermore, the most common cause of neonatal seizures, perinatal asphyxia, may be associated with abnormal hepatic and renal function, which also retard drug elimination. Although the neonatal pharmacokinetic effects of intrauterine exposure to drugs that have become available in the 1990s, such as oxcarbazepine, lamotrigine, gabapentin, and topiramate, they are unlikely to have much impact because they do not induce hepatic drug metabolism.

The postnatal maturation of renal function and hepatic systems for drug conjugation is well recognized. Renal function increases rapidly in the first day of life and reaches nearly adult capacity by age 3 weeks. Immature hepatic phase II conjugation of nonpolar compounds to water soluble glucuronides is one reason for slow elimination of AEDs, especially valproate, by newborns and infants (29). The maturation of hepatic phase I biotransformation of drugs via the cytochrome P-450 system of enzymes varies according to the particular enzymatic pathway.

Different components of the cytochrome P-450 system mature at different times during gestation and postnatally. The capacity to carry out aromatic oxidations (the principle metabolic pathway for phenytoin and phenobarbital) develops early in gestation. No significant differences have been found between premature and full-term newborns in the development of aromatic oxidations. Postnatally this pathway is induced extensively and has very high capacity by the end of the neonatal period. In fact, infants who have been treated for neonatal seizures have the greatest relative capacity to oxidize these drugs. However, N-dealkylation is more variable (30). Premature newborns have less capacity than full-term newborns to metabolize drugs such as diazepam and methylxanthines via this pathway. Both of these pathways, aromatic oxidations and N-dealkylation, are induced by intrauterine drug exposure to drugs such as phenobarbital and phenytoin but not by exposure to valproate. In the absence of prior drug treatment, the newborn's relative capacity for N-dealkylation is approximately 20 percent of adult values at birth and gradually increases to adult capacity by age 2 years (31).

The pharmacokinetics of AEDs change during the neonatal period. After loading doses have been given and maintenance drug therapy is under way, several factors act simultaneously to reduce drug concentrations during the neonatal period. These include accelerating drug elimination, changing routes of drug administration, and recovery from hepatic, renal, or GI dysfunction related to systemic disease. Newborns with seizures experience dramatic increases in the clearance of most of the AEDs during the neonatal period (18). Increases of two- to fourfold are common for phenobarbital and phenytoin, causing drug levels to decline by 50 percent to 75 percent if constant doses are given. The effects of perinatal disease on drug dose requirements are subtle but can be identified in groups of newborns. For example, newborns with perinatal asphyxia have lower relative clearance for phenobarbital than newborns with seizures due to other causes. The relative clearance of phenobarbital of 4.1 ml/kg/h by asphyxiated newborns is approximately 50 percent lower than the average phenobarbital clearance of 8.7 ml/kg/h by nonasphyxiated newborns (32). This predicts that at equivalent doses the levels in asphyxiated newborns will be twice as high.

Switching from IV to oral drug administration leads to slower drug absorption, reducing and delaying peak concentrations. In the case of phenytoin, slowed absorption causes a reduction in the apparent bioavailability of 20 percent to 30 percent (22).

Because drug clearance increases during the neonatal period, it is necessary to increase the dose to sustain uniform drug concentrations. However, most neonatal seizures are symptomatic of disorders that are abating during the neonatal period. Therefore, declining drug levels create fewer problems than might be expected because the intensity of the epileptic process tends to abate concurrently.

After the neonatal period, there are two major differences in the pharmacokinetics of AEDs among children and adults: children have higher relative clearance, and children have greater within-group variability in elimination kinetics (18,28). The effect of age on relative clearance is similar for most of the AEDs. Infants have the highest relative clearances, which are three- to fourfold greater than adult values. The relative clearance declines with advancing age until adult values are reached in late childhood or adolescence (Figure 23-6). Among specific age groups the standard deviation of the average clearance is relatively greater in younger patients. For example, the coefficient of variation* for relative clearance of phenytoin is more than 50 percent of the average value for children who are younger than 5 years old (33). For this reason, the relationship between drug doses and levels are more unpredictable in children than in adults. Considerable trial and error are often required to adjust children's drug levels.

Drug levels are surprisingly stable during the middle and later years of childhood because increases in body mass are offset by declining relative drug clearance. This means that children do not outgrow their drug doses frequently. Although the adolescent

---

* The coefficient of variation is the standard deviation divided by the mean times 100.

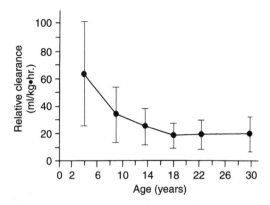

Figure 23-6. Effect of age on relative clearance of phenytoin. The vertical bars indicate one standard deviation. Drawn from data reported by Guelen (30). Reproduced with permission from Dodson WE. Kinetics of antiepileptic drugs in children. In: Schoolar JC, Claghorn JL, eds. *The Kinetics of Psychiatric Drugs.* New York: Brunner/Mazel, 1979:227–242.

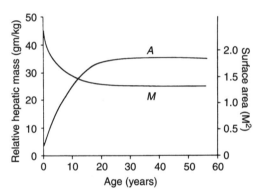

Figure 23-7. Relationship between age and body surface area (A) and between age and relative hepatic mass. Data from Korenchevsky (34) were used to create the figure.

growth spurt does occasionally necessitate dosage adjustments, dramatic changes in relative drug clearance are scarce during adolescence. Noncompliance is far more common and causes drug levels to vary erratically.

The factors that underlie the age-related changes in drug clearance of all of the AEDs correlate with the changes that occur in relative hepatic mass, relative caloric requirements, and surface area relative to body mass during growth to adult size. Compared with adults, children have larger surface area relative to body mass and they are hypermetabolic in order to maintain constant body temperature. With growth and increasing body mass, the surface area relative to body mass decreases, reducing the relative area that is available for radiant heat loss. Concomitantly, the relative hepatic mass and relative production of heat both decline (34) (Figure 23-7). Since most AEDs are eliminated by hepatic biotransformation, the declining relative hepatic mass coincides with the decline in drug clearance that occurs with growth. Thus, the

age-related pattern of declining relative drug clearance seems to be a by-product of growth in warm-blooded homeotherms and results from size-related differences in metabolic rate.

ANTIEPILEPTIC DRUGS IN BREAST MILK

Maternal treatment with AEDs is not a contraindication to breast-feeding (35,36). However, the issue of maternal drug administration and breast feeding is somewhat controversial because of conflicting opinions and recommendations in the literature. Data regarding transplacental partition ratios and breast milk to maternal serum concentration ratios are limited largely to case reports. The anecdotal data that are available, however, are consistent with expectations. Furthermore, newborns who were exposed chronically to inducing drugs in utero are born with induced drug elimination and may be tolerant to sedative drug actions. If questions arise about the contribution of the AED to a specific symptom in the infant, measuring drug levels in the infant may provide some insight (37).

The amounts of phenytoin, carbamazepine, lamotrigine, vigabatrin, and valproate that are acquired via nursing are generally insignificant (37–44) (Table 23-5). Although isolated case reports describe both neonatal sedation and withdrawal symptoms after prenatal intrauterine and postnatal breast milk–acquired barbiturate exposures, maternal barbiturate therapy is not an absolute contraindication to nursing. Highly lipid-soluble drugs such as diazepam readily penetrate breast milk and theoretically could lead the newborn to accumulate sedating levels, but this rarely occurs. Although the concentration of ethosuximide in breast milk is approximately 90 percent of the maternal levels, the significance of ingesting this amount is not known (39,45)

Table 23-5. Pharmacokinetics of Antiepileptic Drugs Acquired from Maternal Sources (18,52)

Drug	Half-Life of Transplacental AEDs in Newborn (hours)	Percent of Serum Level in Breast Milk Average	S.D.
Carbamazepine	6–44	41	16.8
Ethosuximide	41	94	6
Lamotrigine		56–62	
Phenobarbital	41–628	41	15
Phenylethylmalonamide	35 (6)	76	15
Phenytoin	7–69	18.6	15.7
Primidone	8-83	72	15
Valproic acid	47 (15)	27	15

REFERENCES

1. Gibaldi M, Perrier D. *Pharmacokinetics*. New York: Marcel Dekker, 1975.

2. Greenblatt DJ, Koch-Weser J. Clinical pharmacokinetics. *New Engl J Med* 1975; 293:702–705.

3. Greenblatt DJ, Koch-Weser J. Clinical pharmacokinetics. *New Engl J Med* 1975; 293:964–970.

4. Greenblatt DJ, Shader RI. *Pharmacokinetics in Clinical Practice*. Philadelphia: WB Saunders, 1985.

5. Riegelman S, Loo J, Rowland M. Shortcomings in pharmacokinetic analysis by conceiving the body to exhibit properties of a single compartment. *J Pharm Sci* 1968; 57:117–123.

6. Levy RE, Unadkat JD. General principles. Drug absorption, distribution, and elimination. In: Levy R, Mattson R, Meldrum B, Penry JK, Dreifuss FE, eds. *Antiepileptic Drugs*. 3rd ed. New York: Raven Press, 1989:1–22.

7. Brachet-Lierman A, Goutieres F, Aicardi J. Absorption of phenobarbital after intramuscular administration of single large doses. *J Pediatr* 1975; 87:624–626.

8. Woody RC, Golladay ES, Fiedorek-SC. Rectal anticonvulsants in seizure patients undergoing gastrointestinal surgery. *J Pediatr Surg* 1989; 24:474–477.

9. de Boer AG, Moolenaar F, de Leede LG, Breimer DD. Rectal drug administration: clinical pharmacokinetic considerations. *Clin Pharmacokinet* 1982; 7:285–311.

10. Graves NM, Kreil RL, Jones-Saete C. Bioavailability of rectally administered lorazepam. *Clin Neuropharmacol* 1987; 10:555.

11. Dulac O, Aicardi J, Rey E, Olive G. Blood levels of diazepam after single rectal administration. *J Pediatr* 1978; 31:1047–1050.

12. Franzoni E, Carboni C, Lambertini A. Rectal diazepam: a clinical and EEG study after a single dose in children. *Epilepsia* 1983; 24:35–41.

13. Graves NM, Kriel RL. Rectal administration of antiepileptic drugs in children. *Pediatr Neurol* 1987; 3:321–326.

14. Graves NM, Kriel RL, Jones-Saete C, Cloyd JC. Relative bioavailability of rectally administered carbamazepine suspension in humans. *Epilepsia* 1985; 26:429–433.

15. Gustavson LE, Boellner SW, Granneman GR, et al. A single-dose study to define tiagabine pharmacokinetics in pediatric patients with complex partial seizures. *Neurology* 1997; 48:1032–1037

16. Riva R, Albani F, Contin M, Baruzzi A. Pharmacokinetic interactions between antiepileptic drugs. Clinical considerations. *Clin Pharmacokinet* 1996; 31:470–493.

17. Arnold K, Gerber N. The rate of decline of diphenylhydantoin in human plasma. *Clin Pharmacol Ther* 1970; 11:121–135.

18. Dodson, WE. Special pharmacokinetic considerations in children. *Epilepsia* 1987; 8(Suppl 1):S56–S70.

19. Dodson, WE. Nonlinear kinetics of phenytoin in children. *Neurology* 1982; 32:42–48.

20. Mullen PW, Foster RW. Comparative evaluation of six techniques for determining Michaelis-Menten parameters relating phenytoin dose and steady-state concentrations. *J Pharm Pharmacol* 1979; 31:100–104.

21. Martis L, Levy RH. Bioavailability calculations for drugs showing simultaneous first-order and capacity-limited elimination kinetics. *J Pharmacokinet Biopharmaceut* 1973; 1:381–383.

22. Dodson WE, Bourgeois BF. Changing kinetic patterns of phenytoin in newborns. In: Wasterlain CG, Vert P, eds. *Neonatal Seizures*. New York: Raven Press, 1990:271–276.

23. Koch-Wesser J, Sellers EM. Binding of drugs of serum albumin (first of two parts). *New Engl J Med* 1976; 294:311–316.

24. Koch-Wesser J, Sellers EM. Binding of drugs of serum albumin (second of two parts). *New Engl J Med* 1976; 294:526–531.

25. Dodson WE. Aspects of antiepileptic drug treatment in children. *Epilepsia* 1988; 29(Suppl 3):S10–S14.

26. Krasner J, Yaffe SJ. Drug-protein binding in the neonate. In: Morselli PL, Garattini S, and Sereni F, eds. *Basic and Therapeutic Aspects of Perinatal Pharmacology*. New York: Raven Press, 1975:357–366.

27. Riva R, Albani F, Franzoni E, et al. Valproic acid free fraction in epileptic children under chronic monotherapy. *Ther Drug Mon* 1983; 5:197–200.

28. Dodson, WE. Antiepileptic drug utilization in children. *Epilepsia* 1984; 25(Suppl 2):S132–S139.

29. Gal P, Oles KS, Gilman JT, Weaver R. Valproic acid 1. efficacy, toxicity, and pharmacokinetics in neonates with intractable seizures. *Neurology* 1988; 38:467–471.

30. Aranda JV, MacLeod SM, Renton KW, Eade NR. Hepatic microsomal drug oxidation and electron transport in newborn infants. *J Pediatr* 1974; 85:534–542.

31. Rating D, Jager-Roman E, Nau H, Kuhnz W, Helge H. Enzyme induction in neonates after fetal exposure to antiepileptic drugs. *Ped Pharmacol* 1983; 3:209–218.

32. Gal P, Toback J, Erkan NV, Boer HR. The influence of asphyxia on phenobarbital dosing requirements in neonates. *Dev Pharmacol Ther* 1984; 7:145–152.

33. Guelen PJM. General discussion. In: Schneider J, Janz D, Gardner-Thorpe C, Meinardi H, Sherwin AL, eds. *Clinical Pharmacology of Anti-epileptic Drugs*. New York: Springer-Verlag, 1974:2–45.

34. Korenchevsky V. *Physiological and Pathological Aging*. New York: Hafner Publishing Company, 1961:160–162.

35. Roberts RJ. *Drug Therapy in Infants*. Philadelphia: WB Saunders, 1984:346–372.

36. Yerby MS. Problems and management of the pregnant woman with epilepsy. *Epilepsia* 1987; 28(Suppl 3):S29–S36.

37. Wong SH. Monitoring of drugs in breast milk. *Ann Clin Lab Sci* 1985; 15:100–105.

38. Nau H, Kuhnz W, Egger HJ, Rating D, Helge H. Anticonvulsants during pregnancy and lactation. Transplacental, maternal and neonatal pharmacokinetics. *Clin Pharmacokinet* 1982; 7:508–543.

39. Rating D, Nau H, Kuhnz W, Jager-Roman E, Helge H. Antiepileptika in der neugeborenenperiode. *Monatsschr Kinderheilkd* 1983; 131:6–12

40. Tomson T, Ohman I, Vitols S. Lamotrigine in pregnancy and lactation: a case report. *Epilepsia* 1997; 38: 1039–1041.

41. Tran A, O'Mahoney T, Rey E, et al. Vigabatrin: placental transfer in vivo and excretion into breast milk of the enantiomers. *Br J Clin Pharmacol* 1998; 45:409–411.

42. Brodie MJ. Management of epilepsy during pregnancy and lactation. *Lancet* 1990; 336:426–427.

43. Johannessen SI. Pharmacokinetics of valproate in pregnancy: mother-foetus-newborn. *Pharm Weekbl Sci* 1992; 14:114–117.

44. Rambeck B, Kurlemann G, Stodieck SR, May TW, Jurgens U. Concentrations of lamotrigine in a mother on lamotrigine treatment and her newborn child. *Eur J Clin Pharmacol* 1997; 51:481–484.

45. Tomson T, Villen T. Ethosuximide enantiomers in pregnancy and lactation. *Ther Drug Monit* 1994; 16:621–623.

46. Levy RH. Cytochrome P450 isozymes and antiepileptic drug interactions. *Epilepsia* 1995; 36(Suppl 5):S8–S13.

47. Sproule BA, Naranjo CA, Brenmer KE, Hassan PC. Selective serotonin reuptake inhibitors and CNS drug interactions. A critical review of the evidence. *Clin Pharmacokinet* 1997; 33:454–471.

48. Glue P, Banfield CR, Perhach JL, et al. Pharmacokinetic interactions with felbamate. In vitro-in vivo correlation. *Clin Pharmacokinet* 1997; 33:214–224.

49. Nakasa H, Nakamura H, Ono S, et al. Prediction of drug-drug interactions of zonisamide metabolism in humans from in vitro data. *Eur J Clin Pharmacol* 1998; 54:177–183.

50. Natsch S, Hekster YA, Keyser A, et al. Newer anticonvulsant drugs: role of pharmacology, drug interactions and adverse reactions in drug choice. *Drug Saf* 1997; 17:228–240.

51. Rambeck B, Kurlemann G, Stodieck SR, May TW, Jurgens U. Concentrations of lamotrigine in a mother on lamotrigine treatment and her newborn child. *Eur J Clin Pharmacol* 1997; 51:481–484.

52. Tomson T, Ohman I, Vitols S. Lamotrigine in pregnancy and lactation: a case report. *Epilepsia* 1997; 38:1039–1041.

53. Riggs DS. *The Mathematical Approach to Physiological Problems.* Baltimore: Williams and Wilkins, 1972.

54. Dodson WE. Kinetics of antiepileptic drugs in children. In: Schoolar JC, Claghorn JL, eds. *The Kinetics of Psychiatric Drugs.* New York: Brunner/Mazel, 1979:227–242.

CHAPTER 24

Dosage Form Considerations in the Treatment of Pediatric Epilepsy

William R. Garnett, Pharm.D., and James C. Cloyd, Pharm.D.

Drugs are rarely administered in their pure form. Because of the difficulties in accurately administering small quantities of the pure chemical, drugs are compounded into dosage forms that facilitate administration. These dosage forms offer the ability to individualize drug administration; however, ignoring the differences among dosage forms can result in a failure of the patient to receive full therapeutic benefit of the medication.

THEORETICAL ASPECTS IN ANTIEPILEPTIC DOSAGE FORM SELECTION

Intravenous Formulations

When an antiepileptic drug (AED) is administered intravenously, high blood drug concentrations may be reached very quickly, allowing the drug to rapidly distribute throughout the body (1,2). Only drugs that are water-soluble or that are soluble in a solvent that has little or no pharmacologic activity can be formulated for an intravenous (IV) dosage form. In some cases (e.g., phenytoin), the solvent may contribute to the toxicity that results from excessively rapid infusion (3). Intravenous dosage forms usually are more expensive than oral formulations. The IV administration of AEDs requires the presence of trained medical personnel and specialized equipment, such as infusion pumps and monitoring equipment, which also add to the cost of therapy. Therefore, IV drug administration is indicated only when rapid attainment of blood levels is needed, as in status epilepticus or when the patient is unable or unwilling to take medications by mouth.

Oral Formulations

Following oral administration, capsules or tablets first must disintegrate, liberating the drug, which then must dissolve in an un-ionized state into intraintestinal fluids before being absorbed (Figure 24-1). While immediate-release drugs are designed to be liberated in the stomach, other drugs, such as Depakote, are formulated to delay drug liberation until the drug reaches the small intestine. Other medications, such as Tegretol and Carbatrol, are liberated throughout the gastrointestinal (GI) tract at controlled rates providing sustained release. The dissolution time, the time to dissolve in GI fluids, may be altered by the surface area of the particles. The smaller the particle size, the faster the rate of dissolution. Liquid dosage forms, such as solution in which the drug is already dissolved, and suspension in which the drug is suspended as very small particles, generally display more rapid absorption than solid dosage forms. The rate of absorption for

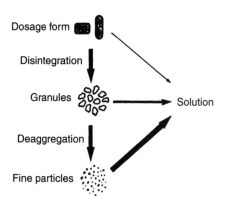

Figure 24-1. Drug disintegration and absorption. (Reproduced from ref. 1 by permission.)

oral formulations usually conforms to the following order: solutions > suspensions > capsules > tablets.

Immediate-release oral solids are designed to disperse all of the medication quickly after ingestion. This usually is followed by rapid absorption. If the drug has a short half-life, multiple daily doses are required to prevent peak concentrations, which may result in side effects, and trough concentrations, which may be associated with seizures. Multiple daily doses may result in poor compliance. There is a trend in pharmaceutical development to develop dosage forms that release drug slowly over time rather than all at once.

Dosage forms that are designed to release their drug content slowly have been referred to as controlled-release, prolonged release, time-release, slow-release, sustained-release, prolonged-action, or extended-action. Although some interchange these terms, there are technical differences. A controlled-release dosage form is a system in which the rate of release is regulated and is supposed to be constant during GI transit. A sustained-release dosage form releases its contents over an extended period of time. Sustained-release dosage forms provide for the immediate release of an amount of drug that is immediately absorbed and then gradual and continual release of additional drug over the dosing interval. The advantages of controlled-release and sustained-release dosage formulations are (1) reduction in blood drug level fluctuations, (2) enhanced patient convenience and adherence, (3) reduction in adverse side effects, and (4) reduction in health care costs. Potential disadvantages to controlled-release and sustained-release formulations are (1) prolonged effects if the patient develops an adverse drug reaction or is accidentally intoxicated, and (2) interactions may occur with the contents of the GI tract, and (3) changes in GI motility resulting in "dose dumping," or all of the drug being absorbed at once (4).

Most drugs are weak acids or weak bases and exist in solution as an equilibrium between the ionized and the un-ionized forms. In these cases, it is the un-ionized form in the gut that passively crosses the GI membrane. A continuous flow of blood to the GI tract ensures movement of drug from an area of high concentration in the gut to an area of relatively low concentration in the blood. Once a drug is dissolved, the rate of absorption is determined by the ratio of ionized to un-ionized forms because it is the un-ionized form that can diffuse across membranes. Weak acids are absorbed more rapidly at pH 1.0 than at pH 8.0, and the converse is true for weak bases because there is more of the un-ionized form present. The formulation of poorly soluble drugs as salts may enhance solubility and result in better absorption. Physiologic or pharmacologically induced changes in the GI pH may affect the disintegration

of tablets or capsules, the dissolution time, and/or the equilibrium between the ionized and un-ionized forms, which, alters the rate and/or amount of drug absorption.

Some drugs are absorbed by active transport processes. For example, gabapentin is carried across the GI membrane via a transport enzyme (5). Absorption may became saturated with this type of process. When the amount of drug in the GI tract is low relative to the number of transport enzyme-binding sites, the extent of absorption is high and constant. As the amount of drug approaches the capacity limits of the transport enzymes, the fraction of the dose that is absorbed per unit of time decreases. As a result, increases in dose produce less than proportional increases in serum concentration.

Some of the drug may be metabolized as it passes across the gut wall. Further metabolism may take place in the liver before the drug reaches the systemic circulation. This phenomenon is known as first-pass metabolism. Systemic bioavailability depends on the amount of drug absorbed across the gut wall and the degree of first-pass metabolism occurring in the GI tract and the liver before the drug reaches the systemic circulation. If a drug has extensive first-pass metabolism, it may not be suitable for oral administration.

The manufacturing process of the dosage form may affect absorption. There are no legal requirements for the excipients used in solid dosage formulations. Excipients may vary from manufacturer to manufacturer and cause different absorption rates that in vitro dissolution tests do not detect. A change in the excipients of a phenytoin capsule in Australia resulted in greater bioavailability and an epidemic of phenytoin toxicity (6,7). Other aspects of manufacturing may differ, such as tablet hardness and friability. The particle size of the active ingredient may also be different. Thus, there may be different rates and amounts of drug absorbed from the same dosage form made by different manufacturers. Sometimes there may be differences in absorption between lots of the same manufacturer.

Oral absorption may be altered by a variety of physiologic and pharmacologic phenomena. For example, food decreases the rate but not the extent of absorption of valproic acid, which results in a delayed time to peak (8). Food enhances the bioavailability of carbamazepine (9). Achlorhydria or the coadministration of drugs that reduce or neutralize gastric acid may alter disintegration and dissolution and affect absorption. Antacids in large doses decrease the absorption of phenytoin (10). For drugs with significant first-pass metabolism, food may alter hepatic blood flow and compete with liver enzymes to increase the systemic bioavailability of drugs. Foods and drugs may affect gastric emptying time and drug absorption.

Absorption usually is greater in the small intestine than in the stomach because the surface area is larger, the permeability is higher, and the blood flow is greater. Therefore, absorption may be altered by changes in gastric emptying and GI transient times. Diarrhea may decrease the absorption of phenytoin and other slowly absorbed drugs because GI transient time is increased and reduces drug contact time at intestinal absorption sites (3).

Age per se may alter absorption. In the newborn the intragastric pH and the efficiency of gut enzymes change rapidly (11,12). Because of relative achlorhydria in the newborn and infant, there should be an increased absorption of acid-labile drugs such as penicillin (13). Age effects on pharmacokinetics are discussed in Chapter 23.

Generic Formulations

When the patent of a drug expires, companies other than the innovator of the drug may manufacture the generic equivalent. The U.S. Food and Drug Administration (FDA) is concerned about generic equivalency, and generic manufacturers must compare their product with that of the innovator. This usually is done by administering equal doses of the brand-name formulation and the generic drug to a population of between 24 and 36 normal healthy adults. Multiple blood samples are collected to determine the amount of drug absorbed as assessed by the total area under the concentration time curve (AUC), the peak concentration (C_{max}), and the rate of drug absorption (time to C_{max}). The generic formulation must be within ± 20 percent of these values. Individual generic drugs do not have to be compared with each other. One drug (drug A) may have a 15 percent higher AUC than the innovator (drug B), and the other generic drug (drug C) may have a 15 percent lower AUC than the innovator. Therefore, two generic drugs might be considered bioequivalent to the innovator but would not be bioequivalent to each other. For drugs with a wide therapeutic index this should not cause a problem. However, most AEDs have a narrow therapeutic index, and these differences may be significant. For this reason, The American Academy of Neurology has cautioned against switching suppliers for carbamazepine and phenytoin (14).

Since generic drugs often are less expensive, they may offer an advantage for many patients. When generic drugs are prescribed, the patient should remain on the formulation from one supplier. Problems may arise when one generic product is used for 1 month and then another supplier is used for another month. Unfortunately, in some facilities the source of drug supply is determined by someone other than a pharmacist or physician. Clinicians should know when the source of an AED is being changed.

Intramuscular Formulations

Absorption of drugs from muscle and subcutaneous tissue is dependent on solubility, ionization, and tissue perfusion. Increases in tissue blood flow increase absorption. Physical activity that changes blood flow rates alters the rate of drug absorption from intramuscular (IM) injections. The locations of the injection site also influences the rate of absorption. A standard part of nursing care is to rotate the sites of injection to prevent damage to a particular area. Because different muscle tissues have varying perfusion rates, the rotation of injection sites may result in varying rates of absorption. Injections into muscle tissue have different rates of absorption than injections into fatty tissue. In contrast, the extent of absorption is 100 percent unless drug is degraded in the tissue. The injection of IM drugs always causes some degree of discomfort, may be irritating to the tissue, and in some cases may result in muscle damage. IM injections require skilled personnel, which limits their use. Therefore, IM injections should be limited to short-term situations.

Rectal Formulations

The rectum is a useful route of administration, although there is little intraluminal fluid and the absorptive surface is only 1/10,000 that of the upper GI tract. The disintegration and dissolution problems associated with oral dosage formulations also occur with rectal dosage formulations (15). Solutions and suppositories are the most commonly used rectal dosage forms. Suppositories usually are formulated with a quick-melting base such as cocoa butter. Adequate retention time in the rectum is essential for complete absorption from the rectal dosage forms. Highly lipid-soluble compounds are more rapidly absorbed than less soluble, ionized drugs. The inability to retain the suppository or solution diminishes the usefulness of this route of administration. In contrast to oral administration, first-pass metabolism is significantly reduced with rectal administration, particularly when drug is absorbed from the lower two-thirds of the rectum, where venous drainage bypasses the liver.

SELECTION OF PARENTERAL AND ORAL ANTIEPILEPTIC DOSAGE FORMS IN PEDIATRIC PATIENTS

The factors that influence the selection of a particular dosage form for a child include the need for rapid attainment of therapeutic blood concentrations, the importance of maintaining therapeutic concentrations throughout a dosing interval, the ability to swallow, the ability to retain a rectal dosage form, the palatability of the oral dosage form, and cost.

Ideally, the drug should be available in a parenteral form for IV and IM administration as well as in oral solid and liquid formulations. The availability of a rectal formulation would allow greater flexibility in dosing. Among the AEDs used for maintenance therapy, only phenytoin, phenobarbital, and valproic acid are available as parenteral formulations. Diazepam is now available in a gel formulation specifically designed for rectal administration.

For maintenance therapy, oral dosage forms are preferable because they are relatively inexpensive and easy to administer. Therefore, when the patient is able to swallow, the AED should be given orally. If the patient is not able to take a tablet or capsule, consideration should be given to chewable tablets or liquids. Patients with a nasogastric tube may be given liquid AEDs, which negates the need for chronic parenteral therapy. Obviously, liquid medicines should be palatable or capable of being mixed with beverages without interactions so that the patient is able to ingest the medicine. It is possible to give loading doses of oral medications to attain therapeutic concentrations more quickly. However, this is often neither rapid enough nor feasible when dealing with an emergency such as status epilepticus.

Phenytoin

Phenytoin is available in parenteral, capsule, chewable tablet, and suspension formulations. Phenytoin is poorly soluble in water; thus, the parenteral formulation contains propylene glycol and ethanol and is buffered to a pH of 12 to keep the drug in solution. The solvents have inherent pharmacologic activity, including cardiac arrhythmias and hypotension. The combination of co-solvent effects and the alkaline pH commonly cause pain and inflammation at the infusion site. Therefore, phenytoin infusions are limited to a rate no faster than 1 to 3 mg/kg/min in otherwise healthy children (3). Because of the high ionization constant (pK_a) of phenytoin, it is not stable in every IV solution. Phenytoin may be mixed with normal saline in concentration ranges of 2 to 20 mg/ml. Use of an in-line 20-micron filter is recommended to reduce the risk of infusing small particle precipitants. Admixtures should be stored for no longer than 24 hours (16).

Although the parenteral formulation of phenytoin may be given by IM injection, this route is not recommended. The high pK_a of phenytoin results in crystallizing in muscle tissue. This results in slow and erratic absorption (17). In addition, IM phenytoin is quite painful and may cause muscle damage (18).

Fosphenytoin is a phenytoin prodrug formed by the addition of a phosphate ester to the phenytoin molecule. The phosphate ester significantly increases the water solubility of fosphenytoin. The phosphate ester must be cleaved and the compound converted to phenytoin to exert pharmacologic activity. The conversion is done by systemic phosphatases that are found throughout the body. The conversion of fosphenytoin to phenytoin is rapid and complete. The phosphatases are not affected by age, gender, race, hepatic impairment, or renal function. An ex vivo study using blood obtained from premature infants and neonates demonstrated that fosphenytoin is converted to phenytoin in these populations (19).

Because fosphenytoin is more water-soluble than phenytoin, it does not require propylene glycol or ethanol to increase solubility. Fosphenytoin is compatible with all IV fluids, whereas phenytoin should only be admixed with normal saline. Fosphenytoin does not require an in-line filter as phenytoin does (20). Fosphenytoin may be given at a much faster IV infusion rate than phenytoin, and the infusion rate does not need to be altered because of age or underlying cardiac disease. The maximum rate of infusion of fosphenytoin is 150 mg/min compared with 50 mg/min for phenytoin. This means that the patient can be loaded in less time. Fosphenytoin is rapidly converted to phenytoin after administration, with a conversion half-life of approximately 15 minutes. Fosphenytoin is highly protein-bound, as is phenytoin. Therefore, fosphenytoin competes with phenytoin for binding sites, which increases the "free" or unbound portion of phenytoin. When both drugs are given at the maximum rate of administration, fosphenytoin achieves bioequivalency with phenytoin in 7 minutes. If the rate of phenytoin is slowed, higher concentrations of phenytoin may be achieved with the administration of fosphenytoin (21). Another advantage of fosphenytoin is that in comparative studies it causes less thrombophlebitis and less burning, pain, or irritation at the injection site. This results in fewer changes in the site of administration (22). The decreased venous irritation is a particular advantage in premature infants, neonates, and children, in whom venous access is a serious problem. The primary side effects of fosphenytoin are pruritus and paresthesias, which are common to phosphate esters and disappear with a reduction in the infusion rate or when the infusion is completed.

Fosphenytoin can safely be given intramuscularly. Peak phenytoin concentrations occur about 3 hours following IM fosphenytoin. However, free phenytoin concentrations in the accepted target range occur in approximately 30 minutes after an IM injection of fosphenytoin (22a). There is no pain or necrosis associated with fosphenytoin after IM administration, and the absorption is rapid and complete. Loading doses

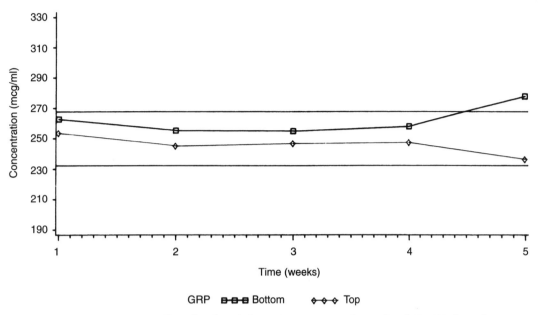

Figure 24-2. Long-term concentration vs. time effect of packaged phenytoin suspension. "Bottom" and "Top" indicate that concentrations were measured in suspensions taken from the bottom and top of the bottle, respectively. (Reproduced from *Neurology* February 1990 by permission.)

of 20 mg/kg have been safely given intramuscularly. In adults, volumes exceeding 20 mL have been safely given as a single injection (22b). When given as replacement therapy, fosphenytoin is completely converted to phenytoin, whereas oral phenytoin capsules are 92 percent phenytoin. Therefore, the trough concentrations may increase. If the patient is at the point of enzyme saturation for phenytoin metabolism, there may be a significant increase in blood concentrations (23).

As noted in Chapter 29, the various formulations of phenytoin differ in content of phenytoin (Table 24-1). The capsule and parenteral formulations of phenytoin contain sodium phenytoin and are only 92 percent phenytoin. The suspension and chewable tablet formulations of phenytoin contain phenytoin acid and

are 100 percent phenytoin. Because of the Michaelis-Menten kinetics of phenytoin, these salt differences should be considered when switching dosage forms. Although it would be anticipated that the rate of absorption of the phenytoin suspension would be faster than the rate of absorption from the capsule, a single-dose study in normal volunteers demonstrated that the time to peak concentration, C_{max}, and AUC time curve for phenytoin extended-release capsules were not different from these parameters for phenytoin suspension when the dose of the suspension was adjusted for the difference in salt concentration (24). It was postulated that the rate of absorption is more dependent on particle size than on formulation. There are also differences in the rate of absorption among the various manufacturers of phenytoin capsules. The innovator's formulation (Dilantin) provides an extended release. Some of the generic formulations provide faster release. Phenytoin is thus labeled as either prompt-release or extended-release capsules. The FDA recommends that only the extended-release capsules be used for once-a-day dosing (25). The difference in the rate and extent of absorption between the prompt-release and extended-release capsules may affect how rapidly peak concentrations of phenytoin can be obtained. The extended-release capsules display a slower rate and extent of absorption as the dose is increased. This suggests that oral doses need to be larger than IV doses to achieve the same concentration (26). However, if prompt-release capsules are used, phenytoin concentrations are achieved more rapidly, and the prompt-release capsule has been suggested as an alternative in situations in which an

Table 24-1. Phenytoin Content of Various Products

Product	Listed Strength	Phenytoin Content
Phenytoin capsule (phenytoin sodium)	100 mg	92 mg
Phenytoin capsule (phenytoin sodium)	30 mg	27.5 mg
Fosphenytoin parenteral (fosphenytoin sodium)	50 mg PE/mL	46 mg PE/mL
Phenytoin suspension (phenytoin)	125 mg/5 mL	125 mg/5 mL
Phenytoin chewable tablet (phenytoin)	50 mg	50 mg
Phenytoin parenteral (phenytoin sodium)	50 mg/mL	46 mg

PE = phenytoin equivalent

IV injection is not possible or practical (27). The chewable tablet seems to have an absorption profile similar to that of phenytoin extended-release capsules when adjusted for salt content.

Although the suspension dosage form has been considered to have rapid settling properties, a report measuring settling rates in bottles of phenytoin suspension that were well shaken and then left untouched revealed no differences in concentration between the top of the bottle and the bottom of the bottle from 15 minutes to 4 weeks after resuspension. Beyond 5 weeks after resuspension was there a difference between the aliquots taken from the top and the bottom of the bottle (28) (Figure 24-2). In the same study, a dose (5.0 ml) was measured every day simulating patient use by a well-shaken technique (vigorous shaking), a poorly shaken technique (inverted once), and an unshaken technique until the bottle was depleted. Only the unshaken technique demonstrated differences in the doses taken (Figure 24-3). It was concluded that phenytoin suspension requires minimal agitation to be uniformly mixed and that it has a slow rate of settling. The problems reported with phenytoin suspension in the past possibly reflect inaccurate measurement by the patient or a failure to understand the Michaelis-Menten kinetics of phenytoin. This dosage form may be very acceptable for young children or for patients with difficulty in swallowing. An accurate measuring device should be used for administration.

Carbamazepine

Carbamazepine is available as a chewable tablet, tablet, and suspension. A single-dose study in normal volunteers demonstrated that the bioavailability of chewable tablets is comparable to the bioavailability of swallowed tablets (29). The rate of absorption of carbamazepine suspension is faster than carbamazepine tablets in single-dose studies in normal volunteers (30). A multidose bioavailability study in epileptic patients comparing equal total daily doses of carbamazepine suspension administered three times a day to tablets administered twice a day also demonstrated that the suspension is absorbed faster than the tablets (Figure 24-4). However, there were no differences in the C_{max}, the AUC time curve, or the peak to trough fluctuations for either the parent drug or the 10,11-epoxide metabolite (31) (Table 24-2). If the faster absorption rate is not considered in scheduling dosage administration times, the suspension will produce higher peaks (greater chance of side effects) and lower troughs (greater chance of loss of efficacy) than a comparable dose using carbamazepine tablets.

There are controlled-release and sustained-release dosage forms of carbamazepine. The controlled-release formulation is Tegretol-XR®, which utilizes an osmotic release delivery system. The formulation is provided in a wax matrix with a permeable membrane. This allows water from gastric contents to enter the matrix and increase the osmotic pressure. This forces the drug out at a constant rate. For the 100-mg tablet, 10 mg

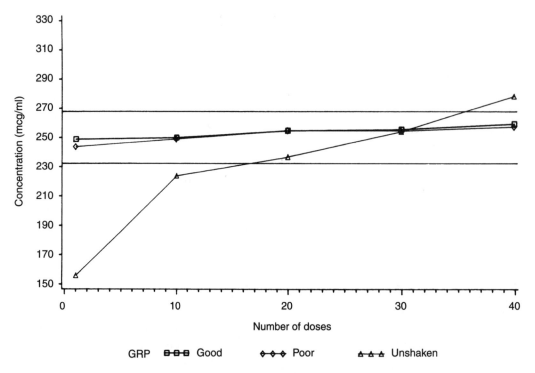

Figure 24-3. Effect of shaking techniques on concentration of dose of phenytoin. (Reproduced from *Neurology*, February 1990 by permission.)

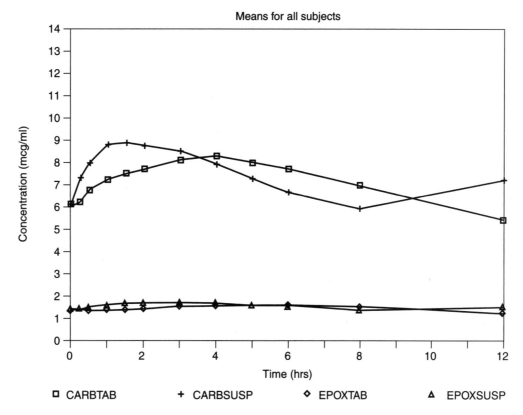

Figure 24-4. Twelve-hour concentration vs. time profile of carbamazepine tablets vs. suspension.

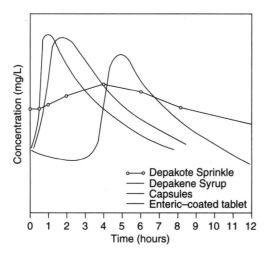

Figure 24-5. The effect of formulation on the time course of valproate absorption.

of drug is released per hour for the first 7 or 8 hours and then the rest of the drug is released. The casing of the tablet is excreted in the feces. Patients should be told that although casings will appear in the stool, the drug is being absorbed. Any disruption to the tablet results in a loss of the controlled-release design. Therefore, this controlled-release formulation must not be crushed, chewed, or opened (32). The sustained-release

formulation is Carbatrol®, which uses three different types of beads: immediate-release, extended-release, and enteric-release. This formulation is a capsule, and it may be opened and mixed with food. The ability to use this formulation as a "sprinkle" is an advantage in pediatric patients (33).

Both controlled-release and sustained-release dosage forms have been compared with immediate-release carbamazepine in patients with epilepsy. Patients were converted from four-times-a-day dosing with immediate-release carbamazepine to twice-a-day dosing with both formulations in separate studies. In both studies twice-a-day dosing with controlled-release or sustained-release tablets was bioequivalent to the four-times-a-day dosing with immediate-release tablets (32,33). The controlled-release formulation was compared with the sustained-release formulation in a randomized cross-over study in normal volunteers who were dosed for 5 days on each formulation. The two dosage formulations were found to be bioequivalent, although the sustained-release formulation had larger confidence intervals (34).

The advantage of controlled-release and sustained-release carbamazepine is that either may be given twice a day. This optimizes convenience and promotes compliance. In a pediatric patient who cannot or will not swallow oral solids, the sustained-release formulation can be opened and mixed with food.

Table 24-2. Pharmacokinetic Comparison of Carbamazepine Tablets and Suspension

Parameter	Tablet	Suspension	Statistical Significance	Power	CI (percent)
AUC $0- < 24$	192.1	196.9	NS	0.73	12.8
C_{max}	8.5	9.4	NS	0.97	18.4
T_{max}	3.7	1.5	$p < 0.05$	—	196.0
C_{min}	5.3	5.7	NS	<0.99	14.0
C_{max}					
C_{min}	1.7	1.7	NS	0.92	12.9
$Conc_{ss}$	8.0	8.2	NS	0.73	12.8

AUC = area under the curve; NS = not significant

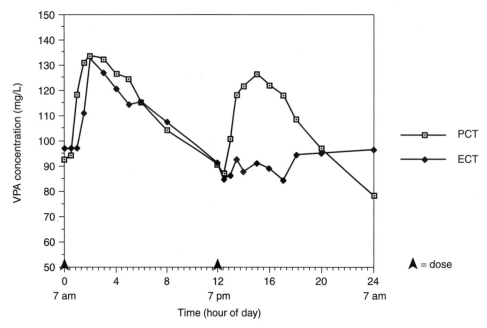

Figure 24-6. Twenty-four hour total valproate concentration-time profile following particle and enteric coated tablets. (Reproduced from ref. 30 by permission.)

Valproic Acid

Valproic acid is available as a soft gelatin capsule containing a liquid, an enteric-coated tablet, a coated particle (sprinkle) capsule, a syrup, and an IV solution. The bioavailability of the soft gelatin capsule formulation is comparable to the solution. The enteric-coated tablet was developed to delay dissolution of the drug until after it leaves the stomach, thereby reducing the incidence of nausea, vomiting, and other types of GI distress. Although the enteric coating does delay and slow absorption, it does not result in true sustained release of valproic acid. For most drugs the minimum (trough) concentration occurs just before the next dose. In contrast, the delayed absorption of enteric-coated valproic acid produces trough concentrations 2 to 4 hours after the dose when given on an empty stomach (Figure 24-7). Coadministration with food extends the time to the trough concentration from 2 to 8 hours

after administration, and peak concentrations may occur just before the next dose (35). These changes in normal absorption profiles must be considered in evaluating blood concentrations, particularly if the timing between drug administration and meals varies. Recently, a diurnal effect on valproic acid absorption from the enteric-coated tablet was also shown (36) (Figure 24-8). Valproic acid is absorbed more slowly, and the amount of drug absorbed is reduced at night. The enteric-coated dosage form should not be crushed before administering.

A coated particle (sprinkle) formulation of valproic acid is available. The sprinkle formulation is designed to provide slow consistent input, which minimizes peak to trough fluctuations (see Figure 24-5) (37). This dosage form allows the patient or parent to open the capsule and sprinkle the particles over food. It is intended for pediatric use and for patients who have difficulty swallowing solid dosage forms. This dosage

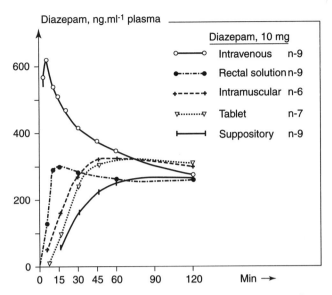

Figure 24-7. Plasma concentrations of diazepam following administration in different dosage forms. (Reproduced from ref. 30 by permission.)

form also is particularly useful for patients with large fluctuations between doses who require frequent dosing or who may experience distress with enteric-coated tablets.

The IV formulation, valproate sodium injection, is approved for use when initiating therapy or as replacement therapy for patients on maintenance valproate. Valproate sodium injection should not be given as an IM injection because tissue damage may result (38).

Phenobarbital and Primidone

Phenobarbital is available in a parenteral form, a tablet, and a solution. The parenteral form can be given by rapid IV infusion or by IM injection. Absorption from the oral formulations seems to be complete and relatively rapid. Primidone is available as a tablet and an oral suspension. Absorption from both formulations appears complete with peak concentrations occurring 2 to 6 hours after the dose (39).

Ethosuximide

Ethosuximide is available as a capsule and a solution. Absorption appears to be complete from both formulations. Ethosuximide has a long half-life even in children. However, some patients may develop GI side effects with once-a-day dosing and require twice-a-day dosing (39).

Newer Antiepileptic Drugs

The newer AEDs have been studied primarily in adults and administered primarily as oral solid dosage forms.

However, felbamate is approved for use in the Lennox-Gastaut syndrome and is available as a suspension formulation and a tablet formulation. Lamotrigine has recently received approval for use in the Lennox-Gastaut syndrome and is available in a tablet that readily disperses in water and can be easily given to children. Topiramate comes as a sprinkle as well as a tablet. Although gabapentin is very water-soluble, it has a very bad taste when given as a solution. Undoubtedly, new pediatric dosage forms will be developed for the newer AEDs as use in this population is approved.

RECTAL ADMINISTRATION OF ANTIEPILEPTIC DRUGS

Overview

The rectal route of administration is a practical alternative when oral or parenteral routes are not available (15) (Table 24-3). Rectal administration is often useful in the treatment of emergent conditions such as prolonged seizures or clusters of seizures and status epilepticus when access to a vein is delayed or when therapy is started at home. Additionally, rectal administration can substitute for oral administration of maintenance AEDs when the latter route is temporarily unavailable because of upper GI illnesses, dental procedures, abdominal surgery, or transient GI intolerance to medication (40). Occasionally, rectal administration is indicated when psychiatric or mentally handicapped patients refuse or are unable to take their medications. A commercial diazepam rectal formulation is available in the United States, and the parenteral solution can also be administered rectally.

Clonazepam

The injectable solution of clonazepam has been administered rectally to volunteers and patients (41,42). Doses in patients have ranged from 0.05 to 0.1 mg/kg, which produce peak serum concentrations 10 to 120 minutes after administration of the dose. There is no information on the extent of absorption.

Carbamazepine

Carbamazepine has been given rectally as a suspension, a suppository, and a viscous gel solution (30,43,44). The commercially available suspension, when diluted and given rectally, is bioequivalent to the tablet given orally but the peak concentration occurs later than when taken by mouth (30). The suspension is hypertonic, causing a strong urge to defecate. An extemporaneously prepared suppository has been evaluated in both healthy subjects and patients (43). It

Table 24-3. Antiepileptic Drugs Available for Rectal Administration

Drug	Treatment Usefulness	Dosage (mg/kg/dose)	Preparation	Pharmacokinetics	Comments
Carbamazepine	Maintenance	Same as oral	Oral suspension (dilute with equal volume of water) Suppository gel (CBZ powder dissolved in 20% alcohol and methyl hydroxy cellulose)	Peak concentration 4–8 h; 80% absorbed	Definite cathartic effect
Clonazepam	?Acute	0.02–0.1 mg	Suspension	Peak concentration 0.1–2 h	Onset may be too slow for acute use
Diazepam	Acute	0.2–0.5 mg	Parenteral solution	Effect in 2–10 min; peak concentration 2–30 min	Well tolerated; nordiazepam accumulates with repeated doses
Lorazepam	Acute	0.05–0.1 mg	Parenteral solution	Peak concentration 0.5–2 h	Well tolerated
Paraldehyde	Acute	0.3 mL	Oral solution (dilute with equal volume of mineral oil)	Effect in 20 min, peak concentration 2.5 h	Moderate cathartic effect; use glass syringe
Valproic acid	Acute	5–25 mg	Oral solution (dilute with equal volume of water)	Peak concentration 1–3 h	Definite cathartic effect
	Maintenance	Same as oral	VPA liquid from capsule mixed into Supocire C lipid base	Peak concentration 2–4 h; 80% absorbed	Well tolerated

was more consistently absorbed than the commercial tablet, with a mean bioavailability of 67 percent and a T_{max} of 12 hours. A viscous gel containing 200 mg of carbamazepine and 250 mg of methylhydroxycellulose dissolved in 5 mL of 20% alcohol was administered in a single patient and produced therapeutic serum concentrations (44). Rectal carbamazepine is absorbed too slowly to be useful in treating status epilepticus, but it may be tried as temporary replacement therapy when the oral route is not available.

Diazepam

Diazepam has been given rectally as a solution and a suppository. Rectal administration of diazepam solutions in children results in rapid and complete absorption, with peak concentrations attained within 5 to 15 minutes after administration (45–47) (Figure 24-8). Given the time needed to establish an IV line, the rectal administration of diazepam solution or gel is a practical alternative to IV diazepam in the acute management of severe seizures (48,49). A recently completed double-blind, placebo-controlled trial demonstrated that a rectal diazepam gel (Diastat) administered by parents or other caregivers was highly effective in interrupting

clusters of seizures and reducing subsequent emergent care (50). Another study has shown that home use of a rectally administered diazepam solution was safe and effective in controlling prolonged seizures and preventing febrile convulsions (51). Although suppositories are commercially available in some countries other than the United States, they are not recommended because absorption is slow and erratic.

Gabapentin

A recent report involving two children found that the bioavailability of a gabapentin solution given rectally ranged from 17 percent to 29 percent (52). Therefore, it should not be administered rectally.

Lorazepam

The commercially available parenteral formulation of lorazepam has been given rectally to volunteers and patients (53,54). Doses of 0.05 mg/kg stopped seizures in eight children. The bioavailability of rectally administered lorazepam was assessed in six volunteers who were given 2 mg of the parenteral solution. The T_{max} was 67 minutes, and the fraction absorbed averaged

86 percent with a range of 51 percent to 118 percent. The slow absorption of the parenteral solution limits the usefulness of rectal lorazepam for treatment of emergent conditions. Diazepam is absorbed more rapidly and is preferred for rectal administration.

Paraldehyde

Rectally administered paraldehyde has been widely used to control severe seizures, particularly in children (55,56). However, information on the efficacy, toxicity, and pharmacokinetics is limited. Rectal bioavailability is 75 percent to 90 percent versus 90 percent to 100 percent for the oral route. Time to peak concentrations after rectal or oral administration is 2.5 hours versus 0.5 hours. Paraldehyde should be diluted with an equal volume of olive oil or vegetable oil to reduce mucosal irritation.

Phenobarbital

There is no commercially available rectal dosage form for phenobarbital. Graves and coworkers gave seven volunteers phenobarbital sodium parenteral solution rectally and intramuscularly (57). After rectal administration absorption was 90 percent complete, with a time to peak concentration of 4.4 hours versus 2.1 hours for the IM injection. Suppositories containing phenobarbital sodium are more rapidly absorbed than phenobarbital acid given either orally or intramuscularly (58,59).

Phenytoin

Occasionally, there arises a need to administer phenytoin rectally, although no commercial rectal dosage form is available. Several studies of investigational suppository formulations have failed to demonstrate absorption. Rectal administration of phenytoin sodium parenteral solution in dogs produced low but measurable serum concentrations, but absorption was slow (60). Rectal administration of phenytoin is not recommended.

Valproic Acid

Valproic acid absorption has been studied after rectal administration of diluted syrup and suppositories. Rectal absorption of the commercially available syrup is complete, with peak concentrations occurring approximately 2 hours after a dose (61–63). High osmolality necessitates 1:1 dilution of the syrup to minimize catharsis. The syrup has been used to treat status epilepticus when other therapy is ineffective. Various suppository formulations are absorbed well, albeit more slowly than the syrup, with time to peak concentration occurring in 2 to 4 hours (64,65).

SUMMARY

The selection of AED dosage forms is very important in pediatric epilepsy. Patients may be unwilling or unable to take oral solid dosage forms. Therefore, the availability of alternative oral dosage forms such as suspensions, solutions, and sprinkles is important. Patients who experience concentration-dependent side effects or breakthrough seizures may realize improved control by switching to an alternative dosage form.

Although it has been the practice to crush oral solids and mix the contents with food, this is not always desirable. Some products, such as Depakote® and Tegretol-XR®, lose the properties they were designed to provide if the structure of the preparation is disrupted. In some cases, the rate or extent of absorption may be altered when the drug is given with food. It also has been a custom to extemporaneously compound pediatric dosage forms. This is an important way to provide drug in a form that young children can take. However, clinicians should be cautious about extemporaneous compounding of pediatric formulations unless they can determine the amount of drug in the formulation, the stability of the product, and the bioavailability. This requires an assay for the compounded product and an assay of the drug in blood. In addition, with compounded drugs, someone should taste the preparation before it is given to the patient. For example, gabapentin has a very bitter taste when it is put into solution. Therefore, when a drug is compounded for pediatric delivery, the new formulation should be tested to ensure that it is being delivered properly. Specialized dosage forms generally are more expensive.

Caregivers should be thoroughly educated in drug administration techniques for children. When carefully instructed, caregivers can properly administer medications (66). Drug administration techniques are summarized in Tables 24-4, 24-5, and 24-6. When doses are given as "teaspoonfuls," caregivers should have a calibrated device for measuring the dose rather than using a common utensil. The volume of standard teaspoons varies up to fourfold. Drugs given rectally, such as diazepam, require special caregiver education.

Clinical assessment, selection of a drug, and determination of the dose require special attention in the

Table 24-4. Medication Administration Guidelines for Infants

Use a calibrated dropper or oral syringe.
Support the infant's head while holding the infant in lap.
Give small amounts of medication to prevent choking.
If desired, crush non–enteric-coated tablets to a powder and sprinkle on small amounts of food.
Provide physical comforting while administering medications to calm the infant.

Table 24-5. Medication Administration Guidelines for Toddlers

Allow child to choose a position in which to take medications.

Disguise the taste with a small volume of flavored drink or food. Rinse mouth with flavored drink to remove aftertaste.

Use simple commands in the toddler's jargon to obtain cooperation.

Allow the toddler to choose which medications to take first.

Allow toddler to become familiar with the oral dosing device.

Table 24-6. Medication Administration Guidelines for Preschool Children

Place tablet or capsule near back of tongue and provide water or a flavored liquid to aid in swallowing.

Do not use chewable tablets if the child's teeth are loose.

Use a straw to administer medications that may stain teeth.

Use a rinse with a flavored drink to minimize aftertaste.

Allow child to help make decisions about dosage forms, place of administration, which medication to take first, and the type of flavored drink to use.

pediatric patient, as does the selection of the appropriate formulation and dosage form. This last step in the therapeutic plan plays a pivotal role in the ultimate success of therapy. The objective is to ensure the regular and consistent delivery of drug to the brain. When conventional oral tablets and capsules are inappropriate or impractical, alternate formulations, dosages forms, and routes of administration should be considered. The clinician also must assess the ability of the caregiver to correctly prepare, measure, and administer medications and instruct caregivers about proper drug administration.

REFERENCES

1. Rowland M, Tozer TN. *Clinical Pharmacokinetics: Concepts and Applications*. 2nd ed. Philadelphia: Lea & Febiger, 1989.

2. Gibaldi M. *Biopharmaceutics and Clinical Pharmacokinetics*. 3rd ed. Philadelphia: Lea & Febiger, 1984.

3. Winter ME, Tozer TN. Phenytoin. In: Evans WE, Schentag JJ, Jusko WJ, eds. *Applied Pharmacokinetics: Principles of Therapeutic Drug Monitoring*. 3rd ed. Spokane: Applied Therapeutics, Inc.,

4. Ansel HC, Popovich NG. *Pharmaceutical Dosage Forms and Drug Delivery Systems*. 5th ed. Philadelphia: Lea & Febiger, 1990.

5. Stewart BH, Kugler AR, Thompson PR, Bockbrader HN. A saturable transport mechanism in the intestinal absorption of gabapentin is the underlying cause of lack of proportionality between increasing dose and drug levels in plasma. *Pharm Res* 1993; 10:276–281.

6. Tyrer JH, Eadie MJ, Sutherland JM, Hooper WD. Outbreak of anticonvulsant intoxication in an Australian city. *Br. Med J [Clin Res]* 1970; 4:271–273.

7. Bochner F, Hooper WD, Tyrer JH, Eadie MJ. Factors involved in an outbreak of phenytoin intoxication. *J Neurol Sci* 1972; 16:481–487.

8. Hamilton RA, Garnett WR, Kline BJ, et al. The effect of food on valproic acid absorption. *Am J Hosp Pharm* 1981; 38:1490–1493.

9. Levy R, Pitlick W, Troupin A, et al. Pharmacokinetics of carbamazepine in normal man. *Clin Pharmacol Ther* 1975; 17:657–668.

10. Carter BL, Garnett WR, Pellock JM, et al. Interaction between phenytoin and three commonly used antacids. *Ther Drug Monit* 1981; 3:333–340.

11. Stewart CG, Hampton EM. Effect of maturation on drug disposition in pediatric patients. *Clin Pharm* 1987; 6:548–564.

12. Painter MJ, Pippenger C, MacDonald H, et al. Phenobarbital and diphenylhydantoin levels in neonates with seizures. *J Pediatr* 1978; 92:315–319.

13. Kearns GL, Reed MD. Clinical pharmacokinetics in infants and children: a reappraisal. *Clin Pharmacokinet* 1989; 17(Suppl):29–67.

14. American Academy of Neurology. Assessment: generic substitution for antiepileptic medication. *Neurology* 1990; 40:1641–1643.

15. deBoer AG, Moolenaar F, deLeed LGJ, et al. Rectal drug administration: Clinical pharmacokinetic considerations. *Clin Pharmacokinetics* 1982; 7:285–311.

16. Carmichael RR, Mahoney DC, Jeffrey LP. Solubility and stability of phenytoin sodium when mixed with intravenous solutions. *Am J Hosp Pharm* 1980; 37:95–98.

17. Kostenbauder HD, Rapp RP, McGovern JP, et al. Bioavailability and single-dose pharmacokinetics of intramuscular phenytoin. *Clin Pharmacol Ther* 1975; 18:449–456.

18. Serrano EE, Wilder BJ. Intramuscular administration of diphenylhydantoin. Histologic follow-up. *Arch Neurol* 1974; 31:276–8.

19. Leppik IE, et al. Phenytoin prodrug: preclinical and clinical studies. *Epilepsia* 1989; 30(Suppl):S22–S26.

20. Fisher JH, Cwik MS, Sibley CB, Doyo K. Stability of fosphenytoin sodium with intravenous solutions in glass bottles, polyvinyl chloride, and polypropylene syringes. *Ann Pharmacother* 1997; 31:553–559.

21. Eldon MA, Loewen GR, Viogtman RE, et al. Pharmacokinetics and tolerance of fosphenytoin and phenytoin administered intravenously to healthy subjects. *Can J Neurol Sci* 1993; 20(Suppl 4):S180.

22. Jamerson BD, Dukes GE, Grouwer KLR, et al. Venous irritation related to intravenous administration of phenytoin versus fosphenytoin. *Pharmacotherapy* 1994; 14:47–52.

22a. Garnett WR, Kugler AR, O'Hara KA, Driscoll SM, Pellock JM. Pharmacokinetics of fosphenytoin following intramuscular administration of fosphenytoin substituted for oral phenytoin in epileptic patients. *Neurology* 1995; 45:A248.

22b. Ramsay RE, Wider BJ, Uthman BM, et al. Intramuscular fosphenytoin (Cerebyx) in patients requiring a loading dose of phenytoin. *Epilepsy Res* 1997; 181–187.

23. Wilder BJ, Campbell K, Ramsey RE, et al. Safety and tolerance of multiple doses of intramuscular fosphenytoin substituted for oral phenytoin in epilepsy and neurosurgery. *Arch Neurol* 1996; 53:764–768.

24. Fitzsimmons WE, Garnett WR, Comstock TJ, et al. Comparison of the single dose bioavailability and pharmacokinetics of extended phenytoin sodium capsules and phenytoin oral suspension. *Epilepsia* 1986; 27:464–468.

25. Food and Drug Administration. New prescribing directions for phenytoin. *FDA Drug Bull* 1978; 8:27–28.

26. Jung D, Powell JR, Walson P, Perrier D. Effect of dose on phenytoin absorption. *Clin Pharmacol Ther* 1980; 28:479–485.

27. Goff DA, Spunt KAL, Jung D, Bellur SN, Fischer JH. Absorption characteristics of three phenytoin sodium products after administration of oral loading doses. *Clin Pharmacol* 1984; 3:634–638.

28. Sarkar MA, Karnes HT, Garnett WR. Effects of storage and shaking on the settling properties of phenytoin suspension. *Neurology* 1989; 39:202–209.

29. Maas B, Garnett WR, Comstock TJ, et al. A comparison of the relative bioavailability and pharmacokinetics of carbamazepine tablets and chewable tablet formulations. *Ther Drug Monit* 1987; 9:28–33.

30. Graves NG, Kriel RL, Jones-Saete C, et al. Relative bioavailability of rectally administered carbamazepine suspension in humans. *Epilepsia* 1985; 26:429–433.

31. Garnett WR, Carson, Pellock JM, et al. Comparison of carbamazepine and 10-11 diepoxide carbamazepine plasma levels in children following chronic dosing with Tegretol suspension and Tegretol tablets. *Neurology* 1987; 37(Suppl):93.

32. Thakker KM, Mangat S, Garnett WR, et al. Comparative bioavailability and steady state fluctuations of Tegretol commercial and carbamazepine OROS tablets in adult and pediatric patients. *Biopharm Drug Dispos* 1992; 13:559–569.

33. Garnett WR, Levy B, McLean AM, et al. A pharmacokinetic evaluation of twice-daily extended-release carbamazepine and four-times daily immediate-release carbamazepine in patients with epilepsy. *Epilepsia* 1998; 39:274–279.

34. Stevens RE, Limsakun T, Evans G, Mason DH. Controlled, steady-state, pharmacokinetic evaluation of two-extended release carbamazepine formulations (Carbatrol and Tegretol-XR). *Neurology* 1998 (abstract).

35. Fischer JH, Barr AN, Palovcek FP, et al. Effect of food on the serum concentration profile of enteric-coated valproic acid. *Neurology* 1988; 38:1319–20.

36. Cloyd JC. Pharmacokinetic pitfalls of present antiepileptic medications. *Epilepsia* 1991; 32(Suppl 5):S53–S65.

37. Cloyd JC, Kriel RL, Janes-Saete CM, et al. Comparison of sprinkle vs syrup formulations of valproate for bioavailability, tolerance and preference. *J Pediatr* 1992; 120:634–638.

38. Granneman GR, Lamm JE, Cavanaugh JH. Assessment of pharmacokinetics of sodium valproate injectable. *Epilepsia* 1989; 30:668.

39. Garnett WR. Antiepileptics. In: Schumacher GE, ed. *Therapeutic Drug Monitoring*. Norwalk, Conn: Appleton and Lange, 1995:345–395.

40. Graves NM, Kriel RL. Rectal administration of antiepileptic drugs in children. *Pediatr Neurol* 1987; 3:321–326.

41. Jensen PK, Abild K, Poulsen MN. Serum concentration of clonazepam after rectal administration. *Acta Neurol Scand* 1983; 68:417–420.

42. Rylance GW, Poulton J, Cherry RC, et al. Plasma concentrations of clonazepam after single rectal administration. *Arch Dis Child* 1986; 61:186–188.

43. Johannessen SI, Henriksen O, Munthe-Kaas AW, et al. Serum concentration profile studies of tablets and suppositories of valproate and carbamazepine in healthy subjects and patients with epilepsy. In: Levy RH, Pitlick WH, Eichelbaum M, Meijer J, eds. *Metabolism of Antiepileptic Drugs*. New York: Raven Press, 1984:61–71.

44. Brouard A, Fonta JE, Masselin S, et al. Rectal administration of carbamazepine gel. *Clin Pharm* 1990; 9:13–14.

45. Moolenaar F, Bakker S, Visser J, et al. Biopharmaceutics of rectal administration of drugs in man. IX: comparative biopharmaceutics of diazepam after single rectal, oral, intramuscular and intravenous administration in man. *Int J Pharm* 1980; 5:127–137.

46. Lombroso CT. Intermittent home treatment of status and clusters of seizures. *Epilepsia* 1989; 30(Suppl):S11–S14.

47. Dhillon S, Oxley J, Richens A. Bioavailability of diazepam after intravenous, oral and rectal administration in adult epileptic patients. *Br J Clin Pharmacol* 1982; 13:427–432.

48. Hoppu K, Santavuori P. Diazepam rectal solution for home treatment of acute seizures in children. *Acta Paediatr Scand* 1981; 70:369–372.

49. Albano A, Reisdorff J, Wiegenstein JG. Rectal diazepam in pediatric status epilepticus. *Am J Emerg Med* 1989; 70:168–172.

50. Dreifuss FE, Rosman NP, Cloyd JC, et al. A comparison of rectal diazepam gel and placebo for acute repetitive seizures. *N Engl J Med* 1998 (in press).

51. Kriel RL, Cloyd JC, Hadsall RS, et al. Home use of rectal diazepam for cluster and prolonged seizures: efficacy adverse reactions, quality of life, and cost analysis. *Pediatr Neurol* 1991; 7:13–17.

52. Kriel RL, Birnbaum AK, Cloyd JC, et al. Failure of absorption of gabapentin after rectal administration. *Epilepsia* 1997; 38:1242–1244.

CHAPTER 25

Adverse Effects of Antiepileptic Drugs

L. James Willmore, M.D, James W. Wheless, M.D., and John M. Pellock, M.D.

Once a child with seizures is known to have epilepsy and a classification has been developed, commonly a drug for treatment must be selected. Although efficacy for some specific seizure types sometimes drives drug selection, the side-effect profile of drugs and the potential for toxicity become important considerations. Parents and patients must receive adequate data so they may participate in their treatment. This process is known as providing informed consent. Treatment must balance the need for seizure control with drug toxicity during both acute and chronic treatment (1). Antiepileptic drugs (AEDs) may cause nonspecific dose-related responses, unique effects specific to a given drug, or rare but potentially dangerous idiosyncratic reactions. In the absence of a specific history of allergy, drug administration is a task of trial and error. However, specific cellular mechanisms or metabolic abnormalities may account for some adverse drug effects.

Treatment planning begins with accurate diagnosis followed by knowledgeable use of drugs based on pharmacokinetics and pharmacodynamics. Symptoms of drug toxicity caused by high plasma drug levels can be useful for patient management. Although the commonly used AEDs are effective in many patients, efficacy of any selected drug for a specific patient cannot be predicted. Therefore, sequencing of treatment using several drugs may be required. Plasma levels guide treatment in some cases, but a titration of dose using the development of dose-related symptoms should be completed before a drug is declared ineffective.

Common problems can be anticipated, but dangerous, unexpected, and rare individual responses and reactions require physicians to provide most of the information during the process of informed consent. Thus, all people involved in the care of a patient must be informed in explicit terms about the potential for serious or even fatal reactions to drugs.

Adverse drug reactions (ADRs) are noxious effects occurring at doses of drugs used appropriately in humans for prophylaxis, diagnosis, or therapy (2). Drug-induced toxic reactions by class are listed in Table 25-1 (3). Some of these reactions depend on pharmacokinetic effects, with dose-dependent responses that correlate with plasma blood levels of a drug.

Pharmacodynamic effects occur when target organ responses are altered in a way that is independent of plasma concentration; such effects may be unique to a drug or to an individual patient. Serious non–dose-related ADRs cause drug-induced disease that may be acute or may occur following chronic treatment. Potentially fatal idiosyncratic reactions are listed in Table 25-2 (4).

Neurotoxicity, either dependent on dose or pharmacodynamic in nature, may occur at the time of drug initiation, during dose escalation, or at the time of the peak in plasma levels. These mild and reversible effects include sedation, changes in behavior, tremor, vertigo, diplopia, nystagmus, ataxia, or even dysarthria (1,4,5). Dose-related neurotoxicity becomes a more commonly encountered problem if two or more AEDs are used in combination. Monotherapy allows achievement of higher plasma levels of a drug than would be achieved if combined with other agents. Monotherapy improves compliance, reduces total cost of medication, and may eliminate interactions that could cause additive adverse effects (6,11). Monotherapy use of the commonly available AEDs results in seizure control in 50 percent to 80 percent of patients with epilepsy (12,13).

Almost all AEDs have caused idiosyncratic reactions or drug allergy. Such reactions may be severe, unpredictable, and, although rare, life-threatening (3). Idiosyncratic responses to AEDs in a given patient are associated with cellular, immunologic, or enzymatic characteristics that are unique to that patient. Drug clearance by oxidation requires catalyzed effects of the microsomal membrane-bound mixed function oxidases that contain cytochrome P-450 (14). The P-450 terminal oxidases receive electrons from reduced nicotinamide adenine dinucleotide phosphate (NADPH) and reduced nicotinamide adenine dinucleotide (NADH). The heterogenicity of the P-450 system causes apparent specificity, with isozyme families produced by the same gene family. AEDs are metabolized through such mixed-function oxidases, yielding stable, unstable, or potentially reactive molecular species. The accumulation of reactive and toxic intermediates as a result of drug treatment is determined by genetically derived enzyme activities. Thus, metabolism of a ring compounds via arene oxidase with impairment of metabolism of the arene oxide product could occur with deficiency of the enzyme epoxide hydrolase. The arene form of phenytoin has been implicated as a cause of hepatotoxicity, teratogenicity, bone marrow toxicity, and allergic skin reactions (15,19).

AED hypersensitivity syndrome occurs early in the treatment with aromatic antiepileptic compounds. Components of this syndrome include rash, fever, and eosinophilia and may include lymphadenopathy and life-threatening hepatic necrosis (20). Skin rash may or may not be pruritic and is in the form of an exanthema. More severe reactions include exfoliative dermatitis, erythema multiforme, Stevens-Johnson syndrome, or even toxic epidermal necrolysis (21). Adverse reactions of the idiosyncratic type tend to be immune-mediated effects in a person susceptible to such effects (22).

Mechanisms are not completely understood, but most rash and hypersensitivity syndromes are related to pharmacogenetic variation in drug biotransformation (23). Immune involvement is suggested by the occurrence of a sensitization period of 7 to 10 days after first use (24). In fact, T lymphocytes have been found in the perivascular infiltrate and epidermis (CD8+ and CD4+) of a patient with carbamazepine-induced toxic dermal necrolysis (25). Reactive metabolites produced by bioactivation are cytotoxic by binding to microsomal proteins. Such covalent adducts are formed in hepatic cytochrome P-450–mediated reactions (22). An alternate mechanism may involve impaired capacity for detoxification, with implication that the microsomal enzyme epoxide hydrolase is impaired (25,26).

As summarized by Leeder (22) in a useful model for understanding, antibodies to P-450 enzymes, with epitopes such as anti-CYP2D6 and anti-CYP3A have amino acid sequences similar to those of viral or fungal origin that suggest prior host-dependent immune responses to infection that are unique to an individual's human lymphocyte antigen (HLA) genotype. With

exposure to a bioactivated AED, a chemical modification of the P-450 enzyme occurs. These effects may be from formation of reactive drug metabolites, free radical species, or impairment of detoxification enzymes. These changes in enzyme function yield altered peptide structures that result in the immune response (22).

SPECIFIC DRUGS

Phenobarbital

Phenobarbital (see Chapter 28) has been in continual use for at least 85 years. Common side effects in children include behavioral changes with hyperactivity and irritability; adults experience drowsiness. Altered attention, effects on cognition, and even depression may be dose-related or may occur in specific patients without relationship to plasma level (27–29). Dose-related neurotoxicity includes nystagmus, ataxia, incoordination, dyskinesia, and altered sleep patterns. Idiosyncratic reactions include allergic dermatitis, Stevens-Johnson syndrome, serum sickness, and hepatic failure. Agranulocytosis and aplastic anemia have been reported (3,4). Folate deficiency in patients treated with AEDs is claimed to be associated with behavioral changes (30). Phenobarbital is known to exacerbate acute intermittent porphyria (31).

Induction of hepatic oxidative metabolism by phenobarbital is a fundamental mechanism for drug interactions. Vitamin D metabolism is induced by phenobarbital, thus multihandicapped and bedridden children receiving this drug or other AEDs may develop osteoporosis; vitamin D supplementation is important in these children (32). Phenobarbital alters absorption and induces metabolism of vitamin K as well. Neonates of mothers treated with phenobarbital or other barbiturates need vitamin K supplementation to prevent neonatal hemorrhagic disease. Prophylactic vitamin K must be given during the last month of gestation, at the beginning of labor, and to the infant at birth.

Chronic phenobarbital treatment may cause connective tissue changes, with coarsened facial feature, Dupuytren's contracture, Ledderhose syndrome (plantar fibromas), and frozen shoulder (33). Sedative effects of phenobarbital may cause exacerbation of absence, atonic, and myoclonic seizures, although other mechanisms may be operant (6). Sudden withholding of doses of short-acting barbiturates may precipitate drug withdrawal seizures or even status epilepticus. Given the slow rate of clearance of phenobarbital, such acute withdrawal seizures are less problematic, but it is wise to taper the dose of phenobarbital if the drug is to be discontinued. Some children, and even adults, may experience mild withdrawal symptoms that include tremor, sweating, restlessness, irritability, weight loss, disturbance of sleep, and even psychiatric symptoms. Mothers treated with phenobarbital may deliver infants who have withdrawal symptoms, including irritability, hypotonia, and vomiting for several days after delivery (34).

Phenytoin

Phenytoin (PHT) is a weak organic acid, poorly soluble in water, and available as free acid and as a sodium salt (see Chapter 29). Absorption occurs in the intestines. Peak concentration occurs at 3 to 12 hours after administration. Approximately 90 percent of PHT is protein-bound. The drug is eliminated by metabolic transformation, mostly via parahydroxylation. The pattern of elimination kinetics of PHT is nonlinear. PHT is metabolized by hepatic enzymes that are capacity-limited. This system is saturated at serum concentrations of 8 to 10 µg/mL. Because of the saturation kinetics of PHT, small changes in the maintenance dose produce large changes in the total serum concentration (35). Therefore, the half-life of the drug increases with higher plasma concentrations. The usual maintenance dose is 4 to 6 mg/kg/day. Because of saturation kinetics, dose changes must be made with care. One challenge to PHT use is alteration of steady state by interaction with other drugs (36).

Dose-related effects of PHT include nystagmus, ataxia, altered coordination, cognitive changes, and dyskinesia (3). Infrequently, children may become irritable or hyperactive (37). Children seldom develop nystagmus even when they are overtly ataxic and have elevated serum levels of PHT. A constellation of anorexia, weight loss, and vomiting should suggest PHT toxicity in a child (37). Although not strictly a pharmacologic problem, PHT causes some drug-specific effects that do not appear to be related to dose. Facial features may coarsen, and body hair changes in texture and becomes dark in color. Acne may worsen, and gingival hypertrophy is common, although careful dental hygiene may limit gum changes. Other effects of chronic PHT use are osteoporosis and lymphadenopathy (38). Folate deficiency may be severe enough to cause megaloblastic anemia; a transient encephalopathy is said to occur by a similar mechanism (30). Prolonged exposure to high plasma levels of PHT has been associated with cerebellar atrophy (37,39). Idiosyncratic reactions that may be fatal include allergic dermatitis, hepatotoxicity (40), serum sickness reaction, and aplastic anemia (3,38). Drug-induced lupus erythematosus reactions have been observed (41).

Ethosuximide

Ethosuximide (see Chapter 32) causes nausea, gastric distress, and abdominal pain unless the drug is given with meals. Rash and headaches, and on rare occasion leukopenia, pancytopenia, and aplastic anemia, have occurred (4). Neurologic effects include headache that may be severe, lethargy, agitation, aggressiveness, depression, and memory problems. Psychiatric disorders were attributed to normalization of the electroencephalogram (EEG) by this drug, but such reactions have been described with other drugs as well, making this hypothesis less tenable (42,43). Drug-induced lupus has been reported to occur in children (44).

Carbamazepine

Carbamazepine (CBZ) (see Chapter 30) is insoluble in aqueous solutions, behaving as a neutral lipophilic substance (45). CBZ is biotransformed, forming CBZ-10,11-epoxide (46). This epoxide is formed at the 10,11 double bond of the azepine ring when CBZ is catalyzed by the hepatic monooxygenases (47). The epoxide is hydrated by the microsomal epoxide hydrolase. Because of the problem with solubility, GI absorption of CBZ is both slow and unpredictable (48). Peak plasma levels occur at 4 to 8 hours after ingestion, so multiple dosing is required (45).

Elimination of CBZ follows linear kinetics. Although the single-dose half-life ranges from 18 to 55 hours, the half-life in most children is 6 to 12 hours and about 15 hours in adults. Elimination of CBZ varies greatly with age (48,49). CBZ also is has problematic interactions with other AEDs as well as with various other medications. Since CBZ induces its own metabolism, any drug that increases activity of P-450 enzymes causes a fall in CBZ blood levels. Inhibition of the activity of epoxide hydrolase, which occurs with concomitant administration of valproic acid, will increase the quantity of the epoxide (50). Both CBZ and the epoxide have effects as anticonvulsants (51,52).

Carbamazepine causes mild dose-related neurotoxic effects. Most are concentration-dependent. Transient effects include nausea, drowsiness, vertigo, ataxia, and speech slurring. Diplopia is a common concentration-dependent effect that is useful for clinical titration (5). Tremor and headache have been reported. Nausea, vomiting, diarrhea, and abdominal pain occur, albeit infrequently. Hyponatremia is common but rarely is of clinical consequence (53). These transient adverse effects may be markedly decreased by administering one of the extended-release formulations that result in less peak-to-trough variations in blood levels.

Severe reactions to CBZ cause alteration of hematopoietic, skin, hepatic, and cardiovascular systems (5). Rash occurs in 5 percent to 8 percent of patients and rarely may progress to exfoliative dermatitis or even a bullous reaction such as Stevens-Johnson syndrome (54). Hematologic changes are common, with leukopenia observed in 10 percent to 12 percent of patients treated with CBZ. However, fatal reactions such as aplastic anemia are rare, with death in 1.1 per 500,000 treated patients per year (55). Patients and parents must be informed about these serious reactions and reassured that frequent monitoring of blood cell counts and liver studies are unnecessary. Communication with the patient and informed consent are the best methods for long-term monitoring (56).

Valproate

Gastrointestinal effects commonly accompanying initiation of valproic acid (VPA) (see Chapter 31) treatment include nausea, diarrhea, abdominal pain, and even vomiting (57). Use at meal time or administration of an enteric-coated form of the drug abates these symptoms in most patients. Three dose-related effects require informing patients because they occur commonly. Tremor with sustention and at rest is dose-related (58). Weight gain is another common side effect, with 20 percent to 54 percent of patients reporting this problem (59). Patients report appetite stimulation. Weight change may require discontinuation of this drug. Hair loss is common and transient. Hair appears to be fragile; regrowth of the broken hair results in a curlier shaft (60). Supplementation with multivitamins containing zinc protects hair.

Thrombocytopenia occurs in a pattern that appears to be dose-related. Platelet counts vary without dose changes necessarily and are commonly asymptomatic. Petechial hemorrhage and ecchymoses do occur, necessitating lowering the dose or even discontinuing the drug (61,62).

Other less frequently encountered effects include sedation or encephalopathy (63,64). Acute encephalopathy and even coma may develop on initial exposure to VPA (63). Upon investigation, patients receiving VPA may be severely acidotic and have elevated urinary organic acid excretion. Because VPA is known to sequester co-enzyme A (65), such patients are suspect of having a partially compensated defect in the mitochondrial beta oxidation enzymes (64,66). Dermatological abnormalities are unusual, but may be severe (67).

Acute hemorrhagic pancreatitis may develop in younger patients. Fatal outcome has been reported. If patients experience abdominal pain after receiving VPA, lipase and amylase levels should be measured (68).

Hepatic failure is a rare but serious problem in children. Early reports of changes in hepatic enzymes (69) were soon followed by observation of fatal hepatotoxicity (70). Risk is greatest in young patients receiving several medications. Further risk factors include children with genetic metabolic diseases, a history of hepatic disorders in the family, particularly in siblings, and

mental retardation (71–73). Histopathological inspection of abnormal liver shows microvesicular steatosis (74). Children younger than 2 years of age receiving multiple AEDs are at greatest risk for a fatal reaction. An estimate for rate fatal outcome is 1 per 60,000 patients, regardless of age with the highest risk of 1 in 500 to 800 in children younger than 2 years old receiving AED adjunctive therapy.

Clinical risk assessments suggest the use of VPA as monotherapy whenever possible and the establishment of good clinical monitoring (75) because symptoms of nausea, vomiting, anorexia, and loss of seizure control are more effective in signaling a problem than routine blood studies (56,76,77). Furthermore, be cautious about giving VPA to patients with liver disease or a family history of hepatic dysfunction. Obtain urinary organic acid measurement and metabolic evaluation in high-risk patients as indicated previously, or any patient without an established reason for mental retardation and seizures (76).

Hyperammonemia may occur in the absence of hepatic dysfunction (78,79). This effect may be caused by inhibition of nitrogen elimination or inhibition of urea synthesis (80,81). In rare instances, patients may have deficiency in urea cycle enzymes such as ornithine transcarbamylase (82).

Age-related changes in pharmacokinetics of VPA should be anticipated because of the high percentage of drug that is protein bound (83). VPA is a branched chain carboxylic acid that may be metabolized either through mitochondrial mechanisms or via cytoplasmic enzymes. Dehydrogenation of VPA results in the accumulation of 2-en, 3-en, and 4-en-VPA compounds. The 4-en metabolites are highest in infants and decline with age. The 2-en compound had anticonvulsant potency (84). VPA binds to albumin at high and low affinity sites. This binding is saturable causing, free fraction increases with dose.

RECENTLY AVAILABLE DRUGS

Felbamate

Felbamate (FBM) is a dicarbamate compound that is related to meprobamate. Its sedative and tranquilizing action is obviated by substitution at the 2-carbon of a phenyl group for an aliphatic side chain. Pharmacokinetic profiles show linear, first-order kinetics. The elimination half-life ranges from 14 to 22 hours, with a mean of 20 hours. The T_{max} averages 2 hours. Plasma concentrations of FBM are also linear with regard to the oral dose. Drug interactions are vigorous and may cause clinically significant toxicity or seizure exacerbation. When FBM is added to CBZ, levels of the parent compound decline by 20 percent to 25 percent, but the metabolite CBZ-10,11-epoxide increases by as much as 50 percent (85,86). These effects suggest induction of cytochrome P-450 along with inhibition of some of the action of epoxide hydrolase. This interaction induces CBZ side effects; the combination also causes headache. PHT levels increase by approximately 20 percent when FBM is added (87). Although FBM causes about 20 percent increase in valproate levels, no specific clinical problem results. Conversely, PHT and CBZ cause a decrease in FBM levels of about 15 percent, whereas VPA increases the FBM level by 40 percent. The pharmacokinetic characteristics described here all help explain some dose-related interactions that induce adverse effects.

Felbamate (see Chapter 35) was evaluated in patients from 4 to 36 years of age with Lennox-Gastaut syndrome. The drug was given as adjunctive treatment at 45 mg/kg/day in a double-blind, placebo-controlled trial. Efficacy was demonstrated, with overall seizure frequency reduced by 19 percent, with atonic seizures reduced 34 percent and generalized tonic-clonic seizures reduced by 28 percent. Although these changes were of statistical interest, no practical effect was demonstrated. However, when global evaluation scores from parents were evaluated there was uniform endorsement of the salutatory effects on patients with Lennox-Gastaut syndrome.

Following the identification of aplastic anemia and hepatotoxicity and notification of physicians by the U.S. Food and Drug Administration (FDA) in August and September 1994, the number of persons being treated with FBM decreased drastically. Kaufman and coworkers (88) reviewed cases of aplastic anemia reported in the United States and suggested an incidence of aplastic anemia of 27 to 209 per million in those receiving FBM versus 2 to 2.5 per million persons in the general population. The aplastic anemia risk with FBM treatment is perhaps up to 20 times greater than that for CBZ. No case of aplastic anemia has been reported in children less than 13 years old. The mean time to presentation is 154 days, with very few cases being reported after 6 months of exposure. Similarly, severe hepatotoxicity associated with FBM has been reported, but this risk seems to be similar to that of VPA. Although there is no predilection for age, children have been effected by severe, life-threatening hepatotoxicity associated with FBM.

Recommended guidelines for the use of FBM now stress that this agent should be used for adults and children with severe epilepsy refractory to other therapy, especially for patients with Lennox-Gastaut syndrome and other encephalopathic epilepsies. A careful history concerning past indications of hematologic disorder, hepatotoxicity, and autoimmune diseases should be sought before beginning treatment. Women with autoimmune disease account for the largest portion of those who developed aplastic anemia. Baseline routine hematologic and liver function tests should be performed, and patients and their families must be fully informed of the potential risks; written consent is recommended in the United States. Dose escalation should be made slowly, and doses of adjunctive medication must be corrected for known interactions where possible. Monotherapy with FBM leads to fewer systemic side effects, but it is not known whether the rare but potentially life-threatening side effects are decreased by using FBM alone. Clinical monitoring rather than specific scheduled blood testing should be done frequently, and patients should be educated regarding symptoms that may possibly signify either hematologic disorder or hepatotoxicity.

It has been proposed that an intermediate FBM metabolite is formed as a reactive compound. The formation of an atropaldehyde has been confirmed in human liver tissue (89). One hypothesis is that FBM toxicity may be correlated with the amount of atropaldehyde produced or the ability to detoxify the compound through glutathione conversion. At present the clinical profile of patients at highest risk seems more useful than the testing for potential metabolic abnormalities in patients who are receiving FBM. Future studies and experience should further determine which method is superior.

Gabapentin

The agent 1-(aminomethyl)cyclohexaneacetic acid) is structurally related to gamma-aminobutyric acid (GABA). The drug crosses the blood–brain barrier; peak plasma concentrations are achieved 2 to 3 hours after an oral dose. Unique for an AED, gabapentin is not bound to plasma proteins and is not metabolized. The bland pharmacokinetic properties of gabapentin include no hepatic enzyme induction and little effect on plasma levels of other AEDs. Adverse events were detected in treated patients and were typically neurotoxic, but withdrawal from studies was infrequent.

Gabapentin is effective in partial seizures like most other recent drugs (90–92). Children have adverse events profiles similar to those noted in adults. However, particularly in mentally retarded children, there is an increase in the incidence of hyperactivity and aggressive behavior (93) (see Chapter 33).

Lamotrigine

Lamotrigine was identified through screening of drugs being evaluated for efficacy in antagonizing folate (see Chapter 34). The study designs have depended on use in patients with refractory partial seizures and the

Lennox-Gastaut syndrome. Dosing at twice daily is an advantage regarding compliance. No serious adverse events occurred during assessment, although some reports of Stevens-Johnson dermatological responses when combined with valproate warrant caution. Central nervous system (CNS)-related side effects included lethargy, fatigue, and mental confusion (94–99).

Side-effect assessment in the add-on trials showed drowsiness and headache to be common minor problems, but, overall, lamotrigine seems less sedating that other drugs. Serious rashes have occurred; the rate of dose ascension appears to be correlated with this type of adverse event. Rash was suspected to be a drug interaction with valproate, but that drug inhibits metabolism of lamotrigine, causing diminished clearance with resultant high blood levels (100). Serious rash may be more common in children, but current guidelines in the United States require that this drug be discontinued if a rash develops. Lamotrigine does not induce hepatic enzymes to any great extent, so this drug may be useful in treating the elderly (99,101). Lamotrigine is eliminated mostly by hepatic glucuronide conjugation. Concomitant use with hepatic enzyme–inducing drugs accelerates elimination of lamotrigine.

Of most concern, however, is the potentially life-threatening rash associated with lamotrigine. The overall rash rate is 10 percent to 12 percent. Lamotrigine-associated rash was initially described as being macular-papular or erythematous in its typical appearance, displaying characteristics of a delayed hypersensitivity reaction. This rash typically appears within the first 4 weeks of therapy and is rarely seen after 8 weeks. Subsequently, several patients developed much more serious rash, an erythema multiforme–type eruption that sometimes progressed to desquamation with involvement of mucous membranes to resemble Stevens-Johnson syndrome or Lyell's syndrome. In some patients this was accompanied by a general hypersensitivity reaction, whereas in others it was more limited to skin. Recent information confirms that the incidence is slightly greater in children and with concomitant valproate therapy. Rapid increase in the rate of titration of lamotrigine may increase the risk of rash. Approximately 1 in 1,000 adult patient and 1 in 100 to 200 children may be at risk for this potentially life-threatening dermatological reaction. The FDA has issued a warning in the lamotrigine package insert. It is recommended in the United States that the medication be discontinued when rash appears, but this recommendation may not be followed internationally because of the benign nature of most episodes of rash, even those associated with lamotrigine. Careful attention to titration and dose schedule is mandatory. As always with children, the clinician's challenge is to work with the family and patient to determine which skin changes indicate a possible serious dermatological complication (102).

Topiramate

Topiramate has a monosaccharide-type structure. This drug appears to influence sodium channels, block non-NMDA glutamate receptors, have an effect on a portion of chloride channels, and inhibit carbonic anhydrase. Adverse cognitive effects occur at high doses (103). Bioavailability is high, ranging from 80 percent to 95 percent, and elimination mostly is by renal mechanisms.

In adults with partial seizures, doses of 200 to 1000 mg/day showed an overall responder rate for 50 percent or greater reduction in seizures of 44 percent (104–108). Assessment in patients with generalized seizures and with monotherapy use showed similar patterns of efficacy (see Chapter 36).

Treatment-emergent adverse effects with add-on studies showed ataxia, impaired concentration, confusion, dizziness, fatigue, paresthesias, somnolence, and abnormal thinking related to topiramate treatment. Nephrolithiasis and dose-related weight loss are potential problems that require discussion with patients. Many side effects detected in the studies were caused by forced titration to high doses. Adverse cognitive effects occur at high doses in adults (103). Slowing the pace of dose ascension reduces the impact on cognitive function.

Tiagabine

Tiagabine is a derivative of nipecotic acid that enhances GABA-mediated inhibition by reducing cellular uptake of GABA through an effect on transporter proteins (109). Oral bioavailability is about 90 percent, and protein binding in plasma is 96 percent (110). Clearance is rapid and accelerated by concomitant use of enzyme-inducing drugs; the drug is almost completely metabolized, and the products are not biologically active. Although renal disease does not appear to have an effect on tiagabine excretion (111), altered hepatic function does prolong clearance (see Chapter 37)

Placebo-controlled, double-blind trials (five being multicenter and two having crossover design) used doses from 16 mg/day up to 56 mg/day. As with most such studies, efficacy was reported as the 50 percent responder rate, along with the median reduction of seizures from baseline. Doses of 32 to 56 mg/day were associated with significant reduction of the seizure rate when compared with placebo. While the responder rate for complex partial seizures was 24 percent (8% placebo), the responder rate for secondarily generalized tonic-clonic seizures was 45 percent (30% placebo) (112).

Most commonly identified side effects in the pivotal trials included somnolence, asthenia, and headache. These occurred during dose titration. Reasons for withdrawal from the trials included occurrence of confusion, somnolence, ataxia, and dizziness (112).

Oxcarbazepine

Oxcarbazepine is a keto analogue of CBZ that is rapidly converted to a 10-monohydroxy active metabolite. Oxcarbazepine is available around the world; studies have been completed in the United States, and the drug has been approved for use. Oxcarbazepine is rapidly and completely absorbed after oral intake. Conversion by cytosol arylketone reductase to the monohydroxy form is rapid and complete; autoinduction of metabolism does not occur, but concomitant use with inducing drugs results in the need to increase the oxcarbazepine dose to maintain stable blood levels. Renal clearance of the active metabolite correlates with measured creatinine clearance.

Controlled clinical trials showed efficacy patterns similar to those of CBZ (113,114). Use in newly diagnosed or previously untreated patients with partial seizures showed equal efficacy with CBZ (115), PHT (116), and VPA (117). Dizziness, sedation, and fatigue were side effects that may be dose-related. Hyponatremia has occurred with this drug, and some vigilance may be required in that regard (118).

Vigabatrin

Vigabatrin, also known as gamma-vinyl GABA, is an analogue of GABA that acts to increase tissue concentration of that inhibitory transmitter by irreversible inhibition of GABA-transaminase, the enzyme that degrades GABA. This effect on a specific enzyme makes traditional pharmacokinetics less relevant. However, absorption is rapid and proportional to dose, with peak plasma concentration occurring around 90 minutes. Vigabatrin is hydrophilic, not protein-bound, and widely distributed in body water (119,120). Elimination is by renal excretion of the unchanged drug. There are changes in pharmacokinetics in the elderly, with longer T_{max} and higher mean maximum concentration consistent with longer half-life for that age group (119). Lack of protein binding and metabolism, as expected, means vigabatrin does not have any vigorous interactions with established drugs such as PHT or CBZ.

Pivotal trials from studies in the United States have not been published, but extensive information is available from other countries (121). Blinded, placebo-controlled trials treating patients with complex partial seizures show 50 percent responder rates ranging from 45 percent to 55 percent (122). This approximate pattern of efficacy has been observed over many trials (122).

In general, adverse effects are those expected with an AED: drowsiness, irritability, ataxia, and headache. Of concern are severe changes in behavior with agitation, hallucinations, and altered thinking, effects that are thought to be dose-related (43). Depression is an important potential problem in treating all patients (123).

Loss of peripheral retinal visual function is of major concern (124,125). One report compared 32 adults treated with vigabatrin with 18 patients treated with CBZ. Up to 40 percent of the vigabatrin-treated patients had concentrically constricted visual fields (125).

Zonisamide

Zonisamide is a sulfonamide drug that has a wide spectrum of activity. Zonisamide is rapidly absorbed by oral intake; protein binding is about 50 percent, but the drug accumulates in erythrocytes. Plasma half-life is prolonged at around 55 hours but is reduced to about 30 hours in patients being treated with enzyme-inducing drugs. This drug is extensively metabolized (111).

Efficacy as measured in U.S. trials by the 50 percent responder rate showed up to 45 percent and without loss of efficacy over time (126). Adverse effects of drowsiness and altered thinking are not unexpected. Due to its inhibition of carbonic anhydrase, this drug can cause nephrolithiasis; appropriate history needs to be obtained, and advice must be given to patients to maintain fluid intake.

MECHANISMS OF ADVERSE EFFECTS

Antiepileptic drugs can induce either expected or unique changes. Carbamazepine may cause changes in levels of serum sodium (127–128). This drug-induced hyponatremia seldom causes symptoms and usually responds to gentle restriction of fluids. Valproate causes dose-related tremor, weight gain, and transient alopecia. Hand tremor seldom causes difficulty, but this cosmetic problem can be ameliorated by low doses of beta-adrenergic blocking agents. The precise mechanism for weight gain during valproate treatment is not known; however, patients do complain of an increase in appetite. Management requires prospective intervention; patients must be forewarned of this side effect and counseled to be mindful of their diet. The transient alopecia that occurs in some patients taking VPA may be related to its tendency to chelate trace metals. Trace metal insufficiency can result in fragility of the hair shaft. Addition of a vitamin with zinc supplement usually results in an abatement of this hair loss. Sequestration of selenium may play a role as well.

The epoxide that forms with the metabolism of CBZ is stable and less reactive than the PHT compound. Carbamazepine 10-11 epoxide accumulates in plasma and has its own an antiepileptic effects. Accumulation of the epoxide following impairment of the epoxide hydrolase by drug interaction has been associated with symptoms of toxicity (129).

A transient elevation of circulating amylase has been observed in some patients during VPA therapy. In addition, symptomatic cases of pancreatitis and even fatalities have been observed in children and adults during VPA treatment (68,130,131). The mechanism of these rare idiosyncratic reactions remains unconfirmed, but reexposure to VPA has caused recurrent symptoms (132). Physicians must be alert for the development of abdominal pain among patients being treated with VPA.

Hyperammonemia has been observed in patients treated with most of the AEDs. Although most patients with elevated plasma ammonia are asymptomatic, some patients have developed lethargy, stupor, hypotonia, or increased seizure activity. Underlying metabolic abnormalities have been associated with some deaths attributed to VPA use. For example, the urea cycle defects (81), including ornithine carbamoyl transferase deficiency (133,134), have been associated with fatal outcome following VPA administration. The clinical presentation of these patients was apparently not appreciably different from the sequence of symptoms in patients without identified metabolic defects.

Hypersensitivity reactions may cause cellular changes that resemble the cytotoxic effects of viral hepatitis. This type of hepatic injury is a common component of systemic reactions involving rash, lymphadenopathy, and eosinophilia. Toxic injury at the cellular level may be related to the formation of arene oxide (18).

Even though routine monitoring may detect alterations in liver function, clinical problems are often not apparent (69). Such findings, however, create a dilemma for the physician regarding plans for ongoing assessment, and the need for specific action. Biochemical changes observed in patients being treated with VPA seldom herald the development of a fatal reaction. The first detailed report of VPA-induced hepatotoxicity included one patient with symptomatic hepatic dysfunction and three patients with isolated biochemical changes (69). The observation of transient, dose-related hepatotoxicity was followed in 1979 by reports of fatalities associated with VPA treatment (70,135). Unfortunately, although metabolic abnormalities are occasionally discovered by VPA administration (64,81,133), most patients with mild to moderate symptoms caused by a dose-related side effect cannot be differentiated from those with serious idiosyncratic responses in any way other than by outcome. The idiosyncratic effects on liver function include hyperammonemia (136–138), severe hepatic dysfunction with recovery, and fulminant hepatic failure (71,133,139). VPA occasionally causes stupor or coma (63). It is known to affect mitochondrial function, causing elevations in serum levels of some branched chain fatty acids (140). Decreased serum carnitine levels observed with VPA administration (65,141) are accompanied by increased excretion of acetylcarnitine (140). Valproate reduces levels of both free coenzyme A (CoASH) and acetyl-CoA in rat liver (142,143). This reduction in CoASH is accompanied by an increase in the intrahepatic medium chain acyl-CoA fraction, identified as valproyl-CoA (142). Although VPA increases activity of the medium chain fraction of acyl-CoA hydrolase, valproyl-CoA itself is hydrolyzed poorly (144). Since VPA-induced inhibition of in vitro fatty acid oxidation is reversed by addition of CoASH and carnitine to the reactants (145), it would appear that VPA causes sequestration of CoASH.

Sequestration of CoASH and formation of valproyl-CoA could impair or block several steps in fatty acid oxidation. Because fatty acid is esterified to acyl-CoA in the cytosol before carnitine-mediated transport across the mitochondrial membrane, decreased CoASH would impair formation of acyl-CoA or conversion of acyl-carnitine to acyl-CoA, favoring omega oxidation with resultant dicarboxylic aciduria. Coenzyme A deficiency also could impair cleavage of 3-ketoacyl-CoA by thiolase activity, causing accumulation of acetoacetyl-CoA, butyryl-CoA, and hexanoyl-CoA, producing ketosis with excretion of ethylmalonic and adipic acids. Because butyryl-CoA and hexanoyl-CoA dehydrogenases are inhibited by an acyl-CoA metabolite of hypoglycin (146) valproyl-CoA may inhibit these dehydrogenases (64,66,76).

Drug-induced effects on the hematopoietic system may be caused by hypersensitivity reactions with antibody-mediated peripheral destruction, by secondary effects such as occurs in a lupus-like syndrome, or by toxic marrow inhibition (147–149). Hypersensitivity reactions may be associated with the drug acting as a hapten with a protein. The net result is that IgE is produced. Another possibility is that there may be a direct drug effect by activation of the complement cascade or by a change in the function of lymphocytes. Direct cellular effects may alter lymphocyte populations or reactivity. For example, it has been postulated that PHT may alter lymphocytes because 21 percent to 25 percent of patients chronically treated with this drug have decreased circulating levels of IgA along with depressed lymphocyte phytohemagglutinin transformation (150,151). PHT hypersensitivity includes characteristic hepatic involvement and lymphadenopathy (152–155). Potential mechanisms include hapten formation, formation of an arene compounds (18), conversion of the aromatic ring by oxidation to phenol metabolites, or chlorination of nitrogen components on the hydantoin ring (149). Indeed, a metabolite of PHT from hepatic microsomes appears to be toxic to lymphocytes. A similar mechanism has been proposed for CBZ. Indeed, CBZ is oxidized to several metabolites that may cause toxic effects on granulocytes (156). Lymphocytes from a patient with sequential aplastic anemia had challenge of those cells with metabolites derived from murine hepatocytes; the sensitivity of the lymphocytes suggested an arene oxide metabolite formation as a mechanism (157).

Serious toxic effects that result from the use of AEDs are usually discovered during the course of treatment. Hence, patients need to be informed and freely communicate with their physician It takes a joint effort to use medications to control seizures. Good therapeutic alliances between patient and physician will serve until such time that screening assays are developed to identify patients likely to develop serious adverse drug effects (56).

REFERENCES

1. Pellock JM. Efficacy and adverse effects of antiepileptic drugs. *Pediatr Clin North Am* 1989; 345–348.
2. Karsh FE, Lasagna L. Adverse drug reactions. A critical review. *JAMA* 1975; 234:1236–1241.
3. Plaa GI, Willmore LJ. General principles: toxicology. In: Levy RH, Mattson RH, Meldrum BS, eds. *Antiepileptic Drugs*. 4 ed. New York: Raven Press, 1998:51–60.
4. Schmidt D. *Adverse Effects of Antiepileptic Drugs*. New York: Raven Press, 1982:
5. Pellock JM. Carbamazepine side effects in children and adults. *Epilepsia*. 1987; 28:S64–S70.
6. Lerman P. Seizures induced or aggravated by anticonvulsants. *Epilepsia* 1986; 27:706–710.
7. Callaghan N, Kenny RA, O'Neill B, Crowley M, Goggin T. A prospective study between carbamazepine, phenytoin and sodium valproate as monotherapy in previously untreated and recently diagnosed patients with epilepsy. *J Neurol Neurosurg Psychiatry* 1985; 48:639–644.
8. Dulac O, Steru D, Rey E, Perret A, Arthuis M. Sodium valproate monotherapy in childhood epilepsy. *Brain Dev* 1986; 8:47–52.
9. Chadwick DW. Valproate monotherapy in the management of generalized and partial seizures. *Epilepsia* 1987; 28 (Suppl. 2):S12–S17.
10. Dean JC, Penry JK. Carbamazepine/valproate therapy in 100 patients with partial seizures failing carbamazepine monotherapy: long-term follow-up. *Epilepsia* 1988; 29:687–687.
11. Herranz JL, Armijo JA, Artega R. Clinical side effect of phenobarbital, primidone, phenytoin, carbamazepine and valproate during monotherapy in children. *Epilepsia* 1988; 29:794–804.
12. Mattson RH, Cramer JA, Collins JF, et al. Comparison of carbamazepine, phenobarbital, phenytoin, and primidone in partial and secondarily generalized tonic-clonic seizures. *N Engl J Med* 1985; 313:145–151.
13. Elwes RDC, Johnson AL, Shorvon SD, Reynolds EH. The prognosis for seizure control in newly diagnosed epilepsy. *N Engl J Med* 1984; 311:944–947.
14. Galbraith RA, Michnovicz JJ. The effects of cimetidine on the oxidative metabolism of estradiol. *N Engl J Med* 1989; 321:269–274.
15. Gerson WT, Fine DG, Spielberg SP, et al. Anticonvulsant-induced aplastic anemia: increased susceptibility to toxic drug metabolites in vitro. *Blood* 1983; 61:889–893.
16. Moustafa MA, Claesen M, Adline J, Vandervorst D, Poupaert JH. Evidence for an arene-3,4-oxide as a metabolic intermediate in the meta- and para-hydroxylation of phenytoin in the dog. *Drug Metab Dispos* 1983; 11:574–580.
17. Shear NH, Spielberg SP. Anticonvulsant hypersensitivity syndrome. In vitro assessment of risk. *J Clin Invest* 1988; 82:1826–1832.
18. Spielberg SP, Gordon GB, Blake DA, et al. Predisposition to phenytoin hepatotoxicity assessed in vitro. *N Engl J Med* 1981; 305:722–727.
19. Strickler SM, Miller MA, Andermann E, et al. Genetic predisposition to phenytoin-induced birth defects. *Lancet* 1985; 2:746–749.
20. Schlienger RG, Shear NH. Antiepileptic drug hypersensitivity syndrome. *Epilepsia* 1998; 39(Suppl.7):S3–S7.
21. Licata AL, Louis ED. Anticonvulsant hypersensitivity syndrome. *Comprehens Ther* 1996; 22:152–155.
22. Leeder JS. Mechanisms of idiosyncratic hypersensitivity reactions to antiepileptic drugs. *Epilepsia* 1998; 39(Suppl.7):S8–S16.
23. Shear NH, Spielberg SP. Pharmacogenetics and adverse drug reactions in the skin. *Pediatr Dermatol* 1983; 1:165–173.
24. Pohl LR, Satoh H, Christ DD, et al. The immunologic and metabolic basis of drug hypersensitivities. *Annu Rev Pharmacol* 1988; 28:367–387.
25. Pirmohamed M, Kitteringham NR, Guenthner TM, et al. An investigation of mechanisms in toxic epidermal necrolysis induced by carbamazepine. *Arch Dermatol* 1992; 130:598–604.
26. Pirmohamed M, Graham A, Roberts P, et al. Carbamazepine-hypersensitivity: assessment of clinical and in vitro chemical cross-reactivity with phenytoin and oxcarbazepine. *Br J Clin Pharmacol* 1991; 32:741–749.
27. Meador KJ, Loring DW, Huh K, Gallagher BB, King DW. Comparative cognitive effects of anticonvulsants. *Neurology* 1990; 40:391–394.
28. Pellock JM, Culbert JP, Garnett WR, et al. Significant differences of AEDs cognitive and behavioral effects in children. *Ann Neurol* 1988; 24:325.

29. Vining EPG, Mellits ED, Dorsen MM, et al. Psychologic and behavioral effects of antiepileptic drugs in children, a double-blind comparison between phenobarbital and valproic acid. *Pediatrics* 1987; 80:165–174.

30. Reynolds EH, Chanarin I, Milner G, Matthews DM. Anticonvulsant therapy, folic acid and vitamin B12 metabolism and mental symptoms. *Epilepsia* 1966; 7:261–270.

31. Granick S. Hepatic porphyria and drug-induced or chemical porphyria. *Ann NY Acad Sci* 1965; 123:197.

32. Hunt PA, Wu-Chen ML, Handal JM, et al. Bone disease induced by anticonvulsant therapy and treatment with calcitrol (1, 25-dihydroxy-vitamin D3). *Am J Dis Child* 1986; 140:715–718.

33. Mattson RH, Cramer JA, McCutchen CB. Barbiturate related connective tissue disorders. *Arch Intern Med* 1989; 149:911–914.

34. Morselli PL, Franco-Morselli R, Bossi L. Clinical pharmacokinetics in newborns and infants: age related differences and therapeutic implications. *Clin Pharmacokinet* 1980; 5:485–527.

35. Bender AD, Post A, Meier JP, Higson JE, Reichard G Jr. Plasma protein binding of drugs as a function of age in adult human subjects. *J Pharmaceut Sci* 1975; 64:1711–1713.

36. Kutt H. Interactions between anticonvulsants and other commonly prescribed drugs. *Epilepsia* 1984; 25(Suppl 2):S118–S131.

37. Pellock JM. Seizures and epilepsy. In: Kelley VC, ed. *Practice in Pediatrics*. Philadelphia: Harper & Row, 1987.

38. Haruda F. Phenytoin hypersensitivity: 38 cases. *Neurology* 1979; 29:1480–1485.

39. Rapport RL, Shaw CM. Phenytoin-related cerebellar degeneration without seizures. *Ann Neurol* 1977; 2:437.

40. Horowitz S, Patwardhan R, Marcus E. Hepatotoxic reactions associated with carbamazepine therapy. *Epilepsia* 1988; 29:149–154.

41. Gleichmann H. Systemic lupus erythematosus triggered by diphenylhydantoin. *Arthritis Rheum* 1982; 25:1387.

42. Wolf P, Inoue Y, Roder-Wanner U, et al. Psychiatric complications of absence therapy and their relation to alteration of sleep. *Epilepsia* 1984; 25:S56–S59.

43. Brodie MJD, McKee PJW. Vigabatrin and psychosis. *Lancet* 1990; 335:1279–1279.

44. Jacobs JC. Systemic lupus erythematosus in childhood. Report of 35 cases, with discussion of seven apparently induced by anticonvulsant medication and the prognosis and treatment. *Pediatrics* 1963; 32:257.

45. Leppik IE. Metabolism of antiepileptic medication: newborn to elderly. *Epilepsia* 1992; 33(Suppl.4):S32–S40.

46. Patsalos PN, Stephenson TJ, Krishna S, Elyas AA, Lascelles PT, Wiles CM. Side-effects induced by carbamazepine-10,11-epoxide. *Lancet* 1985; 2:496.

47. Riley RJ, Kitteringham NR, Park BK. Structural requirements for bioactivation of anticonvulsants to cytotoxic metabolites in vitro. *Br J Clin.Pharmacol.* 1989; 28:482–487.

48. Morselli PL, Bossi L. Carbamazepine absorption, distribution and excretion. In: Woodbury DM, Penry JK, Pippenger CE, eds. Antiepileptic drugs. 2 ed. New York: Raven Press, 1982:465–482.

49. Hockings N, Pall A, Moody APJ, Davidson AVM, Davidson DLW. The effects of age on carbamazepine pharmacokinetics and adverse effects. *Br J Clin Pharmacol* 1986; 22:725–728.

50. Pisani F, Caputo M, Fazio A, et al. Interaction of carbamazepine-10,11-epoxide, an active metabolite of carbamazepine, with valproate: a pharmacokinetic study. *Epilepsia* 1990; 31:339–342.

51. Albright PS, Bruni J. Effects of carbamazepine and its epoxide metabolites on amygdala-kindled seizures in rats. *Neurology* 1984; 34:1383–1386.

52. Bourgeois BFD, Wad N. Individual and combined antiepileptic and neurotoxic activity of carbamazepine and carbamazepine-10,11-epoxide in mice. *J Pharmacol Exp Ther* 1984; 231:411–415.

53. Lahr MB. Hyponatremia during carbamazepine therapy. *Clin Pharmacol Ther* 1985; 37:693–696.

54. Coombes BW. Stevens-Johnson syndrome associated with carbamazepine. *Med J Aust* 1965; 1:895–896.

55. Bertolino JG. Carbamazepine. What physicians should know about its hematologic effects. *Postgrad Med* 1990; 88:183–186.

56. Pellock JM, Willmore LJ. A rational guide to routine blood monitoring in patients receiving antiepileptic drugs. *Neurology* 1991; 41:961–964.

57. Dreifuss FE, Langer DH. Side effects of valproate. *Am J Med* 1988; (Suppl 1A):34–41.

58. Hyuman NM, Dennis PD, Sinclair KG. Tremor due to sodium valproate. *Neurology* 1979; 29:1177–1180.

59. Dinesen H, Gram L, Andersen T, Dam M. Weight gain during treatment with valproate. *Acta Neurol Scand* 1984; 70:65–69.

60. Jeavons PM, Clark JE, Hirdme GA. Valproate and curly hair. *Lancet* 1977; 1:359–359.

61. Loiseau P. Sodium valproate, platelet dysfunction and bleeding. *Epilepsia* 1981; 22:141–146.

62. Sandler RM, Emberson C, Roberts GE, Voak D, Darnborough J, Heeley AF. IgM platelet autoantibody due to sodium valproate. *Br Med J* 1978; 2:1683–1684.

63. Sackellares JC, Lee SI, Dreifuss FE. Stupor following administration of valproic acid to patients receiving other antiepileptic drugs. *Epilepsia* 1979; 20:697–703.

64. Triggs WJ, Bohan TP, Lin S-N, Willmore LJ. Valproate induced coma with ketosis and carnitine insufficiency. *Arch Neurol* 1990; 47:1131–1133.

65. Millington DS, Bohan TP, Roe CR, Yergey AL, Liberato DJ. Valproylcarnitine: a novel drug metabolite identified by fast atom bombardment and thermospray liquid chromatography- mass spectrometry. *Clin Chim Acta* 1985; 145:69–76.

66. Triggs WJ, Roe CR, Rhead WJ, et al. Neuropsychiatric manifestations of defect in mitochondrial beta oxidation response to riboflavin. *J Neurol Neurosurg Psychiatry* 1992; 55:209–211.

67. Roujeau JC, Stern RS. Severe adverse cutaneous reactions to drugs. *N Engl J Med* 1994; 331:1272–1285.

68. Wyllie E, Wyllie R, Cruse RP, Erenberg G, Rothner AD. Pancreatitis associated with valproic acid therapy. *Am J Dis Child* 1984; 138:912–914.

69. Willmore LJ, Wilder BJ, Bruni J, Villarreal HJ. Effect of valproic acid on hepatic function. *Neurology* 1978; 28:961–964.

70. Suchy FJ, Balistreri WF, Buchino JJ, et al. Acute hepatic failure associated with the use of sodium valproate. *N Engl J Med* 1979; 300:962–966.

71. Dreifuss FE, Santilli N, Langer DH, et al. Valproic acid hepatic fatalities: a retrospective review. *Neurology* 1987; 37:379–385.

72. Dreifuss FE, Langer DH, Moline KA, Maxwell JE. Valproic acid hepatic fatalities. II. U.S. experience since 1984. *Neurology* 1989; 39:201–207.

73. Bryant AE, Dreifuss FE. Valproic acid hepatic fatalities. III. U.S. experience since 1986. *Neurology* 1996; 46:465–469.

74. Zimmerman HJ, Ishak KG. Valproate-induced hepatic injury: analysis of 23 fatal cases. *Hepatology* 1982; 2:591–597.

75. Willmore LJ. Clinical risk patterns: summary and recommendations. In: Levy RH, Penry JK, eds. *Idiosyncratic Reactions to Valproate: Clinical Risk Patterns and Mechanisms of Toxicity.* New York: Raven Press, 1991:163–165.

76. Willmore LJ, Triggs WJ, Pellock JM. Valproate toxicity: risk-screening strategies. *J Child Neurol* 1991; 6:3–6.

77. Willmore LJ. Clinical manifestations of valproate hepatotoxicity. In: Levy RH, Penry JK, eds. *Idiosyncratic Reactions to Valproate: Clinical Risk Patterns and Mechanisms of Toxicity.* New York: Raven Press, 1991:3–7.

78. Thom H, Carter PE, Cole GF, Stevenson KL. Ammonia and carnitine concentrations in children treated with sodium valproate compared with other anticonvulsant drugs. *Dev Med Child Neurol* 1991; 33:795–802.

79. Zaret B, Beckner RR, Marini AM, Wagle W, Passarelli C. Sodium valproate-induced hyperammonemia without clinical hepatic dysfunction. *Neurology* 1982; 32:206–208.

80. Hjelm M, Oberholzer V, Seakins J, Thomas S, Kay JDS. Valproate-induced inhibition of urea synthesis and hyperammonemia in healthy subjects. *Lancet* 1986; 2:859–859.

81. Hjelm M, de Silva LKV, Seakins JWT, Oberholzer VG, Rolles CJ. Evidence of inherited urea cycle defect in a case of fatal valproate toxicity. *Br Med J* 1986; 292:23–24.

82. Volzke E, Doose H. Dipropylacetate (Depakine, Ergenyl) in the treatment of epilepsy. *Epilepsia* 1973; 14:185–193.

83. Perucca E, Grimaldi R, Gatti G, et al. Pharmacokinetics of valproic acid in the elderly. *Br J Clin Pharmacol* 1984; 17:665–669.

84. Loscher W, Nau H. Pharmacological evaluation of various metabolites and analogues of valproic acid: anticonvulsant and toxic potencies in mice. *Neuropharmacology* 1985; 24:427–435.

85. Graves NM, Holmes GB, Fuerst RH, Leppik IE. Effect of felbamate on phenytoin and carbamazepine serum concentrations. *Epilepsia* 1989; 30:225–229.

86. Theodore WH, Raubertas RF, Porter RJ, et al. Felbamate: a clinical trial for complex partial seizures. *Epilepsia* 1991; 32:392–397.

87. Sheridan PH, Ashworth M, Milne K, et al. Open pilot study of felbamate (ADD 03055) in partial seizures. *Epilepsia* 1986; 27:649–650.

88. Kaufman DW, Kelly JP, Anderson T, et al. Evaluation of case reports of aplastic anemia among patients treated with felbamate. *Epilepsia* 1997; 38:1265–1269.

89. Thompson CD, Gulden PH, Macdonald TL. Identification of modified atropaldehyde mercapturic acids in rat and human urine after felbamate administration. *Chem Res Toxicol* 1997; 10:457–462.

90. The US Gabapentin Study Group No.5. Gabapentin as add-on therapy in refractory partial epilepsy. *Neurology* 1993; 43:2292–2298.

91. Bauer G, Bechinger D, Castell E, et al. Gabapentin in the treatment of drug resistant epileptic patients. In: Manelis J, Benral E, Loeber JN, Dreifuss FE, eds. *Advances in Epileptology.* 17th ed. New York: Raven Press, 1989:219–221.

92. Crawford P, Ghadiali E, Lane R, Blumhardt L, Chadwick D. Gabapentin as an antiepileptic drug in man. *J Neurol Neurosurg Psychiatry* 1987; 50:682–686.

93. Pellock JM. Utilization of new antiepileptic drugs in children. *Epilepsia* 1996; 37(Suppl 1):S66–S73.

94. Binnie CD, Debets RM, Engelsman M, et al. Double-blind crossover trial of lamotrigine (Lamictal) as add-on therapy in intractable epilepsy. *Epilepsy Res* 1989; 4:222–229.

95. Matsuo F, Bergen D, Faught E, et al. Placebo-controlled study of the efficacy and safety of lamotrigine in patients with partial seizures. *Neurology* 1993; 43:2284–2291.

96. Warner T, Patsalos PN, Prevett M, Elyas AA, Duncan JS. Lamotrigine-induced carbamazepine toxicity: an interaction with carbamazepine-10,11 epoxide. *Epilepsy Res* 1992; 11:147–150.

97. Jawad S, Richens A, Goodwin G, Yuen WC. Controlled trial of lamotrigine (Lamictal) for refractory partial seizures. *Epilepsia* 1989; 30:356–363.

98. Schapel GJ, Beran RG, Vajda FJE, et al. Double-blind, placebo-controlled, crossover study of lamotrigine in treatment resistant partial seizures. *J Neurol Neurosurg Psychiatry* 1993; 56:448–453.

99. Messenheimer JA, Ramsay RA, Willmore LJ, et al. Lamotrigine therapy for partial seizures: a multicenter placebo-controlled, double-blind, crossover trial. *Epilepsia* 1994; 35:113–121.

100. Willmore LJ, Messenheimer JA. Adult experience with lamotrigine. *J Child Neurol* 1997; 12:S16–S18.

101. Brodie MJ, Richens A, UK Lamotrigine/Carbamazepine Monotherapy Trial Group. Lamotrigine versus carbamazepine: a double-blind comparative study in newly diagnosed epilepsy. *Epilepsia* 1994; 35(Suppl 8):31–31.

102. Garnett L, et al. Adverse effects of lamotrigine. *J Child Neurol* 1997; 12:S10–S15.

103. Stables JP, Bialer M, Johannessen SI, et al. Progress report on new antiepileptic drugs: a summary of the second Eilat conference. *Epilepsy Res* 1995; 22:235–246.

104. Sharief M, Viteri C, Ben-Menachem E, et al. Double-blind, placebo controlled study of topiramate in patients with refractory partial epilepsy. *Epilepsy Res* 1996; 37:217–224.

105. Tassinari CA, Michelucci R, Chauvel P, et al. Double-blind, placebo-controlled trial of topiramate (600 mg daily) for the treatment of refractory partial epilepsy. *Epilepsia* 1996; 37:763–768.

106. Ben-Menachem E, Henricksen O, Dam M, et al. Double-blind, placebo-controlled trial of topiramate as add-on therapy in patients with refractory partial seizures. *Epilepsia* 1996; 37:539–543.

107. Faught E, Wilder BJ, Ramsay RA, et al. Topiramate placebo-controlled dose-ranging trial in refractory partial epilepsy using 200-, 400-, and 600-mg daily dosages. *Neurology* 1996; 46:1648–1690.

108. Privitera M, Fincham R, Penry JK, et al. Topiramate placebo-controlled dose-ranging trial in refractory partial epilepsy using 600-, 800-, and 1,000-mg daily dosages. *Neurology* 1996; 46:1678–1683.

109. Braestrup C, Nielsen EB, Sonnewald U, et al. (R)-N-[4,4-bis(3-methyl-7-thienyl) but-3-en-1-yl] Nipecotic acid binds with high affinity to the brain gamma (symbol)-aminobutyric acid uptake carrier. *J Neurochem* 1990; 54:639–647.

110. Adkins JC, Noble S. Tiagabine. A review of its pharmacodynamic and pharmacokinetic properties and therapeutic potential in the management of epilepsy. *Drugs* 1998; 55:437–460.

111. Perucca E, Bialer M. The clinical pharmacokinetics of the newer antiepileptic drugs. *Clin Pharmacokinet* 1996; 1:29–46.

112. Schachter SC. Tiagabine. *Epilepsia* 1999; 40:S17–S22.

113. Friis ML, Kristensen O, Boas J, et al. Therapeutic experiences with 947 epileptic out-patients in oxcarbazepine treatment. *Acta Neurol Scand* 1993; 87:224–227.

114. Schachter SC, Vasquez B, Fisher RS, et al. Oxcarbazepine: a double-blind, placebo-controlled, monotherapy trial for partial seizures. *Neurology* 1999; 52:732–737.

115. Dam M, Ekberg R, Loyning Y, Waltimo O, Jakobsen K. A double-blind study comparing oxcarbazepine and carbamazepine in patients with newly diagnosed, previously untreated epilepsy. *Epilepsy Res* 1989; 3:70–76.

116. Bill PA, Vigonius U, Pohlmann H, et al. A double-blind controlled clinical trial of oxcarbazepine versus phenytoin in adults with previously untreated epilepsy. *Epilepsy Res* 1997; 27:195–204.

117. Christe W, Kramer G, Vigonius U, et al. A double-blind controlled clinical trial: oxcarbazepine versus sodium valproate in adults with newly diagnosed epilepsy. *Epilepsy Res* 1997; 26:451–460.

118. Dam M. Practical aspects of oxcarbazepine treatment. *Epilepsia* 1994; 35(Suppl 3):S23–S25.

119. Haegele KD, Huebert ND, Ebel M, et al. Pharmacokinetics of vigabatrin: implications of creatinine clearance. *Clin Pharmacol Ther* 1988; 44:558–565.

120. Reynolds EH. Vigabatrin. *Br Med J* 1990; 300:277–278.

121. Reynolds EH, Ring H, Heller A. A controlled trial of gamma-vinyl-GABA (vigabatrin) in drug-resistant epilepsy. *Br J Clin Pract Symp* 1988; 61(Suppl):33–33.

122. Kurland AH, Browne TR. Vigabatrin (Sabril). *Clin Neuropharmacol* 1994; 17:560–568.

123. Levinson DF, Devinsky O. Psychiatric adverse events during vigabatrin therapy. *Neurology* 1999; 53:1503–1511.

124. Krauss GL, Johnson MA, Miller NR. Vigabatrin-associated retinal cone system dysfunction. *Neurology* 1998; 50:614–618.

125. Kalviainen R, Nousiainen I, Mantyjarvi M, et al. Vigabatrin, a gabaergic antiepileptic drug, causes concentric visual field defects. *Neurology* 1999; 53:922–926.

126. Leppik IE, Willmore LJ, Homan RW, et al. Efficacy and safety of zonisamide: results of a multicenter study. *Epilepsy Res* 1993; 14:165–173.

127. Perucca E, Garratt A, Hebdige S, Richens A. Water intoxication in epileptic patients receiving carbamazepine. *J Neurol Neurosurg Psychiatry* 1978; 41:713–718.

128. Ringel RA, Brick JF. Perspective on carbamazepine-induced water intoxication: reversal by demeclocycline. *Neurology* 1986; 36:1506–1507.

129. Brodie MJ, Forrest G, Rapeport WG. Carbamazepine 10, 11 epoxide concentrations in epileptics on carbamazepine alone and in combination with other anticonvulsants. *Br J Clin Pharmacol* 1983; 16:747–749.

130. Camfield PR, Bagnell P, Camfield CS, Tibbles JAR. Pancreatitis due to valproic acid. *Lancet* 1979; 1:1198–1199.

131. Rosenberg HK, Ortega W. Hemorrhagic pancreatitis in a young child following valproic acid therapy. Clinical and ultrasonic assessment. *Clin Pediatr* 1987; 26:98–101.

132. Parker PH. Recurrent pancreatitis induced by valproic acid. *Gastroenterology* 1981; 80:826–828.

133. Kay JDS, Hilton-Jones D, Hyman N. Valproate toxicity and ornithine carbamoyltransferase deficiency. *Lancet* 1986; 2:1283–1284.

134. Tripp JH, Hargreaves T, Anthony PP, et al. Sodium valproate and ornithine carbamyl transferase deficiency. *Lancet* 1981; 1:1165–1166.

135. Gerber N, Dickinson G, Harland RC, et al. Reye-like syndrome associated with valproic acid therapy. *J Pediatr* 1979; 95:142–144.

136. Stolz A, Kaplowitz N. Biochemical tests for liver disease. In: Zakim D, Boyer TD, eds. *Hepatology*. 2nd ed. Philadelphia: WB Saunders, 1990:637–667.

137. Williams C, Tiefenbach S, McReynolds J. Valproic acid-induced hyperammonemia in mentally retarded adults. *Neurology* 1984; 34:550–553.

138. Zaccara G, Paganini M, Campostrini R, Arnetoli G, Zappoli R. Hyperammonemia and valproate induced alterations of the state of consciousness: a report of eight cases. *Eur Neurol* 1984; 23:104–112.

139. Zarfani ES, Berthelot P. Sodium valproate in the induction of unusual hepatotoxicity. *Hepatology* 1982; 2:648–649.

140. Coude FX, Grimer G, Pelet A, Benoit Y. Action of the antiepileptic drug, valproic acid, on fatty acid oxidation in isolated rat hepatocytes. *Biochem Biophys Res Comm* 1983; 115:730–736.

141. Murphy JV, Marquardt KM, Shug AL. Valproic acid associated abnormalities of carnitine metabolism. *Lancet* 1985; 1:820–821. Letter.

142. Becker CM, Harris RA. Influence of valproic acid on hepatic carbohydrate and lipid metabolism. *Arch Biochem Biophys* 1983; 223:381–382.

143. Thurston JH, Carroll JE, Hauhart RE, Schiro JA. A single therapeutic dose of valproate affects liver carbohydrate, fat, adenylate, amino acid, coenzyme A, and carnitine metabolism in infant mice: possible clinical significance. *Life Sci* 1985; 36:1643–1651.

144. Moore KH, Decker BP, Schreefel FP. Hepatic hydrolysis of octanoyl-CoA and valproyl-CoA in control and valproate-fed animals. *Int J Biochem* 1988; 20:175–178.

145. Thurston JH, Carroll JE, Norris BJ, et al. Acute in vivo and in vitro inhibition of palmitic acid and pyruvate oxidation by valproate and valproyl-coenzyme a in livers of infant mice. *Ann Neurol* 1983; 14:384–385.

146. Kean EA. Selective inhibition of acyl-CoA dehydrogenases by a metabolite of hypoglycin. *Biochim Biophys Acta* 1976; 422:8–14.

147. Pisciotta AV. Hematological toxicity of carbamazepine. *Adv Neurol* 1975; 11:355–368.

148. Pisciotta AV. Phenytoin: Hematological toxicity. In: Woodbury DM, Penry JK, Pippenger CE, eds. *Antiepileptic Drugs.* 2nd ed. New York: Raven Press, 1982:257–268.

149. Utrecht J. Drug metabolism by leukocytes and its role in drug-induced lupus and other idiosyncratic drug reactions. *Crit Rev Toxicol* 1990; 20:213–235.

150. Aarli JA, Tonder O. Effect of antiepileptic drugs on serum and salivary IgA. *Scand J Immunol* 1975; 4:391.

151. Sorrell TC, Forbes IJ. Depression of immune competence by phenytoin and carbamazepine. *Clin Exp Immunol* 1975; 20:273–285.

152. Weisberg LA, Shamsnia M, Elliott D. Seizures caused by nontraumatic parenchymal brain hemorrhages. *Neurology* 1991; 41:1197–1199.

153. Brown M, Schubert T. Phenytoin hypersensitivity hepatitis and mononucleosis syndrome. *J Clin Gastroenterol* 1986; 8:469–477.

154. Kahn HD, Faguet GB, Agee JF, Middleton HM. Drug-induced liver injury: in vitro demonstration of hypersensitivity to both phenytoin and phenobarbital. *Arch Intern Med* 1984; 144:1677.

155. Taylor JW, Stein MN, Murphy MJ, Mitros FA. Cholestatic liver dysfunction after long-term phenytoin therapy. *Arch Neurol* 1984; 41:500.

156. Hart RG, Easton JD. Carbamazepine and hematological monitoring. *Ann Neurol* 1982; 11:309–312.

157. Middleton E Jr, Reed CE, Ellis EF, Adkinson NF, Yunginger JW. *Allergy: Principles and Practice.* 3rd ed. St. Louis: CV Mosby, 1988.

CHAPTER 26

Teratogenicity of Anticonvulsant Medication

Mark S. Yerby, M.D.

Epilepsy is a common neurologic disorder with a prevalence of approximately 6 per 1,000 (1). Between 680,000 and 1.1 million women with epilepsy of childbearing age live in the United States today. The repeal of discriminatory legislation prohibiting marriage, development of more effective therapies, and changing social attitudes have encouraged more women with epilepsy to consider childbearing. Despite the medical advances, such women are considered high-risk patients because of the greater risk of complications of pregnancy and labor and adverse pregnancy outcomes.

Low birth weight (<2,500 g) and prematurity occur more often in infants of mothers with epilepsy (IMEs), ranging from 7 percent to 10 percent and 4 percent to 11 percent, respectively (2–7). Microcephaly has been demonstrated with increased frequency in IMEs (4,8). Stillbirth rates are higher in IMEs (1.3%–14%) compared with controls (1.2%–7.8%) (3,4,9,10). Other studies have also demonstrated increased rates of neonatal and perinatal death. The rates have ranged from 1.3 percent to 7.8 percent for IMEs compared with 1.0 percent to 3.9 percent for controls (2,4,9,11–14).

Congenital malformations are the most widely reported and dramatic adverse outcomes of pregnancy. Malformations are defined as a physical defect requiring medical or surgical intervention and causing major functional disturbance. Infants of mothers with epilepsy exposed to antiepileptic drugs (AEDs) in utero are twice as likely to develop birth defects as infants not exposed to these drugs (15,16).

HISTORICAL ASPECTS

The first report of a malformation associated with AEDs described a child exposed to mephenytoin in utero who developed microcephaly, cleft palate, malrotation of the intestine, a speech defect, and an IQ of 60 (17). The pregnancy had been complicated by vaginal bleeding.

In 1964 Janz and Fuchs conducted a retrospective survey to evaluate the problem of AED-associated malformations at the University of Heidelberg (9). A total of 426 pregnancies in 246 mothers with epilepsy were studied. The rates of miscarriages and stillbirths were increased for these patients, but the malformation rate was only 2.2 percent, not significantly different from that of the general population of what was then West Germany. The authors concluded that AEDs were not associated with an increased risk of malformations.

Pantarotto described a newborn with aplasia of the bone marrow after phenytoin exposure in utero (18). Centa and Rasore-Quartino reported the first case of congenital heart disease with in utero exposure to phenytoin and phenobarbital (19). Melchior and coworkers described orofacial clefts with exposure to primidone or phenobarbital (20).

In a letter to *Lancet* in 1968, S.R. Meadow reported six cases of children with orofacial clefts, four of whom had additional abnormalities of the heart and dysmorphic facial features (21). All of these children had been exposed to AEDs in utero. He noted that similar abnormalities had been reported following the unsuccessful use of abortifacient folic acid antagonists. Because some AEDs act as folic acid antagonists, he postulated that this might account for AED teratogenicity and asked for other clinicians to inform him of similar cases. The first report of malformations associated with a specific AED was published two years later (22.) Trimethadione was implicated as a teratogen in 8 of 14 patients who took it in the first trimester.

Meadow's 1968 inquiry concerning AED-associated malformations resulted in the collection of 30 additional cases. This prompted a retrospective survey of 427 pregnancies in 186 women with epilepsy. For the first time, a clear increase in the malformation rates

Table 26-1. Malformation Rates in the Offspring of Mothers with Epilepsy and Control Mothers

Authors	Malformation Rate (%)	No. of Pregnancies	Control Rate (%)	Epileptic Malformation Pregnancies
Sabin and Oxorn (151)			5.4	56
Janz and Fuchs (9)			2.3	225
Germanetal (22)			5.3	243
Elshove and VanEck (35)	1.9	12,051	15.0	65
Speidel and Meadow (15)	1.6	483	5.2	427
South (26)	2.4	7,892	6.4	31
Spellacy (152)		50	5.8	51
Bjerkdal and Bahna (2)	2.2	12,530	4.5	311
Fedrick (16)	5.6	649	13.8	217
Koppe et al. (153)	2.9	12,455	6.6	197
Kuenssberg and Knox (154)	3.0	14,668	10.0	48
Lowe (27)	2.7	31,877	5.0	245
Meyer (155)	2.7	110	18.6	593
Millar and Nevin (156)	3.8	32,227	6.4	110
Monson et al. (28)	2.4	50,591	4.7	306
Niswander and Wertelecki (157)	2.7	347,097	4.1	413
Biale and Lewenthal (113)			16.0	56
Knight and Rhind (13)	3.65	69,000	4.3	140
Starreveld-Zimmerman et al. (158)			7.0	372
Visser et al. (159)	2.3	9,869	3.7	54
Weber et al. (160)	2.2	5,011	4.0	731
Annegers et al. (29)	3.5	748	8.1	259
Seino and Miyakoshi (161)			13.7	272
Dieterich et al. (41)				37
Majewski et al. (33)			16.0	111
Nakane et al. (10)			11.5	700
Hiilesmaa et al. (75)	2.0	5,613	7.7	4,795
Stanley et al. (162)	3.4	62,265	3.7	244
Beaussart-Defaye et al. (163)			7.8	295
Rating et al. (164)	3.7	162	5.3	150
Gaily (165)	2.9	105	9.1	153
Dravet et al. (166)	1.4	117,183	7.0	281
Kaneko et al. (167)			6.2	145
Koch et al. (168)	4.3	116	6.9	116
Lindhout et al. (34)			7.6	172
Tanganelli and Regesta (134)	2.6	140	3.6	138

among IMEs was demonstrated. Speidel and Meadow concluded that (1) congenital malformations are twice as common in IMEs exposed to AEDs; (2) no single abnormality was specific for AED exposure; and (3) a group of these children would have a characteristic pattern of anomalies, which at its fullest expression consisted of trigonocephaly, microcephaly, hypertelorism, low-set ears, short neck, transverse palmer creases, and minor skeletal abnormalities.

Congenital malformations remain the most commonly reported adverse outcomes in the pregnancies of epileptic mothers. Malformation rates in the general population range from 2 percent to 3 percent (23,24). Reports of malformation rates in various populations of IMEs range from 1.25 percent to 11.5 percent (10,21,25). Among women with epilepsy who are taking AEDs

these combined estimates yield a risk of malformations in an individual epileptic pregnancy of 4 percent to 6 percent, approximately twice the risk in the general population. Table 26-1 reviews the various studies that compare malformation rates in the offspring of mothers with and without epilepsy.

CURRENT CONCEPTS

The increased rate of malformations in the offspring of mothers with epilepsy appears to be related to AED exposure in utero. Evidence to support this association comes from four observations.

1. Comparisons of the malformation rates in the offspring of epileptic mothers treated with AEDs

Table 26-2. Malformation Rates in the Offspring of Treated and Nontreated Mothers with Epilepsy

| Authors | Malformation Rate (%) | |
	Anticonvulsants	No Anticonvulsants
Janz and Fuchs (9)	2.2	0
Speidel and		
Meadow (15)	5.0	0
South (26)	9.0	0
Lowe (27)	6.7	2.7
Monson (28)	5.3	2.9
Annegers et al. (130)	7.1	1.8
Annegers et al. (29)	10.7	2.4
Nakane (31)	11.5	2.3
Nakane (3)	13.8	8.5
Robert et al. (169)	7.2	0
Rating et al. (164)	5.3	5.9

with those with no AED treatment reveal consistently higher rates in the children of the treated group (Table 24-2) (10,11,26–29).

2. Mean plasma AED concentrations are higher in mothers who give birth to malformed infants than in mothers whose offspring are healthy (30).

3. Infants of mothers taking multiple AEDs have higher malformation rates than those who take a single AED (31,32).

4. Although the results are mixed, maternal seizures during pregnancy do not appear to increase the risk of congenital malformations (16).

Majewski and coworkers described increased malformation rates and central nervous system (CNS) injury in IMEs whose mothers had seizures during pregnancy (33). More recently, Lindhout and coworkers described a marked increase in malformations among infants whose mothers had seziures in the first trimester (12.3%) compared with infants whose mothers did not have seizures (4%) (34). Malformations were more often observed in infants exposed to partial seizures than to generalized tonic-clonic seizures. However, several investigators have found that maternal seizures during pregnancy had no impact on the frequency of malformations, development of epilepsy, or febrile convulsions (10,29).

Virtually every type of congenital malformation has been reported in children of mothers with epilepsy, and every anticonvulsant medication has been implicated in the development of malformations. Cleft lip and palate and congenital heart disease account for a majority of all reported cases (29,35,36). Orofacial clefts are relatively common malformations in the general population, occurring with a frequency of 1.5 per 1,000 live births. Infants of mothers with epilepsy have a rate of orofacial clefting of 13.8 per 1,000, a ninefold increase in risk (7,24). Early observations that people with cleft

lip or palate were twice as likely to have family members with epilepsy as controls suggested that orofacial clefts were associated with epilepsy (37). Subsequent studies of the prevalence of facial clefts in the siblings and children of 2,072 people with epilepsy found observed to expected ratios increased only for maternal epilepsy. The risk was greater if AEDs were taken during pregnancy (4.7) than if no AED treatment was used (2.7). The authors concluded that there was no evidence that epilepsy itself contributed to the development of orofacial clefts (38). Israeli researchers have found that children with cleft lip or palate are four times as likely to have a mother with epilepsy as the general population, and mothers with epilepsy are six times as likely to bear a child with an orofacial cleft as nonepileptic women (39). Orofacial clefts account for 30 percent of the excess of congenital malformations in IMEs.

Congenital heart defects are the second most frequently reported teratogenic abnormality associated with AEDs. IMEs have a 1.5 percent to 2 percent prevalence of congenital heart disease, a relative risk of threefold over the general population (7). Anderson prospectively studied maternal epilepsy and AED use in 3,000 children with heart defects at the University of Minnesota (36). Eighteen IMEs were identified. Twelve of these had ventricular septal defects; nine of the 18 children had additional noncardiac defects, eight of which were orofacial clefts.

No AED can be considered absolutely safe in pregnancy, but no specific pattern of major malformations has been identified for the vast majority of drugs (14). This lack of a particular or characteristic pattern of defects has been cited as evidence that AEDs are not teratogenic. When phenobarbital is given during pregnancy for conditions other than epilepsy, no increase in malformation rates has been demonstrated (40).

Some investigators have found increased malformation rates in the infants of fathers with epilepsy and suggest that epilepsy per se is associated with birth defects and not AED exposure (41,42). Others have failed to demonstrate an increased malformation rate in IMEs (43). However, these studies have been retrospective, and case ascertainment has been uncertain. The weight of the evidence supports some teratogenic effect of AEDs. Furthermore, in addition to major malformations, a variety of anomaly syndromes associated with AED exposure (7).

SYNDROMES OF ANOMALIES

Distinct from malformations, which are deformities of anatomy requiring medical or surgical intervention to maintain a functionally healthy person, anomalies are abnormalities of structure, which, although they vary from the norm, do not constitute a threat to health. Patterns of anomalies in IMEs have been linked to exposure to certain AEDs. Five clinical syndromes have been reported in IMEs: fetal trimethadione syndrome, fetal hydantoin syndrome, primidone embryopathy, fetal valproate syndrome, and fetal carbamazepine syndrome. The clinical features of these syndromes are outlined in Table 26-3.

Table 26-3. Syndromes of Anomalies Associated with Anticonvulsants

Fetal trimethadione syndrome
Developmental delay
V-shaped eyebrows
Low-set ears IUGR
Cardiac anomalies
Speech difficulties
Epicanthal folds
Irregular teeth
Microcephaly
Inguinal hernia
Simian creases

Fetal hydantoin syndrome
Craniofacial anomalies
Broad nasal bridge
Short upturned nose
Low-set ears
Prominent lips
Epicanthal folds
Hypertelorism
Wide mouth
Ptosis or strabismus
Distal digital hypoplasia
IUGR
Mental deficiency

Fetal valproate syndrome
Craniofacial anomalies
Epicanthal folds inferiorly
Small antiverted nose
Shallow philtrum
Flat nasal bridge
Long upper lip
Downturned mouth
Thin vermillion border

Primidone embryopathy
Hirsute forehead
Thick nasal root
Distal digital hypoplasia
Antiverted nostrils
Long philtrum
Straight thin upper lip
Psychomotor retardation

Fetal carbamazepine syndrome
Upslanting palpebral fissures
Epicanthal folds
Short nose
Long philtrum
Hypoplastic nails
Microcephaly
Developmental delay

Fetal Trimethadione Syndrome

In 1970 German and colleagues described a case of a woman with epilepsy treated with trimethadione who had had four unsuccessful pregnancies (22). She went on to have two healthy children after trimethadione was discontinued. Her physician then surveyed trimethadione-exposed infants delivered at New York Hospital between 1946 and 1968. The records of 278 women with epilepsy were reviewed, and of these, 14 had taken trimethadione during pregnancy. Only two of these 14 resultant children were normal. One had multiple hernias and diabetes, eight had developmental defects, three spontaneously aborted, and only three of the 14 survived infancy.

The peculiar facial characteristics of these children were delineated by Zachai and coworkers, who noted that not only were these children short in stature and suffering from microcephaly, but also they had V-shaped eyebrows, epicanthal folds, low-set ears, anteriorly forled helices, and irregular teeth (44). Other common abnormalities include inguinal hernias, hypospadias, and simian creases. Feldman and colleagues reviewed 53 pregnancies in which trimethadione was used (45). In 46 of these (87%) there was fetal loss or the development of a congenital malformation. Follow-up studies of the surviving children have reported significant rates of mental retardation (46).

Fetal Hydantoin Syndrome

The most controversial of the dysmorphic syndromes associated with AEDs is the fetal hydantoin syndrome (FHS). It was first reported by Loughnan and coworkers, who described seven infants exposed to hydantoin in combination with a barbiturate in utero (47). The children displayed hypoplasia and irregular ossification of the distal phalanges. In 1974 Barr and coworkers reported distal digital hypoplasia (DDH) in eight children exposed to phenytoin and phenobarbital (48). The syndrome was given its name by Hanson and Smith, who reported on five IMEs who had been exposed to hydantoin in utero (49). The infants had multiple systemic abnormalities of the face, cranium, and nails; DDH; intrauterine growth retardation; and mental deficiencies. Only one of the five was exposed to phenytoin monotherapy. Of the others, three were exposed to phenobarbital, one to mephobarbital, and one to a combination of phenobarbital, phensuximide, and mephenytoin. Despite the multiplicity of exposure, the authors noted the resemblance to fetal alcohol syndrome (FAS) and described their patients as suffering from FHS.

Subsequent work by Hanson's group found that approximately 11 percent of infants exposed to hydantoin in utero demonstrated the complete syndrome, and an additional 30 percent had some anomalous components (50). Many of the features of the syndrome appear to be subjective, but some investigators believe that DDH is a unique and relatively constant feature (51).

The prevalence and significance of the dysmorphic features of FHS remain unclear. Researchers at the University of Virginia followed up 98 women with epilepsy who took phenytoin during pregnancy and found that 30 percent of their offspring had DDH with no other features of FHS (52). Gaily and coworkers reported a prospective study of 121 IMEs at the University of Helsinki, 82 of whom were exposed to phenytoin (53). None of the children had FHS. Hypertelorism and DDH were the only dysmorphic features associated with phenytoin exposure. In our own experience following 64 IMEs, no children with FHS were seen. Dysmorphic features could be seen with any drug exposure (54).

Hanson described three components to the syndrome: (1) abnormal growth, (2) abnormal performance, and (3) dysmorphic cranial facial features (55). An unexpected sequela of the syndrome may be an increased risk of cancer. Four cases of neuroblastoma associated with FHS have been described since 1976, although all children were also exposed in utero to primidone or phenobarbital. There have also been reports of carcinoma, ganglioneuroblastoma, Wilms' tumor, a melanotic neuroectodermal tumor, and a malignant mesenchymona in children with FHS (56).

The contention that FHS results in abnormal performance or mental deficiency is not supported by subsequent research. Of 103 IMEs exposed to phenytoin, only 1.4 percent displayed mental deficiency on the Wechsler Preschool and Primary Scale of Intelligence or Leiter International Performance Scale, not significantly different from the general population (57).

Gaily's work suggests that there is a genetic component that permits expression of the FHS. Children of mothers with epilepsy who are not exposed to AEDs in utero have frequencies of dysmorphic abnormalities intermediate to those children exposed to AEDs and controls. Dizygotic twins exposed to hydantoins in utero have been shown to display discordant dysmorphism (58,59). If the first child in a family has FHS, the chance of a second such child is 90 percent, compared with the 2 percent chance that a second-born child will have FHS if the first is normal (60). Such observations suggest that hydantoin exposure may be a necessary but not sufficient cause of FHS.

To make matters even more confusing, Krauss and coworkers described four siblings with features of FHS (61). The first two were exposed to both phenytoin and primidone in utero. In an attempt to prevent further fetal injury, Krauss discontinued the phenytoin

and the patient was treated with primidone monotherapy. Two subsequent pregnancies resulted in children with dysmorphic features that were similar to those in their elder siblings.

Primidone Embryopathy

Five years before Krauss's report, Rudd and Freedom had described craniofacial abnormalities in children exposed to primidone in utero (62). These children had hirsute foreheads, thick nasal roots, antiverted nostrils, a long philtrum, straight thin upper lips, and hypoplastic nails. They were also likely to be small for their gestational age and to have psychomotor retardation and heart defects (63).

Fetal Valproate Syndrome

Several investigators had reported dysmorphic children after exposure to valproate in utero (64,65), but it was DiLiberti and coworkers who proposed a specific fetal valproate syndrome (66). They reported seven infants exposed to valproic acid in utero who had facial abnormalities characterized by interiorepicanthal folds, a flat nasal bridge, an upturned nose, a long upper lip, a thin vermillion border, a shallow philtrum, and a downturned mouth. These children also had abnormalities of their distal digits, and they tended to have long, thin, overlapping fingers and toes and hyperconvex nails. Subsequent reports have also been made of valproate exposed infants having radial ray aplasia.

The prevalence of this syndrome has not yet been established. Jager-Roman and coworkers described it in 5 of 14 children exposed to valproate monotherapy (67). In this same group, 43 percent of the children were distressed at labor and 28 percent had low Apgar scores and other major malformations. High doses of valproate were associated with drug withdrawal, hypotonia, and motor and language delay. In a review of 344 women who took valproate during the first trimester of pregnancy, Jeavons described a 19.8 percent rate of abnormal deliveries but no evidence of a dose-response effect with valproate exposure (68).

Felding and Rane described an infant with severe congenital liver disease after in utero exposure to valproic acid and phenytoin (69). Ardinger and coworkers reported craniofacial dysmorphism in 19 children exposed to valproate in utero and confirmed the features described by DiLiberti (70). They also found that a large proportion of these infants had postnatal growth deficiency and microcephaly, particularly if the children were exposed to polytherapy in utero. The association of valproate with spina bifida is discussed subsequently.

Benzodiazepine Syndrome

Infants exposed to benzodiazepines in utero are at greater risk for intrauterine growth retardation, dysmorphic features, and neurologic dysfunction. Seven of 37 infants exposed to benzodiazepines in utero were described as hypotonic and hyperexcitable and exhibited dystonic postures and choreoathetotic movements (71) Delayed hand-eye coordination, psychomotor slowing, and a learning disability were also noted. Four infants had major malformations and dysmorphic faces with wide-set eyes, epicanthal folds, upturned noses, dysplastic ears, high-arched palates, webbed necks, and wide-spaced nipples (71). In a survey of 278 women whose infants had congenital malformations, children with a history of diazepam exposure in the first trimester had a fourfold increase in cleft lip or palate (72).

Carbamazepine Syndrome

The most recently described syndrome of anomalies associated with AED exposure is the carbamazepine syndrome. One group of investigators has described craniofacial defects (upslanting palpebral fissures, epicanthal folds, short nose, long philtrum), hypoplastic nails, and microcephaly in 37 IMEs exposed to carbamazepine monotherapy (73). A case of DDH in an IME exposed to carbamazepine monotherapy had been described earlier, but that child was otherwise normal (74). Based on testing with the Bayley Scale of Infant Development, the Stanford-Binet IV, and the Wechsler Scale of Preschool and Primary Intelligence in their evaluations, 20 percent of 25 children born to mothers taking carbamazepine monotherapy scored one standard deviation or more below the mean.

Low birth weight has been reported with in utero exposure to carbamazepine monotherapy (14). A reduction in fetal head circumference has been noted in IMEs exposed to carbamazepine (75). Although smaller than control children, the head sizes were still within the normal range. Subsequent studies on the same clinical population failed to find differences in head circumference as the children matured (76).

CURRENT CONCEPTS OF ANOMALIES — ANTIEPILEPTIC DRUG EMBRYOPATHY

Clinical and laboratory evidence clearly links certain anticonvulsants with teratogenic effects, especially facial and distal digital anomalies; however, the existence of drug-specific syndromes is doubtful. Facial dysmorphism is difficult to quantify and clearly is not drug-specific. In the preanticonvulsant era, infants of mothers with epilepsy were described who had similar dysmorphic features (25,77). Follow-up of these

infants into adult life has yet to be accomplished, and therefore the significance of these anomalies is unclear. Gaily and coworkers followed up a cohort of IMEs to 5.5 years of age (53). These children had more minor anomalies characteristic of FHS than control children, but so did their mothers. Only hypertelorism and digital hypoplasia were associated with phenytoin exposure. Certain anomalies, particularly epicanthal folds, appeared to be associated with maternal epilepsy, not to AED exposure.

The hypothetical association of dysmorphic features with mental retardation (24) has not been confirmed (78,79). In the few cases that have been followed up into early childhood, the dysmorphic features become less apparent as the child grows older (80). In one study mental deficiency was found in only 1.4 percent of IMEs followed up to 5.5 years of age (57). Exposure to AEDs below the toxic concentration range or to maternal seizures did not increase the risk of lower intelligence. No association between features of FHS and mental retardation could be demonstrated.

The primary abnormalities in AED-related syndromes involve the midface and distal digits. A retrospective study spanning 10 years of deliveries in Israel found hypertelorism to be the only anomaly seen more often in IMSe than in controls (8). This was associated with all AEDs except primidone. A prospective study of 172 deliveries of IMEs that evaluated eight specific AEDs and other potential confounding factors found no dose-dependent increase in the incidence of malformations associated with any individual AED. Furthermore, no specific defect could be associated with individual AED exposure (81). It has been suggested that, because a variety of similar anomalies of the midface and distal digits are seen in a small proportion of children exposed to anticonvulsants in utero, a better term for the entire group of abnormalities would be *fetal anticonvulsant syndrome* or *AED embryopathy* (41,82,83).

MECHANISMS OF TERATOGENICITY

Over the last 10 years, a body of evidence has accumulated supporting the hypotheses that (1) an arene oxide metabolite of phenytoin or another AED is the ultimate teratogen, (2) a genetic defect in epoxide hydrolase (arene oxide detoxifying enzyme system) increases the risk of fetal toxicity, (3) free radicals produced by AED metabolism are cytotoxic, and (4) a genetic defect in free radical scavenging enzyme activity (FRSEA) increases the risk of fetal toxicity.

Epoxides

Many drugs and chemicals are converted to epoxide intermediates by reactions that are catalyzed by the microsomal monoxygenase system (84,85). Arene oxides are unstable epoxides formed from aromatic compounds. Toxic epoxides elicit carcinogenic, mutagenic, and other toxic effects by covalent binding to vital cell macromolecules (86,87). Epoxides are detoxified by two types of processes: (1) conversion to dihydrodiols catalyzed by epoxide hydrolase in the cytoplasm, and (2) conjugation with glutathione in the microsomes (spontaneously or mediated by glutathione transferase). Epoxide hydrolase activity has been found in the cytosol and the microsomal subcellular fraction of adult and fetal human hepatocytes. Interestingly, epoxide hydrolase activity in fetal livers is much lower than that in adult livers (88). One-third to one-half of fetal circulation bypasses the liver, resulting in higher direct exposure of extrahepatic fetal organs to potential toxic metabolites (89).

Arene oxides are obligatory intermediates in the metabolism of aromatic compounds to *trans*-dihydrodiols. For over 15 years, it has been known that phenytoin forms a transdihydrodiol metabolite in several species (90). This metabolite is also formed by neonates exposed to phenytoin in utero (91). In vitro studies have shown that an oxidative metabolite of phenytoin binds irreversibly to rat liver microsomes by a process that is nicotinamide-adenine dinucleotide phosphase (NADPH)/O_2-dependent (92). This reaction product is increased by an inhibitor of epoxide hydrolase [trichloroponene oxide (TCPO)] and decreased by glutathione (92–94). Using a mouse hepatic microsomal system to produce phenytoin metabolites, and human lymphocytes to assess cellular toxicity, Spielberg and coworkers (1981) showed that cytotoxicity was enhanced by inhibitors of epoxide hydrolase (95). Similarly, in a study in mice, Martz and coworkers (1977) showed that treatment with an inhibitor of epoxide hydrolase led to an increased rate of orofacial anomalies in animals exposed to phenytoin (92). Furthermore, there was a correlation between the teratogenic effect and the amount of covalently bound toxin in fetal tissue.

Subsequently, lymphocytes from 24 children exposed to phenytoin during gestation and lymphocytes from their families using the Spielberg test of cytotoxicity have given more insight into the likely teratogenic mechanism (95,96). In this system, a positive response was highly correlated with major birth defects. Cells from 15 children gave a positive response, and each positive child had a positive parent (as many mothers as fathers). The authors concluded that a genetic defect in arene oxide detoxification seems to increase the risk of the baby's having major birth defects (96).

Variations in epoxide hydrolase activity may explain why some dizygotic twins are discordant for FHS. In 1985 Buchler reported epoxide hydrolase activity in skin fibroblasts from a pair of dizygotic twins exposed to phenytoin in utero. The infant who had more features of FHS showed lower epoxide hydrolase activity.

Intersubject Variability in Epoxide Hydrolase Activity

Since 1977 several studies have documented the degree of intersubject variability in epoxide hydrolase activity measured in various organs obtained at autopsy or from biopsies (97–102). Generally, a large degree of variability was found. In a recent study, Mertes and coworkers measured microsomal and cytosolic epoxide hydrolase activity in liver biopsy samples from 166 subjects (103). Microcytosolic epoxide hydrolase activity was found to vary by a factor of 64, whereas the cytosolic activity varied 539-fold.

The evidence that epoxide metabolites of phenytoin are teratogenic can be summarized as follows. Phenytoin has an epoxide metabolite that binds to tissues. Inhibition of the detoxifying enzyme epoxide hydrolase increases the rate of orofacial clefts in experimental animals, lymphocyte cytotoxicity, and the binding of epoxide metabolite to liver microsomes.

Questions remain about the mechanism of AED-associated teratogenicity. The lymphocyte cytotoxicity mediated by epoxide metabolites correlates with major but not minor malformations (104). Dysmorphic abnormalities have been described in siblings exposed to ethotoin in utero even though ethotoin is not metabolized through an arene oxide intermediate (105). Embryopathies have been described with exposure to mephenytoin, which does not form an arene oxide intermediate (106). Trimethadione is clearly teratogenic but has no phenyl rings and thus cannot form an arene oxide metabolite; therefore, alternate mechanisms must exist.

Free Radical Intermediates of AEDs and Teratogenicity

Some drugs are metabolized or bioactivated by cooxidation during prostaglandin synthetase (PGS) catalyzed synthesis of prostaglandins. Such drugs serve as electron donors to peroxidases, resulting in electron-deficient free radicals. In the search for additional electrons to complete their outer ring, free radicals can covalently bind to cell macromolecules, including nucleic acids (DNA, RNA), proteins, cell membranes, and lipoproteins to produce cytotoxicity.

Phenytoin is cooxidated by PGS, thyroid peroxidase, and horseradish peroxidase producing reactive free radical intermediates that bind to proteins (10). Phenytoin teratogenicity can be modulated by substances that reduce the formation of phenytoin-free radicals. Acetylsalicylic acid (ASA) irreversibly inhibits PGS, caffeic acid is an antioxidant, and alpha-phenyl-*N-t*-butylnitrone (PBN) is a free radical spin-trapping agent. Pretreatment of pregnant mice with these compounds reduces the number of cleft lip and palates caused by phenytoin in their offspring (108).

Reduced glutathione (GSH) is believed to detoxify free radical intermediates by forming a nonreactive conjugate. N-acetylcysteine, a glutathione precursor, decreases phenytoin-induced orofacial clefts and fetal weight loss in rodents (109). BCNU inhibits GSH reductase, an enzyme necessary to maintain adequate cellular glutathione concentrations, and increases phenytoin embryopathy at doses at which BCNU alone has no embryopathic effect (110). The metabolism of phenytoin or other AEDs to free radical intermediates may be responsible for the teratogenicity seen in IMEs.

Other Potential Mechanisms of AED Teratogenicity

It has been proposed that the glucocorticoid receptor mediates the teratogenicity of phenytoin. Arachiodonic acid reverses clefting induced by glucocorticoids in rats. Phospholipase inhibitory proteins (PLIPs) inhibit arachiodonic acid release. Glucocorticoid receptors mediate the induction of PLIPs. Infants of mothers with epilepsy exposed to phenytoin with the stigmata of FHS have increased levels of glucocorticoid receptors (111).

Deficiencies of folate have been implicated in the development of birth defects. Dansky and coworkers found significantly lower blood folate concentrations in women with epilepsy with abnormal pregnancy outcomes (104). Cotreatment of mice with folic acid, with or without other vitamins and amino acids, reduced malformation rates and increased fetal weight and length in mice pups exposed to phenytoin in utero (112). Biale and Lewenthal reported a 15 percent malformation rate in IMEs with no folate supplementation, whereas none of 33 folate-supplemented children had congenital abnormalities (113).

A group of European researchers have demonstrated fetal injury in in vitro rodent models. In these systems antiarrhythmic drugs inhibit potassium channels resulting in fetal bradycardia and cardic arrest. The fetal hypoxia is then followed by reoxygenation and generation of reactive oxygen species The resulting reduction in oxygen saturation causes fetal injury. Low doses of phenytoin administration in combination with brief periods of clamping the uterine artery result in DDH in animal models. Thus an alternate mechanism of anticonvulant teratogenicity has been proposed (114–116). It may well be that a variety of mechanisms may operate on an individual fetus at any one time.

Valproic Acid Teratogenicity

A specific adverse outcome is necessary to classify a substance as a teratogen. Phocomelia associated with

exposure to thalidomide is a good example. Although orofacial clefts are the most common malformations associated with AED exposure, they are clearly not the majority of malformations. This has led some investigators to contend that true teratogenicity is not associated with AEDs.

The introduction of valproic acid (VPA) to the anticonvulsant armamentarium has modified our thinking in this regard. Dysmorphism has been associated with in utero exposure to VPA. The first such case was reported by Dalens and coworkers, who described an infant exposed to VPA in utero who was born with low birth weight, hypoplastic nose and frontoorbital ridges, and levocardia (64). The baby died at 19 days old. Subsequent reports of dysmorphism followed up by Clay and coworkers (65), and a child with lumbosacral meningocele was described by Gomez (117). Dickinson and coworkers had previously demonstrated the ability of VPA to cross the placenta (118). Kaneko and coworkers found VPA to result in the highest malformation rate of any AED utilized in 172 pregnancies (81). As already noted, a fetal valproate syndrome has been described (66,68,119).

A report in *Morbidity and Mortality Weekly Report* (MMWR) in October 1982 associated VPA with a specific malformation — neural tube defects — for the first time. The Institute European de Genomutations in Lyon, France, developed a system of birth defect surveillance and registered 145 cases of spina bifida between 1976 and 1982. They noted that of IMEs exposed to VPA, 34 percent had malformations, and five of nine exposed to VPA monotherapy had spine bifida, a rate 20 times that expected (120).

Subsequent reports confirmed the linkage between intrauterine VPA exposure and spina bifida. Robert and coworkers sent questionnaires to 646 women with epilepsy, aged 15 to 45 years (121). Of 280 responses they collected, there were 74 deliveries, to which they added 74 cases collected from women delivering in Lyon, France. The malformation rate of the entire group was 13 percent, with a higher than expected rate of neural tube defects in children exposed to VPA.

Stanley and Chambers reported an infant exposed to VPA in utero with spina bifida whose two normal siblings were not exposed to the drug (122). Lindhout and Schmidt surveyed 18 epilepsy groups and collected 12 cases of infants and epileptic mothers with neural tube defects (123). A higher rate was seen in children exposed to VPA monotherapy (2.5%) than polytherapy (1.5%). The increased risk appears to be limited to spina bifida rather than other neural tube defects with an overall risk of an infant exposed to VPA in utero of 1.5 percent.

Along with VPA, carbamazepine has been implicated as a cause of spina bifida apperta as opposed to other neural tube defects (34). Methodological difficulties make prevalence estimates imprecise becausemmost of the data published are in the form of case reports, case series, or very small cohorts from registries that were not designed to evaluate pregnancy outcomes, (124).

It has been estimated that the prevalence of spina bifida aperta following VPA exposure is 1 percent to 2 percent (123), and following carbamazepine 0.5 percent (124). A prospective study in Holland, however, demonstrated a prevalence rate of spina bifida aperta with VPA exposure of 5.4 percent. This increased rate was associated with higher average daily doses (1,640 ± 136 mg/day) of valproate in the affected than in the unaffected IME (941 ± 48 mg/day). The authors suggest that the dose be reduced whenever VPA must be used in pregnancy (126).

The mechanism of VPA teratogenicity is not known. The risk of spina bifida with VPA monotherapy if greater than with than polytherapy. VPA appears to be embryotoxic to cultured whole rat embryos, but none of the hydroxylated metabolites have exhibited significant embryotoxicity (127). This implies a direct teratogenic effect of the parent drug. VPA and its 4-en metabolite accumulate in embryonic tissue. Nau and Scott have suggested that alterations in intracellular pH may explain the teratogenicity of VPA (128). Lindhout has proposed different mechanisms, such as interference with lipid metabolism, alterations in zinc concentrations, or disruption of folate utilization (129).

Carbamazepine Teratogenicity

An association of carbamazepine and spina bifida has been proposed (73). Data from Michigan Medicaid Registry revealed four cases of spina bifida in 1,490 births to women with epilepsy between 1980 and 1988, or 0.2 percent. Of the four cases, three were exposed to carbamazepine, but all three were also exposed to VPA, phenytoin, or a barbiturate (124). A Danish study of 3,635 children between 1984 and 1986 described six of nine infants exposed to carbamazepine in utero who developed spina bifida (125). No new neural tube defect and carbamazepine cases were described subsequently. While there is a suggestion that carbamazepine may be associated with spina bifida, the data are sparse and and lack statistical significance. Improved prenatal diagnostic techniques and abortion of affected fetuses make documentation of these types of associations more difficult now than before.

Phenobarbital Teratogenicity

Phenobarbital has been implicated in the development of congenital malformations since the 1970s (31). Rates of malformations appear to be similar to that of other "older" AEDs.

OTHER ADVERSE OUTCOMES OF PREGNANCY WITH AED EXPOSURE

Death

Fetal wastage (defined as fetal loss after 20 weeks gestation) is as great a problem as AED-associated congenital malformations and anomalies. Studies comparing stillbirth rates found higher rates in infants for mothers with epilepsy (1.3–14.0%) than unaffected mothers (1.2–7.8%) (Table 26-4). Some reports do not compare rates with general population figures or other controls, making it difficult to establish whether children are at increased risk (13,130). A large Norwegian study failed to demonstrate increased risks of stillbirth in IMEs but clearly demonstrated an increase in neonatal deaths (2).

Spontaneous abortions, defined as fetal loss occurring before 20 weeks of gestation, do not appear to occur more commonly in infants of mothers with epilepsy. A history of previous spontaneous abortions was not found to be significantly different between women with epilepsy (24%) and controls (17.8%) (odds ratio 1.44, 95 percent C.I. 1.03–2.02) (131). In a report by Annegers and coworkers, the gestational age–adjusted rate ratio for spontaneous abortions was no higher when the mothers had epilepsy than when fathers had epilepsy. Nor was there any difference in spontaneous abortion rates for treated women with epilepsy (14.6%) compared with untreated women (15.7%) (132).

Other studies have, however, demonstrated increased rates of neonatal and perinatal death. Perinatal death rates range from 1.3 percent to 7.8 percent compared with 1.0 percent to 3.9 percent for controls (2,7,9,13,15,133,134) (Table 26-4).

Table 26-4. Stillbirth and Neonatal Death Rates in Infants of Epileptic Mothers

Investigator	Percentage			
	Stillbirths		Neonatal Births	
	Cases	Controls	Cases	Controls
Janz and Fuchs (9)	12.1	7.0	1.3	—
Spiedel and Meadow (15)	1.3	1.2	2.7	1.0
Bjenkdal and Bahna (2)	5.3	7.8	3.2	1.5
Fedrick (16)	2.7	1.1	—	—
Higgins and				
Comerford (12)	5.2	—	7.8	3.9
Knight and Rhind (13)	2.0	—	2.9	—
Nakane (31)	13.5	4.3	—	—
Nakane et al. (10)	14.0	6.7	—	—
Nelson and Ellenberg (4)	5.1	1.9	3.5	2.7
Svigos (5)	0	1.3	—	—
Kalen (7)	2.2	—	2.7	—
Tanganelli and				
Regesta (134)	—	—	2.2	1.4

Hemorrhagic Disease

Infants of mothers with epilepsy are at heightened risk for neonatal hemorrhage, which differs somewhat from other hemorrhagic disorders in infancy in that the bleeding occurs internally during the first 24 hours of life. First described by Van Creveld (135) and delineated as a syndrome by Mountain (136), it was initially associated with exposure to phenobarbital or primidone but has subsequently also been described in children exposed in utero to phenytoin, carbamazepine, diazepam, mephobarbital, amobarbital, and ethosuximide. Prevalence figures average 10 percent. The mortality from this phenomenon is over 30 percent.

The hemorrhage appears to be a result of a deficiency of vitamin K–dependent clotting factors II, VII, IX, and X. Maternal coagulation parameters are invariably normal. The fetus, however, demonstrates diminished clotting factors and prolonged prothrombin and partial thromboplastin times. A prothrombin precursor, protein induced by vitamin K deficiency has been discovered in the serum of mothers taking anticonvulsants (137). Assays for this protein may permit prenatal identification of infants at risk for hemorrhage (138,139).

The risk of hemorrhage can be reduced by maternal ingestion of oral vitamin K1 in the last month of gestation (140). Anticonvulsants can act like warfarin and can inhibit vitamin K transport across the placenta, effects that can be overcome by large concentrations of the vitamin. Despite lower coagulation factor levels, the fetus generally obtains enough maternal vitamin K in utero but after birth must rely on exogenous sources of vitamin K because the newborn gut is sterile. Routine administration of vitamin K at birth is not adequate to prevent hemorrhage if any two of the coagulation factors fall below 5 percent of normal values (141). Successful treatment requires fresh frozen plasma intravenously.

Low Birth Weight and Microcephaly

Rates of low birth weight (less than 2,500 gm) and prematurity in IMEs range from 7 percent to 10 percent and 4 percent to 11 percent, respectively (2,4,5,10, 130,142). Microcephaly has been demonstrated in these infants and associated with all anticonvulsants (4,8). A Finnish study found a stronger association between carbamazepine exposure in utero and small head circumference than with other anticonvulsant drugs (75).

Developmental Delay

Infants of mothers with epilepsy have been reported to have twofold to sevenfold higher rates of mental retardation than controls (4,15,143). None of the studies controlled for parental intelligence, and while IQ scores at age 7 between groups of children exposed [full-scale intelligence quotient (FSIQ) = 91.7] or not exposed (FSIQ = 96.8) to phenytoin reached statistical significance, the clinical ramifications of such a difference is not known (4). Children exposed prenatally to phenytoin score lower on performance, IQ, FSIQ, and visual motor integration tests, (144).

We have found that IMEs score lower on measures of verbal development at both 2 and 3 years of age. Although there was no difference in physical growth parameters between IMEs and controls, IMEs scored significantly lower in the Bailey Scale of Infant Development mental developmental index (MDI) at 2 and 3 years. They also performed significantly less well on the Bates Bretherton early language inventory ($p \leq 0.02$), in the Peabody Picture Vocabulary test scales of verbal reasoning ($p \leq 0.001$), and composite IQ ($p \leq 0.01$) and displayed significantly shorter mean lengths of utterance ($p \leq 0.001$), (145).

A prospective Canadian study found that AED polytherapy and maternal seizures during pregnancy have adverse effects on a child's cognitive development. Children of mothers with epilepsy tested during their school-age years were found to have lower scores than age-matched controls in verbal information, picture completion, block design, object assembly, and digit symbol ($p < 0.01$). Their mean IQ scores were 8.8 points lower than controls (104.1 and 112.9, respectively), and even lower 100.3 when their mothers had seizures during pregnancy. Although these average values are normal or above, the investigators found that 8.6 percent of children of mothers with epilepsy had intellectual deficiency (146).

Feeding Difficulties

In anecdotal reports perinatal lethargy, irritability, and feeding difficulties have been attributed to intrauterine exposure to anticonvulsants, especially phenobarbital and phenytoin (5,147). Nursing children often become sleepy and stop feeding before satiation. Shortly thereafter they awaken, hungry and irritable, to repeat the process. Some investigators have found no relationship between type of anticonvulsant drug, concentration, or disappearance from plasma despite a twofold increase in frequency of sedation and drug withdrawal symptoms in infants of epileptic mothers (148). Virtually all anticonvulsants are excreted in breast milk, and, hence breast-fed infants may continue to be exposed.

INHERITANCE OF EPILEPSY

The risk of epilepsy in children of parents with epilepsy is higher than that in the general population. This risk is higher (relative risk of 3.2) for children of mothers with epilepsy (29). Paternal epilepsy appears to have less impact on the development of seizures in children. The presence of maternal seizures during pregnancy, but not AED use, is associated with an increased risk of seizures in the offspring (relative risk of 2.4) (149).

AEDS INTRODUCED SINCE 1990

In animal models felbamate, gabapentin, lamotrigine, and tiagabine have not been found to be mutagenic, teratogenic, or carcinogenic. However, all of these drugs that yield maternal toxicity also produce some secondary embryotoxicty in the form of increased resorptions, reduced numbers of implantation scars, reduced number of live fetuses per litter, and reduced fetal weight. I am aware of only seven human pregnancies with felbamate exposure, all resulted in healthy children. Gabapentin has been reported in only 20 pregnancies and tiagabine in only 29, all with polytherapy. The numbers are too small to evaluate safety.

In rabbits vigabatrin in very high maternal doses — 150 to 200 mg/kg — has been shown to reduce the mean fetal weight and increase cleft lip and palate rate. In rats reduction in mean fetal weight and multiple soft tissue malformations have been reported. In the few reported instances of human fetal exposure in monotherapy no congenital malformations have resulted. Polytherapy is a different story; malformations have occuried in infants exposed to polytherapy with vigabatrin, although the overall rates of malformations are no higher than with conventional AEDs.

A registry to monitor the drug's effect on pregnancy outcomes has been established. To date, there have been over 80 pregnancies. While there have been malformations and facial anomalies reported, they have been in children exposed to polytherapy. The overall malformation rates are no higher that that seen with the older AEDs.

Topiramate is a carbonic anhydrase inhibitor and a feeble hepatic microsomal enzyme inducer. Although carbonic anhydrase inhibitors produce birth defects in animals, they usually do not in humans; however, data with TPM are insufficient to justify any conclusions about safety during pregnancy. One can therefore expect a higher rate of contraceptive failure when topiramate is used in women of childbearing age.

CONCLUSIONS

Exposure to anticonvulsants in utero increases the risk of developing congenital malformations between 4 percent and 6 percent overall. In addition, a subgroup of exposed children have characteristic dysmorphic features of the midface and distal digits of uncertain long-term significance. The prevalence of this AED syndrome is unclear; between 5 percent and 45 percent of IMEs have some minor anomalies (7).

All commonly used AEDs equilibrate across the placenta. Unbound fetal and maternal AED concentrations are equivalent (6). All commonly used AEDs have been associated with congenital malformations. Although many different types have been described, orofacial clefts are the most common and account for approximately 30 percent of the excess of malformations seen (38). Specific major malformations associated with AEDs have been described only for VPA, which carries a 1 percent risk of spina bifida in exposed infants. AEDs share many of the features of classic teratogens but generally do not produce a consistent pattern of major malformations.

No single AED has emerged as the safest to use in a pregnant woman. At present there appears to be little to choose among them in terms of risk for birth defects. Both the American Acadmey of Neurology and the American College of Obstetrics and Gynecology recommend using the AED that is most effective in controlling seizures.

Generalized convulsions pose clear risks for maternal injury and miscarriage (12,133,150). They may also increase the risk of impaired cognitive development in offspring. For most women, anticonvulsant therapy needs to be continued during pregnancy to reduce the risk of seizure-related consequences.

For women with epilepsy who are contemplating pregnancy, the most effective risk reduction strategy starts before conception. Patients need to be educated abouot the risks of pregnancy and epilepsy. The diagnosis should be carefully reviewed to determine whether anticonvulsant utilization is still necessary. Many people with childhood-onset epilepsy "outgrow" their disorder and no longer need therapy, while a majority can be controlled by a single AED. Monotherapy should be attempted for all patients. Placing women with epilepsy who are fertile on multivitamins with folate prophylactically should reduce the risks of congenital malformations. The Centers for Disease Control recommend a minimum folate dose of 400 mcg/day.

Changing the AED after conception is unlikely to reduce the risks of malformations and may place the mother at risk for increased seizures. Women with epilepsy should obtain early and consistent prenatal care. Efforts to maintain good seizure control without clinical toxicity and use of prenatal vitamins are also important. I recommend monitoring unbound AED levels monthly and adjusting the dose, aiming to keep the "free" or unbound concentrations in the therapeutic range. Because maternal seizures increase in risk as pregnancy progresses, I particularly want to monitor theraputic levels as the woman nears delivery.

Women taking VPA and possibly carbamazepine should be informed of the additional risks of spina bifida, a defect that can be detected in the prenatal period. Ultrasonography between 16 and 18 weeks gestation detects more than 90 percent of all cases of spine bifida.

Amniocentesis for alpha-fetoprotein concentration increases the diagnostic accuracy to 95 percent. Despite the real risks, well over 90 percent of women with epilepsy taking AEDs deliver children free of congenital malformations.

ACKNOWLEDGMENT

Without the assistance of Drs. Charles Pippenger and Rene Levy, Patrick Friel, and Karen B. McCormick, RM, this chapter would not have been possible.

REFERENCES

1. Hauser WA, Kurland LT. Epidemiology of epilepsy in Rochester, Minnesota, 1935 through 1967. *Epilepsia* 1975; 16:1–66.

2. Bjerkdal T, Bahna SL. The course and outcome of pregnancy in women with epilepsy. *Acta Obstet Gynecol Scand* 1973; 52:245–248.

3. Nakane Y. The teratological problem of antiepileptic drugs. *Folia Psychiatr Neurol Jpn* 1980; 34:277–287.

4. Nelson KB, Ellenberg JH. Maternal seizure disorder outcomes of pregnancy and neurologic abnormalities in the children. *Neurology* 1982; 32:1247–1254.

5. Svigos JM. Epilepsy and pregnancy. *Aust NZ Obstet Gynecol* 1984; 24:182–185.

6. Levy RH, Yerby MS. Effects of pregnancy on antiepileptic drug utilization. *Epilepsia* 1985; 26(Suppl 1):525–557.

7. Kallen B. A register study of maternal epilepsy and delivery outcome with special reference to drug use. *Acta Neurol Scand* 1986; 73:253–259.

8. Neri A, Heifetz L, Nitke S, et al. Neonatal outcomes in infants of epileptic mothers. *Eur J Obstet Gynecol Reprod Biol* 1983; 16:263–268.

9. Janz D, Fuchs U. Are antiepileptic drugs harmful when given during pregnancy? *Ger Med Month* 1964; 9:20–22.

10. Nakane Y, Oltuma T, Takahashi R, et al. Multi-institutional study on the teratogenicity and fetal toxicity of anticonvulsants: a report of a collaborative study group in Japan. *Epilepsia* 1980; 21:663–680.

11. Speidel BD, Meadow SR. Anticonvulsant drugs and congenital anomalies. *Lancet* 1968; 2:1296.

12. Higgins TA, Comerford JB. Epilepsy in pregnancy. *J Irish Med Assoc* 1974; 67:317–329.

13. Knight AH, Rhind KG. Epilepsy and pregnancy: a study of 153 pregnancies in 59 patients. *Epilepsia* 1975; 16:99–110.

14. Kallen B. Maternal epilepsy, antiepileptic drugs and birth defects. *Pathologica* 1986; 78:757–768.

15. Speidel BD, Meadow SR. Maternal epilepsy and abnormalities of the fetus and newborn. *Lancet* 1972; 2:839–843.

16. Fedrick J. Epilepsy and pregnancy: a report from the Oxford record linkage study. *Br Med J* 1983; 2:442–448.

17. Mullers-Kuppers von M. Embryopathy during pregnancy caused by taking anticonvulsants. *Acta Paedopsychiatr* 1963; 30:401–405.

18. Pantarotto ME. A case of bone marrow aplasia in a newborn attributable to anticonvulsant drugs used by the mother during pregnancy. *Quad Clin Obstet Gynecol* 1965; 67:343–348.

19. Centa E, Rasore-Quartino A. La sindrome malformatine "digitocardiaca" forme genetsche e fenocopie. *Probabil Azione Tertog Farm Antiepilep Pathol* 1965; 57:227–232.

20. Melchior IC, Svenswark O, Trolle D. Placental transfer of phenobarbitone in women and elimination in newborns. *Lancet* 1967; 2:860–861.

21. Meadow SR. Anticonvulsant drugs and congenital abnormalities. *Lancet* 1968; 2:1296.

22. German I, Kowal A, Ehlers KH. Trimethadione and human teratogenesis. *Teratology* 1970; 3:349–362.

23. Kalter H, Warkany J. Congenital malformations. *N Engl J Med* 1983; 308:491–497.

24. Kelly TE. Teratogenicity of anticonvulsant drugs. I: Review of literature. *Am J Med Genet* 1984a 19:413–434.

25. Philbert A, Dam M. The epileptic mother and her child. *Epilepsia* 1982; 23:85–99.

26. South J. Teratogenic effects of anticonvulsants. *Lancet* 1972; 2:1154.

27. Lowe CR. Congenital malformations among infants born to epileptic women. *Lancet* 1973; 1:9–10.

28. Monson RR, Rosenberg L, Hartz SC. Diphenylhydantoin and selected congenital malformations. *N Engl J Med* 1973; 289:1049–1052.

29. Annegers JF, Hauser WA, Elveback LR, Anderson VE, Kurland LT. Congenital malformations and seizure disorders in the offspring of parents with epilepsy. *Int J Epidemiol* 1978; 7:241–247.

30. Dansky LV, Andermann E, Sherwin AL, Andermann F, Kinch RA. Maternal epilepsy and congenital malformations: a prospective study with monitoring of plasma anticonvulsant levels during pregnancy. *Neurology* 1980; 3:15.

31. Nakane Y. Congenital malformations among infants of epileptic mothers treated during pregnancy. *Folia Psychiatr Neurol Jpn* 1979; 33:363–369.

32. Lindhout D, Rene JE, Hoppener A, Meinardi H. Teratogenicity of antiepileptic drug combinations with special emphasis on epoxidation (of carbamazepine). *Epilepsia* 1984; 25:77–83.

33. Majewski F, Raft W, Fischer P, Huenges R, Petruch E. Zur tertogenitat von anticonvulsiva. *Dtsch Med Wochenschr* 1980; 105:719–723.

34. Lindhout D, Meinardi H, Meijer JWA, Nau H. Antiepileptic drugs and teratogenesis in two consecutive cohorts: changes in prescription policy paralleled by changes in pattern of malformations. *Neurology* 1992; 42 (Suppl 5):94–110.

35. Elshove J, Van Eck JHM. Aangeboren misvorminge, met name gespleten lipmet zonder gespleten verhemelte, bij kinderen van moeders met epilepsie. *Nederland T Geneesk* 1971; 115 1371–1375.

36. Anderson RC. Cardiac defects in children of mothers receiving anticonvulsant therapy during pregnancy. *J Pediatr* 1976; 89:318–319.

37. Friis ML, Breng-Nielsen B, Sindrup EH, et al. Facial clefts among epileptic patients. *Arch Neurol* 1981; 38:227–229.

38. Friis ML, Holm NV, Sindrup EH, Fogh-Andersen P, Hauge M. Facial clefts in sibs and children of epileptic patients. *Neurology* 1986; 38:346–350.

39. Gatoh N, Millo Y, Taube E, Bechar M. Epilepsy among parents of children with cleft lip and palate. *Brain Dev* 1987; 9:296–299.

40. Shapiro S, Slone D, Hartz SC, et al. Anticonvulsant and parental epilepsy in the development of birth defects. *Lancet* 1976; 1:272–275.

41. Dieterich E, Steveling A, Lukas A, Seyfeddinipur N, Spranger J. Congenital anomalies in children of epileptic mothers and fathers. *Neuropediatrics* 1980; 11:274–283.

42. Friis ML, Hauge M. Congenital heart defects in live born children of epileptic parents. *Arch Neurol* 1985; 42:374–376.

43. Grosse KP, Schwanitz G, Rott HD, Wissmuler HE. Chromosomenuntersuchungen bei behandlung mit anticonvulsiva. *Humangenetik* 1972; 16:209–216.

44. Zachai EH, Mellman WJ, Neideren B, Hanson JW. The fetal trimethadione syndrome. *J Pediatr* 1975; 87:280–284.

45. Feldman GL, Weaver DD, Lovrien EW. The fetal trimethadione syndrome: report of an additional family and further delineation of this syndrome. *Am J Dis Child* 1977; 131:89–92.

46. Goldman AS, Zachai EH, Yaffe SJ. Environmentally induced birth defect risks. In: Sever JL, Brent RL, eds. *Teratogen Update.* New York: Liss, 1986:35–38.

47. Loughnan PM, Gold H, Vance JC. Phenytoin teratogenicity in man. *Lancet* 1973; 1:70–72.

48. Barr M, Pozanski AK, Schmickel RD. Digital hypoplasia and anticonvulsant during gestation: a teratogenic syndrome? *J Pediatr* 1974; 84:254–256.

49. Hanson JW, Smith DW. The fetal hydantoin syndrome. *J Pediatr* 1975; 87:285–290.

50. Hanson JW, Myrianthopoulos NC, Sedgwich MA, Smith DW. Risks to the offspring of women treated with hydantoin anticonvulsants with emphasis on the fetal hydantoin syndrome. *J Pediatr* 1976; 89:662–668.

51. Kelly TE. Teratogenicity of anticonvulsants. III: Radiographic hand analysis of children exposed in utero to diphenylhydantoin. *Am J Med Genet* 1984; 19:445–450.

52. Kelly TE, Edwards P, Rein M, Miller JQ, Dreifuss FE. Teratogenicity of anticonvulsant drugs. II: A prospective study. *Am J Med Genet* 1984; 19:435–443.

53. Gaily E, Granstrom ML, Hiilesmaa V, Bandy A. Minor anomalies in offspring of epileptic mothers. *J Pediatr* 1988; 112:520–529.

54. Yerby MS, Leavitt A, Erickson D, et al. Antiepileptics and the development of congenital anomalies. *Neurology* 1992; 42(Suppl 5):132–140.

55. Hanson JW. Teratogen update: fetal hydantoin effects. *Teratology* 1986; 33:349–353.

56. Ehrenband LT, Chaganti RSK. Cancer in the fetal hydantoin syndrome. *Lancet* 1981; 1:97.

57. Gaily E, Sorsa EK Granstrom ML. Intelligence of children of epileptic mothers. *J Pediatr* 1988; 113:677–684.

58. Phelan MC, Pellock JM, Nance WE. Discordant expression of fetal hydantoin syndrome in heteropaternal dizygotic twins. *N Engl J Med* 1982; 307:99–101.

59. Buchler BA. Epoxide hydrolase activity and the fetal hydantoin syndrome. *Clin Res* 1985; 33:A129.

60. Van Dyke DC, Hodge SE, Heide F, Hill LR. Family studies in fetal phenytoin exposure. *J Pediatr* 1988; 113:301–306.

61. Krauss CM, Holmes LB, Van Lang QC, Keith DA. Four siblings with similar malformations after exposure to phenytoin and primidone. *J Pediatr* 1984; 105:750–755.

62. Rudd NL, Freedom RM. A possible primidone embryopathy. *J Pediatr* 1979; 94:835–837.

63. Gustavson EE, Chen H. Goldenhar syndrome, anteriorencephalocele and aqueductal stenosis following fetal primidone exposure. *Teratology* 1985; 32:13–17.

64. Dalens B, Raynaud EJ, Gaulme J. Teratogenicity of valproic acid. *J Pediatr* 1980; 97:332–333.

65. Clay SA, McVie R, Chen HC. Possible teratogenic effect of valproic acid. *J Pediatr* 1981; 98:828.

66. DiLiberti JH, Farndon PA, Dennis NR, Curry CJR. The fetal valproate syndrome. *Am J Med Genet* 1984; 19:473–481.

67. Jager-Roman E, Deichl A, Jakob S, et al. Fetal growth major malformations and minor anomalies in infants born to women receiving valproic acid. *J Pediatr* 1986; 108:997–1004.

68. Jeavons PM. Non dose related side effects of valproate. *Epilepsia* 1984; 25(Suppl 1):550–555.

69. Felding I, Rane A. Congenital liver damage after treatment of mother with valproic acid and phenytoin? *Acta Pediatr Scand* 1984; 73:565–568.

70. Ardinger HH, Atkin JF, Blackston D, et al. Verification of the fetal valproate syndrome phenotype. *Am J Med Genet* 1988; 29:171–185.

71. Laegreid L, Olegard R, Wahlstrom I, Conradi N. Abnormalities in children exposed to benzodiazepines in utero. *Lancet* 1987; 1:108–109.

72. Safra ML, Oakley GP. Association between cleft lip with or without cleft palate and prenatal exposure to diazepam. *Lancet* 1975; 2:478–480.

73. Jones KL, Lacro RV, Johnson KA, Adams J. Pattern of malformations in the children of women treated with carbamazepine during pregnancy. *N Engl J Med* 1989; 320:1661–1666.

74. Niesen M, Froscher W. Finger and toenail hypoplasia after carbamazepine monotherapy in late pregnancy. *Neuropediatrics* 1985; 16:167–168.

75. Hiilesmaa VK, Teramo K, Granstrom ML, Bardy AH. Fetal head growth retardation associated with maternal antiepileptic drugs. *Lancet* 1981; 2:165–167.

76. Granstrom ML. Early postnatal growth of the children of epileptic mothers. In: Wolf P, Dam M, Janz D, Dreifuss FE, eds. The XVIth Epilepsy International Symposium. New York: Raven Press, 1987:573–577 (Advances in Epileptology, vol. 16).

77. Baptisti A. Epilepsy and pregnancy. *Am J Obstet Gynecol* 1938; 35:818–824.

78. Hutch HC, Steinhouse HC, Helge H. Mental development in children of epileptic parents. *Epilepsia* 1975; 16:1–66.

79. Granstrom ML. Development of the children of epileptic mothers, preliminary results from the prospective Helsinki study. In: Janz D, Dam M, Richens A, Bossi L, Helge H, Schmidt D, eds. *Epilepsy, Pregnancy, and the Child*. New York: Raven Press, 1982:403–408.

80. Janz D. Antiepileptic drugs and pregnancy: Altered utilization patterns and teratogenesis. *Epilepsia* 1982; 23(Suppl 1):853–863.

81. Kaneko S, Otani K, Fukushima Y, et al. Teratogenicity of antiepileptic drugs: analysis of possible risk factors. *Epilepsia* 1988; 29:459–467.

82. Vorhees CV. Developmental effects of anticonvulsants. *Neurotoxicology* 1986; 7:235–244.

83. Huot C, Gauthier M, Lebel M, Larbisseau A. Congenital malformations associated with maternal use of valproic acid. *Can J Neurol Sci* 1987; 14:290–293.

84. Jerina DM, Daly JW. Arene oxides: A new aspect of drug metabolism. *Science* 1974; 185:573.

85. Sims P, Grover PL. Epoxides in polycyclic aromatic hydrocarbon metabolism and carcinogenesis. *Adv Cancer Res* 1974; 20:165.

86. Nebert DW, Jensen NM. The Ah locus: genetic regulation of the metabolism of carcinogens, drugs, and other environmental chemicals by cytochrome P-450 mediated mono-oxygenases. *CRC Crit Rev Biochem* 1979; 6:401–437.

87. Shum S, Jensen NM, Nebert DW. The Ah locus: in utero toxicity and teratogenesis associated with genetic differences in B(a)P metabolism. *Teratology* 1979; 20:365–376.

88. Pacifici GM, Colizzi C, Giuliani L, Rane A. Cytosolic epoxide hydrolase in fetal and adult human liver. *Arch Toxicol* 1983; 54:331.

89. Pacifici GM, Rane A. Metabolism of styrene oxide in different human fetal tissues. *Drug Metab Dispos* 1982; 10:302–305.

90. Chang T, Savory A, Glazko AJ. A new metabolite of 5,5 diphenylhydantoin. *Biochem Res Commun* 1970; 38:444–449.

91. Horning MG, Stratton C, Wilson A, Horning EC, Hill RM. Detection of 5-3,4-diphenylhydantoin in the newborn human. *Anal Lett* 1974; 4:537–582.

92. Martz F, Failinger C, Blake DA. Phenytoin teratogenesis: correlation between embryopathic effect and covalent binding of putative arene oxide metabolite to gestational tissue *J Pharmacol Exp Ther* 1977; 203:231–239.

93. Pantarotto C, Arboix M, Sezzano P, Abbruzzo R. Studies on 5,5-diphenyl hydantoin irreversible binding to rat liver microsomal proteins. *Biochem Pharmacol* 1982; 31:1501–1507.

94. Wells PG, Harbison RD. Significance of the phenytoin reactive arene oxide intermediate, its oxepintantomer, and clinical factors modifying their roles in phenytoin-induced teratology. In: Hussell TM, Johnston MC, Dudley KH, eds. *Phenytoin-Induced Teratology and Gingival Pathology*. New York: Raven Press, 1985:83–112.

95. Spielberg SP, Gordon GB, Blake DA, Mellits ED, Bross DS. Anticonvulsant toxicity in vitro: possible role of arene oxides. *J Pharmacol Exp Ther* 1981; 217:386–389.

96. Strickler SM, Dansky LV, Miller MA, et al. Genetic predisposition to phenytoin induced birth defects. *Lancet* 1985; 1:746–749.

97. Kapitulnik I, Levin W, Lu AYH, et al. Hydration of arene and alkene oxides by epoxide hydrolase in human liver microsomes. *Clin Pharmacol Ther* 1977; 21:158.

98. Guengerick FP, Wang P, Mitchell MB, Mason PS. Rat and human microsomal epoxide hydrolase. *J Biol Chem* 1979; 254:122–488.

99. Glatt HR, Lorenze J, Fleischmann R, et al. Interindividual variations of epoxide hydrolase activity in human liver and lung biopsies, lymphocytes and fibroblast cultures. In: Conn MI, Conney AH, Estabrook RW, et al., eds. *Microsomes, Drug Oxidations and Chemical Carcinogenesis*. New York: Academic Press, 1980:551.

100. Thomas PE, Ryan DE, vonBahr D, Glaumann H, Levin W. Human liver microsomal epoxide hydrolase: correlation of immunochemical quantitation with catalytic activity. *Mol Pharmacol* 1982; 22:190.

101. Lorenz I, Glatt HR, Fleischmann R, Ferlinz R, Oesch R. Drug metabolism in man and its relationship to that in three rodent species: mono-oxygenase, epoxide hydrolase, and glutathione s-transferase activities in subcellular fractions of lung and liver. *Biochem Med* 1984; 32:43.

102. Cresteil T, Beaune P, Kremers P, et al. Immunoquantification of epoxide hydrolase and cytochrome P-450 isozymes in fetal and adult human liver microsomes. *Eur J Biochem* 1985; 151:345.

103. Mertes I, Gleischmann R, Glatt HR, Oesch F. Interindividual variations in the activities of cytosolic and microsomal epaxide hydrolase in human liver. *Carcinogenesis* 1985; 6:219.

104. Dansky LV, Strickler SM, Andermann E, et al. Pharmacogenetic susceptibility to phenytoin teratogenesis. In: Wolf P, Dam M, Janz D, Dreifuss FE, eds. The XVIth Epilepsy International Symposium. New York: Raven Press, 1987:555–559 (Advances in Epileptology, vol. 16).

105. Finnell RH, DiLiberti JH. Hydantoin induced teratogenesis: are arene oxide intermediates really responsible? *Helv Pacdiatr Acta* 1983; 38:171–177.

106. Wells PG, Kuper A, Lawson JA, Harbison RD. Relation of in vivo drug metabolism to stereoselective fetal hydantoin toxicology in mouse: evaluation of mephenytoin and its metabolite, nirvanol. *J Pharmacol Exp Ther* 1982; 221:228–234.

107. Kubow S, Wells PG. In vitro bioactivation of phenytoin to a reactive free radical intermediate by prostaglandin synthetase, horseradish peroxidase, and thyroid peroxidase. *Mol Pharmacol* 1989; 35:504–511.

108. Wells PG, Zubovits JT, Wong ST, Molinari LM, Ali S. Modulation of phenytoin teratogenicity and embryonic covalent binding by acetylsalicylic acid, and alpha-phenyl-*N*-*t*-butylnitrone implications for bioactivation by prostaglandin synthetase. *Toxicol Appl Pharmacol* 1989; 97:192–202.

109. Wong M, Wells PG. Effects of *N*-acetylcysteine on fetal development and on phenytoin teratogenicity in mice. *Teratogenesis Carcinog Mutagen* 1988; 8:65–79.

110. Wong M, Wells PG. Modulation of embryonic glutathione reductase and phenytoin teratogenicity by 1,3-bis(2-chloroethyl)-1-nitrosurea (BCNU). *J Pharmacol Exp Ther* 1989; 250:336–342.

111. Goldman AS, Van Dyke DC, Gupta C, Katsumata M. Elevated glucocorticoid receptor levels in lymphocytes of children with the fetal hydantoin syndrome. *Am J Med Genet* 1987; 28:607–618.

112. Zhu M, Zhou S. Reduction of the teratogenic effects of phenytoin by folic acid and a mixture of folic acid, vitamins, and amino acids: a preliminary trial. *Epilepsia* 1989; 30:246–251.

113. Biale Y, Lewenthal H. Effect of folic acid supplementation on congenital malformations due to anticonvulsant drugs. *Eur J Obstet Gynecol Reprod Biol* 1984; 18:211–216.

114. Leist KH, Grauwiler J. Fetal pathology in rats following uterine vessel clamping on day 14 of gestation. *Teratology* 1974; 10:55–68.

115. Webster WS, Lipson AH, Brown-Woodman PDC. Uterine trauma and limb defects. *Teratology* 1987; 28:1–8.

116. Danielsson BRG, Danielson M, Rundqvist E, Reiland S. Identical phalangeal defects induced by phenytoin and nifedipine suggest fetal hypoxia and vascular disruption behind phenytoin teratogenicity. *Teratology* 1992; 45:247–258.

117. Gomez MR. Possible teratogenicity of valproic acid. *J Pediatr* 1981; 9:508.

118. Dickinson RG, Harland RC, Lynn RK, Brewster-Smith W, Gerber N. Transmission of valproic acid (Depakene) across the placenta: half-life of the drug in motber and baby. *J Pediatr* 1979; 94:832–835.

119. Tein I, MacGregor DL. Possible valproate toxicity. *Arch Neurol* 1985; 42:291–293.

120. Valproic acid and spinal bifida: a preliminary report. *MMWR* 1982; 31:565–566.

121. Robert E, Lodkvist E, Maugiere E. Valproate and spina bifida. *Lancet* 1984; 1:1392.

122. Stanley OH, Chambers TL. Sodium valproate and neural tube defects. *Lancet* 1982; 2:1282–1283.

123. Lindhout D, Schmidt D. In utero exposure to valproate and neural tube defects. *Lancet* 1986; 1:1392–393.

124. Rosa FW. Spina bifida in infants of women treated with carbamazepine during pregnancy. *N Engl J Med* 1991; 324:674–677.

125. Kallen B. Maternal carbamazepine and infant spina bifida. *Reprod Toxicol* 1994; 8:203–205.

126. Omtzigt JG, Los FJ, Hagenaars AM. Prenantal diagnosis of spina bifida aperta after first-trimester valproate exposure. *Prenat Diagn* 1992; 12:893–897.

127. Rettie AK, Rettenmeir AW, Beyer BK, Baile TA, Juchau MR Valproate hydroxylation by human fetal tissues and embryotoxicity of metabolites. *Clin Pharmacol Ther* 1986; 40:172–177.

128. Nau H, Scott WJ. Weak acids may act as teratogens by accumulating in the basic milieu of the early mammalian embryo. *Nature* 1986; 323:276–278.

129. Lindhout D. Commission reviews teratogenesis and genedes in epilepsy. *World Neurol* 1989; 4:3–7.

130. Annegers JR, Elveback LR, Hauser WA, Kurland LT. Do anticonvulsants have a teratogenic effect? *Arch Neurol* 1974; 31:364–373.

131. Yerby M, Koepsell T, and Daling J. Pregnancy complications and outcomes in a cohort of women with epilepsy. *Epilepsia* 1985; 26:631–635.

132. Annegers JF, Baumgartner KB, Hauser WA, Kurland LT. Epilepsy, antiepileptic drugs, and the risk of spontaneous abortion. *Epilepsia* 1988; 29:451–458.

133. Stumpf DA, Frost M. Seizures, anticonvulsants, and pregnancy. *Am J Dis Child* 1978; 132:746–748.

134. Tanganelli P, Regesta G. Epilepsy, pregnancy, and major birth anomalies: an Italian prospective, controlled study. *Neurology* 1992; 42(Suppl 5):89–93.

135. Van Creveld S. Nouveaux aspects de la maladie hemorragique du nouveau ne. *Ned Tijdschr Geneeskd* 1957; 101:2109–2112.

136. Mountain KR, Hirsh J, Gallus AS. Material coagulation defect due to anticonvulsant treatment in pregnancy. *Lancet* 1978; 1:265–268.

137. Davies VA, Rothberg AD, Argent AC, et al. Precursor prothrombin status in patients receiving anticonvulsant drugs. *Lancet* 1985; 19:126–128.

138. Walker NP, Bardlow BA, Atkinson PM. A rapid chromogenic method for the determination of prothrombin precursor in the plasma. *Am J Clin Pathol* 1982; 78:777–780.

139. Argent AC, Rothberg AD, Pienaar N. Precursor prothrombin status in the mother infant pairs following gestational anticonvulsant therapy. *Pediatr Pharmacol* 1984; 4:183–187.

140. Deblay MF, Vert P, Andre M, et al. Transplacental vitamin K prevents hemorrhagic disease of infants of epileptic mothers. *Lancet* 1982; 1:1247.

141. Srinivasan G, Seeler RA, Tiruvury A, et al. Maternal anticonvulsant therapy and hemorrhagic disease of the newborn. *Obstet Gynecol* 1982; 59:250–252.

142. Teramo K, Hiilesmaa VK, Bardy A, et al. Fetal heart rate during a maternal grand mal epileptic seizure. *J Perinat Med* 1979; 7:3–5.

143. Hill RM, Verniaud WM, Horning MG, McCulley LB, Morgan NF. Infants exposed in utero to antiepileptic drugs. A prospective study. *Am J Dis Child* 1974; 127:645–653.

144. Vanderloop D, Schnell RR, Harvey EA, Holmes LB. The effects of prenatal exposure to phenytoin and other anticonvulsants on intellectual function at 4 to 8 years of age. *Neurotoxicol Teratol* 1992; 14:329–335.

145. Leavitt AM, Yerby MS, Robinson N, Sells CJ, Erickson DM. Epilepsy and pregnancy: developmental outcomes at 12 months. *Neurology* 1992; 42(Suppl 5):141–143.

146. Leonard G, Aldermann E, Pitno A, Schopflocher C. Cognitive effects of antiepileptic drug therapy during pregnancy on school age offspring. *Epilepsia* 1997; 38(Suppl 3):170.

147. Bethenod M, Frederich A. Les enfants des antiepileptiques. *Pediatrie* 1975; 30:227–248.

148. Koch S, Gopfert-Geyer I, Hauser A, et al. Neonatal behavior disturbances in infants of epileptic women treated during pregnancy. In: Liss A, ed. *Epidemiology, Early Detection and Therapy, and Environmental Factors.* New York: Alan R. Liss, 1985:453–461.

149. Ottman R, Annegers JF, Hauser WA, Kurland LT. Higher risk of seizures in offspring of mothers than fathers with epilepsy. *Am J Hum Genet* 1988; 43:357–364.

150. Burnett CWF. A survey of the relation between epilepsy and pregnancy. *J Obstet Gynecol* 1946; 53:539–556.

151. Sabin M, Oxorn H. Epilepsy and pregnancy. *Obstet Gynecol* 1956; 7:175–179.

152. Spellacy WN. Maternal epilepsy and abnormalities of the fetus and newborn. *Lancet* 1972; 2:1196–1197.

153. Koppe JG, Bosmon W, Oppers VM, et al. Epilepsie en aangeborn afwijkingen. *Ned Tijdschr Geneesk* 1973; 117:220–224.

154. Kuenssberg EV, Knox JDE. Teratogenic effect of anticonvulsants. *Lancet* 1973; 1:198.

155. Meyer JG. The teratological effects of anticonvulsants and the effects of pregnancy and birth. *Eur Neurol* 1973; 10:179–180.

156. Millar JHD, Nevin NC. Congenital malformations and anticonvulsant drugs. *Lancet* 1973; 2:328.

157. Niswander JD, Wertelecki W. Congenital malformation among offspring of epileptic women. *Lancet* 1973; 1:1062.

158. Starreveld-Zimmerman AAE, Van Der Kolk WJ, Meinardi H. Are anticonvulsants teratogenic? *Lancet* 1973; 2:48–49.

159. Visser GH, Hisjes HI, Elshove J. Anticonvulsants and fetal malformations. *Lancet* 1976; 1:970.

160. Weber M, Schweitzer M, Mur JM, et al. Epilepsie medicaments antiepileptiques et grossesse. *Arch Francais Pediatr* 1977; 34:374–383.

161. Seino M, Miyakoshi M. Teratogenic risks of antiepileptic drugs in respect to the type of epilepsy. *Folia Psychiatr Neurol Jpn* 1979; 33:379–385.

162. Stanley FJ, Priscott PK, Johnston R, Brooks B, Bower S. Congenital malformations in infants of mothers with diabetes and epilepsy in Western Australia, 1980–82. *Med J Aust* 1985; 143:440–442.

163. Beaussart-Defaye J, Bastin M, Demareq C. *Epilepsies and Reproduction.* Grine Lille, France: Grine Nord Epilepsy Research and Information Group, 1985:1–79.

164. Rating D, Jager-Roman E, Koch S, et al. Major malformations and minor anomalies in infants exposed to different anticonvulsants during pregnancy. In: Wolf P, Dam M, Janz D, Dreifuss FE, eds. The XVIth Epilepsy International Symposium. New York: Raven Press, 1987:561–565 (Advances in Epileptology; vol 16).

165. Gaily E, Kantola-Sorsa E, Granstrom ML. Specific cognitive dysfunction in children with epileptic mothers. *Dev Child Neurol* 1990; 32:403–414.

166. Dravet C, Julian C, Legras C, et al. Epilepsy, antiepileptic drugs, and malformations in children of women with epilepsy: a French prospective cohort study. *Neurology* 1992; 42(Suppl 5):75–82.

167. Kaneko S, Otani K, Fukushima Y, et al. Malformation in infants of mothers with epilepsy receiving antiepiletics drugs. *Neurology* 1992; 42(Suppl 5):68–74.

168. Koch S, Losche G, Jager-Roman E, et al. Major and minor birth malformations and antiepileptic drugs. *Neurology* 1992; 42 (Suppl 5):83–88.

169. Robert E, Lolkvist E, Mauguiere F, Robert JM. Evaluadon of drug therapy and teratogenic risk in a Rhone-Alps district population of pregnant epileptic women. *Eur Neurol* 1986; 25:436–443.

CHAPTER 27

Benzodiazepines

Kevin Farrell, M.B.

The antiepileptic activity of benzodiazepines has been demonstrated in seizure models of both partial and generalized epilepsies. Benzodiazepines act by binding to the $GABA_A$ receptor, a macromolecular protein that forms a chloride ion–selective channel and contains binding sites for GABA, benzodiazepines, and barbiturates (1). At high concentrations, they also influence sodium channel function in a similar fashion to phenytoin and carbamazepine (2). Benzodiazepines raise the seizure threshold, decrease the duration of epileptiform discharges, and limit their spread (2).

Based on the position of nitrogen within the molecule, a distinction is made between the 1,4-benzodiazepines and 1,5-benzodiazepines. The 1,4-benzodiazepines, diazepam, lorazepam, and midazolam, have an established role in the treatment of status epilepticus, in which condition parenteral clonazepam and nitrazepam have also been reported to be effective. The 1,4-benzodiazepines, clonazepam, nitrazepam, and clorazepate, and the 1,5-benzodiazepine, clobazam, have been reported to be effective against a wide range of seizure types. However, there have been few well-designed studies of their antiepileptic effect. The intermittent use of benzodiazepines has also been effective in the treatment of febrile seizures (diazepam, nitrazepam), clusters of seizures (diazepam, lorazepam), and catamenial epilepsy (clobazam).

The usefulness of benzodiazepines in the management of epilepsy is compromised by neurotoxicity, which is more prominent with the 1,4-benzodiazepines (3), and by their predilection for tolerance. The phenomenon of tolerance probably occurs with all antiepileptic drugs (AEDs) (4) but has been reported most with benzodiazepines. The development of tolerance to the antiepileptic effect is dependent partly on the type and severity of epilepsy. Thus, tolerance to clonazepam is observed

less often in patients with typical absence seizures than in patients with West syndrome or Lennox-Gastaut syndrome (5). Similarly, the incidence of tolerance in children who received clobazam as their first or second AED (7.5%) was similar to that in children receiving carbamazepine or phenytoin (6) and considerably less than the 18 percent to 65 percent described in studies involving patients with intractable epilepsy (3,7–10).

DIAZEPAM

Clinical Indications

Diazepam has been established for the treatment of status epilepticus and serial seizures. Ideally, diazepam should be administered intravenously for the treatment of status epilepticus. The rapid redistribution of diazepam following a single dose results in an abrupt fall in brain concentration and reduction in the anticonvulsant effect. Consequently, a long-acting anticonvulsant (e.g., phenytoin) should also be administered in children with status epilepticus. Rectal diazepam is absorbed rapidly, and this route of administration is particularly useful in small children in whom the establishment of intravenous (IV) access may be difficult. Rectal formulations of diazepam can also be administered by the parent, which permits treatment of the child to be initiated at home and decreases emergency room visits (11). This is of considerable value in children with a history of prolonged seizures, who are at high risk of a further prolonged seizure (12,13). Rectal diazepam gel, administered by trained caregivers, has also been demonstrated to be an effective and well-tolerated treatment for acute repetitive seizures (14).

Intermittent diazepam at times of fever has been reported to be effective in the prevention of recurrent febrile convulsions. In placebo-controlled studies, both oral diazepam (15) and rectal diazepam (16) have been demonstrated to be effective in the prevention of recurrent febrile convulsions. Furthermore, rectal diazepam, at a dose of 5 mg every 8 hours when the rectal temperature was above 38.4 °C, was as effective as continuous phenobarbital in the prevention of recurrent febrile seizures (17). Finally, rectal diazepam can be used in the acute treatment of recurrent febrile convulsions to prevent prolonged seizures (18–20).

Unwanted Effects

Sedation and ataxia occur commonly when diazepam is used in the treatment of status epilepticus or in the prevention of recurrent febrile convulsions. Intravenous diazepam may cause respiratory depression, particularly if administered rapidly or used in combination with phenobarbital (21). The use of IV diazepam is associated with a higher rate of endotracheal intubation in children than IV lorazepam (22,23). Respiratory depression and apnea are extremely rare following rectal diazepam (24). A mild thrombophlebitis may occur following IV administration, particularly if diazepam is mixed with a saline solution or is injected rapidly (21). Very rarely, diazepam may precipitate tonic status epilepticus in children with symptomatic generalized epilepsy (25).

Pharmacokinetics and Dosage

Plasma concentrations of 500 ng/mL of diazepam, which are necessary for acute seizure control, are achieved in infants and children under 11 years within 2 to 6 minutes following rectal administration of 0.5 to 1 mg/kg (21). Diazepam is absorbed more slowly following oral or intramuscular (IM) administration, and these routes are not recommended. The low pK_a and high lipophilicity results in diazepam crossing the blood–brain barrier rapidly and distributing quickly into fatty tissues. The short duration of action following IV administration relates to the rapid distribution. Diazepam and N-desmethyldiazepam, its major metabolite, are both highly protein bound to albumin (21). The elimination half-life of diazepam is 10 ± 2 hours in infants and 17 ± 3 hours in older children (21).

N-desmethyldiazepam is a major metabolite with significant antiepileptic and sedative properties (26). The elimination half-life of N-desmethyldiazepam is longer than that of diazepam in patients receiving diazepam, and serum concentrations are two to five times higher in patients receiving long-term treatment (21).

Diazepam does not significantly influence the pharmacokinetics of other drugs. The protein binding of diazepam is decreased by valproate (27), which may

Table 27-1. The Use of Benzodiazepines in Status Epilepticus and Serial Seizures

Drug	Dosage	Comments
Diazepam		
Intravenous	0.3 mg/kg; max dose 10 mg; can be repeated after 10 minutes	Administer over 2–5 minutes; rapid administration increases risk of apnea
Rectal	0.5–0.7 mg/kg; max dose 20 mg	
Lorazepam		
Intravenous	0.1 mg/kg; max dose 4 mg; can be repeated after 10 minutes	Administer over 2 minutes
Sublingual	0.05–0.15 mg/kg; max dose 4 mg	Can be used for serial seizures, but should not be used for tonic-clonic status epilepticus
Midazolam		
Intravenous bolus	0.15 mg/kg	Administer over 2–5 minutes; if not effective, continuous infusion should be started
Continuous infusion	1–5 µg/kg/min; max dose 18 µg/kg/min	Initiate treatment at 1 µg/kg/min and increase rate by that amount at 15-minute intervals to achieve seizure control.
Intramuscular	0.2 mg/kg	

explain the increased anticonvulsant effect and sedation observed with valproate comedication (28).

In the treatment of children with status epilepticus, an initial IV dose of 0.3 mg/kg (maximum dose 10 mg) of diazepam should be given slowly over 2 to 5 minutes (21) (Table 27-1). An infusion rate of 3 to 12 mg/kg/day has been used successfully in five infants (29). Rectal doses of 0.5 to 0.7 mg/kg have been used in the treatment of status epilepticus, with a suggested maximum dose of 20 mg (16,18,30). Rectal diazepam, administered at a dose of 5 mg every 8 hours in instances in which the temperature is greater than 38.5 °C, has been demonstrated to reduce the risk of recurrent febrile convulsions (17). Measurement of blood levels of diazepam is not helpful in clinical management.

LORAZEPAM

Clinical Indications

Lorazepam is a 1,4-benzodiazepine that has been demonstrated to be effective in the treatment of status epilepticus and serial seizures. Lorazepam has also been reported to be useful in the treatment of postanoxic myoclonus (31).

Lorazepam is as effective as diazepam in the treatment of status epilepticus, has fewer side effects, and has a longer duration of action. In a prospective comparison of diazepam and lorazepam in 102 children presenting at an emergency department with convulsions, 0.3 to 0.4 mg/kg diazepam or 0.05 to 0.1 mg/kg lorazepam were administered intravenously. When IV access was not possible, the same dose was given rectally. Convulsions were controlled in 76 percent of children who received lorazepam and 51 percent of those who received diazepam. Significantly fewer side effects occurred in those receiving lorazepam. Thus, respiratory depression occurred in 3 percent of who received lorazepam and 15 percent of those who received diazepam (32). Sublingual lorazepam has also been shown to be a convenient and effective treatment of serial seizures in children (33).

Unwanted Effects

Sedation is the most common side effect of lorazepam. Anterograde amnesia and impaired psychomotor function are also observed at usual doses (34). Respiratory depression has occasionally been described in children with status epilepticus who were treated with lorazepam but occurs much less commonly than with diazepam (23,34). Thrombophlebitis occurs less commonly than with IV diazepam (35) and is rare if lorazepam is diluted with an equal volume of sterile water, saline, or 5% dextrose. Lorazepam becomes progressively less effective when serial doses are required in the management of status epilepticus (36). Abrupt discontinuation of lorazepam has been associated with withdrawal seizures, which may occur up to 60 hours following its discontinuation (34). Lorazepam has precipitated tonic seizures in patients being treated for atypical absence status epilepticus, but this is a very rare complication (37,38).

Pharmacokinetics and Dosage

Lorazepam is absorbed more rapidly when administered sublingually than orally or intramuscularly, and peak plasma levels are achieved within 60 minutes (34). The rectal absorption of lorazepam parenteral solution is slow, and peak concentrations may not be reached for 1 to 2 hours (39). In addition, peak concentrations are much lower than those achieved following IV administration, and higher lorazepam doses are required when lorazepam is administered rectally (39). Lorazepam is metabolized rapidly, and hepatic glucuronidation is the major pathway involved (40). First-pass hepatic transformation decreases the absolute systemic availability of lorazepam administered orally to 29 percent when compared with IV administration (41). Lorazepam is 90 percent protein bound and rapidly crosses the blood–brain barrier. Following IV administration, there is a rapid fall in blood levels because of the distribution phase. The elimination half-life is 10.5 ± 2.9 hours in children (42) but is longer in neonates (43). The clearance of lorazepam is not influenced by acute viral hepatitis (44) or renal disease (45). However, valproate reduces the clearance of lorazepam, possibly by inhibition of glucuronidation (46). There are no other significant interactions with AEDs (34), and, unlike other benzodiazepines, the protein binding of lorazepam is not influenced by heparin (47).

The recommended IV dose of lorazepam in children is 0.1 mg/kg (maximum dose 4 mg) (36,48,49). The IV rate of administration should not exceed 2 mg/min. The dose can be repeated if necessary after 10 minutes. Sublingual doses of 0.05 to 0.15 mg/kg have been used in children with serial seizures (33). Higher doses may be required when lorazepam is administered rectally for control of status epilepticus because of the incomplete and slow absorption.

MIDAZOLAM

Midazolam is a 1,4-benzodiazepine that was developed initially as a preanesthetic agent. It is the first water-soluble benzodiazepine and has been administered by the IV, IM, and intranasal routes in children with epilepsy. It has been demonstrated to be effective in the treatment of refractory status epilepticus (50–52), and its relatively short half-life makes it more suitable for continuous infusion than diazepam or lorazepam.

Clinical Indications

Intravenous midazolam was found to be effective in the treatment of refractory status epilepticus in 43 of 44 children in two studies (50,51). The patients received a bolus of 0.15 mg/kg and a continuous infusion starting at 1 g/kg/min. The infusion rate was increased by 1 g/kg/min every 15 minutes until seizures were controlled. The infusion rates that were required to control seizures ranged from 1 to 5 and 1to18 µg/min (mean 2.0 and 2.3 g/min) in the two studies, and the mean times to seizure control were 0.9 and 0.78 hours, respectively. No metabolic derangements or interference with vital functions were observed. Full consciousness was regained approximately 4 to 5 hours after discontinuation of midazolam.

The high water solubility of midazolam permits administration by a variety of routes. IM midazolam (15 mg) had an effect comparable to that of IV diazepam (20 mg) in the suppression of interictal spikes in adults within 5 minutes (53). Intramuscular midazolam at a dose of 0.2 mg/kg was effective in stopping 64 of 69 prolonged seizures in 48 children (54). Intranasal administration of midazolam is a well-established method of sedation in children (55) and may be useful in the treatment of seizures. Intranasal midazolam at a dose of 0.2 mg/kg rapidly suppressed spike activity on the electroencephalogram in a study of 19 children between 1 and 14 years of age (56).

Unwanted Effects

Drowsiness and ataxia are the most common side effects. Apnea and hypotension may occur following rapid IV administration of a bolus of midazolam, but apnea has been reported in only one patient following administration of IM midazolam (57). Bradycardia, hypotension, and involuntary movements, thought to be epileptiform, have been reported in premature neonates below 32 weeks gestation immediately following an IV bolus dose of 0.2 mg/kg (58). Thrombophlebitis occurs less often than with diazepam (57).

Pharmacokinetics and Dosage

Before administration, the benzodiazepine ring of midazolam is open and it water-soluble. However, following administration, the benzodiazepine ring closes at physiologic pH and midazolam becomes lipid-soluble. These characteristics permit absorption via the IM route and rapid transport across the blood–brain barrier. The onset of sedative effects are observed within 1 to 5 minutes of IV administration, and the duration of action is approximately 2 hours (range 1–6 hours) (59). The absorption of IM midazolam is rapid, and 80 percent to 100 percent is absorbed (60). Pharmacologic effects are observed within 5 to 15 minutes but may not be maximal for 20 to 60 minutes (59). Peak blood levels are obtained approximately 25 minutes following an IM injection (60). Oral midazolam is also absorbed rapidly, with peak blood levels being achieved within 1 hour. First-pass metabolism in the liver limits the availability to 40 percent to 50 percent of the oral dose. Midazolam has high lipophilicity, which results in rapid brain penetration (61). It is distributed rapidly and possesses a short elimination half-life (1.5–3 hours) in children. A longer half-life (6.5 hours) has been observed in critically ill neonates (62).

Midazolam is highly protein bound (96–98%) and is metabolized extensively by the cytochrome P-450/3A enzyme system. Its metabolism is induced by phenytoin and carbamazepine (63). A metabolite, α-hydroxymidazolam, has antiepileptic activity but has a shorter half-life, and its serum concentration is approximately one-third that of midazolam (57). Thus, its contribution to the antiepileptic action of midazolam is probably minimal. Renal failure does not influence the pharmacokinetics of midazolam (64).

The initial IV bolus dose is 0.15 mg/kg (50,51), which may be followed by continuous infusion at an initial rate of 1 µg/kg/min, which may be increased subsequently by 1 µg/kg/min every 15 minutes to achieve seizure control. Seizures are controlled at infusion rates less than 3 g/kg/min in most children, but rates up to 18 g/mL may be necessary (50). An IM dose of 0.2 mg/kg has been used effectively in children (54).

CLONAZEPAM

Clonazepam is a benzodiazepine that has been used largely as adjunctive therapy in the treatment of epilepsy. It has a wide spectrum of antiepileptic activity, but its usefulness is limited to some extent by neurotoxicity and tolerance.

Clinical Indications

Clonazepam, a 1,4-benzodiazepine, has been demonstrated in controlled studies to be effective in the treatment of absence (65–67), myoclonic (66), and atonic seizures (66). Open studies have suggested that clonazepam is also effective in the treatment of photosensitive epilepsy and primarily generalized tonic-clonic seizures, both as monotherapy (68) and in combination with valproic acid (69). In patients with juvenile myoclonic epilepsy, clonazepam is more effective in the prevention of myoclonic seizures than tonic-clonic seizures (70). Suppression of the myoclonic component that usually occurs at the onset of the tonic-clonic seizure in that syndrome eliminates the warning to the patient and may result in an increased risk of injury during a seizure (70). Clonazepam is also effective in the treatment of other myoclonic epilepsies, including reflex myoclonic epilepsy, progressive myoclonic epilepsy, posthypoxic intention myoclonus, and epilepsia partialis continua (71). Partial epilepsy may also respond to clonazepam. Clonazepam monotherapy was associated with elimination of rolandic discharges in 8 of 11 children with benign rolandic epilepsy (72). The addition of clonazepam was also effective in the treatment of children with partial seizures resistant to carbamazepine (73).

Unwanted Effects

The most common adverse effects of clonazepam include drowsiness, ataxia, incoordination, and behavioral changes (24,74). Comedication with phenobarbital usually exacerbates the drowsiness (75). Diplopia, nystagmus, dysarthria, excessive drooling, and hypotonia may occur. Initiation of therapy at a low dose and slow increase of the dose may reduce the neurotoxicity, which is the major factor limiting the usefulness of clonazepam. Increased appetite and weight gain of more than 20 percent were reported in 9 of 81 children treated with clonazepam (74).

Tolerance to clonazepam has been demonstrated in both animal and human studies. The development of tolerance to its motor and sedative effects occurs relatively early and is the rationale behind a gradual escalation of the dose. The use of alternate-day clonazepam has been reported in an animal model to be associated with significantly less tolerance (76), and this effect has also been observed in children (77). The development of tolerance to the antiepileptic effect of clonazepam is also dependent on the type of epilepsy. Thus, tolerance did not develop in 23 children with

partial epilepsy who were treated with clonazepam monotherapy or clonazepam and carbamazepine (73). In addition, tolerance to clonazepam is observed less often in patients with typical absence seizures than in patients with West syndrome or Lennox-Gastaut syndrome (5).

Pharmacokinetics and Dosage

The absorption of clonazepam is >80 percent, and peak levels occur between 1 and 4 hours (71). The high lipid solubility results in rapid distribution, with easy passage across the blood–brain barrier. The metabolism of clonazepam involves the hepatic cytochrome P-450 3A4 (78), and comedication with carbamazepine or phenobarbital lowers blood clonazepam levels (71). Acetylation is also a major metabolic pathway, and patients who are rapid acetylators are more likely to require higher doses to achieve a response than slow acetylators (79). The serum half-life in children is 22 to 33 hours (65).

To minimize side effects, clonazepam should be started at a dose of 0.01 to 0.03 mg/kg/day in children under 30 kg and should be given in two or three daily doses (80). The dose can be increased by 0.25 to 0.5 mg/day every 5 to 7 days to a total dose of 0.2 mg/kg/day, which may be required in patients receiving drugs that induce microsomal metabolism, and to 0.1 mg/kg/day in other children (Table 27-2). Clonazepam has been administered to neonates with seizures by slow IV infusion in doses of 0.1 to 0.2 mg/kg. The plasma half-life in this population was 20 to 43 hours (81).

Discontinuation of clonazepam may be complicated by a transient worsening in seizure control, and status epilepticus may occur if the drug is withdrawn abruptly (5). Behavioral changes, including restlessness, dysphoria, sleep disturbance, and tachycardia, may occur during clonazepam withdrawal (5). To minimize these effects, withdrawal should be gradual, and clonazepam should be discontinued within 3 to

Table 27-2. Benzodiazepine Dosages for Prevention of Seizures

Drug	Initial Dose	Dosage Increase	Maximum Dose
Clobazam	2.5 mg/day < 2 years; 5 mg/day if 2–10 years; 10 mg/day > 10 years	2.5–5 mg/day every 5–7 days	Doses over 30 mg/day rarely improve seizure control
Clonazepam	0.01–0.03 mg/kg/day in children under 30 kg	0.25–0.5 mg/day every 5–7 days; bid or tid	0.2 mg/kg/day if on enzyme-inducing drugs; 0.1 mg/kg/day in others
Clorazepate	0.3 mg/kg/day	0.4–3 mg/kg/day (max 60 mg) every 5–7 days; bid	15 mg/kg/day
Nitrazepam	0.1–0.2 mg/kg/day	every 5–7 days; bid or tid	<0.8 mg/kg/day

6 months in patients who do not achieve a clear lasting benefit (5).

NITRAZEPAM

Clinical Indications

Nitrazepam is a 1,4-benzodiazepine that has been reported to be effective in certain types of epilepsy. In a randomized controlled study in patients with infantile spasms, excellent control (75–100% reduction in spasm frequency) was observed in 52 percent of patients receiving nitrazepam and 57 percent of patients receiving adrenocorticotropin (82), but side effects were less severe in the patients who received nitrazepam. In open studies, nitrazepam has been reported to be effective in the treatment of absence and primarily generalized tonic-clonic seizures (83), myoclonic seizures (84), the Lennox-Gastaut syndrome (85), and partial seizures (83). Given intermittently at times of fever, nitrazepam has been reported to be effective in the prevention of recurrent febrile convulsions (86).

Unwanted Effects

Drowsiness, ataxia, and incoordination, which are common side effects, may be diminished by initiation of treatment at a low dose and by slow dose increase. Nitrazepam may cause increased salivation, hypersecretion of the tracheobronchial tree, and abnormal swallowing, which relates to delay of cricopharyngeal relaxation (87). This may result in excessive drooling, feeding difficulties, and aspiration pneumonia (84,88). Caution should be exercised when nitrazepam is used in children under 4 years of age, particularly if they have evidence of mental retardation or cerebral palsy (88a).

Pharmacokinetics and Dosage

Nitrazepam is highly protein bound (85–90%) and has an elimination half-life of 24 to 31 hours (85). There are no clinically significant interactions with other AEDs. Oral contraceptive steroids and cimetidine reduce nitrazepam clearance and rifampin increases nitrazepam clearance (85).

To reduce the risk of side effects, nitrazepam should be started in children at a low dose (0.1–0.2 mg/kg/day), and the dosage should be increased every 5 to 7 days to a maximum of 0.8 mg/kg/day (88). Discontinuation of nitrazepam should be gradual in order to minimize withdrawal seizures.

CLORAZEPATE

Clorazepate, a 1,4-benzodiazepine, was developed initially as an anxiolytic agent, but it has been used as adjunctive therapy in epilepsy. Clorazepate is a prodrug, which is decarboxylated in the stomach to the active medication, N-desmethyldiazepam. Although N-desmethyldiazepam is a metabolite of diazepam, it is not possible to achieve consistently high concentrations using diazepam without marked drug toxicity.

Clinical Indications

Clorazepate was introduced in the 1960s, and there have been no controlled studies in children. Improvement in seizure control has been observed in children with partial (89) and generalized seizures (89–92), including children with Lennox-Gastaut syndrome (89).

Unwanted Effects

Sedation, ataxia, behavioral changes, and drooling, which are the most common side effects of clorazepate in children, often lessen with time. Comedication with phenobarbital increases the probability of behavioral problems (93) and should be avoided. Idiosyncratic reactions are rare (94).

Tolerance limits the usefulness of clorazepate, but animal studies suggest that tolerance occurs less often with clorazepate than with diazepam or clonazepam (94). Withdrawal seizures and behavioral changes may complicate the discontinuation of therapy, which should occur slowly.

Pharmacokinetics and Dosage

Clorazepate is converted rapidly in the stomach to N-desmethyldiazepam. Peak concentrations of N-desmethyldiazepam are normally achieved at 0.5 to 2 hours and after 12 hours with the slow-release preparation (94,95). Serum concentrations of N-desmethyldiazepam rise after meals, and this may result in somnolence (95). N-desmethyldiazepam is 97 percent protein bound, largely to serum albumin (94). Although N-desmethyldiazepam has an elimination half-life of 55 to 100 hours, administration of clorazepate once daily is associated with unacceptable side effects because of the relatively high peak concentrations that follow its rapid absorption (94). N-desmethyldiazepam is metabolized extensively by the liver, and its elimination half-life is prolonged in patients with liver disease. Drugs that induce hepatic microsomal metabolism enhance the clearance of N-desmethyldiazepam, and patients receiving these drugs require higher doses of clorazepate.

The initial dose of clorazepate in children is 0.3 mg/kg/day, and the dose is increased gradually to achieve seizure control or until side effects appear. Doses of 7.5 to 15 mg/kg/day given on a twice-daily basis have been used in children.

CLOBAZAM

Clobazam differs from the 1,4 benzodiazepines by the presence of a nitrogen atom in the 1 and 5 positions of the diazepine ring. The use of clobazam in the treatment of epilepsy was pioneered by Gastaut, who reported its effectiveness in patients with partial seizures, idiopathic generalized epilepsy, reflex epilepsy, and the Lennox-Gastaut syndrome (96). A major advantage of clobazam over the 1,4 benzodiazepines is its much lower incidence of neurotoxicity. Differences in efficacy and side effects between clobazam and the other benzodiazepines are probably related to their influence on the GABA$_A$ receptor.

Clinical Indications

The antiepileptic effect of clobazam has been demonstrated in several placebo-controlled studies (97). In addition, clobazam monotherapy has been demonstrated to be as effective as either carbamazepine or phenytoin in the treatment of children with partial and/or tonic-clonic seizures (6). This double-blind comparison demonstrated that clobazam monotherapy was as effective and safe as phenytoin or carbamazepine monotherapy in children who were previously untreated or who had received only one drug. Clobazam appears to have a broad spectrum of antiepileptic activity. In a large retrospective study consisting of 1,300 refractory epileptic patients, including 440 children, greater than 50 percent reduction in seizure frequency was observed for each seizure type (except tonic seizures) in 40 percent to 50 percent of patients, and complete seizure control was obtained in 10 percent to 30 percent (98). It has also been reported to be effective in the treatment of reflex epilepsies (99–101), startle epilepsy (102,103), epilepsy with continuous spike-waves during slow sleep (104), and eyelid myoclonia with absence (105). Clobazam taken intermittently for 10 days each month has also been demonstrated in a double-blind fashion to be effective in the treatment of catamenial epilepsy (106,107). Intermittent clobazam has also been used successfully by the author in the treatment of seizures that occur periodically in clusters. The lack of microsomal induction by clobazam has been considered an advantage over phenytoin in the prevention of seizures in patients receiving busulfan chemotherapy (108).

Adverse Effects

The side effects of clobazam are generally mild and resolve with dose reduction. Drowsiness, short attention span, mood change, ataxia, and drooling may occur. These occur less commonly than in patients receiving 1,4-benzodiazepines (3). In a double-blind comparison of clobazam with phenytoin and carbamazepine in children, the incidence of side effects was similar (6). Marked worsening of behavior has been reported in some patients in open studies but does not appear to occur more commonly than with carbamazepine or phenytoin (6). Excessive weight gain, which responds to withdrawal of the drug, has been reported (3). Hematologic and hepatic side effects have not been reported. Drug-induced skin rash is extremely rare.

The development of tolerance to the antiepileptic effect of clobazam has limited the use of clobazam. Animal studies have suggested that tolerance occurs more rapidly to clobazam than to clonazepam or diazepam (109,110). Open studies in children have reported tolerance in 18 percent to 65 percent of patients (3,7–10). Most of these studies involved patients who had been intractable to a variety of anticonvulsants. In a controlled study of children who were previously untreated or who had received only one drug, the incidence of tolerance was similar in patients receiving clobazam (7.5%), carbamazepine (4.2%), and phenytoin (6.7%) (6).

Pharmacokinetics and Dosage

Oral clobazam is absorbed rapidly, and peak concentrations are reached in 1 to 4 hours (111). Clobazam is relatively insoluble and cannot be administered intravenously or intramuscularly. It is highly lipophilic, is distributed rapidly, and is approximately 85 percent protein bound. Factors that influence protein binding (e.g., liver disease) may affect the free and total levels of the drug (97). Clobazam is metabolized extensively in the liver to a number of metabolites including N-desmethylclobazam, which also has antiepileptic activity. Although the potency of N-desmethylclobazam appears to be less than that of clobazam, concentrations of N-desmethylclobazam are approximately 10 times those of clobazam following long-term administration of clobazam (112), and N-desmethylclobazam is responsible for most of the antiepileptic effect in patients receiving clobazam (97).

Comedication with phenytoin, phenobarbital, or carbamazepine increases the N-desmethylclobazam to clobazam ratio (113). Increased phenytoin concentration has been observed (114) and may result in clinical phenytoin intoxication (115,116). Clobazam has also been reported to increase valproate levels, which may remain elevated for several weeks after the clobazam has been withdrawn (117). Mild increases in phenobarbital, carbamazepine, and carbamazepine epoxide have also been reported (114). In one retrospective series involving 1,319 adults and children, 5 percent had symptoms attributed to drug interactions and responded to changes in drug dose. These symptoms were associated with concomitant use of valproate in 70 percent of patients (98).

Clobazam should be started at a dose of 2.5 mg/day in infants and 5 mg/day in older children. The dose can be increased at 5- to 7-day intervals until the seizures are controlled or side effects occur. Although doses of up to 3.8 mg/kg/day can be administered to children without undue side effects, doses greater than 1 mg/kg/day are rarely associated with improved seizure control (3). In teenagers and adults, the initial dose is 10 mg/day. The dose can be increased at 5- to 7-day intervals, but those who do not respond to 30 mg/day rarely do so at a higher dose (97). Clobazam is normally administered twice a day. Discontinuation should be done gradually over several weeks to minimize the risk of withdrawal seizures.

REFERENCES

1. MacDonald RL, Olsen RW. GABA$_A$ receptor channels. *Annu Rev Neurosci* 1994; 17:569–602.

2. MacDonald RL. Benzodiazepines: mechanisms of action. In: Levy RH, Mattson RH, Meldrum BS, eds. *Antiepileptic Drugs*. 4th ed. New York: Raven Press, 1995:695–703.

3. Munn R, Farrell K. Open study of clobazam in refractory epilepsy. *Pediatr Neurol* 1993; 9:465–469.

4. Frey H-H. Experimental evidence for the the development of tolerance to anticonvulsant drug effects. In: Frey H-H, Froscher W, Koella WP, Meinardi H, eds. *Tolerance to the Beneficial and Adverse Effects of Antiepileptic Drugs*. New York: Raven Press, 1986:7–16.

5. Specht U, Boenigk HE, Wolf P. Discontinuation of clonazepam after long-term treatment. *Epilepsia* 1989; 30:458–463.

6. Canadian Clobazam Study Group. Clobazam has equivalent efficacy to carbamazepine and phenytoin as monotherapy for childhood epilepsy. *Epilepsia* 1998; 39:952–959.

7. Campos P. Uso de clobazam en epilepsias de dificil control en ninos. *Arq Neuropsiqiatr* 1993; 51:66–71.

8. Keene DL, Whiting S, Humphreys P. Clobazam as an add-on drug in the treatment of refractory epilepsy of childhood. *Can J Neurol Sci* 1990; 17:317–319.

9. Shimuzu H, Abe J, Futagi Y, al e. Antiepileptic effects of clobazam in children. *Brain Dev* 1982; 4:57–62.

10. Bardy AH, Seppala T, Salokorpi T. Monitoring of concentrations of clobazam and norclobazam in serum and saliva of of children with epilepsy. *Brain Dev* 1991; 13:174–179.

11. Kriel RL, Cloyd JC, Hadsall RS, et al. Home use of rectal diazepam for cluster and prolonged seizures: efficacy, adverse reactions, quality of life, and cost analysis. *Pediatr Neurol* 1991; 7:13–17.

12. Berg M, Espezel H. Evaluation of rectal diazepam teaching for home use. *Epilepsia* 1993; 34(Suppl 6):20.

13. Alldredge BK, Wall DB, Ferriero DM. Effect of prehospital treatment on the outcome of status epilepticus in children. *Pediatr Neurol* 1995; 12:213–216.

14. Dreifuss FE, Rosman NP, Cloyd JC, et al. A comparison of rectal diazepam gel and placebo for acute repetitive seizures. *N Engl J Med* 1998; 338:1869–1875.

15. Rosman NP, Colton T, Labazzo J, et al. A controlled trial of diazepam administered during febrile illnesses to prevent recurrence of febrile seizures. *N Engl J Med* 1993; 329:79–84.

16. Knudsen FU. Effective short-term diazepam prophylaxis in febrile convulsions. *J Pediatr* 1985; 186:487–490.

17. Knudsen F, Vestermark S. Prophylactic diazepam or phenobarbitone in febrile convulsions: a prospective controlled study. *Arch Dis Child* 1978; 53:660–663.

18. Hoppu K, Santavuori P. Diazepam rectal solution for home treatment of acute seizures in children. *Acta Paediatr Scand* 1981; 70:369–372.

19. Knudsen FU. Rectal administration of diazepam in solution in the acute treatment of convulsions in infants and children. *Arch Dis Child* 1979; 54:855–857.

20. Ventura A, Basso T, Bortolan G, et al. Home treatment of seizures as a strategy for the long-term management of febrile convulsions in children. *Helv Pediatr Acta* 1982; 37:581–587.

21. Schmidt D. Benzodiazepines: diazepam. In: Levy RH, Mattson RH, Meldrum BS, eds. *Antiepileptic Drugs*. 4th ed. New York: Raven Press, 1995:705–724.

22. Giang DW, McBride MC. Lorazepam versus diazepam for the treatment of status epilepticus. *Pediatr Neurol* 1988; 4:358–361.

23. Chiulli DA, Terndrup TE, Kanter RK. The influence of diazepam or lorazepam on the frequency of endotracheal intubation in childhood status epilepticus. *J Emerg Med* 1991; 9:13–17.

24. Farrell K. Benzodiazepines in the treatment of children with epilepsy. *Epilepsia* 1986; 27(Suppl 1):S45–S51.

25. Tassinari CA, Daniele O, Michelucci R, et al. Benzodiazepines: efficacy in status epilepticus. In: Delgado-Escueta AV, Wasterlain CG, Treiman DM, Porter RJ, eds. *Status Epilepticus: Mechanisms of Brain Damage and Treatment*. New York: Raven Press, 1983:465–475. Advances in Neurology.

26. Dasberg HH, Van der Kleijn E, Guelen PJR, Van Praag HM. Plasma concentrations of diazepam and of its metabolite *N*-desmethyldiazepam in relation to its anxiolytic effect. *Clin Pharmacol* 1974; 15:473–483.

27. Dhillon S, Richens A. Valproic acid and diazepam interaction in vivo. *Br J Clin Pharmacol* 1982; 13:553–560.

28. Kulkarni SK, Jog MV. Facilitation of diazepam action by anticonvulsant agents against picrotoxin induced convulsions. *Psychopharmacology* 1983; 81:332–334.

29. Thong YH, Abramson DC. Continuous infusion of diazepam in infants with severe recurrent convulsions. *Med Ann Dist Columb* 1974; 43:63–65.

30. Knudsen FU. Plasma diazepam in infants after rectal administration in solution and by suppository. *Acta Paediatr Scand* 1977; 66:563–567.

31. Vincent FM, Vincent T. Lorazepam in myoclonic seizures after cardiac arrest. *Ann Intern Med* 1986; 104:586.

32. Appleton R, Sweeney A, Choonara I, Robson J, Molyneux E. Lorazepam versus diazepam in the acute treatment of epileptic seizures and status epilepticus. *Dev Med Child Neurol* 1995; 37:682–688.

33. Yager JY, Seshia SS. Sublingual lorazepam in childhood serial seizures. *Am J Dis Child* 1988; 142:931–932.

34. Homan RW, Treiman DM. Benzodiazepines: lorazepam. In: Levy RH, Mattson RH, Meldrum BS, eds. *Antiepileptic Drugs*. 4th ed. New York: Raven Press, 1995:779–790.

35. Hegarty JE, Dundee JW. Sequelae after the intravenous injection of three benzodiazepines—diazepam, lorazepam, and flunarizine. *Br Med J* 1977; 2:1384–1385.

36. Crawford TO, Mitchell WG, Snodgrass SR. Lorazepam and childhood status epilepticus and serial seizures: effectiveness and tachyphylaxis. *Neurology* 1987; 37.

37. Amand G, Evrard P. Le lorazepam injectable dans les états de mal epileptiques. *Rev Electroencephalogr Neurophysiol Clin* 1976; 6:532–533.

38. Waltregny A, Dargent J. Preliminary study of parenteral lorazepam in status epilepticus. *Acta Neurol Belg* 1975; 75:219–229.

39. Graves NM, Kriel RL, Jones-Saete C. Bioavailability of rectally administered lorazepam. *Clin Neuropharmacol* 1987; 10:555–559.

40. Herman RJ, Van Pham JD, Szakacs CB. Disposition of lorazepam in human beings: enterohepatic recirculation and first-pass effect. *Clin Pharmacol Ther* 1989; 46:18–25.

41. Ochs HR, Greenblatt DJ, Eichelkraut W, et al. Contribution of the gastrointestinal tract to lorazepam conjugation and clonazepam nitroreduction. *Pharmacology* 1991; 42:36–48.

42. Relling MV, Mulhern RK, Dodge RK, et al. Lorazepam pharmacodynamics and pharmacokinetics in children. *J Pediatr* 1989; 114:641–646.

43. McDermott CA, Kowalczyk AL, Schnitzler ER, et al. Pharmacokinetics of lorazepam in critically ill neonates with seizures. *J Pediatr* 1992; 120:479–483.

44. Krauss JW, Desmond PV, Marshall JP, et al. Effects of aging and liver disease on the disposition of lorazepam. *Clin Pharmacol Ther* 1978; 24:411–419.

45. Morrison G, Chiang ST, Koepke HH, Walker BR. Effect of renal impairment and hemodialysis on lorazepam kinetics. *Clin Pharmacol Ther* 1984; 35:646–652.

46. Anderson GD, Gidal BE, Kantor ED, Wilensky AJ. Lorazepam–valproate interaction: studies in normal subjects and isolated perfused rat liver. *Epilepsia* 1994; 35:221–225.

47. Desmond PV, Roberts RK, Wood AJJ, et al. Effect of heparin administration on plasma binding of benzodiazepines. *Br J Clin Pharmacol* 1980; 9:171–175.

48. Epilepsy Foundation of America Working Group on Status Epilepticus. Treatment of convulsive status epilepticus. *JAMA* 1993; 270:854–859.

49. Mitchell WG, Crawford TO. Lorazepam is the treatment of choice for status epilepticus. *J Epilepsy* 1990; 3:7–10.

50. Rivera R, Segnini M, Boltadano A, Perez V. Midazolam in the treatment of status epilepticus in children. *Crit Care Med* 1993; 21:991–994.

51. Koul RL, Aithala GR, Chacko A, Joshi R, Elbualy MS. Continuous midazolam as treatment of status epilepticus. *Arch Dis Child* 1997; 76:445–448.

52. Parent JM, Lowenstein DH. Treatment of refractory generalized status epilepticus with continuous infusion of midazolam. *Neurology* 1994; 44:1837–1840.

53. Jawad S, Oxley J, Wilson J, Richens A. A pharmacodynamic evaluation of midazolam as an antiepileptic compound. *J Neurol Neurosurg Psychiatry* 1986; 49:1050–1054.

54. Lahat E, Aladjem M, Eshel G, Bistritzer T, Katz Y. Midazolam in treatment of epileptic seizures. *Pediatr Neurol* 1992; 8:215–216.

55. Ljung B, Andreasson S. Comparison of midazolam nasal spray to nasal drops for the sedation of children. *J Nucl Med Technol* 1996; 24:32–34.

56. O'Regan ME, Brown JK, Clarke M. Nasal rather than rectal benzodiazepines in the management of acute childhood seizures. *Dev Med Child Neurol* 1996; 38:1037–1045.

57. Shorvon SD. The use of clobazam, midazolam and nitrazepam in epilepsy. *Epilepsia* 1998; 39(Suppl 1):S15–S23.

58. van den Anker JN, Sauer PJJ. The use of midazolam in the preterm neonate. *Eur J Paediatr* 1992; 151:152.

59. Bebin M, Bleck TP. New anticonvulsant drugs: focus on flunarizine, fosphenytoin, midazolam and stiripentol. *Drugs* 1994; 48:153–171.

60. Bell DM, Richards G, Dhillon S, et al. A comparative pharmacokinetic study of intravenous and intramuscular midazolam in patients with epilepsy. *Epilepsy Res* 1991; 10:183–190.

61. Dundee JW, Halliday NJ, Harper KW, Brogden RN. Midazolam: a review of its pharmacological properties and therapeutic use. *Drugs* 1984; 28:519–543.

62. Jacqz-Aigrain E, Wood C, Robieux I. Pharmacokinetics of midazolam in critically ill neonates. *Eur J Clin Pharmacol* 1990; 3:191–192.

63. Backman JT, Olkola KT, Ojala M, Laaksovirta H, Neuvonen PJ. Concentrations and effects of oral midazolam are greatly reduced in patients treated with carbamazepine or phenytoin. *Epilepsia* 1996; 37:253–257.

64. Driessen JJ, Vree TB, Guelen PJ. The effects of acute changes in renal function on the pharmacokinetics of midazolam during long-term infusion in ICU patients. *Acta Anaesthesiol Belg* 1991; 42:149–155.

65. Dreifuss FE, Penry JK, Rose SW, et al. Serum clonazepam concentrations in children with absence seizures. *Neurology* 1975; 25:255–258.

66. Mikkelsen B, Birket-Smith E, Brandt S, et al. Clonazepam in the treatment of epilepsy. *Arch Neurol* 1976; 33:322–325.

67. Sato S, Penry JK, Dreifuss FE, et al. Clonazepam in the treatment of absence seizures: a double-blind clinical trial. *Neurology* 1977; 27:371.

68. Naito H, Wachi M, Nishida M. Clinical effects and plasma concentrations of long-term clonazepam monotherapy in previously untreated epileptics. *Acta Neurol Scand* 1987; 76:58–63.

69. Mireles R, Leppik IL. Valproate and clonazepam comedication in patients with intractable epilepsy. *Epilepsia* 1985; 26:122–126.

70. Obeid T, Panayiotopoulos CP. Clonazepam in juvenile myoclonic epilepsy. *Epilepsia* 1989; 30:603–606.

71. Sato S, Malow BA. Benzodiazepines: clonazepam. In: Levy RH, Mattson RH, Meldrum BS, eds. *Antiepileptic Drugs*. 4th ed. New York: Raven Press, 1995:725–734.

72. Takahashi K, Saito M, Kyo K. The effect of clonazepam on Rolandic discharge of benign epilepsy of children with centro-temporal EEG foci. *Jpn J Psychiatry Neurol* 1991; 45:468–470.

73. Hosoda N, Miura H, Takanashi S, Shirai H, Sunaoshi W. The long-term effectiveness of clonazepam therapy in the control of partial seizures in children difficult to control with carbamazepine monotherapy. *Jpn J Psychiatry Neurol* 1991; 45:471–473.

74. Hanson RA, Menkes JH. A new anticonvulsant in the management of minor motor seizures. *Dev Med Child Neurol* 1972; 14:3–14.

75. Browne TR. Clonazepam: a review of a new anticonvulsant drug. *Arch Neurol* 1976; 33:326–332.

76. Suzuki Y, Edge J, Mimaki T, Walson PD. Intermittent clonazepam treatment prevents anticonvulsant tolerance in mice. *Epilepsy Res* 1993; 15:15–20.

77. Sher PK. Alternate-day clonazepam treatment of intractable seizures. *Arch Neurol* 1985; 42:787–788.

78. Seree EJ, Pisano PJ, Placidi M, Rahamani R, Barra YA. Identification of human and animal cytochromes P450 involved in clonazepam metabolism. *Fundam Clin Pharmacol* 1993; 7:69–75.

79. DeVane CL, Ware MR, Lydiard RB. Pharmacokinetics, pharmacodynamics, and treatment issues of benzodiazepines: alprazolam, adinazolam, and clonazepam. *Psychopharmacol Bull* 1991; 27:463–473.

80. Schmidt D. How to use benzodiazepines. In: Morselli PL, Pippenger CE, Penry JK, eds. *Antiepileptic Drug Therapy in Pediatrics*. New York: Raven Press, 1983:271–282.

81. Andre M, Boutroy MJ, Dubruc C, et al. Clonazepam pharmacokinetics and therapeutic efficacy in neonatal seizures. *Clin Pharmacol* 1986; 30:585–589.

82. Dreifuss F, Farwell J, Holmes G, et al. Infantile spasms: comparative trial of nitrazepam and corticotrophin. *Arch Neurol* 1986; 43:1107–1110.

83. Vanasse M, Geoffroy G. Treatment of epilepsy with nitrazepam. In: Wada JA, Penry JK, eds. *Advances in Epileptology: The Xth Epilepsy International Symposium*. New York: Raven Press, 1980:503.

84. Millichap JG, Ortiz WR. Nitrazepam in myoclonic epilepsies. *Am J Dis Child* 1966; 112:242–248.

85. Baruzzi A, Michelucci R, Tassinari CA. Benzodiazepines: nitrazepam. In: Levy RH, Mattson RH, Meldrum BS, eds. *Antiepileptic Drugs*. 4th ed. New York: Raven Press, 1995:735–749.

86. Vanasse M, Masson P, Geoffroy G, Larbrisseau A, Favid PC. Intermittent treatment of febrile convulsions with nitrazepam. *Can J Neurol Sci* 1984; 11:377–379.

87. Wyllie E, Wyllie R, Cruse RP, Rothner AD, Erenburg G. The mechanism of nitrazepam-induced drooling and aspiration. *N Engl J Med* 1986; 314:35–38.

88. Murphy JV, Sawasky F, Marquardt KM, Harris DJ. Deaths in young children receiving nitrazepam. *J Pediatr* 1987; 111:145–147.

88a. Rintahhaka PJ, Nakagawa JA, Shewmon DA, Kyyronen P, Shields WD. Incidence of death in patients with intractable epilepsy during nitrazepam treatment. *Epilepsia 1999*; 40:492–496.

89. Guggenheim MA, Donaldson J, Hotvedt C. Clinical evaluation of clorazepate. *Ann Neurol* 1987; 22:412–413.

90. Mimaki T, Tagawa T, Ono J, et al. Antiepileptic effect and serum levels of clorazepate in children with refractory epilepsy. *Brain Dev* 1984; 6:539–544.

91. Sobaniek W, Kulac W. Clorazepate in treatment of childhood epilepsy. *Epilepsia* 1993; 34(Suppl 2):7.

92. Graf WD, Rothman SJ. Clorazepate therapy in children with refractory seizures. *Epilepsia* 1987; 28:606.

93. Feldman RG. Clorazepate in temporal lobe epilepsy. *JAMA* 1976; 236:2603.

94. Wilensky AJ. Benzodiazepines: Clorazepate. In: Levy RH, Mattson RH, Meldrum BS, eds. *Antiepileptic Drugs*. 4th ed. New York: Raven Press, 1995:751–762.

95. Wilensky AJ, Ojemann LM, Temkin NR, Troupin AS, Dodrill CB. Clorazepate kinetics in treated epileptics. *Clin Pharmacol* 1978; 24:22–30.

96. Gastaut H, Low MD. Antiepileptic properties of clobazam, a 1,5, benzodiazepine, in man. *Epilepsia* 1979; 20:437–446.

97. Shorvon SD. Benzodiazepines: clobazam. In: Levy RH, Mattson RH, Meldrum BS, eds. *Antiepileptic Drugs*. 4th ed. New York: Raven Press, 1995:763–777.

98. Canadian Clobazam Cooperative Group. Clobazam in the treatment of refractory epilepsy: the Canadian experience. A retrospective study. *Epilepsia* 1991; 32:407–416.

99. Senanayake N. Epilepsia arithmetics revisited. *Epilepsy Res* 1989; 3:167–169.

100. Senanayake N. Epileptic seizures evoked by card games, draughts and similar games. *Epilepsia* 1987; 28:356–361.

101. Senanayake N. "Eating epilepsy"—a reappraisal. *Epilepsy Res* 1990; 5:74–79.

102. Tinuper P, Aguglia U, Gastaut H. Use of clobazam in certain forms of status epilepticus and in startle induced epileptic seizures. *Epilepsia* 1986; 27:S18–S26.

103. Aguglia U, Tinuper P, Gastaut H. Startle-induced epileptic seizures. *Epilepsia* 1984; 25:712–720.

104. DeMarco P. Electrical status epilepticus during slow sleep: one case with sensory aphasia. *Clin Electroencephalogr* 1988; 19:111–113.

105. DeMarco P. Eyelid myoclonia with absences in two monovular twins. *Clin Electroencephalogr* 1989; 20:193–195.

106. Feely M, Gibson J. Intermittent clobazam for catamenial epilepsy: avoid tolerance. *J Neurol Neurosurg Psychiatry* 1984; 47:1279–1282.

107. Feely M, Calvert R, Gibson J. Clobazam in catamenial epilepsy. A model for evaluating anticonvulsants. *Lancet* 1982; 2:71–73.

108. Schwarer A, Sopat S, Watson AL, Cole-Sinclair MF. Clobazam for seizure prophylaxis during busulfan chemotherapy. *Lancet* 1995; 346:1238.

109. DeSarro GB, Rotiroti D, Gratteri S, et al. Tolerance to anticonvulsant effects of clobazam, diazepam and clonazepam in genetically epilepsy prone rats. In: Biggio G, Concas A, Costa E, eds. *GABAergic Synaptic Transmission*. New York: Raven Press, 1992:249–254.

110. Gent JP, Feely MP, Haigh JRM. Differences between the tolerance characteristics of two antiepileptic drugs. *Life Sci* 1985; 37:849–856.

111. Jawad S, Richens A, Oxley J. Single dose pharmacokinetic study of clobazam in normal volunteers and epileptic patients. *Br J Clin Pharmacol* 1984; 18:873–877.

112. Rupp W, Badian M, Christ O, et al. Pharmacokinetics of single and multiple doses of clobazam in humans. *Br J Clin Pharmacol* 1979; 7(Suppl 1):51S–57S.

113. Sennoune S, Mesdjian E, Bonneton J, et al. Interactions between clobazam and standard antiepileptic drugs in patients with epilepsy. *Ther Drug Monit* 1992; 14:269–274.

114. Goggin T, Callaghan N. Blood levels of clobazam and its metabolites and therapeutic effect. In: Hindmarch I, Stonier PD, Trimble MR, eds. *Clobazam: Human Psychopharmacology and Clinical Applications*. London: Royal Society of Medicine, 1985:149–153. Vol. International Congress and Symposium Series; No. 74.

115. Munn R, Camfield P, Camfield C, Dooley J. Clobazam for refractory childhood seizure disorders—a valuable supplementary drug. *Can J Neurol Sci* 1988; 15:406–408.

116. Zifkin B, Sherwin A, Andermann F. Phenytoin toxicity due to interaction with clobazam. *Neurology* 1991; 41:313–314.

117. Cocks A, Critchley EMR, Hayward HW, Thomas D. The effect of clobazam on blood levels of valproate. In: Hindmarch I, Stonier PD, Trimble MR, eds. *Clobazam: Human Psychopharmacology and Clinical Applications*. London: Royal Society of Medicine, 1985:149–153. Vol. International Congress and Symposium Series; No. 74.

CHAPTER 28

Barbiturates and Primidone

Robert S. Rust, M.D.

Although phenobarbital (PB) is the major focus of this chapter, other drugs are reviewed, particularly mephobarbital, pentobarbital, and primidone. Mephobarbital (MPB) is a useful alternative to PB, more widely employed in some other countries, such as Australia, than in the United States. Like primidone, it undergoes biotransformation to PB. Among the more sedative barbiturates, pentobarbital has been useful in the management of severe and persistent seizures that do not respond to more routine anticonvulsant therapy. Primidone (PRM) is not actually a barbiturate, although it is subject to biotransformation into PB and probably exerts most of its anticonvulsant effects in that form. Because the major antiepileptic effects and side effects can be ascribed to the PB metabolite and because of pharmacokinetic and pharmacodynamic similarities, it is quite appropriate to consider PRM in this chapter.

PHENOBARBITAL

Phenobarbital is 5-ethyl-5-phenyl substituted barbituric acid with a molecular weight of 232.23. It is a weakly acidic substance with a pKa that is usually reported as 7.3 (1–4). The free acid has low aqueous and relatively low lipid solubility; however, the sodium salt, which is used for intravenous (IV) and intramuscular (IM) preparations, is freely soluble in slightly alkaline aqueous solutions.

Mechanisms of Action

Phenobarbital exhibits a wide spectrum of anticonvulsant activity, conferring protection to animals subjected either to electroshock or chemically induced (pentylenetetrazol or bicuculline) experimental seizures (5,6). This spectrum is shared by most barbiturates and is consistent with their wide spectrum of activity in clinical seizure disorders.

Understanding of the antiepileptic activity of PB has been limited by the incomplete state of our understanding of the mechanisms of epilepsy. Current views suggest that PB modulates the postsynaptic effects of certain neurotransmitters. The modulation is thought to affect both the inhibitory substance gamma-aminobutyric acid (GABA) and such excitatory amino acids as glutamate. Whether by these or other mechanisms, antiepileptic barbiturates appear to elevate the threshold to chemical or electrical induction of seizures in ways that differ from and are in some respects superior to those of phenytoin (7).

A large body of information has accumulated concerning the ability of barbiturates to depress physiologic excitation in the nervous system and enhance inhibition of synaptic transmission. PB shares with pentobarbital (PnB) the capacity for selective postsynaptic augmentation of GABA-mediated inhibition and depression of glutamate- and quisqualate-mediated excitation in at least some central nervous system (CNS) regions (8–14). Barbiturate augmentation of GABA-stimulated postsynaptic inhibition appears to be due to activation of a subset (alpha-beta) of the $GABA_A$-receptor gated chloride channels (13,15). These receptors differ from those that are activated by benzodiazepines and are differentially expressed in brain (16). These postsynaptic effects are produced at clinically relevant concentrations (12,13).

The reduction of voltage-activated calcium currents may in part account for the sedative and anesthetic effects of barbiturates and may possibly play a role in the efficacy of PnB and very high concentrations of PB in suppressing seizures (13). This is another potential mechanism whereby these agents may work in the setting of intractable status epilepticus with barbiturate coma and may represent one of the mechanisms for production of anesthesia (13).

Pharmacokinetics

Absorption

Phenobarbital is rapidly and nearly completely absorbed after oral or IM administration to infants or children. For most children older than 6 months of age or adults it is likely that peak serum concentrations of PB are achieved by 2 hours after oral and 2 to 4 hours after IM bolus administration of the usual age-appropriate maintenance doses. The bioavailability of most oral and parenteral formulations is essentially quantitative (85–100%) through a wide range of doses in otherwise healthy children (>6 months of age) or adults. Rectally administered parenteral solutions of sodium PB are well absorbed at all ages, although the latency to peak concentration may be slightly longer and the bioavailability slightly lower than after IM administration (17).

Distribution

Phenobarbital disseminates into all body tissues. At lower serum pH the ionized fraction of serum PB is smaller, and therefore diffusion into tissues is enhanced leading to lower serum but higher tissue concentrations. More alkaline serum produces opposite effects (4). Only approximately 50 percent or less of circulating PB is bound to serum proteins in most patients whose ages are greater than 3 to 6 months. Equilibration of PB across the blood–brain barrier is relatively slow. Twelve to 60 minutes are required for maximal brain to plasma PB ratios in adult mammalian brain after IV administration. These data suggest that (1) dosage of PB should be based on lean body mass to prevent overdosing obese individuals (18,19), and (2) sufficient time for maximal brain penetration should be allowed to occur after bolus administration of PB before administration of additional doses.

Phenobarbital readily crosses the placenta and is secreted in breast milk (20,21). Breast milk concentrations were 36 ± 20 percent and 41 ± 16 percent of maternal serum concentrations in two studies (22,23). The newborn infants of mothers treated with PB have levels equivalent to those of their mothers immediately after birth (22,24–27). Estimates of the apparent volume of distribution (Vd) of PB vary over nearly a fourfold range but are generally larger in infants and small children than in older individuals (28–30). The Vds for newborns and infants less than 4 months of age treated with IV PB average approximately 0.9 to 1.0 L/kg, independent of body weight, dose, gestational age, or occurrence of asphyxia (28,31–34). Older children and adults exhibit Vds that range from approximately 0.45 to 0.7 L/kg more or less irrespective of route of administration (35–37).

Metabolism and Elimination

Phenobarbital may be excreted unchanged or may undergo biotransformation before excretion. The most quantitatively important fates for PB metabolism include (1) aromatic hydroxylation to p-hydroxyphenobarbital (PBOH) and (2) N-glucosidation to 9-D-glucopyranosyl phenobarbital (PNG) (38,39). On average (with wide interindividual variation), approximately 20 percent to 30 percent of a daily dose of PB is converted to the pharmacologically unimportant PBOH, apparently by at least one cytochrome P-450 isozyme. In most children and adults, about half of the PBOH is excreted unchanged and about half is excreted as a PBOH-glucuronide conjugate that is formed in liver (40). Although PB is the classic inducer of hepatic microsomal metabolism, it does not appear to induce significant changes in its own metabolic rate or plasma clearance in humans, although slight effects may occasionally be detected (41,42).

Phenobarbital has the longest half-time of elimination of any of the frequently used anticonvulsants. The two-standard-deviation range for half-time of elimination in children and adults is 24 to 140 hours, resulting in the capacity to eliminate between 11 percent and 50 percent of total body PB in 24 hours (41,43–48). Elimination half-time is longest in premature and full-term newborns, with various studies showing mean values of 100 to 200 hours with standard deviations of 30 percent to 80 percent (full range across these studies of 59 to greater than 400 hours) (30,32,49–52). Clearance may vary from day to day in individual babies (52); however, the rate of elimination may double by the second week of life and tends to continue to increase for the ensuing few weeks. Infants 6 weeks to 12 months old have the shortest mean half-times of elimination (30–75 hours) of any age group (30,34,53,54). At age 2 months half-time of elimination is usually in the range of 39 to 55 hours. Children 1 to 15 years of age typically have half-time of elimination of 37 to 73 (68 ± 30) hours, while subjects 15 to 40 years of age have 53 to 141 (100 ± 20) hours half-time of elimination (29,55). Perinatal asphyxia may considerably decrease the clearance by newborns, probably due to the combination of renal and hepatic dysfunction (21,34,37,53,56–65). Clearance of unmetabolized PB may be higher at higher rates of urine formation (66–68) or in more alkaline urine, as both of these conditions reduce the rate of PB resorption in the distal nephron. Eightfold increase in the rate of urine formation may increase PB clearance by three- to fourfold (69,70). This effect may be considerably enhanced by the alkalinization of urine with sodium bicarbonate (4).

Interactions with Other Drugs

Although some drugs affect PB kinetics, most of the pharmacokinetically important interactions encountered with the use of PB are those caused by the effects of PB on the kinetics of other drugs. The most common key encountered effect that PB has on the metabolism of other drugs is to increase their biotransformation, thereby increasing their clearance rate. PB is the prototypical inducer of the hepatic mixed-function oxidase system that is comprised of, among other elements, the numerous isoenzymes of P-450 and of NADPH-cytochrome c reductase.

A list of drugs for which this effect may be clinically important is provided in Table 28-1. In several instances, as indicated in Table 28-1, PB may result in increased concentrations of potentially toxic metabolites. The enhancement of potential valproate toxicity to kidney and liver must be considered in cases in which these drugs are used in combination. Renal tubular injury may be exacerbated by the increased dose of valproate required in some patients taking PB (71,72), while the chance of hepatic injury may be increased because of PB-induced production of the "4-en" metabolite of valproate that appears to be toxic to hepatocytes (73–76).

Although PB induces the metabolism of phenytoin, the degree of that effect is seldom great enough to

Table 28-1. Drug Subject to Kinetic Alteration When Administered to Patients Receiving Phenobarbital

Shortened Half-Time of Elimination and/or Peak Levels
Acetaminophen (231)*
Amidopyrine (42)
Aniline
Antipyrine (232)*
Bishydroxycoumarin (79)
Carbamazepine, 10,11-carbamazepine epoxide (233–235)
Chloramphenicol (236)
Chlorpromazine (237,238)
Cimetidine (239)
Cyclosporine (240)
Doxicycline (241)
Ethylmorphine
Flunarizine (242,243)
Griseofulvin (244)
Haloperidol (245)
Hexobarbital
Meperidine (246)*
Mesoridazine (245)
Methadone (247)*
Methsuximide (248)
Nortriptyline) (249)
Theophylline (250)
Valproic acid (71,72)*
Warfarin (80)

*May result in increased levels of toxic metabolites.

cause an adjustment of phenytoin dosage (77,78). Other important potential effects of comedication with PB include inadequate anticoagulation with warfarin (42, 79,80), reduction of serum levels of exogenously administered prednisone or dexamethasone (81,82), or failure of oral contraception (83,84). Coadministration of PB with coumadin or other medications can be managed when the combination is essential. In such cases, care must be taken to adjust anticoagulants with any changes in PB discontinuation (85). The effect of PB on these various drugs may become manifest within days to weeks of initiation of comedication.

Less commonly, other drugs affect PB kinetics. The most important of these in everyday practice is the interaction of PB and valproic acid. Accumulation of PB occurs in most patients who are comedicated with PB and valproate, accompanied by a lower than expected serum level to dosage ratio of valproate. The rate and magnitude of these effects are variable but generally require lowering of PB and increasing of valproate dosages as compared with what might be expected with monotherapy (86). Valproate-related weight gain and thrombocytopenia may also be dose-related. Elevation of PB levels may occur within days of initiation of valproate, but more typically the increase occurs slowly over a number of weeks.

Pharmacodynamic Interactions

Little is known about the pharmacodynamic interactions of PB and other drugs. It was long argued that PB potentiated the antiepileptic effects of phenytoin; therefore, the two drugs were coadministered in many patients for several decades. There is no scientific data upon which such a contention, or the view that PB may potentiate the antiepileptic potency of carbamazepine, can be based (87,88). Currently, it is more widely held that the combination of these and other antiepileptic drugs more often exacerbate side effects than enhance desirable effects, although there are few objective data to support this clinical impression. The combination of PB with other sedative medications, such as benzodiazepines, may provoke status epilepticus, including tonic motor status in patients with Lennox-Gastaut syndrome (89).

Adverse Effects

Experience has demonstrated that PB generally is a very safe and predictable medication. Nonetheless, it does produce various undesirable effects. The majority of these are reversible effects that can be tolerated but reduce the attractiveness of PB therapy. Serious side effects also occur, but they are rare. The most frequently encountered adverse characteristics of PB are (1) sedation, (2) disturbances of mood and behavior and possibly cognition, and (3) induction of hepatic metabolism producing various effects on the disposition of a wide variety of other drugs (previously considered). Exacerbation of seizures may possibly occur with weaning and discontinuation of phenobarbital maintenance. Serious allergic reactions may occur.

Sedation and Behavior

Although phenobarbital has the most favorable ratio of antiepileptic potency to sedative properties among the antiepileptic barbiturates, it is certainly more sedating than most other anticonvulsants (90). Drowsiness is most common at the initiation of therapy, afflicting as many as one-third of newly treated patients. Sedation may occur even at very low doses and may persist for several days, occasionally as long as several weeks (44). Sedation may return with dose increases, and there may be a dose-related increment in difficulty awakening in the morning or increase in the frequency with which a nap is required. However, many patients do not experience significant sedation after initially becoming accustomed to the medication despite many-fold increases in dose (91,92). Patients receiving chronic PB therapy are least likely to feel drowsy if their serum level falls between 15 and 30 µg/mL, but there is considerable individual variation in tolerance. Some patients complain of little sedation with levels as high as 50 µg/mL, while others find levels of 10 to 15 µg/ml intolerable because of lethargy (93).

Mood Disturbance

Studies have shown that 30 percent to 42 percent of children with febrile seizures treated with PB prophylaxis experience deterioration in behavior, the majority having relatively low PB levels (i.e., less than 15 µg/mL). Hyperactivity, irritability, belligerence, intermittent agitation, disruptive and defiant behavior, insomnia, and uncharacteristic episodic sedation are among the most frequent troublesome manifestations—effects that are not related to dose or serum level (94–96). Hyperkinetic characteristics have occurred in as many as 79 percent of children treated with any drug for epilepsy (97), and the disturbances of behavior similar to those noted occur in at least 18 percent of children that have had at least one febrile seizure without any prophylactic anticonvulsant (98).

Several well-designed studies have failed to find a significant incidence of behavioral deterioration of children treated with PB (99,100). In a particularly well-designed, double-blind, placebo-controlled study of toddlers, the rate of hyperactivity was no different whether treated with PB or placebo. There were few significant PB-related side effects, and those that did occur (irritability and sleep disturbance) responded to dose reduction (99). The prospective, double-blind, randomized, crossover study of Young and coworkers

(101) showed no significant worsening of behavior with either PB or mephobarbital. Drugs that are converted into PB, such as methylphenobarbital and primidone, are regarded by some as less likely to produce behavioral side effects than PB; however, these hypotheses have not been subjected to careful trials in children. One study of the *treatment* of childhood behavioral disturbances with PB or PRM has shown these drugs to be *beneficial* in 33 percent and 11 percent of children, respectively (102).

Higher Cortical Function

Very early in what has been nearly nine decades of clinical use of PB, the intellectual function of many epileptic patients improved as their seizures came under better control with PB. With a wider choice of antiepileptic medications and other treatments now available, disturbances of cognition, especially attention and memory, and of skilled motor functions may occur in patients as a consequence of the medication rather than of the epilepsy. In an era of quite limited antiepileptic medication choices, Lennox (103) noted the additional toll that medications might take on epileptic patients with brain injuries, changes readily observed by patients, families, and teachers that were "often subtle and difficult to measure." Nearly 60 percent of the epileptic patients treated with PB that Lennox studied did not appear to have such difficulties.

Hillesmaa and coworkers (104) found decreased rate of fetal head growth for human infants of mothers taking PB. Although some early studies documented changes in various measures of intelligence and learning in patients of various ages with some onset of epilepsy, no patterns of deterioration attributable to PB treatment were found. In individual cases IQ measurements increased, while others decreased with PB treatment (105,106). Dosage in many of these early cases was lower than is now typical, and these studies did not address issues of compliance or attempt to relate intellectual dysfunction to drug levels. A subsequent study suggested, but did not prove, that the everyday intellectual performance of children on PB was deficient as compared with what might be expected given their performance on standardized tests of intellectual function (107). Schain and coworkers (108) found improvement in intelligence subtest scores, attentiveness, and impulse control in children who had their PB replaced with carbamazepine, although these children exhibited the simultaneous and potentially confounding variable of improved seizure control. Subtle but statistically significant lowering of performance- and full-scale IQ, verbal and nonverbal task subtest scores, and deterioration of behavior were found to be a consequence of PB as compared with valproate therapy of epilepsy in a more recent double-blind crossover study (109). Similar results were obtained in another study

(110) that also provided evidence on repeat testing for impairment of learning and cognitive development while on PB compared with valproate-treated or untreated control groups.

Several additional studies have aroused concern, especially in the setting of febrile seizure prophylaxis with PB. Hirtz and coworkers (111) and Farwell and colleagues (112) demonstrated that mean IQ scores of large cadres of such children were 5.2 to 8.4 points lower than anticipated, compared with untreated or placebo-treated control groups. A disparity of at least 5 points was shown to persist for as long as 6 months after PB prophylaxis had been discontinued in both studies. Various concerns have been raised about certain aspects of the design of these studies, including low enrollment rates of eligible children, incomplete testing of significant fractions of enrolled children, and particularly the "intention to treat" design. Thus, in the case of one study (112), some children in the placebo group actually received PB while less than two-thirds of those in the PB-treated group received PB throughout the entire study period (2 years), and one-third of the treatment group had little if any PB exposure or low drug levels during follow-up. An earlier, smaller, but particularly well designed and executed study did not show any such significant effect of PB prophylaxis on infant developmental scales over an 8 to 12 month follow-up interval. However, Stanford-Binet Intelligence scale assessment suggested that in some of these children there were negative effects of PB on performance of certain memory tasks that were drug concentration–related, but the effect was not statistically significant (99).

Dependence and Withdrawal

Prolonged administration of PB produces both habituation and dependence; therefore, significant withdrawal signs and symptoms may be provoked by abrupt discontinuation of the drug. Patients may experience anxiety, irritability, insomnia, mood disturbance, emotional lability, hyperexcitability, and tremulousness, various gastrointestinal disturbances, confusion, or delirium. Therefore, chronically administered PB should be withdrawn slowly to prevent these various reactions as well as withdrawal seizures. Seizures that occur during withdrawal of PB (whether suggested by the physician or undertaken by the noncompliant patient) do not necessarily indicate that the drug remains therapeutically indispensable. In many cases slower rates of withdrawal permit the drug to be withdrawn without seizure recurrence (91,113,114). A similar abstinence syndrome may occur in newborn infants of mothers treated with PB given the ease with which PB crosses the placenta, rendering a level in the neonate that is close to that found in the mother (50). The abstinence syndrome of the newborn may persist for days to weeks and is likely to be better tolerated and of shorter duration in infants whose mothers received the usual antiepileptic doses of PB compared with PB-abusing mothers.

Overdosage

Intoxication with PB can occur because of dosing errors, coadministration of valproic acid, accidental ingestion, and suicide attempts. We have observed several instances in which IV PB boluses have been administered in the emergency department to patients on chronic primidone therapy that have presented to the emergency room in status epilepticus with failure to recognize that primidone is metabolized into PB. Rapid administration of a full loading dose of PB (20 mg/kg) to patients with PB levels of 30 to 40 µg/mL is particularly likely to prompt the development of pulmonary edema and respiratory failure. More frequently encountered are cases in which valproate is added to chronic PB therapy and patients developed progressive lethargy 3 to 5 weeks later with elevated PB levels. Inattention, drowsiness, and dysarthric slurring of speech that may resemble drunkenness are often exhibited by patients acutely intoxicated with PB. Curiously, plasma levels similar to those that produce such effects acutely may be tolerated without evident ill effects after slowly increasing the dose with chronic therapy. Other findings observed in patients that have toxic plasma concentrations (usually >40 µg/mL) include dizziness, constricted pupils, nystagmus, ataxia, or coma (generally with levels above 60 µg/mL).

Phenobarbital levels in excess of 80 µg/mL, although well tolerated in carefully monitored patients with appropriate cardiorespiratory intervention, are potentially lethal if such support is not provided. Such high levels, particularly if acutely achieved, may occasionally produce both cardiac and respiratory dysfunction (115). However, cardiac dysfunction is significantly less likely to occur with PB than with PnB. Indeed, levels in excess of 130 µg/mL appear to be tolerated reasonably well by patients receiving appropriate intensive care support and requiring burst suppression for the management of intractable seizures.

Other Adverse Effects

Phenobarbital therapy has been associated with hypocalcemia more commonly than vitamin D–deficient osteomalacia (116). This may be the result of mixed-function oxidase induction with enhanced clearance of 25-hydroxy-cholicalciferol (117). The patients who are particularly vulnerable to "phenobarbital rickets" are those who have received many years of PB therapy, are poorly mobile, and have limited exposure to sunlight; diet also may play a role. Symptomatic patients may respond to the administration of 4000 units of vitamin D each day or 125 μg of vitamin D3 each week. Prophylactic administration of vitamin D is not recommended (118–121).

Such serious consequences as Stephens-Johnson syndrome, erythema multiforme, or toxic epidermal necrolysis are rare, but they do occur. Malaise, fatigue, fever, and eosinophilia typically accompany allergic rash, which may start centrally and spread to the face and extremities. Variable degrees of hepatic inflammation may accompany the hypersensitivity reaction in children, including fulminant fatal liver necrosis (122–124). Connective tissue disorders including Dupuytren's contracture, Ledderhose's syndrome (plantar fibromatosis), Peyronie's disease, frozen shoulder, and aching joints have been associated with PB.

Clinical Use

Phenobarbital is indicated in the treatment of partial, simple, or complex seizures, as well as primary or secondarily generalized motor seizures (tonic, clonic, tonic-clonic) in all age groups. It is the drug of choice in the treatment of most forms of neonatal seizures and for prophylaxis of febrile seizures, and it is among the most valuable agents for the management of status epilepticus. Well-designed studies of adults have shown that PB, PRM, phenytoin, and carbamazepine are equally effective in the management of generalized motor seizures (125), and although there may be differences in efficacy in treatment of partial seizures, they are slight. The cooperative VA study showed complete control of primary generalized tonic-clonic seizures in 43 percent of men receiving PB or phenytoin, 45 percent of those receiving primidone, and 48 percent of those receiving carbamazepine. Only 16 percent achieved complete control of partial or secondarily generalized seizures with PB compared with 43 percent with carbamazepine (126). Other studies of adults have demonstrated similar results (127,128). One large noncrossover study of 3- to 14-year-old children with generalized tonic-clonic seizures showed a 22 percent rate of remission with PB monotherapy compared with 34 percent for phenytoin, 40 percent for carbamazepine, and 16 percent for valproate. One study showed that localization-related seizures with secondary generalization were completely controlled in only 3 percent of patients on PB, as compared with 21 percent with phenytoin, 25 percent with carbamazepine, and 4 percent with valproate (129).

Plasma concentrations of PB required for control of generalized tonic-clonic seizures may be bimodally distributed. Schmidt (130) found that the majority of responding patients achieved control at PB levels of 18 ± 10 μg/mL but that a significant minority achieved

control at levels of 38 ± 6 μg/mL. One-third of patients considered to have intractable partial complex seizures (e.g., with PB levels less than 20 μg/mL) were found to improve significantly if "adequate" PB or PRM levels were achieved (i.e., levels high enough to achieve control without intolerable side effects). An additional 16 percent responded if either of these drugs at higher concentrations were combined with phenytoin or carbamazepine (130,131).

For the management of children under 1 year of age who present with focal or generalized motor seizures excepting infantile spasms, PB represents an attractive "first choice" agent because of its relative ease of administration, reliable kinetics, wide therapeutic window, and safety as compared with phenytoin or valproate. It is less frequently chosen in older children because of sedative qualities and potential effects on behavior. Nonetheless, it remains a valuable reserve agent for older children who cannot be managed effectively with other drugs. There is no clear indication that PB is any less effective than any other major anticonvulsant as alternative therapy for the management of anticonvulsant drug–resistant localization-related seizures, and it should be among the drugs that are tried in succession in those difficult cases (128,132). The use of PB as part of polytherapy for such resistant seizures may introduce difficulties because of sedative effects and induction of hepatic enzymes. One study showed that one-third of patients receiving combinations containing PB had improved seizure control when PB was eliminated from the regimen (133).

Initiation of PB Therapy

Phenobarbital loading can be achieved by IV or oral administration. IV loading typically requires administration of 15 to 20 mg/kg for newborns or very young infants and 10 to 20 mg/kg for older infants and children. The drug may be administered as a single dose or in two doses divided by a few hours (33,134,135). A number of different approaches to oral loading have been described. Administration of 6 to 8 mg/kg/day for 2 days followed by an age-appropriate daily maintenance dose will quickly render plasma levels of at least 10 μg/mL (127,136). Bourgeois (137) demonstrated that the PB dose could be increased over 4 days as total daily doses of 3, 3.5, 4, and 5 mg/kg/day on successive days to achieve, in a linear fashion and without significant interim sedation, a serum level of approximately 20 μg/mL at 96 hours. The maintenance dose must be adjusted thereafter to prevent toxic accumulation of PB. Without some form of initial loading, as many as 30 days may be necessary to achieve maximal steady-state PB concentrations (138). Obese adolescent patients may have a volume of distribution of 0.5 mg/L or less, and suitable adjustment in their loading dose must be considered in some cases.

Daily maintenance dose requirements for children are higher, on a weight basis, than those for adults, averaging 2 to 4 mg/kg/day (134,139). To maintain plasma levels of 10 to 25 µg/ml, Rossi (140) recommended oral maintenance doses of 4.79 ± 1.3 mg/kg in infants aged 2 to 12 months, 3.5 ± 0.99 mg/kg in children aged 1 to 3 years, and 2.31 ± 0.74 mg/kg in those 3 to 6.5 years. The data of others would suggest that for children older than 3 years who weigh less than 40 kg, doses of 1.5 to 3 mg/kg/day are appropriate, whereas doses no greater than 1 to 1.5 mg/kg/day may maintain satisfactory levels for adolescents and adults who weigh more than 40 kg (127,136). The PB dose may be administered entirely at bedtime or divided throughout the day, depending on degree of sleep disturbance and susceptibility to behavioral abnormalities or sedative effects. Once-daily administration is beneficial to some but not all patients. Multiple daily administration may in some cases improve compliance for forgetful parents.

Neonatal Seizures

Phenobarbital is the most widely employed drug for the management of neonatal seizures. This practice reflects familiarity with the agent and widely shared confidence in the efficacy and safety of PB in neonates rather than any well-established evidence for the superiority of this agent over other anticonvulsants. The choice of PB may be based more on the dosing inconvenience or potential risks associated with other drugs rather than on any demonstrated superiority of PB (141,142). Thus, the second most commonly employed agent, phenytoin, carries risks for tissue injury if tissues are infiltrated at the site of IV line placement or for adverse cardiac effects if the rate of administration is excessive, problems that are less frequently encountered with fosphenytoin. However, nonlinear kinetics make oral administration of phenytoin a problem in very small infants.

The initiation of PB therapy for seizures in newborns should start with IV administration of a loading dose of 16 to 20 mg/kg delivered as a single bolus or as two divided boluses. Volume of distribution of an administered bolus of PB to a neonate has been variously estimated at 0.81 to 0.97 L/kg, with 15 percent to 20 percent deviation of such mean values and does not vary as a result of gestational age of the newborn infant (143,144). From a practical vantage point, a volume of distribution of approximately 1.0 L/kg can safely be presumed in most cases, a loading dose of 20 mg/kg resulting in a peak serum level of 20 µg/mL. Plasma protein binding of phenobarbital averages 22 percent to 25 percent in neonates, approximately half the value that is anticipated in older children and adults (145).

Successful control of neonatal seizures is seldom achieved with serum levels less than 16 µg/mL; initial loading should attempt to achieve serum levels ranging from 15 to 25 µg/mL. Electrographic monitoring has shown that many clinically responding newborns show persistence of electrographic seizures after routine loading doses (146). Although the significance of electrographic activity in the newborn without clinical seizures remains uncertain, infants with recalcitrant *clinical* seizures require additional loading boluses delivered as 10 mg/kg at intervals of one to several hours. At plasma concentrations of at least 40 µg/mL as many as 77 percent to 85 percent of neonates respond (147,148). Serum levels as high as 60 to 80 µg/mL appear to be tolerated by most newborns, although such high levels may necessitate greater degrees of cardiorespiratory support, compromise clinical examination, and interfere with feeding. Svenningson and coworkers (149) found that plasma PB concentrations in excess of 50 µg/mL in newborns were associated with slowing of heart rate to less than 100 beats per minute. This is a potentially serious matter because the neonate lacks the reflexive capacity to alter stroke volume in compensation for bradycardia.

Newborns respond to an initial loading dosage of 20 mg/kg, a serum level of 20 µg/mL with oral or IV total daily maintenance dose 2.25 to 4 mg/kg. Although doses of 5 mg/kg/day are widely recommended, the continuation of such a dose through the first few weeks of life generally results in accumulation to serum levels significantly in excess of 20 mg/dL (33,52,150). Plasma clearance of PB usually increases after 1 to 2 weeks of life and may require modification of maintenance dosage in some but not all cases.

Status Epilepticus

The ease and relative safety of administration, wide therapeutic window, and long duration of action combine to make PB a particularly attractive choice in the treatment of status epilepticus. Negative aspects of the use of this drug include the relatively low lipid solubility, sedative effects, and the possible provocation of respiratory depression, hypotension, or pulmonary edema. Thus, benzodiazepines and phenytoin are the usual first-line treatments for status epilepticus in children of most ages. On the other hand, PB can be administered more rapidly and in higher concentration than phenytoin, and it can be administered intramuscularly if necessary. IM administration of a full loading dose to a well-perfused location may achieve brain levels adequate for the control of some seizures in less than an hour and is indicated if no better access can be achieved.

The rate of administration of sequential boluses of PB determines the risk for cardiopulmonary complications, which is lower for PB than for PnB or too rapidly administered phenytoin. In general, the rate of IV administration of PB for treatment of status epilepticus should be 2 mg/kg/min for children who weigh less than 40 kg. The rate should be 100 mg/min for children and adults who weigh more than 40 kg. Slower rates may be required in special cases, such as in patients with acute cardiac disease (e.g., tricyclic overdose). In general, respiratory depression is not seen below plasma levels of 60 µg/mL, and hypotension may not arise as a complication of PB until after even higher levels are achieved. Pulmonary edema is an uncommon complication and usually requires very massive PB bolusing over short time intervals to high levels. The most widely accepted practice for PB administration in treatment of status epilepticus in the PB-naive patient is to administer at total loading dose of 20 mg/kg. This quite reliably produces a plasma level close to 20 µg/mL. It is clear that the administration of only a partial loading dose (e.g., 10 mg/kg) to the anticonvulsant-naive patient usually is inadequate. Seizures may well diminish or stop, but they often recur as the PB becomes distributed throughout the body. Respiratory support is usually required as the plasma level rises above 50 to 70 µg/mL, and pressor support may be required above levels of 70 to 90 µg/mL, whether as the result of PB, the causative illness, or both.

Febrile Seizures

Phenobarbital has been the most commonly employed prophylactic agent for prevention of febrile seizures. As febrile seizures are generally without significant immediate or long-term serious medical consequences, there has been significant momentum away from providing prophylactic treatment. Enthusiasm for prophylactic treatment has diminished because (1) approximately two-thirds of children have just one febrile seizure, (2) recurrent febrile seizures have exceedingly low risk for untoward consequences, (3) PB and other agents introduce a risk for various drug-related side effects (94), and (4) it has been difficult to provide convincing proof that prophylaxis is effective. Although there is some evidence supporting the effectiveness of treatment with PB, sodium valproate, or benzodiazepines, it is not conclusive proof. PB is usually judged a safer choice than valproate for administration to very young children, and long-term prophylaxis with benzodiazepines poses unacceptable problems with sedation and tachyphylaxis. However, it is not without risk, as the death of one child has been ascribed to the use of PB for prophylaxis against febrile seizures (123). The efficacy of PB as prophylactic therapy has recently come into question (151).

There is evidence to suggest that if PB prophylaxis is to be effective, steady-state serum concentrations of 16 to 30 µg/mL are required (152). This study demonstrated a 4 percent risk for recurrence in children with such levels compared with approximately 20 percent rates of recurrence for untreated children

and for those with PB levels of 8 to 15 µg/mL. Several more recent studies have failed to demonstrate a difference in outcome between groups of children at risk for febrile seizures who received either PB or valproate for prophylaxis compared with children who received no prophylactic anticonvulsant medication (112,153,154). However, these studies did not control for the important element of compliance by assessing serum PB levels at time of recurrence. Compliance with PB prophylactic regimens for febrile seizures is notoriously low (155). Herranz (156) found that 20 percent of children treated with PB prophylaxis for febrile seizures had recurrences at mean levels of 16.4 ± 2.8 µg/mL compared with 88 percent of those treated with PRM (mean PB levels 14.1 ± 3.7 µg/mL) and 92 percent of those treated with valproate (mean levels 35.2 ± 5.9 µg/mL). Side effects were experienced by 7 percent of those on PB, 53 percent of those on PRM, and 45 percent of those on valproate, although most side effects were tolerable.

PB is discontinued gradually in most cases. This is based on evidence that dependence on PB results in provocation of seizures if the rate of decline of PB levels is too rapid. This presumption has been placed in question in one study of patients with partial complex seizures that appeared to demonstrate that the risk for seizures was not dependent on rate of withdrawal but on the achievement of a concentration below 15 to 20 µg/mL (157).

OTHER BARBITURATES

The N-methylbarbiturates (methylphenobarbital and metharbital) and the anesthetic pentobarbital have all been used as anticonvulsants.

Methylphenobarbital

Methylphenobarbital (Mebaral, MBL), although infrequently used in the United States, is widely employed in some countries, such as Australia. A considerable portion of the administered dose is rapidly cleared as the R-enantiomer; therefore, the dose of racemic MBL should be approximately twice the PB dose required to achieve satisfactory clinical effects (158–160). The single oral dose half-time of elimination for the R-enantiomer has been estimated at 7.5 ± 1.7 hours compared with 69.8 ± 19.7 hours for the S-enantiomer and 98.0 ± 19.7 hours for the PB metabolite (161).

MBL clearance is almost entirely by biotransformation with urinary excretion of the major metabolites, which are PB and parahydroxymethyl PB (as a phenolic glucuronide conjugate) (159,162,163). PB is the only pharmacologically important biotransformation product. The capacity to generate this product may increase with chronic therapy because of increased rate of MBL clearance with faster rates of appearance and higher peak levels of PB. Naive subjects may excrete less than 11 percent of their MBL dose as PB, while subjects exposed to MBL or PB may increase that amount to more than 50 percent (162). Because PB has a smaller volume of distribution and is cleared more slowly than MBL, plasma PB levels may accumulate over time to much higher values than simultaneous serum MBL values. Many or most of the drug interactions experienced with chronic MBL therapy are thought to be due to PB, and any interaction or side effect that has been described for PB can occur with MBL therapy.

The experimental and clinical spectrum of MBL is similar to that of PB (164). It may be administered once or twice daily. Because of the tendency for PB levels to accumulate to higher serum levels than MBL levels over the long term and greater availability of PB level determinations, most clinicians follow up only the PB level in patients taking MBL. Doses that are calculated to produce therapeutic steady-state PB levels may result in unacceptable drowsiness during the initial phases of therapy, and therefore compliance may be poor. Starting with half the expected dose and accelerating the dose over 1 to 2 weeks avoids this problem but delays the achievement of the desired steady-state peak PB concentrations to as long as 4 to 5 weeks after initiation of therapy. Full initial doses may be started in patients who have recently been treated with PB or other "inducing" anticonvulsants. At steady state, PB concentration is generally 7 to 10 times greater than the total (R + S) MBL in serum.

Pentobarbital

Pentobarbital (PnB) is a 5-ethyl-5 (1-methylbutyl) barbiturate that is clinically employed as a sodium salt (Nembutal). It is a short-acting barbiturate. The half-time of elimination in adults ranges from 18 to 50 hours and is dose-dependent. The partition coefficient for PnB is approximately 11 times greater than that for PB. This reflects much faster lipid solubility, accounting for shorter latency in onset of activity, shorter duration of action, and faster metabolic degradation. The superior lipid solubility may be in part responsible for the fact that PnB is much more potently sedative and hypnotic than PB. Acutely achieved blood concentrations of 0.5 to 3 µg/mL produce approximately the same degree of sedation as PB levels of 5 to 40 µg/mL. PnB levels $\geq$10 to 18 µg/mL usually induce coma. When employed as a constant infusion of 0.3 to 4.0 mg/kg/hr after bolus administration of 15 mg/kg over 1 hour, the serum half-time of elimination ranges from approximately 11 to 23 hours in adults (165).

Pentobarbital is indicated for the treatment of status epilepticus that is unresponsive to such first-line therapies as benzodiazepines, phenytoin, or PB. The aim of PnB therapy is to produce coma with suppression-burst pattern on EEG; therefore, the sedative properties of this drug are not deleterious. On the other hand, PnB is more likely than PB to have negative effects on cardiac contractility and to require the addition of cardiotonic medications to support blood pressure and perfusion when employed in the usual doses. Particular caution should be used in the management of patients who have cardiac disease and those whose seizures are the result of hypoxic-ischemic injury or tricyclic overdose, as the negative effects on cardiac function may be particularly deleterious in such settings. Barbiturate anesthesia (PnB more commonly than thiopental or methohexital) is considered by many neurologists to be the ultimate form of therapy for status epilepticus that has proved intractable to the usual combinations and dosages of short- and long-acting anticonvulsants, including PB (166,167). Treatment with PnB has not been proved to be superior to the use of very high doses of PB to achieve burst suppression or control seizures.

Lowenstein and associates (165) reviewed their results with eight retrospectively studied and six prospectively enrolled patients treated with PnB, thiopental, or methohexital anesthesia; only one of these patients was a child. PnB loading with 15 mg/kg over 1 hour to the prospective group resulted in prompt cessation of seizures in patients treated with this protocol. Infusion of PnB at rates that varied from 0.3 to 4.0 mg/kg/hr and additional boluses as needed of 5 mg/kg (maximum of 30 mg/kg of bolus drug in the first 12 hours) to achieve and maintain burst suppression. The median peak serum PnB level for patients treated in this fashion was 10.8 µg/mL (range 6.5–21.2 µg/mL). Treatment resulted in a favorable outcome for three of these six adults, whereas one had a poor outcome and two had indeterminate outcomes. Only two of these six required pressors. Significant drop in blood pressure occurred within a few hours of initiation of therapy in 9 of the 14 patients of the entire group reported by these investigators.

Lowenstein and colleagues stopped PnB after approximately 12 hours of treatment, restarting therapy if seizures recurred. Duration of infusion ranged (in the prospective group) from 11 to 77 hours. For those patients who recovered function after cessation of anesthesia, brain stem functions returned in 6 to 24 hours, and various forms of motor activity returned in 1 to 72 hours. Some possible withdrawal phenomena occurred, including repetitive twitching of the extremities, resembling activity observed in some cases of barbiturate overdose and difficult to distinguish on a clinical basis from seizure activity (165,168,169). Patients receiving particularly high doses of PnB were found in some instances to have profound weakness and areflexia that persisted for as long as 2 weeks (including as many as 5 days of complete paralysis after cessation of infusion) despite much more rapid recovery of alertness and intellectual interactiveness. This effect may have been the result of PnB-induced dysfunction of peripheral nerve function or release of neurotransmitter in the peripheral synaptic cleft, as has been observed experimentally (170,171). These transient forms of dysfunction may introduce confusion when attempting to assess patients for "brain death" or to estimate prognosis.

PRIMIDONE

Primidone (PRM), 5-ethyldihydro-5-phenyl-4,6 (1H, 5H) pyrimidine-dione or 2-desoxy-phenobarbital, was synthesized in 1949 and was shown to be effective in the treatment of major motor epilepsy shortly thereafter (172). It is therefore the third oldest anticonvulsant that continues in regular use (173). It has just two rather than three carbonyl substituents of the pyrimidine ring that are characteristic of barbiturates. Hepatic biotransformation renders two main metabolites of PRM: phenylethylmalonamide (PEMA) and PB. The identification of PB as a metabolite raised questions as to the importance of the other substances in control of seizures, a subject that remains controversial. Although it has remained difficult to clearly demonstrate the contribution that PRM and PEMA make to clinical management of epilepsy independent of the effects of PB, there are both experimental and clinical data that support the view that they are pharmacodynamically important.

Anticonvulsant Activity

The fact that PRM has anticonvulsant properties is suggested by several lines of evidence, including the facts that (1) administration of PRM lowers the plasma level of PB required to protect animals against experimental forms of seizure, and (2) protection against seizures is afforded in the few hours after a single PRM dose is administered before the achievement of significant levels of PEMA or PB (5,6,174–176). The potency of PRM is equal to or possibly superior to that of PB in the prevention of electroshock-induced seizures, but it has much less activity against chemically induced (pentylenetetrazol or bicuculline) seizures (6,173,174,176). This is similar to the spectrum of activity exhibited by phenytoin and carbamazepine.

Baumel and coworkers (175) roughly estimated the potency (ED_{50} for prevention of maximal electroshock seizures) of PRM to be 25 percent more and of PEMA to be 90 percent less than PB. They also found that PRM had no detectable antichemoconvulsant activity, while PEMA is approximately 0.025 as potent as PB

for prevention of that form of experimental seizure. Other researchers in a variety of animal lines have found somewhat different potency ratios of these compounds (5,176,177), but PRM and PB generally have had similar antielectroshock potency while PEMA has been 12- to 18-fold less potent. Experimental evidence (5) suggests that PRM is approximately 2.5 times less neurotoxic than PB and that the two substances are synergistic in seizure control, possibly exerting different mechanisms of action. Bourgeois and coworkers established that a ratio of 1:1 brain concentration of PRM to PB achieved the best therapeutic index (ratio of therapeutic efficacy to toxicity) in control of seizures (5). A therapeutic range for PRM trough concentration of 3 to 12 µg/mL has been suggested (178), but somewhat higher levels may be tolerated. Although PEMA also has anticonvulsant properties, the potency appears to be too low to contribute much to the antiepileptic effects or toxicity of PRM at the usually encountered plasma concentrations of clinical practice (137). Monitoring of serum PEMA levels in patients treated with PRM has no practical value.

Pharmacokinetics

Peak serum PRM levels are achieved in approximately 3 hours in adults and 4 to 6 hours in children after single-dose ingestion of tablets in doses of 12.5 to 20 mg/kg (179). Brand-name tablets probably have nearly complete bioavailability, with 72 percent to 100 percent of a single oral dose excreted in urine as PRM or its metabolites (179–181). Absorption of generic preparations may be less reliable (182). Absorption of PRM tablets is reduced by concurrent acetazolamide administration (183). Volume of distribution of PRM and of PEMA after single oral dose has been estimated at 0.86 L/kg and 0.69 L/kg, respectively. There is less than 10 percent plasma protein binding of either PRM or of PEMA (184,185).

Biotransformation of PRM is very complicated. PEMA and PB are the two major metabolites with antiepileptic potency. It has been difficult to estimate the relative contribution of PEMA and PB to the pharmacodynamic properties of PRM, including both antiepileptic potency and toxicity, although these properties have been studied carefully in animals (5,6). Zadavil and Gallagher (186) showed that, on average, approximately 65 percent of a single IV PRM dose is excreted unchanged in the urine within 5 days of administration to adults, while 7 percent is secreted as PEMA and 2 percent is excreted as PB. The rate of conversion of PRM to PB is much slower than that to PEMA. Under steady-state conditions of chronic administration, approximately 25 percent of monotherapeutically administered PRM can be relied on to be converted to PB (187). The bioconversion of

PRM to PB shows age-related variation. In general, the more complete transformation of PRM to PB by children aged 0.5 to 6.5 years often results in disappointingly low PRM to PB serum ratios, although there is considerable individual variability (188,189).

PRM and its various metabolites are primarily (at least 75–77%) renally excreted (186). The half-time for elimination of orally administered PRM ranges from 10 to 15 hours in adults on monotherapy, but comedication with antiepileptic inducers of hepatic biotransformation enzymes lowers this time to 6.5 to 8.3 hours (180,183,186,190). On average, half-time of elimination for PRM in children ranges from 4. 5 to 11 hours, lower with phenytoin comedication than PRM monotherapy (179). The hepatic immaturity of newborns accounts for half-times of PRM elimination that vary from 8 to 80 hours.

In one study of steady-state PRM monotherapy, the average trough serum concentration to total daily dose of PRM for PRM, PEMA, and PB were 0.78 ± 0.25, 0.64 ± 0.39, and 1.47 ± 0.53, respectively (191). At steady state, PB levels are almost always higher than PRM levels. Because PB is probably responsible for many of the toxic effects of PRM, especially sedation, attempts have been made to diminish the biotransformation of PRM to PB. As noted previously, a brain ratio of 1 : 1 for PRM and PB concentrations has been established experimentally as ideal for the achievement of maximal therapeutic efficacy with minimal toxicity (5). Both nicotinamide and isoniazid have been tried for this purpose, but gastrointestinal, hepatic, and other possible toxicities have limited the usefulness of such approaches (192–194). In most clinical situations, PRM levels are of relatively little value as management tools. They may be useful in two situations, however: (1) assigning a cause for possible drug side effects or (2) establishing that the conversion rate of PRM to PB is unfavorably rapid and therefore that the use of the more expensive and inconvenient to administer PRM is poorly justified.

Drug Interactions

Coadministration of PRM and some other major antiepileptic drugs to adults decreases excretion of unchanged PRM after a single dose by more than one-third. This is the result of fourfold increase in the conversion rate to PEMA and 50 percent increase in conversion to PB. Interactions with various anticonvulsants may result in considerable changes in the ratios of PRM, PEMA, and PB. Phenytoin is the most potent accelerator of PRM biotransformation, while carbamazepine has a lesser effect (183,188,195,196). Bourgeois (137) showed that, on average, coadministration of PRM with either phenytoin or carbamazepine, or both, resulted in 50

percent reduction in the trough PRM level at steady state compared with that expected with monotherapy. PEMA levels increased by 17 percent and PB levels by 60 percent under those polytherapeutic conditions, and the trough ratio of PB to PRM increased by as much as threefold. Application of the data obtained in Bourgeois's study predicts that with PRM monotherapy, a steady-state PB level of 16.5 µg/mL can be expected to be associated with an average PRM level of 10 µg/mL, but that the coadministration of phenytoin or carbamazepine, or both, increases the average PB level to a level of 26.5 µg/mL, while the average PRM level falls to 5 µg/mL. If the total daily dose were increased by approximately 100 percent to maintain the serum PRM level at 10 µg/mL, the PB level at steady state could be expected to rise to as much as 58.3 µg/mL. Thus, polytherapy with these agents can be expected to significantly lower the therapeutic index of PRM because of the unfavorable ratio of PRM to PB in brain compared with the experimentally ideal 1 : 1 ratio.

When polytherapy is considered necessary, problems of enzymatic induction are avoided by combining PRM with noninducing agents such as valproate, gabapentin, lamotrigine, topiramate, tiagabine, or benzodiazepines (197). However, combination with valproate produces the unfavorable kinetic problems encountered when PB and valproate are combined (197). Combination with benzodiazepines may produce intolerable sedation. Coadministration of PRM and valproate tends to produce lesser degrees of PB accumulation than are observed with PB and valproate coadministration (as stated previously). This may be because valproate inhibits not only PB clearance but also the conversion of PRM to PB (198). Thus, if it is judged necessary to coadminister valproate with PB, it might be better to administer it as PRM. Acetazolamide may diminish the gastrointestinal absorption of PRM, and carbamazepine may in some cases inhibit biotransformation of PRM to PB (194).

Toxicity

Animal studies demonstrate that PRM has less toxicity to the nervous system and other organs than PB (5,173). Nonetheless, toxic effects, particularly those of the CNS, are common. They are reported at some point in their therapy by one-half to two-thirds of patients who are treated with this drug (126,199–201). PRM therapy is unsuccessful and is discontinued in 10 percent to 30 percent of patients. Discontinuation is much more commonly the result of intolerable side effects than lack of therapeutic efficacy (126,200). Side effects of PRM therapy closely resemble those seen with PB. It has been difficult to distinguish the contributions of

PRM compared with PB in the elicitation of these problems. Time of onset of side effects and the development of tolerance assist in making this determination.

Sensations variously characterized as sleepiness, light-headedness, dizziness, weakness, or intoxication are very common, if not universal, at the initiation of PRM therapy (190,202). They develop within a few hours of ingestion of PRM, but there is considerable individual variability in susceptibility to these dose-related effects, which range from mild to severe and incapacitating affectation (203,204). Cross-tolerance occurs in patients who are in the process of changing from PB to PRM therapy, but those changing from phenytoin or carbamazepine do not experience such cross-tolerance (202). These very early effects are due to PRM as they occur before any significant accumulation of PB and usually wane within a few days, despite the fact that that is the time at which PB levels begin to rise (205,206). The severe effects can be avoided by administration of a small "test dose" at the onset of therapy to determine whether the individual patient is highly susceptible. These effects can be minimized in all patients by careful attention to the speed and amplitude of the acceleration of the dosing schedule to achieve full doses (190,204).

There is a second family of more persistent sedative side effects that develop during the chronic phase of PRM therapy. These chronic side effects are quite similar, if not identical, to those reported by some patients treated with PB. Patients and families report abnormalities of energy level, attentiveness, behavior, and learning. The frequency with which they are reported and their amelioration in at least some cases when PRM is discontinued suggest that the medication may be in part or entirely responsible. Rodin and coworkers (207) compared the effects of PRM and carbamazepine as adjuncts to phenytoin therapy and found that PRM produced more significant impairment of performance in a cognitive-perceptual test battery than carbamazepine, especially with regard to concentration and fine motor performance (208). The fact that these types of difficulties are quite similar, if not identical, to the problems reported during PB therapy, and the observation that they are most troublesome during the chronic phase of therapy when the PB to PRM ratio is highest, suggest that PB is the likely culprit. It is unlikely that PEMA, which contributes little to the anticonvulsant potency of PRM, plays any significant role in CNS or other forms of PRM-related toxicity (184).

Virtually all of the other PB-related side effects can occur with PRM therapy, including the various connective tissue problems such as contracture formation, joint problems, and Peyronie's disease. One study has suggested that in children, PRM is less likely to produce any more significant side effects than phenytoin or PB (96). Transient nausea, vomiting, dizziness, and drowsiness may occur with initiation of PRM therapy, a peculiar combination of side effects that are seldom seen in patients who start on PB (126).

Overdosage

Little is known about the relationship between peak PRM concentrations and short-term toxic effects. Acute PRM overdosage (PRM levels exceeding 80–100 µg/mL in tolerant patients) may produce varying degrees of CNS depression ranging from somnolence or lethargy to deep coma, flaccidity, and loss of deep tendon reflexes (206,209,210). The degree of these abnormalities tends to correlate with PRM levels rather than PB or PEMA levels in the acute interval, although the ensuing rise in PB levels produces additional CNS depression (206,211).

Massive overdosage may result in hypotension and acute renal failure in association with crystalluria, especially when serum PRM levels exceed 200 µg/mL (212). Fatal cases of PRM ingestion have been reported. However, with appropriate management (gastric lavage, administration of activated charcoal, forced diuresis, and supportive measures) patients have recovered without permanent sequelae from ingestion of as much as 22 grams of PRM (204). Crystalluria (largely crystallized PEMA) after administration of large amounts of PRM was first observed in rats (173) and is an almost constant feature of serious PRM overdosage in humans (213). It has not been shown to result in chronic renal failure even after massive overdosage with acute renal dysfunction (210). Massive overdosage can be effectively treated with hemoperfusion (212).

Clinical Use

Early uncontrolled, retrospective studies demonstrated that PRM could be used with considerable success as an adjuvant drug in the management of generalized tonic-clonic seizures, localization-related seizures, and myoclonus epilepsies (199,214–218); however, some more recent controlled studies have shown less favorable results. These data, combined with the availability of a wider range of major anticonvulsants and decreased enthusiasm for polytherapy have reduced the popularity of this agent. Early comparison studies failed to demonstrate that PRM had some unique value in the treatment of any particular type of epilepsy or population of patients compared with PB or phenytoin, drugs that were less expensive and in some ways easier to use (187,219,220). Therefore, it appears that the benefits of PRM therapy and the potential toxicity do not support the use of this agent as first-line therapy for any seizure type or syndrome (93).

One possible exception is the treatment of epilepsy occurring in patients with long QT syndrome because

PRM may have some value in the treatment of the cardiac dysrhythmia (221). However, most patients who have seizures in association with the long QT syndrome have them only in association with cardiac decompensation, which may be effectively treated with other medications. On the other hand, PRM continues to be useful as a third-line agent for treatment of occasional patients affected with almost any form of epilepsy for which PB is indicated, including age groups ranging from the neonate (222) to the adult. The exception to this principle is the fact that PRM has little value in the management of status epilepticus because there is no commercially available parenteral formulation. PRM may be effective in the prophylaxis of febrile seizures (153).

Various direct comparisons of PRM to PB, phenytoin, or carbamazepine treatment in patients of various ages have shown these drugs to have similar efficacy for oral treatment of partial, secondarily generalized, and generalized tonic-clonic seizures (126,187,207,220,223). However, most of these studies do not control for PB levels. Reinterpretation of one of the best of these studies (187) has suggested that a subgroup of patients may enjoy better control at any given PB level if that level is achieved as the result of PRM rather than PB oral therapy (224). One crossover comparison showed that PRM was superior to orally administered PB in the management of generalized tonic-clonic seizures (225). The VA Epilepsy Cooperative study comparison of PRM to PB, phenytoin, and carbamazepine showed the highest rate of failures in treatment of partial or secondarily generalized seizures occurred with PRM therapy, failure that usually was due to drug discontinuation or poor compliance early in the course of treatment because of intolerable side effects (126). Sapin and coworkers (226) found that PRM exerted antiepileptic effects in neonates that were independent of the effects of PB.

Two potential benefits of the choice of PRM compared with PB are (1) the possibility of achieving seizure control in a given subject at lower serum PB levels than are required with the administration of PB itself, and (2) the possibility that in certain settings PRM is a "better" drug than PB. Others have argued that most or all of the clinically significant antiepileptic effect of PRM is simply due to its conversion into PB (227,228). This is particularly likely to be true when PRM is administered too infrequently during the day to achieve the most favorable serum ratio of PRM to PB. In most patients this requires administration every 6 hours, which may be inconvenient. Because of unfavorable effects in the PRM to PB ratio, there are reasons I believe that there is no advantage to employing PRM in combination with phenytoin, acetazolamide, or carbamazepine. Unfortunately, most patients who now receive PRM are patients with intractable epilepsy on polytherapy with complicated dosing schedules.

When administered to adults as monotherapy, PRM can be administered twice daily because the half-time of elimination for PRM typically is 10 to 15 hours. However, the shorter elimination half-time that is typical of most children and most patients on polytherapy mandates administration of this drug at 6-hour intervals if advantage is to be taken of the presumed antiepileptic potency of PRM. Administration to newborns is little studied, but in the event that administration of PRM were judged important, once-daily dosing is theoretically possible. So great is the variation of elimination half-times observed in the newborn (22) that individualization of dosage for newborns would be prudent, as would careful follow-up to ensure that toxic accumulation of metabolites does not occur.

Treatment Guidelines

If there are no coadministered drugs that interfere with metabolism or distribution, an initial daily PRM dose of approximately 20 mg/kg/day will result, after 2 to 3 weeks, in a steady-state PB level ranging from 10 to 30 µg/mL. Neonates typically require maintenance doses of 15 to 25 mg/kg/day, infants 10–25 mg/kg/day, and children 10–20 mg/kg/day (22). The total daily dose should be divided into three or four times of administration, as noted previously, given the short half-time of elimination of PRM; the peak serum concentration typically is achieved 3 to 5 hours after each dose. Initiation of PRM monotherapy in patients who are not already receiving barbiturates should in many cases start with a low single daily dose at bedtime (e.g., 1/4 of a 250-mg tablet for patients who weigh more than 20 kg) with subsequent upward titration at 3-day intervals (137). Not every patient will require or tolerate steady-state dosage at 20 mg/kg/day. In some cases, relatively large initial doses may be tried to more rapidly achieve serum levels that are effective in controlling seizures. For example, it has been shown that the administration to neonates of 25 mg/kg/day divided into three doses produces a serum PRM level of approximately 10 mg/dL by day 3, a level that is sufficient to control the seizures of many neonates independent of the associated PB level (226). Monitoring PRM or PEMA levels confers little therapeutic advantage in most clinical situations.

Changing patients from chronic oral PB therapy to PRM is usually easily accomplished by administering four to five times as much PRM each day as the discontinued total daily PB dose. In patients who are not on PB, rapid initiation of PRM therapy can be achieved by first loading with PB (229). Rapid escalation of oral PB loading can be achieved using PB doses of 3 mg/kg/day on the first day of treatment, 3.5 mg/kg/day on the second day, 4 mg/kg/day on the third day, and 5 mg/kg/day on the fourth day.

This approach results in a linear accumulation of PB in the serum to approximately 20 μg/mL on day 4 without significant sedation. The PB can be discontinued on the following day and replaced with a full maintenance PRM dose of between 12.5 and 20 mg/kg/day (137).

Immediate initiation of PRM at an amount expected to produce serum concentration of 20 to 30 μg/mL can be undertaken by IV loading of 20 mg/kg of PB (producing a serum concentration of 20 μg/mL and initiation of 20 mg/kg/day of PRM divided into three or four doses. Any patient loaded with enough PB to achieve serum PB concentrations of at least 20 μg/mL within 3 days after initiation will experience significant degrees of sedation (229).

Discontinuation

In general, the considerations that arise with regard to drug discontinuation are similar to those previously noted for PB. One small study suggested that withdrawal-related seizures may be more likely with PRM than with PB (230). Theodore and coworkers (157) found no relationship between the peak dose or rate of withdrawal of PRM or PB and the occurrence of seizures. In their study, seizures were most likely to occur as the PB level fell between 15 and 20 μg/mL.

REFERENCES

1. Butler TC. Metabolic oxidation of phenobarbital to *p*-hydroxyphenobarbital. *Science* 1954; 120:494.

2. Bush MT. Sedatives and hypnotics: absorption, fate and excretion. In: Rot WS, Hofmann FG, eds. *Physiological Pharmacology*. New York: Academic Press, 1963:185–218.

3. Nishihara K, Katsuyoski U, Saitoh Y, et al. Estimation of plasma unbound phenobarbital concentration by using mixed saliva. *Epilepsia* 1979; 20:37–45.

4. Wade A. *Barbiturates. Pharmaceutical Handbook*. London: The Pharmaceutical Press, 1980.

5. Bourgeois BF, Dodson WE, Ferrendelli JA. Primidone, phenobarbital, and PEMA: I. Seizure protection, neurotoxicity, and therapeutic index of individual compounds in mice. *Neurology* 1983; 33:283–290.

6. Bourgeois BF, Dodson WE, Ferrendelli JA. Primidone, phenobarbital, and PEMA: II. Seizure protection, neurotoxicity, and therapeutic index of varying combinations in mice. *Neurology* 1983; 33:291–295.

7. Morrell F, Bradley W, Ptashne M. Effects of drugs on discharge characteristics of chronic epileptogenic lesions. *Neurology* 1959; 9:492–498.

8. Nicoll RA. Pentobarbital: actions on frog motor neurons. *Brain Res* 1975; 96:119–123.

9. Macdonald RL, Barker JL. Different actions of anticonvulsant and anesthetic barbiturates resolved by use of cultured mammalian neurons. *Science* 1978; 200:775–777.

10. Ransom BR, Barker JL. Pentobarbital modulates transmitter effects of mouse spinal neurones grown in tissue culture. *Nature* 1975; 254:703–705.

11. Ransom BR, Barker JL. Pentobarbital selectivity enhances GABA-mediated postsynaptic inhibition in tissue cultured mouse spinal neurons. *Brain Res* 1976; 114:530–535.

12. Schulz DW, MacDonald RL. Barbiturate enhancement of GABA-mediated inhibition and activation of chloride ion conductance. *Brain Res* 1981; 209:177–188.

13. French-Mullen JMH, Barker JL, Rogawski MA. Calcium current block by (−)-pentobarbital, phenobarbital, and CHEB but not (+)-pentobarbital in acutely isolated hippocampal CA1 neurons: Comparison with effects on GABA-activated Cl⁻ current. *J Neurosci* 1993; 13:3211–3221.

14. Sawada S, Yamamoto C. Blocking action of pentobarbital on receptors for excitatory amino acids in the guinea pig hippocampus. *Exp Brain Res* 1985; 59:226–231.

15. Newberry NR, Nicoll RA. Comparison of the action of baclofen with gamma-aminobutyric acid on rat hippocampal pyramidal cells. *J Physiol* 1984; 360:161–185.

16. Pritchett DB, Sontheimer H, Shivers BD, et al. Importance of a novel GABA-A receptor subunit for benzodiazepine pharmacology. *Nature* 1989; 338:582–585.

17. Graves NM, Holmes GB, Kriel RL, et al. Relative bioavailability of rectally administered phenobarbital sodium parenteral solution. *DICP* 1989; 23:565–568.

18. Svensmark O, Buchthal F. Accumulation of phenobarbital in man. *Epilepsia* 1963; 4:199–206.

19. Svensmark O, Buchthal F. Dosage of phenytoin and phenobarbital in children. *Dan Med Bull* 1963; 10:234–235.

20. Fouts JR, Hart LG. Hepatic drug metabolism during the perinatal period. *Ann NY Acad Sci* 1965; 123:245–251.

21. Langset A, Meberg A, Bredesen JE, Lunde PKM. Plasma concentrations of diazepam and *N*-dimethyldiazepam in newborn infants after intravenous, intramuscular, rectal and oral administration. *Acta Paediatr Scand* 1978; 67:699–704.

22. Nau H, Rating D, Hauser I, et al. Placental transfer and pharmacokinetics of primidone and its metabolites phenobarbital, PEMA and hydroxyphenobarbital in neonates and infants of epileptic mothers. *Eur J Clin Pharmacol* 1980; 18:31–42.

23. Kaneko S, Suzuki K, Sato T, Ogawa Y, Nomura Y. The problems of antiepileptic medication in the neonatal period: is breastfeeding advisable? In: Janz D, Dam M, Richens A, et al., eds. *Epilepsy, Pregnancy, and the Child*. New York: Raven Press, 1982:343–348.

24. Boreus LO, Jalling B, Kallberg N. Phenobarbital metabolism in adults and in newborn infants. *Acta Paediatr Scand* 1978; 67:193–200.

25. Boreus LO, Jalling B, Wallin A. Plasma concentrations of phenobarbital in mother and child after combined prenatal and postnatal administration of prophylaxis of hyperbilirubinemia. *J Pediatr* 1978; 93:695–698.

26. Bossi L, Battino D, Caccamo ML, et al. Pharmacokinetics and clinical effects of antiepileptic drugs in newborns of chronically treated epileptic mothers. In: Janz D,

Dam M, Richens A, et al., eds. *Epilepsy, Pregnancy, and the Child.* New York: Raven Press, 1982:373–381.

27. Rating D, Nau H, Kuhnz W, Jager-Rom E, Helge H. Antiepileptika in der neugeborenenperiode. *Monatsschr Kinderheilkd* 1983; 131:6–12.

28. Boreus LO, Jalling B, Kallberg N. Clinical pharmacology of phenobarbital in the neonatal period. In: Morselli PL, Garattini S, Sereni F, eds. *Basic and Therapeutic Aspects of Perinatal Pharmacology.* New York: Raven Press, 1975:331–340.

29. Dodson WE. Antiepileptic drug utilization in pediatric patients. *Epilepsia* 1984; 25:S132–S139.

30. Heinze E, Kampffmeyer HG. Biological half-life of phenobarbital in human babies. *Klin Wochenschr* 1971; 49:1146–1147.

31. Ehrnebo M, Agurell S, Jalling B, Boreus LO. Age differences in drug binding by plasma proteins: studies on human foetuses, neonates and adults. *Eur J Clin Pharmacol* 1971; 3:189.

32. Painter MJ, Pippenger C, MacDonald H, Pitlick W. Phenobarbital and diphenylhydantoin levels in neonates with seizures. *J Pediatr* 1978; 92:315–319.

33. Lockman LA, Kriel R, Zaske D. Phenobarbital dosage for control of neonatal seizures. *Neurology* 1979; 29:1445–1449.

34. Pitlick W, Painter M, Pippenger C. Phenobarbital pharmacokinetics in neonates. *Clin Pharmacol Ther* 1978; 23:346–350.

35. Strandjord RE, Johannessen SI. Serum levels of phenobarbitone in healthy subjects and patients with epilepsy. In: Gardner-Thorpe C, Janz D, Meinardi H, Pippenger CE, eds. *Antiepileptic Drug Monitoring.* Tunbridge Wells (Kent), U.K.: Pitman Medical, 1977:89–103.

36. Brachet-Lierman A, Gouteres F, Aicardi J. Absorption of phenobarbital after the intramuscular administration of single doses in infants. *J Pediatr* 1975; 87:624–626.

37. Jalling B. Plasma and cerebrospinal fluid concentrations of phenobarbital in infants given single doses. *Dev Med Child Neurol* 1974; 11:781–793.

38. Butler TC, Waddell WJ. Metabolic conversion of primidone (Mysoline) to phenobarbital. *Proc Soc Exp Biol Med* 1956; 93:544–546.

39. Tang BK, Kalow W, Grey AA. Metabolic fate of phenobarbital in man. *N*-glucoside formation. *Drug Metab Dispos* 1979; 7:315–318.

40. Whyte MP, Dekaban AS. Metabolic fate of phenobarbital. A quantitative study of *p*-hydroxyphenobarbital elimination in man. *Drug Metab Dispos* 1977; 5:63–70.

41. Wilensky AJ, Friel PN, Levy RH, Comfort CF, Kaluzny SP. Kinetics of phenobarbital in normal subjects and epileptic patients. *Eur J Clin Pharmacol* 1982; 23:87–92.

42. Conney AH. Pharmacological implications of microsomal enzyme induction. *Pharmacol Rev* 1967; 19:317–366.

43. Butler TC, Mahafee C, Waddell WJ. Phenobarbital: studies of elimination, accumulation, tolerance, and dosage schedules. *J Pharmacol Exp Ther* 1954; 111:425–435.

44. Butler TC, Mahafee C, Waddell WJ. Studies of elimination accumulation, tolerance and dosage schedules. *J Pharmacol Exp Ther* 1954; 111:425–435.

45. Lous P. Blood serum and cerebrospinal fluid levels and renal clearance of phenemal in treated epileptics. *Acta Pharmacol Toxicol* 1954; 10:166–177.

46. Lous P. Plasma levels and urinary excretion of three barbituric acids after oral administration to man. *Acta Pharmacol Toxicol* 1954; 10:147–165.

47. Morselli PL, Rizzo M, Garrattini S. Interaction between phenobarbital and diphenylhydantoin in animals and in epileptic patients. *Ann NY Acad Sci* 1971; 179:88–107.

48. Patel IH, Levy RH, Cutler RE. Phenobarbital-valproic acid interaction. *Clin Pharmacol Ther* 1980; 27:515–521.

49. Domek NS, Barlow CF, Roth LJ. An ontogenetic study of phenobarbital-C 14 in cat brain. *J Pharmacol Exp Ther* 1960; 130:285–293.

50. Melchior JC, Svensmark O, Trolle D. Placental transfer of phenobarbitone in epileptic women, and elimination in newborns. *Lancet* 1967; 11:860–861.

51. Painter MJ, Pippenger CE, MacDonald H, Pitlick WH. Phenobarbital and phenytoin blood levels in neonates. *Pediatrics* 1977; 92:315–319.

52. Painter MJ, Pippenger C, Wasterlain C, Barmada M. Phenobarbital and phenytoin in neonatal seizures: metabolism and tissue distribution. *Neurology* 1981; 31:1107–1112.

53. Heimann G, Gladtke E. Pharmacokinetics of phenobarbital in childhood. *Eur J Clin Pharmacol* 1977; 12:305–310.

54. Jalling B. Plasma concentrations of phenobarbital in the treatment of seizures in the newborn. *Acta Paediatr Scand* 1975; 64:514–524.

55. Dodson WE, Prensky AL, DeVivo D, Goldring S, Dodge PR. Management of seizure disorders: selected aspects. Part I. *J Pediatr* 1976; 89:527–540.

56. Baumel I, DeFeo JJ, Lal H. Effects of acute hypoxia on brain-sensitivity and metabolism of barbiturates in mice. *Psychopharmacologia* 1970; 17:1983–1987.

57. Dauber IM, Krauss AN, Symchych PS, Auld PA. Renal failure following perinatal anoxia. *J Pediatr* 1976; 88:851–855.

58. Gal P, Toback J, Erkan NV, Boer HR, Henry R. The influence of asphyxia on phenobarbital dosing requirements in neonates. *Dev Pharmacol Ther* 1984; 7:145–152.

59. Morselli PL. Antiepileptics. In: Morselli PL, ed. *Drug Disposition During Development.* New York: Spectrum, 1977:311–360.

60. Neuvonen PJ, Elonen E. Effect of activated charcoal on absorption and elimination of phenobarbitone, carbamazepine and phenylbutazone in man. *Eur J Clin Pharmacol* 1980; 17:51–57.

61. Viswanathan CT, Booker HE, Welling PG. Bioavailability of oral and intramuscular phenobarbital. *J Clin Pharmacol* 1978; 18:100–105.

62. Yaffe SJ. Developmental factors influencing interactions of drugs. *Ann NY Acad Sci* 1976; 281:90–97.

63. Neimann G, Gladtke E. Pharmacokinetics of phenobarbital in childhood. *Eur J Clin Pharmacol* 1977; 12:305.

64. Garrettson LK, Dayton PG. Disappearance of phenobarbital and diphenylhydantoin from serum of children. *Clin Pharmacol Ther* 1970; 11:674–679.

65. Dodson WE. Special pharmacokinetic considerations in children. *Epilepsia* 1987; 28:S56–S70.

66. Waddell WJ, Butler TC. Distribution and excretion of phenobarbital. *J Clin Invest* 1957; 36:1217–1226.

67. Kapetanovic IM, Kupferberg HJ. Inhibition of microsomal phenobarbital metabolism by valproic acid. *Biochem Pharmacol* 1981; 30:1361–1363.

68. Kapetanovic IM, Kupferberg HJ, Porter RJ, et al. Mechanism of valproate-phenobarbital interaction in epileptic patients. *Clin Pharmacol Ther* 1981; 29:480–486.

69. Giotti A, Maynert EW. The renal clearance of barbital and the mechanism of its reabsorption. *J Pharmacol Exp Ther* 1951; 101.

70. Myschetzky A, Lassen NA. Forced diuresis in treatment of acute barbiturate poisoning. In: Matthew H, ed. *Acute Barbiturate Poisoning*. Amsterdam: Excerpta Medica, 1971:223–232.

71. May T, Rambeck B. Serum concentrations of valproic acid: influence of dose and co-medication. *Ther Drug Monit* 1985; 7:387–390.

72. Perruca E, Gatti G, Frigo GM, et al. Disposition of sodium valproate in epileptic patients. *Br J Clin Pharmacol* 1978; 5:495–499.

73. Rettie AE, Rettenmeier AW, Howald WN, Baillie TA. Cytochrome P-450-catalyzed formation of delta-four VPA, a toxic metabolite of valproic acid. *Science* 1987; 235:890–893.

74. Kesterson JW, Granneman GR, Machinist JM. The hepatotoxicity of valproic acid and its metabolites in rats. I. Toxicologic, biochemical and histopathologic studies. *Hepatology* (Baltimore) 1984; 4:1143.

75. Kochen W, Schneider A, Ritz A. Abnormal metabolism of valproic acid in fatal hepatic failure. *Eur J Pediatr* 1983; 141:30–35.

76. Prickett KS, Baillie TA. Metabolism of unsaturated derivatives of valproic acid in rat liver microsomes and destruction of cytochrome P-450. *Drug Metab Dispos* 1986; 14:221–229.

77. Booker HE, Tormey A, Toussaint J. Concurrent administration of phenobarbital and diphenylhydantoin: lack of interference effect. *Neurology* (Minneap) 1971; 21:383–385.

78. Browne TR, Szabo GK, Evans JE, et al. Phenobarbital does not alter phenytoin steady-state serum concentration or pharmacokinetics. *Neurology* 1988; 38:639–642.

79. Cucinell SA, Conney AH, Sansur MS, Burns JJ. Drug interactions in man. I. Lowering effect of phenobarbital on plasma levels of bishydroxycoumarin (Dicumarol) and diphenylhydantoin (Dilantin). *Clin Pharmacol Ther* 1965; 6:420–429.

80. MacDonald MG, Robinson DS. Clinical observations of possible barbiturate interference with anticoagulation. *JAMA* 1968; 204:95–100.

81. Brooks SM, Werk EE, Ackerman SJ, Sullivan I, Thrasher K. Adverse effects of phenobarbital on corticos-

teroid metabolism in patients with bronchial asthma. *N Engl J Med* 1972; 286:1125–1128.

82. Burstein S, Klaiber E. Phenobarbital induced increase in 6β-hydroxycortisol excretion: clue to its significance in human urine. *J Clin Endocrinol Metab* 1965; 25:293–296.

83. Janz D, Schmidt D. Antiepileptic drugs and failure of oral contraceptives. *Lancet* 1974; 1:1113.

84. Levin W, Kuntzman R, Conney AH. Stimulatory effect of phenobarbital on the metabolism of the oral contraceptive 17α-ethylnylestradiol-3-methyl ether (Mestranol) by rat liver microsomes. *Pharmacology* 1979; 19:255–294.

85. Kleinman PD, Griner PF. Studies of the epidemiology of anticoagulant drug interactions. *Arch Intern Med* 1970; 126:522–523.

86. Bourgeois BF. Pharmacologic interactions between valproate and other drugs. *Am J Med* 1988; 84:29–33.

87. Leppik IE, Sherwin A. Anticonvulsant activity of phenobarbital and phenytoin in combination. *J Pharmacol Exp Ther* 1977; 200:570–575.

88. Bourgeois BFD, Wad N. Combined administration of carbamazepine and phenobarbital: effect on anticonvulsant activity and neurotoxicity. *Epilepsia* 1988; 29:482–487.

89. Bittencourt PR, Richens A. Anticonvulsant-induced status epilepticus in Lennox-Gastaut syndrome. *Epilepsia* 1981; 22:129–134.

90. Vining EP. Use of barbiturates and benzodiazepines in treatment of epilepsy. *Neurol Clin* 1986; 4:617–632.

91. Buchthal F, Svensmark O, Simonsen H. Relation of EEG and seizures to phenobarbital in serum. *Arch Neurol* 1968; 19:567–572.

92. Hutt SJ, Jackson PM, Belsham A, Higgins G. Perceptual motor behavior in relation to blood phenobarbitone level: a preliminary report. *Dev Med Child Neurol* 1968; 10:626–632.

93. Mattson RH, Cramer JA, Collins JF, VA Epilepsy Cooperative Study #264 Group. Comparison between carbamazepine and valproate for complex partial and secondarily generalized tonic-clonic seizures. *Epilepsia* 1991; 32:S18.

94. Addy DT. Phenobarbitone and febrile convulsions. *Arch Dis Child* 1990; 65:921.

95. Sylvester CE, Marchlewski A, Manaligod JM. Primidone or phenobarbital use complicating disruptive behavior disorders. *Clin Pediatr* 1994; 33:252–253.

96. Herranz JL, Armijo JA, Arteaga R. Clinical side effects of phenobarbital, primidone, phenytoin, carbamazepine, and valproate during monotherapy in children. *Epilepsia* 1988; 29:794–804.

97. Ounsted C. The hyperkinetic syndrome in epileptic children. *Lancet* 1955; 1:303–311.

98. Wolf S, Forsythe A. Behavior disturbance, phenobarbital and febrile seizures. *Pediatrics* 1978; 61:729–731.

99. Camfield CS, Chaplin S, Doyle A. Side effects of phenobarbital in toddlers: behavioral and cognitive aspects. *J Pediatr* 1979; 95:361–365.

100. Mitchell W, Chavez J. Carbamazepine versus phenobarbital for partial onset seizures in children. *Epilepsia* 1987; 28:56–60.

101. Young RSK, Alger PM, Bauer L, Lauderbaugh D. A randomized double-blind crossover study of phenobarbital and methobarbital. *J Child Neurol* 1986; 1:361–363.

102. Hayes SG. Barbiturate anticonvulsants in refractory affective disorders. *Ann Clin Psychiatry* 1993; 5:35–44.

103. Lennox WG. Brain injury, drugs and environment as causes of mental decay in epilepsy. *Am J Psychiatry* 1942; 99:174–180.

104. Hillesmaa VK, Teramo K, Granstrom ML, Bardy AH. Fetal head growth retardation associated with maternal antiepileptic drugs. *Lancet* 1981; 1:165–167.

105. Somerfeld-Ziskind E, Ziskind E. Effect of phenobarbital on the mentality of epileptic patients. *Arch Neurol Psychol* 1940; 43:70–79.

106. Wapner I, Thurston DL, Holowach J. Phenobarbital: its effect on learning in epileptic children. *JAMA* 1962; 182:937.

107. Stores G. Behavioral effects of antiepileptic drugs. *Dev Med Child Neurol* 1975; 17:647–658.

108. Schain RJ, Ward JW, Guthrie D. Carbamazepine as an anticonvulsant in children. *Neurology* 1977; 27:476–480.

109. Vining EPG, Mellits ED, Dorsen MM, et al. Psychologic and behavioral effects of antiepileptic drugs in children: a double-blind comparison between phenobarbital and valproic acid. *Pediatrics* 1987; 80:165–174.

110. Calandre EP, Dominguez-Granados R, Gomez-Rubio M, Molina-Font JA. Cognitive effects of long-term treatment with phenobarbital and valproic acid in school children. *Acta Neurol Scand* 1990; 81:504–506.

111. Hirtz DG, Sulzbacher SI, Ellenberg JH, Nelson KB. Phenobarbital for febrile seizures—effects on intelligence and on seizure recurrence. *N Engl J Med* 1990; 322:364–369.

112. Farwell J, Young J, Hartz D, et al. Phenobarbital for febrile seizures: effects on intelligence and on seizure recurrence. *N Engl J Med* 1990; 322:364–369.

113. Hollister LE. Nervous system reactions to drugs. *Ann NY Acad Sci* 1965; 123:342–353.

114. Isbell H, Fraser HF. Addiction to analgesics and barbiturates. *Pharmacol Rev* 1959; 2:355–397.

115. Berman LB, Jeghers HJ, Schreiner GE, Pallotta AJ. Hemodialysis, an effective therapy for acute barbiturate poisoning. *JAMA* 1956; 161:820–827.

116. Christiansen C, Rodbro P, Lund M. Incidence of anticonvulsant osteomalacia and effect of vitamin D: controlled therapeutic trial. *Br Med J* 1973; 4:695–701.

117. Richens A, Rowe DJF. Disturbance of calcium metabolism by anticonvulsant drugs. *Br Med J* 1970; 4:73–76.

118. Hahn TJ, Birge SJ, Shapp CR, Avioli LV. Phenobarbital-induced alterations in vitamin D metabolism. *J Clin Invest* 1972; 51:741–748.

119. Hunter J. Effects of enzyme induction on vitamin D3 metabolism in man. In: Richens A, Woodford FP, eds. *Anticonvulsant Drugs and Enzyme Induction*. New York: Elsevier, 1976:77–84.

120. Offermann G, Pinto V, Kruse R. Antiepileptic drugs and vitamin D supplementation. *Epilepsia* 1979; 20:3–15.

121. Perruca E. Clinical implications of hepatic microsomal enzyme induction by antiepileptic drugs. *Pharmacol Ther* 1987; 33:139–144.

122. Welton DG. Exfoliative dermatitis and hepatitis due to phenobarbital. *JAMA* 1950; 143:232–234.

123. Mockli G, Crowley M, Stern R, Warnock ML. Massive hepatic necrosis in a child after administration of phenobarbital. *Am J Gastroenterol* 1989; 84:820–822.

124. Morkunas AR, Miller MB. Anticonvulsant hypersensitivity syndrome. *Crit Care Clin* 1997; 13:727–739.

125. Smith DB, Mattson RH, Cramer JA, et al. Results of a nationwide Veterans Administration Cooperative Study comparing the efficacy and toxicity of carbamazepine, phenobarbital, phenytoin, and primidone. *Epilepsia* 1987; 28 Suppl 3.

126. Mattson RH, Cramer JA, Collins JF, et al. Comparison of carbamazepine, phenobarbital, phenytoin, and primidone in partial and secondarily generalized tonic-clonic seizures. *N Engl J Med* 1985; 313:145–151.

127. Feely M, O'Callaghan M, Duggan G, Callagan N. Phenobarbitone in previously untreated epilepsy. *J Neurol Neurosurg Psychiatry* 1980; 43:364–368.

128. Schmidt D, Richter K. Alternative single anticonvulsant drug therapy for refractory epilepsy. *Ann Neurol* 1986; 19:85–87.

129. Forsythe WI. One drug for childhood grand mal: medical audit for three-year remissions. *Dev Med Child Neurol* 1984; 26:742–748.

130. Schmidt D. Two antiepileptic drugs for intractable epilepsy with complex-partial seizures. *J Neurol Neurosurg Psychiatry* 1982; 45:1119–1124.

131. Schmidt D. Single drug therapy for intractable epilepsy. *J Neurol* 1983; 229:221–226.

132. Cornaggia CM, Canevini MP, Giuccioli D, Pruneri C, Canger R. Carbamazepine, phenytoin and phenobarbital in drug-resistant partial epilepsies. *Ital J Neurol Sci* 1986; 7:113–117.

133. Callaghan N, O'Dwyer R, Keating J. Unnecessary polypharmacy in patients with frequent seizures. *Acta Neurol Scand* 1984; 69:15–19.

134. Painter MJ. How to use phenobarbital. In: Morselli PL, Pippinger CE, Penry JK, eds. *Antiepileptic Drug Therapy in Pediatrics*. New York: Raven Press, 1983:245–252.

135. Painter MJ. Phenobarbital clinical use. In: Levy RH, Dreifuss FE, Mattson RH, Meldrum BS, Penry JK, eds. *Antiepileptic Drugs*. 3rd ed. New York: Raven Press, 1989:329–340.

136. Elwes RDS, Johnson AL, Shorvon SC, Reynolds EH. The prognosis for seizure control in newly diagnosed epilepsy. *N Engl J Med* 1984; 311:944–947.

137. Bourgeois BFD. Primidone. In: Wyllie E, ed. *The Treatment of Epilepsy: Principles and Practices*. Philadelphia: Lea & Febiger, 1993:909–913.

138. Tokola RA, Neuvonen PJ. Pharmacokinetics of antiepileptic drugs. *Acta Neurol Scand Suppl* 1983; 97:17–27.

139. Alix D, Berthou F, Riche C, Castel Y. Concentrations plasmatiques de phenobarbital et posologie en function de l'âge. *Dev Pharmacol Ther* 1984; 7:164–170.

140. Rossi LN. Correlation between age and plasma level dosage for phenobarbital in infants and children. *Acta Paediatr Scand* 1979; 68:431–434.

141. Mizrahi E, Kelloway P. Characterization and classification of neonatal seizures. *Neurology* 1987; 37:1837–1844.

142. Painter MJ, Gaus LM. Neonatal seizures: diagnosis and treatment (review). *J Child Neurol* 1991; 6:101–108.

143. Fischer J, Lockman L, Zoske D, Kriel R. Phenobarbital maintenance dose requirements in treating neonatal seizures. *Neurology* 1982; 31:1042–1044.

144. Donn S, Grasela T, Goldstein G. Safety of a higher loading dose of phenobarbital in the term newborn. *Pediatrics* 1985; 75:1061–1064.

145. Painter MJ, Gaus LM. Phenobarbital. In: Wyllie E, ed. *The Treatment of Epilepsy: Principles and Practices.* Philadelphia: Lea & Febiger, 1993:900–908.

146. Connell J, Oozeer R, DeVries L, Dubowitz L, Dubowitz V. Clinical and EEG response to anticonvulsants in neonatal seizures. *Arch Dis Child* 1989; 64:459–464.

147. Gal P, Boer HR, Toback J, Erkan NV. Phenobarbital dosing in neonates and asphyxia. *Neurology* 1982; 32:788–789.

148. Gilman J, Gal P, Duchowny M, Weaver R, Ransom J. Rapid sequential phenobarbital treatment of neonatal seizures. *Pediatrics* 1989; 83:674–678.

149. Svenningson NW, Blennow G, Landroth M, Gaddlin P, Ahlstrom H. Brain oriented intensive care treatment in severe neonatal asphyxia. *Arch Dis Child* 1982; 57:176–183.

150. Grasela TH, Donn SM. Neonatal population pharmacokinetics of phenobarbital derived from routine clinical data. *Dev Pharmacol Ther* 1985; 8:374–383.

151. Siemes H. New aspects in prevention of febrile convulsions. *Klinische Padiatrie* 1992; 204:67–71.

152. Faero O, Kastrup KW, Nielsen E, Melchior JC, Thorn I. Successful prophylaxis of febrile convulsions with phenobarbital. *Epilepsia* 1972; 13:279–285.

153. Minagawa K, Miura H. Phenobarbital, primidone and sodium valproate in the prophylaxis of febrile convulsions. *Brain Dev* 1981; 3:385–393.

154. McKinlay I, Newton R. Intention to treat febrile convulsions with rectal diazepam, valproate or phenobarbitone. *Dev Med Child Neurol* 1989; 31:617–625.

155. Schmidt D. Pharmacotherapy of epilepsy — current problems and controversies. *Fortschritte der Neurologie-Psychiatrie* 1983; 51:363–386.

156. Herranz JL, Armijo JA, Arteaga R. Effectiveness and toxicity of phenobarbital, primidone, and sodium valproate in the prevention of febrile convulsions, controlled by plasma levels. *Epilepsia* 1984; 25:89–95.

157. Theodore WH, Porter RJ, Raubertas RF. Seizures during barbiturate withdrawal: relation to blood level. *Ann Neurol* 1987; 22:644–647.

158. Butler TC, Waddell WJ. N-methylated derivatives of barbituric acids, hydantoin and oxazolidine used in the treatment of epilepsy. *Neurology* 1958; 8(Suppl 1):106–112.

159. Hooper WD, Kunze HE, Eadie MJ. Pharmacokinetics and bio-availability of methylphenobarbital in man. *Ther Drug Monit* 1981; 3:39–44.

160. Hooper WD, Qing MS. The influence of age and gender on the stereoselective metabolism and pharmacokinetics of methylphenobarbital in humans. *Clin Pharmacol Ther* 1990; 48:633–640.

161. Lim W, Hooper WD. Stereoselective metabolism and pharmacokinetics of methylphenobarbitone in humans. *Drug Metab Dispos* 1989; 17:212–217.

162. Eadie MJ, Bochner F, Hooper WD, Tyrer JH. Preliminary observations on the pharmacokinetics of methylphenobarbitone. *Clin Exp Neurol* 1978; 15:131–144.

163. Kunze HE, Hooper WD, Eadie MJ. High performance liquid chromatographic assay of methylphenobarbital and metabolites in urine. *Ther Drug Monit* 1981; 3:45–49.

164. Craig CR, Shideman FE. Metabolism and anticonvulsant properties of mephobarbital and phenobarbital in rats. *J Pharmacol Exp Ther* 1971; 176:35–42.

165. Lowenstein DH, Aminoff MJ, Simon RP. Barbiturate anesthesia in the treatment of status epilepticus: clinical experience with 14 patients. *Neurology* 1988; 38:395–400.

166. Delgado-Escueta AV, Wasterlain C, Treiman DM, Porter RJ. Current concepts in neurology: management of status epilepticus. *N Engl J Med* 1982; 306:1337–1340.

167. Simon RP. Management of status epilepticus. In: Pedley TA, Meldrum BS, eds. *Recent Advances in Epilepsy.* London: Churchill Livingstone, 1985.

168. Fraser HF, Wikler A, Essig CF, Isbell H. Degree of physical dependence induced by secobarbital or pentobarbital. *JAMA* 1958; 166:126–129.

169. Essig CF. Clinical and experimental aspects of barbiturate withdrawal convulsions. *Epilepsia* 1967; 8:21–30.

170. Narahashi T, Moore JW, Postron RN. Anesthetic blocking of nerve membrane conductances by internal and external applications. *J Neurobiol* 1969; 1:3–22.

171. Proctor WR, Weakly JN. A comparison of the presynaptic and postsynaptic actions of pentobarbitone and phenobarbitone on the neuromuscular junction of the frog. *J Physiol* (Lond) 1976; 258:257–268.

172. Handley R, Stewart ASR. Mysoline: a new drug in the treatment of epilepsy. *Lancet* 1952; 1:742–744.

173. Bogue JY, Carrington HC. The evaluation of Mysoline — a new anticonvulsant drug. *Br J Pharmacol* 1953; 8:230–235.

174. Frey HH, Hahn I. Untersuchungen uber die Bedeutung des durch Biotransformation gebildeten Phenobarbital fur die antikonvulsive Wirkung von Primidon. *Arch Int Pharmacodyn Ther* 1960; 128:281–290.

175. Baumel IP, Gallagher BB, DiMicco D, Goico H. Metabolism and anticonvulsant properties of primidone in the rat. *J Pharmacol Exp Ther* 1973; 186:305–314.

176. Leal KW, Rapport RL, Wilensky AJ, Friel PN. Single dose pharmacokinetics and anticonvulsant efficacy of primidone in mice. *Ann Neurol* 1979; 5:470–474.

177. Frey HH, Loscher W. Is primidone more efficient than phenobarbital? An attempt at a pharmacological evaluation. *Nervenarzt* 1980; 51:359–362.

178. Schottelius DD, Fincham RW. Clinical application of serum primidone levels. In: Pippenger CE, Penry JK, Kutt H, eds. *Antiepileptic Drugs: Quantitative Analysis and Interpretation.* New York: Raven Press, 1978:273–282.

179. Kauffman RE, Habersang R, Lansky J. Kinetics of primidone metabolism and excretion in children. *Clin Pharmacol Ther* 1977; 22:200–205.

180. Gallagher BB, Baumel IP, Mattson RH. Metabolic disposition of primidone and its metabolites in epileptic subjects after single and repeated administration. *Neurology* 1972; 22:1186–1192.

181. Gallagher BB, Baumel IP. Primidone. Absorption, distribution and excretion. In: Woodbury DM, Penry JK, Schmidt RP, eds. *Antiepileptic Drugs.* New York: Raven Press, 1972:357–359.

182. Wyllie E, Pippenger CE, Rothner AD. Increased seizure frequency with generic primidone. *JAMA* 1987; 258:1216–1217.

183. Cloyd JC, Miller KW, Leppik IE. Primidone kinetics: effects of concurrent drugs and duration of therapy. *Clin Pharmacol Ther* 1981; 29:402–407.

184. Baumel IP, Gallagher BB, Mattson RH. Phenylethylmalonamide (PEMA). An important metabolite of primidone. *Arch Neurol* 1972; 27:34–41.

185. Pisani F, Richens A. Pharmacokinetics of phenylethylmalonamide (PEMA) after oral and intravenous administration. *Clin Pharmacol* 1983; 8:272–276.

186. Zavadil P, Gallagher BB. Metabolism and excretion of 14C-primidone in epileptic patients. In: Janz D, ed. *Epileptology.* Stuttgart: Georg Thieme, 1976:129–139.

187. Oleson OV, Dam M. The metabolic conversion of primidone to phenobarbitone in patients under long-term treatment. *Acta Neurol Scand* 1967; 43:348–356.

188. Battino D, Avanzini G, Bossi L, et al. Plasma levels of primidone and its metabolite phenobarbital: Effect of age and associated therapy. *Ther Drug Monit* 1983; 5:73–79.

189. Armijo JA, Herranz JL, Arteaga R, Valiente R. Poor correlation between single-dose data and steady-state kinetics for phenobarbitone, primidone, carbamazepine and sodium valproate in children during monotherapy. Possible reasons for lack of correlation. *Clin Pharmacokinet* 1986; 11:323–335.

190. Booker HE, Hosokowa K, Burdette RD, Darcey B. A clinical study of serum primidone levels. *Epilepsia* 1970; 11:395–402.

191. Bourgeois BFD. Primidone. In: Resor SR, Kutt H, eds. *The Medical Treatment of Epilepsy.* New York: Marcel Dekker, 1992:371–378.

192. Sutton G, Kupferberg HJ. Isoniazid as an inhibitor of primidone metabolism. *Neurology* 1975; 25:1179–1181.

193. Bourgeois BF, Dodson WE, Ferrendelli JA. Isoniazid and other drugs. *Pediatrics* 1982; 70:824–825. Letter.

194. Bourgeois BF, Dodson WE, Ferrendelli JA. Interactions between primidone, carbamazepine, and nicotinamide. *Neurology* 1982; 32:1122–1126.

195. Fincham RW, Schottelius DD, Sahs AL. The influence of diphenylhydantoin on primidone metabolism. *Arch Neurol* 1974; 30:259–262.

196. Reynolds EH, Fenton G, Fenwick P, Johnson AL, Laundy M. Interaction of phenytoin and primidone. *Br Med J* 1975; 2:594–595.

197. Bruni J. Valproic acid and plasma levels of primidone and derived phenobarbital. *Can J Neurol Sci* 1981; 8:91–92.

198. Windorfer JA, Sauer W. Drug interactions during anticonvulsant therapy in childhood: diphenylhydantoin, primidone, phenobarbitone, clonazepam, nitrazepam, carbamazepine and dipropylacetate. *Neuropediatrie* 1977; 8:29–41.

199. Smith BH, McNaughton FL. Mysoline, a new anticonvulsant drug. Its value in refractory cases of epilepsy. *Can Med Assoc J* 1953; 68:464–467.

200. Sciarra D, Carter S, Vicale CT, Merrit HH. Clinical evaluation of primidone (Mysoline), a new anticonvulsant drug. *JAMA* 1954; 154:827–829.

201. Gallagher BB, Baumel IP, Mattson RH, Woodbury SG. Primidone, diphenylhydantoin and phenobarbital: aspects of acute and chronic toxicity. *Neurology* 1973; 23:145–149.

202. Leppik IE, Cloyd JC, Miller K. Development of tolerance to the side effects of primidone. *Ther Drug Monit* 1984; 6:189–191.

203. Ajax ET. An unusual case of primidone intoxication. *Dis Nerv Syst* 1966; 27:660–661.

204. Leppik IE, Cloyd JC. Primidone: toxicity. In: Levy RH, Mattson RH, Meldrum BS, eds. *Antiepileptic Drugs.* 4th ed. New York: Raven Press, 1995:487–490.

205. Goldin S. Toxic effects of primidone. *Lancet* 1954; 1:102–103.

206. Brillman J, Gallagher BB, Mattson RH. Acute primidone intoxication. *Arch Neurol* 1974; 30:255–258.

207. Rodin EA, Rim CS, Kitano H, Lewis R, Rennick PM. A comparison of the effectiveness of primidone versus carbamazepine in epileptic outpatients. *J Nerv Ment Dis* 1976; 163:41–46.

208. Hartlage LC, Stovall K, Kocack B. Behavioral correlates of anticonvulsant blood levels. *Epilepsia* 1980; 21:185.

209. Dotevall G, Herner B. Treatment of acute primidone poisoning with bemegride and amphenazole. *Br Med J* 1957; 3:451–452.

210. Matzke GR, Cloyd JC, Sawchuk RJ. Acute phenytoin and primidone intoxication: a pharmacokinetic analysis. *J Clin Pharmacol* 1981; 21:92–99.

211. Lin SL, Chung MY. Acute primidone intoxication: report of a case. *J Formosan Med Assoc* 1989; 88:1053–1055.

212. van Heijst AN, de Jong W, Seldenrijk R, van Dijk A. Coma and crystalluria: a massive primidone intoxication treated with haemoperfusion. *J Toxicol Clin Toxicol* 1983; 20:307–318.

213. Lehman DF. Primidone cystalluria following overdose. A report of a case and an analysis of the literature. *Med Toxicol Adverse Drug Exp* 1987; 2:383–387.

214. Butter AJM. Mysoline in treatment of epilepsy. *Lancet* 1953; 1:1024.

215. Calnan WL, Borrell YM. Mysoline in the treatment of epilepsy. *Lancet* 1953; 2:42–43.

216. Jorgenson G. Mysoline in the treatment of epilepsy. *Lancet* 1953; 2:835.

217. Smith B, Forster FM. Mysoline and Milontin: two new medicines for epilepsy. *Neurology* (Minneap) 1954; 4:137–142.

218. Livingston S, Petersen D. Primidone (Mysoline) in the treatment of epilepsy. *N Engl J Med* 1956; 254:327–329.

219. Millichap JC, Aymat F. Controlled evaluation of primidone and diphenylhydantoin sodium. Comparative anticonvulsant efficacy and toxicity in children. *JAMA* 1968; 204:738–739.

220. White PT, Pott D, Norton J. Relative anticonvulsant potency of primidone. *Arch Neurol* 1966; 14:31–35.

221. DeSilvey DL, Moss AJ. Primidone in the treatment of the long QT syndrome: QT shortening and ventricular arrhythmia suppression. *Ann Intern Med* 1980; 93:53–54.

222. Powell C, Painter MJ, Pippenger CE. Primidone therapy in refractory neonatal seizures. *J Pediatr* 1984; 105:651–654.

223. Gruber CM, Brock JT, Dyken M. Comparison of the effectiveness of primidone, mephobarbital, diphenylhydantoin, ethotoin, metharbital, and methylphenylethylhydantoin in motor seizures. *Clin Pharmacol Ther* 1962; 3:23–28.

224. Booker HE. Primidone toxicity. In: Woodbury DM, Penry JK, Schmidt RP, eds. *Antiepileptic Drugs*. 1st ed. New York: Raven Press, 1972:377–383.

225. Oxley J, Hebdige S, Laidlaw J, Wadsworth J, Richens A. A comparative study of phenobarbitone and primidone in the treatment of epilepsy. In: Johannessen SI, Morselli PL, Pippenger CE, et al., eds. *Advances in Drug Monitoring*. New York: Raven Press, 1980:237–245.

226. Sapin JI, Riviello JJJ, Grover WD. Efficacy of primidone for seizure control in neonates and young infants. *Pediatr Neurol* 1988; 4:292–295.

227. Shorvon S. The treatment of epilepsy by drugs. In: Hopkins A, ed. *Epilepsy*. New York: Demos, 1987:229–282.

228. Eadie MJ. Formation of active metabolites of anticonvulsant drugs. A review of their pharmacokinetic and therapeutic significance. *Clin Pharmacokinet* 1991; 21:27–41.

229. Bourgeois BFD, Lüders H, Morris H, et al. Rapid introduction of primidone using phenobarbital loading: acute primidone toxicity avoided. *Epilepsia* 1989; 30:667.

230. Coulter DL. Withdrawal of barbiturate anticonvulsant drugs: prospective controlled study. *Am J Ment Retard* 1988; 93:320–327.

231. Davis M, Simmons C, Harrison NG, Williams R. Paracetamol overdose in man: relationship between pattern of urinary metabolites and severity of liver damage. *Q J Med* 1976; 45:181–191.

232. Vesell ES, Page JG. Genetic control of the phenobarbital-induced shortening of plasma antipyrine half-lives in man. *J Clin Invest* 1969; 48:2202–2209.

233. Christiansen J, Dam M. Influence of phenobarbital and diphenylhydantoin on plasma carbamazepine levels in patients with epilepsy. *Acta Neurol Scand* 1973; 49:543–546.

234. Lander CM, Eadie MJ, Tyrer JH. Factors influencing plasma carbamazepine concentration. *Clin Exp Neurol* 1977; 14:184–193.

235. Spina E, Martines C, Fazio A, et al. Effect of phenobarbital on pharmacokinetics of carbamazepine-10,11-epoxide, an active metabolite of carbamazepine. *Ther Drug Monit* 1991; 13:109–112.

236. Krasinski K, Kusmiesz H, Nelson JD. Pharmacologic interactions among chloramphenicol, phenytoin and phenobarbital. *Pediatr Infect Dis* 1982; 1:232–235.

237. Lader M. Drug interactions and the major tranquilizers. In: Grahame-Smith DG, ed. *Drug Interactions*. Baltimore: University Park Press, 1977:159–170.

238. Loga S, Curry S, Lader M. Interactions of orphenadrine and phenobarbitone with chlorpromazine: plasma concentrations and effects in man. *Br J Clin Pharmacol* 1975; 2:197–208.

239. Somogyi A, Gugler R. Drug interaction with cimetidine. *Clin Pharmacokinet* 1982; 7:23–41.

240. Carststensen H, Jacobsen N, Dieperink H. Interaction between cyclosporin and phenobarbitone. *Br J Clin Pharmacol* 1986; 21:550–551.

241. Neuvonen PJ, Penttila O, Lehtovaara R, Aho K. Effects of antiepileptic drugs on the elimination of various tetracycline derivatives. *Eur J Clin Pharmacol* 1975; 9:147–154.

242. Fonne R, Meyer UA. Mechanisms of phenobarbital-type induction of cytochrome P-450 isozymes. *Pharmacol Ther* 1987; 33:19–22.

243. Treiman DM, Pledger GW, DeGiorgio C, Tsay J-Y, Cereghino JJ. Increasing plasma concentration tolerability study of flunarizine in comedicated patients. *Epilepsia* 1993; 34:944–953.

244. Beaurey J, Weber M, Vignaud JM. Treatment of tinea capitis: metabolic interference of griseofulvin with phenobarbital. *Ann Dermatol Venereol* 1982; 109:567–570.

245. Linnoila M, Viukari M, Vaisanen K, Auvinen J. Effect of anticonvulsants on plasma haloperidol and thioridazine levels. *Am J Psychiatry* 1980; 137:819–821.

246. Stambaugh JE, Hemphill DM, Wainer IW, Schwartz I. A potentially toxic drug interaction between pethidine (meperidine) and phenobarbital. *Lancet* 1977; 1:398–399.

247. Liu SJ, Wang RIH. Case report of barbiturate-induced enhancement of methadone metabolism and withdrawal syndrome. *Am J Psychiatry* 1984; 141:1287–1288.

248. Rambeck B. Pharmacological interactions of mesuximide with phenobarbital and phenytoin in hospitalized epileptic patients. *Epilepsia* 1979; 20:147–156.

249. Braithwaite RA, Flanagan RA, Richens A. Steady state plasma nortriptyline concentrations in epileptic patients. *Br J Clin Pharmacol* 1975; 2:469–471.

250. Jonkman JHG, Upton RA. Pharmacokinetic drug interactions with theophylline. *Clin Pharmacokinet* 1984; 9:309–334.

CHAPTER 29

Phenytoin and Related Drugs

W. Edwin Dodson, M.D.

Since phenytoin was introduced for the treatment of epilepsy by Merritt and Putnam in 1938, it has become one of the most widely used and extensively investigated antiepileptic drugs (AEDs). It has been administered to patients of all ages and thus provides a good model for evaluating the effects of age on pharmacokinetics. In addition, phenytoin is unique among the commonly prescribed AEDs because of its nonlinear elimination kinetics [1,2]. (Figure 29-1.)

Phenytoin is a weak acid having a pKa of 8.06 [3] (Table 29-1). Phenytoin sodium is approximately 92 percent phenytoin, a difference that is sometimes important because of phenytoin's nonlinear elimination kinetics. It has limited aqueous solubility of

Table 29-1. Phenytoin Reference Information

Molecular weight of sodium phenytoin	274.25
Molecular weight of phenytoin	252.26
pKa of phenytoin	8.06
Conversion factor: $CF = \dfrac{1000}{252.3} = 3.96$	
Conversion:	
$\mu g/ml$ (or mg/L) $\times 3.96 = \mu moles/L$	
Formulations	
Phenytoin suspension (Dilantin)	50 mg/mL
Phenytoin (Dilantin Infatabs)	50 mg
Phenytoin sodium (Dilantin Capseals)	30, 60, or 100 mg
Type of elimination kinetics	Nonlinear

approximately 20 mg/L unless solubilizing agents are added to the solution. Parenteral formulations of phenytoin are strongly basic and contain the alcohols propylene glycol and ethanol. These formulations are potentially cardiotoxic and should be administered slowly intravenously to avoid bradyarrhythmia and hypotension. The phenytoin prodrug fosphenytoin has enhanced solubility and circumvents this hazard; although it is considerably safer for intravenous (IV) administration, it is also considerably more expensive.

SPECTRUM OF ACTIVITY

The spectrum of activity of phenytoin includes status epilepticus, partial seizures, partial seizures secondarily generalized, tonic seizures, and generalized tonic-clonic seizures [4,5]. Increasing doses and levels of phenytoin are associated with progressive reduction of seizures in adults [6] and children [7]. Although the therapeutic range is widely quoted at 10 to 20 mg/L, individual patients may require lower or higher levels for successful treatment. Phenytoin is not effective

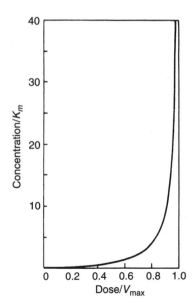

Figure 29-1. Dose versus concentration curve for drugs with nonlinear elimination kinetics. Reproduced with permission from Dodson WE. The nonlinear kinetics of phenytoin in children. *Neurology* 1982; 32:42–48.

against generalized absence seizures and may increase their frequency; it is also ineffective in preventing recurrent febrile seizures. Phenytoin has been widely used to treat neonatal seizures including neonatal status epilepticus (8–10). After phenobarbital fails to control neonatal seizures, the chance that phenytoin will succeed is approximately 50 percent (11,12). However, the response of neonatal seizures caused by hypoxia, ischemia, or hemorrhage is poor (13). Phenytoin is also used to treat kinesigenic choreoathetosis (14).

PHENYTOIN ADMINISTRATION

Phenytoin is available for parenteral and oral administration (Table 29-1). Although IV phenytoin is effective in stopping status epilepticus and preventing recurrent seizures, it is slower acting in stopping acute convulsions than a benzodiazepine (15). However, when status has been interrupted by a short-acting drug such as diazepam, phenytoin can be administered next to prevent seizure recurrence. When phenytoin is administered intravenously, it must be given slowly to reduce the risk of cardiovascular toxicity (Table 29-2). For this reason the safer formulation fosphenytoin is preferred because of the desirability of stopping status epilepticus as rapidly as possible.

Phenytoin has several advantages in the acute treatment of seizures. It is not sedating and thus does not potentiate sedation and respiratory depression like benzodiazepines and barbiturates do. When seizures persist after administration of phenytoin in status, cumulative doses of up to 30 mg/kg can be given initially but should not be exceeded unless it is documented that phenytoin levels are not excessive, because high phenytoin levels can cause seizures. Intramuscular (IM) phenytoin is not effective in the acute treatment of seizures.

In chronic oral therapy, phenytoin usually can be administered twice daily. Because of the nonlinear kinetics of phenytoin, it is best to begin with a low average dose and increase the dose stepwise until the desired clinical result is obtained. In young children initial doses of 8–10 mg/kg/day are reasonable, whereas older children, adolescents, and young adults should begin with 6–8 mg/kg/day (16). As the dose is

raised, progressively smaller increases should be made to avoid disproportionate increases in phenytoin level and resultant toxicity. If precise adjustment of phenytoin levels is necessary, the distinction between phenytoin and phenytoin sodium becomes an important consideration when mixing or switching to different phenytoin-containing products. The concentration of phenytoin in contemporary suspensions remains fairly uniform, but in the past suspensions were ill-advised because of the tendency for phenytoin to precipitate. Doses from the top of the bottles were lower than expected, whereas those from the bottom were higher than expected, as the suspension became more concentrated. In all instances when the phenytoin dose has been changed, patients should be reexamined to evaluate whether the dose is correct.

PHARMACOKINETICS

Phenytoin is largely eliminated by enzymatic biotransformation in the liver to 5-parahydroxyphenyl, 5-phenyl hydantoin (HPPH), which is the major metabolite, and to a dihydrodiol that accounts for approximately 10 percent of phenytoin metabolites in urine. Both of these metabolites are thought to be derived from a highly reactive arene oxide (epoxide) intermediate (17). Negligible amounts of unmetabolized phenytoin are excreted in urine.

Phenytoin is metabolized by the cytochrome P-450 enzymes CYP2C9 and CYP2C19 (18,19). In some families who metabolize phenytoin slowly, mutations have been identified that account for these pharmacokinetic differences (20). Odani and coworkers identified a mutation of CYP2C9 due to a substitution of leucine for isoleucine at position 359 that results in a 33 percent reduction in maximal capacity to metabolize (V_{MAX}) phenytoin among Japanese people. Mutations in CYP2C19 reduced V_{MAX} by up to 14 percent.

Phenytoin has nonlinear kinetics in all age groups (1,21–28). As the dose and concentration of phenytoin increase, the eliminating mechanism becomes progressively saturated, reducing the fraction of phenytoin that is eliminated per unit of time. This leads to a nonlinear relationship between phenytoin dose and concentration (Figure 29-1). Because increasing doses cause disproportional rises in the phenytoin level, smaller increments in dose should be made as the phenytoin level approaches the therapeutic range. Phenytoin kinetics are best characterized by Michaelis-Menten equations. However, the concept of half-life is widely used in clinical pharmacokinetics and therefore merits discussion (Table 29-3).

Phenytoin Half-Life

Phenytoin elimination kinetics are concentration-dependent. Although the half-life of phenytoin is

Table 29-2. Aspects of Phenytoin Administration

Intravenous dose	15–20 mg/kg*
Intravenous administration rates	
Adults	<50 mg/min
Children	<3 mg/kg/min
Maintenance dose	6–20 mg/kg/day
Therapeutic concentration range	10–20 mg/L

*Administer slowly to avoid cardiovascular toxicity.

Table 29-3. Phenytoin Pharmacokinetics

Protein binding	90%
Volume of distribution	
Newborns	0.8–1.2 L/kg
Older children and adults	0.7–0.9 L/kg
Half-life	Concentration-dependent
Nonlinear kinetic parameters*	
K_M	5 mg/L
V_{MAX}	10–20 mg/kg/day

*See text for details.

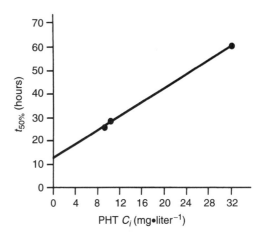

Figure 29-3. Relationship of the initial concentration (Ci) to the apparent half-life ($t_{50\%}$) that was observed in an infant taking phenytoin. The apparent half-life was prolonged as the concentration increased.

widely quoted and discussed, applying the concept of a half-life to phenytoin kinetics is technically improper because phenytoin does not have first-order elimination kinetics. The apparent half-life ($t_{50\%}$) of phenytoin changes depending on the concentration range over which it is measured. As a consequence of phenytoin's nonlinear elimination kinetics, increasing concentrations lead to prolongation of the $t_{50\%}$. The apparent half-lives can be quite prolonged when phenytoin levels are high (23,28). As the level declines, the clearance of phenytoin elimination increases and the $t_{50\%}$ becomes shorter (Figure 29-2). At different concentrations, therefore, different half-lives can be measured in a single patient. As was shown in equation 5 in Chapter 23, the $t_{50\%}$ is directly related to the concentration at which the $t_{50\%}$ is determined (Figure 29-3).

Because the $t_{50\%}$ of phenytoin varies, it takes longer than expected for patients to reach a steady state. This is particularly a problem when patients take relatively high doses that are close to their maximal phenytoin eliminating capacity (V_{MAX}). As a rule of thumb, at least two weeks should be allowed before phenytoin levels are considered to be at steady state after the dose is changed. Even more time may be required in some patients who have very high levels.

The changing $t_{50\%}$ of phenytoin is occasionally useful in clinical situations. For example, small increases in the average phenytoin level can be achieved by giving the total daily dose as a single dose (29). This increases the average level slightly because the large single dose produces a higher initial phenytoin concentration, thereby prolonging the $t_{50\%}$. Dividing the daily dose into more frequent daily doses has the opposite effect and slightly lowers the average concentration.

Nonlinear Kinetics, K_M and V_{MAX}

Phenytoin kinetics are best characterized by Michaelis-Menten kinetic parameters K_M and V_{MAX}. Children and adults have similar K_M values of approximately 5 mg/L; however, children have higher capacity to eliminate phenytoin than adults resulting in higher V_{MAX} (2,21,22,30). Much of the variation in K_M is due to drug interactions.

There are several methods for calculating the K_M and V_{MAX}. The easiest and most reliable method is the direct linear plot (31). This is a graphic solution that can be performed at the bedside. The method depends on knowing the patient's phenytoin level at two or more pairs of doses and steady-state concentrations. The concentrations should be obtained at consistent times after doses. When phenytoin is given twice daily, the best times to measure the level are either just before a dose or 8 hours after a dose (32). Once K_M and V_{MAX} are known, it is possible to estimate the relationship between future doses and concentrations.

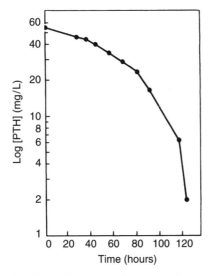

Figure 29-2. Log phenytoin concentration versus time curve that was obtained in a 14-month-old child who ingested a large dose of phenytoin. Note that the observed half-life becomes progressively shorter as the concentration declines. Reproduced with permission from Dodson WE. Phenytoin elimination in childhood: effect of concentration dependent kinetics. *Neurology* 1980; 30:196–199.

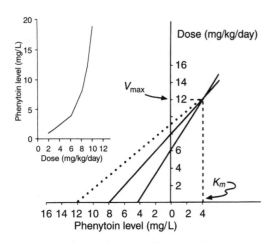

Figure 29-4. Direct linear plot (31). In this example $K_M = 4$ mg/L and $V_{MAX} = 12$ mg/kg/day. Predicted values are indicated by the dotted line. Insert indicates the shape of the dose versus concentration curve. See text for details.

The direct linear plot technique for calculating K_M and V_{MAX} is fairly simple and is illustrated in Figure 29-4 (33). The negative value of the phenytoin level is plotted on the horizontal axis, and the dose is plotted on the vertical axis. The dose and level pairs are connected by lines that are extended up and to the right where they intersect. This point of intersection is used as a fulcrum for determining K_M, V_{MAX} and other dose-level relationships. A horizontal line drawn from the point of intersection to the vertical axis is V_{MAX}. A vertical line drawn from the intersection indicates K_M on the horizontal axis. The relationships between other doses and levels are solved by drawing additional lines from the point of intersection as shown in the figure.

There are many nomograms and related methods for predicting the relationship between phenytoin dose and concentration in various groups of patients (27). Although these provide excellent exercises in clinical pharmacology, they are untrustworthy guides to phenytoin dosing. In one study significant errors in predicted levels occurred in 21 percent to 38 percent of subjects (34). Large errors are most likely among patients who need high phenytoin levels. For this reason, every patient whose phenytoin dose is changed should be reevaluated after an appropriate time interval (27). Although nomograms can reduce trial and error in estimating phenytoin doses, they are no substitute for patient follow-up.

Phenytoin Absorption

As indicated in Chapter 23, the nonlinear kinetics of phenytoin can affect the apparent extent of phenytoin absorption (bioavailability). Slowing the absorption rate has the practical result of reducing the apparent bioavailablilty (36). Computer simulations indicate that at average values of K_M and V_{MAX}, increasing

the absorption half-life from 0 to 1.2 hours causes the apparent bioavailability to decrease by approximately 25 percent (36). If the actual fraction that is absorbed also decreases slightly, the reduction in apparent bioavailability is greater. For example, with 90 percent absorption and an absorption half-life of 0.9 hour, the apparent bioavailability declines to 69 percent.

Although phenytoin is well absorbed after oral administration, the rate of absorption depends on the formulation. Changing excipients has been associated with changes in steady-state levels (37). But even without changes in excipients other aspects of tablet formulation can affect the absorption rate. Thus, switching formulations can significantly change the phenytoin levels. Generic substitution of phenytoin should be prohibited for this reason.

In infants peak phenytoin concentrations occur 2 to 6 hours after oral dosing (38). In older children peak concentrations occur 3 to 10 hours following oral doses. The administration of phenytoin with food further delays the time to peak concentrations in patients of all ages (39). However, taking phenytoin postprandially produces 40 percent higher concentrations than when it is taken before meals (40). The relationship between phenytoin doses and meals should be consistent.

Intramuscular administration of phenytoin is associated with slow and erratic absorption (41). Because of the low solubility of phenytoin, it can crystallize and precipitate at the injection site. Although absorption is eventually complete, IM administration of phenytoin is unreliable and should be avoided (42). If IM administration is needed, fosphenytoin should be given.

Phenytoin Drug-protein Binding

The unbound drug concentration, not the total drug concentration, determines the drug's action. Phenytoin is normally 90 percent bound to constituents of serum, mainly to albumin. In diseases with hypoalbuminemia such as renal disease, hepatic disease, severe malnutrition, burns, and pregnancy (43,44), the unbound phenytoin fraction increases such that the total phenytoin levels no longer provide reliable indicators of the unbound levels. In these situations, measuring the unbound phenytoin level is sometimes indicated.

Phenytoin binding is also reduced by bilirubin and acidic compounds such as fatty acids, including valproic acid and salicylate, which displace phenytoin from protein binding sites (45). When the unbound phenytoin increases chronically, hepatic metabolism compensates such that the unbound concentration is readjusted to the previous level. This leads to a decline in the total phenytoin level, but the effect on unbound levels is insignificant. Thus, chronic changes in binding have a negligible effect on the unbound concentration unless the phenytoin dose is changed (46). On the other hand, acute changes in phenytoin binding may cause transient and symptomatic changes in unbound phenytoin levels. For example, valproate can increase the unbound phenytoin level transiently when valproate levels fluctuate widely between doses. This can cause transient phenytoin toxicity (47).

Effect of Age on Phenytoin Pharmacokinetics

The maximal capacity to eliminate phenytoin is affected by genetic factors, age, and drug interactions. However, the nonlinear kinetics of phenytoin have confounded most clinical investigations of the effect of age on phenytoin kinetics. When linear kinetic parameters such as half-life or relative clearance are used, the nonlinear kinetics often obscure age-related pharmacokinetic differences (23,48). In a practical sense, the nonlinear kinetics of phenytoin influence relative dosage requirements more than age.

Newborns

Newborns who are exposed to phenytoin in utero usually eliminate transplacentally acquired phenytoin at rates that are comparable to those in adults. Studies of urinary metabolites indicate that these newborns rapidly metabolize phenytoin (49). On the other hand, newborns with seizures eliminate phenytoin slowly at first, but later during the neonatal period they eliminate it rapidly after their drug eliminating mechanisms have matured (24).

Among all age groups, premature and full-term newborns who were not exposed to inducing agents in utero have the lowest relative capacity to eliminate phenytoin, and therefore they require the lowest doses on average. Phenytoin concentrations and apparent half-lives vary extensively in newborns with seizures, more so than in any other age group. Newborns with seizures have several factors that act simultaneously to produce unstable phenytoin levels. These include nonlinear phenytoin kinetics, postnatal maturation of hepatic function, induction of phenytoin elimination by phenobarbital and other drugs, and slowed phenytoin absorption, which occurs after switching from IV to oral dosing. Most newborns who receive phenytoin have been treated with phenobarbital previously. Phenobarbital affects the hepatic biotransformation of phenytoin increasing both V_{MAX} and K_M (2,50). For this reason, the changing phenytoin kinetics during the neonatal period preclude the use of steady-state methods for analyzing the nonlinear kinetics of phenytoin. These changes make it necessary to increase the phenytoin dose during the neonatal period if consistently high phenytoin levels are needed.

High phenytoin concentrations occur after IV loading doses, often leading to very long apparent half-lives

in the first and second week of life. The phenytoin half-lives that have been reported in newborns vary widely, with extremes of 6 hours to more than 200 hours after IV therapy (9,24,51). Bourgeois and Dodson (24) found that the phenytoin $t_{50\%}$ ranged from 6.9 to 140 hours, with an average value of 57.3 ± 48.2 hours. By age 3 to 5 weeks, the $t_{50\%}$ decreased by two-thirds.

After the first week of life, shorter phenytoin half-lives have been reported, but some newborns continue to have prolonged half-lives if phenytoin levels are high (9,51). Painter and coworkers (9) reported an average value of 104 ± 17 hours during the second week of life. In a different group of 16 newborns with seizures, half-lives diminished considerably after the first week of life (24). Among children more than one week old there was good correlation ($r = 0.88$ to 0.93) between the apparent half-life and the initial phenytoin concentration (24). Correcting for initial concentration revealed that newborns aged 3 to 5 weeks had the shortest half-life, averaging 19.7 and 12 hours at initial phenytoin concentrations of 18 and 10 mg/L, respectively.

After the first or second weeks of life, phenytoin elimination capacity increases and phenytoin concentrations often decline. Older newborns and young infants require doses as high as 18 to 20 mg/kg/day to achieve therapeutic levels (39). If declining concentrations occur when phenytoin administration is switched from the IV to the oral route, the changing dose requirements give the appearance of malabsorption of phenytoin (9,10).

Newborns absorb phenytoin slowly but completely after oral administration with less than 3 percent of administered phenytoin found in feces (52). Studies using stable isotope-labeled phenytoin also indicate complete absorption (53). Similarly, comparisons of levels obtained after IV and oral doses indicate complete absorption of orally administered suspensions (54). Thus, the decline in phenytoin levels that takes place in the second or third week of life is due to an increasing capacity for phenytoin biotransformation plus the unique consequences of nonlinear elimination kinetics. Despite numerous statements to the contrary, newborns do not malabsorb phenytoin. Reliable concentrations can be produced by oral administration even in premature newborns (54).

It is technically difficult to measure phenytoin bioavailability in newborns because of the changing elimination kinetics during the newborn period. For this reason, computer simulations have been used to provide insight into the problem. These simulations indicate that the changing phenytoin elimination kinetics (V_{MAX} and K_M) and the slower absorption rates that occur after phenytoin administration is switched from IV to oral routes both affect the phenytoin level (36). For example, slowing the absorption rate of phenytoin decreases the apparent bioavailablilty by up to 26 percent.

The effects of varying the absorption rate and K_M on the apparent extent of phenytoin absorption are modest compared with the large changes that occur when V_{MAX} increases. Based on computer simulations, increasing V_{MAX} is expected to produce sizable reductions in apparent bioavailability even when absorption is complete (36). For example, increasing V_{MAX} threefold from 5 mg/kg/day to 15 mg/kg/day causes the apparent bioavailability to decrease by 77 percent. Variations in K_M cause smaller changes in apparent bioavailability; changing K_M from 5 mg/L to 1 mg/L decreases the apparent bioavailability to 67 percent. Increasing K_M from 5 to 10 mg/L, such as might occur because of the interaction with phenobarbital, has the opposite effect.

Infants and Children

Among all age groups infants have the highest relative capacity to eliminate phenytoin, causing them to have average dosage requirements that are fourfold greater than adults. V_{MAX} but not K_M changes with increasing age (2,22) (Figure 29-5). After phenytoin eliminating capacity peaks during infancy, it declines during childhood to adult values (21). In one study the V_{MAX} in infants ranged from 11 to 30 mg/kg/day and averaged 17.9 mg/kg/day (2). The average values in older children and adults are approximately 8 to 10 mg/kg/day in various studies. Although most of the variation in K_M is due to drug interactions, K_M does vary independently as well. In one study, 28 percent of children had a K_M of 2.5 mg/L or less (2). This low value of K_M makes it technically difficult to adjust phenytoin levels when levels are above 10 mg/L because the dose versus concentration curve becomes progressively steep and nonlinear (Figure 29-6).

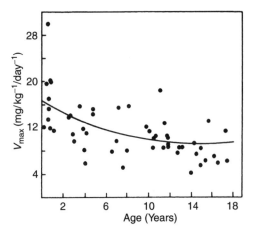

Figure 29-5. Relationship between age and V_{MAX} for phenytoin elimination. Reproduced with permission from Dodson WE. The nonlinear kinetics of phenytoin in children. *Neurology* 1982; 32:42–48.

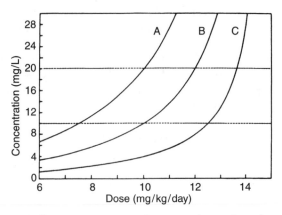

Figure 29-6. Dose versus concentration curves for varying values of K_M when V_{MAX} is held constant at 15 mg/kg/day. Note that as the values for K_M decline from 10 to 2 mg/L, the curve becomes more nearly vertical through the concentration range of 10 to 20 mg/L.

The higher relative clearance for phenytoin seen in children gradually declines until adult values are reached around age 10 to 15 (see Figure 23-6). During this period, changes in body weight are offset by declining relative drug clearance such that dosage changes are less frequent than expected. However, within any age group, individual patients deviate significantly from the group average. There are several causes for this variation, and foremost among them are drug interactions and intercurrent illness.

Adolescents

No major changes in phenytoin kinetics have been described in adolescence. However, phenytoin concentrations fluctuate during the menstrual cycle. Although these fluctuations are usually modest, concentrations are higher at midcycle, when ovulation occurs, than at the time of menstruation. This suggests that increased concentrations of estrogen and progesterone interfere with phenytoin biotransformation (55). The fluctuations in phenytoin levels are most extensive in patients who have the highest concentrations.

Drug Interactions and Nonlinear Kinetics of Phenytoin

Phenytoin is both the instigator and the victim of pharmacokinetic drug interactions. First, it is a potent inducer of many enzymes in the cytochrome P-450 drug metabolizing system (56). By this mechanism, the addition of phenytoin increases the clearance and decreases the concentrations of most other antiepileptics that are eliminated by hepatic metabolism. Examples include carbamazepine, methsuximide, primidone, valproate, and most of the AEDs that have been introduced in the 1990s, including felbamate, topiramate, lamotrigine, and tiagabine. Besides enhancing the clearance of these compounds, phenytoin also stimulates the clearance of steroids, including oral contraceptives, and the clearance of vitamins, including vitamin D, folic acid, and vitamin K (56,57).

Phenytoin elimination is extremely vulnerable to drug interactions by virtue of its dependence on hepatic metabolism for elimination and its nonlinear kinetics (58). Even though general trends can be described, the direction and extent of these interactions are highly unpredictable. For this reason, diligent clinical follow-up is required whenever a comedication is added to or deleted from treatment regimens that include phenytoin.

Phenobarbital consistently increases both the V_{MAX} and K_M of phenytoin elimination (2). Therefore, phenobarbital has conflicting effects, acting simultaneously as an inducer and as a competitive inhibitor of phenytoin elimination. In groups of patients the addition of phenobarbital to phenytoin regimens produces no change in the average phenytoin level in groups of patients, but phenytoin levels can change significantly in individual patients.

Drug interactions can make the adjustment of phenytoin easier or more difficult depending on the drug that is involved. The phenobarbital-phenytoin interaction facilitates the titration of phenytoin levels in the upper part of therapeutic range (Figure 29-5). This pharmacokinetic benefit is due to the increased value of K_M for phenytoin elimination, which leads to a mild degree of flattening of the phenytoin dose versus concentration curve. As a result, the dose to concentration relationship becomes more linear and more predictable. Carbamazepine interacts with phenytoin elimination by inducing cytochrome P-450 enzymes CYP2C9 and CYP219 (18,59,60). The net effect of this interaction is to reduce both the K_M and V_{MAX} for phenytoin elimination (2,61), which is a complex interaction that usually leads to a reduction in phenytoin level. This interaction makes readjustment of phenytoin levels technically difficult because of the reduced K_M value and increased nonlinearity of the dose to concentration relationship. Valproate interacts with phenytoin by displacing it from binding sites on albumin and increasing the unbound phenytoin fraction. Valproate reduces the K_M of phenytoin elimination but has no effect on V_{MAX} (2). However, switching from the standard formulation of sodium valproate to a slow-release formulation can cause the phenytoin level to increase. Suzuki and coworkers (62) found that the average phenytoin level increased from 14.4 to 18.7 mg/L when the valproate formulation was switched to the slow-release formulation.

Certain drug interactions usually increase the phenytoin level. Chloramphenicol consistently inhibits phenytoin elimination, thus increasing phenytoin levels (63). Conversely, discontinuing chloramphenicol causes phenytoin levels to decline dramatically. Isoniazide also usually increases phenytoin levels. According to the Boston Collaborative Drug Surveillance Program, 27 percent of the patients who take isoniazide plus phenytoin develop phenytoin toxicity if the phenytoin dose is not adjusted (64).

Effect of Illness on Phenytoin Pharmacokinetics

Intercurrent illness can cause changes both in seizure threshold and in drug levels. Among all AEDs, phenytoin levels are most liable to change during intercurrent illness. Infectious mononucleosis, influenza immunization, streptococcal pharyngitis, and any illness that causes fever can cause reduced phenytoin levels (65–67). One study indicated that phenytoin levels decrease during febrile illness by approximately 50 percent, declining from 16 to 8 mg/L on average (67). Changes of this magnitude are expected to contribute to seizure recurrence in some patients.

Chronic renal disease is usually associated with alterations of phenytoin binding. In nephrotic syndrome, phenytoin binding is reduced to 80 percent, doubling the unbound phenytoin fraction (68). In addition, the half-life of phenytoin is decreased in uremia (69). Phenytoin binding returns to normal after successful renal transplantation (70). Although dialysis removes relatively little phenytoin, dialysis can remove significant amounts of water, thereby altering the patient's serum albumin concentration (71). This in turn can reduce the unbound fraction of phenytoin following dialysis even though the total phenytoin level does not change (72). Measuring the unbound phenytoin concentration may be necessary in such situations.

Significant hepatic disease is associated with hypoalbuminemia and increased concentrations of bilirubin and bile acids in serum, which can alter phenytoin binding. In addition, the hepatic biotransformation of phenytoin is variably impaired if hepatic parenchymal function is reduced, such as occurs in hepatitis or passive hepatic congestion caused by heart failure. Again, measuring the unbound phenytoin level is sometimes indicated.

ADVERSE EFFECTS

Phenytoin is one of the best tolerated antiepileptic medications. It causes some degree of side effects in the majority of patients, but only an estimated 10 percent to 40 percent of patients require a change of medication (73). In a study conducted among children in India, the risk of more than one side effect was 32 percent, 40 percent, and 19 percent for children treated with either phenobarbital, phenytoin, or sodium valproate, respectively. However, most of the side effects that were associated with phenytoin disappeared after phenytoin dosage adjustment (74).

In a British randomized comparison of phenytoin with carbamazepine, phenobarbital, and sodium valproate, all four drugs had equivalent efficacy, but there were substantial differences in side effects. Phenobarbital was withdrawn from the study after a high percentage of the children who were assigned to that medicaton developed side effects. Among the remaining agents, phenytoin was withdrawn in 9 percent of children compared with 4 percent withdrawal rates because of unacceptable side effects for carbamazepine and valproate (75).

Overall, the incidence of side effects with phenytoin is similar to that of carbamazepine, but the nature of the side effects differs. In children, the cosmetic side effects of gingival hyperplasia and hirsutism are notably common and aggravating after chronic phenytoin therapy.

Idiosyncratic side effects of phenytoin include blood dyscrasia, allergic reactions, and certain forms of neurotoxicity. Idiosyncratic neurotoxicity is a problem primarily in patients who are abnormal neurologically and who do not manifest the usual signs of phenytoin toxicity. Immune-mediated reactions to phenytoin usually occur within the first two months of therapy. These include rashes, fever, lymphadenopathy, eosinophilia, serum sickness with hepatic and renal dysfunction, and polymyositis (76). Pseudolymphoma consisting of rash, fever, and lymphadenopathy is rare.

Phenytoin is one of many drugs that can cause the AED hypersensitivity syndrome. This syndrome consists of rash, fever, lymphadenopathy, and visceral organ involvement, especially involvement of the liver and/or kidneys. The estimated incidence is 1 per 3,000 phenytoin exposures. Approximately 70 percent to 80 percent of patients demonstrate cross-reactivity with phenobarbital, primidone, and carbamazepine (77). The risk of serious skin rashes, defined as rashes that are extensive enough to require hospitalization, has been estimated to be 2.3 to 4.5 per 10,000 for phenytoin compared with 1 to 4.1 per 10,000 for carbamazepine (78). Other forms of rash such as fixed drug eruptions also have been linked to phenytoin (79).

Rarely, movement disorders are caused by phenytoin. These disorders usually occur in patients who are neurologically abnormal (80). Both bradykinesia and choreoathetosis have been described. Both may occur on either an idiosyncratic basis or a dose-related basis, although the latter is more common, with most affected patients having levels above 20 mg/L (81–83). Choreoathetosis has occurred after IV therapy and may be long-lasting (84,85). Choreoathetosis can also be caused by carbamazepine and ethosuximide (83,86,87).

Dose-related adverse effects of phenytoin may be either acute or delayed, appearing only after chronic treatment. The acute dose-related neurotoxicity of phenytoin was well described by Kutt and cowokers more than three decades ago (50). Nystagmus occurs at levels of 15–25 mg/L, ataxia occurs at levels greater than 30 mg/L, and mental changes with lethargy and mental clouding occur at levels above 40 mg/L. Most patients with levels above 20 mg/L have nystagmus. Blood levels above 60 mg/L cause difficulty sitting up. Although rare, ophthalmoplegia is also dose-related (88). Paradoxically, seizure frequency increases at phenytoin levels above 30 mg/L in some patients (89,90). This becomes a thorny management issue among patients with severe epilepsy because certain patients require equally high levels for seizure control. The adverse effect of seizure exacerbation has been linked to several other drugs besides phenytoin, especially carbamazepine, gabapentin, phenobarbital, vigabatrin, and lamotrigine (91,92). However, carbamazepine-exacerbated seizures may be controlled by replacing carbamazepine with phenytoin (93).

Phenytoin-induced encephalopathy with dementia is also rare. Usually subacute and insidious, it is more likely to occur in neurologically abnormal patients who do not manifest the usual progression of concentration-related toxic signs. It is usually reversible after phenytoin is discontinued (94–96).

Delayed adverse effects of phenytoin include peripheral neuropathy, reduced vitamin D levels, bone demineralization, and cosmetic changes. The cosmetic side effects of hirsutism and gingival hyperplasia are more common with phenytoin than with other AEDs. The incidence of gingival hyperplasia is approximately 40 percent, but figures as high as 69 percent have been reported in Indian patients with tuberculous meningitis treated chronically with phenytoin (97). Although not all study results agree, the risk of gingival hyperplasia appears to be directly related to the phenytoin dose and level and inversely related to age (98,99). Factors that are unrelated to increased risk of this side effect include sex, age at onset of treatment, and duration of treatment (99). Other factors include genetic predisposition, plaque-induced gingival inflammation, immunologic status, and the induction of growth factors. Overall, gingival hyperplasia is more common in children than in adults. Poor oral hygiene further increases the risk; preventive dental hygiene programs reduce the incidence and severity of this problem (100,101).

The pathogenesis of gingival hyperplasia has not been completely elucidated; reactive intermediates are thought to play a role. Microsomes from gingival tissue do have the capacity to metabolize phenytoin (102). Phenytoin also increases serum concentrations of basic fibroblast growth factor threefold. Furthermore, basic fibroblast growth factor levels have correlated better with the extent of gingival overgrowth than age, phenytoin dose, duration of phenytoin administration, and serum phenytoin level (103).

The question of whether chronic phenytoin therapy at ordinary levels causes cerebellar and brain stem atrophy remains unanswered despite years of concern. The problem is complicated because cerebellar atrophy also occurs in patients with severe epilepsy who have not received phenytoin. In one study of mentally retarded patients, the incidence of cerebellar atrophy (28%) was similar in phenytoin-treated and untreated patients (104). Most cases of persistent ataxia and cerebellar and brain stem atrophy have occurred after chronically high levels of phenytoin and clinical signs of intoxication. However, brief periods of intoxication and even single episodes of severe phenytoin intoxication have been followed by cerebellar atrophy with permanent disability (105,106). The issue is especially complex in mentally handicapped patients who may not show the usual signs of phenytoin intoxication despite levels that would ordinarily be considered toxic (107). Nonetheless, high phenytoin levels have been temporally linked to the permanent loss of locomotion in mentally handicapped patients who had high levels chronically.

ADVANTAGES AND DISADVANTAGES OF PHENYTOIN THERAPY

In the balance, phenytoin ranks among the best tolerated and most widely used AEDs in childhood epilepsy. It has several special features that should be borne in mind when comparing it with other AEDs (Table 29-4). Advantages of phenytoin in the treatment of childhood epilepsy include the following:

1. It is available for parenteral administration and is effective in status epilepticus.
2. Pediatric physicians have extensive experience with phenytoin, and most are familiar with administering it to children.
3. Phenytoin is nonsedating and can be coadministered with sedative anticonvulsants if necessary.

Table 29-4. Summary of Special Features Regarding Phenytoin Administration in Childhood Epilepsy

Nonlinear elimination kinetics
Frequent drug interactions
Fosphenytoin is preferred for IV and IM administration
Slow IV administration of phenytoin is necessary
Unreliable intramuscular absorption
High concentrations paradoxically cause seizures
Cosmetic and cognitive side effects
Generic substitution prohibited

Disadvantages include the pharmacokinetic issues and cognitive side effects that are discussed elsewhere. The major adverse cognitive effects include slowing of motor and mental processes and variable impairment of memory. Cosmetic side effects are also more common with phenytoin than with other anticonvulsants. Finally, the nonlinear kinetics of phenytoin are complicated and make phenytoin levels vulnerable to change because of drug interactions and intercurrent illness.

FOSPHENYTOIN

The IV administration of phenytoin has long been hazardous because of the need for alkaline pH and high concentrations of solvents (propylene glycol) to keep phenytoin in solution. The formulation of fosphenytoin, the disodium phosphate ester of phenytoin, has circumvented both of these problems, resulting in a safer phenytoin formulation for parenteral administration (108). Unfortunately, fosphenytoin is far more expensive, pharmacoeconomic arguments not withstanding (109,110).

Fosphenytoin can be administered intravenously and intramuscularly and can be used to administer phenytoin parenterally for extended periods if necessary (111–113). The phosphate ester is hydrolyzed rapidly by nonspecific hepatic phosphatases releasing phenytoin. Although the half-life of the hydrolysis is on the order of 8 to 15 minutes (114), the concentration of unbound phenytoin increases more rapidly because fosphenytoin displaces phenytoin from binding sites in blood (115). As a result, the newly liberated phenytoin is largely unbound until the fosphenytoin concentration declines.

The fosphenytoin dose is prescribed and administered as equimolar amounts of phenytoin called phenytoin equivalents; therefore, the loading and maintenance dose of fosphenytoin in phenytoin equivalents are identical to the phenytoin dose (116). Fosphenytoin infusion causes fewer adverse effects than IV phenytoin (113). Unique side effects compared with phenytoin are pruritus and perineal paresthesias (108). Hypotension occurs less often following fosphenytoin IV infusion than with phenytoin but may occur later after the infusion (117,118). Compared with IV phenytoin, fosphenytoin infusion is less likely to be painful or to cause erythema, irritation at the infusion site, or venous cording (118,119). It has not been reported to cause purple glove syndrome as IV phenytoin does. Purple glove syndrome, which occurs mainly in elderly patients, consists of progressive edema, pain, and discoloration of the limb following IV phenytoin infusion (120).

OTHER ANTIEPILEPTIC COMPOUNDS RELATED TO PHENYTOIN

The other hydantoins in clinical use include mephenytoin (Mesantoin), a *N*-methlylated compound, and ethotoin (Peganone), which is *N*-ethylated (121). Whereas phenytoin has two phenyl groups in the 5 position of the hydantoin ring, mephenytoin has both a phenyl and an ethyl group like phenobarbital; ethotoin has a single phenyl group in the same position. Like other *N*-alkylated compounds, both ethotoin and mephenytoin are dealkylated in the body. The spectrum of activity of these compounds is similar to that of phenytoin, but their side effects differ, with both compounds having a lower incidence of gingival hyperplasia and hirsutism. The genetic basis for variability in mephenytoin metabolism has been described (121).

Information about the use of these drugs in children is scant. Mephenytoin use has been discouraged by reports of potentially fatal blood dyscrasia occurring in an estimated 1 percent of patients. The *N*-demethylated metabolite nirvanol is a racemic mixture of dextro- and levorotary isomers and accumulates in serum. Nirvanol, possibly the dextrorotary isomer, is responsible for most of the anticonvulsant activity of mephenytoin. Nirvanol has a long half-life in adults ranging from 77 to 176 hours (121,122). Among adults, levels of 25–40 mg/L have been associated with improved seizure control (123).

Ethotoin has nonlinear kinetics with one study reporting V_{MAX} to range from 50 to 95 mg/kg/day and K_M to range from 9 to 43 mg/L in children (124). Among patients switched from phenytoin to ethotoin, gingival hyperplasia recedes. The incidence of hirsutism and ataxia is also said to be lower with ethotoin. Doses have ranged from approximately 20 to 50 mg/kg/day.

REFERENCES

1. Arnold K, Gerber N. The rate of decline of diphenylhydantoin in human plasma. *Clin Pharmacol Ther* 1970; 11:121–135.

2. Dodson WE. The nonlinear kinetics of phenytoin in children. *Neurology* 1982; 32:42–48.

3. Glazko AJ. Phenytoin: chemistry and methods of determination. In: Levy R, Mattson RH, Meldrum BS, Penry JK, eds. *Antiepileptic Drugs*. 3rd ed. New York: Raven Press, 1989:159–176.

4. Cranford RE, Leppik IE, Patrick B, Anderson CB, Kostick B. Intravenous phenytoin in acute treatment of seizures. *Neurology* 1979; 29:1474–1479.

5. Cloyd JC, Gumnit RJ, McLain W. Status epilepticus. The role of intravenous phenytoin. *JAMA* 1980; 244:1479–1481.

6. Lund L. Anticonvulsant effect of diphenylhydantoin relative to plasma levels. *Arch Neurol* 1974; 31:289–294.

7. Borofsky LG, Louis S, Kutt H. Diphenylhydantoin in children. *Neurology* 1973:23:967–972.

8. Koren G, Brand N, Halkin H, Dany S, Shahar E, Barzilay Z. Kinetics of intravenous phenytoin in children. *Pediatr Pharmacol* 1984; 4:31–38.

9. Painter MJ, Pippenger C, MacDonald H, Pitlick W. Phenobarbital and diphenylhydantoin levels in neonates with seizures. *J Pediatr* 1978; 92: 315–319.

10. Painter MJ, Pippenger C, Wasterlain C, et al. Phenobarbital and phenytoin in neonatal seizures: metabolism and tissue distribution. *Neurology* 1981; 31:1107–1112.

11. Gilman JT, Gal P, Duchowny MS, Weaver RL, Ransom JL. Rapid sequential phenobarbital treatment of neonatal seizures. *Pediatrics* 1989; 83:674–678.

12. Camfield PR, Camfield CS, Gordon K, Dooley JM. If a first antiepileptic drug fails to control a child's epilepsy, what are the chances of success with the next drug? *J Pediatr* 1997; 131:821–824.

13. Connell J, Oozeer R, de Vries L, Dubowitz L-M, Dubowitz V. Clinical and EEG response to anticonvulsants in neonatal seizures. *Arch Dis Child* 1989; 64:459–464.

14. Homan RW, Vasko MR, Blaw M. Phenytoin plasma concentration in paroxysmal kinesigenic choreoathetosis. *Neurology* 1980; 30:673–676.

15. Treiman DM, Meyers PD, Walton NY, et al. A comparison of four treatments for generalized convulsive status epilepticus. Veterans Affairs Status Epilepticus Cooperative Study Group. *N Engl J Med* 1998; 339:792–798.

16. O'Mara NB, Jones PR, Anglin DL, Cox S, Nahata MC. Pharmacokinetics of phenytoin in children with acute neurotrauma. *Crit Care Med* 1995; 23:1418–1424.

17. Browne TR, LeDuc B. Phenytoin: chemistry and biotransformation. In: Levy RH, Mattson RH, and Meldrum BS, eds. *Antiepileptic Drugs*. 4th ed. New York: Raven Press, 1995:283–300.

18. Levy RH. Cytochrome P450 isozymes and antiepileptic drug interactions. *Epilepsia* 1995; 36(Suppl 5):S8–S13.

19. Nakasa H, Nakamura H, Ono S, et al. Prediction of drug-drug interactions of zonisamide metabolism in humans from in vitro data. *Eur J Clin Pharmacol* 1998; 54:177–183.

20. Odani A, Hashimoto Y, Otsuki Y, et al. Genetic polymorphism of the CYP2C subfamily and its effect on the pharmacokinetics of phenytoin in Japanese patients with epilepsy. *Clin Pharmacol Ther* 1997; 62:287–292.

21. Chiba K, Ishiizaki T, Muri H, Minagawa K. Michaelis-Menten pharmacokinetics of diphenylhydantoin and application in the pediatric age patient. *J Pediatr* 1980; 96:479–484.

22. Chiba K, Ishiizaki T, Muri H, Minagawa K. Apparent Michaelis-Menten kinetic parameters of phenytoin in pediatric patients. *Pediatr Pharmacol* 1980; 1:171–180.

23. Dodson, WE. Phenytoin elimination in childhood: effect of concentration dependent kinetics. *Neurology* 1980; 30:196–199.

24. Bourgeois BFD, Dodson WE. Phenytoin elimination in newborns. *Neurology* 1983; 33:173–178.

25. Bauer LA, Blouin RA. Phenytoin Michaelis-Menten pharmacokinetics in Caucasian paediatric patients. *Clin Pharmacokinet* 1983; 8:545–549.

26. Yukawa E. Higuchi S. Aoyama T. Population pharmacokinetics of phenytoin from routine clinical data in Japan. *J Clin Pharm Ther* 1989; 14:71–77.

27. Yuen GJ, Latimer PT, Littlefield LC, Mackey RW. Phenytoin dosage predictions in paediatric patients. *Clin Pharmacokinet* 1989; 16:254–260.

28. Jacobsen D. Alvik A. Bredesen JE. Brown RD. Pharmacokinetics of phenytoin in acute adult and child intoxication. *J Toxicol Clin Toxicol* 1986–87; 24:519–531.

29. Zaccara G, Galli A. Effectivness of simplified dosage schedules on management of ambulant epileptic patients. *Eur Neurol* 1979; 18:341–344.

30. Eadie MJ, Tyrer JH, Bochner F, Hooper WD. The elimination of phenytoin in man. *Clin Exp Pharmacol Ther* 1976; 3:217–224.

31. Mullen PW, Foster RW. Comparative evaluation of six techniques for determining Michaelis-Menten parameters relating phenytoin dose and steady-state concentrations. *J Pharm Pharmacol* 1979; 31:100–104.

32. Dodson WE. Phenytoin kinetics in children. *Clin Pharmacol Ther* 1980; 27:704–707.

33. Mullen PW. Optimal phenytoin therapy: a new technique for individualizing dosage. *Clin Pharmacol Ther* 1978; 23:228–232.

34. Chan E. Single-point phenytoin dosage predictions in Singapore Chinese. *J Clin Pharm Ther* 1997; 22:47–52.

35. Martis L, Levy RH. Bioavailability calculations for drugs showing simultaneous first-order and capacity-limited elimination kinetics. *J Pharmacokinet Biopharmaceut* 1973; 1:381–383.

36. Dodson WE, Bourgeois BF. Changing kinetic patterns of phenytoin in newborns. In: Wasterlain CG, Vert P, eds. *Neonatal Seizures*. New York: Raven Press, 1990:271–276.

37. Tryer JH, Eadie MJ, Sutherland JM, et al. Outbreak of anticonvulsant intoxicaton in an Australian city. *Br Med J* 1970; 4:271–273.

38. Albani M. Phenytoin in infancy and childhood. In: Delgado-Escuata AV, Wasterlain CG, Treiman DM, Porter RJ, eds. *Status Epilepticus*. New York: Raven Press, 1983:457–464. (Advances in Neurology, vol. 34).

39. Albani M, Wernicke I. Oral Phenytoin in infancy: dose requirement, absorption, and elimination. *Pediatr Pharmacol* 1983; 3:229–236.

40. Melander A, Brante G, Johansson O, Lindberg T, Wahlin-Boll E. Influence of food on the absorption of phenytoin in man. *Eur J Clin Pharmacol* 1979; 15:269–274.

41. Serrano EE, Roye DB, Hammer RH, Wilder BJ. Plasma diphenylhydantoin values after oral and intramuscular adminstration of diphenylhydantoin. *Neurology* 1973, 23:311–317.

42. Kostenbauder HB, Rapp RP McGovern JP, et al. Bioavailability and single-dose pharmocokinetics of intramuscular phenytoin. *Clin Pharmacol Ther* 1975; 18:449–456.

43. Koch-Weser J, Sellers EM. Binding of drugs to serum albumin (second of two parts). *N Engl J Med* 1976; 294:526–31.

44. Reidenberg MM, Odar-Cdearlof I, von Bahr C, Borga O, Sjoqvist F. Protein binding of diphenylhydantoin and desmethylimiporamine in plasma from patients with poor renal function. *N Engl J Med* 1971; 285:264–267.

45. Fredholm BB, Rane A, Persson B. Diphenylhydantoin binding to proteins in plasma and its dependence on free fatty acid and bilirubin concentration in dogs and newborn infants. *Pediatr Res* 1075; 9:26–30.

46. Olanow CW, Finn AL, Prussak C. The effects of salicylate on the pharmacokinetics of phenytoin. *Neurology* 1981; 31:341–342.

47. Rodin EA, DeSousa G, Haidkewych D, Lodhi R, Berchou RC. Dissociation between free and bound phenytoin levels in presence of valproate sodium. *Arch Neurol* 1981; 38:240–242.

48. Houghton GW, Richens A, Leighton M. Effect of age, height, weight, and sex on serum phenytoin concentration in epileptic patients. *Br J Clin Pharmacol* 1975; 2:251–256.

49. Rane A. Urinary excretion of diphenylhydantoin metabolites in newborn infants. *J Pediatr* 1974; 85:534–545.

50. Kutt H, Winters W, Kokenge R, McDowell F. Dipheylyhydantoin metabolism, blood levels, and toxicity. *Arch Neurol* 1964; 11:642–648.

51. Loughnan PM, Greenwald A, Purton WW, et al. Pharmacokinetic observations of phenytoin disposition in the newborn and young infant. *Arch Dis Child* 1977; 52:302–309.

52. Leff RD, Fischer LJ, Roberts RJ. Phenytoin metabolism in infants following intravenous and oral administration. *Dev Pharmacol Ther* 1986; 9:217–223.

53. Painter MJ. Personal communication.

54. Frey OR, von Brenndorff AI, Probst W. Comparison of phenytoin serum concentrations in premature neonates following intravenous and oral administration. *Ann Pharmacother* 1998; 32:300–303.

55. Shavit G, Korczyn AD, Kivity S, Bechar M, Gitter S. Phenytoin pharmacokinetics in catamennial epilepsy. *Neurology* 1984; 34:959–961.

56. Kutt H. Phenytoin: interactions with other drugs: clinical aspects. In: Levy RH, Mattson RH, and Meldrum BS, eds. *Antiepileptic Drugs*. 4th ed. New York: Raven Press, 1995:315–328.

57. Howe AM, Lipson AH, Sheffield LJ, et al. Prenatal exposure to phenytoin, facial development, and a possible role for vitamin K. *Am J Med Genet* 1995; 58:238–244.

58. Kutt H. Interactions between anticonvulsants and other commonly prescribed drugs. *Epilepsia* 1984; 25(Suppl 2):S118–S131.

59. Sproule BA, Naranjo CA, Brenmer KE, Hassan PC. Selective serotonin reuptake inhibitors and CNS drug

interactions. A critical review of the evidence. *Clin Pharmacokinet* 1997; 33:454–471.

60. Nakasa H, Nakamura H, Ono S, et al. Prediction of drug-drug interactions of zonisamide metabolism in humans from in vitro data. *Eur J Clin Pharmacol* 1998; 54:177–183.

61. Leppik IE, Pepin SM, Jacobi J, Miller KW. Effect of carbamazepine on the Michaelis-Menten parameters of phenytoin. In: Levy RH, et al., eds. *Metabolism of Antiepileptic Drugs*. New York: Raven Press, 1984:217–222.

62. Suzuki Y, Nagai T, Mano T, et al. Interaction between valproate formulation and phenytoin concentrations. *Eur J Clin Pharmacol* 1995; 48:61–63.

63. Rose JQ, Choi HK, Schentag JJ, Kinkel WR, Jusko WJ. Intoxication caused by interaction of chloramphenicol and phenytoin. *JAMA* 1977; 237:2630–2631.

64. Miller RR, Porter J, Greenblatt DJ. Clinical importance of the interaction of pheytoin and isoniazid. *Chest* 1979, 75:356–358.

65. Braun CW, Goldstone JM. Increased clearance of phenytoin as the presenting feature of infectious mononucleoisis. *Ther Drug Mon* 1980; 2:355–357.

66. Leppik IE, Ramani V, Sawchuk RJ, Gumnit RJ. Increased clearance of phenytoin during infectious mononucleosis. *N Engl J Med* 1979; 300:481–482.

67. Leppik IE, Fisher J, Kreil R, Sawchuck RJ. Altered phenytoin clearance with febrile illness. *Neurology* 1986, 36:1367–1370.

68. Gugler R, Azarnoff DL, Shoeman DW. Diphenylhydantoin: correlation between protein binding and albumin concentration. *Klin Wshcr* 1975; 53:445–446.

69. Letteri JM, Mellik H, Louis S, et al. Diphenylhydantoin metabolism in uremia. *N Engl J Med* 1971; 285:648–652.

70. Kang H, Leppik IL. Phenytoin binding and renal transplantation. *Neurology* 1984; 34:83–86.

71. Martin E, Gambertoglio JG, Adler DS, et al. Removal of phenytoin by hemodialysis in uremic patients. *JAMA* 1977; 238:1750–1753.

72. Dodson WE, Loney LC. Hemodialysis reduces the unbound phenytoin in plasma. *J Pediatr* 1982; 101:465–468.

73. Herranz JL, Armijo JA, Arteaga R. Clinical side effects of phenobarbital, primidone, phenytoin, carbamazepine, and valproate during monotherapy in children. *Epilepsia* 1988; 29:794–804.

74. Thilothammal N, Banu K, Ratnam RS. Comparison of phenobarbitone, phenytoin with sodium valproate: randomized, double-blind study. *Indian Pediatr* 1996; 33:549–555.

75. de Silva M, MacArdle B, McGowan M, et al. Randomised comparative monotherapy trial of phenobarbitone, phenytoin, carbamazepine, or sodium valproate for newly diagnosed childhood epilepsy. *Lancet* 1996; 347:709–713.

76. Haruda F. Phenytoin hypersensitivity: 38 cases. *Neurology* 1979; 29:1480–1485.

77. Schlienger RG, Shear NH. Antiepileptic drug hypersensitivity syndrome. *Epilepsia* 1998; 39(Suppl 7):S3–S7.

78. Tennis P, Stern RS. Risk of serious cutaneous disorders after initiation of use of phenytoin, carbamazepine, or sodium valproate: a record linkage study. *Neurology* 1997; 49:542–546.

79. Sharma VK, Dhar S, Gill AN. Drug related involvement of specific sites in fixed eruptions: a statistical evaluation. *J Dermatol* 1996; 23:530–534.

80. Luhdorf K, Lund M. Phenytoin-induced hyperkinesia. *Epilepsia* 1977; 18:409–415.

81. Prensky AL, DeVivo DC, Palkes H. Severe bradykinesia as a manfestation of toxicity to antiepileptic medications. *J Pediatr* 1971; 78:700–704.

82. Challub EG, DeVivo DC, Volpe JJ. Phenytoin-induced dystonia and choreoathetosis in two retarded epileptic children. *Neurology* 1976; 26:494–498.

83. Krishnamoorthy KS, Zaleraitis EL, Young RSK, Bermad PG. Phenytoin-induced choreoathetosis in infancy: case reports and a review. *Pediatrics* 1983; 72:831–834.

84. Kurata K, Kido H, Kobayashi K, Yamaguchi N. Long-lasting movement disorder induced by intravenous phenytoin administration for status epilepticus. A case report. *Clin Neuropharmacol* 1988; 11:467–471.

85. Howrie DL, Crumrine PK. Phenytoin-induced movement disorder associated with intravenous administration for status epilepticus. *Clin Pediatr* 1985; 24:467–469.

86. Chaudhary N, Ravat SH, Shah PU. Phenytoin induced dyskinesia. *Indian Pediatr* 1998; 35:274–276.

87. Koukkari MW, Vanefsky MA, Steinberg GK, Hahn JS. Phenytoin-related chorea in children with deep hemispheric vascular malformations. *J Child Neurol* 1996; 11:490–491.

88. Spector RH, Davidoff RA, Schwartzman RJ. Phenytoin-induced ophthalmoplegia. *Neurology* 1976; 26: 1031–1034.

89. Levy LL, Fenichel GM. Diphenylhydantoin activated seizures. *Neurology* 1965:15:716–722.

90. Stilman N, Masdeu JC. Incidence of seizures with phenytoin toxicity. *Neurology* 1985; 35:1769–1772.

91. Wallace SJ. A comparative review of the adverse effects of anticonvulsants in children with epilepsy. *Drug Safety* 1996; 15:378–393.

92. Perucca E, Gram L, Avanzini G, Dulac O. Antiepileptic drugs as a cause of worsening seizures. *Epilepsia* 1998; 39:5–17.

93. Miyamoto A, Takahashi S, Oki J, Itoh J, Cho K. Exacerbation of seizures by carbamazepine in four children with symptomatic localization related epilepsy. *No To Hattatsu* 1995; 27:23–28.

94. Logan WJ, Freeman JM. Pseudodegenerative disease due to diphenylhydantoin intoxication. *Arch Neurol* 1969; 21:631–637.

95. Vallarta JM, Bell DB, Reichert A. Progressive encephalopathy due to chronic hydantoin intoxication. *Am J Dis Child* 1974; 128:27–34.

96. Tindall RSA, Willerson J. Subacute phenytoin intoxication syndrome. *Arch Intern Med* 1978; 138:1168–1169.

97. Patwari AK, Aneja S, Chandra D, Singhal PK. Long-term anticonvulsant therapy in tuberculous meningitis — a four-year follow-up. *J Trop Pediatr* 1996; 42:98–103.

98. Seymour RA, Thomason JM, Ellis JS. The pathogenesis of drug-induced gingival overgrowth. *J Periodontol* 1996; 23:165–175.

99. Casetta I, Granieri E, Desidera M, et al. Phenytoin-induced gingival overgrowth: a community-based cross-sectional study in Ferrara, Italy. *Neuroepidemiology* 1997; 16:296–303.

100. Addy V, McElnay JC, Eyre DG, Campbell N, Darcy PF. Risk factors in phenytoin-induced gingival hyperplasia. *J Periodontol* 1983; 54:373–377.

101. Stinnett E, Rodu B, Grizzle WE. New developments in understanding phenytoin-induced gingival hyperplasia. *J Am Dent Assoc* 1987; 114:814–816.

102. Zhou LX, Pihlstrom B, Hardwick JP, et al. Metabolism of phenytoin by the gingiva of normal humans: the possible role of reactive metabolites of phenytoin in the initiation of gingival hyperplasia. *Clin Pharmacol Ther* 1996; 60:191–198.

103. Sasaki T, Maita E. Increased bFGF level in the serum of patients with phenytoin-induced gingival overgrowth. *J Clin Periodontol* 1998; 25:42–47.

104. Botez MI, Attig E, Vezina JL. Cerebellar atrophy in epileptic patients. *Can J Neurol Sci* 1988; 15:299–303.

105. Masur H, Elger CE, Ludolph AC, Galanski M. Cerebellar atrophy following acute intoxication with phenytoin. *Neurology* 1989; 39:432–433.

106. Lindvall O, Nilsson B. Cerebellar atrophy following phenytoin intoxication. *Ann Neurol* 1984; 16:258–260.

107. Iivanainen M, Viukari M, Helle EP. Cerebellar atrophy in phenytoin-treated mentally retarded epileptics. *Epilepsia* 1977; 18:375–386.

108. Ramsay RE, DeToledo J. Intravenous administration of fosphenytoin: options for the management of seizures. *Neurology* 1996; 46(Suppl 1):S17–S19.

109. Marchetti A, Magar R, Fischer J, Sloan E, Fischer P. A pharmacoeconomic evaluation of intravenous fosphenytoin (Cerebyx) versus intravenous phenytoin (Dilantin) in hospital emergency departments. *Clin Ther* 1996; 18:953–966.

110. Miller MH. Fosphenytoin: worth the cost? *Ann Emerg Med* 1997; 29:823.

111. Wilder BJ, Campbell K, Ramsay RE, et al. Safety and tolerance of multiple doses of intramuscular fosphenytoin substituted for oral phenytoin in epilepsy or neurosurgery. *Arch Neurol* 1996; 53:764–768.

112. Pellock JM. Fosphenytoin use in children. *Neurology* 1996; 46(Suppl 1):S14–S16.

113. Boucher BA, Feler CA, Dean JC, et al. The safety, tolerability, and pharmacokinetics of fosphenytoin after intramuscular and intravenous administration in neurosurgery patients. *Pharmacotherapy* 1996; 16:638–645.

114. Browne TR, Kugler AR, Eldon MA. Pharmacology and pharmacokinetics of fosphenytoin. *Neurology* 1996; 46(Suppl 1):S3–S7.

115. Lai CM, Moore P, Quon CY. Binding of fosphenytoin, phosphate ester pro drug of phenytoin, to human serum proteins and competitive binding with carbamazepine, diazepam, phenobarbital, phenylbutazone, phenytoin, valproic acid or warfarin. *Res Commun Mol Pathol Pharmacol* 1995; 88:51–62.

116. Fierro LS, Savulich DH, Benezra DA. Safety of fosphenytoin sodium. *Am J Health Syst Pharm* 1996; 53:2707–2712.

117. Browne TR. Fosphenytoin (Cerebyx). *Clin Neuropharmacol* 1997; 20:1–12.

118. Luer MS. Fosphenytoin. *Neurol Res* 1998; 20:178–182.

119. Jamerson BD, Dukes GE, Brouwer KL, et al. Venous irritation related to intravenous administration of phenytoin versus fosphenytoin. *Pharmacotherapy* 1994; 14:47–52.

120. O'Brien TJ, Cascino GD, So EL, Hanna DR. Incidence and clinical consequence of the purple glove syndrome in patients receiving intravenous phenytoin. *Neurology* 1998; 51:1034–1039.

121. Kupferberg HJ. Other hydantoins: mephenytoin and ethotoin. In: Levy RH, Mattson RH, and Meldrum BS, eds. *Antiepileptic Drugs*. 4th ed. New York: Raven Press, 1995:351–357.

122. Bourgeois BF, Kupfer A, Wad N, Egli M. Pharmacokinetics of R-enantiomeric normephenytoin during chronic administration in epileptic patients. *Epilepsia* 1986; 27:412–418.

123. Troupin AS, Ojemann LM, Dodrill CB. Mephenytoin: a reappraisal. *Epilepsia* 1976; 17:403–414.

124. Carter CA. Helms RA. Boehm R. Ethotoin in seizures of childhood and adolescence. *Neurology* 1984; 34:791–795.

CHAPTER 30

Carbamazepine and Oxcarbazepine

W. Edwin Dodson, M.D.

Since it was introduced in 1962 for the treatment of trigeminal neuralgia, carbamazepine (CBZ) has been found to be effective for the treatment of epilepsy. It has also been reported to benefit neuropathic pain, certain behavior disorders, and affective disorders. At first CBZ was used to replace sedating antiepileptic drugs (AEDs), but it soon became the initial therapy for many patients who have either localization-related epilepsy with partial (focal) seizures or epilepsy with generalized tonic-clonic seizures. Although CBZ produces side effects in many patients, the relative lack of sedation and the low incidence of cosmetic, cognitive, and behavioral side effects are advantages. The major disadvantages have been its propensity to cause rash and to aggravate absence and astatic seizures in patients with generalized epilepsy.

ACTIONS

Carbamazepine is effective in partial (focal seizures), especially complex partial (psychomotor) seizures and generalized tonic-clonic (grand mal) seizures (1,2). It is ineffective in febrile seizures and absence seizures. Furthermore, children with the Lennox-Gastaut syndrome sometimes have CBZ-induced worsening of several types of seizures, especially atypical absence seizures and astatic seizures or drop attacks (3–7). Nonetheless, numerous studies have shown that CBZ is just as effective as other major anticonvulsants when prescribed for the appropriate type of seizure (8–18). For example, in benign rolandic epilepsy, a pediatric epileptic syndrome that is characterized by partial seizures, CBZ is effective in 94 percent of patients and produces complete control in 65 percent. Given its comparable efficacy to other first-line anticonvulsants, the somewhat unique spectrum of adverse effects associated with CBZ differentiates it from other AEDs.

Although different rates of response to CBZ have been linked to age and gender, these differences appear to be small.

Carbamazepine has been reported to be more effective in girls than in boys (19) and is more effective in older patients than in children (19,20). The causes of these differences are most likely pharmacokinetic, although they may also relate to distribution of seizure types in various age groups. For example, lower CBZ concentrations have been found among nonresponding children (21). Furthermore, young children have accelerated relative clearance of CBZ compared with older children. Partial or generalized tonic-clonic seizures are the predominant seizure types in 55 percent and 90 percent of children and adults, respectively (22,23).

Carbamazepine limits use-dependent increases in sodium conductance and restricts neuronal high-frequency discharges, a mechanism similar to that of phenytoin but different from that of barbiturates, benzodiazepines, valproate, and suximides (24). This profile of activity correlates with clinical efficacy against partial and generalized tonic-clonic seizures. In experimental animal brains CBZ concentrations of $3.5–4.5\,\mu g/g$ prevent maximal electroshock-induced seizures (25).

Carbamazepine in therapeutic concentrations has few effects on the electroencephalogram (EEG). It does not produce frontal low-voltage fast activity like that caused by barbiturates and benzodiazepines (26). High concentrations of CBZ produce generalized slowing. The effect of CBZ on seizure activity in the EEG varies depending on its efficacy. When CBZ is effective in preventing seizures, focal spikes at first become more brief and sharp and eventually may disappear (27). Discontinuation of CBZ is associated with an increase in the mean dominant rhythm frequency (28). Generalized spike and spike-wave abnormalities either are unaffected by carbamazepine or worsen (20).

Other uses of CBZ include the treatment of chronic neurogenic pain (29,30), affective disorders (31), and hemifacial spasm (32). CBZ also has psychotropic actions and has been used in affective disorders, to treat attention deficit hyperactivity disorder in children, and in other psychiatric conditions (33–37). Among impulsive hyperkinetic children with attention deficit disorder, the administration of CBZ is preferred over barbiturates, benzodiazepines, and vigabatrin and other GABA agonists because the latter cause worsening of behavior in a substantial percentage of patients (38–44).

When patients who have side effects caused by other anticonvulsants are switched to CBZ, overall functioning often improves. Subjectively, these changes are described as less dulling of mentation, a steadier gait, and improved attention and alertness (41,44). The improvement is most dramatic among patients who are switched from multidrug regimens that include barbiturates to monotherapy with CBZ. On the other hand, CBZ does not enhance cognitive function or behavior in otherwise normal patients unless seizures are occurring frequently enough to impair thinking.

Carbamazepine is also beneficial in affective disorders—both depression and mania—an important consideration in many patients with epilepsy (33, 45–48). CBZ has been used in combination with lithium to treat refractory depression, refractory mania, and rapid cycling depression (49–51). It also may be beneficial in the dyscontrol syndrome, a disorder characterized by episodic aggressive outbursts (52,53).

CHEMISTRY AND METABOLISM

Carbamazepine is a tricyclic compound that is related to iminostilbene (54). Although the two-dimensional structure of CBZ resembles that of tricyclic antidepressants, its three-dimensional conformation is more akin to that of phenytoin. CBZ is a hydroscopic, neutral, lipophilic chemical that is soluble in organic solvents but possesses low water solubility. Because of its limited aqueous solubility, CBZ has been impossible to formulate for parenteral administration thus far. The crystal structure and dissolution rate of CBZ are sensitive to the degree of hydration. Exposure to high humidity leads to increasing hydration of CBZ, causing the progressive development of a crystalline lattice that resists dissolution and is thereby insoluble. Thus, patients who take CBZ that has been crystallized by high humidity and warmth are likely to experience a drop in CBZ levels.

Carbamazepine is eliminated largely by hepatic metabolism. Unique among unsaturated heterocyclic chemicals, the predominant elimination pathway in humans results in the formation of a stable epoxide that accumulates in serum. This compound, carbamzepine-10-11 epoxide (CBZE) has actions similar to those of CBZ, but it is less potent in experimental models of epilepsy (54). The epoxide is subsequently hydrolyzed to form an inactive 10,11-dihydroxide, the principal urinary metabolite. Lesser amounts of CBZ are metabolized by aromatic hydroxylation of the lateral rings. CBZ also induces hepatic cytochrome P-450 enzymes, which are responsible for the metabolism of several other antiepileptic drugs.

PHARMACOKINETICS

Carbamazepine has linear, predictable elimination kinetics. In individual patients, but not in groups of patients, the relationship between CBZ dose and concentration is linear and predictable (56–58). However, when standardized doses of CBZ are given to a large group, there is a wide scatter in the concentrations because of individual differences in CBZ elimination. Therefore, little or no correlation is found between CBZ doses and concentrations in groups (58,59). For this reason, measurement of CBZ concentrations in blood is an important aspect of individualizing CBZ doses.

Elimination

Carbamazepine induces its own metabolism by simulating the activity of the CYP3A4 component of cytochrome P-450 (60). This process of inducing its own metabolism is called *autoinduction* (55,61). Autoinduction causes the elimination rate of CBZ to increase in the days that follow the initiation or modification of doses. Because this process takes several weeks to evolve fully, CBZ pharmacokinetics have also been described as *time-dependent kinetics*. Among both children and adults who have not previously taken hepatic enzyme–inducing drugs, the half-life of CBZ decreases approximately 50 percent as autoinduction takes place. In adults the half-life declines from approximately 36 hours after the first dose to 18 to 20 hours following chronic monotherapy (55,61). Similarly, studies in children indicate that CBZ clearance doubles (0.028 L/kg/hr to 0.056 L/kg/hr) after two or three weeks of therapy (62). Therefore, in all age groups, autoinduction causes levels to be approximately 50 percent of what would be predicted from first-dose pharmacokinetics. Autoinduction is usually complete three to six weeks after the CBZ dose is changed.

It is important to recognize autoinduction and not to mistake it for noncompliance. If consistent doses are given during the first weeks of treatment, the concentration of CBZ increases at first and then declines. When seizures are initially controlled but then recur, autoinduction causing reduced CBZ levels may be the explanation. Measuring serum drug levels can help clarify the situation.

The half-life of the epoxide metabolite has been estimated to range from 10 to 20 hours in patients who stopped taking CBZ (61,63). When CBZE was administered to normal volunteers, a shorter half-life of 6.1 ± 0.9 hours was found (64). Among this same group of subjects, the half-life of CBZ was 26 ± 4.6 hours, but autoinduction probably was incomplete.

Carbamazepine elimination is influenced by age, pregnancy, and drug interactions (65). As with other AEDs, the clearance of CBZ is much higher in young children but declines to adult values in the later years of childhood. Younger patients and pregnant women in their last trimester have higher clearance rates and require higher relative doses than other patients (66). They also have higher ratios of CBZE to CBZ (67,68).

The ratio of CBZE to CBZ is 10 percent to 15 percent in adults. The ratio is higher in children and pregnant women, ranging up to 20 percent. The ratio can exceed 50 percent in certain drug interactions involving valproate. Valproate elevates the ratio because it inhibits epoxide hydrolase and increases the epoxide concentration.

Absorption Rate Varies with Formulation

The bioavailability of CBZ has been estimated to be 75 percent to 85 percent (55,69). Food variably increases the rate of absorption (55). Larger doses may be absorbed more slowly than smaller ones. Slow absorption facilitates once-daily administration in some patients. However, most authorities recommend more frequent administration to minimize the chance of side effects (44,70) and to counteract the effect of forgotten doses.

Carbamazepine is absorbed slowly after oral administration of tablets, with peak concentrations occurring 4–8 hours after ingestion (25). This slow absorption results from the slow dissolution of CBZ tablets. For this reason, CBZ absorption has been described as dissolution-rate-limited (55). Variations in the CBZ formulation significantly affects the tablet rate of dissolution and thus the absorption rate. Newer formulations have been designed to slow

absorption even more . Suspensions and certain generic formulations are absorbed more rapidly than proprietary Tegretol. For some patients, especially children in whom CBZ has a short half-life, rapid absorption confounds the problem.

Slow absorption of CBZ is preferred for most patients. Generic formulations tend to be absorbed more rapidly than Tegretol or other formulations designed for slow absorption. For patients who require high, nearly toxic concentrations of CBZ for seizure control, switching to a more rapidly absorbed generic formulation can cause both seizure relapse and side effects because of wider fluctuations in CBZ concentrations between doses. Thus, substitution of generic CBZ must be considered on a case-by-case basis. Generic CBZ is suitable mainly for those patients with mild epilepsy who are treated adequately with low levels.

Rapid elevation of the CBZ concentration is desirable for certain patients such as those who have completed video-EEG recording to determine whether they are candidates for epilepsy surgery or those who need their drugs switched rapidly. The administration of 8 mg/kg of CBZ suspension or tablets produces therapeutic levels in 2 and 5 hours, respectively (71,72).

Recognizing the desirability of slow formulations of CBZ, manufacturers have introduced slowly absorbed formulations that retard drug release in the gastrointestinal (GI) tract. A crystalline matrix formulation has been used in Europe, whereas an osmotically released formulation (Tegretol-XR) is available in the United States. This formulation consists of an osmotic core surrounded by a semipermeable membrane. When water enters the chamber in the center of the drug delivery system, it forces the drug out of the delivery orifice into the GI tract. Crystalline matrix "retard" formulations (marketed as Timonil Retard or Tegretol Retard in Europe) also significantly attenuate the fluctuation index between doses (73,74). In some patients this allows twice daily dosing, which is more convenient, encourages compliance, and reduces the chance of side effects (74).

Carbatrol is yet another slow-release formulation of CBZ. This formulation is a mixture of CBZ beads with three different coatings that dissolve at different rates. The so-called immediate coating dissolves quickly and initiates absorption. A slow-release coating of other beads is removed more slowly and releases the CBZ later. Finally, a pH-sensitive coating triggers dissolution in the alkaline pH of the small intestine (75). Both Tegretol-XR and Carbatrol can be substituted mg for mg for other CBZ formulations, including each other. Tegretol-XR is available in 100-mg, 200-mg, and 400-mg tablets. Carbatrol comes in 200-mg and 300-mg capsules (77–79). For more information about CBZ formulations, see Chapter 24.

Distribution

Carbamazepine and CBZE distribute throughout the body. The volume of distribution for CBZ ranges from 0.93 to 1.28 L/kg (25). The brain to plasma ratio of both CBZ and CBZE is approximately 1, with a range of 0.8 to 1.6 (25,79). Approximately 75 percent and 50 percent of CBZ and CBZE are bound to albumin, respectively (25). Concentrations of CBZ and CBZE in cerebrospinal fluid (CSF) are consistent with the protein-binding values in serum, and CSF concentrations equal the unbound fractions in plasma. The CSF to plasma concentration ratios average 0.25 and 0.50 for CBZ and CBZE, respectively. The binding of these compounds is low enough that unless CBZ levels are high, the consequences of altered CBZ binding to constituents of plasma are usually trivial and do not justify routine measurement (80). Salivary concentrations of CBZ also approximate the unbound concentrations in plasma, although the ratio of CBZ levels in plasma versus saliva varies during the day (81).

Carbamazepine crosses the placenta and penetrates breast milk. Transplacentally acquired CBZ concentrations in newborns at birth correlate highly with those found in maternal plasma (58). Newborns who have been exposed to CBZ in utero experience autoinduction of CBZ metabolism and eliminate CBZ at rates comparable to those of adults. Among newborns acquiring CBZ transplacentally, the reported half-lives have ranged from 8.2 to 28.1 hours (58). Among mothers taking CBZ, concentrations in breast milk are so low that nursing infants rarely ingest a substantial dose.

Drug Interactions

Pharmacokinetic drug interactions involve both CBZ metabolism and CBZ binding to serum protein (82). Numerous drugs, including other anticonvulsants, alter the enzymatic metabolism of CBZ. Phenytoin, phenobarbital, and primidone usually induce CBZ biotransformation (83). Phenobarbital has the greatest effect, reducing the average half-life to 10–11 hours in adults. Phenytoin has an intermediate effect, lowering the half-life to 14 hours. Adult patients taking all three together have an average half-life of 10.6 hours (63). Among patients receiving polytherapy, CBZ half-lives may be as short as 5 hours (84), considerably shorter than the average values of 18–20 hours reported for adults on CBZ monotherapy.

Valproate increases the unbound fraction of both CBZ and CBZE, and it inhibits the hydrolysis of CBZE by epoxide hydrolase, thereby increasing the ratio of

CBZE to CBZ (67,68). Under these circumstances, the valproate concentration correlates with the unbound CBZ fraction (85). Valproate and valpromide reduce the clearance of CBZE by inhibiting hepatic microsomal epoxide hydrolase (86,87). The highest CBZE concentrations, which sometimes exceed 50 percent of the CBZ level, occur when CBZ is administered simultaneously with both an inducing agent, such as phenytoin, and valproate. In these situations, CBZE levels may be high enough to contribute to neurotoxicity. Routine CBZ levels do not include CBZE.

Patients with "therapeutic" concentrations of both phenytoin and CBZ sometimes develop side effects (61). There also is evidence of a pharmacodynamic interaction between CBZ and phenytoin in experimental animals (88). Pharmacodynamic interactions take place in the target organ and are not secondary to changes in drug concentrations. Morris and coworkers (88) found that in mice the therapeutic index of combined CBZ and phenytoin was no better than either drug given alone. Both efficacy in prevention of seizures and neurotoxicity increased when these drugs were given simultaneously. Although comparable data in humans are lacking, it is highly likely that the toxicities of CBZ and phenytoin are additive.

A toxic pharmacodynamic interaction has also been described between CBZ and lamotrigine (89). Patients who had CBZ concentrations greater than 8 μg/mL developed diplopia and dizziness after lamotrigine was added, even though the CBZ concentration did not change and lamotrigine levels were in the nontoxic range. The side effects abated after the CBZ dose was decreased.

Carbamazepine also accelerates the metabolism of folic acid and biotin (90). Folic acid deficiency can cause psychiatric symptoms and should be considered when patients who have been treated chronically with inducing AEDs develop psychiatric symptoms (91). Even more critical, folate deficiency during pregnancy has been linked to neural tube defects, and folate supplementation has been recommended for all women of childbearing potential. (92,93). Needless to say, folate supplementation is twice as important for women with epilepsy. Although CBZ has significant effects on folate levels, it has not been linked to abnormal bone or calcium metabolism as other AEDs have (94).

Several drugs inhibit CBZ elimination and cause CBZ levels to increase (Table 30-1). Isoniazid and CBZ increase the concentration of each other (95). Among the macrolide antibiotics, erythromycin, triacetyloleandomycin, and clarithromycin inhibit the biotransformation of CBZ, causing predictable increases in CBZ levels and neurotoxicity if the CBZ dose is not reduced (97–101). Other macrolide antibiotics have weaker and inconsistent effects on CBZ levels. Several antidepressants and selective sertonin reuptake

Table 30-1. Reference Information

Carbamazepine (CBZ)

Molecular weight	236.26
Conversion factor	

$$CF = \frac{1000}{236.26} = 4.23$$

Conversion: μg/mL or mg/L × 4.32 = μmoles/L

Carbamazepine-10,11-Epoxide (CBZE)

Molecular weight	252.3
Conversion factor	

$$CF = \frac{1000}{252.3} = 3.96$$

Conversion: μg/mL (or mg/L) × 3.96 = μmoles/L

Ratio of CBZE to CBZ	
Monotherapy	0.10–0.20
Polytherapy	0.15–0.66

Source: Morselli PL. Carbamazepine absorption, distribution and excretion. In: Levy RH, Mattson RH, Meldrum BS, eds. *Antiepileptic Drugs.* 4th ed. New York: Raven Press, 1995:515–528. Faigle JW, Feldman KF. Carbamazepine: chemistry and biotransformation. In: Levy RH, Mattson RH, Meldrum BS, eds. *Antiepileptic Drugs.* 4th ed. New York: Raven Press, 1995:499–513.

inhibitors are competitive substrates with CBZ for CYP3A4 (101). Dextropropoxyphene and the antidepressant viloxazine increase CBZ levels after chronic administration (87,102). Nicotinamide, which is chemically related to isoniazid, also inhibits CBZ elimination, causing CBZ concentrations to increase (103). CBZ does not interact with disulfiram (104) or cimetidine (105), which are metabolized by CYP2C9 and CYP2C19 but not by CYP3A4 (107–109).

Add-on therapy with CBZ reduces the concentrations of other anticonvulsants that are eliminated by hepatic metabolism because it is a potent inducer of cytochrome P-450 (106). CBZ causes ethosuximide levels to decline by an average of 17 percent (109) and lowers valproate levels twice as much, increasing the

clearance of valproate by one-third or more (110). The addition of CBZ to phenytoin usually decreases phenytoin concentrations, but the mechanism of the interaction is complex, with CBZ decreasing both the V_{MAX} and the K_M of phenytoin elimination (111) because it stimulates the activity of cytochromes CYP2C9 and CYP2C19, both of which catalyze phenytoin elimination (106).

The induction of CBZ elimination by other drugs changes the relationship between CBZ dose and concentration. Among children on monotherapy each 2-mg/kg/day dose increases the CBZ concentration by 1 μg/mL. When other AEDs are given simultaneously, more than 3 mg/kg/day are required to increase the CBZ concentration by 1 μg/mL (58). Typically, patients on polytherapy have lower concentrations despite higher doses (112). Furthermore, patients on polytherapy need more frequent doses to avoid intermittent side effects that occur because of wide fluctuations in serum levels (70).

Changes of Drug Regimens That Involve CBZ

When adding or deleting CBZ, remember that other inducers of hepatic cytochrome P-450 enhance CBZ metabolism and vice versa. Therefore, when CBZ is added to an AED regimen, it usually lowers the concentration of other AEDs that are subject to hepatic biotransformation. For this reason, the dose of the first drug should be held constant as CBZ is added until the concentration of the CBZ exceeds 4 μg/L. Then the original drug can be tapered over a period of three or more weeks, depending on the drug. After this is completed, the CBZ level usually increases if the drug that was replaced was a cytochrome P-450 inducer. This process in which discontinuation of an inducing drug leads to an increase in drug level is called *disinduction* (71,113). The autoinduction of CBZ is also subject to disinduction when CBZ is discontinued (113).

Table 30-2. Carbamazepine Administration and Pharmacokinetics

Type of elimination kinetics	Linear
Special pharmacokinetic features	Autoinduction; dissolution rate-limited absorption
Maintenance dose	10–20 mg/kg/day
Therapeutic concentration range	4–12 mg/L
Half-life (range)	5–36 hours*
Formulations	
Suspension (Tegretol)	50 mg/mL
Chewable tablet (Tegretol)	100 mg
Tablet (Tegretol, generic)	200 mg
Sustained-release granules (Carbitrol)	200, 400
Sustained-release (Tegretol XR)	100, 200, 400

*Half-life varies with duration of therapy (autoinduction), age, pregnancy, and comedication.
Source: Morselli PL. Carbamazepine absorption, distribution and excretion. In: Levy RH, Mattson RH, Meldrum BS, eds. *Antiepileptic Drugs.* 4th ed. New York: Raven Press, 1995:515–528.

Table 30-3. Pharmacokinetic Drug Interactions Involving CBZ

Decrease CBZ Action
Phenytoin
Phenobarbital
Primidone

Increase CBZ Action
Danazole
Diltiazem
Erythromycin
Isoniazid
Nicotinamide
Propoxyphene
Triacetyloleandomycin
Valproic acid
Verapamil
Viloxazine

Drugs Whose Actions Are Decreased by CBZ
Clonazepam
Doxycycline
Ethosuximide
Felbamate
Haloperidol
Lamotrigine
Phenytoin*
Steroid contraceptives
Tiagabine
Topiramate
Valproic acid
warfarin

*Interaction is variable. CBZ usually decreases phenytoin levels, but the opposite sometimes occurs (189).
Source: Delcker A, Wilhelm H, Timmann D, Diener HC. Side effects from increased doses of carbamazepine on neuropsychological and posturographic parameters of humans. *Eur Neuropsychopharmacol* 1997; 7:213–218.

This disinduction occurs rather rapidly, and if CBZ is restarted at the same dose after having been stopped for only a few days, this can result in toxic CBZ levels. Because discontinuation of benzodiazepines may evoke withdrawal seizures, they should be reduced quite slowly, usually over several months to years. Furthermore, patients with severe epilepsy who are having frequent seizures may need to be hospitalized while their regimens are simplified because of the risk of provoking convulsive status epilepticus by changing the medications.

ADVERSE EFFECTS OF CBZ

Carbamazepine is one of the best-tolerated anticonvulsants (115–117). Although some authorities report side effects in as many as 63 percent of patients (117,118), most of the side effects do not warrant discontinuation of therapy. In one pediatric study, 43 percent had side effects; however, these were usually mild and tolerable such that only 3 percent discontinued the medication and another 3 percent required a dose reduction (115). The most frequent neurologic side effect, drowsiness, occurred in 11 percent. GI complaints were uncommon. Tolerance to the neurologic side effects of CBZ develops in chronic therapy, and many of them abate completely (114). As with most other AEDs, starting at a low dose and slowly escalating to the desired maintenance dose causes fewer side effects than rapidly raising the dose or starting at full maintenance dose (119).

Side effects are increasingly common at concentrations above 12 µg/mL. Unbound CBZ levels correlate better with neurotoxicity than total CBZ levels in serum (70). Unbound CBZ concentrations of 1.7 µg/mL or more usually produce side effects. High levels of CBZ cause sedation, vertigo, and ophthalmoplegia resulting in the "3-D" triad of drowsiness, dizziness, and diplopia (8,10,26,120). Brief episodes of toxicity can result from transient elevations of CBZ concentrations because of fluctuations between doses (74,118–121). In these situations it is necessary to administer smaller, more frequent doses or, better yet, switch to a slow-release CBZ formulation. When concentrations are below 8 µg/mL, dose-related side effects are uncommon unless therapy has been initiated rapidly with high doses or unless the patient is taking other medications that have side effects that are additive to the side effects of CBZ (59,122). Overdoses have been associated with symptoms resembling the central anticholinergic syndrome similar to that caused by tricyclic antidepressants (123,124).

Whereas high concentrations consistently cause neurologic side effects, at usual concentrations CBZ appears to have few if any effects on cognitive function (125–127). See Chapter 50 or more information about the cognitive side effects of CBZ and other drugs.

Hyponatremia caused by CBZ occurs in patients of any age (128) but is more common among the elderly (129,130). It is usually mild and asymptomatic in children (130). Oxcarbazepine is much more likely to cause hyponatremia than CBZ, and this can be problematic (131). Hyponatremia is not a side effect of other anticonvulsant drugs. Interestingly, CBZ-induced hyponatremia is said to be reversed by phenytoin (132).

Chronic side effects of CBZ differ from those of other anticonvulsants. In contrast to phenobarbital and phenytoin, CBZ monotherapy has not been associated with anticonvulsant-induced osteomalacia (133–135). Similarly, among the AEDs CBZ is one of the least likely to cause cosmetic side effects. Gingival hyperplasia is not a problem with CBZ monotherapy (136).

Carbamazepine variably affects other laboratory tests. It lowers the plasma concentrations of thyroid-binding globulin and both bound and unbound T3 and T4 (137), but clinical hypothyroidism is rare among patients taking CBZ. Among the anticonvulsants used to treat major seizures, CBZ is least likely to elevate the gamma-glutamyl transpeptidase (138).

Idiosyncratic neurologic adverse reactions include behavioral reactions, tics, asterixis, dystonia, and worsening of seizures, especially atonic or astatic seizures in children with Lennox-Gastaut syndrome (3,140–143). Dystonia induced by CBZ at usual doses in brain-damaged children is rare and apparently idiosyncratic (143); it is more common with CBZ poisoning and high levels (144). Patients with cerebellar atrophy develop gaze-evoked nystagmus, dizziness, and ataxia at lower CBZ doses and levels than patients who have normal magnetic resonance imaging (). Acute idiosyncratic, adverse behavioral reactions have occurred among children with psychiatric disorders. Silverstein and coworkers (146) reported episodic bizarre behavior in seven pediatric patients after CBZ was added; however, five of the seven children tolerated CBZ when it was reintroduced later.

Hematological Side Effects

Severe idiosyncratic hematological toxicity, such as aplastic anemia, agranulocytosis, or thrombocytopenia, is rare among patients taking CBZ (148–152). The incidence of these complications has been estimated to be less that 1 per 50,000 (151). Thus, is spite of previous concerns, experience has shown CBZ to be safe.

On the other hand, CBZ is associated with a dose-dependent reduction in neutrophil counts in 10 percent to 20 percent of patients. Leukopenia occurred in 2.1 percent of adult psychiatric patients who took CBZ and was approximately seven times more likely with CBZ than with valproate or antidepressants (152). For example, in one study of 200 children taking CBZ, leukopenia (white blood count $< 4,000$ per mm^3) occurred in 17 percent of patients less than 12 years old and 8 percent of children aged 12 to 17 years (153). These changes sometimes persist but usually do not forebode serious problems (9). Rarely does the neutrophil count decline below 1,200 per mm^3 (152). For this reason, the justification for costly, routine monitoring of blood counts has been questioned (151).

Although there is agreement about obtaining baseline blood counts, there is no consensus about how often blood counts should be determined during CBZ therapy (147,148). Some authorities almost never perform blood counts; others obtain them weekly at the onset of CBZ therapy and then monthly. Emphasizing that many factors influence the white blood count simultaneously, Silverstein and coworkers recommended doing blood counts monthly during the first six months of therapy and every three months thereafter (153).

When starting CBZ, I check blood counts at baseline and after six weeks, three months, and six months if the counts are adequate. If the leukocyte count is consistently at or above 3,500 per mm^3 and granulocytes are higher than 1,200, the frequency of the measurements can be reduced. Because of the possibility of a spurious laboratory result, neutrophil counts below 1,200 per mm^3 and leukocyte counts lower than 3,500 per mm^3 should be repeated to confirm the finding before therapy is modified. If the neutrophil count is confirmed to be less than 1,200 per mm^3, the frequency of the observations should be increased. The dose should be reduced or stopped if the neutrophil count is persistently below 900 per mm^3.

If both anemia and neutropenia occur, obtaining a reticulocyte count, serum iron concentration, and iron-binding capacity provides an indirect indication of hematopoietic activity. The combination of a normal or elevated reticulocyte count with a normal or low iron level is reassuring that the bone marrow is active. On the other hand, a low reticulocyte count plus an increased serum iron concentration indicate that hematopoietic activity is reduced. CBZ should be stopped promptly if this occurs, and a hematologist should be consulted regarding a bone marrow evaluation.

Allergic rash is the most common reason that patients are intolerant of CBZ. The incidence of rash has varied from 4 percent to 10 percent in various series (14,21,118) and may result from the intradermal production of reactive CBZ metabolites (154). Data from a Saskatchewan study indicate that the risk of serious rash is about the same with CBZ as with phenytoin, approximately 1 to 4 per 10,000 (155). Most CBZ-induced rashes abate after CBZ is discontinued, but severe rashes have been described (156,157) Approximately 1 in 3,000 patients who are treated for epilepsy will develop hypersensitivity to multiple drugs. AEDs that have aromatic structures include phenytoin, primidone, and phenobarbital along with CBZ, and in some cases sulfonamides (159–162). Valproate and clobazam have been recommended when multiple drug sensitivities occur (162).

Hypersensitivity reactions characterized by fever and, renal and hepatic toxicity are very rare (150, 164–166). Hepatotoxicity caused by CBZ, like that caused by phenytoin, usually has occurred in the setting of a generalized hypersensitivity response (166). Most of the patients who have developed CBZ-induced hepatic dysfunction have taken it for less than one month and usually have associated fever or rash (167,168). The hepatic histopathology usually indicates an inflammatory granulomatous infiltrate, but a different pathologic picture consistent with chemical hepatic insult also occurs (169). Furthermore, some cases have occurred when CBZ was administered with other potentially hepatotoxic agents such as isoniazid (170). In either case, fatalities are uncommon if the drug is stopped promptly (171,172).

Other rare idiosyncratic reactions include systemic lupus erythematosus and pseudolymphoma (174–178). Most of the cases of pseudolymphoma seem to be manifestations of the CBZ hypersensitivity syndrome.

MONOTHERAPY

Monotherapy with CBZ is often superior to polytherapy. Approximately 80 percent of patients with only generalized tonic-clonic seizures (grand mal) can be controlled with CBZ alone, as can 69 percent of patients with partial seizures of certain types (20). The most difficult patients are those who have both partial and secondarily generalized seizures, in whom single drug therapy succeeds in less than half. Although most authorities agree that such patients deserve a trial of therapy with drug combinations, all patients should have a diligent trial of monotherapy before resorting to polytherapy. Among patients with severe epilepsy, combinations of CBZ, phenytoin, and phenobarbital are more efficacious than monotherapy, but severe side effects are prevalent. Cereghino and coworkers (178) found that 68 percent of adults who took these drugs concurrently had excessive sleepiness, malaise, and impaired abilities to conduct their daily activities.

In the end, the impairment caused by neurotoxicity must be weighed against the handicap caused by the seizures. The regimen that allows the patient to function optimally is best. Many patients with persistent seizures and side effects on polytherapy are better off after having their regimens simplified (179,180). Schmidt was able to switch 83 percent of patients with intractable complex partial seizures from two medications to CBZ monotherapy with fewer side effects but no increase in seizure frequency; 36 percent had fewer seizures (181). In another series, 75 percent of 280 patients had adequate seizure control with monotherapy (118). In yet another series involving mentally retarded institutionalized patients, seizure control was no different with monotherapy than with polytherapy (182). Thus, many patients who are having both side effects and seizures benefit from a simplified regimen.

OXCARBAZEPINE

This compound is the 10-keto analogue of CBZ and is preferred over CBZ in Scandinavia. Oxcarbazepine (Trileptal) is rapidly metabolized to an active 10-hydroxy metabolite, which is responsible for most of the antiepileptic effect. Whereas the half-life of oxcarbazepine is 1 to 2.5 hours, the half-life of the hydroxy metabolite is 8 to 10 hours (183,184). Both oxcarbazepine and its metabolite have a spectrum of activity that is similar to that of CBZ. In contrast to CBZ, oxcarbazepine does not induce hepatic drug metabolism in humans and autoinduction is not an issue. Oxcarbazepine has a lower incidence of allergic reactions and is less neurotoxic (186–189); however, it causes symptomatic hyponatremia more frequently than does CBZ.

Oxcarbazepine is effective as add-on therapy in refractory seizures and as initial therapy in new-onset seizures (189). In a double-blind, randomized study that compared oxcarbazepine with phenytoin in 193 children aged 5 to 18 years with new-onset or partial generalized tonic-clonic seizures, efficacy was equivalent, with approximately 60 percent of subjects in each group becoming seizure-free (190). Oxcarbazepine was better tolerated, however, because more subjects discontinued phenytoin because of adverse effects.

REFERENCES

1. Loiseau P, Duche B. Carbamazepine clinical use. In: Levy RH, Mattson RH, Meldrum BS, eds. *Antiepileptic Drugs*. 4th ed. New York: Raven Press, 1995:555–566.
2. Dodson WE. Carbamazepine efficacy and utilization in children. *Epilepsia* 1987; 28(Suppl 3):S17–S24.
3. Snead OC, Hosey LC. Exacerbation of seizures in children by carbamazepine. *N Engl J Med* 1985; 313:916–921.
4. Bauer J. Seizure-inducing effects of antiepileptic drugs: a review. *Acta Neurol Scand* 1996; 94:367–377.
5. Guerrini R, Belmonte A, Genton P. Antiepileptic drug-induced worsening of seizures in children. *Epilepsia* 1998; 39(Suppl 3):S2–S10.
6. Berkovic SF. Aggravation of generalized epilepsies. *Epilepsia* 1998; 39(Suppl 3):S11–S14.
7. Parker AP, Agathonikou A, Robinson RO, Panayiotopoulos CP. Inappropriate use of carbamazepine and vigabatrin in typical absence seizures. *Dev Med Child Neurol* 1998; 40:517–519.
8. Livingston S, Villamatar C, Sakata Y, Pauli LL. Use of carbamazepine in epilepsy. *JAMA* 1967; 200:116–119.
9. Livingston S, Pauli LL, Berman W. Carbamazepine (Tegretol) in epilepsy. *Dis Nerv Sys* 1974; 35:103–107.
10. Cereghino JJ, Brock JT, Van Meter JC, et al. Carbamazepine for epilepsy. *Neurology* 1974; 24:401–410.
11. Gram L, Bentsen KD, Parnas J, Flachs H. Controlled trials in epilepsy: a review. *Epilepsia* 1982; 23:491–519.
12. Simonsen N, Zander-Olsen P, Kuhl V, et al. A comparative controlled study between carbamazepine and diphenylhydantion in psychomotor epilepsy. *Epilepsia* 1976; 17:169–176.

13. Kosteljanetz M, Christiansen J, Dam AM, et al. Carbamazepine versus phenytoin. A controlled clinical trial in focal motor and generalized epilepsy. *Arch Neurol* 1979; 36:22–24.

14. Ramsey, RE, Wilder BJ, Berger JR, Bruni J. A double-blind study comparing carbamazepine with phenytoin as initial seizure therapy in adults. *Neurology* 1983; 33:904–910.

15. Mitchell WG, Chavez JM. Carbamazepine versus phenobarbital for partial onset seizures in children. *Epilepsia* 1987; 28:56–60.

16. Mattson RH, Cramer JA, Collins JF, et al. Comparison of carbamazepine, phenobarbital, phenytoin, and primidone in partial and secondarily generalized tonic-clonic seizures. *N Engl J Med* 1985, 313:145–151.

17. Verity CM, Hosking G, Easter DJ. A multicentre comparative trial of sodium valproate and carbamazepine in paediatric epilepsy. The Paediatric EPITEG Collaborative Group. *Dev Med Child Neurol* 1995; 37:97–108.

18. Ramsay RE, DeToledo J. Tonic-clonic seizures: a systematic review of antiepilepsy drug efficacy and safety. *Clin Ther* 1997; 19:433–446.

19. Rett A. The so-called psychotropic effect of Tegretol in the treatment of convulsions of cerebral origin in children. In: Birkmayer W, ed. *Epileptic Seizures-Behavior-Pain.* Baltimore: University Park Press, 1976:194–208.

20. Scheffner D, Schiefer I. The treatment of epileptic children with carbamazepine. *Epilepsia* 1972; 13:819–828.

21. Huf R, Schain RJ. Long-term experiences with carbamazepine (Tegretol) in children with seizures. *J Pediatr* 1980; 97:310–312.

22. Gastaut H, Gastaut GE, Silva GEG, Sanchez GFR. Relative frequency of different types of epilepsy: a study employing the classification of the International League Against Epilepsy. *Epilepsia* 1975; 16:457–461.

23. Cavazutti GB. Epidemiology of different types of epilepsy in school age children of Modena, Italy. *Epilepsia* 1980; 21:57–62.

24. Macdonald RL. Carbamazepine mechanisms of action In: Levy RH, Mattson RH, Meldrum BS, eds. *Antiepileptic Drugs.* 4th ed. New York: Raven Press, 1995:491–498.

25. Morselli PL. Carbamazepine absorption, distribution and excretion. In: Levy RH, Mattson RH, Meldrum BS, eds. *Antiepileptic Drugs.* 4th ed. New York: Raven Press, 1995:515–528.

26. Rodin EA, Rim CS, Rennick PM. The effects of carbamazepine on patients with psychomotor epilepsy: results of a double-blind study. *Epilepsia* 1974; 15:547–561.

27. Frost JD Jr, Kellaway P, Hrachovy RA, Glaze DG, Mizrahi EM. Changes in epileptic spike configuration associated with attainment of seizure control. *Ann Neurol* 1986; 20:723–726.

28. Duncan JS, Smith SJ, Forster A, Shorvon S, Trimble MR. Effects of the removal of phenytoin, carbamazepine, and valproate on the electroencephalogram. *Epilepsia* 1989; 30:590–596.

29. Swederlow M. Anticonvulsant drugs and chronic pain. *Clin Neuropharmacol* 1984; 7:51–82.

30. Leijon G, Boivie J. Central post-stroke pain—a controlled trial of amitriptyline and carbamazepine. *Pain* 1989, 36:27–36

31. Keck PE Jr, McElroy SL. Outcome in the pharmacologic treatment of bipolar disorder. *J Clin Psychopharmacol* 1996; 16(2 Suppl 1):15S–23S.

32. Shaywitz BA. Hemifacial spasm in childhood treated with carbamazepine. *Arch Neurol* 1974; 31:63.

33. Ballenger JC. The use of anticonvulsants in manic-depressive illness. *J Clin Psychiatry* 1988; 49(Suppl):21–25.

34. Silva RR, Munoz DM, Alpert M. Carbamazepine use in children and adolescents with features of attention-deficit hyperactivity disorder: a meta-analysis. *J Am Acad Child Adolesc Psychiatry* 1996; 35:352–358.

35. Hernandez-Avila CA, Ortega-Soto HA, Jasso A, Hasfura-Buenaga CA, Kranzler HR. Treatment of inhalant-induced psychotic disorder with carbamazepine versus haloperidol. *Psychiatr Serv* 1998; 49:812–815.

36. Greil W, Ludwig-Mayerhofer W, Erazo N, et al. Lithium vs carbamazepine in the maintenance treatment of schizoaffective disorder: a randomised study. *Eur Arch Psychiatry Clin Neurosci* 1997; 247:42–50.

37. Greil W, Ludwig-Mayerhofer W, et al. Lithium versus carbamazepine in the maintenance treatment of bipolar disorders—a randomised study. *J Affect Disord* 1997; 43:151–161.

38. Huf R, Schain RJ. Long-term experiences with carbamazepine (Tegretol) in children with seizures. *J Pediatr* 1980; 97:310–312.

39. Camfield CS, Chaplin S, Doyle A, et al. Side effects of phenobarbital in toddlers: behavioral and cognitive aspects. *J Pediatr* 1979; 95:361–365.

40. Wolf SM, Forsythe A. Behavior disturbance, phenobarbital and febrile seizures. *Pediatrics* 1978; 61:728–731.

41. Troupin AS, Green JR, Levy RH. Carbamazepine as an anticonvulsant: a pilot study. *Neurology* 1974; 24:863–869.

42. Vining EP, Mellitis ED, Dorsen MM, et al. Psychologic and behavioral effects of antiepileptic drugs in children: a double-blind comparison between phenobarbital and valproic acid. *Pediatrics* 1987; 80:165–174.

43. Trimble MR, Cull C. Children of school age: the influence of antiepileptic drugs on behavior and intellect. *Epilepsia* 1988; 29(Suppl 3):S15–S19.

44. Schain RJ, Ward JW, Guthrie D. Carbamazepine as an anticonvulsant in children. *Neurology* 1977; 27:476–480.

45. Trimble MR. Carbamazepine and mood: evidence from patients with seizure disorders. *J Clin Psychiatry* 1988; 49(Suppl):7–12.

46. Kobayashi T, Kishimoto A, Inagaki T. Treatment of periodic depression with carbamazepine. *Acta Psychiatr Scand* 1988; 77:364–367.

47. Post RM, Uhde TW, Rubinow DR, et al. Biochemical effects of carbamazepine: relationship to its mechanisms of action in affective illness. *Prog Neuropsychopharmacol Biol Psychiatry* 1983; 7:263–271.

48. Wunderlich HP, Grunes JU, Neumann J, et al. Antidepressive therapie mit carbamazepin (Finlepsin). *Schweiz Arch Neurol Neurochir Psychiatr* 1983; 133:363–371.

49. Arana GW, Santos AB, Knax EP, Ballenger JC. Refractory rapid cycling unipolar depression responds to lithium and carbamazepine treatment. *J Clin Psychiatry* 1989; 50:356–357.

50. Kramlinger KG, Post RM. The addition of lithium to carbamazepine. Antidepressant efficacy in treatment-resistant depression. *Arch Gen Psychiatry* 1989; 46:794–800.

51. Spurkland I, Vandvik IH. Rapid cycling depression in adolescence. A case treated with family therapy and carbamazepine. *Acta Psychiatr Scand* 1989; 80:60–63.

52. Tunks ER, Dermer SW. Carbamazepine in the dyscontrol syndrome associated with limbic system dysfunction. *J Nerv Ment Dis* 1977; 164:56–63.

53. Foster HG, Hillbrand M, Chi CC. Efficacy of carbamazepine in assaultive patients with frontal lobe dysfunction. *Prog Neuropsychopharmacol Biol Psychiatry* 1989; 13:865–874.

54. Faigle JW, Feldman KF. Carbamazepine: chemistry and biotransformation. In: Levy RH, Mattson RH, Meldrum BS, eds. *Antiepileptic Drugs.* 4th ed. New York: Raven Press, 1995:499–513.

55. Levy RH, Pitlick WH, Troupin AS, Green JR, Neal JM. Pharmacokinetics of carbamazepine in normal man. *Clin Pharmacol Ther* 1975; 17:657–668.

56. Perucca E, Bittencourt P, Richens A. Effect of dose increments on serum carbamazepine concentration in epileptic patients. *Clin Pharmacokinet* 1980, 5:576–582.

57. Kerr BM, Levy RH. Carbamazepine: carbamazepine epoxide. In: Levy RH, Mattson RH, Meldrum BS, eds. *Antiepileptic Drugs.* 4th ed. New York: Raven Press, 1995:529–541.

58. Rane A, Bengt H, Wilson JT. Kinetics of carbamazepine and its 10,11-epoxide metabolite in children. *Clin Pharmacol Ther* 1976; 19:276–283.

59. Tomson T, Tybring G, Bertilsson L, Ekbom K, Rane A. Carbamazepine therapy in trigeminal neuralgia. *Arch Neurol* 1980; 37:699–703.

60. Levy RH. Cytochrome P450 isozymes and antiepileptic drug interactions. *Epilepsia* 1995; 36(Suppl 5):S8–S13.

61. Eichelbaum M, Ekbom K, Bertilsson L, Ringberger VA, Rane A. Plasma kinetics of carbamazepine and its epoxide metabolite in man after single and multiple doses. *Clin Pharmacol* 1975; 8:337–341.

62. Bertilsson L, Bengt H, Gunnel T, et al. Autoinduction of carbamazepine metabolism in children examined by a stable isotope technique. *Clin Pharmacol Ther* 1980; 27:83–88.

63. Westenberg HGM, van der Kleijn E, Oei TT, de Zoeuw RA. Kinetics of carbamazepine and carbamazepine-epoxide determined by use of plasma and saliva. *Clin Pharmacol Ther* 1978; 23:320–328.

64. Tomson T, Tybring G, Bertilsson E, Bertilsson L. Single-dose kinetics and metabolism of carbamazepine-10,11-epoxide. *Clin Pharmacol Ther* 1983; 33:58–65.

65. Battino D, Bossi L, Croci D, et al. Carbamazepine plasma levels in children and adults: influence of age, dose, and associated therapy. *Ther Drug Mon* 1980; 2:315–322.

66. Pynnonen S, Sillanpaa M, Frey H, Iisalo E. Carbamazepine and its 10,11-epoxide in children and adults with epilepsy. *Eur J Clin Pharmacol* 1977; 11:129–133.

67. Brodie MJ, Forrest G, Papeport WG. Carbamazepine 10,11 epoxide concentrations in epileptics on carbamazepine alone and in combination with other anticonvulsants. *Brit J Clin Pharmacol* 1983; 16:747–749.

68. Robertson IG, Donnai D, DSouza S. Cranial nerve agenesis in a fetus exposed to carbamazepine. *Dev Med Child Neurol* 1983; 25:540–541.

69. Wada JA, Troupin AS, Friel P, Remick R, Leal K, Pearmain J. Pharmacokinetic comparison of tablet and suspension dosage forms of carbamazepine. *Epilepsia* 1978; 19:251–255.

70. Riva R, Albani F, Ambrosetto G, et al. Diurnal fluctuations in free and total steady-state plasma levels of carbamazepine and correlation with intermittent side effects. *Epilepsia* 1984; 25:476–481.

71. Cohen H, Howland MA, Luciano DJ, et al. Feasibility and pharmacokinetics of carbamazepine oral loading doses. *Am J Health Syst Pharm* 1998; 55:1134–1140.

72. Kanner AM, Bourgeois BF, Hasegawa H, Hutson P. Rapid switchover to carbamazepine using pharmacokinetic parameters. *Epilepsia* 1998; 39:194–200.

73. Jensen PK, Moller A, Gram L, Jensen NL, Dam M. Pharmacokinetic comparison of two carbamazepine slow-release formulations. *Acta Neurol Scand* 1990; 82:135–137.

74. Canger R, Altamura AC, Belvedere O, et al. Conventional vs controlled-release carabamazepine: a multicentre, double-blind, crossover study. *Acta Neurol Scand* 1990; 82:9–13.

75. Garnett WR, Levy B, McLean AM, et al. Pharmacokinetic evalution of twice daily extended-release carbamazepine (CBZ) in patients with epilepsy. *Epilepsia* 1998; 39:274–279.

76. The Tegretol OROS Osmotic Release Delivery System Study Group. Double-blind crossover comparison of Tegretol-XR and Tegretol in patients with epilepsy. *Neurology* 1995; 45:1703–1707.

77. Stevens, RE, Limsakun T, Evans G, Mason DH. Controlled, multidose, pharmacokinetic evaluation of two extended-release carbamazepine formulations (Carbatrol and Tegretol-SR). *J Pharm Sci* 1998; 87:1531–1534.

78. Mirza WU, Rak IW, Thadani VM, et al. Six-month evaluation of Carbatrol (extended-release carbamazepine) in complex partial seizures. *Neurology* 1998; 19:1727–1729.

79. Friis ML, Christiansen J. Carbamazepine, carbamazepine-10,11-epoxide and phenytoin concentrations in brain tissue of epileptic children. *Acta Neurol Scand* 1978; 58:104–108.

80. Warner A, Privitera M, Bates D. Standards of laboratory practice: antiepileptic drug monitoring. National Academy of Clinical Biochemistry. *Clin Chem* 1998; 44:1085–1095.

81. Paxton JW, Aman MG, Werry JS. Fluctuations in salivary carbamazepine and carbamazepine-10,11-epoxide concentrations during the day in epileptic children. *Epilepsia* 1983; 24:716–724.

82. Baciewicz AM. Carbamazepine drug interactions. *Ther Drug Monit* 1986; 8:305–317.

83. Lander CM, Eadie MJ, Tyrer JH. Factors influencing plasma carbamazepine concentrations. *Clin Exp Neurol* 1977; 14:184–193.

84. Eichelbaum M, Kothe KW, Hoffman F, von Unruh GE. Kinetics and metabolism of carbamazepine during combined antiepileptic drug therapy. *Clin Pharmacol Ther* 1979; 26:366–371.

85. Haidukewych D, Zielinski JJ, Rodin EA. Derivation and evaluation of an equation for prediction of free carbamazepine concentrations in patients comedicated with valproic acid. *Ther Drug Monit* 1989; 11:528–532.

86. Kerr BM, Rettie AE, Eddy AC, et al. Inhibition of human liver microsomal epoxide hydrolase by valproate and valpromide: in vitro/in vivo correlation. *Clin Pharmacol Ther* 1989; 46:82–93.

87. Pisani F, Narbone MC, Fazio A, et al. Effect of viloxazine on serum carbazmazepine levels in epileptic patients. *Epilepsia* 1984; 25:482–485.

88. Morris JC, Dodson, WE, Hatelid JM, Ferrendelli JA. Phenytoin and carbazazepine, alone and in combination: anticonvulsant and neurotoxic effects. *Neurology* 1987; 37:1111–1119.

89. Besag FM, Berry DJ, Pool F, Newbery JE, Subel B. Carbamazepine toxicity with lamotrigine: pharmacokinetic or pharmacodynamic interaction? *Epilepsia* 1998; 39:183–187.

90. Kishi T, Fujita N, Eguchi T, Ueda K. Mechanism for reduction of serum folate by antiepileptic drugs during prolonged therapy. *J Neurol Sci* 1997; 145:109–112.

91. Froscher W, Maier V, Laage M, et al. Folate deficiency, anticonvulsant drugs, and psychiatric morbidity. *Clin Neuropharmacol* 1995; 18:165–182.

92. Lewis DP, Van Dyke DC, Stumbo PJ, Berg MJ. Drug and environmental factors associated with adverse pregnancy outcomes. Part I: Antiepileptic drugs, contraceptives, smoking, and folate. *Ann Pharmacother* 1998; 32:802–817.

93. Chang SI, McAuley JW. Pharmacotherapeutic issues for women of childbearing age with epilepsy. *Ann Pharmacother* 1998; 32:794–801.

94. Sheth RD, Wesolowski CA, Jacob JC, et al. Effect of carbamazepine and valproate on bone mineral density. *J Pediatr* 1995; 127:256–262.

95. Wright JM, Stokes EF, Sweeney VP. Isoniazid-induced carbamazepine toxicity and vice versa. *N Engl J Med* 1982; 307:1325–1327.

96. Mesdjian E, Dravert C, Cenraud B, Roger J. Carbamazepine intoxication due to triacetyloleandomycin administration in epileptic patients. *Epilepsia* 1980; 21:489–496.

97. Goulden KJ, Camfield P, Dooley JM, et al. Severe carbamazepine intoxication after administration of erythromycin. *J Pediatr* 1986; 109:135–138.

98. Hedrick R, Williams F, Morin R, et al. Carbamazepine-erythromycin interaction leading to carbamazepine toxicity in four epileptic children. *Ther Drug Monit* 1983; 5:405–407.

99. von Rosensteil NA, Adam D. Macrolide antibacterials. Drug interactions of clinical significance. *Drug Safety* 1995; 13:105–122.

100. Yasui N, Otani K, Kaneko S, et al. Carbamazepine toxicity induced by clarithromycin coadministration in psychiatric patients. *Int Clin Psychopharmacol* 1997; 12:225–229.

101. Nemeroff CB, DeVane CL, Pollock BG. Newer antidepressants and the cytochrome P450 system. *Am J Psychiatry* 1996; 153:311–320.

102. Hansen BS, Dam M, Brandt J, et al. Influence of dextropropoxyphene on steady state levels and protein binding of three anti-epileptic drugs in man. *Acta Neurol Scand* 1980; 61:357–367.

103. Bourgeois BFD, Dodson WE, Ferrenedelli JA. Interaction between primidone, carbamazepine and nicotinamide. *Neurology* 1982; 32:1122–1126.

104. Krag B, Dam M, Angelo H, Christensen JM. Influence of disulfiram on the serum concentraion of carbamazepine in patients with epilepsy. *Acta Neurol Scand* 1981; 63:395–398.

105. Sonne J, Luhdorf K, Larsen NE, Andreasen PB. Lack of interaction between cimetidene and carbamazepine. *Acta Neurol Scand* 1983, 68:253–256.

106. Levy RH. Cytochrome P450 isozymes and antiepileptic drug interactions. *Epilepsia* 1995; 36(Suppl 5):S8–S13.

107. Nakasa H, Nakamura H, Ono S, et al. Prediction of drug-drug interactions of zonisamide metabolism in humans from in vitro data. *Eur J Clin Pharmacol* 1998; 54:177–183.

108. Bertilsson L, Tybring G, Widen J, Chang M, Tomson T. Carbamazepine treatment induces the CYP3A4 catalyzed sulphoxidation of omeprazole, but has no or less effect on hydroxylation via CYP2C19. *Br J Clin Pharmacol* 1997; 44:186–189.

109. Warren JW, Benmaman JD, Wannamaker BB, Levy RH. Kinetics of a carbamazepine-ethosuximide interaction. *Clin Pharmacol Ther* 1980; 28:646–651.

110. Bowdle TA, Levy RH, Cutler RE. Effects of carbamazepine on valproic acid kinetics in normal subjects. *Clin Pharmacol Ther* 1979; 26:629–634.

111. Dodson, WE. The nonlinear kinetics of phenytoin in children. *Neurology* 1982; 32:42–48.

112. Pippenger CE. Clinically significant carbamazepine drug interactions: an overview. *Epilepsia* 1987; 28(Suppl 3):S71–S76.

113. Schäffler L. Bourgeois BFD, Lüders HO. Rapid reversibility of autoinduction of carbamazepine after temporary discontinuation. *Epilepsia* 1994; 35:195–198.

114. Collaborative Group for Epidemiology of Epilepsy. Adverse reaction to antiepileptic drugs: a follow-up study of 355 patients with chronic antiepileptic drug treatment. *Epilepsia* 1988; 29:787–793.

115. Herranz JL, Armijo JA, Arteaga R. Clinical side effects of phenobarbital, primidone, phenytoin, carbamazepine, and valproate during monotherapy in children. *Epilepsia* 1988; 29:794–804.

116. Wallace SJ. A comparative review of the adverse effects of anticonvulsants in children with epilepsy. *Drug Safety* 1996; 15:378–393.

117. Ramsey, RE, Wilder BJ, Berger JR, Bruni J. A double-blind study comparing carbamazepine with phenytoin as initial seizure therapy in adults. *Neurology* 1983; 33:904–910.

118. Andersen EB, Philbert A, Klee JG. Carbamazepine monotherapy in epileptic outpatients. *Acta Neurol Scand* 1983; 67(Suppl):29–34.

119. Delcker A, Wilhelm H, Timmann D, Diener HC. Side effects from increased doses of carbamazepine on neuropsychological and posturographic parameters of humans. *Eur Neuropsychopharmacol* 1997; 7:213–218.

120. Keranen T, Silvenius J. Side effects of carbamazepine, valproate and clonazepam during long-term treatment of epilepsy. *Acta Neurol Scand* 1983, 97(Suppl):69–80.

121. Hoppener RJ, Kuyer A, Meijer JW, Hulsman J. Correlation between daily fluctuations of carbamazepine serum levels and intermittent side effects. *Epilepsia* 1980; 21:341–350.

122. Dulac O, Bouguerra L, Rey E, de Lauture D Arthuis M. Monotherapie par la carbamazepine dans les epilepsies de l'enfant. *Arch Fr Pediatr* 1983; 40:415–419.

123. Sullivan JB, Rumack BH, Peterson RG. Acute carbamazepine toxicity resulting from overdose. *Neurology* 1981; 31:621–624.

124. Fisher R-S, Cysyk B. A fatal overdose of carbamazepine: case report and review of literature. *J Toxicol Clin Toxicol* 1988; 26:477–486.

125. Aldenkamp AP, Vermeulen J. Phenytoin and carbamazepine: differential effects on cognitive function. *Seizure* 1995; 4:95–104.

126. Wallace SJ. A comparative review of the adverse effects of anticonvulsants in children with epilepsy. *Drug Safety* 1996; 15:378–393

127. Sabers A, Moller A, Dam M, et al. Cognitive function and anticonvulsant therapy: effect of monotherapy in epilepsy. *Acta Neurol Scand* 1995; 92:19–27.

128. Koivikko MJ, Valikangas SL. Hyponatremia during carbamazepine therapy in children. *Neuropediatrics* 1983; 14:93–96.

129. Rado JP, Juhos E, Sawinsky I. Dose-response relations in drug-induced inappropriate secretion of ADH: effects of clofibrate and carbamazepine. *Int J Clin Pharmacol* 1975; 12:315–319.

130. Kalff R, Houtkooper MA, Meyer JW, et al. Carbamazepine and serum sodium levels. *Epilepsia* 1984; 25:390–397.

131. Borusiak P, Korn-Merker E, Holert N, Boenigk HE. Hyponatremia induced by oxcarbazepine in children. *Epilepsy Res* 1998; 30:241–246.

132. Perucca E, Richens A. Water intoxication produced by carbamazepine and its reversal by phenytoin. *Br J Clin Pharmacol* 1980; 9:302–304.

133. Tjellesen L, Gotfredsen A, Christiansen C. Effect of vitamin D2 and D3 on bone-mineral content in carbamazepine-treated epileptic patients. *Acta Neurol Scand* 1983; 68:424–428.

134. Tjellesen L, Nilas L, Christiansen C. Does carbamazepine cause disturbances in calcium metabolism in epileptic patients? *Acta Neurol Scand* 1983; 68:13–19.

135. Wolschendorf K, Vanselow K, Moller WD, Schulz H. A quantitative determination of anticonvulsant-induced bone demineralization by an improved X-ray densitometry technique. *Neuroradiology* 1983; 25:315–318.

136. Lundstrom A, Eeg-Olofsson O, Hamp SE. Effects of antiepileptic drug treatment with carbamazepine or phenytoin on the oral state of children and adolescents. *J Clin Periodontol* 1982; 9:482–488.

137. Bentsen KD, Gram L, Veje A. Serum thyroid hormones and blood folic acid during monotherapy with carbamazepine or valproate. A controlled study. *Acta Neurol Scand* 1983; 67:235–241.

138. Deisenhammer E, Schwarzbach H, Sommer R. Erhohung der gamma-GT bei anticonvulsiver theapie. *Wien Klin Whenschr* 1982; 92:584–585.

139. Silverstein FS, Parrish MA, Johnston MV. Adverse behavioral reactions in children treated with carbamazepine (Tegretol). *J Pediatr* 1982; 101:785–787.

140. Ambrosetti G, Riva R. Hyperammonemia in asterixis induced by carbamazepine: two case reports. *Acta Neurol Scand* 1984; 69:186–189.

141. Bimping-Bita K, Froscher W. Carbamazepine-induced choreoathetoid dyskinesia. *J Neurol Neurosurg Psychiatry* 1982; 45:560.

142. Neglia JP, Glaze DG, Zion TE. Tics and vocalizations in children treated with carbamazepine. *Pediatrics* 1984; 73:841–844.

143. Crosley CJ, Swender PT. Dystonia associated with carbamazepine administration: experience in brain-damaged children. *Pediatrics* 1979; 63:612–615.

144. Stremski ES, Brady WB, Prasad K, Hennes HA. Pediatric carbamazepine intoxication. *Ann Emerg Med* 1995; 25:624–630.

145. Specht U, May TW, Rohde M, et al. Cerebellar atrophy decreases the threshold of carbamazepine toxicity in patients with chronic focal epilepsy. *Arch Neurol* 1997; 54:427–431.

146. Silverstein FS, Parrish MA, Johnston MV. Adverse reactions to carbamazepine (Tegretol) in children with epilepsy. *Ann Neurol* 1982; 12:198–199.

147. Holmes GL. Carbamazepine: toxicity. In: Levy RH, Mattson RH, Meldrum BS, eds. *Antiepileptic Drugs.* 4th ed. New York: Raven Press, 1995:567–579.

148. Mattson RH. Carbamazepine. In: Engel J Jr, Pedley T, eds. *Epilepsy: A Comprehensive Textbook.* Philadelphia: Lippincott-Raven, 1997:1491–1502.

149. Luchins DJ. Fatal agranulocytosis in a chronic schizophrenic patient treated with carbamazepine. *Am J Psychiatry* 1984; 141:687–688.

150. Ponte CD. Carbamazepine-induced thrombocytopenia, rash, and hepatic dysfunction. *Drug Intell Clin Pharm* 1983; 17:642–644.

151. Hart RG, Easton JD. Carbamazepine and hematological monitoring. *Ann Neurol* 1981; 11:309–312.

152. Tohen M, Castillo J, Baldessarini RJ, Zarate C Jr, Kando JC. Blood dyscrasias with carbamazepine and valproate: a pharmacoepidemiological study of 2,228 patients at risk. *Am J Psychiatry* 1995; 152:413–418.

153. Silverstein FS, Boxer L, Johnston MV. Hematological monitoring during therapy with carbamazepine in children. *Ann Neurol* 1983; 13:685–686.

154. Wolkenstein P, Tan C, Lecoeur S, et al. Covalent binding of carbamazepine reactive metabolites to P450 isoforms present in the skin. *Chem Biol Interact* 1998; 113:39–50.

155. Tennis P, Stern RS. Risk of serious cutaneous disorders after initiation of use of phenytoin, carbamazepine, or sodium valproate: a record linkage study. *Neurology* 1997; 49:542–546.

156. Roujeau JC, Kelly JP, Naldi L, et al. Medication use and the risk of Stevens-Johnson syndrome or toxic epidermal necrolysis. *N Engl J Med* 1995; 333:1600–1607.

157. Jarrett P, Rademaker M, Havill J, Pullon H. Toxic epidermal necrolysis treated with cyclosporin and granulocyte colony stimulating factor. *Clin Exp Dermatol* 1997; 22:146–147.

158. Morkunas AR, Miller MB. Anticonvulsant hypersensitivity syndrome. *Crit Care Clin* 1997; 13:727–739.

159. Mauri-Hellweg D, Bettens F, Mauri D, et al. Activation of drug-specific CD4+ and CD8+ T cells in individuals allergic to sulfonamides, phenytoin, and carbamazepine. *J Immunol* 1995; 155:462–472.

160. Schlienger RG, Shear NH. Antiepileptic drug hypersensitivity syndrome. *Epilepsia* 1998; 39(Suppl 7):S3–S7.

161. De Vriese AS, Philippe J, Van Renterghem DM, et al. Carbamazepine hypersensitivity syndrome: report of 4 cases and review of the literature. *Medicine* 1995; 74:144–151.

162. Hyson C, Sadler M. Cross sensitivity of skin rashes with antiepileptic drugs. *Can J Neurol Sci* 1997; 24:245–249.

163. Hogg RJ, Sawyer M, Hecox K, Eigenbrodt. Carbamazepine-induced acute tubulointersitial nephritis. *J Pediatr* 1981; 98:830–832.

164. Stewart CR, Vengrow MI, Riley TL. Double quotidian fever caused by carbamazepine. *N Engl J Med* 1980; 302:1262–1264.

165. Eijgenraam JW, Buurke EJ, van der Laan JS. Carbamazepine-associated acute tubulointerstitial nephritis. *Neth J Med* 1997; 50:25–28.

166. Gram L, Bentsen KD. Hepatic toxicity of antiepileptic drugs: a review. *Acta Neurol Scand* 1982; 97(Suppl): 81–90.

167. Mitchell MC, Boitnott, JK, Arregui A, Maddrey WC. Granulomatous hepatitis associated with carbamazepine therapy. *Am J Med* 1981; 71:733–735.

168. Levy M, Goodamn MW, Van Dyne BJ, Sumner HW. Granulomatous hepatitis secondary to carbamazepine. *Ann Intern Med* 1981; 95:64–65.

169. Soffer EE, Taylor RJ, Bertram PD, Haggitt RC, Levinson MJ. Carbamazepine-induced liver injury. *South Med J* 1983; 76:681–683.

170. Berkowitz FE, Henderson SL, Fajman N, et al. Acute liver failure caused by isoniazid in a child receiving carbamazepine. *Int J Tuberc Lung Dis* 1998; 2:603–606.

171. Hopen G, Nesthus I, Laerum OD. Fatal carbamazepine-associated hepatitis. Report of two cases. *Acta Med Scand* 1981; 210:333–335.

172. Zucker P, Daum F Cohen MI. Fatal carbamazepine hepatitis. *J Pediatr* 1977; 91:667.

173. Toepfer M, Sitter T, Lochmuller H, Pongratz D, Muller-Felber W. Drug-induced systemic lupus erythematosus after 8 years of treatment with carbamazepine. *Eur J Clin Pharmacol* 1998; 54:193–194.

174. Nathan DL, Belsito DV. Carbamazepine-induced pseudolymphoma with CD-30 positive cells. *J Am Acad Dermatol* 1998; 38:806–809.

175. Reiffers-Mettelock J, Hentges F, Humbel RL. Syndrome resembling systemic lupus erythematosus induced by carbamazepine. *Dermatology* 1997; 195:306.

176. Milesi-Lecat AM, Schmidt J, Aumaitre O, et al. Lupus and pulmonary nodules consistent with bronchiolitis obliterans organizing pneumonia induced by carbamazepine. *Mayo Clin Proc* 1997; 72:1145–1147.

177. Yeo W, Chow J, Wong N, Chan AT, Johnson PJ. Carbamazepine-induced lymphadenopathy mimicking Ki-1 (CD30+) T-cell lymphoma. *Pathology* 1997; 29:64–66.

178. Cereghino JJ, Brock JT, Van Meter JC, et al. The efficacy of carbamazepine combinations in epilepsy. *Clin Pharmacol Ther* 1975; 18:733–741.

179. Lesser RP, Pippenger CE, Luders H, Dinner DS. High dose monotherapy in treatment of intractable seizures. *Neurology* 1984; 34:707–711.

180. Callaghan N, O'Dwyer R, Keating J. Unnecessary polypharmacy in patients with frequent seizures. *Acta Neurol Scand* 1984, 69:15–19.

181. Schmidt D. Reduction of two drug therapy in intractable epilepsy. *Epilepsia* 1983; 24:368–376.

182. Bennett HS, Dunlop T, Ziring P. Reduction of polypharmacy for epilepsy in an institution for the retarded. *Dev Med Child Neurol* 1983; 25:735–737.

183. Hooper WD, Dickinson RG, Dunstan PR, et al. Oxcarbazepine: preliminary clinical and pharmacokinetic studies on a new anticonvulsant. *Clin Exp Neurol* 1987; 24:105–112.

184. Dickinson RG, Hooper WD, Dunstan PR, Eadie MJ. First dose and steady-state pharmacokinetics of oxcarbazepine and its 10-hydroxy metabolite. *Eur J Clin Pharmacol* 1989; 37:69–74.

185. Dam M, Ekberg R, Lyning Y, et al. A double-blind study comparing oxcarbazepine and carbamazepine in patients with newly diagnosed, previously untreated epilepsy. *Epilepsy Res* 1989; 3:70–76.

186. Editorial. Oxcarbazepine. *Lancet* 1989; 2:196–198.

187. Nielsen OA, Johannessen AC, Bardrum B. Oxcarbaze-pine-induced hyponatremia, a cross-sectional study. *Epilepsy Res* 1988; 2:269–271.

188. Pendlebury SC, Moses DK, Eadie MJ. Hyponatraemia during oxcarbazepine therapy. *Hum Toxicol* 1989; 8:337–344.

189. Beydoun A. Monotherapy trials of new antiepileptic drugs. *Epilepsia* 1997; 38(Suppl):S21–S31.

190. Guerreiro MM, Vigonius U, Pohlmann H, et al. A dou-ble-blind controlled clinical trial of oxcarbazepine versus phenytoin in children and adolescents with epilepsy. *Epilepsy Res* 1997; 27:205–213.

191. Levy RH, Wurden CJ. Carbamazepine: interactions with other drugs. In: Levy RH, Mattson RH, Meldrum BS, eds. *Antiepileptic Drugs.* 4th ed. New York: Raven Press, 1995:543–551.

CHAPTER 31

Valproate

Blaise F.D. Bourgeois, M.D.

Valproic acid, or valproate (VPA), has been used in the treatment of epilepsy for well over 30 years (1). During this time, it undoubtedly has established itself as one of the major antiepileptic drugs (AEDs), distinguishing itself from previously released drugs by its broad spectrum of activity against very different seizure types and by its relatively low sedative effect. In addition to being the first drug to be highly effective against several primarily generalized seizure types, such as absences, myoclonic seizures, and generalized tonic-clonic seizures, VPA also was found to be effective in the treatment of partial seizures, Lennox-Gastaut syndrome, infantile spasms, neonatal seizures, and febrile seizures. Thus, VPA has become particularly popular among pediatric neurologists. In addition to its place in the treatment of epilepsy, VPA has gained acceptance in the treatment of affective disorders in psychiatry and in the prophylaxis of migraine headaches. Effectiveness in the treatment of Sydenham's chorea has also been suggested (2). These indications are not included in this chapter. Several reviews have addressed the clinical profile of VPA as an AED (3–7).

CHEMISTRY, ANIMAL PHARMACOLOGY, AND MECHANISM OF ACTION

Valproic acid (Figure 31-1) is a colorless liquid (MW 144.21) with low solubility in water. Sodium valproate (MW 166.19) is a highly water-soluble

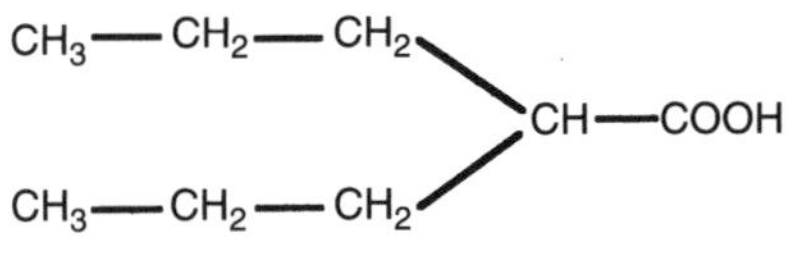

Figure 31-1. Structural formula of valproic acid (*N*-dipropylacetic acid).

and highly hygroscopic, white, crystalline material. Sodium hydrogen divalproate (divalproex sodium) is a compound composed of equal parts of valproic acid and sodium valproate. Being a short-chain branched fatty acid, VPA differs chemically from all other known AEDs. The anticonvulsant effect of valproic acid was discovered serendipitously when it was used as a solvent for compounds being tested in an animal model of seizures (8). The antiepileptic activity of VPA has been well demonstrated in several animal models (9–11). The effects of VPA include protection against maximal electroshock (MES)–induced seizures; seizures induced chemically by pentylenetetrazol (PTZ), bicuculline, glutamic acid, kainic acid, strychnine, ouabain, nicotine, and intramuscular penicillin; and seizures induced by kindling (12). The potency of VPA is somewhat lower against MES than against PTZ. This broad spectrum of efficacy of VPA in animal models suggests that VPA is effective in both preventing the spread and lowering the threshold of seizures, and this is consistent with the broad spectrum of antiepileptic activity of VPA in humans.

Extensive studies have been carried out to elucidate the mechanism of action of VPA. Several effects of VPA have been demonstrated at the cellular level, but the precise mechanism underlying the antiepileptic effect of VPA has not been identified, and more than one mechanism may be involved (13). VPA raises brain levels of the inhibitory neurotransmitter gamma-aminobutyric acid (GABA) (10,14,15). This may be due to the inhibition of GABA-transaminase, the first step in GABA deactivation (16), inhibition of succinic semialdehyde dehydrogenase, the second step in GABA deactivation (17), and an increase in glutamic acid decarboxylase activity, an enzyme involved in the synthesis of GABA (15). However, because it occurs at much higher than usual therapeutic doses and because its time course lags behind the anticonvulsant effect (18), elevation of GABA is unlikely to be the predominant mechanism of the antiepileptic effect of VPA. In addition to its effect on GABA levels, VPA reduces sustained repetitive high-frequency firing by blocking voltage-sensitive sodium channels (19) or by activating calcium-dependent potassium conductance (20). A decrease by VPA of brain levels of the excitatory amino acid aspartate was also demonstrated in mice (21). It is not known to what extent these actions contribute to the clinical effect of VPA.

BIOTRANSFORMATION AND PHARMACOKINETICS IN HUMANS

Biotransformation

The main pathways of VPA biotransformation in humans include glucuronidation of VPA itself, beta-oxidation, hydroxylation, ketone formation, and desaturation. Both beta-oxidation and desaturation can result in the formation of double bonds. By far the most abundant metabolites are VPA glucuronide and 3-oxo-VPA, which represent about 40 percent and 33 percent, respectively, of the urinary excretion of a VPA dose (22). Two desaturated metabolites of VPA, 2-ene-VPA, and 4-ene-VPA have anticonvulsant activity that is similar in potency to that of VPA itself (23). Because there is delayed but significant accumulation of 2-ene-VPA in the brain and it is cleared more slowly than VPA itself (24), the formation of 2-ene-VPA may provide a possible explanation for the discrepancy between the time courses of VPA concentrations and the antiepileptic activity of VPA (25). It appears that 2-ene-VPA does not possess the pronounced embryotoxicity (26) and hepatotoxicity (27) of 4-ene-VPA. The metabolite 2-ene-VPA may thus represent a better AED than VPA itself. In addition to being strongly hepatotoxic, 4-ene-VPA is produced under the action of cytochrome P-450 enzymes. These enzymes are induced by other AEDs such as phenobarbital, phenytoin, and carbamazepine (22,28), and this may explain the increased risk of hepatotoxicity in patients receiving these drugs together with VPA (29). However, elevation of 4-ene-VPA levels has not yet been documented in patients with VPA hepatotoxicity or in conjunction with short-term adverse effects or hyperammonemia (30).

Pharmacokinetics

Many different preparations of VPA are available, although not all preparations are available in any given country. Preparations of VPA include valproic acid capsules, tablets, and syrup (immediate release), enteric-coated tablets of sodium valproate or

Table 31-1. Pharmacokinetic Parameters of Valproate

Bioavailability	>90%
Time to peak level[a]	1–8 hours
Volume of distribution	0.16 L/kg
Serum protein binding[b]	70–93%
Elimination half-life[c]	5–15 hours
Therapeutic range	50–100 (–150) mg/L
	350–700 (–1000) μmol/l

[a]The longer values are for enteric-coated and slow-release preparations.
[b]Concentration-dependent; lower at higher total concentrations.
[c]Shorter values are for comedication with inducing drugs.

sodium hydrogen divalproate (divalproex sodium), divalproex sodium enteric-coated sprinkles, slow-release oral preparations, magnesium valproate and valpromide (the amide of VPA) for oral administration, valproate suppositories, and a parenteral formulation of sodium valproate for intravenous (IV) use. The main pharmacokinetic parameters of VPA are summarized in Table 31-1. The bioavailability of oral preparations of valproate is virtually complete when compared with the IV route (31). The purpose of the enteric coating of tablets is to prevent the gastric irritation associated with release of valproic acid in the stomach. When valproic acid syrup was administered rectally, it was found to have the same bioavailability as the oral preparation (32,33). Compared with oral syrup, the relative bioavailability of VPA suppositories was found to be 80 percent in volunteers (34). The time to peak levels was longer for the suppositories than for the syrup (3.1 hours versus 1.0 hour). In a study in patients treated chronically with valproate, administration of valproate suppositories was well tolerated for several days, and the bioavailability was the same as for the oral preparations (35). The available evidence suggests that there is no need for a dosage change or a change in regimen when oral VPA administration is transiently replaced by rectal administration.

The rate of absorption of VPA after oral administration is quite variable depending on the formulation. Administration of syrup or uncoated regular tablets or capsules is followed by rapid absorption and peak levels within 2 hours. Absorption from enteric-coated tablets is delayed, but once absorption begins, it is rapid. The onset of absorption varies as a function of the state of gastric emptying at the time of ingestion, and peak levels may be reached only 3 to 8 hours after oral ingestion of enteric-coated tablets (36–38). Figure 31-2 shows the serum levels of a patient who received a first oral dose of 500 mg of enteric-coated divalproex sodium. No VPA was detectable in serum until 8 hours after the oral intake, and this was followed by a rapid rise of levels (39). Because of this delayed absorption, serum levels of VPA in patients taking VPA chronically (twice or three times daily) continue to decrease for 2 or

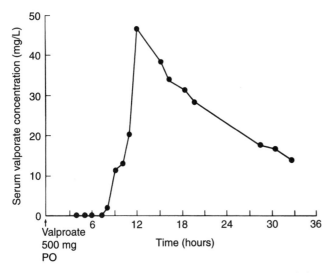

Figure 31-2. Valproate serum concentrations after a 500-mg single first oral dose of enteric-coated divalproex sodium in a 60.4-kg woman. (Reproduced with permission from Bourgeois BFD. Pharmacokinetics and pharmacodynamics in clinical practice. In: Wylie E, ed. *The Treatment of Epilepsy: Principles and Practice.* 2nd ed. Baltimore: Williams & Wilkins, 1997:728–736.

more hours after drug ingestion. Therefore, the lowest VPA levels of a 24-hour cycle are not the assumed "trough levels" before the morning dose but actually occur in the late morning or early afternoon (35). A newer oral formulation of VPA are the sprinkles, which consist of capsules containing enteric-coated particles of divalproex sodium. The capsules can be swallowed as such or they can be opened and the contents can be sprinkled on food. This is a convenient formulation for younger children. The absorption of enteric-coated sprinkles was compared with the absorption of VPA syrup in 12 children, and this showed no difference in overall bioavailability between the two formulations. However, the absorption of VPA was slower from the sprinkles, with an average time to maximal VPA concentrations of 4.2 hours after ingestion of sprinkles, as compared with 0.9 hours after ingestion of syrup (40). With the recently available IV formulation of sodium valproate, peak VPA serum levels are reached at the end of the recommended infusion time of 60 minutes.

The volume of distribution of VPA is relatively small (0.13–0.19 L/kg in adults and 0.20–0.30 L/kg in children). This suggests that VPA has less affinity for binding outside the blood compartment than for binding to serum proteins. Indeed, VPA is highly bound to serum proteins. This binding appears to be saturable at therapeutic concentrations, and the free fraction of VPA increases as the total concentration increases. For instance, Cramer and coworkers (41) found that the average free serum fraction of VPA in adults was only 7 percent at 50 mg/L and 9 percent at 75 mg/L, increasing to 15 percent at 100 mg/L, 22 percent at 125 mg/L, and 30 percent at 150 mg/L. Based on these values, the

free level of VPA would increase more than 10 times from 3.5 mg/L to 45 mg/L with a threefold increase in the total concentration of VPA from 50 to 150 mg/L. Because the clearance of VPA is related to the free concentration, there is a linear relationship between the daily maintenance dose of VPA and steady-state free levels. But, as expected, on the basis of saturable binding, a curvilinear relationship between VPA maintenance dose and total steady-state concentrations was found by Gram and coworkers (42) with relatively smaller increases in concentrations at higher doses.

The elimination half-life of VPA varies as a function of comedication. In the absence of inducing drugs, the half-life in adults is 13 to 16 hours (37,43), whereas the half-life in adults on polytherapy with inducing drugs averaged 9 hours (31); half-lives in children are slightly shorter. Cloyd and coworkers (44) found an average half-life of 11.6 hours in children on monotherapy and 7.0 hours with polytherapy. Hall and coworkers (45) determined that VPA half-life was significantly related to age, but volume of distribution and clearance were not. Newborns eliminate VPA slowly, with half-lives that are longer than 20 hours (46).

Interactions

Various pharmacokinetic interactions occur when VPA is administered concomitantly with other medications. These interactions fall into three categories based on the fact that (1) the metabolism of VPA is sensitive to enzymatic induction, (2) VPA itself can inhibit the metabolism of other drugs, and (3) VPA has a high affinity for serum proteins and can displace other drugs or can itself be displaced from proteins. Pharmacokinetic interactions with valproate have been the object of several reviews (47–49).

Concomitant administration of enzyme-inducing AEDs such as carbamazepine, phenytoin, phenobarbital, and primidone has been repeatedly shown to result in lower VPA levels in relation to the maintenance dose (50). Both carbamazepine (51–53) and phenytoin (52) significantly lower VPA levels, usually by at least one-third to one-half. These interactions are particularly pronounced in children, resulting in VPA level reductions of 50 percent or more (54–56). When children receiving polytherapy had other drugs discontinued, VPA levels rose 122 percent after withdrawal of phenytoin, 67 percent after withdrawal of phenobarbital, and 50 percent after withdrawal of carbamazepine (57). In general, when an inducing drug is added or withdrawn in a patient taking VPA, the dose of VPA has to be increased or decreased, respectively, by a factor of about 2. Inversely, levels of VPA are raised by felbamate (58,59). The increase in VPA levels was found to be 28 percent at a felbamate dose of 1200 mg/day and 54 percent at a dose of 2400 mg/day.

When VPA affects the kinetics of other drugs, the interaction is either an enzymatic inhibition or a displacement from serum proteins. Levels of phenobarbital have been found to increase by 57 percent (60) to 81 percent (61) after the addition of VPA. Levels of ethosuximide can also be raised by the addition of VPA, mostly in the presence of additional AEDs (62). Although VPA does not raise levels of carbamazepine itself, levels of the active metabolite, carbamazepine-10, 11-epoxide may double (63,64). Elimination of lamotrigine is markedly inhibited by VPA, with a resulting two- to threefold prolongation of the lamotrigine half-life (65). Consequently, lamotrigine must be introduced at low doses in patients taking VPA.

A pharmacokinetic interaction occurs between VPA and phenytoin because both drugs have a high affinity for serum proteins. VPA increases the free fraction of phenytoin (66,67). Because the free serum level of phenytoin determines the brain concentration, total phenytoin concentrations in the usual therapeutic range may, in the presence of VPA, be associated with clinical toxicity. Other pharmacokinetic interactions involving VPA have little or no clinical significance. In contrast to inducing AEDs, VPA is not associated with failure of oral contraceptives (68). Acetylsalicylic acid can both displace VPA from serum proteins and alter its metabolism (69). It appears that this interaction can be sufficient to cause clinical VPA toxicity (70).

CLINICAL EFFICACY

Absence Seizures

During the first years of routine clinical use of VPA, it soon became apparent that it is a highly effective first-line drug in the treatment of primarily generalized idiopathic seizures such as absence seizures, generalized tonic-clonic seizures, and myoclonic seizures (71). The primary indication of VPA when it was first released in North America in 1978 was the treatment of absence seizures. When VPA was administered to patients with typical and atypical absence seizures, a reduction of spike-and-wave discharges was repeatedly demonstrated (72–76). Nineteen of 25 patients with absence seizures who were treated with VPA for 10 weeks experienced a reduction in seizure frequency, and a reduction in the total duration of spike-and-wave discharges was seen in 21 patients (77). In 11 of these patients, the reduction in spike-and-wave discharges was greater than 75 percent. Comparison of the efficacy of VPA and ethosuximide in the treatment of absence seizures revealed equal efficacy in at least two studies (78,79). Sixteen patients not previously treated for absence seizures and 29 refractory patients were enrolled in a double-blind cross-over study of VPA

and ethosuximide, in which the measure of efficacy was the frequency and duration of generalized spike-wave bursts on electroencephalogram (EEG) telemetry (79). Ethosuximide and VPA were equally effective in previously untreated patients. Simple absence seizures could be completely controlled by VPA monotherapy in 11 of 12 patients (80), in 10 of 12 patients (57), in 14 of 17 patients (81), and in 20 of 21 patients (82). It appears that absence seizures are more likely to be fully controlled if they occur alone than if they are mixed with another seizure type (57,82). Overall, treatment with VPA appears to be somewhat less effective against atypical or "complex" absences than against simple absences (80,83). VPA can also be used effectively in patients with recurrent absence status. In 25 patients who were enrolled in an open evaluation, episodes of absence status decreased from a yearly average of 5.7 to an average of 0.6 (84). In this study, patients who had primary generalized epilepsy experienced a more dramatic response to VPA.

Generalized Tonic-Clonic Seizures

In addition to establishing itself as a first-line drug in the treatment of absence seizures, VPA was found to be highly effective in the treatment of certain generalized convulsive seizures (85–88). In 36 patients with primarily generalized tonic-clonic seizures, of whom 24 had been treated previously with other AEDs, VPA was used in monotherapy (80). In 33 of these patients, seizures were fully controlled. Among 42 patients with intractable seizures, the generalized tonic-clonic seizures were fully controlled by add-on VPA in 14 patients (57). VPA was compared with phenytoin in 61 previously untreated patients with generalized tonic-clonic, clonic, or tonic seizures (89). The seizures came under control during the time of observation in 73 percent of patients receiving VPA and in 47 percent of patients treated with phenytoin. When seizures occurring before therapeutic plasma drug levels had been reached were discounted, this response increased to 82 percent for VPA and 76 percent for phenytoin. In another randomized study comparing valproate and phenytoin in patients with previously untreated tonic-clonic seizures, a two-year remission was achieved in 27 of 37 patients with VPA and in 22 of 39 patients with phenytoin (86). Monotherapy with VPA was assessed in two studies of patients with primary (or idiopathic) generalized epilepsies (81,82). Among patients who had only generalized tonic-clonic seizures, complete seizure control was achieved in 51 of 70 patients (81) and in 39 of 44 patients (82), respectively. Monotherapy with VPA in children with generalized tonic-clonic seizures was also found to be highly effective (90).

Myoclonic Seizures

VPA is currently the drug of first choice for most myoclonic seizures, particularly those occurring in patients with primary or idiopathic generalized epilepsies (80–82). In a group of 23 patients with myoclonic epilepsy of adolescence, 16 came under full control with VPA monotherapy (80). In the same study, 22 patients with myoclonic epilepsy of adolescence and abnormality on intermittent photostimulation, of whom 17 had failed to respond to previous medications, full seizure control was achieved in 17 patients. Photosensitivity on the EEG is easily suppressed by valproate, regardless of the associated clinical seizure type (91). Among a group of patients with primary generalized epilepsies treated with VPA monotherapy, 22 patients had myoclonic seizures and 20 of those had at least one other seizure type, either absence or tonic-clonic seizures. The myoclonic seizures were controlled by VPA monotherapy in 18 of these 22 patients (82). Patients with juvenile myoclonic epilepsy have an excellent response to VPA (92), which probably still remains the drug of first choice for this condition in most patients. Benign myoclonic epilepsy of infancy, which belongs to the group of primary or idiopathic generalized epilepsies, also responds well to treatment with VPA (90). Postanoxic intention myoclonus is usually quite refractory to treatment, but some success has been achieved with VPA (93–95). A combination of VPA and clonazepam is often used with some success in the treatment of the myoclonic and tonic-clonic seizures of severe progressive myoclonus epilepsy (96).

Infantile Spasms and Lennox-Gastaut Syndrome

The available information on the use of VPA in the treatment of generalized encephalopathic epilepsies of infancy and childhood, such as infantile spasms and Lennox-Gastaut syndrome, is much less extensive than for the more benign idiopathic primary generalized epilepsies. Like all other antiepileptic medications, VPA is less effective in the treatment of these more severe forms of generalized epilepsy. In a larger series of patients treated with VPA, 38 had myoclonic astatic epilepsy, a term used by the authors synonymously with Lennox-Gastaut syndrome. Of these patients, seven became and remained seizure-free with VPA. In addition, a 50 percent to 80 percent improvement was achieved after the addition of VPA in one third of these patients, and other AEDs were withdrawn or reduced (80). In the same series, seizures were fully controlled in three of six patients with myoclonic absence epilepsy, all of them on combination therapy. In another series involving 100 children treated with VPA (57), seizure control was achieved in 12 of 27 children with "absences and other seizures" and in 9 of 39 children with atonic seizures.

The majority of reports on the use of VPA for the treatment of infantile spasms include small numbers of patients (97–99), or they include patients receiving corticotropin and VPA simultaneously (100,101). VPA was not used simultaneously with corticotropin in one series of 19 infants with infantile spasms (102). With VPA as their first drug, 8 of these 19 infants experienced good seizure control and did not require corticotropin. These patients received VPA doses ranging from 20 to 60 mg/kg/day. The patients who experienced an initial failure with either VPA or corticotropin were subsequently switched to the other drug. Comparison of the two groups revealed a tendency toward a better response to corticotropin, but the incidence and severity of side effects was lower with VPA. A low dose of 20 mg/kg/day of VPA was used in a series of 18 infants with infantile spasms not previously treated with corticotropin (103). In 12 of these patients, the short-term results were described as good to excellent. On follow-up, 7 patients had residual seizure activity, and moderate to severe mental retardation was diagnosed in 16. The authors concluded that efficacy of VPA was similar to the efficacy of corticotropin and that VPA was associated with fewer side effects.

Partial Seizures

Systematic assessment of the efficacy of VPA against partial seizures began only after its role in the treatment of generalized seizures had been established. Preliminary information had been provided by subgroups of patients in studies not dealing primarily with partial seizures, all of which suggested some benefit (57,80,104). Probably the first direct comparison of VPA with carbamazepine in the treatment of partial seizures was an open study in 31 previously untreated adults (105). Eleven patients on VPA and 8 patients on carbamazepine were controlled, but follow-up was less than 1 year in 12 of the 31 patients. Comparison among carbamazepine, phenytoin, and VPA in monotherapy in a prospective study of 79 patients with previously untreated simple partial or complex partial seizures revealed no difference in efficacy among the three drugs (106). A group of 140 adults with previously untreated seizures were randomized to monotherapy with phenytoin or VPA (107). The seizures were tonic-clonic in 76 patients and predominantly complex partial in 64. Determination of 2-year remission rate or time to first seizure revealed no difference between the two drugs in either subgroup. A retrospective study of VPA monotherapy in 30 patients with simple partial and complex partial seizures in whom previous drugs had failed revealed a remarkable response (108). Seizure control was achieved in 12 patients, a more than

50 percent seizure reduction occurred in 10 patients, and only 9 patients were not improved.

Mattson and coworkers (109) carried out the most comprehensive controlled comparison of VPA and carbamazepine monotherapy in the treatment of partial and secondarily generalized seizures. This multicenter, double-blind, randomized trial included 480 adult patients in whom several seizure indicators, as well as neurotoxicity and systemic neurotoxicity, were assessed quantitatively. Four of five efficacy indicators were significantly in favor of carbamazepine in the treatment of complex partial seizures, and a combined composite score for efficacy and toxicity was higher for carbamazepine than for VPA at 12 months but not at 24 months. Outcomes for secondarily generalized seizures did not differ between the two drugs. Two comparative studies of VPA were carried out specifically in children (110,111). A total of 260 children with newly diagnosed primary generalized or partial epilepsy were randomized to VPA or carbamazepine and followed up for 3 years (110). The doses were titrated as needed and as tolerated according to clinical response. Equal efficacy was found for the two drugs against generalized and partial seizures, and adverse events were mostly mild for both drugs. The four drugs, phenobarbital, phenytoin, carbamazepine, and VPA, were compared in 167 children with untreated tonic-clonic or partial seizures entered into a randomized, unblinded study (111). Based on time to first seizure and to 1-year remission, there was no difference in efficacy at 1, 2, or 3 years. Unacceptable side effects necessitating withdrawal occurred in 6 of 10 patients on phenobarbital, which was prematurely eliminated from the study; in 9 percent of children on phenytoin; and in 4 percent each of children taking carbamazepine or VPA. More recently, VPA was evaluated in 143 adult patients with poorly controlled partial epilepsy randomized to monotherapy with VPA at low levels (25–50 mg/L) or high levels (80–150 mg/L) (112). The reduction in the frequency of both complex partial and secondarily generalized tonic-clonic seizures was significantly higher among patients in the high-level group.

Other Uses

Several studies have assessed the efficacy of VPA in the prevention of febrile seizures (113–119). In some studies VPA was found to be as effective as phenobarbital, and in other studies it was more effective than phenobarbital, placebo, or no treatment in reducing the risk of seizure recurrence. Nevertheless, based on risk versus benefit ratio considerations, VPA cannot be recommended for this indication. Treatment with intermittent diazepam during febrile episodes was as effective as prophylactic VPA in children with a high risk of recurrence of febrile seizures (120). A

small group of newborns with seizures have also been treated with VPA either rectally (121) or orally (46). Overall results were favorable. A loading dose of 20 to 25 mg/kg was followed by a maintenance dose of 5 to 10 mg/kg every 12 hours (46). Newborns treated with VPA were found to have a longer elimination half-life (26.4 hours) and higher levels of ammonia.

ADVERSE EFFECTS

Although adverse effects of AEDs are commonly divided into those that are dose-related and those that are idiosyncratic, the distinction is not always clear-cut, particularly with VPA. Not all adverse effects of VPA are strictly dose-related or idiosyncratic. Some reactions, such as tremor, are indeed fairly predictable and dose-related. However, certain adverse events that only occur in a small fraction of patients, and therefore appear to be idiosyncratic, may be more likely to occur at high doses or levels of VPA, such as thrombocytopenia, certain cases of confusion or stupor, and neural tube defects. Finally, certain side effects that are too common to be considered idiosyncratic could never be clearly shown to be dose-related, such as hair changes and weight gain. The main adverse effects of VPA are summarized in Table 31-2.

Table 31-2. Adverse Effects of Valproate

Neurologic
Tremor
Drowsiness, lethargy, confusion
Reversible dementia, brain atrophy
Stupor and coma

Gastrointestinal
Nausea, vomiting, anorexia
Gastrointestinal distress
Hepatic failure
Pancreatitis

Hematologic
Thrombocytopenia
Decreased platelet aggregation
Fibrinogen depletion

Metabolic/Endocrinologic
Hyperammonemia
Hypocarnitinemia
Menstrual irregularities
Polycystic ovaries

Teratogenicity
Neural tube defect

Miscellaneous
Hair loss
Edema
Nocturnal enuresis

Neurologic Adverse Effects

A tremor with the characteristics of essential tremor is relatively common with VPA (122,123). It is dose-related and occurs in about 10 percent of patients. If it does not improve sufficiently with dose reduction, propranolol may be tried (123). Asterixis (124) and reversible parkinsonism (125,126) have also been described. Drowsiness, lethargy, and confusional states are uncommon with VPA but may occur in some patients, usually at levels above 100 mg/L. There have also been well-documented case reports of reversible dementia (125,127,128) and pseudoatrophy of the brain (128–130). Treatment with VPA has been associated with a rather specific and unique adverse effect characterized by an acute mental change that can progress to stupor or coma (131,132). It is usually associated with generalized delta slowing of the EEG tracing. The mechanism is not known with certainty, and it is probably not due to hyperammonemia or carnitine deficiency. This encephalopathic picture is more likely to occur when VPA is added to another AED, and it is usually reversible within 2 to 3 days upon discontinuation of VPA or of the other antiepileptic drug. Overall, VPA does not appear to have significant dose-related effects on cognition or behavior (133–137). A possible psychotropic effect of VPA (138) was not found in a controlled study (139).

Gastrointestinal Adverse Effects

The most frequent adverse effects of VPA are nausea, vomiting, gastrointestinal distress, and anorexia. They may be due in part to direct gastric irritation by VPA, and the incidence is lower with enteric-coated tablets. Excessive weight gain is another common problem (140,141). It is not due entirely to increased appetite, and decreased beta-oxidation of fatty acids has been postulated as a mechanism (142). Despite recommendations for diet and exercise, weight gain tends to be a bothersome side effect, especially in young women. Excessive weight gain seems to be less of a problem in children, and a recent report suggests that VPA does not cause more weight gain than carbamazepine in children (143).

Fatal hepatotoxicity remains the most feared adverse effect of VPA (29,144–147). The two main risk factors are young age and polytherapy (147). The risk of fatal hepatotoxicity on polytherapy with VPA is approximately 1 in 600 below the age of 3 years, 1 in 8,000 from 3 to 10 years, 1 in 10,000 from 11 to 20 years, 1 in 31,000 between 21 and 40 years, and 1 in 107,000 above the age of 41 years. The risk is much lower on monotherapy and varies between 1 in 16,000 (3–10 years old) and 1 in 230,000 (21–40 years old). No fatalities have been reported for certain age

groups. Because a benign elevation of liver enzymes is common with VPA, and the severe hepatotoxicity is not preceded by a progressive elevation of liver enzymes, laboratory monitoring is of little value, although it is commonly done routinely. The diagnosis of hepatotoxicity from VPA depends mostly on recognition of the clinical features, which include nausea, vomiting, anorexia, lethargy, and at times loss of seizure control, jaundice, or edema. Although increased production of toxic metabolites has been considered as a cause of VPA hepatotoxicity, this has not yet been documented (148,140). There also has been no documentation of a protective effect of carnitine administration against VPA hepatotoxicity.

Another serious complication of VPA treatment is the development of acute hemorrhagic pancreatitis (150–154). Suspicion should be raised by the occurrence of vomiting and abdominal pain. Serum amylase and lipase are the most helpful diagnostic tests, and abdominal ultrasound may be considered also. However, amylase may be elevated in 20 percent of asymptomatic patients on VPA (155), and pancreatitis has been described in a patient with normal amylase but elevated lipase (156).

Hematologic Adverse Effects

Hematologic alterations are relatively common with VPA therapy, but they seldom lead to discontinuation of the drug (157,158). By far the most frequently diagnosed hematologic adverse event is thrombocytopenia (159,160), which can fluctuate and tends to improve with dosage reductions. The thrombocytopenia, in conjunction with other VPA-mediated disturbances of hemostasis, such as impaired platelet function, fibrinogen depletion, and coagulation factor deficiencies (161,162), may cause excessive bleeding. The common practice of withdrawing VPA before elective surgery is therefore recommended, although several recent reports have found no objective evidence of excessive operative bleeding in patients maintained on VPA (163–165). In addition to the described hematologic changes, VPA can also occasionally cause neutropenia (166), bone marrow suppression (167), and systemic lupus erythematosus (168).

Metabolic, Endocrinologic Changes, and Teratogenicity

Hyperammonemia is a very common finding in asymptomatic patients on chronic VPA therapy, and routine monitoring of ammonia is not warranted. Because ammonia levels were initially measured in symptomatic patients, their elevation was thought to be the cause of the symptoms (169–171). It was later found that hyperammonemia is very common in asymptomatic patients, particularly in those taking VPA together with an enzyme-inducing AED (172,173). The origin of the excessive ammonium may be renal (174). Although hyperammonemia can be reduced by L-carnitine supplementation (175), there is no documentation that this is necessary or clinically beneficial (176). Chronic treatment with VPA, especially in polytherapy, also tends to lower carnitine levels (177,178). A role for carnitine deficiency in the development of severe adverse effects of VPA has never been established. One patient who developed an acute encephalopathy and cerebral edema after acute administration of VPA was found to have low carnitine levels (179). A beneficial role of L-carnitine supplementation in acute VPA overdoses has been suggested (180,181), but in the absence of documented carnitine deficiency there is no evidence to support routine supplementation with L-carnitine in patients taking VPA.

VPA can cause menstrual irregularities (182), hormonal changes (183–185), and pubertal arrest in women (186). A recent concern has been the increasing recognition of the frequent association between VPA therapy and polycystic ovaries (183–185,187).

Treatment with VPA during the first trimester of pregnancy is associated with an estimated 1 percent to 2 percent risk of neural tube defect in the newborn (188–190). Folate supplementation appears to reduce the risk (191), and a daily dose of at least 1 mg should be considered in all female patients of childbearing age who are taking VPA (see Chapter 26).

Miscellaneous Adverse Effects

Excessive hair loss may be seen early during treatment with VPA, and, although the hair tends to grow back, it may become different in texture (192) or color (193). Facial or limb edema can occur in the absence of VPA-induced hepatic injury (194). Children may develop secondary noctural enuresis after the introduction of VPA therapy (117,140,195–197). Hyponatremia (198) has also been reported in one patient. The occurrence of rashes with VPA is extremely rare (199).

ADMINISTRATION AND LABORATORY MONITORING

An initial VPA dose of approximately 15 mg/kg/day is recommended, with subsequent dose increases, as necessary and as tolerated, by 5 to 10 mg/kg/day at weekly intervals. The optimal VPA dose of concentration may vary according to the patient's seizure type (200). Daily doses between 10 and 20 mg/kg are often sufficient for VPA monotherapy in primary generalized epilepsies (57,81,82,89). Children may require higher doses in milligrams per kilogram per day (61,80). Doses of 30 to 60 mg/kg/day (in children even more than 100 mg/kg/day) may be necessary

to achieve adequate VPA levels in patients who are also taking enzyme-inducing AEDs. If therapeutic levels of VPA are to be achieved rapidly or in patients who are unable to take oral medications, VPA can now be administered intravenously (201). This route has also been suggested for the treatment of status epilepticus, with an initial dose of 15 mg/kg followed by 1 mg/kg/hour (202), but more rapid administration, up to 6 mg/kg/min, has been successfully given (203). In those receiving IV replacement therapy or bolus dosing, subsequent administration should be given within 6 hours because of the precipitous fall in levels and return of clinical symptoms. Because of the short elimination half-life of VPA, it is common practice to divide the daily dose into two or three single doses. However, the pharmacodynamic profile of VPA may explain why equally good results were achieved with a single daily dose of VPA (80,204,205).

The value of serum levels of VPA is relatively limited. First, there is a considerable fluctuation in VPA levels because of the short half-life, and the reproducibility in a given patient is not good. Second, there seems to be a poor correlation between VPA serum levels and clinical effect at a given time, and the pharmacodynamic effect of VPA may lag significantly behind its blood concentrations (5,82,100,206,207). Although the recommended therapeutic range for VPA serum levels is usually 50 to 100 mg/L (350–700 μmol/L), levels up to 150 mg/L are often both necessary and well tolerated. In selected cases, and particularly during combination therapy with enzyme-inducing drugs, serum VPA levels can be valuable, but the result of a single measurement has limited value and needs to be interpreted cautiously (208). In patients on chronic VPA therapy, it is common practice to monitor routinely liver enzymes and complete blood count with platelets. Severe hepatotoxicity is unlikely to be detected by routine monitoring of liver enzymes, but hematologic abnormalities are more likely to be discovered.

REFERENCES

1. Carraz G, Gau R, Chateau R, Bonnin J. Communication a propos des premiers essais cliniques sur l'activite anti-epileptique de l'acide n-dipropylacetique (sel de Na+). *Ann Med Psychol* 1964; 122:577–585.

2. Daoud AS, Zaki M, Shakir R, Al-Saleh Q. Effectiveness of sodium valproate in the treatment of Sydenham's chorea. *Neurology* 1990; 40:1140–1141.

3. Simon D, Penry JK. Sodium di-n-propylacetate (DPA) in the treatment of epilepsy: a review. *Epilepsia* 1975; 22:1701–1708.

4. Pinder RM, Brodgen RN, Speight TM. Sodium valproate: a review of its pharmacological properties and therapeutic efficacy in epilepsy. *Drugs* 1977; 13:81–123.

5. Bruni J, Wilder BJ. Valproic acid. Review of a new antiepileptic drug. *Arch Neurol* 1979; 36:393–398.

6. Gram L, Bentsen KD. Valproate: an update review. *Acta Neurol Scand* 1985; 72:129–139.

7. Bourgeois BFD. Valproic acid: clinical use. In: Levy RH, Mattson RH, Meldrum BS, eds. *Antiepileptic Drugs.* 4th ed. New York: Raven Press, 1995:633–639.

8. Meunier H, Carraz G, Meunier V, Eymard M. Proprietes pharmacodynamiques de l'acide n-propylacetique. *Therapie* 1963; 18:435–438.

9. Pellegrini A, Gloor P, Sherwin AL. Effect of valproate sodium on generalized penicillin in the cat. *Epilepsia* 1978; 19:351–360.

10. Chapman A, Keane PE, Meldrum BS, Simiand J, Vernieres JC. Mechanism of anticonvulsant action of valproate. *Prog Neurobiol* 1982; 19:315–399.

11. Frey HH, Loscher W, Reiche R, Schultz D. Antiepileptic potency of common antiepileptic drugs in the gerbil. *Pharmacology* 1983; 27:330–335.

12. Leveil V, Naquet R. A study of the action of valproic acid on the kindling effect. *Epilepsia* 1977; 18:229–234.

13. Fariello RG, Varasi M, Smith MC. Valproic acid: mechanisms of action. In: Levy R, Mattson R, Meldrum B, eds. *Antiepileptic Drugs.* 4th ed. New York: Raven Press, 1995:581–588.

14. Godin Y, Heiner L, Mark J, Mandel P. Effects of di-n-propylacetate, an anticonvulsive compound, on GABA metabolism. *J Neurochem* 1969; 16:869–873.

15. Löscher W. Correlation between alterations in brain GABA metabolism and seizure excitability following administration of GABA aminotransferase inhibitors and valproic acid — a reevaluation. *Neurochem Int* 1981; 3:397–404.

16. Fowler LJ, Beckford J, John RA. An analysis of the kinetics of the inhibition of rabbit brain GABA-transaminase by sodium *N*-dipropylacetate and some other simple carboxytic acids. *Biochem Pharmacol* 1975; 24:1267–1270.

17. Harvey PKB, Bradford HF, Davisson AN. The inhibitory effect of sodium n-dipropylacetate on the degradative enzymes of the GABA shunt. *FEBS Lett* 1975; 52F:251–254.

18. Kerwin RW, Olpe HR, Schmutz M. The effect of sodium-n-dipropylacetate on GABA dependent inhibition on rate cortex *in vivo. Br J Pharmacol* 1980; 71:545–551.

19. McLean MJ, MacDonald RL. Sodium valproate, but not ethosuximide, produces use and voltage-dependent limitation of high frequency repetitive firing of action potentials of mouse central neurons in cell culture. *J Pharmacol Exp Ther* 1986; 237:1001–1011.

20. Franceschetti S, Hamon B, Heinemann U. The action of valproate on spontaneous epileptiform activity in the absence of synaptic transmission and on evoked changes on [Ca+] AND [K+] in the hippocampal slice. *Brain Res* 1986; 386:1–11.

21. Schechter PJ, Trainer Y, Grove J. Effect of *N*-dipropylacetate on amino acid concentration in mouse brain: correlations with anticonvulsant activity. *J Neurochem* 1978; 3:1325–1327.

22. Levy RH, Rettenmeier AW, Anderson GD. Effects of polytherapy with phenytoin, carbamazepine, and stiripentol on formation of 4-ene-valproate, a hepatotoxic metabolite of valproic acid. *Clin Pharmacol Ther* 1990; 48:225–235.

23. Löscher W, Nau H. Pharmacological evaluation of various metabolites and analogues of valproic acid. *Neuropharmacology* 1985; 24:427–435.

24. Pollack GM, McHugh WB, Gengo FM, Ermer JC, Shen DD. Accumulation and washout kinetics of valproic acid and its active metabolites. *J Clin Pharmacol* 1986; 26:668–676.

25. Nau H, Löscher W. Valproic acid: brain and plasma levels of the drug and its metabolites, anticonvulsant effects and γ-aminobutyric acid (GABA) metabolism in the mouse. *J Pharmacol Exp Ther* 1982; 220:654–659.

26. Nau H, Hauck RS, Ehlers K. Valproic acid-induced neural tube defects in mouse and human: aspects of chirality, alternative drug development, pharmacokinetics, and possible mechanisms. *Pharmacol Toxicol* 1991; 69:310–321.

27. Kesterson JW, Granneman GR, Machinist JM. The hepatotoxicity of valproic acid and its metabolites in rats. I. Toxicologic, biochemical and histopathologic studies. *Hepatology* 1984; 4:1143–1152.

28. Rettie AE, Rettenmeier AW, Howald WN, Baillie TA. Cytochromie P450-catalyzed formation of D^4-VPA, a toxic metabolite of valproic acid. *Science* 1987; 235:890–893.

29. Dreifuss FE, Langer DH, Moline KA, Maxwell JE. Valproic acid hepatic fatalities. II. U.S. experience since 1984. *Neurology* 1989; 39:201–207.

30. Paganini M, Zaccara G, Moroni F, et al. Lack of relationship between sodium valproate-induced adverse effects and the plasma concentration of its metabolite 2-propylpenten-4-oic acid. *Eur J Clin Pharmacol* 1987; 32:219–222.

31. Perucca E, Gatti G, Frigo GM, et al. Disposition of sodium valproate in epileptic patients. *Br J Clin Pharmacol* 1978; 5:495–499.

32. Cloyd JC, Kriel RL. Bioavailability of rectally administered valproic acid syrup. *Neurology* 1981; 31:1348–1352.

33. Thorpy MJ. Rectal valproate syrup and status epilepticus. *Neurology* 1980; 30:1113–1114.

34. Holmes GB, Rosenfeld WE, Graves NM, et al. Absorption of valproic acid suppositories in human volunteers. *Arch Neurol* 1989; 46:906–909.

35. Issakainen J, Bourgeois BFD. Bioavailability of sodium valproate suppositories during repeated administration of steady-state in epileptic children. *Eur J Pediatr* 1987; 146:404–407.

36. Klotz U, Antonin KH. Pharmacokinetics and bioavailability of sodium valproate. *Clin Pharmacol Ther 1 977*; 21:736–743.

37. Gugler R, Schell A, Eichelbaum M, Froscher W, Schulz HU. Disposition of valproic acid in man. *Eur J Clin Pharmacol* 1977; 12:125–132.

38. Levy RH, Conraud B, Loiseau P, et al. Meal-dependent absorption of enteric-coated sodium valproate. *Epilepsia* 1980; 21:273–280.

39. Bourgeois BFD. Pharmacokinetics and pharmacodynamics in clinical practice. In: Wyllie E, ed. *The Treatment of Epilepsy: Principles and Practice.* 2nd ed. Baltimore: Williams & Wilkins, 1997:728–736.

40. Cloyd J, Kriel R, Jones-Saete C, et al. Comparison of sprinkle versus syrup formulations of valproate for bioavailability, tolerance, and preference. *J Pediatr* 1992; 120:634–638.

41. Cramer JA, Mattson RH, Bennett DM, Swick CT. Variable free and total valproic acid concentrations in sole- and multidrug therapy. *Ther Drug Monit* 1986; 8:411–415.

42. Gram L, Flachs H, Wnrtz-Jorgensen A, Parnas J, Andersen B. Sodium valproate, serum level and clinical effect in epilepsy: a controlled study. *Epilepsia* 1979; 20:303–312.

43. Perucca E, Grimaldi R, Gatti G, et al. Pharmacokinetics of valproic acid in the elderly. *Br J Clin Pharmacol* 1984; 17:665–669.

44. Cloyd JC, Fischer JH, Kriel RL, Kraus DM. Valproic acid pharmacokinetics in children. IV. Effects of age and antiepileptic drugs on protein binding and intrinsic clearance. *Clin Pharmacol Ther* 1993; 53:22–29.

45. Hall K, Otten N, Johnston B, et al. A multivariable analysis of factors governing the steady-state pharmacokinetics of valproic acid in 52 young epileptics. *J Clin Pharmacol* 1985; 2:261–268.

46. Gal P, Oles KS, Gilman JT, Weaver R. Valproic acid efficacy, toxicity and pharmacokinetics in neonates with intractable seizures. *Neurology* 1988; 38:467–471.

47. Levy RH, Koch KM. Drug interactions with valproic acid. *Drugs* 1982; 24:543–556.

48. Bourgeois BFD. Pharmacologic interactions between valproate and other drugs. *Am J Med* 1988; 84(Suppl 1A):29–33.

49. Scheyer RD, Mattson RH. Valproic acid—Interactions with other drugs. In: Levy RH, Mattson RH, Meldrum BS, eds. *Antiepileptic Drugs.* 4th ed. New York: Raven Press, 1995:621–631.

50. May T, Rambeck B. Serum concentrations of valproic acid: influence of dose and comedication. *Ther Drug Monit* 1985; 7:387–390.

51. Bowdle TA, Levy RH, Cutler RE. Effect of carbamazepine on valproic acid kinetics in normal subjects. *Clin Pharmacol Ther* 1979; 26:629–634.

52. Reunanen MI, Luoma P, Myllyla V, Hokkanen E. Low serum valproic acid concentrations in epileptic patients on combination therapy. *Curr Ther Res* 1980; 28:456–462.

53. Hoffmann F, von Unruh GE, Jancik BC. Valproic acid disposition in epileptic patients during combined antiepileptic maintenance therapy. *Eur J Clin Pharmacol* 1981; 19:383–385.

54. De Wolff FA, Peters ACB, van Kempen GMJ. Serum concentrations and enzyme induction in epileptic children treated with phenytoin and valproate. *Neuropediatrics* 1982; 13:10–13.

55. Sackellares JC, Sato S, Dreifuss FE, Penry JK. Reduction of steady-state valproate levels by other antiepileptic drugs. *Epilepsia* 1981; 22:437–441.

56. Cloyd JC, Kriel RL, Fischer JH. Valproic acid pharmacokinetics in children. II. Discontinuation of concomitant antiepileptic drug therapy. *Neurology* 1985; 35:1623–1627.

57. Henriksen O, Johannessen SI. Clinical and pharmacokinetic observations on sodium valproate—a 5-year follow-up study in 100 children with epilepsy. *Acta Neurol Scand* 1982; 65:504–523.

58. Wagner ML, Graves NM, Leppik IE, et al. The effect of felbamate on valproate disposition. *Epilepsia* 1991; 32:15.

59. Hooper WD, Franklin ME, Glue P, et al. Effect of felbamate on valproic acid disposition in healthy volunteers: inhibition of B-oxidation. *Epilepsia* 1996; 37:91–97.

60. Suganuma T, Ishizaki T, Chiba K, Hori M. The effect of concurrent administration of valproate sodium on phenobarbital plasma concentration/dosage ratio in pediatric patients. *J Pediatr* 1981; 99:314–317.

61. Redenbaugh JE, Sato S, Penry JK, Dreifuss FE, Kupferberg HJ. Sodium valproate: pharmacokinetics and effectiveness in treating intractable seizures. *Neurology* 1980; 30:1–6.

62. Mattson RH, Cramer JA. Valproic acid and ethosuximide interaction. *Ann Neurol* 1980; 7:583–584.

63. Levy RH, Moreland TA, Morselli PL, et al. Carbamazepine/valproic acid interaction in man and rhesus monkey. *Epilepsia* 1984; 25:338–345.

64. Pisani F, Fazio A, Oteri G, et al. Sodium valproate and valpromide: differential interactions with carbamazepine in epileptic patients. *Epilepsia* 1986; 27:548–552.

65. Yuen AWC, Land G, Weatherley BC, Peck AW. Sodium valproate acutely inhibits lamotrigine metabolism. *Br J Clin Pharmacol* 1992; 33:511–513.

66. Rodin EA, De Sousa G, Haidukewych D, et al. Dissociation between free and bound phenytoin levels in presence of valproate sodium. *Arch Neurol* 1981; 38:240–242.

67. Pisani FD, Di Perri RG. Intravenous valproate: effects on plasma and saliva phenytoin levels. *Neurology* 1981; 31:467–470.

68. Mattson RH, Cramer JA, Darney PD, Naftolin F. Use of oral contraceptives by women with epilepsy. *JAMA* 1986; 256:238–240.

69. Abbott FS, Kassam J, Orr JM, Farrell K. The effect of aspirin on valproic acid metabolism. *Clin Pharmacol Ther* 1986; 40:94–100.

70. Goulden KJ, Dooley JM, Camfield PR, Fraser AD. Clinical valproate toxicity induced by acetylsalicylic acid. *Neurology* 1987; 37:1392–1394.

71. Jeavons PM, Clark JE, Maheshwari MC. Treatment of generalized epilepsies of childhood and adolescence with sodium valproate (Epilim). *Dev Med Child Neurol* 1977; 19:9–25.

72. Adams DJ, Luders H, Pippenger CE. Sodium valproate in the treatment of intractable seizure disorders: a clinical and electroencephalographic study. *Neurology* 1978; 28:152–157.

73. Bergamini L, Mutani R, Fulan PM. The effect of sodium valproate (Epilim) on the EEG. *Electroencephalogr Clin Neurophysiol* 1975; 39:429.

74. Braathen G, Theorell K, Persson A, Rane A. Valproate in the treatment of absence epilepsy in children. *Epilepsia* 1988; 29:548–552.

75. Maheshwari MC, Jeavons PM. The effect of sodium valproate (Epilim) on the EEG. *Electroencephalogr Clin Neurophysiol* 1975; 39:429.

76. Mattson RH, Cramer JA, Williamson PD, Novelly R. Valproic acid in epilepsy: clinical and pharmacological effects. *Ann Neurol* 1978; 3:20–25.

77. Villareal HJ, Wilder BJ, Willmore LJ, et al. Effect of valproic acid on spike and wave discharges in patients with absence seizures. *Neurology* 1978; 28:886–891.

78. Callaghan N, O'Hare J, O'Driscoll D, O'Neill B, Dally M. Comparative study of ethosiximide and sodium valproate in the treatment of typical absence seizures (petit mal). *Dev Med Child Neurol* 1982; 24:830–836.

79. Sato S, White BG, Penry JK, et al. Valproic acid versus ethosuximide in the treatment of absence seizures. *Neurology* 1982; 32:157–163.

80. Covanis A, Gupta AK, Jeavons PM. Sodium valproate: monotherapy and polytherapy. *Epilepsia* 1982; 23: 693–720.

81. Feuerstein J. A long-term study of monotherapy with sodium valproate in primary generalized epilepsy. *Br J Clin Pract* 1983; 27(Suppl 1):17–23.

82. Bourgeois B, Beaumanoir A, Blajev B, et al. Monotherapy with valproate in primary generalized epilepsies. *Epilepsia* 1987; 28(Suppl 2):S8–S11.

83. Erenberg G, Rothner AD, Henry CE, Cruse RP. Valproic acid in the treatment of intractable absence seizures in children. A single-blind clinical and quantitative EEG study. *Am J Dis Child* 1982; 136:526–529.

84. Berkovic SF, Andermann F, Guberman A, Hipola D, Bladin PF. Valproate prevents the recurrence of absence status. *Neurology* 1989; 39:1294–1297.

85. Dulac O, Steru D, Rey E, Perret A, Arthuis M. Monothérapie par le valproate de sodium dans les épilepsies de l'enfant. *Arch Fr Pediatr* 1982; 39:347–352.

86. Turnbull DM, Howel D, Rawlins MD, Chadwick DW. Which drug for the adult epileptic patient: phenytoin or valproate? *Br Med J* 1985; 290:816–819.

87. Spitz MC, Deasy DN. Conversion to valproate monotherapy in nonretarded adults with primary generalized tonic-clonic seizures. *J Epilepsy* 1991; 4:33–38.

88. Ramsey RE, Wilder BJ, Murphy JV, Holmes GL, Uthman B. Efficacy and safety of valproic acid versus phenytoin as sole therapy for newly diagnosed primary generalized tonic-clonic seizures. *J Epilepsy* 1992; 5:55–60.

89. Wilder BJ, Ramsey RE, Murphy JV, et al. Comparison of valproic acid and phenytoin in newly-diagnosed tonic-clonic seizures. *Neurology* 1983; 33:1474–1476.

90. Dulac O, Steru D, Rey E, Arthius M. Sodium valproate monotherapy in childhood epilepsy. *Brain Dev* 1986; 8:47–52.

91. Jeavons PM, Bishop A, Harding GFA. The prognosis of photosensitivity. *Epilepsia* 1986; 27:569–575.

92. Delgado-Escueta AV, Enrile-Bacsal F. Juvenile myoclonic epilepsy of Janz. *Neurology* 1984; 34:285–294.

93. Fahn S. Post-anoxic action myoclonus: improvement with valproic acid. *N Engl J Med* 1978; 299:313–314.

94. Bruni J, Willmore LJ, Wilder BJ. Treatment of post-anoxic intention myoclonus with valproic acid. *Can J Neurol Sci* 1979; 6:39–42.

95. Rollinson RD, Gilligam BS. Post-anoxic action myoclonus (Lance-Adams syndrome) responding to valproate. *Arch Neurol* 1979; 36:44–45.

96. Iivanainen M, Himberg JJ. Valproate and clonazepam in the treatment of severe progressive myoclonus epilepsy. *Arch Neurol* 1982; 39:236–238.

97. Barnes SE, Bower BD. Sodium valproate in the treatment of intractable childhood epilepsy. *Dev Med Child Neurol* 1975; 17:175–181.

98. Olive D, Tridon P, Weber M. Action du dipropylacTtate de sodium sur certaines variétés d'encéphalopathies épileptogènes du nourrisson. *Schweiz Med Wochenschr* 1969; 99:87–92.

99. Rohmann E, Arndi R. The efficacy of Ergenyl (dipropyl acetate) in clonic-, jackknife-, and salaam spasms. *Kinderaerztl Prax* 1976; 44:109–113.

100. Brachet-Liermain A, Demarquez JL. Pharmacokinetics of dipropylacetate in infants and young children. *Pharm Weekbl* 1977; 112:293–297.

101. Yokoyama S, Kodama S, Ogini H. Study of the treatment of infantile spasms. *Brain Dev* 1976; 8:447–453.

102. Bachman DS. Use of valproic acid in treatment of infantile spasms. *Arch Neurol* 1982; 39:49–52.

103. Pavone L, Incorpora G, LaRosa M, LiVolti S, Mollica F. Treatment of infantile spasms with sodium dipropylacetic acid. *Dev Med Child Neurol* 1981; 23:454–461.

104. Bruni J, Albright P. Valproate acid therapy for complex partial seizures: its efficacy and toxic effects. *Arch Neurol* 1983; 40:135–137.

105. Loiseau P, Cohadon S, Jogeix M, Legroux M, Artigues J. Efficacité du valproate de sodium dans les épilepsies partielles. *Rev Neurol (Paris)* 1984; 140:434–437.

106. Callaghan N, Kenny RA, O'Neill B, Crowley M, Goggin T. A prospective study between carbamazepine, phenytoin and sodium valproate as monotherapy in previously untreated and recently diagnosed patients with epilepsy. *J Neurol Neurosurg Psychiatry* 1985; 48:639–644.

107. Turnbull DM, Rawlins MD, Weightman D, Chadwick DW. A comparison of phenytoin and valproate in previously untreated adult epileptic patients. *J Neurol Neurosurg Psychiatry* 1982; 45:55–59.

108. Dean JC, Penry JK. Valproate monotherapy in 30 patients with partial seizures. *Epilepsia* 1988; 29:140–144.

109. Mattson RH, Cramer JA, Collins JF, Dept. of VA Epilepsy Cooperative Study No. 264 Group. A comparison of valproate with carbamazepine for the treatment of complex partial seizures and secondarily generalized tonic-clonic seizures in adults. *N Engl J Med* 1992; 327:765–771.

110. Verity CM, Hosking G, Easter DJ. A multicentre comparative trial of sodium valproate and carbamazepine in pediatric epilepsy. The Paediatric EPITEG Collaborative Group. *Dev Med Child Neurol* 1995; 37(2):97–108.

111. deSilva M, MacArdle B, McGowan M, et al. Randomised comparative monotherapy trial of phenobarbitone, phenytoin, carbamazepine, or sodium valproate for newly diagnosed childhood epilepsy. *Lancet* 1996; 347:709–713.

112. Beydoun A, Sackellares JC, Shu V. Safety and efficacy of divalproex sodium monotherapy in partial epilepsy: a double-blind, concentration-response design clinical trial. Depakote monotherapy for partial seizures study group. *Neurology* 1997; 48:182–188.

113. Cavazzutti GB. Prevention of febrile convulsions with dipropylacetate (Depakine). *Epilepsia* 1975; 16:645–648.

114. Ngwane E, Bower B. Continuous sodium valproate or phenobarbital in the prevention of "simple" febrile convulsions. *Arch Dis Child* 1980; 55:171–174.

115. Minagawa K, Miura H. Phenobarbital, primidone and sodium valproate in the prophylaxis of febrile convulsions. *Brain Dev* 1981; 3:385–393.

116. Lee K, Melchoir JC. Sodium valproate versus phenobarbital in the prophylactic treatment of febrile convulsions in childhood. *Eur J Pediatr* 1981; 137:151–153.

117. Herranz JL, Armijo JA, Arteaga R. Effectiveness and toxicity of phenobarbital, primidone and sodium valproate in the prevention of febrile convulsions, controlled by plasma levels. *Epilepsia* 1984; 25:89–95.

118. Mamelle N, Mamelle JC, Plasse JC, Revol M, Gilly R. Prevention of recurrent febrile convulsions — a randomized therapeutic assay: sodium valproate, phenobarbital and placebo. *Neuropediatrics* 1984; 15:37–42.

119. Rantala H, Tarkka R, Uhari M. A meta-analytic review of the preventive treatment of recurrences of febrile seizures. *J Pediatr* 1997; 131(6):922–925.

120. Lee K, Taudorf K, Hvorslev V. Prophylactic treatment with valproic acid or diazepam in children with febrile convulsions. *Acta Paediatr Scand* 1986; 75:593–597.

121. Steinberg A, Shaley RS, Amir N. Valproic acid in neonatal status convulsion. *Brain Dev* 1986; 8:278–279.

122. Hyuman NM, Dennis PD, Sinclar KG. Tremor due to sodium valproate. *Neurology* 1979; 29:1177–1180.

123. Karas BJ, Wilder BJ, Hammond EJ, Bauman AW. Treatment of valproate tremors. *Neurology* 1983; 33:1380–1382.

124. Bodensteiner JB, Morris HH, Golden GS. Asterixis associated with sodium valproate. *Neurology* 1981; 31:186–190.

125. Armon C, Miller P, Carwile S, et al. Valproate-induced dementia and parkinsonism: prevalence in actively ascertained epilepsy clinic population. *Neurology* 1991; 41:22.

126. Sasso E, Delsoldato S, Negrotti A, Mancia D. Reversible valproate-induced extrapyramidal disorder. *Epilepsia* 1994; 35:391–393.

127. Zaret BS, Cohen RA. Reversible valproic acid-induced dementia: a case report. *Epilepsia* 1986; 27(Suppl 3):234–240.

128. Shin C, Gray L, Armond C. Reversible cerebral atrophy: radiologic correlate of valproate-induced parkinson-dementia syndrome. *Neurology* 1992; 42(Suppl 3):277.

129. McLachlan RS. Pseudoatrophy of the brain with valproic acid monotherapy. *Can J Neurol Sci* 1987; 14:294–296.

130. Papazian O, Canizales E, Alfonso I, et al. Reversible dementia and apparent brain atrophy during valproate therapy. *Ann Neurol* 1995; 38:687–691.

131. Sackellares JC, Lee SI, Dreifuss FE. Stupor following administration of valproic acid to patients receiving other antiepileptic drugs. *Epilepsia* 1979; 20:697–703.

132. Marescaux C, Warter JM, Micheletti G, et al. Stuporous episodes during treatment with sodium valproate: report of seven cases. *Epilepsia* 1982; 23:297–305.

133. Sonnen AEH, Zelvelder WH, Bruens JH. A double blind study of the influence of dipropylacetate on behaviour. *Acta Neurol Scand* 1975; 60(Suppl):43–47.

134. Aman M, Werry J, Paxton J, Turbott S. Effect of sodium valproate on psychomotor performance in children as a function of dose, fluctuations in concentration and diagnosis. *Epilepsia* 1987; 28:115–125.

135. Vining EPG, Mellits ED, Dorsen MM, et al. Psychologic and behavioral effects of antiepileptic drugs in children: a double-blind comparison between phenobarbital and valproic acid. *Pediatrics* 1987; 80:165–174.

136. Gallassi R, Morreale A, Lorusso S, et al. Cognitive effects of valproate. *Epilepsy Res* 1990; 5:160–164.

137. Stores G, Williams PL, Styles E, Zaiwalla Z. Psychological effects of sodium valproate and carbamazepine in epilepsy. *Arch Dis Child* 1992; 67:1330–1337.

138. Betts TA, Crowe A, Alford C. Psychotropic effect of sodium valproate. *Br J Clin Pract* 1982; 18:145–146.

139. Sommerbeck KW, Theilgaard A, Rasmussen KE, et al. Valproate sodium: evaluation of so-called psychotropic effect. A controlled study. *Epilepsia* 1977; 18:159–167.

140. Dinesen H, Gram L, Anderson T, Dam M. Weight gain during treatment with valproate. *Acta Neurol Scand* 1984; 70:65–69.

141. Dean JC, Penry JK. Weight gain patterns in patients with epilepsy: comparison of antiepileptic drugs. *Epilepsia* 1995; 36(Suppl 4):72.

142. Breum L, Astrup A, Gram L, et al. Metabolic changes during treatment with valproate in humans: implications for weight gain. *Metabolism* 1992; 41:666–670.

143. Easter D, O'Bryan-Tear CG, Verity C. Weight gain with valproate or carbamazepine — a reappraisal. *Seizure* 1997; 6(2):121–125.

144. Dreifuss FE, Santilli N, Langer DH, et al. Valproic acid hepatic fatalities: a retrospective view. *Neurology* 1987; 37:379–385.

145. Scheffner D, König S, Rauterberg-Ruland I, et al. Fatal liver failure in 16 children with valproate therapy. *Epilepsia* 1988; 29(Suppl 5):530–542.

146. König SA, Siemes H, Bläker F, et al. Severe hepatotoxicity during valproate therapy: an update and report of eight new fatalities. *Epilepsia* 1994; 35:1005–1015.

147. Bryant A, Dreifuss FE. Valproic acid hepatic fatalities. III. U.S. experience since 1986. *Neurology* 1996; 46:465–469.

148. Sugimoto T, Muro H, Woo M, Nishida N, Murakami K. Valproate metabolites in high-dose valproate plus phenytoin therapy. *Epilepsia* 1996; 37:1200–1203.

149. Sugimoto T, Muro H, Woo M, Nishida N, Murakami K. Metabolite profiles in patients on high-dose valproate monotherapy. *Epilepsy Res* 1996; 25:107–112.

150. Camfield PR. Pancreatitis due to valproic acid. *Lancet* 1979; 1:1198–1199.

151. Coulter DL, Allen RJ. Pancreatitis associated with valproic acid therapy for epilepsy. *Ann Neurol* 1980; 7:693–720.

152. Williams LHP, Reynolds RP, Emery JL. Pancreatitis during sodium valproate treatment. *Arch Dis Child* 1983; 58:543–544.

153. Wyllie E, Wyllie R, Cruse R, Erenberg G, Rothner AD. Pancreatitis associated with valproic acid therapy. *AJDC* 1984; 138:912–914.

154. Asconapé JJ, Penry JK, Dreifuss FE, Riela A, Mirza W. Valproate-associated pancreatitis. *Epilepsia* 1993; 34:177–183.

155. Bale JF, Gay PE, Madsen JA. Monitoring of serum amylase levels during valproic acid therapy. *Ann Neurol* 1982; 11:217–218.

156. Otusbo S, Huruzono T, Kobae H, Yoshimi S, Miyata K. Pancreatitis with normal serum amylase associated with sodium valproate case report. *Brain Devel* 1995; 17(3):219–221.

157. May RB, Sunder TR. Hematologic manifestations of long-term valproate therapy. *Epilepsia* 1993; 34:1098–1101.

158. Hauser E, Seidl R, Freilinger M, Male C, Herkner K. Hematologic manifestations and impaired liver synthetic function during valproate monotherapy. *Brain Devel* 1996; 18(2):105–109.

159. Neophytides AN, Nutt JG, Lodish JR. Thrombocytopenia associated with sodium valproate treatment. *Ann Neurol* 1978; 5:389–390.

160. Barr RD, Copeland SA, Stockwell ML, Morris N, Kelton JC. Valproic acid and immune thrombocytopenia. *Arch Dis Child* 1982; 57:681–684.

161. Gidal B, Spencer N, Maly M, et al. Valproate-mediated disturbances of hemostasis: relationship to dose and plasma concentration. *Neurology* 1994; 44:1418–1422.

162. Kreuz W, Linde M, Funk R, et al. Valproate therapy induces von Willebrand disease Type I. *Epilepsia* 1991; 33:178–184.

163. Winter SL, Kriel RL, Novachec TF, et al. Perioperative blood loss: the effect of valproate. *Ped Neurol* 1996; 15:19–22.

164. Ward MM, Barbaro NM, Laxer KD, Rampil IJ. Preoperative valproate administration does not increase blood loss during temporal lobectomy. *Epilepsia* 1996; 37:98–101.

165. Anderson GD, Lin YX, Berge C, Ojemann G. Absence of bleeding complications in patients undergoing cortical surgery while receiving valproate treatment. *J Neurosurg* 1997; 87(2):252–256.

166. Jaeken J, van Goethem C, Casaer P, Devlieger H, Eggermont E. Neutropenia during sodium valproate treatment. *Arch Dis Child* 1979; 54:985–986.

167. Smith FR, Boots M. Sodium valproate and bone marrow suppression. *Ann Neurol* 1980; 8:197–199.

168. Asconapé JJ, Manning KR, Lancman ME. Systemic lupus erythematosus associated with use of valproate. *Epilepsia* 1994; 35:162–163.

169. Coulter DL, Allen RJ. Hyperammonemia with valproic acid therapy. *J Pediatr* 1981; 99:317–319.

170. Batshaw ML, Brusilow SW. Valproate-induced hyperammonemia. *Ann Neurol* 1982; 11:319–321.

171. Zaret BS, Beckner RR, Marini AM, Wagle W, Passarelli C. Sodium valproate-induced hyperammonemia without clinical hepatic dysfunction. *Neurology* 1982; 32:206–208.

172. Haidukewych D, John G, Zielinski JJ, Rodin EA. Chronic valproic acid therapy in incidence of increases in venous plasma ammonia. *Ther Drug Monit* 1985; 7:290–294.

173. Zaccara G, Paganini M, Campostrini R, et al. Effect of associated antiepileptic treatment on valproate-induced hyperammonemia. *Ther Drug Monit* 1985; 7:185–190.

174. Warter JM, Brandt C, Marescaux C, et al. The renal origin of sodium valproate-induced hyperammonemia in fasting humans. *Neurology* 1983; 33:1136–1140.

175. Gidal BE, Inglese CM, Meyer JF, et al. Diet- and valproate-induced transient hyperammonemia: effect of L-carnitine. *Ped Neurol* 1997; 16(4):301–305.

176. Bohles H, Sewell AC, Wenzel D. The effect of carnitine supplementation in valproate-induced hyperammonaemia. *Acta Paediatr* 1996; 85(4):446–449.

177. Laub MC, Paetake-Brunner I, Jaeger G. Serum carnitine during valproate acid therapy. *Epilepsia* 1986; 27(Suppl 5):559–562.

178. Coulter DL. Carnitine deficiency in epilepsy: risk factors and treatment. *J Child Neurol* 1995; 10(Suppl 2):S32–S39.

179. Triggs WJ, Gilmore RL, Millington DS, et al. Valproate-associated carnitine deficiency and malignant cerebral edema in the absence of hepatic failure. *Int J Clin Pharmacol Therap* 197; 35(9):353–356.

180. Ishikura H, Matsuo N, Matsubara M, et al. Valproic acid overdose and L-carnitine therapy. *J Anal Toxicol* 1996; 20(1):55–58.

181. Murakami K, Sugimoto T, Woo M, Nishida N, Muro H. Effect of L-carnitine supplementation on acute valproate intoxication. *Epilepsia* 1996; 37(7):687–689.

182. Margraf JW, Dreifuss FE. Amenorrhea following initiation of therapy with valproic acid. *Neurology* 1981; 31:159.

183. Isojarvi JI, Laatikainen TJ, Pakarinen AJ, Juntunen KT, Myllyla VV. Polycystic ovaries and hyperandrogenism in women taking valproate for epilepsy. *N Engl J Med* 1993; 19:1383–1388.

184. Isojarvi JI, Laatikainen TJ, Knip M, Pakarinen AJ, Juntunen KT, Myllyla VV. Obesity and endocrine disorders in women taking valproate for epilepsy. *Ann Neurol* 1996; 39:579–584.

185. Isojarvi JI, Rattya J, Myllyla VV, et al. Valproate, lamotrigine, and insulin-mediated risks in women with epilepsy. *Ann Neurol* 1998; 43:446–451.

186. Cook JS, Bale JF, Hoffman RP. Pubertal arrest associated with valproic acid therapy. *Ped Neurol* 1992; 8:229–231.

187. Sharma S, Jacobs HS. Polycystic ovary syndrome associated with treatment with the anticonvulsant sodium valproate. *Curr Opinion Obst Gynecol* 1997; 9(6):391–392.

188. Bjerkedal T, Czeizel A, Goujard J, et al. Valproic acid and spina bifida. *Lancet* 1982; 2:1096.

189. Lindhout D, Meinardi H. Spina bifida and in utero exposure to valproate. *Lancet* 1984; 2:396.

190. Omtzigt JGC, Los FJ, Grobbee DE, et al. The risk of spina bifida aperta after first-trimester exposure to valproate in a prenatal cohort. *Neurology* 1992; 42(Suppl 5):119–125.

191. Wegner C, Nau H. Alteration of embryonic folate metabolism by valproic acid during organogenesis. *Neurology* 1992; 42(Suppl 5):17–24.

192. Jeavons PM, Clark JE, Harding GFA. Valproate and curly hair. *Lancet* 1977; 1:359.

193. Herranz JL, Arteaga R, Armijo JA. Change in hair colour induced by valproic acid. *Dev Med Child Neurol* 1987; 23:386–387.

194. Ettinger A, Moshe S, Shinnar S. Edema associated with long-term valproate therapy. *Epilepsia* 1990; 31:211–213.

195. Herranz JL, Arteaga R, Armijo JA. Side effects of sodium valproate in monotherapy controlled by plasma levels: a study in 88 pediatric patients. *Epilepsia* 1982; 23:203–214.

196. Panayiotopoulos CP. Nocturnal enuresis associated with sodium valproate. *Lancet* 1985; 1:980–981.

197. Choonra IA. Sodium valproate and enuresis. *Lancet* 1985; 1:1276.

198. Branten AJ, Wetzels JF, Weber AM, Koene RA. Hyponatremia due to sodium valproate. *Ann Neurol* 1998; 43(2):265–267.

199. Hyson C, Sadler M. Cross sensitivity of skin rashes with antiepileptic drugs. *Can J Neurol* 1997; 24(3):245–249.

200. Lundberg B, Nergardh A, Boreus LO. Plasma concentrations of valproate during maintenance therapy in epileptic children. *J Neurol* 1982; 228:133–141.

201. Devinsky O, Leppik I, Willmore LJ, et al. Safety of intravenous valproate. *Ann Neurol* 1995; 38(4):670–674.

202. Giroud M, Gras D, Escousse A, Dumas R, Venaud G. Use of injectable valproic acid in status epilepticus: a Pilot Study. *Drug Invest* 1993; 5:154–159.

203. Wheless J, Venkataraman V. Safety of high intravenous valproate loading doses in epilepsy patients. *J Epilepsy* 1998; 11:319–324.

204. Gjerloff I, Arentsen J, Alving J, Secher BG. Monodose versus 3 daily doses of sodium valproate: a controlled trial. *Acta Neurol Scand* 1984; 69:120–124.

205. Stefan H, Burr W, Fichsel H, Fröscher W, Penin H. Intensive follow-up monitoring in patients with once daily evening administration of sodium valproate. *Epilepsia* 1974; 25:152–160.

206. Rowan AJ, Binnie CD, Warfield CA, Meinardi H, Meijer JWA. The delayed effect of sodium valproate on the photoconvulsive response in man. *Epilepsia* 1979; 20:61–68.

207. Burr W, Fröscher W, Hoffmann F, Stefan H. Lack of significant correlation between circadian profiles of valproic acid serum levels and epileptiform electroencephalographic activity. *Ther Drug Monit* 1984; 6:179–181.

208. Chadwick DW. Concentration-effect relationships of valproic acid. *Clin Pharmacokinet* 1985; 10:155–163.

CHAPTER 32

Clinical Use of Ethosuximide, Methsuximide, and Trimethadione

Sanford Schneider, M.D.

ETHOSUXIMIDE

Ethosuximide (2-ethyl-2-methyl succinimide, Zarontin) is remarkably effective in controlling childhood absence epilepsy (CAE). Since its introduction in 1958, it remains the initial drug of choice for CAE. Its infrequent side effects, long half-life, and lack of behavioral alterations constitute a near-ideal antiepileptic drug (AED) for CAE. However, not all absence epilepsy in children is CAE, so failure of seizure control in patients with "petit mal" frequently reflects errant diagnosis rather than ethosuximide failure.

Clinical Use

Long-term follow-up of children with absence epilepsy reveals that only two-thirds have complete remission of their epilepsy (1).The remaining one-third usually do not have CAE but are manifesting absence seizures as the presenting feature of either juvenile myoclonic epilepsy (JME) or atypical absence (usual onset is in adolescence).

Childhood absence epilepsy generally presents in either sex between the ages of 4 and 7 years. CAE patients are almost always neurologically normal and frequently have positive CAE family histories. The diagnosis is often first suspected by a teacher even though parents may have observed, but disregarded, staring spells for months. Neurologic examination is normal, and 3 minutes of hyperventilation almost always produces an absence paroxysm. Minimal automatisms (finger fumbling, lip smacking, blinking) may be observed during a seizure but usually are overlooked unless the patient is videotaped. The electroencephalogram (EEG) typically demonstrates bilaterally synchronous 3 cycle per second spike-and-wave paroxysms, particularly during hyperventilation, interrupting a normal background.

History of rare generalized tonic-clonic seizures, parental awakening myoclonus, a 4 to 6 cycle per second spike-and-wave ("fast spike-and-wave") EEG, and a later age of onset should alert the clinician to the correct diagnosis of JME. Onset in adolescence, particularly in girls, with occasional generalized tonic-clonic seizures and a EEG pattern of 2.5 to 3 cycle per second spike-and-wave ("slow spike-and-wave"), admixed with minimal multispikes should suggest atypical absence. Neurologic examination usually is normal, and the patient frequently can be hyperventilated into an absence seizure. JME is treated with valproate, while atypical absence is difficult to control, frequently requiring a combination of valproate and lamotrigine.

Many nonneurologists tend to lump seizures into two categories: generalized and petit mal. This tendency to label and lump all seizures of short duration as "petit mal" usually results in therapeutic failure.

Ethosuximide is effective in controlling 80 percent to 90 percent of CAE, which fulfills the aforementioned diagnostic guidelines. The patient is often not fully aware that a seizure has occurred (although the patient is aware of a "lapse"), but parents and teachers often report complete cessation of staring episodes. School performance frequently improves, and a repeat EEG generally shows resolution of spike-and-wave activity. Repeat provocative hyperventilation almost always shows resolution if the patient is controlled; however, inability to induce hyperventilation does not always indicate total seizure cessation, as even inadequate dosing blocks seizure induction by hyperventilation. Ethosuximide should be minimally increased if near control has been achieved or if hyperventilation still provokes a seizure (2). A steady state is achieved in 7 to 10 days. Further medication increases should occur in 2-week intervals. Clinical impression is usually more valuable than serum levels, but obtaining levels, as with most anticonvulsants, confirms that the patient is receiving medication, severe drug malabsorption or hypermetabolism is not occurring, or seizure control has not occurred despite therapeutic or even toxic levels. If seizure control is not forthcoming despite biweekly medication increases or unacceptable side effects (usually vomiting or nausea), a 10 percent to 20 percent reduction in medication coupled with the introduction of acetazolamide (Diamox) at a dose of 30 mg/kg divided into two daily doses should be considered. If this combination fails, valproate should be substituted for the combination and both medications tapered (3). In extremely refractory patients, combining valproate and ethosuximide is often effective (4), or the combination of valproate and lamotrigine (which will result in an extraordinary lengthening of lamotrigine's half-life) might be considered.

Other than its typical excellent control, without side effect in CAE, ethosuximide has a limited role as an adjunctive anticonvulsant. In children with multiple seizure types, frequent astatic episodes ("drop attacks") with traumatic consequences, the addition of ethosuximide to the existing drug regimen may result in substantial, or evenly rarely complete, control of drop attacks (5).

Ethosuximide therapy occasionally may be used as add-on therapy in myoclonic epilepsy after other major anticonvulsants either singly or in combination have failed. Although valproate is the drug of choice for photic-induced epilepsy, ethosuximide may be effective either alone or combined with valproate. Although there is little support in the literature, some clinicians use adjunctive ethosuximide to control generalized tonic-clonic seizure activity. A rare patient with infantile spasms refractory to adrenocorticotropic hormone (ACTH), clonazepam, and valproate demonstrate clinical and EEG improvement after adding ethosuximide to the drug combinations.

Automatic multiyear maintenance on ethosuximide in CAE is often not necessary. The immediate stigmata of epilepsy and possibly the adult psychological burden of childhood absence should direct the clinician to plan strategies for relatively short ethosuximide treatment protocols (6). Most CAE patients in complete remission (no clinical absence and normalized EEG) following a year of ethosuximide can be safely tapered off medication over 6 weeks (7).

Dosage

The goal of administrating ethosuximide, as with all AEDs, is cessation of seizure activity without side effects. Ethosuximide is relatively unique among anticonvulsant medications in that this goal can usually be obtained. Parents and teachers usually report disappearance of staring spells several weeks after the introduction of ethosuximide. The clinician is no longer able to induce a seizure by hyperventilation, and the EEG normalizes. The initial pediatric dose of ethosuximide is 20 to 30 mg/kg/day (Table 32-1). Rather than initiating the full dose, experienced clinicians start one-third of the dose after the evening meal and in 5 days increase by an additional one-third after breakfast, and 5 days later, add the remaining one-third after lunch. Medication should be given during or after meals to lessen the possibility of gastric upset.

Absorption is nearly complete after oral administration with peak levels in 3 to 7 hours. Ethosuximide is not protein-bound and serum, saliva, and cerebrospinal fluid levels approximate each other (8). Ethosuximide readily passes into breast milk and across the placenta (9). It is not stored in body fat. Although the usual therapeutic level of ethosuximide is 40 to 100 μg/mL, many patients will be controlled with levels of 15 to 20 g/mL. Occasionally it is necessary to increase the serum level to 150 μg/mL, which seldom results in patient toxicity. A typical 10-year-old usually is maintained on 250 mg three times a day, and a 4-year-old usually receives 125 mg twice a day. Because of its extremely long half-life, blood sampling is valid throughout the day. The well-controlled patient rarely needs monitoring of the serum level. However, serum levels are useful if compliance is questionable, especially in the self-medicating adolescent, reporting of seizure activity is not clarified, or for the occasional patient who requires excessive amounts for maintenance.

Ethosuximide is available in 250-mg capsules and as a 250-mg/5 mL suspension. Children should take the capsules rather than the suspension for convenience and accuracy of dose, although some children accept only liquid. Freezing capsules often eases swallowing and allows the capsules to be easily halved for 125-mg dosing.

Initial therapy should be three times a day after meals. After 2 months of control, the dosing should be altered to twice a day, after breakfast and dinner, to simplify the schedule and eliminate dosing during school hours. Despite the long half-life of 30 or more hours, some children inexplicably have loss of seizure control on twice-a-day dosing; these children should be restored to three-times-a-day dosing.

Pharmacokinetics

Ethosuximide decreases membrane excitability by reducing a low threshold (T-type) calcium-channel current (10). The hypothesis is that hypermetabolic, hyperexcitable nervous tissue is more vulnerable to the

Table 32-1. Clinical Features of Ethosuximide, Methsuximide, and Trimethadione

Drug	Pharmaco-kinetics	Typical Dose/Day Pediatric (mg/kg)	Adult (mg)	Therapeutic Serum Concentration (mg/L)	Development of Steady State (days)	Serum Half-Life (h) Children	Adults	Side Effects	Dispensed As
Ethosuximide (Zarontin)	Linear	20–30	1000	40–100	7–10	30	40–60	Gastrointestinal upset, vomiting, headache, depression	250 mg caps 250 mg/5 mL suspension
Methsuximide (Celontin)	Linear	20	1200	Active metabolite N-desmethyl methsuximide 20–40	8–16	N/A	Methsuximide 1.4 N-desmethyl-methsuximide 30–50	Drowsiness, gastrointestinal upset hiccups, depression	150 mg caps 300 mg caps
Trimethadione (Tridione)	Linear	30–60	1200–2400	Trimethadione 20–35	14–28	N/A	Trimethadione 16 Dimethadione 240 (10 days)	Day blindness (hemeralopia), photophobia, dermatitis, Stevens-Johnson syndrome, pancytopenia, nephrotic syndrome, known teratogen (fetal trimethadione syndrome)	300 mg caps 150 mg tabs 200 mg/5 mL suspension

N/A = not applicable.

depressing effects of ethosuximide (11). Animal models suggest the site of action may be localized to hindbrain structures (12).

Ethosuximide is transformed to glucoronide by hepatic hydroxylation (13). Approximately 25 percent of the drug is excreted in the liver. Ethosuximide is not known to significantly interfere with the metabolism of other drugs. The clearance of ethosuximide is delayed by valproic acid, which may cause a mild, rarely a marked rise, in serum ethosuximide levels (14). Carbamazepine, primidone, and phenytoin may mildly enhance ethosuximide clearance (15), whereas isoniazid and rifampin may cause a significant elevation of ethosuximide levels (16). Oral contraceptives do not alter serum levels. Ethosuximide is dialyzable, which may be clinically important for treatment of a massive overdose or for the seizure patient on chronic dialysis.

Steady state occurs 7 to 10 days after the recommended maintenance dose is obtained. Ethosuximide elimination kinetics are linear; change in the dose produces a proportional change in serum level. However, predicting the serum level to dose (L/D) ratio is difficult as large study populations demonstrate wide scatter (17).

Toxicity

Ethosuximide is relatively free of side effects at routine dosing, but patients occasionally complain of nausea and gastrointestinal upset. This can usually be resolved by taking the medication after eating and by slightly reducing the dose. Headache can also be usually controlled by a modest reduction in dose. The medication seldom causes sedation, behavioral changes, or cognitive alteration. The most serious association is aplastic anemia, with fewer than a 12 cases suggesting a chance occurrence (18). It is doubtful that routine blood counts would detect early anemia. Systemic lupus erythematosus has also rarely been associated with ethosuximide administration (19,20). Thyroiditis, Stevens-Johnson syndrome, and urticaria have been reported as isolated cases. Teratogenicity has been suggested but not confirmed (21).

METHSUXIMIDE

Methsuximide (N-2-dimethyl-2-phenyl-succinimide, Celontin), which has been available since 1956, initially was introduced for control of absence epilepsy. Although it is moderately effective in controlling absence seizures, ethosuximide is superior. The present-day usefulness of methsuximide is as an adjunct in complex partial epilepsy and, to a lesser extent, in generalized epilepsies. When combined with carbamazepine or phenytoin in refractory patients with

partial complex epilepsy or valproate in generalized epilepsy, methsuximide may substantially improve seizure control (22).

Early studies of methsuximide indicate that only 20 percent to 30 percent of patients with absence epilepsy achieve seizure control. Thus, in order, methsuximide, ethosuximide with acetazolamide, valproate, and clonazepam should be instituted before a trial of methsuximide in refractory absence patients.

Epileptologists have recognized that methsuximide is of adjunctive value in controlling refractory complex partial epilepsy. Approximately one-third of patients who have achieved only partial control on phenytoin or carbamazepine demonstrate significant improvement to complete control with the addition of methsuximide (23). It usually is preferable to introduce methsuximide as an adjunctive agent before trying phenobarbital or primidone because of their frequent behavioral and cognitive side effects. Comparison adjunctive studies of lamotrigine or gabapentin and methsuximide have not been undertaken, but clinical experience indicates similar effectivity. If the partial complex epilepsy patient is already maintained on a barbiturate with incomplete control, methsuximide can also be introduced as an adjunctive anticonvulsant.

Methsuximide should be initiated with a 150-mg capsule, increasing by 150 mg weekly until NDM, the active metabolite, has reached 20 to 40 µg/mL (the average adult is generally maintained on a total dose of 600–1200 mg daily). The serum half-life of NDM varies from 38 to 80 hours (Table 32-1). Other concomitant anticonvulsant levels should be measured simultaneously as both phenytoin and phenobarbital compete for hydroxylation of their phenyl rings. Side effects of increasing methsuximide, such as ataxia, lethargy, diplopia, and dysarthria, may be related to the elevations of companion drugs rather than methsuximide intolerance (23). Occasionally, in patients with primary generalized seizures, a similar methsuximide trial, particularly combined with valproate, may reward the patient with improved or complete control.

Rarely, methsuximide is successful in controlling myoclonic epilepsy or myoclonic atonic seizures. One small study of adolescent females with JME reported complete control on up to 1,200 mg of methsuximide monotherapy (24).

Dosage

Methsuximide is supplied only in 150-mg or 300-mg capsules which limit pediatric dosage adjustments. Generally, it is introduced as a single capsule after the evening meal and is increased weekly until the dose approximates 20 mg/kg. The active metabolite has a long half-life, so methsuximide can be taken twice a day in children.

Pharmacology

Methsuximide is rapidly and nearly completely absorbed from the gastrointestinal tract. It distributes throughout all body tissues and is completely and rapidly metabolized within 2 hours to N-demethyl-methsuximide. NDM subsequently is conjugated and competes with other anticonvulsants for biotransformation. This results in increased serum levels of NDM, phenytoin, phenobarbital, and primidone in polytherapy.

Although serum levels of methsuximide are commonly measured along with NDM, only the latter serum level is clinically important (methsuximide levels frequently approach 0 g/mL). The usual therapeutic range of NDM is 20 to 40 µg/mL, but this is based on limited patient study populations. Frequently, seizure control is achieved with levels as low as 10 µg/mL.

Toxicity

Clinical toxicity is similar to ethosuximide and in order includes nausea, gastrointestinal upset, headache, and dizziness. Idiosyncratic reactions include skin rash, depression, and pancytopenia. The drug is not known to be teratogenic, but the usual pharmacologic precautions in women of childbearing age and pregnancy should be observed.

TRIMETHADIONE

Trimethadione (3,5,5-trimethyl-oxozolidine-2,4-dione, Tridione), which was introduced in 1945, was the first medication to significant control absence epilepsy (25). Its use has been largely supplanted by newer and far less toxic medications. Neurologists, should only consider trimethadione, when all other absence AEDs have been thoroughly exhausted and the physician and patient are fully aware of the potential side effects of the medication. Trimethadione is one of a handful of drugs that are unequivocally confirmed as a teratogen, which severely limits its use by females of childbearing age. The prescribing physician should carefully record the side effects with the patient and parents. In this litigious climate, the physician should consider recording or videotaping this discussion.

Although trimethadione is generally useful only in absence epilepsy, older studies report value in patients with refractory photic-induced epilepsy and the Lennox-Gastaut syndrome (26). The legal caveat noted would also apply to clinical trials in these patients.

Dosage

Trimethadione is available in 150-mg tablets, 300-mg capsules, and a 40-mg/mL suspension. Therapy in children is initiated at 20 mg/kg with the adult maximum being 2,400 mg daily. The dose in children should be increased every 2 weeks until a maximum of 60 mg/kg is achieved or side effects are intolerable.

The active metabolite, dimethadione, has a half-life exceeding a week. Each 1 mg/kg increase in medication results in a serum dimethadione level of approximately 12 µg/mL Clinicians commonly divide dosing into two or three daily doses, although once-a-day administration should suffice. The drug has had a recent rebirth of interest because of its ability to dissolve some renal stones so that urologists and internists are prescribing the drug.

Pharmacokinetics

Trimethadione is absorbed nearly completely from the gastric mucosa, and peak serum levels occur within 2 hours of ingestion. It is widely distributed throughout all body tissues. In the liver, it is demethylated to dimethadione, which has a half-life of 10 days. Dimethadione is excreted without further degradation in urine and bile.

Increasing doses results in linear increases in serum concentration although a dimethadione steady state may not be achieved for 4 to 10 weeks. Therefore, dose increases should be in small increments at 3-week intervals. Therapeutic serum level studies are limited but suggest a trimethadione level of 35 µg/mL 2 hours after ingestion and dimethadione levels between 500 and 1200 µg/mL. Drug interactions are not reported except that metarbital, which competes for demethylization, elevates serum levels.

Toxicity

The potential toxicity of this drug is extensive. Side effects include sedation, fatigue, ataxia, and visual deterioration. Heralopia (day blindness) can be controlled by dose reduction. Skin rash is relatively common and occasionally progresses to erythema multiforme or the Stevens-Johnson syndrome. A mild leukopenia is typical but can progress to aplastic anemia. There are rare reports of a reversible myasthenic syndrome, systemic lupus erythematosus, and nephrotic syndrome. Severe overdose results in significant metabolic acidosis. Complete blood counts, urinalysis, and hepatic and renal studies should be monitored weekly for the first 6 weeks after initiating therapy and biweekly for the next 6 weeks, with monthly monitoring thereafter for the first year of therapy. Trimethadione has been documented as a teratogen in a number of studies (27,28). More than two-thirds of pregnant women taking the drug have an abnormal fetus with some or all features of the "fetal trimethadione syndrome," including intrauterine growth retardation, microcephaly, cardiac malformation, malformed ears (low-set, posterior rotation, anteriorly folded helices), and mental retardation in over 50 percent of exposed fetuses. Less frequent fetal anomalies include genitourinary malformation, epicanthal folds, broad nasal bridge, and cleft palate. Potential childbearing adolescents and young women should be extensively counseled and highly educated in the near-universal fetal risks while on trimethadione.

REFERENCES

1. McDonald RL, Kelly KM. Antiepileptic drug mechanisms of action. *Epilepsia* 1995; 36(Suppl 2):S2–S12.

2. Krenz NR, Cooper RM. A combined cobalt and C-14 2-deoxyglucose approach to antiepileptic drug assessment. *Int J Neurosci* 1996; 86:55–66.

3. Mares P, Pohl M, Kubova H, Zelizko M. Is the site of action of ethosuximide in the hindbrain? *Physiol Res* 1994; 43:51–56.

4. Evans E, Schentag J, Jusko W. *Applied Pharmacokinetics, Other Antiepileptic Drugs.* Spokane: Applied Therapeutics, 1986.

5. Tomson T, Villen T. Ethosuximide enantiomers in pregnancy and lactation. *Ther Drug Monit* 1994; 16:621–623.

6. Millership JS, Mifsud J, Collier PS. The metabolism of ethosuximide. *Eur J Drug Metab Pharmacokinet* 1993; 18:349–353.

7. Battino D, Costi C, Francesshett S. Ethosuximide plasma concentrations: influence of age and associated concomitant therapy. *Clin Pharm* 1982; 7:176–180.

8. Mattson RH, Cramer SA. Valproic acid and ethosuximide interaction. *Ann Neurol* 1980; 7:583–584.

9. Giaccone M, Bartoli A, Gatti G, et al. Effect of enzyme inducing anticonvulsants on ethosuximide pharmacokinetics in epileptic patients. *Brit J Clin Pharmacol* 1996; 41:575–579.

10. Bachman KA, Jauregvi L. Use of single sample clearance estimates of cytochrome P450 substrates to characterize human hepatic CYP status in vivo. *Xenobiotica* 1993; 23:307–315.

11. Wirrel EC, Camfield CS, Camfield PR, Gordon KE, Dooley JM. Long-term prognosis of typical childhood absence epilepsy. *Neurology* 1996; 47:912–918.

12. Blomquist H, Zeiterund B. Evaluation of treatment in the typical absence seizures. *Acta Paediatr Scand* 1985; 74:409–415.

13. Wallace SJ. Use of ethosuximide and valproate in the treatment of epilepsy. *Neurol Clin* 1986; 4:601–616.

14. Rowan AJ, Meiser JW, De-Beer-Pawlikowski N. Valproate-ethosuximide combination therapy for refractory absence seizures. *Arch Neurol* 1983; 40: 797–802.

15. Snead OC, Horsey L. Treatment of epileptic falling spells with ethosuximide. *Brain Dev* 1987; 9:602–604.

16. Olsson I, Campenhausen G. Social adjustment in young adults with absence epilepsies. *Epilepsia* 1993; 34:846–851.

17. Amit R, Vitale S, Maytal S. How long to treat childhood absence epilepsy. *Clin Electroencephalogr* 1995; 20:163–165.

18. Massey GV, Dunn NL, Heckel JL, Myer EC, Russell EC. Aplastic anemia following therapy for absence seizures with ethosuximide. *Ped Neurol* 1994; 11:59–61.

19. Takeda S, Koizumi F, Takazakura E. Ethosuximide-induced lupus-like syndrome with renal involvement. *Intern Med* 1996; 35:587–591.

20. Ansell BM. Drug-induced lupus erythematosus in a 9-year-old boy. *Lupus* 1993; 2:193–194.

21. Kuhnz W, Koch S, Jakob S. Ethosuximide in epileptic women during pregnancy and lactation. *Br J Clin Pharmacol* 1984; 18:671–677.

22. Wilder BJ, Buchanan RA. Methsuximide for refractory complex partial seizures. *Neurology* 1981; 31:741–744.

23. Browne TR, Feldman RG, Buchanan RA. Methsuximide for complex partial seizures: efficacy, toxicity, clinical pharmacology, and drug interactions. *Neurology* 1983; 33:414–418.

24. Hurst DL. The use of methsuximide for juvenile myoclonic epilepsy. *Ann Neurol* 1995; 38:517.

25. Lennox MG. The petit mal epilepsies: their treatment with tridione. *JAMA* 1945; 129:1069–1075.

26. Dreiffus FI. *Pediatric Epileptology.* Boston: Wright, 1983.

27. Nichols MM. Fetal anomalies following maternal trimethadione ingestion. *J Pediatr* 1973; 82:885–886.

28. Rosen RC, Lightner EW. Phenotypic malformations in association with maternal methadione therapy. *J Pediatr* 1978; 92:240–244.

CHAPTER 33

Gabapentin

Gregory L. Holmes, M.D., and Phillip L. Pearl, M.D.

Gabapentin [GBP, 1-(aminomethyl)cyclohexaneacetic acid] is a structural analogue of gamma-aminobutyric acid (GABA), which has been available in the United States since 1994 (1). It currently is marketed under the trade name Neurontin and currently has indications for add-on treatment of partial seizures in patients 12 years and older. However, GBP is now being widely used in younger patients, both as adjunctive therapy and as monotherapy. The drug has structural similarities to GABA, the major inhibitory neurotransmitter in the human brain (Figure 33-1). Whereas GABA does not cross the blood–brain barrier, conformational restriction of the GABA molecule with binding into a cyclohexane system confer lipid solubility to the molecule and facilitates the penetration of the blood–brain barrier.

ANIMAL STUDIES

Testing in animals has demonstrated that GBP had considerable antiepileptic properties (2,3). It is effective in the maximal electroshock test in rodents, protects against aspartate- and strychnine-induced and audiogenic tonic-clonic seizures, and prevents seizures

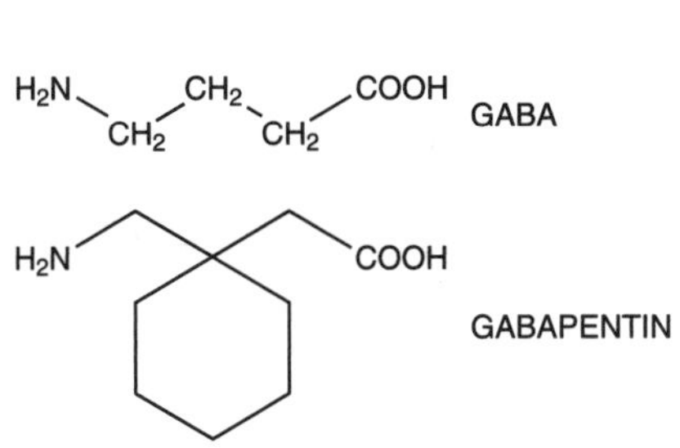

Figure 33-1. Graphic formula of gamma-aminobutyric acid (GABA) and gabapentin.

in the Mongolian gerbil, a model of reflex epilepsy (2,3). GBP prolongs time to clonic activity, tonic extension of the extremities, and death in mice after injections of N-methyl-D-aspartate (NMDA) but not of kainic acid or quinolinic acid (4). When these drugs or glutamate were injected into the lateral ventricles of rats, there were no clear effects of GBP on the seizures (5). Gabapentin reduces after-discharge duration in the kindling model (3,6). These animal studies suggest that GBP should be clinically useful for partial seizures.

While GBP protects mice from clonic convulsions in both the subcutaneous pentylenetetrazol test and the intravenous threshold test (7), in a rat genetic model of absence epilepsy, GBP actually increased spike-and-wave bursts (8). In the lethargic (*lh/lh*) model of absence seizures, Hosford and Wang (9) found that GBP had no effect on absence seizure frequency. Although efficacy against pentylenetetrazol seizures suggests that the drug should be useful in absence seizures, the finding that it is not effective in these animal models of absence seizures raises concerns about the efficacy of the drug in this seizure type. As is described subsequently, GBP has not been demonstrated to be effective in the treatment of childhood absence seizures. The drug does not prevent photosensitive, myoclonic epilepsy in baboons.

In a developmental study, Mares and Haugvicova (10) administered GBP before pentylenetetrazol to rats starting at 7 days. GBP suppressed or at least restricted the tonic phase of generalized tonic-clonic seizures at all the developmental stages studied. In unpublished work from our laboratory, we have also found that GBP increases latency and decreases intensity of flurothyl-induced seizures in immature rats.

Gabapentin exhibits low acute toxicity in mice, rats, and monkeys and no significant systemic toxicity in four species after multidose administration for up to 52 weeks. GBP is not teratogenic and does not affect fertility or general reproductive parameters (6,11). Pancreatic acinar cell tumors have been found in male Wistar rats receiving very large doses of GBP (2,000 mg/kg). These tumors were not observed in female rats or male or female mice. The tumors were low-grade malignancies, did not metabolize, and did not alter survival. The rat pancreatic tumor is not a generally accepted model of human pancreatic cancer, and human pancreatic tumors have not been reported in patients taking GBP (12).

MECHANISM OF ACTION

Despite the similarity of GBP to GABA, binding experiments in rat brain and spinal cord have shown that GBP has no significant affinity for the $GABA_A$ or $GABA_B$ binding sites as measured by [^{3}H]muscimol and [^{3}H] baclofen displacement, respectively. GBP does not inhibit binding of [^{3}H]diazepam at the GABA receptor, has only modest inhibitory effects on the GABA-degrading enzyme GABA-aminotransferase, does not elevate GABA content in nerve terminals, and does not effect the GABA uptake inhibitor. However, GABA concentrations do appear to increase with administration of GBP. Petroff and coworkers (13) used magnetic resonance spectroscopy to estimate GABA brain concentrations. GABA was elevated in patients with partial seizures taking GBP compared with patients matched for antiepileptic drug (AED) treatment. There appeared to be a dose-related response; patients taking high-dose gabapentin had higher levels of GABA than those taking standard doses.

Gabapentin also does not have any significant action at the NMDA receptors, non-NMDA glutamate receptors, or strychnine-insensitive glycine receptors. Based on the lack of a GBP-effect on sustained repetitive firing of action potentials in mouse spinal cord neurons, it does not appear that the drug has an effect on voltage-dependent Na^+ channels (6,14). While GBP was not found to have any significant affect on any Ca^{++} channel current subtype (T, N, or L) (14), studies have demonstrated that the drug may act by binding to the $alpha_2$ delta subunit of the calcium channel (15).

Because the maximal anticonvulsant effect in the maximal electroshock threshold model is not seen until 2 hours after intravenous (IV) administration, the anticonvulsant effects is probably a result of delayed or indirect pharmacologic action (6,16). GBP appears to bind to a high-affinity site in membrane fractions of rat brain tissue (17,18) and is predominately located on neurons in the brain (17). Binding of GBP is highest in the superficial layers of neocortex and dendritic layers of the hippocampus, with low levels of binding in the white matter and brain stem (17). GBP binding is not affected by valproate, phenytoin, carbamazepine, phenobarbital, dizaepam, ethosuximide, or any other neuroactive substance (19). Binding of radiolabeled GBP to this protein is inhibited by leucine, isoleucine, valine, and phenylalanine, which indicates that GBP may bind to a site in the brain that resembles the large neutral amino acid transporter described in other tissues (20). It is possible that this may result in a decrease in the uptake of branch-chain amino acids into neurons; consequently, decreased neuronal glutamate synthesis may occur (21).

PHARMACOKINETIC PROPERTIES

Although most of the available information regarding pharmacokinetics is from adult studies, there do not appear to be any unexpected pharmacokinetic differences between children and adults.

The absorption of GBP is dose-dependent. Sixty percent of a 300-mg dose of GBP is absorbed compared with 35 percent of a 1600-mg dose (22,23). The drug is transported from the blood into the gut by a saturable transport mechanism, the L-system transporter of amino acids (24,25). Because of this dose-dependent bioavailiability, plasma concentrations of the drug are not directly proportional to dose throughout the range of doses studied (26). In adults, mean steady-state maximal and minimal concentrations (C_{min} and C_{max}, respectively) of GBP were proportional with doses up to approximately 1.8 g daily. At higher doses, however, C_{max} and C_{min} continued to increase, but the rate of increase was less than expected (24).

Maximum GBP concentrations occur 2–3 hours after administration of the drug. GBP absorption pharmacokinetics are not altered following multiple-dose administration, and accumulation of the drug following multiple-dose administration is predictable from single-dose data. While food has no effect on absorption (22), aluminum hydroxide–magnesium hydroxide antacid decreases the extent of GBP bioavailability by 20 percent when administered simultaneously or 2 hours after GBP ingestion (27).

Once absorbed, the drug is widely distributed throughout the body. GBP does not bind to plasma proteins to any clinically relevant extent, and protein displacement of drugs is not a concern with GBP. GBP readily crosses the blood–brain barrier in rodents and humans (28). GBP concentrations in cerebrospinal fluid and brain tissue are approximately 20 percent and 80 percent of corresponding serum concentrations (29). After 3 months of treatment with 900 or 1200 mg/day of GBP, brain concentrations of GBP in spinal fluid varied from 6 percent to 34 percent of those in plasma (30). There does not appear to be a linear relationship between plasma and cerebral spinal fluid concentrations (31).

Table 33-1.: Chemical and Pharmacokinetic Features of Gabapentin

Pharmacokinetic Properties	Clinical Significance
Bioavailability is dose-dependent. With a 300-mg dose the absorption is 68% versus 46% absorption with 1200 mg.	There is a progressive reduction in percentage of the drug absorbed with increasing dosage. Drug should be given three times daily
T_{max} is 2–3 hours	Reasonably rapid absorption
Half-life of 5–7 hours	Drug should be given at least three times daily
Not metabolized	Half-life not affected by other drugs
No protein binding	No interaction with bound drugs
No metabolites	No concern about toxic metabolites
Excreted by kidneys	Creatinine clearance determines clearance
No hepatic induction/inhibition	Once a steady state is reached blood levels should not fluctuate

Because GBP is not metabolized but is excreted unchanged through the kidneys, clearance of the drug is related to creatinine clearance (21,32). Renal clearance of the drug approximates glomerular filtration rate with an elimination half-life ($t_{1/2}$) in normal healthy adults of 5–9 hours (24). In patients with normal renal function, steady-state can be achieved within 2 days. Autoinduction does not occur with this drug.

Because of the increased creatinine clearance in children, clearance of GBP is greater than adults. In 12 children treated with GBP as add-on therapy Khurana and coworkers (33) found apparent clearance rates to range from 115 mL/kg/hr to 1446 mL/kg/hr with a mean of 372 ± 105 and a median of 292 mL/kg/hr. In this small population the authors did not find a correlation of clearance rates with age.

Doses of GBP should be decreased in patients with renal impairment in whom the peak plasma concentration of GBP are increased and occur later than in patients with normal renal function (34,35). GBP is removed by hemodialysis, and patients undergoing this therapy need to be placed on maintenance doses of the drug. Guidelines are provided in the package insert by the manufacturers. A summary of chemical and pharmacokinetic properties of GBP is provided in Table 33-1.

Serum Concentrations

The usefulness of GBP serum levels has not yet been established (4,21,36,37). The U.K. GBP Study Group found that "mean and median plasma GBP concentrations were higher in responders than in non-responders" but did not provide any specific data (38). Sevenius and coworkers found seizure frequency to be significantly decreased in patients with serum GBP concentrations above 2 mg/L. Crawford and coworkers (37) reported a significant therapeutic benefit from 900 mg GBP per day, which resulted in plasma GBP levels of 2–6 µg/mL. It is likely that with further experience with GBP that a better understanding of the relationship between serum GBP levels, efficacy, and toxicity will be established. Of interest is a patient

described by Brodie (36) with renal impairment who reported a 67 percent reduction in seizure number without side effects while taking 6000 mg of GBP daily. The patient had a plasma GBP level of 61.2 mg/L. In an open-label study of efficacy of GBP in a pediatric population, Khurana and colleagues (33) found that patients with a greater than 50 percent reduction in seizures had a mean serum concentration of 3.7 µg/mL.

Drug Interactions

Because GBP is not protein-bound or metabolized in the liver, there are no significant drug interactions with the other commonly used AEDs, carbamazepine, phenytoin, or valproate (7,39) In addition, GBP pharmacokinetics have not been significantly changed by concomitant administration of other AEDs (32). Studies of the effects of GBP on oral contraceptives report no changes in concentration of the contraceptive components (22,34). Cimtidine use modestly reduces oral and renal clearance of GBP; however, this is of minimal clinical significance and requires no adjustment in GBP dosages (22).

CLINICAL STUDIES

As with most of the recently released AEDs, GBP has been primarily studied in partial seizures in adults. While there are a number of on-going studies, to date there are no published double-blind, placebo-controlled studies evaluating the efficacy of GBP in children with partial seizures. Because partial seizures in children are quite similar to those in adults, however, it is likely that the results of efficacy and safety studies in adults with partial seizures also pertain to children.

Add-On Therapy — Partial Seizures

A total of 792 patients with refractory partial seizures with or without secondary generalization were studied in five double-blind, placebo-controlled, parallel-group studies in adults (40). A minimum of four partial seizures were required per month. Patients received GBP or placebo as add-on therapy for 12 weeks after a 12-week baseline phase, during which concurrent AED therapy was maintained at prestudy levels and baseline seizure frequency was obtained. A total of 307 patients received placebo and 485 received GBP doses of 600, 900, 1200, or 1800 mg/day.

The primary efficacy variable was responder rate, which is defined as the percentage of patients experiencing at least a 50 percent reduction in seizure frequency from baseline to treatment. In this series of placebo-controlled trials, the responder rate in the placebo group was approximately 10 percent compared with 20 percent to 25 percent in the patients who received placebo. The greatest seizure reduction was seen among patients receiving 1800 mg/day of GBP.

In a study of 129 patients with refractory generalized seizures Chadwick and colleagues (41) randomized patients to either placebo or 1200 mg/day of GBP as add-on therapy. While gabapentin provided greater reduction in the frequency of generalized tonic-clonic seizures than placebo, the results were not statistically significant. Gabapentin was tolerated well in this study.

Open-Label Studies

A large number of patients on GBP have been followed up for many years in open-label trials (42–45). Sivenius (43) treated patients with GBP for more than 4 years and found a significant reduction in seizures frequency (>50%) during the follow-up period in five of the seven patients. Likewise, Handforth and Treiman (44) entered 23 patients with intractable epilepsy into an open-label treatment study after a blinded, placebo-controlled, add-on efficacy study. Nine patients had no improvement in seizure control and discontinued the GBP, whereas the remaining 14 patients continued on the GBP. Seven patients on GBP were followed up for 4 years. Maintenance of the efficacy of GBP was investigated in five long-term, open-label studies in a total of 774 patients (42). A majority of these patients had previously participated in a placebo-controlled study and subsequent short-term, open-label extension, reflecting a retention rate of 66 percent. The responder rate remained relatively stable over time, and patients who were responders in early phases continued to respond in later phases (12–18 months). The authors also noted that GBP discontinuation did not cause a rebound increase in seizures.

Leiderman and colleagues (46) presented data on 240 patients who entered an open-label trial after completion of a double-blind, placebo-controlled trial of GBP for partial seizures. GBP was continued in 78 (33%) patients for 3 years, 65 (27%) for 4 years, and 40 (17%) for 5 years. The maximum treatment period was

7 years with a mean treatment duration of 843 days. This study demonstrates that GBP can be tolerated for long periods of time.

Patients who have a response to GBP with add-on therapy may be converted to monotherapy. In an on-going study of an open-label extension of a double-blind, multicenter trial of GBP in partial seizures, 54 of 250 (22%) patients were able to have concurrent AEDs discontinued (47). The patients were allowed to take up to 4800 mg/day.

In a study of the efficacy of GBP in children with refractory partial seizures, Khurana and colleagues (33) reviewed their results in 32 children with refractory partial seizures in which GBP was added to the drug regimen. GBP was given in a dose ranging from 10 to 50 mg/kg/day with a mean dose of 26.7 mg/kg/day for children with partial seizures with or without secondary generalization. Compared to baseline, eleven patients (34.4%) had a greater than 50 percent reduction in seizure frequency, and four patients (12.5%) had a 25 percent to 50 percent decrease.

Comparison of Gabapentin with Other AEDs in Partial Seizures

There are few studies comparing GBP with other AEDs in adults and none that directly compare the antiepileptic efficacy of GBP with other AEDs in children. Anhut and coworkers (48) randomized newly diagnosed patients with a minimum of two partial seizures to one of four parallel fixed-dose treatment groups: 136 patients received one of three GBP doses — 300, 900, or 1800 mg/day, and 46 patients received 600 mg/day of carbamazepine (CBZ). The authors found similar efficacy of the two drugs: 42 percent of the GBP-treated group and 48 percent of the CBZ-treated group were responders.

Other Seizure Types

Gabapentin has been used in one double-blind study of absence seizures in children (49). Unfortunately, a small dose of GBP (15–20 mg/kg/day) was used in the study. In this study of 33 children, GBP was not effective in reducing seizure frequency. No children had an exacerbation of seizure frequency. There is no information available regarding the usefulness of GBP in neonatal seizures, atonic, or tonic seizures. In rare cases GBP may exacerbate myoclonic seizures.

ADVERSE EFFECTS

In general, GBP is very well tolerated in children. Adverse effects with GBP are uncommon and typically consist of somnolence, dizziness, ataxia, fatigue, nystagmus, headache, tremor, diplopia, and nausea and vomiting (12,50). In the five placebo-controlled trials in adults, 76 percent experienced at least one adverse event, compared with 57 percent of patients treated with placebo. Most of the side effects were mild and transient, and few patients have withdrawn from studies because of adverse side effects (12,50). In a review of adverse events with GBP, Ramsay (12) noted that in controlled clinical trials approximately 7 percent of patients receiving GBP withdraw compared with 3 percent of those receiving placebo, with the most common complaints in the GBP-treated patients being somnolence and ataxia. Urinary and fecal incontinence have been reported with GBP (51). As with a number of other AEDs, GBP rarely exacerbates seizures (52).

Side effects do not appear to have a strong relationship to dose. In a study of 245 patients randomized to placebo or GBP, Anhut and colleagues (51) found that 69 percent of patients receiving 900 mg/kg/day and 64 percent of those receiving 1200 mg/kg/day had adverse events compared with 52 percent in the group that received placebo. Weight gain has been reported in some women but has not been a major issue in children. Severe, life-threatening adverse events have not been reported (12). The most significant serious side effects include rash (0.54%), decreased white blood count (0.19%), increased blood urea nitrogen (0.09%), decreased platelets (0.09%), and angina or electrocardiographic changes (0.04%) (12). Changes in clinical laboratory values during GBP therapy are usually transient, isolated occurrences, most of which have not been considered significant or related to GBP therapy (12,40). The incidence of rash compares quite favorably with other AEDs. As with many other AEDs, GBP may exacerbate seizures on rare occasions (52).

Gabapentin has been associated with behavioral disturbances in some children (53–55) For the most part, these disturbances appear to be most prominent in children with preexisting behavioral disturbances. Wolf and coworkers (53) described three children with learning disabilities who developed behavioral problems with hyperactive behavior and explosive outbursts consisting of aggressive and oppositional behavior. The behavior improved once GBP was stopped. Lee and colleagues (55) from Children's Hospital in Boston described seven children who received GBP as adjunctive medication and subsequently developed an intensification of baseline behaviors as well as some new behavioral disturbances. These behaviors included tantrums, directed aggression, defiance, and hyperactivity. All of the children had attention deficit hyperactivity disorder and developmental delays before institution of GBP. The exacerbation of GBP-associated behaviors may be dose-related in some patients since reduction of the dose results in improvement in some children. It is not always necessary to discontinue GBP in children with adverse behavioral

changes if it has been useful in reducing seizure frequency (54,55). The behavioral problems do not appear to be totally confined to children since hypomania with GBP in an adult patient has been reported (56).

No disturbances of memory or learning have been reported with GBP. In a study of normal subjects, a psychotropic effect characterized by improvement in concentration, numerical memory, complex reactions, and reaction time test was reported with GBP (44). Because of the excellent safety profile and lack of interactions, the drug is increasingly being used in the treatment of epilepsy in children with other medical conditions who are receiving medications.

DOSAGE

Dosing for children is not yet well established because the drug has not been approved by the U.S. Food and Drug Administration for a pediatric indication. Nevertheless, the drug is widely used in children, primarily because it is easy to use and is well tolerated by most children.

The drug comes in 100-, 300-, 400-, 600-, and 800-mg capsules. There is no liquid or IV form of the drug. Because clearance of GBP is greater in children than in adults, higher doses, on a milligram per kilogram basis, are needed in children (33). GBP can be started at 10 mg/kg/day and increased weekly, if necessary, until the child is receiving a dose of 30–40 mg/kg/day. The maximum daily dose has not been established. However, we have had children who tolerated and required over 60 mg/kg/day. Because of the dose-dependent bioavailability and short half-life, most children should take the medication three times a day. GBP has a saturable, dose-dependent absorption; however, this becomes a problem with dosing only when high doses of GBP are required. Gidal and coworkers found that there were minimal differences in bioavailability between 3600 mg/day tid and qid. When the dose was increased to 4800 mg/day, a 22 percent increase in absorption was found with qid compared with tid dosing (57).

Because there are no drug interactions, doses of other AEDs do not need to be adjusted. However, if the patient does well on GBP, it is recommended that other AEDs be reduced and eliminated. As mentioned previously, withdrawal of GBP has not been associated with rebound increases of seizures (44). Nevertheless, GBP be tapered over several months once the decision is made to withdraw the drug.

SUMMARY

Gabapentin was initially released as adjunctive therapy for the treatment of partial seizures in adults.

Since the drug has been released, there have been a number of studies demonstrating its efficacy and safety in children. In addition to its antiepileptic properties, the drug has been found to be useful in pain management. GBP has a number of highly desirable properties. There is no protein binding, the drug is not metabolized, and it is excreted unchanged through the urine. There are no significant drug interactions with other AEDs, and other AEDs do not alter the pharmacokinetics of GBP. The drug appears to have a narrow therapeutic profile. It is effective against partial seizures, although the majority of studies have used the drug as add-on therapy, and it has some efficacy in primarily generalized convulsive seizures. The drug is not effective in the treatment of absence or myoclonic seizures. The side-effect profile of the drug is quite attractive. No significant idiosyncratic reactions have been reported. The most common side effects have included dizziness, fatigue, and headache. Rarely, children have adverse behavioral effects such as hyperactivity and agitated behavior. These children usually have preexisting behavioral disturbances. While the full spectrum of GBP effectiveness remains to be determined, it is likely to have a major beneficial impact on the treatment of childhood epilepsy.

ACKNOWLEDGMENT

Supported by a grant from the NINDS (NS27984) to GLH.

REFERENCES

1. Holmes GL. Gabapentin for treatment of epilepsy in children. *Sem Pediatr Neurol* 1997; 4:244–250.

2. Andrews CO, Fischer JH. Gabapentin: a new agent for the management of epilepsy. *Ann Pharmacother* 1994; 28:1188–1196.

3. Goa KL, Sorkin EM. Gabapentin. A review or its pharmacological properties and clinical potential in epilepsy. *Drugs* 1993; 46:409–427.

4. Macdonald RL, Kelly KM. Mechanisms of action of currently prescribed and newly developed antiepileptic drugs. *Epilepsia* 1994; 35:S41–S50

5. Bartoszyk GD, Meyerson N, Reimann W, Satzinger G, Von Hodenberg A. Gabapentin. In: Meldrum BS, Porter RJ, eds. *Current Problems in Epilepsy: New Anticonvulsant Drugs.* London: John Libbey, 1986:147–164.

6. Taylor CP. Gabapentin. Mechanisms of action. In: Levy RH, Mattson RH, Meldrum BS, eds. *Antiepileptic Drugs.* 4th ed. New York: Raven Press, 1995:829–841.

7. Bourgeois BFD. Important pharmacokinetic properties of antiepileptic drugs. *Epilepsia* 1995; 36:S1–S7

8. Foot M, Wallace J. Gabapentin. In: Pisani F, Perucca E, Avanzini G, Richon A, eds. *New Antiepileptic Drugs.* Amsterdam: Elsevier, 1991:109–114.

9. Hosford DA, Wang Y. Utility of the lethargic *(lh/lh)* mouse model of absence seizures in predicting the effects of lamotrigine, vigabatrin, tiagabine, gabapentin, and topiramate against human absence seizures. *Epilepsia* 1997; 38:408–414.

10. Mares P, Haugvicova R. Anticonvulsant action of gabaapentin during postnatal development in rats. *Epilepsia* 1997; 38:893–896.

11. Taylor CP. Emerging perspectives on the mechanism of action of gabapentin. *Neurology* 1994; 44(Suppl 5): S10–S16.

12. Ramsay RE: Gabapentin. Toxicity. In: Levy RH, Mattson RH, Meldrum BS, eds. *Antiepileptic Drugs.* 4th ed. New York: Raven Press, 1995:857–860.

13. Petroff OA, Rothman DL, Behar KL, Lamoureux D, Mattson RH. The effect of gabapentin on brain gamma-aminobutyric acid in patients with epilepsy. *Ann Neurol* 1996; 39:95–99.

14. Rock DM, Kelly KM, Macdonald RL. Gabapentin actions on ligand- and voltage-gated responses in cultured rodent neurons. *Epilepsy Res* 1993; 16:89–98.

15. Gee NS, Brown JP, Dissanayake VUK, et al. The novel anticonvulsant drug, gabapentin (Neurontin), binds to the $\alpha_2\delta$ subunit of a calcium channel. *J Biol Chem* 1996; 271:5776

16. Welty DF, Schielke GP, Vartanian MG, Taylor CP. Gabapentin anti-convulsant action in rats: disequilibrium with peak drug concentrations in plasma and brain microdialysate. *Epilepsy Res* 1993; 14:175–181.

17. Hill DR, Suman-Chauhan N, Woodruff GN. Localization of (^{3}H)gabapentin to a novel site in rat brain: autoradiographic studies. *Eur J Pharmacol* 1993; 244:303–309.

18. Suman-Chauhan N, Webdale L, Hill DR, Woodruff GN. Characterization of [^{3}H]gabapentin in binding to a novel site in rat brain: homogenate binding studies. *Eur J Pharmacol* 1993; 244: 293–301.

19. Chadwick D, Browne TR. Gabapentin. In: Engel J Jr, Pedley TA, eds. *Epilepsy: A Comprehensive Textbook.* Philadephia: Lippincott-Raven, 1997:1521–1530.

20. Thurlow RJ, Brown JP, Gee NS, Hill DR, Woodruff GN. [^{3}H]Gabapentin may label a system-L-like neutral amino acid carrier in brain. *Eur J Pharmacol* 1993; 247: 341–345.

21. Walker MC, Patsalos PN. Clinical pharmacokinetics of new antiepileptic drugs. *Pharmac Ther* 1995; 67:351–384.

22. Richens A. Clinical pharmacokinetics of gabapentin. In: Chadwick D, ed. *New Trends in Epilepsy Management: The Role of Gabapentin.* London: Royal Society of Medicine Services, 1993:41–46.

23. Vollmer KO, Anhut H, Thomann P, Wagner F, Jähnchen D. Pharmacokinetic model and absolute bioavailability of the new anticonvulsant gabapentin. In: Manelis J, Bental E, Loeber JN, Dreifuss FE, eds. *Advances in Epileptology.* Vol. 17. New York: Raven Press, 1987: 209–211.

24. McLean MJ. Gabapentin. Chemistry, absorption, distribution, and excretion. In: Levy RH, Mattson RH, Meldrum BS, eds. *Antiepileptic Drugs.* 4th ed. New York: Raven Press, 1995:843–849.

25. Stewart BH, Kugler AR, Thompson PR, Bockbrader HN. A saturable transport mechanism in the intestinal absorption of gabapentin is the underlying cause of the lack of proportionality between increasing dose and drug levels in plasma. *Pharm Res* 1993; 10:276–281.

26. Elwes RD, Binnie CD. Clinical pharmacokinetics of newer antiepileptic drugs. Lamotrigine, vigabatrin, gabapentin and oxcarbamazepine. *Clin Pharmacokinet* 1996; 30:403–415.

27. Busch JA, Radulovic LL, Bockbrader HN, et al. Effect of Maalox TC on single-dose pharmoacokinetics of gabapentin capsules in healthy subjects. *Pharm Res* 1992; 9(Suppl):S135.

28. Ben-Menachem E, Persson LI, Hedner T. Selected CSF biochemistry and gabapentin concentrations in the CSF and plasma in patients with partial seizures after a single oral dose of gabapentin. *Epilepsy Res* 1992; 11:45–49.

29. Vollmer KO, Türck D, Bockbrader HN, et al. Summary of Neurontin (gabapentin) clinical pharmacokinetics. *Epilepsia* 1992; 33:77.

30. Ben-Menachem E, Hedner T, Persson LI. Seizure frequency and CSF gabapentin, GABA, and monoamine metabolite concentrations after 3 months treatment with 900 mg or 1200 mg gabapentin daily in patients with intractable complex partial seizures. *Neurology* 1990; 40(Suppl 1):158.

31. Ben-Menachem E, Soderfelt B, Hamberger A, Hedner T, Persson LI. Seizure frequency and CSF parameters in a double-blind, placebo-controlled trial of gabapentin in patients with intractable complex partial seizures. *Epilepsy Res* 1995; 21:231–236.

32. McLean MJ. Gabapentin. *Epilepsia* 1995; 36(Suppl 2):S73–S86.

33. Khurana DS, Riviello J, Helmers S, et al. Efficacy of gabapentin in children with refractory partial seizures. *J Pediatr* 1996; 128:829–833.

34. Comstock TJ, Sica DA, Bockbrader HN, Underwood BA, Sedman AJ. Gabapentin pharmacokinetics in subjects with various degrees of renal function. *J Clin Pharmacol* 1990; 30:862.

35. Blum RA, Comstock TJ, Sica DA, et al. Pharmacokinetics of gabapentin in subjects with various degrees of renal function. *Clin Pharmacol Ther* 1994; 56:154–159.

36. Brodie MJ. Routine measurement of new antiepileptic drug concentrations: a critique and a prediction. In: French JA, Leppik I, Dichter M, eds. *Antiepileptic Drug Development.* Advances in Neurology, vol. 76. Philadelphia: Lippincott-Raven, 1998:223–230.

37. Sivenius J, Kälviäinen R, Ylinen A, Riekkinen P. Double-blind study of gabapentin in the treatment of partial seizures. *Epilepsia* 1991; 32:539–542.

38. U.K. Gabapentin Study Group. Gabapentin in partial epilepsy. *Lancet* 1990; 335:1114–1117.

39. Radulovic LL, Wilder BJ, Leppik IE, et al. Lack of interaction of gabapentin with carbamazepine or valproate. *Epilepsia* 1994; 35:155–161.

40. Leiderman DB. Gabapentin as add-on therapy for refractory partial epilepsy: results of five placebo-controlled trials. *Epilepsia* 1994; 35:S74–S76.

41. Chadwick D, Leiderman DB, Sauermann W, Alexander J, Garofalo E. Gabapentin in generalized seizures. *Epilepsy Res* 1996; 25:191–197.

42. Chadwick D. Gabapentin. Clinical use. In: Levy RH, Mattson RH, Meldrum BS, eds. *Antiepileptic Drugs.* 4th ed. New York: Raven Press, 1995:851–856.

43. Sivenius J, Ylinen A, Kalviainen R, Riekkinen PJ. Long-term study with gabapentin in patients with drug-resistant epileptic seizures. *Arch Neurol* 1994; 51:1047–1050.

44. Handforth A, Treiman DM. Efficacy and tolerance of long-term, high-dose gabapentin: Additional observations. *Epilepsia* 1994; 35:1032–1037.

45. Ojemann LM, Wilensky AJ, Temkin NR, et al. Long-term treatment with gabapentin for partial epilepsy. *Epilepsy Res* 1992; 13:159–165.

46. Leiderman DB, Koto EM, LaMoreaux LK, McLean MJ, U.S. GBS Study Group. Long-term therapy with gabapentin (Neurontin): 5-year experience from a US open-label trial. *Epilepsia* 1995; 36:68.

47. Garaofalo E, Hayes A, Greeley C, et al. Gabapentin (Neurontin) monotherapy in patients with medically refractory partial seizures: an open-label extension study. *Epilepsia* 1995; 36:S119–S120.

48. Anhut H, Greiner M, Möckel V, Murray G. Gabapentin (Neurontin) as monotherapy in newly diagnosed patients with partial epilepsy. *Epilepsia* 1995; 36:S119.

49. Trudeau V, Myers S, LaMoreaux L, et al. Gapabentin in naive childhood absence epilepsy: results from two double-blind, placebo-controlled, multicenter studies. *J Child Neurol* 1996; 11:470–475.

50. Ramsay RE. Clinical efficacy and safety of gabapentin. *Neurology* 1994; 44(Suppl 5):S23–S30.

51. Anhut H, Ashman P, Feuerstein TJ, et al. Gabapentin (Neurontin) as add-on therapy in patients with partial seizures: a double-blind, placebo-controlled study. *Epilepsia* 1994; 35:795–801.

52. Mikati M, Khurana D, Riviello J, et al. Efficacy of gabapentin in children with refractory partial seizures. *Neurology* 1995; 45(Suppl 4):A201–A202.

53. Wolf SM, Shinnar S, Kang H, Gil KB, Moshé SL. Gabapentin toxicity in children manifesting as behavioral changes. *Epilepsia* 1995; 36:1203–1205.

54. Tallian KB, Nahata MC, Lo W, Tsao C-Y. Gabapentin associated with aggressive behavior in pediatric patients with seizures. *Epilepsia* 1996; 37:501–502.

55. Lee DO, Steingard RJ, Cesena M, et al. Behavioral side effects of gabapentin in children. *Epilepsia* 1996; 37:87–90.

56. Short C, Cook L. Hypomania induced by gabapentin. *Br J Psychiatr* 1995; 166:679–680.

57. Gidal BE, De Cerce J, Brockbrader HN, et al. Gabapentin bioavailability: effect of dose and frequency of administration in adult patients with epilepsy. *Epilepsy Res* 1998; 31:91–99.

CHAPTER 34

Lamotrigine

John M. Pellock, M.D.

Lamotrigine was first approved for marketing in Ireland in 1993 and soon thereafter in most other countries, including the United Kingdom and the United States. It was initially recommended for use as adjunctive therapy in the treatment of partial seizures, but it was soon identified as possessing a much broader scope of antiepileptic action. It is one of the new broad-spectrum antiepileptic drugs (AEDs), resembling valproate in its multiple uses. Lamotrigine is nonsedating and offers several advantages, but it must be used correctly, especially in children (1–3).

MECHANISM OF ACTION

Lamotrigine was initially developed on the basis of a probably mistaken hypothesis that some AEDs were efficacious because of an antifolate effect. A series of phenyltriazines were investigated by the Wellcome Foundation and led to the development of lamotrigine. Although it has significant antiepileptic action, its action as an antifolate is minimal (4). The identified mechanisms of action of this drug do not explain its broad range of therapeutic efficacy (5). The sole documented cellular mechanism of action is sodium channel block, a mechanism shared by phenytoin and carbamazepine. These drugs are, however, ineffective against absence seizures, and unless the sodium channel block from lamotrigine is quite unique, other mechanisms should explain its broad clinical efficacy (5). This block is both voltage- and use-dependent. Lamotrigine abolishes hind limb extension in the maximal electroshock model in both mouse and rat, and no tolerance is found after 28 days of dosing. Similar median effective dose (ED_{50}) values are obtained in maximal seizure tests with picrotoxin and bicuculline, but it has no effect on leptazol threshold or clonus latency after leptazol administration, as is shown with

ethosuximide and valproate, and would be expected because of its efficacy in absence seizures. Lamotrigine delays the development of electrical kindling in the rat and modifies seizures. A feature that clearly distinguishes it from phenytoin and carbamazepine is its inhibition of visually evoked after-discharges in the rat, a model in which valproate and ethosuximide are also efficacious. Studies suggest that lamotrigine reduces the effects of glutamate on the rat's spinal cord. The use- and voltage-dependent aspects of lamotrigine interactions at the sodium channel may be hypothesized to be responsible both for lamotrigine's effects in blocking veratridine-induced, but not potassium-induced glutamate release and in reducing epileptic activity in hippocampal neurons. Coulter suggests that there are as yet undefined mechanisms through which lamotrigine works in addition to the sodium channel effects, which would be primarily responsible for the efficacy observed clinically in partial and generalized tonic-clonic seizures (5).

CHEMISTRY, METABOLISM, AND PHARMACOKINETICS

Lamotrigine is the name given to 3,5-diamino-6-(2,3-dichloraphenyl)-1,2,4-triazine. It is a stable white powder with solubility of less than 1 mg/mL in water and 1 mg/mL in ethanol. Lamotrigine is well absorbed, and there is a negligible first-pass metabolic effect so that its bioavailability is virtually 100 percent. It is uniformly distributed throughout the body with the volume of distribution of 1.1 L/kg in volunteers. It is excreted in urine primarily as glucuronide conjugates with only 8 percent of the compound unchanged in humans. Metabolites are not thought to be active. Lamotrigine is approximately 55 percent bound to plasma proteins, which is of little clinical significance (4,6).

The pharmacokinetics of lamotrigine in children are similar to those in adults (6). Lamotrigine exhibits first-order linear pharmacokinetics. Lamotrigine absorption is unaffected by food. In patients, the volume of distribution is between 1.25 and 1.47 L/kg. The serum half-life of lamotrigine is between 24.1 and 35 hours in drug-naive adults, but it is significantly altered by enzyme-inducing and enzyme-inhibiting drugs, including AEDs in particular. Clinical trials have demonstrated no evidence of autoinduction or saturable metabolism. Young children, less than 5 years, eliminate lamotrigine somewhat faster than older children and adults. A half-life of 7.7 ± 1.8 hours was noted in young children receiving enzyme-inducing AEDs as cotherapy (7).

The most clinically significant pharmacokinetic finding regarding lamotrigine is that metabolism of the agent can be affected by concurrent drugs. The dosing schedule therefore must be altered whenever enzyme-inducing or enzyme-inhibiting agents are being administered before the addition of lamotrigine. Similarly, alterations in dose may be required whenever one of these AEDs is added or removed as lamotrigine is continued. The half-life of 24.1 to 35 hours in healthy adult volunteers is decreased to approximately 14 hours (6.4–32.2 hours) in those receiving enzyme-inducing drugs, such as phenytoin, carbamazepine, phenobarbital, and primidone, and increased to 30.5–88.8 hours in volunteers receiving valproate (6,8). Whereas valproic acid decreases the clearance of lamotrigine, lamotrigine has been reported to increase the clearance of valproic acid by up to 25 percent in healthy volunteers. Lamotrigine has no significant interaction on carbamazepine or carbamazepine epoxide levels. Lamotrigine has little effect on the plasma levels of oral contraceptives (9).

Because of concomitant AED interactions and the potential to increase life-threatening rash (see "Adverse Effects"), the dosing of lamotrigine must be carefully approached. Table 34-1 lists the recommended doses for children and adults (6). Initial dosing, using the 2-mg, 5-mg, or 25-mg tablets, is frequently appropriate in children, especially those receiving valproate. The 2-mg or 5-mg dispersible tablets allows for correct dosing to be accomplished even in most infants. It is recommended that titration of dosage be done every 2 weeks until the desired clinical effect, usual maintenance dose, or clinical toxicity occurs. It is imperative that one prescribe the initial dose in children on enzyme-inducing AEDs at 0.6 mg/kg/day, but this initial dose must be decreased to 0.15 mg/kg/day if valproic acid is being administered (10). Note that the usual maintenance dose while on valproate is approximately one-third that otherwise required if enzyme-inducing AEDs continue to be administered without valproate. Although there is no noted pharmacokinetic interaction with carbamazepine or other AEDs, we have found that as lamotrigine doses are increased in some patients to over 600 mg/day, increased neurotoxicity is observed. This pharmacodynamic interaction can be alleviated by reducing existing higher doses and levels, particularly of carbamazepine, slightly (typically by only 100–200 mg/day) to allow further escalation of lamotrigine.

Initial blood level determination in those experiencing improved seizure control were below 5 µg/mL. Subsequent experience would suggest that levels at least 12–15 µg/mL are well tolerated by some people, especially when lamotrigine is used as monotherapy, with continued seizure improvement as doses are titrated upward. Nevertheless, more neurotoxicity is to be expected at levels in this upper range or above.

ACTIONS

The initial trials of lamotrigine were performed in adults with refractory partial onset epilepsy. Using double-blind, add-on, placebo-controlled trials of either crossover or parallel design, data from 457 adult patients with refractory partial epilepsy were used

Table 34-1. Lamotrigine Dose Recommendations in Children and Adults

Concurrent AED	Weeks 1 and 2	Weeks 3 and 4	Usual Maintenance Dose
Children			
EIAED	0.6 mg/kg/day	1.2 mg/kg/day	5–15 mk/kg/day
Monotherapy	0.3 mg/kg/day	0.6 mg/kg/day	2–8 mg/kg/day
Valproic Acid	0.15 mg/kg/day	0.3 mg/kg/day	1–5 mg/kg/day
Adults			
With EIAEDs but no VPA	50 mg/day (once a day)	100 mg/day (2 divided doses)	300–500 mg/day (2 divided doses). Escalate dose by 100 mg/day every week
With EIAEDs and VPA	25 mg every other day	25 mg/day	100–400 mg/day (2 divided doses). Escalate dose by 25–50 mg/day every 1 or 2 weeks

EIAED = enzyme-inducing antiepileptic drug. Modified from references 6 and 10.

as the basis of the initial efficacy reports (10–18). Five of these six studies with crossover design showed significant reduction in seizure frequency with an overall 50 percent reduction in 25 percent of the patients. In these patients, who were formerly primarily on enzyme-inducing concomitant AED therapy, doses of lamotrigine ranged from 200 to 500 mg/day, with a suggestion that doses of 400 to 500 mg were more efficacious than lower doses. In addition to the seizure efficacy, nearly half of the patients reported positive global opinions regarding therapy with lamotrigine versus 22 percent receiving placebo. Efficacy as monotherapy in adults with partial seizures has also been established in follow-up studies and in two trials comparing monotherapy lamotrigine to that with carbamazepine or phenytoin (19,20). Forty-three percent of patients treated with lamotrigine and 36 percent of patients treated with phenytoin were seizure-free at the end of 24 weeks, and similar efficacy was noted with carbamazepine as 39 percent of patients on lamotrigine and 38 percent on carbamazepine became seizure-free. The rates of withdrawal were greater for those treated with phenytoin and carbamazepine than for patients treated with lamotrigine (18–20).

In children, lamotrigine has shown utility in a broad range of pediatric epilepsy syndromes in addition to similar efficacy for partial seizures (21). It has been used to treat juvenile myoclonic epilepsy (22), infantile spasms (23), Rett syndrome (24), absence seizures (25), and seizures associated with the Lennox-Gastaut syndrome (26,27). Myoclonic seizures, however, may not respond as well to lamotrigine therapy (28). In five open-label trials involving 285 pediatric patients, aged 1–13 years, with treatment-resistant epilepsy, 34 percent of all evaluable patients experienced at least a 50 percent decrease in seizure frequency at 12 weeks and 41 percent experienced the same improvement at 48 weeks (21). Children with absence seizures, both typical and atypical, appeared to have the best response. In addition, the global evaluations reported improvement in 69 percent of children at 12 weeks and 74 percent at 48 weeks of follow-up. Rash accounted for a 7.4 percent discontinuation rate, whereas the overall safety data revealed a 30 percent discontinuation rate. In a long-term continuation study (29), similar results were noted, with 73 percent maintaining improvement during the follow-up period of up to 4 years. The improved global functioning, which includes increased attention and alertness, has been reported in both pediatric and adult trials, and this is especially pronounced in children with concomitant developmental and/or attentional problems (21,30). More recently, positive and negative psychotropic effects have been noted during the treatment of mentally retarded persons with epilepsy (31).

The double-blind, placebo-controlled trial of lamotrigine in the treatment of 169 patients with Lennox-Gastaut syndrome, aged 3–25 years, clearly establishes the drug as being efficacious in this difficult to treat encephalopathic epilepsy of childhood (26). Patients received either lamotrigine 50–400 mg/day (1–15 mg/kg/day), based on weight and the absence or presence of valproate coadministration or placebo as add-on therapy for 16 weeks. At the time of final evaluation, 33 percent of patients taking lamotrigine and 16 percent of patients taking placebo achieved a seizure reduction of at least 50 percent ($p = 0.01$). Figure 34-1 reveals the median change from baseline and the frequency of all major seizures, drop attacks, and tonic-clonic seizures during this trial. This controlled study clearly demonstrates that lamotrigine may be one of the most effective AEDs in the treatment of patients with the Lennox-Gastaut syndrome.

A double-blind, randomized, placebo-controlled trial of lamotrigine add-on therapy for partial seizures in children and adolescents was performed with 201 treatment-resistant patients (32). Lamotrigine significantly reduced the frequency of all partial and secondarily generalized seizures versus placebo (44% vs. 12.8%). Neurotoxicity was only slightly more common in the lamotrigine-treated group. Although the overall rash rate was equal in the placebo group and the actively treated group, two patients receiving lamotrigine developed serious rash that resulted in hospitalization. A similar number of patients from each treatment group withdrew from the study. Thus, lamotrigine was effective for the treatment of partial seizures in children, and the safety profile was similar to that seen in adults.

ADVERSE EFFECTS

The toxicity profile of lamotrigine includes common adverse events seen with other AEDs, including dizziness, diplopia, headache, ataxia, blurred vision, nausea, somnolence, and vomiting (1,2,4,18,33). These classic neurotoxic adverse effects were more commonly seen in trials using adjunctive therapy and less frequently noted when lamotrigine was administered as monotherapy (Table 34-2). During the clinical trials, rash was the most common reason for discontinuation of lamotrigine and subsequently has become the most feared adverse effect as the potential for developing a life-threatening rash associated with lamotrigine administration has been recognized.

The overall rash rate during the administration of lamotrigine is approximately 10 percent to 12 percent (33). The rash associated with lamotrigine was initially described as maculopapular or erythematous in appearance, displaying characteristics of a

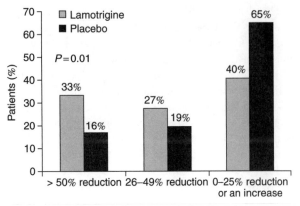

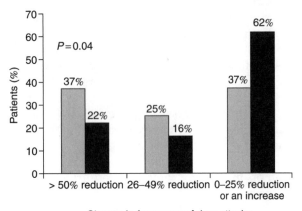

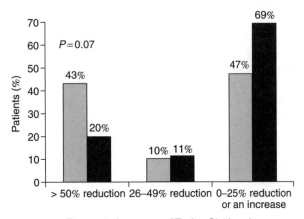

Figure 34-1. Median change from base line in the frequency of all types of major seizures, drop attacks, and tonic-clonic seizures during the 16-week treatment period. The values above the bars are the percentages of patients. Because of rounding, not all percentages total 100. From reference 27.

Table 34-2. Pooled Tolerability from Controlled Comparative Trials of Lamotrigine Monotherapy

Adverse Event[a]	Incidence, % of Patients		
	Lamotrigine ($n = 443$)	Carbamazepine ($n = 246$)	Phenytoin ($n = 95$)
Headache	20	17	19
Asthenia[b]	16	24	29
Rash	12	14	9
Nausea[c]	10	10	4
Dizziness[b]	8	14	13
Somnolence[b]	8	20	28
Insomnia[c]	6	2	3
Flulike syndrome	5	4	3
Rhinitis	4	4	2
Vomiting	4	4	1

[a]Indicates incidence of the most frequently reported adverse events in patients with newly diagnosed or recurrent epilepsy.
[b]Indicates statistically less common with lamotrigine than with carbamazepine or phenytoin or both.
[c]Indicates statistically more common with lamotrigine than with carbamazepine or phenytoin.
(Glaxo Wellcome, data on file)

the first 4 weeks of therapy and is rarely seen after 8 weeks. Subsequently, several children and adults have developed a more severe erythema multiforme-type eruption, sometimes progressing to desquamation with involvement of mucous membranes resembling Stevens-Johnson or Lyell's syndrome. Some patients clearly had a generalized hypersensitivity reaction, but in others the reaction was limited to the skin. A recent review of information concerning the incidence of lamotrigine-associated rash confirms that it is slightly higher in children and when lamotrigine is initiated during concomitant therapy with valproate (35). It also has been suggested that rapid increases in rate of titration of lamotrigine will increase the risk of rash (16,31,35). At present, it is estimated that approximately one adult in 1,000 and one child in 100–200 treated with lamotrigine may be at risk for this potentially life-threatening dermatologic reaction (35).

The U.S. Food and Drug Administration has issued a warning concerning rash within the drug information distributed with lamotrigine. It is recommended that treatment be discontinued when rash appears. However, this recommendation may not be followed outside the United States because of the benign nature of most episodes of rash, even those associated with lamotrigine. When rash is associated with flulike symptoms and malaise, myalgia, lymphadenopathy, or eosinophilia, this suggests a hypersensitivity reaction. The development of these reactions is more common in those who have experienced prior allergic symptoms to medications, particularly those who have experienced allergic or hypersensitivity reactions to AEDs. It is unclear that the present recommendations suggesting

delayed hypersensitivity reaction. It was thought to be self-limited, and no alterations in dosing were suggested. Recent work indicates that the immunologic changes associated with lamotrigine-induced rash may be considered an immune-mediated hypersensitivity reaction (34). This rash typically appears within slower dosage titration truly reduce the rate of rash, but recognizing the risk patterns and paying careful attention to titration and dose schedule is mandatory. The clinician's challenge is to work with the family and patient to determine which possible skin changes indicate a serious dermatologic complication. The time course of appearance (within 4–8 weeks), associated symptoms, distribution over the body, and rash characteristics may significantly help in making a decision to discontinue therapy.

The adverse-effect profile of lamotrigine must be balanced against its broad spectrum efficacy and seemingly positive effects on cognition and behavior (36). Despite the neurobehavioral toxicity noted, it is well tolerated in most adults and children. Direct comparisons reveal positive behavioral and quality of life ratings of patient perceptions. In healthy young adult volunteers, lamotrigine and gabapentin had no performance or other changes, whereas topiramate demonstrated neurocognitive interference after acute and chronic dosing (37). The term *brightening* has been used as patients seem to become less sedated and more alert and attentive. Autistic behaviors showed noted improvements in nearly two-thirds of children with that diagnosis (38).

CONCLUSION

Lamotrigine is a broad-spectrum AED that is effective against both partial and generalized convulsive and nonconvulsive seizures. Its efficacy has been demonstrated in numerous studies in both adult and childhood epilepsy. It joins valproate, felbamate, and topiramate as broad-spectrum agents. Each agent differs slightly in efficacy profiles and reported adverse effects. Improved behavior and brightening has been commonly reported in those taking lamotrigine, whether adjunctive AEDs have been removed or continued. Careful dose titration should be followed during the initiation of this agent, and removal of concomitant agents will allow optimization of monotherapy and total dosing.

REFERENCES

1. Pellock JM, ed. Lamotrigine. *J Child Neurol* 1997; 12(Suppl 1):S1–S52.

2. Fitton A, Goa KL. Lamotrigine: an update of its pharmacology and therapeutic use in epilepsy. *Drugs* 1995; 50:691–713.

3. Goa KL, Ross SR, Chrisp P. Lamotrigine. A review of its pharmacological properties and clinical efficacy in epilepsy. *Drugs* 1993; 46:152–176.

4. Binnie CD. Lamotrigine. In: Engel J, Pedley TA, eds. *Epilepsy: A Comprehensive Textbook.* Philadelphia: Lippincott-Raven, 1997:1531–1540.

5. Coulter DA. Antiepileptic drug cellular mechanisms of action: where does lamotrigine fit in? *J Child Neurol* 1997; 12(Suppl 1):S2–S9.

6. Garnett WR. Lamotrigine: pharmacokinetics. *J Child Neurol* 1997; 12(Suppl 1):S10–S15.

7. Vauzelle-Kervdroedan F, Rey E, Cieuta C, et al. Influence of concurrent antiepileptic medication on the pharmacokinetics of lamotrigine as add-on therapy in epileptic children. *Br J Clin Pharmacol* 1996; 41:325–330.

8. Ramsey RE, Pellock JM, Garnett WR, et al. Pharmacokinetics and safety of lamotrigine (Lamictal) in patients with epilepsy. *Epilepsy Res* 1991; 10:191–200.

9. Holdrich T, Whiteman P, Orme M, et al. Effect of lamotrigine on the pharmacology of the combined oral contraceptive pill. *Epilepsia* 1991; 32(Suppl 1):96.

10. Messenheimer JA, Guberman AH. Rash with lamotrigine: dosing guidelines. *Epilepsia* 2000; 41:488.

11. Binnie CD, Debets RM, Engelsman M, et al. Double-blind, crossover trial of lamotrigine (Lamictal) as add-on therapy in intractable epilepsy. *Epilepsy Res* 1989; 4:222–229.

12. Jawad S, Richens A, Goodwin G, Yuen WC. Controlled trial of lamotrigine (Lamictal) for refractory partial seizures. *Epilepsia* 1989; 30:356–363.

13. Loiseau P, Yuen AWC, Duche B, et al. A randomised double-blind placebo-controlled crossover add-on trial of lamotrigine in patients with treatment-resistant partial seizures. *Epilepsy Res* 1990; 7:136–145.

14. Sanders J, Patsalos P, Oxley J, et al. A randomized, double blind, placebo-controlled, add-on trial of lamotrigine in patients with severe epilepsy. *Epilepsy Res* 1990; 6:221–226.

15. Matsuo F, Bergen D, Faught E, et al. Placebo-controlled study of the efficacy and safety of lamotrigine in patients with partial seizures. *Neurology* 1993; 43:2284–2291.

16. Schapel GJ, Beran RG, Vajda FJE, et al. Double-blind, placebo-controlled, crossover study of lamotrigine in treatment resistant partial seizures. *J Neurol Neurosurg Psychiatry* 1993; 56:448–453.

17. Messenheimer JA, Ramsay RA, Willmore LJ, et al. Lamotrigine therapy for partial seizures: a multicenter placebo-controlled, double-blind, crossover trial. *Epilepsia* 1994; 35:113–121.

18. Smith D, Baker G, Davies G, et al. Outcome of add-on treatment with lamotrigine in partial epilepsy. *Epilepsia* 1993; 34:312–322.

19. Willmore LJ, Messenheimer JA. Adult experience with lamotrigine. *J Child Neurol* 1997; 12(Suppl 1):S16–S18.

20. Brodie Mj, Richens A, Yuen AWC. Double-blind comparison of lamotrigine and carbamazepine in newly diagnosed epilepsy. *Lancet* 1995; 345:476–479.

21. Steiner TJ, Silviera C, Yuen AWC. Comparison of lamotrigine (Lamictal) and phenytoin monotherapy in newly diagnosed epilepsy. *Epilepsia* 1994; 35(Suppl 3):S82.

22. Besag FMC, Wallace SJ, Dulac O, et al. Lamotrigine for the treatment of epilepsy in childhood. *J Pediatrics* 1995; 127:991–997.

23. Timmings PL, Richens A. Efficacy of lamotrigine as monotherapy for juvenile myoclonic epilepsy: pilot study results [abstract]. *Epilepsia* 1993; 34(Suppl 2):S160.

24. Veggiotti P, Cieuta C, Rey E, et al. Lamotrigine in infantile spasms. *Lancet* 1994; 344:1375–1376.

25. Uldall P, Hansen FJ, Tonnby B. Lamotrigine in Rett syndrome. *Neuropediatrics* 1993; 24:339–340.

26. Ferrie CD, Robinson RO, Knott C, et al. Lamotrigine as an add-on drug in typical absence seizures. *Acta Neurol Scand* 1995; 91:200–202.

27. Motte J, Trevathan E, Arvidsson JFV, et al. Lamotrigine for generalized seizures associated with the Lennox-Gastaut syndrome. *N Engl J Med* 1997; 337:1807–1812.

28. Ericksson A-S, Nergardh A, Hoppu K. The efficacy of lamotrigine in children and adolescents with refractory generalized epilepsy: a randomized, double-blind, crossover study. *Epilepsia* 1998; 39:495–501.

29. Guerrini R, Dravet C, Genton P, et al. Lamotrigine and seizure aggravation in severe myoclonic epilepsy. *Epilepsia* 1998; 39:508–512.

30. Besag FMC, Dulac O, Alving J, et al. Long-term safety and efficacy of lamotrigine (Lamictal) in pediatric patients with epilepsy. *Seizure* 1997; 6:51–56.

31. Pellock JM: Overview of lamotrigine and the new antiepileptic drugs: the challenge. *J Child Neurol* 1997; 12(Suppl 1):S48–S52.

32. Ettinger AB, Weisbrot DM, Saracco J, et al. Positive and negative psychotropic effects of lamotrigine in patients with epilepsy and mental retardation. *Epilepsia* 1998; 39(8):874–877.

33. Duchowny M, Pellock JM, Graf WD, et al. A double blind, randomized, placebo- controlled trial of lamotrigine add-on therapy for partial seizures in children and adolescents. *Neurology* 1999; 53:1724–1731.

34. Iannetti P, Raucci U, Zuccaro P, Pacifici R. Lamotrigine hypersensitivity in childhood epilepsy. *Epilepsia* 1998; 39:502–507.

35. Guberman AH, Besag F, Brodie MJ, et al. Lamotrigine-induced rash: risk/benefit considerations in adults and children. *Epilepsia* 1999; 40:985–991.

36. Meador KJ, Baker GA. Behavioral and cognitive effects of lamotrigine. *J Child Neurol* 1997; 12(Suppl 1):S44–S47.

37. Mortin R, Kuzniecky R, Ho S, et al. Cognitive effects of topiramate, gabapentin, and lamotrigine in healthy young adults. *Neurology* 1999; 52:321–327.

38. Uvebrant P, Bauziene R. Intractable epilepsy in children. The efficacy of lamotrigine treatment, including non–seizure-related benefits. *Neuropediatrics* 1994; 25:284–289.

CHAPTER 35

Felbamate

Blaise F.D. Bourgeois, M.D.

At the time of its release in North America in 1993, felbamate was the first new antiepileptic drug (AED) in 15 years. Several relatively unique features characterize the development and release of felbamate. The clinical trials of felbamate were innovative and unconventional. Felbamate was the first AED to undergo a double-blind trial in hospitalized patients withdrawn from AEDs for presurgical long-term monitoring. It was also the first AED submitted to double-blind monotherapy trials. Finally, felbamate was the object of the first placebo-controlled trial conducted in children with the Lennox-Gastaut syndrome. After 1 year of very successful marketing as a drug with no serious toxicity, felbamate came very close to being completely withdrawn from the market because of several cases of severe bone marrow and liver toxicity, some of which were fatal. The main indication for felbamate at the present time is as a third or fourth drug in children with the Lennox-Gastaut syndrome and similar forms of epilepsy who failed to respond to other AEDs.

CHEMISTRY, ANIMAL PHARMACOLOGY, AND MECHANISM OF ACTION

Like the minor tranquilizer meprobamate, felbamate is a dicarbamate. However, felbamate appears to have no sedative or tranquilizing properties at therapeutic levels. Felbamate was found to have a relatively wide spectrum of activity in experimental seizure models. It is effective against seizures produced by systemically administered chemical convulsants, such as pentylenetetrazole and bicucullin, but it is even more potent against seizures elicited by maximal electroshock (1). Felbamate was also shown to possess antiepileptic activity in kindling models (2) and in monkeys with epileptic foci created by injection of aluminum hydroxide (3). The neurotoxicity of felbamate has been found to be exceedingly low in animal models, which resulted in a very high protective index (efficacy to toxicity ratio) (1). In various animal species, repeated administration of felbamate suggested an excellent safety profile on various body systems, and no tolerance to the antiepileptic effect could be demonstrated after repeated administration in animals.

Several potential mechanisms of action for the antiepileptic effect of felbamate have been identified. Inhibition of glycine-enhanced N-methyl-D-aspartate (NMDA)–induced intracellular calcium currents was shown in mice (4). Findings regarding the effect of felbamate on the gamma-aminobutyric acid (GABA) receptor have been contradictory; both a lack of effect on ligand binding to the GABA receptor (5) and potentiation of GABA responses at high felbamate concentrations (6) have been reported. In addition, inhibition of excitatory NMDA responses was demonstrated at high felbamate levels (6). This suggests that felbamate has a dual action on excitatory and on inhibitory brain mechanisms.

METABOLISM, PHARMACOKINETICS, AND INTERACTIONS

After a single dose of felbamate in humans, approximately 50 percent of the drug is excreted in the urine unmetabolized and unconjugated. Approximately 12 percent is excreted in the urine as para-hydroxyfelbamate and 2-hydroxyfelbamate, and most of the remainder of the dose is recovered in urine as unidentified polar metabolites, some of them being glucuronides or sulfate esters (7). Only 2-hydroxyfelbamate and a monocarbamate metabolite could be quantified in plasma during chronic therapy (8). The concentration of these metabolites is too low (approximately 10% of the felbamate concentration) to contribute to the clinical effect, even if they were pharmacologically active. Because of possible pharmacokinetic interactions, these values for the quantitative aspect of felbamate biotransformation may be different in patients taking other AEDs concurrently with felbamate. More recently, evidence has been found in humans suggesting the formation of atropaldehyde (2-phenylpropenal) as a potentially cytotoxic metabolite of felbamate (9,10).

The pharmacokinetics of felbamate have been studied in adults (7,11–15) and in children (16). Based on the administration of ^{14}C-labeled felbamate in adults, an oral bioavailability of at least 90 percent was estimated (7). Linear absorption at least up to doses of 1200 mg was demonstrated in single-dose pharmacokinetic studies (11,12). This linearity was also found during chronic administration at doses of 400 to 3600 mg/day (14). The time to peak concentration is 2 to 6 hours. Felbamate binding to serum proteins is approximately 25 percent and is independent of the felbamate concentration (17). The elimination half-life of felbamate in adult volunteers not taking other medications ranged from 16 to 22 hours (13). The volume of distribution was calculated to be 0.76 L/kg in adults and 0.91 L/kg in children, and, as for most drugs, the clearance of felbamate was found to be higher in children (16). Brain concentrations of felbamate have been measured in humans and were found to correspond to 60 percent to 70 percent of concurrent plasma concentrations (8).

The potential pharmacokinetic interactions between felbamate and other AEDs have been studied quite extensively, and it has been found that felbamate is the cause as well as the object of several pharmacokinetic interactions. When felbamate is added to phenytoin monotherapy, phenytoin levels are raised in a dose-dependent manner (18). Felbamate at a dose of 1200 mg/day raised phenytoin levels by an average of 24 percent, and phenytoin levels were raised further by 20 percent at a felbamate dose of 1800 mg/day. The addition of felbamate also raises valproate levels, probably through an inhibition of the β-oxidation pathway of valproate metabolism (19). Valproate levels were found to be increased by 28 percent at a felbamate dose of 1200 mg/day and by 54 percent at a felbamate dose of 2400 mg/day (17). Inversely, felbamate decreases carbamazepine levels by 20 percent to 25 percent; however, the level of the active metabolite of carbamazepine (carbamazepine-10,11-epoxide) was found to be raised by 57 percent after the addition of felbamate (20). In a group of healthy volunteers, felbamate increased the area under the phenobarbital plasma concentration-time curve by 22 percent (21), and an elevation of methsuximide levels by felbamate was also described (22). No conclusive data are available regarding the effect of felbamate on the levels of other AEDs. The clearance of warfarin was shown to be decreased by approximately 50 percent by the addition of felbamate (23).

Other AEDs also affect the elimination of felbamate. The apparent total body clearance of felbamate is doubled by phenytoin, a known potent enzyme inducer (24). This observation suggests that the felbamate dosage requirements are doubled by the concomitant administration of phenytoin, if the same steady-state serum concentration of felbamate is to be maintained. Carbamazepine also seems to increase the clearance of felbamate but only by about 40 percent (20). No clinically significant effect of valproate on the clearance or elimination half-life of felbamate was demonstrated (13). A recent observation suggests that gabapentin may decrease the clearance of felbamate by approximately one third, with a corresponding 50 percent prolongation of the felbamate half-life (25). If confirmed, this would represent the only known pharmacokinetic interaction involving gabapentin. Significant pharmacokinetic interactions between felbamate and drugs other than AEDs have not been reported.

EFFICACY AND CLINICAL USE

Four pivotal double-blind controlled trials provided most of the the available clinical antiepileptic efficacy data for felbamate: a placebo-controlled trial in patients withdrawn from AEDs for presurgical monitoring, two felbamate monotherapy trials comparing felbamate monotherapy with low-dose valproate monotherapy, and a placebo-controlled trial in children with the Lennox-Gastaut syndrome. The so-called presurgical trial was a novel study design. At the end of a period of seizure monitoring with partial or complete withdrawal from their conventional AEDs, 64 adult patients with documented partial-onset seizures were randomized to felbamate or placebo (26). In addition to their anticonvulsant regimen at the conclusion of the presurgical evaluation, the patients were either rapidly titrated to felbamate 3600 mg/day over 3 days or they received placebo. The predetermined efficacy variable of the study was the time to the fourth seizure or completion of a total of 28 days with less than four seizures, with an initial 8-day inpatient period. At the end of the inpatient period, the dose of one AED was adjusted to the premonitoring dose. Thus, patients were discharged neither on placebo alone nor on placebo with only a low dose of anticonvulsant. Patients experiencing four seizures within 28 days were restarted on the full dose of the medications they were taking before monitoring. For patients receiving felbamate, the time to the fourth seizure was significantly longer than for those receiving placebo. Four seizures within 28 days occurred in 46 percent of the patients taking felbamate as opposed to 88 percent of the patients randomized to placebo. These results clearly established that felbamate has antiepileptic activity in humans with epilepsy, but they did not demonstrate the ability of felbamate to reduce seizure frequency over a longer period in outpatients not withdrawn from AEDs.

The monotherapy studies were designed to compare felbamate with low-dose valproate (15 mg/kg/day) against partial seizures (27,28). The design of these studies was also novel and unique. After felbamate, 3600 mg/day, or low-dose valproate were added in a double-blind parallel manner to the previously administered AED, this drug was withdrawn over 28 days. Because 50 percent of the patients were to be converted to 15 mg/kg/day of valproate alone, the predetermined endpoint and primary efficacy variable consisted of escape criteria (a predefined degree of seizure exacerbation). The number of patients meeting the escape criteria during the observation period of 112 days was significantly higher in the low-dose valproate group than in the felbamate monotherapy group in both studies, showing that felbamate alone has unequivocal efficacy over 112 days against focal onset seizures in adults. However, it is difficult to derive a quantitative assessment of the efficacy. These two studies do not represent a comparison between felbamate and valproate, which was used as a relatively safe placebo. One advantage of such monotherapy studies is that they provide an exclusive assessment of side effects of the new drug being tested. Adverse experiences were mild to moderate, and their incidence was lower during the monotherapy portion of the trial. However, the monotherapy phase was after day 28. Most drugs cause more side effects during the first month of treatment; therefore, the lower incidence of side effects observed after day 28 may also be attributed to tolerance and not to the fact that the drug regimen had been reduced to monotherapy.

A double-blind, placebo-controlled, add-on study of felbamate was carried out in 73 patients with the Lennox-Gastaut syndrome (mean age 13 years, range 4–36 years) (29). An observation period of 56 days was preceded by a 14-day titration period. The previous AED doses remained unchanged, and felbamate was titrated to 45 mg/kg/day or a maximum of 3600 mg/day. The total number of seizures during a 4-hour period of video-EEG recording, the total number of atonic seizures (drop attacks) as reported by the parents or guardians, and the global evaluations of the patients' quality of life were chosen as the primary efficacy variables. In terms of the total frequency of seizures, felbamate was significantly superior to placebo and was particularly effective in reducing drop attacks, the most debilitating seizure type in these patients (Figure 35-1). There was an inverse correlation

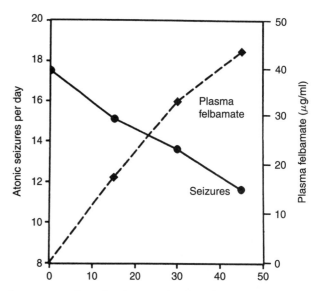

Figure 35-1. Relationship between the daily dose of felbamate and the number of atonic seizures and the plasma felbamate concentration in 28 patients with the Lennox-Gastaut syndrome Reproduced with permission from The Felbamate Study Group in Lennox-Gastaut syndrome. Efficacy of felbamate in childhood epileptic encephalopathy (Lennox-Gastaut syndrome). *N Engl J Med* 1993; 328:29–33.

between felbamate plasma levels and daily number of drop attacks. Additionally, in patients receiving felbamate, the global evaluation scores were significantly higher than in those receiving placebo. When the total number of seizures during a 4-hour period of video-EEG recording was compared, no significant difference between felbamate and placebo was found. The most likely cause of this lack of difference is probably the high spontaneous day-to-day variability in seizure frequency in patients with the Lennox-Gastaut syndrome. This study is of particular interest for two reasons: the Lennox-Gastaut syndrome is notoriously refractory to treatment, and there had been no previous double-blind controlled study of any therapeutic modality in this syndrome. Significant positive behavioral effects in children with Lennox-Gastaut syndrome treated with felbamate have also been reported (30).

A double-blind monotherapy study of felbamate in children with partial seizures was initiated, but it was interrupted when the emergence of serious side effects led to marked restrictions on the use and the promotion of felbamate. The effectiveness of felbamate as an AED that was demonstrated by controlled trials was clearly confirmed by clinical experience during its widespread use after its release. Physicians who have used felbamate in many patients with epilepsy agree that felbamate achieved remarkable seizure control, even in some patients who had been previously refractory to AEDs. In addition, uncontrolled reports have suggested that felbamate may be effective in the treatment of absence seizures (31), juvenile myoclonic epilepsy (32), infantile spasms (33–35), and acquired epileptic aphasia (36).

To minimize the occurrence of initial adverse reactions, felbamate must be introduced cautiously. Titration of the felbamate dose usually must occur simultaneously with a reduction in the dose of concomitant AEDs because of both pharmacokinetic and pharmacodynamic drug interactions. Although precise guidelines have been provided, a slower titration than the one recommended may at times be advisable. A felbamate dose of 1200 mg/day is recommended during the first week in adults, with a reduction of concomitant AED dose(s) by one-fifth to one-third. During the second week of treatment, the dose is to be increased to 2400 mg/day. If monotherapy is the goal, the concomitant AED dose is reduced by another one-third during the second week. During the third week of treatment, if necessary and if tolerated, the felbamate dose is to be increased to 3600 mg/day. In adult patients, doses of 5000 to 6000 mg/day have been commonly used. If felbamate is introduced in a patient who is not taking an enzyme-inducing AED, a slower titration is recommended. After an initial dose of 1200 mg/day, the dose is increased by increments of 600 mg/day at intervals of 2 weeks. Titration is similar in children, the doses corresponding to 1200, 2400, and 3600 mg/day in adults being 15, 30, and 45 mg/kg/day, respectively. Although it is generally better to keep the titration doses below rather than above the recommended doses, maintenance doses may often safely exceed 45 mg/kg/day in children. No definite therapeutic range for plasma felbamate levels has been established. In adults taking 3600 mg/day of felbamate in monotherapy, plasma levels were 65 to 80 mg/L (27,28). In children, the values for felbamate levels in milligram per liter were found to be approximately the same as the dose in mg/kg/day (Figure 35-1). Felbamate levels in 41 adult patients were analyzed by Harden and coworkers (37) and divided into low range (9–36 mg/L), midrange (37–54 mg/L), and high range (44–134 mg/L). Anorexia and complaints of severe side effects occurred significantly more often in the high-level group, but significantly more patients in this group also reported decreased seizure frequency.

TOXICITY

Almost exactly a year after its release, it became evident that the fate of felbamate would be determined much more by its side effects than by its antiepileptic efficacy. Felbamate was initially intensely and broadly marketed as a safe AED that did not display the toxic features of established AEDs and did not require laboratory monitoring. The more common side effects

of felbamate in adults and in children, in monotherapy and with concomitant AEDs, are summarized in Table 35-1 (38). The higher incidence of side effects during adjunctive therapy is likely to be due to pharmacokinetic and pharmacodynamic interactions with other AEDs. The gastrointestinal side effects, including anorexia with weight loss, have been by far the most prominent of these side effects. The quoted numbers of 2 percent to 3 percent probably underestimate the true incidence of weight loss. The weight loss occurs mostly during the first 3 months of treatment, with subsequent stabilization, and represents approximately 2 percent to 5 percent of the body weight. In one series of patients, 34 percent lost more than 4 kg and 11 percent lost more than 8 kg (40). Another significant and rather persistent problem in children has been insomnia and irritability. Two children developed involuntary movements, consisting of choreoathetosis in one child and an acute dystonic reaction in the other child (41).

The first year of postmarketing use revealed that felbamate was associated with a relatively high incidence of life-threatening side effects. In August of 1994, almost a year after the release of felbamate, the number of cases of aplastic anemia that had accumulated was such that the drug came close to being withdrawn from the market (42,43). The aplastic anemias were diagnosed between 2.5 and 6 months after the onset of felbamate therapy. A warning was mailed to all physicians in the United

Table 35-1. Adverse Events Associated with Felbamate Used as Adjunctive Therapy and in Monotherapy in Adults and in Children

Adverse Event	% Patients with Adverse Event	
	Adjunctive Therapy	Monotherapy
Adults		
Nausea	11	4
Anorexia	7	3
Dizziness	6	3
Vomiting	5	2
Weight loss	4	2
Insomnia	4	4
Diplopia	3	0.5
Somnolence	3	1
Headache	3	1
Dyspepsia	2	1
Children		
Anorexia	6	3
Somnolence	6	3
Insomnia	6	1
Vomiting	3	0
Weight loss	2	3
Nausea	2	0
Gait abnormal	2	0

Source: Bourgeois BFD. Felbamate. *Semin Pediatr Neurol* 1997; 4:3–8.

States. In addition, several cases of severe and occasionally fatal hepatotoxicity were reported (44). Promotion of felbamate came to a virtual standstill, all ongoing clinical trials were suspended, and a warning was included in the package insert requiring frequent laboratory monitoring of patients treated with felbamate. Although exact numbers are difficult to determine in such cases, and some degree of underreporting has to be assumed, the reported numbers of cases are as follows (43,45): 31 patients with aplastic anemia were reported and 13 have died; 23 cases were confirmed, of whom 7 have died; among 23 reported patients with hepatotoxicity, felbamate was considered to be the likely cause in 10, 5 of whom have died (Table 35-2). The estimated denominator is a total of 110,000 patients treated with felbamate in the United States after its release. Using this denominator, the calculated risk of developing either one of these two complications is approximately 1 in 4,600, with a risk of death of approximately 1 in 9,300 (Table 35-3). The risk of aplastic anemia could be as much as 10 to 100 times higher than in the general population and 20

times higher than with carbamazepine (45). Although many children have been treated with felbamate, aplastic anemia was not reported in any child under the age of 13 years. The only other patient under 20 years was 18 years of age, and this patient was also the youngest death from aplastic anemia. If the risk of aplastic anemia is discounted, the calculated risk of death from a severe felbamate complication in prepubertal children would be approximately 1 per 22,000. This number is somewhat lower than the rate of valproate hepatic fatalities for monotherapy patients over the age of 2 years and definitely lower than the rate of hepatic fatalities from valproate polytherapy for patients under the age of 10 years (46). This comparison provides a perspective that should help us define the current and future place of felbamate in the treatment of epilepsy. Valproate and carbamazepine have also raised significant concerns of serious idiosyncratic toxicity.

Just as risk factors were identified for valproate, there may also be identifiable risk factors for felbamate toxicity. They may include a history of allergy or cytopenia with previous AEDs, polytherapy, and clinical or serological evidence of a concomitant immune disorder. Individuals in whom abnormally high amounts of the felbamate metabolite atropaldehyde accumulate are at higher risk of toxicity. This and other hypotheses are being explored to identify patients at risk of a severe reaction (47). Felbamate may then regain a more important role in the treatment of epilepsy. Its main indication at the present time is in children with the Lennox-Gastaut syndrome whose seizures remain uncontrolled despite trials with other AEDs such as valproate, clonazepam, lamotrigine, and topiramate. Especially in children, felbamate can also be considered as a third-line drug in patients with refractory focal-onset seizures. If felbamate fails to demonstrate marked seizure reduction after a 2 to 3 month trial, it should be discontinued without delay to reduce or avoid unnecessary exposure of the patient to the risk of a severe reaction.

Table 35-2. Cases of Aplastic Anemia and Hepatotoxicity Associated with Felbamate Therapy (No new cases reported since November 1994)

	Total Number	Number of Deaths
Aplastic anemia		
Reported	31	13
Confirmed	23	7
FBM only cause	3	
FBM most likely cause	11	
FBM possible cause	9	
Hepatotoxicity		
Reported	23	10
FBM likely cause	10	5
FBM unlikely cause	13	5

Sources: Kaufman DW, Kelly JP, Anderson T, Harmon DC, Shapiro S. Evaluation of case reports of aplastic anemia among patients treated with felbamate. *Epilepsia* 1997; 38:1265–1269; and Pellock JM, Brodie MJ. Felbamate: 1997 update. *Epilepsia* 1997; 38:1261–1264.

Table 35-3. Risk of Aplastic Anemia and Hepatotoxicity Associated with Felbamate Therapy (Denominator is 110,000 patients)

	Overall Risk	Risk of Death
Aplastic anemia		
Lower limit ($N = 3$)	1 : 37,000	
Upper limit ($N = 23$)	1 : 4,800	1 : 16,000
Most probable ($N = 14$)	1 : 7,900	
General population	1 : 500,000	
Hepatotoxicity	1 : 11,000	1 : 22,000
Combined risk	1 : 4,600	1 : 9,300

REFERENCES

1. Swinyard EA, Sofia RD, Kupferberg HJ. Comparative anticonvulsant activity and neurotoxicity of felbamate and four prototype antiepileptic drugs in mice and rats. *Epilepsia* 1986; 27:27–34.

2. White HS, Wolf HH, Swinyard EA, et al. A neuropharmacological evaluation of felbamate as a novel anticonvulsant. *Epilepsia* 1992; 33:564–572.

3. Lockard JS, Levy RH, Moore DF. Drug alteration of seizure cyclicity. In Wolf P, Dam M, Janz D, Dreifuss FE, eds. *XVIth Epilepsy International Symposium.* New York:

Raven Press, 1987:725–732. Advances in Epileptology, vol. 16.

4. White HS, Harmsworth WL, Sofia RD, et al. Felbamate modulates the strychnine-insensitive glycine receptor. *Epilepsy Res* 1995; 20:41–48.

5. Ticku MK, Kamatchi GL, Sofia RD. Effect of anticonvulsant felbamate on $GABA_A$ receptor system. *Epilepsia* 1991; 32:389–391.

6. Rho JM, Donevan DC, Rogawski MA. Mechanism of action of the anticonvulsant felbamate: opposing effects on NMDA and $GABA_A$ receptors. *Ann Neurol* 1994; 35:229–234.

7. Shumaker RC, Fantel C, Kelton E, et al. Evaluation of the elimination of [^{14}C]felbamate in healthy men. *Epilepsia* 1990; 31:642.

8. Adusumalli VE, Wichmann JK, Kucharczyk N, et al. Drug concentration in human brain tissue samples from epileptic patients treated with felbamate. *Drug Metab Dispos* 1994; 22:168–170.

9. Thompson CD, Kinter MT, Macdonald TL. Synthesis and in vitro reactivity of 3-carbamoyl-2-phenyl-propionaldehyde and 2-phenylpropenal: putative reactive metabolites of felbamate. *Chem Res Toxicol* 1996; 9:1225–1229.

10. Thompson CD, Gulden PH, Macdonald TL. Identification of modified atropaldehyde mercapturic acids in rat and human urine after felbamate administration. *Chem Res Toxicol* 1997; 10:457–462.

11. Perhach JL, Weliky I, Newton JJ, et al. Felbamate. In: Meldrum BS, Porter RJ, eds. *New Anticonvulsant Drugs*. London-Paris: John Libbey, 1986:117–123.

12. Ward DL, Shumaker RC. Comparative bioavailability of felbamate in healthy men. *Epilepsia* 1990; 31:642.

13. Ward DL, Wagner ML, Perhach JL, et al. Felbamate steady-state pharmacokinetics during co-administration of valproate. *Epilepsia* 1991; 32(Suppl 3):8.

14. Sachdeo RC, Narang-Sachdeo SK, Howard JR, et al. Steady-state pharmacokinetics and dose proportionality of felbamate after oral administration of 1200, 2400, and 3600 mg/day of felbamate. *Epilepsia* 1993; 34:80.

15. Sachdeo R, Narang-Sachdeo SK, Shumaker RC, et al. Tolerability and pharmacokinetics of monotherapy felbamate doses of 1200–6000 mg/day in subjects with epilepsy. *Epilepsia* 1997; 38:887–892.

16. Kelley MT, Walson PD, Cox S, Dusci LJ. Population pharmacokinetics of felbamate in children. *Ther Drug Monit* 1997; 19:29–36.

17. Wagner ML, Graves NM, Leppik IE, et al. The effect of felbamate on valproate disposition. *Epilepsia* 1991; 32:15.

18. Sachdeo R, Wagner M, Sachdeo S, et al. Steady-state pharmacokinetics of phenytoin when co-administered with Felbatol™ (felbamate). *Epilepsia* 1992; 33(Suppl 3):84.

19. Hooper WD, Franklin ME, Glue P, et al. Effect of felbamate on valproic acid disposition in healthy volunteers: inhibition of β-oxidation. *Epilepsia* 1996; 37:91–97.

20. Howard JR, Dix RK, Shumaker RC, et al. Effect of felbamate on carbamazepine pharmacokinetics. *Epilepsia* 1992; 33(Suppl 3):84–85.

21. Reidenberg P, Glue P, Banfield CR, et al. Effects of felbamate on the pharmacokinetics of phenobarbital. *Clin Pharmacol Ther* 1995; 58:279–287.

22. Patrias J, Espe-Lillo J, Ritter FJ. Felbamate-methsuximide interaction. *Epilepsia* 1992; 33:84.

23. Tisdel KA, Israel DS, Kolb KW. Warfarin-felbamate interaction: first report (letter). *Ann Pharmacol* 1994; 28:805.

24. Wagner ML, Graves NM, Marineau K, et al. Discontinuation of phenytoin and carbamazepine in patients receiving felbamate. *Epilepsia* 1991; 32:398–406.

25. Hussein G, Troupin AS, Montouris G. Gabapentin interaction with felbamate. *Neurology* 1996; 47:1106.

26. Bourgeois B, Leppik IE, Sackellares JC, et al. Felbamate: a double-blind controlled trial in patients undergoing presurgical evaluation of partial seizures. *Neurology* 1993; 43:693–696.

27. Sachdeo R, Kramer LD, Rosenberg A, Sachdeo S. Felbamate monotherapy: controlled trial in patients with partial onset seizures. *Ann Neurol* 1992; 32:386–392.

28. Faught E, Sachdeo RC, Remler MP, et al. Felbamate monotherapy for partial-onset seizures: an active-control trial. *Neurology* 1993; 43:688–692.

29. The Felbamate Study Group in Lennox-Gastaut syndrome. Efficacy of felbamate in childhood epileptic encephalopathy (Lennox-Gastaut syndrome). *N Engl J Med* 1993; 328:29–33.

30. Gay PE, Mecham GF, Coskey JS, Sadler T, Thompson JA. Behavioral effects of felbamate in childhood epileptic encephalopathy (Lennox-Gastaut syndrome). *Psychol Reports* 1995; 77:1208–1210.

31. Devinski O, Kothari M, Rubin R, et al. Felbamate for absence seizures. *Epilepsia* 1992; 33(Suppl 3):84.

32. Sachdeo RC, Murphy JV, Kamin M. Felbamate in juvenile myoclonic epilepsy. *Epilepsia* 1992; 33(Suppl 3):118.

33. Hurst DL, Rolan TD. The use of felbamate to treat infantile spasms. *J Child Neurol* 1995; 10:134–136.

34. Stafstrom CE. The use of felbamate to treat infantile spasms. *J Child Neurol* 1996; 11:170–171.

35. Hosain S, Nagarajan L, Carson D, et al. Felbamate for refractory infantile spasms. *J Child Neurol* 1997; 12:466–468.

36. Glauser TA, Olberding LS, Titanic MK, Piccirillo DM. Felbamate in the treatment of acquired epileptic aphasia. *Epilepsy Res* 1995; 20:85–89.

37. Harden CL, Trifiletti R, Kutt H. Felbamate levels in patients with epilepsy. *Epilepsia* 1996; 37:280–283.

38. Wallace Laboratories, Inc., Cranbury, New Jersey: Data on file.

39. Bourgeois BFD. Felbamate. *Semin Pediatr Neurol* 1997; 4:3–8.

40. Bergen D, Ristanovic RK, Waikosky K, Kanner A, Hoeppner TJ. Weight loss in patients taking felbamate. *Clin Neuropharmacol* 1995; 18:23–27.

41. Kerrick JM, Kelley BJ, Maister BH, Graves NM, Leppik IE. Involuntary movement disorders associated with felbamate. *Neurology* 1995; 45:185–187.

42. Pennell PB, Ogaily MS, Macdonald RL. Aplastic anemia in a patient receiving felbamate for complex partial seizures. *Neurology* 1995; 45:456–460.

43. Kaufman DW, Kelly JP, Anderson T, Harmon DC, Shapiro S. Evaluation of case reports of aplastic anemia among patients treated with felbamate. *Epilepsia* 1997; 38:1265–1269.

44. O'Neil MG, Perdun CS, Wilson MB, McGown ST, Patel S. Felbamate-associated fatal acute hepatic necrosis. *Neurology* 1996; 46:1457–1459.

45. Pellock JM, Brodie MJ. Felbamate: 1997 update. *Epilepsia* 1997; 38:1261–1264.

46. Bryant AE, Dreifuss FE: Valproic acid hepatic fatalities. III. U.S. experience since 1986. *Neurology* 1996; 46:465–469.

47. Pellock JM. The place of felbamate in epilepsy therapy: evaluating the risks. *Drug Safety* 1999 (in press).

CHAPTER 36

Topiramate

Tracy A. Glauser, M.D.

Topiramate (TPM) is a new antiepileptic drug (AED) that has recently become available for use in many countries. Evidence of its efficacy was initially demonstrated in multicenter, double-blind, placebo-controlled studies of TPM adjunctive therapy for refractory partial-onset seizures with or without secondary generalization (1–6). Topiramate has also demonstrated efficacy as monotherapy in adults with refractory partial-onset seizures after conversion from one or more standard AEDs (7,8). Based on its broad spectrum of anticonvulsant activity in preclinical studies in vivo and in vitro (9) and favorable results of well-controlled studies in adults, TPM was tested in children with Lennox-Gastaut syndrome, partial-onset seizures, generalized tonic-clonic seizures of nonfocal origin, and infantile spasms (West syndrome) (10–14). Results show that TPM is both well tolerated and effective in reducing seizure frequency in a variety of pediatric epilepsies.

CHEMISTRY

Topiramate, a sulfamate-substituted monosaccharide derived from the *D*-enantiomer of fructose, is structurally distinct from other anticonvulsant drugs (Figure 36-1) (15,16). Topiramate is a white crystalline powder with a molecular weight of 339 and a pK_a of 8.7 at 25 °C (9).

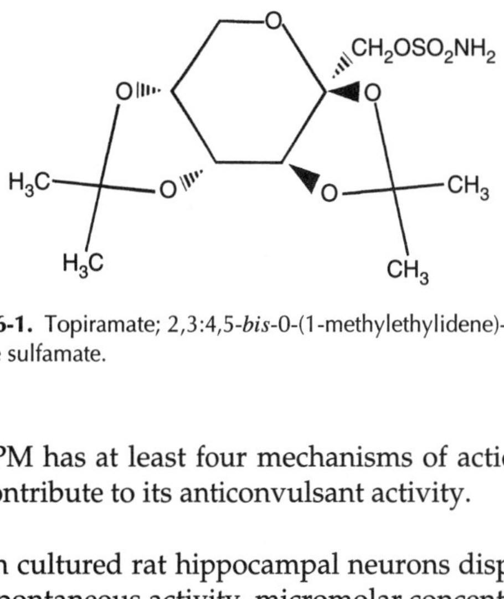

PRECLINICAL IN VITRO STUDIES

In vitro, TPM demonstrates an ability to modulate ionic channels, enhance inhibitory neurotransmission, and reduce excitatory transmission processes involved in the generation of seizures. Preclinical studies indicate

Figure 36-1. Topiramate; 2,3:4,5-*bis*-0-(1-methylethylidene)-β-fructo-pyranose sulfamate.

that TPM has at least four mechanisms of action that may contribute to its anticonvulsant activity.

1. In cultured rat hippocampal neurons displaying spontaneous activity, micromolar concentrations of TPM reduced the duration and frequency of action potentials associated with sustained repetitive firing (17). Topiramate also blocked action potentials induced by depolarizing electric currents. These effects on action potentials may be credited to TPM blockade of voltage-dependent Na^+ channels (17).

2. In cultured murine cerebellar granule cells, micromolar concentrations of TPM in combination with gamma-aminobutyric acid (GABA) augmented GABA-stimulated chloride flux into chloride-depleted neurons compared with GABA alone (i.e., enhanced inhibitory neurotransmission) (18,19). The effect of TPM on $GABA_A$ receptors was not blocked by the benzodiazepine antagonist flumazenil, suggesting that a novel or nonbenzodiazepine modulatory site may be involved (18,20).

3. In other studies, TPM produced concentration-dependent decreases in kainate-evoked inward

currents (excitatory currents) in cultured hippocampal neurons without affecting the activity of glutamate receptors of the N-methyl-D-aspartate (NMDA) subtype (those modulated by benzodiazepines) (17,21).

4. Topiramate's sulfamate moiety is structurally similar to the carbonic anhydrase inhibitor acetazolamide. However, the potency of TPM as an inhibitor of erythrocyte carbonic anhydrase is much lower than that of acetazolamide (15). In vitro, TPM does not appear to exert an anticonvulsant effect through inhibition of carbonic anhydrase (15).

This broad activity profile in vitro suggests that TPM may be effective against a number of seizure types. In particular, two potentially unique mechanisms of action demonstrated with TPM, that is, GABA potentiation and antagonism of a kainate subtype of the glutamate receptor at novel binding sites, suggest that TPM may be effective in patients refractory to other AEDs.

PRECLINICAL IN VIVO STUDIES

Efficacy

Topiramate was initially tested in two traditional animal models of epilepsy, the maximal electroshock test (MES) and the pentylenetetrazol (PTZ) seizure test. The MES test has been hypothesized to identify agents effective against partial-onset and generalized tonic-clonic seizures and those that have the capacity to prevent the spread of seizures (22,23). In rats and mice, TPM blocked MES seizures with a potency similar to that of phenytoin (PHT), carbamazepine (CBZ), phenobarbital (PB), and acetazolamide (15). In the subcutaneous PTZ test, a chemically induced seizure model hypothesized to identify agents that raise the seizure threshold, TPM, like PHT, was either ineffective or only weakly effective (15). This activity profile suggests that TPM exerts its anticonvulsant effects by blocking the spread of seizures rather than by raising seizure threshold. However, TPM did increase seizure threshold in response to an intravenous infusion of PTZ in mice (18), suggesting that TPM possesses an even broader spectrum of action than was originally thought.

Topiramate was effective in blocking seizures in four other rodent models of epilepsy:

1. In rats, TPM inhibited amygdala-kindled seizures indicating a potential for activity against complex partial seizures (22,24).
2. In the DBA/2 mouse, a strain genetically prone to seizures, TPM blocked sound-induced clonic seizures when administered before the auditory stimulus (25).
3. In the spontaneously epileptic rat (SER), a hereditary model of epilepsy, TPM inhibited tonic and absence-like seizures (25).
4. Topiramate was also effective in a rat model of posttraumatic epilepsy (26).

Topiramate's profile of activity in experimental models of epilepsy suggests a multifactorial mechanism of action.

The MES test in rats was used to study the development of tolerance to the anticonvulsant effects of TPM. No tolerance was noted after 14 days of TPM administered at nearly twice the effective dose (ED_{50}) (15,27).

Toxicity

Acute Studies

Topiramate was well tolerated following acute administration in mice, rats, and dogs (9,14). The estimated LD_{50} after oral TPM administration in mice and rats ranged from 2338 to 3745 mg/kg. Dogs were more sensitive than mice or rats to the acute toxic effects of TPM, which were primarily central nervous system (CNS)-related.

Multiple-Dose Studies

Multiple-dose (3- and 12-month) toxicity studies were performed in rats and dogs. In these studies, reversible gastric mucosal hyperplasia changes were seen that were similar to those reported with carbonic anhydrase inhibitors (28–30). No evidence of dysplasia, aplasia, or any change that would suggest tumor formation was apparent. In studies of rats and mice, urinary microcalculi formation associated with TPM use was also consistent with carbonic anhydrase inhibition (31).

Reproductive Studies

Fertility was not affected by TPM in male or female rats (R. Reife, personal communication), and TPM did not affect pup survival at doses up to 100 mg/kg/day (9).

Teratology Studies

In teratology studies, TPM caused right-sided ectrodactyly (congenital absence of all or part of a digit) in rats and rib and vertebral malformations in rabbits (R. Reife, personal communication). These effects of TPM are similar to those reported with acetazolamide and other carbonic anhydrase inhibitors (32–34). The effects of TPM during pregnancy in humans are not yet known.

Protective Index

TPM was selected for development as an AED based on its high protective index (PI) and its potency and duration of action in tests in rodents (15,16). The PI can be determined from the ratio of the median toxic dose (TD_{50}) from a neurotoxicity test, such as the rotorod test or the loss of righting reflex test, to the MES ED_{50}. A higher, more advantageous, ratio was obtained in rats and mice with TPM than with PHT, CBZ, or PB. For example, with oral doses the PI for TPM in rats was above 116, while the values for PB, CBZ and PHT were 3.5, 20.8, and greater than 60.8, respectively (15).

CLINICAL PHARMACOKINETICS

Extensive pharmacokinetic data in adults are available.

Absorption

In adults, TPM has linear pharmacokinetics with low intersubject variability and is rapidly absorbed from the gastrointestinal tract after administration of single, oral doses ranging from 100 to 1200 mg (35). Its estimated bioavailability is 81 percent to 95 percent (36). The volume of distribution of TPM ranges from 0.6 to 0.8 L/kg, consistent with a distribution in total body water (37). For most patients, 90 percent of the maximal plasma concentration (C_{max}) is achieved within 2 hours after oral administration (35), although this can range from 1.4 to 4.3 hours (35), depending on the dose. Mean values for C_{max} and area under the concentration-time curve (AUC), reflections of drug absorption and clearance, increase linearly with respect to dose in adults (Table 36-1) (38).

Table 36-1. Topiramate Mean (SD) Plasma and Urine Pharmacokinetics in Healthy Males — Multiple-Dose Studies

	Twice-Daily Dose for 14 Days	
Variables	50 mg ($n = 9$)	100 mg ($n = 10$)
C_{max} (µg/mL)	3.61 (0.68)	6.76 (2.81)
T_{max} (h)	1.9 (0.9)	3.0 (2.0)
$AUC_{0-12\ h}$ (µg·h/mL)	31.6 (6.6)	57.2 (15.8)
$t_{1/2}$ (h)	21.8 (3.6)	20.6 (2.4)
CL/F (mL/min)	27.5 (6.4)	31.0 (7.9)
CL_R (mL/min)	17.8 (6.6)	16.7 (6.5)

Source: Johannessen SI. Pharmacokinetics and interaction profile if topiramate: review and comparison with newer antiepileptic drugs. *Epilepsia* 1997; 38(Suppl 1):S18–S23; with permission.
$AUC_{0-12\ h}$ = area under the concentration vs. time curve from 0–12 hours; C_{max} = maximum concentration; CL/F = oral clearance; CL_R = renal clearance; T_{max} = time of maximum concentration; $t_{1/2}$ = plasma elimination half-life.

When TPM is taken with food, the rate of absorption is slightly decreased, although this minimal difference is not felt to be clinically significant. Therefore, TPM can be administered without regard to food (35).

Elimination

Renal excretion is a major route of TPM elimination. In adults, within a dose range of 200 to 1200 mg, at least 51 percent of the dose is estimated to be excreted by the kidney (35). The renal clearance of TPM is much lower than its glomerular filtration rate (35), suggesting that the drug may undergo tubular reabsorption. In adults, the elimination half-life ($t_{1/2}$) values for TPM, calculated from plasma (mean, 21.5 hr) and urinary (mean, 18.5 hr) data, appear to be independent of dose (35). In patients with renal failure (creatinine clearance <30 mL/min/1.73 m^2), an approximately twofold increase in AUC and $t_{1/2}$ occurs (39). Therefore, adults with renal impairment may require reduced TPM dosages.

Metabolism

Topiramate is not extensively metabolized (38). Six trace metabolites of TPM were identified that represented less than 5 percent of the sample radioactivity (40). The metabolites, formed by hydroxylation, hydrolysis, and glucuronidation, do not display significant antiepileptic activity (38,40). TPM is poorly bound to plasma proteins (9–17 percent) (41).

Drug Interactions

TPM and AEDs

In general, administration of TPM does not have major effects on the plasma concentrations of other AEDs. Topiramate decreased PHT clearance in some patients (42). When TPM was administered concomitantly with CBZ, there were no significant changes in total or unbound CBZ plasma concentrations (43). A study of potential interactions between TPM and valproic acid (VPA) showed that a TPM dose of 400 mg every 12 hours produced only a minor (11–12 percent) decrease in the average plasma concentration of plasma VPA (44). Topiramate had no effect on plasma PB concentrations (45). No studies are available on the effects of TPM on felbamate (FBM), lamotrigine (LTG), gabapentin (GBP), or tiagabine (TGB).

In contrast, studies have shown that administration of concomitant AEDs may affect plasma concentrations of TPM. Conversion of patients to TPM monotherapy from concomitant therapy with TPM and PHT (an enzyme-inducing AED) resulted in appreciably higher mean steady-state values for TPM C_{max} and AUC (42). Similarly, withdrawal of CBZ from patients receiving concomitant TPM and CBZ resulted in an approximately twofold increase in TPM plasma levels (43). Therefore, there is a potential need for TPM dosage adjustment when enzyme-inducing AEDs are either added or discontinued. On the other hand, simultaneous administration of TPM and VPA (an inhibitor of hepatic enzymes) resulted in slightly (17 percent) higher values for TPM C_{max} and AUC (44).

TPM and Non-AEDs

Studies using oral contraceptives indicate that TPM reduces ethinyl estradiol serum levels by approximately 30 percent without affecting norethindrone levels, suggesting that TPM may decrease the effectiveness of concomitantly administered low-dose oral contraceptives (46). Coadministration of TPM and digoxin in healthy adults results in a small reduction in digoxin C_{max} (16 percent) and AUC (12 percent) (47). The apparent oral clearance of digoxin increased by 13 percent without a corresponding change in the renal clearance, suggesting that TPM may affect the systemic availability of digoxin.

Children and Adolescents

Information on TPM pharmacokinetics in children and adolescents was determined from a single-center, open-label outpatient trial of 18 patients with epilepsy (14,48). Patients aged 4 to 17 years received an oral TPM dose of up to 9 mg/kg/day in addition to their standard regimen of AEDs. As in adults, pharmacokinetics were linear in children, and plasma clearance was not affected by TPM dose. Compared with adults, clearance values were 54 percent greater in children when TPM was administered in the presence of enzyme-inducing drugs, and 44 percent greater in the absence of enzyme-inducing drugs. Because overall TPM clearance was approximately 50 percent greater in children than in adults, for any given dose based on weight (mg/kg), steady-state TPM plasma concentrations would be predicted to be approximately 33 percent lower in children than in adults.

Infants

In a cohort of five infants (<4 years old) with refractory infantile spasms, the mean plasma clearance was slightly higher than that reported for children and adolescents and higher in infants on concomitant enzyme-inducing AEDs than in those on non–enzyme-inducing concomitant AEDs (49).

TOPIRAMATE CLINICAL EFFICACY AND TOXICITY IN ADULTS

Partial-Onset Seizures in Adults

TPM has been extensively studied as adjunctive therapy in adults with refractory partial-onset seizures with or without secondary generalization. The results of six double-blind, placebo-controlled trials conducted in the United States and Europe involving 743 patients indicate that TPM significantly improves seizure control in adults with refractory partial seizures (1–6). In these studies, TPM was administered in doses of 200 to 1000 mg/day on a twice-daily basis. The study design for each trial varied slightly depending on dose. In general, these studies consisted of an 8-week baseline period, followed by a 3- to 11-week titration period, and then 8 to 12 weeks of stabilization. During the baseline period, patients continued to receive their background regimen of no more than two concomitant AEDs at constant dosage levels and had at least one seizure per week. The results were pooled and analyzed on an intent-to-treat basis. Overall, 44 percent of the TPM-treated patients showed at least 50 percent reduction in seizure rate, compared with 12 percent for the placebo-treated controls (Figure 36-2) (6,14). In addition, 21 percent of the TPM-treated patients showed at least 75 percent seizure rate reduction compared with 4 percent of the placebo-treated group. Five percent of TPM-treated patients became seizure-free during the study compared with none of placebo-treated patients (50). Results of the pooled analysis indicate that the median percent reduction in monthly seizure rate was significantly higher ($p \leq 0.001$) in the TPM group than was the reduction in the placebo group for simple partial (57% vs. −25%), complex partial (43% vs. 2%), and secondarily generalized seizures (58% vs. −3%) (Figure 36-3) (6).

Pooled analyses of placebo-controlled studies in adults indicate that TPM is effective regardless of race, gender, baseline seizure rate, or concomitant AEDs (51). A dose of 200 mg/day was the lowest dosage studied as adjunctive therapy in clinical trials and is considered to be the minimally effective dosage. No appreciable increase in responder rate was found at dosages above 400 mg/day (1,4). It is possible, however, that individual patients may benefit from higher dosages. An initial target dose of 200 to 400 mg/day is recommended for adults.

In two types of meta-analyses of the efficacy and tolerability of new AEDs as add-on therapy for the treatment of partial epilepsy in adults, TPM compared favorably with GBP, LTG, TGB, vigabatrin, and zonisamide (52,53). In one report, estimation of efficacy was evaluated in terms of odds ratios based on the proportion of patients showing at least 50 percent reduction in seizure frequency in the active-treatment group versus

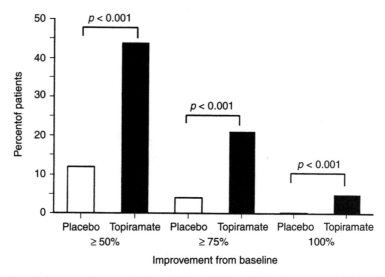

Figure 36-2. Adult patients with partial-onset seizures achieving ≥50%, ≥75%, or 100% seizure-rate reduction during adjunctive therapy with topiramate (*n* = 527) or placebo (*n* = 216).

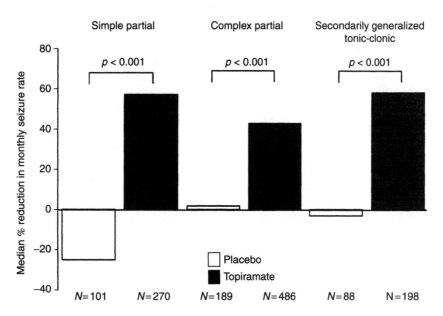

Figure 36-3. Overview of six multicenter, placebo-controlled studies in adults.

the placebo group (the higher the ratio, the greater the efficacy). Tolerability was estimated based on rates of patient withdrawal for any reason from a given study drug versus from placebo (the higher the ratio, the higher the toxicity). Using this approach, TPM had the highest overall odds ratio for efficacy among the newer AEDs analyzed (52). Although TPM showed an intermediate odds ratio for tolerability, this analysis included doses above 600 mg/day, which have not been shown to improve efficacy but which may affect tolerability. An alternative meta-analysis compared the new AEDs by the "number needed to treat," that is, the number of patients that need to be treated to expect to have one patient with at least 50 percent reduction

in baseline seizure rate (54). The lower the number needed to treat, the more effective the treatment. Based on the same data used by Marson and coworkers, the number needed to treat was the lowest and best for TPM (approximately three patients) and was significantly lower for TPM than for zonisamide, TGB, GBP, and LTG.

Topiramate Monotherapy in Adults

The usefulness of TPM as monotherapy was evaluated in a double-blind study of 48 adult patients with recurrent partial-onset seizures (8). A proposed minimally effective dose of 100 mg/day TPM was

Table 36-2. Incidence of Most Common Treatment-Emergent Adverse Events in Adults by Assigned Topiramate Dose in Five Double-Blind, Placebo-Controlled Trials[a]

Event	Placebo (n = 174)	200 (n = 45)	400 (n = 68)	600 (n = 124)	800 (n = 76)	1000 (n = 47)
Dizziness	13.2	35.6	22.1	31.5	31.6	40.4
Fatigue	15.5	13.3	17.6	31.5	48.7	31.9
Diplopia	6.3	6.7	19.1	8.1	18.4	29.8
Nystagmus	11.5	17.8	13.2	10.5	15.8	27.7
Somnolence	10.3	26.7	26.5	16.9	19.7	27.7
Confusion	5.2	8.9	14.7	17.7	14.5	27.7
Abnormal thinking	2.3	20.0	11.8	29.0	27.6	25.5
Ataxia	7.5	20.0	22.0	16.9	15.8	21.3
Anorexia	3.4	4.4	4.4	8.1	9.2	21.3
Impaired concentration	1.1	11.1	8.8	12.1	14.5	21.3
Headache	25.9	28.9	25.0	29.8	25.0	17.0

Header: Assigned topiramate dose (mg/day)

Source: Shorvon SD. Safety of topiramate: adverse events and relationships to dosing. *Epilepsia* 1996; 38)Suppl 2):S18–S22.
[a]Experienced by at least 20 percent of patients in any dose group.

compared with a proposed high TPM dose of 1000 mg/day following withdrawal of background AEDs. The double-blind phase of the study, consisting of a 5-week conversion and an 11-week monotherapy period, was designed so that patients exited the trial if significant seizure deterioration occurred. Treatment effect, defined in terms of time to exit, significantly favored the TPM 1000-mg/day arm ($p = 0.002$). The study indicates that TPM is safe and effective as monotherapy in adults after its substitution for standard AEDs.

Further evidence of the efficacy of TPM monotherapy was provided by a recent retrospective analysis that utilized data from open-extension TPM trials conducted at five centers (7). Of 136 patients still receiving TPM, 33 percent were successfully converted to TPM monotherapy with a mean duration of 22 months. At the time of the most recently analyzed visit, 62 percent percent of these patients were seizure-free for at least the last 3 months of observation.

Generalized Tonic-Clonic Seizures of Nonfocal Origin

To further define its usefulness in the management of epilepsy, TPM was evaluated in a combined population of adults and children with generalized tonic-clonic seizures of nonfocal origin. The study will be described in detail in the section on generalized tonic-clonic seizures in children.

Topiramate Side-Effect Profile in Adults

In adults, a profile of treatment-emergent adverse events resulting from TPM doses of 200 to 1000 mg/day based on data from five placebo-controlled double-blind trials includes 360 patients

treated with TPM (Table 36-2) (55). In these studies, all patients received at least one other AED, and 60 percent received two or three concomitant AEDs. The most commonly reported treatment-emergent adverse events were CNS-related, and most were rated as mild or moderate in severity. Across the five trials, adverse events considered to be related to study medication that occurred in at least 5 percent of TPM-treated patients included ataxia, impaired concentration, confusion, dizziness, fatigue, paresthesia, somnolence, and abnormal thinking. Other clinically important side effects resulting from TPM use include nephrolithiasis, paresthesias, and mild, dose-related weight loss (55,56). Weight loss was typically observed during the first 3 months of TPM treatment, peaked by 15 to 18 months of treatment, and was partially reversible after prolonged therapy (55). Many adverse events were observed with greater frequency at the higher doses (600–1000 mg/day) than at the target 200 to 400 mg/day doses. An unusually rapid titration schedule used to achieve the higher TPM doses in these studies may account for the greater incidence of adverse events (55,57). Overall, 51 patients (14%) treated with TPM and 6 patients (3%) receiving placebo prematurely discontinued study medication because of an adverse event. Of patients who discontinued TPM because of limiting adverse events, approximately 75 percent dropped out during the first 2 months of treatment, often during the rapid titration period (55).

A 1.5 percent incidence of nephrolithiasis during TPM treatment is similar to that seen during treatment with another carbonic anhydrase inhibitor, acetazolamide (14,56). Most cases of nephrolithiasis resolved by the spontaneous passage of renal stones, and 83 percent of the 18 patients with stones elected to continue TPM treatment (55). Like acetazolamide, TPM has a sulfamate moiety; however, carbonic anhydrase inhibition by TPM is relatively weak. Paresthesias have also been reported during treatment with carbonic anhydrase inhibitors. No other clinically relevant changes in laboratory parameters, neurologic, electrocardiographic, ophthalmologic, or audiologic tests were associated with TPM treatment in clinical studies.

TOPIRAMATE CLINICAL EFFICACY AND TOXICITY IN CHILDREN

Although the incidence of epilepsy is higher in children than in adults (58,59), the safety and efficacy of new AEDs are typically investigated first in adults. Following the establishment of TPM's efficacy and tolerability in adults, three randomized, double-blind, placebo-controlled studies investigated its clinical profile as adjunctive therapy in children with epilepsy. These studies showed that TPM is efficacious and well-tolerated as add-on therapy in children with partial-onset seizures, Lennox-Gastaut syndrome, and generalized tonic-clonic seizures of nonfocal origin (10–12).

Partial-Onset Seizures in Children

The efficacy and tolerability of adjunctive TPM in children with refractory partial-onset seizures with or without secondary generalization were tested in a multicenter, double-blind, placebo-controlled trial conducted at 16 sites (11). Eligibility requirements included age between 1 and 16 years, weight over 16 kg, an electroencephalogram (EEG) documenting the diagnosis of partial epilepsy, at least six partial-onset seizures with or without generalization during an 8-week baseline period while being maintained on at least one but no more than two AEDs at a constant dose. Patients were then randomized to adjunctive therapy with either TPM or placebo. The subsequent double-blind, 16-week treatment phase had an 8-week titration period followed by an 8-week stabilization period. TPM was titrated to weight-based target doses of approximately 6 mg/kg/day.

A total of 41 TPM-treated and 45 placebo-treated children between the ages of 2 and 16 years were randomized and completed treatment. The mean age was 9 years, and the mean weight was 35 kg in each treatment group. The median average monthly seizure frequency was 19 in the placebo group and 22 in the TPM group. The median average TPM dose during the stabilization period was 5.9 mg/kg/day.

For partial-onset seizures, the median percent reduction from baseline in the average monthly seizure

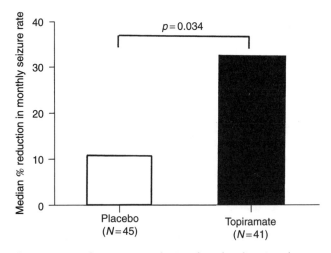

Figure 36-4. Median percent reduction from baseline in refractory partial-onset seizures in children.

rate in the TPM-treated group was 33 percent compared with 11 percent in the placebo group ($p = 0.034$) (Figure 36-4). A total of 39 percent of patients in the TPM group experienced at least 50 percent reduction in average monthly seizure rate compared with 20 percent of the placebo group ($p = 0.080$). TPM was significantly more effective than placebo in reducing the frequency of seizures by 75 percent or more (17% vs. 2%, respectively; $p = 0.02$). During the double-blind phase of this study, seizure freedom was achieved by 5 percent of the TPM-treated patients, while no patient in the placebo group was seizure-free. The adverse experiences that were noted in more than 15 percent of the TPM group were upper respiratory tract infection (41%), fever (29%), injury (20%), sinusitis (17%), fatigue (15%), coughing (15%), viral infection (15%), and bleeding/purpura (15%). The incidence of CNS adverse experiences ranged from 10 percent to 12 percent. The only adverse experiences that occurred in at least 10 percent more patients in the TPM group than in the placebo group were viral infection, bleeding and purpura, and injury.

In retrospect, the TPM target dose used may have been suboptimal. In the presence of concomitant AEDs, mean plasma clearance of TPM may be up to 54 percent higher in children than in adults (14,48). Steady-state TPM plasma concentrations would be expected to be approximately 33 percent lower in children than in adults for the same mg/kg/day dose. Therefore, a 6 mg/kg/day dose of TPM in children is approximately equivalent to a dose of 200 to 300 mg/day in adults, a minimally effective dose. In adults with refractory partial-onset seizures, greater efficacy was seen among patients receiving a TPM dose of 400 mg/day than with the 200 mg/day dose (4).

The double-blind portion of this study demonstrated the effectiveness of TPM as adjunctive therapy in pediatric partial-onset seizures. However, the expected pediatric TPM clearance suggests that a higher TPM dose may have an increased therapeutic effect in children with partial-onset seizures.

In an open-label extension of this study, 83 children (2–16 years of age; mean age, 11 years) received TPM at a mean dose of 9 mg/kg/day (range, 4–22 mg/kg/day) for a mean duration of 441 days (range, 96–923 days). At the last study visit, partial-onset seizures were reduced by at least 50 percent in 57 percent of patients and by at least 75 percent in 42 percent of patients in patients on open-label topiramate for more than 3 months. Seizure freedom for 6 months or more was achieved by 14 percent of TPM-treated patients. The most commonly reported adverse events during the extension were CNS-related effects similar to those observed during the double-blind portion of the study (60).

Lennox-Gastaut Syndrome

A multicenter, double-blind, placebo-controlled trial was conducted at 12 centers to determine the efficacy of TPM as adjunctive therapy in patients with Lennox-Gastaut syndrome (10). Eligibility requirements included age over 1 year but less than 30 years old, weight over 11.5 kg, a prior EEG showing a slow spike-and-wave pattern and seizure types including drop attacks (i.e., tonic or atonic seizures) and a history of or active atypical absence seizures, more than 60 seizures during the month before entering the 4-week baseline phase, and maintenance on one or two standard AEDs. Patients were randomized to either TPM or placebo adjunctive therapy. During a 3-week titration period, TPM dosage was increased at weekly intervals from an initial dose of 1 mg/kg/day to 3 mg/kg/day and then 6 mg/kg/day. Treatment was then continued for an 8-week maintenance period.

Ninety-eight patients ranging in age from 2 to 42 years (mean age of 11 years), with a mean weight of 32 kg in the placebo group and 37 kg in the TPM group, were studied. One patient in the placebo group and two in the TPM group were taking more than two AEDs during the baseline period, whereas the majority of patients in each group were taking two AEDs. During the baseline period, the median monthly drop attack frequencies were 90 in the TPM group and 98 in the placebo group, and the median monthly frequencies of all types of seizures were 267 in the TPM group versus 244 in the placebo group. The median average TPM dose during the maintenance period was 5.8 mg/kg/day.

Patients treated with TPM demonstrated a significantly greater median percent reduction from baseline in drop attacks (15%) as compared with placebo-treated controls (−5%; $p = 0.041$) (Figure 36-5). Twenty-eight

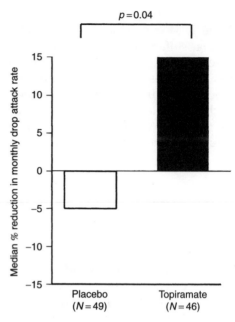

Figure 36-5. Median percent reduction from baseline in drop attacks (tonic-atonic seizures) in children with Lennox-Gastaut syndrome.

percent of the TPM group had at least 50 percent reduction in the monthly drop attack rate compared with 14 percent of the placebo group ($p = 0.071$). The median percent reduction from baseline in the average monthly rate of all seizures was 21 percent for the TPM group and 9 percent for the placebo group ($p = 0.430$). Based on parental global evaluations conducted at the conclusion of the double-blind phase, TPM-treated patients were nearly twice as likely to show an improvement in seizure severity compared with controls (53% vs. 28%; $p = 0.037$).

The most common adverse experiences were somnolence, anorexia, nervousness, behavioral problems, fatigue, dizziness, and weight loss. These adverse events occurred in at least 10 percent more patients in the TPM group than in the placebo group. Most adverse events were rated by the parent as mild to moderate in severity.

In this study, as in the study with children with partial-onset seizures, the target dose of TPM may have been too low because of the high clearance in children. A 6 mg/kg/day dose in pediatric patients would be approximately equivalent to 200 to 300 mg/day in adults, a minimally effective dose. Nonetheless, the double-blind portion of this study demonstrated that TPM is effective as adjunctive therapy in Lennox-Gastaut syndrome and is without serious toxicity.

In an open-label extension of this study, 97 patients have received a mean TPM dose of 10 mg/kg/day for a mean duration of 539 days (range, 44–1225 days) (61). At the last clinical visit, the frequency of drop attacks was at least 50 percent lower than baseline in 58 percent of patients and at least 75 percent lower than baseline in 37 percent of patients on open-label topiramate for more than 3 months. A total of 15 percent of patients were free of drop attacks for at least 6 months at their last visit. During the extension study, the most commonly reported adverse experiences were CNS-related effects (61).

Generalized Tonic-Clonic Seizures of Nonfocal Origin

A double-blind, placebo-controlled, multicenter study was conducted at 17 centers to investigate the effects of TPM in children and adults with uncontrolled generalized tonic-clonic (GTC) seizures of nonfocal origin (12). Eligible patients had to be at least 4 years old, weigh more than 25 kg, be receiving no more than two standard AEDs, experience three GTC seizures during an 8-week baseline phase with at least one seizure in each 4-week period of this phase, and have EEG findings consistent with generalized epilepsy. Following an 8-week baseline phase, patients were randomized to double-blind adjunctive treatment with TPM or placebo. During an initial 4-week interval, 50 mg of TPM or matching placebo was administered once daily in the evening. During the second and third intervals (2 weeks each), TPM or matching placebo was titrated to target doses of 6 mg/kg/day in two divided doses. Patients were then treated for a 12-week maintenance period. Doses of concomitant AEDs were constant during the double-blind treatment period.

In this study, a total of 80 patients between the ages of 3 and 59 years were randomized to receive up to 6 mg/kg/day TPM or placebo as adjunctive therapy. In the placebo group, the mean age was 26 years (13 of 41 patients were 16 years of age or younger), and the mean weight was 61 kg. In the TPM group, the mean age was 27 years (8 of 39 were 16 years of age or younger), and the mean weight was 72 kg. The median average monthly rate of GTC seizures was 4.5 in the placebo group and 5.0 in the TPM group. During the baseline phase, 10 patients in the placebo group and 11 patients in the TPM group received a regimen that included more than two AEDs, while the majority of patients were on a regimen of two AEDs. The mean TPM dose during the stabilization period was 5.0 mg/kg/day.

After a 20-week double-blind phase, the median percent reduction from baseline in average monthly GTC seizure rate was 57 percent for the TPM group compared with 9 percent for the placebo group ($p = 0.019$) (Figure 36-6). Fifty-six percent of the TPM-treated patients experienced at least 50 percent reduction in GTC seizures, compared with 20 percent of the placebo-treated controls ($p = 0.001$). Moreover, 33 percent of TPM-treated patients versus 13 percent of placebo patients had at least 75 percent reduction in GTC seizures ($p = 0.037$), and seizure freedom was achieved in 13 percent of TPM-treated patients compared with 5 percent of placebo patients. The most common adverse experiences, reported with at least a 10 percent greater incidence in the TPM group compared with the placebo group included somnolence, difficulty with memory, nervousness, fatigue, and weight loss.

This study demonstrates that in comparison to placebo, adjunctive therapy of GTC seizures with TPM is effective and well-tolerated in pediatric and adult patients in doses up to 400 mg/day (approximately 6 mg/kg/day in children).

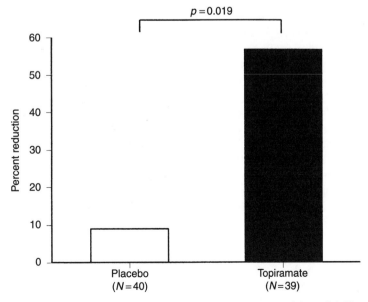

Figure 36-6. Median percent reduction from baseline in average monthly (GTC) seizure rate in adults and children with GTC seizures of non-focal origin.

West Syndrome

TPM also demonstrated efficacy in a pilot study of patients with refractory infantile spasms (West syndrome) (13). During a 2-week baseline period, eligible patients demonstrated features consistent with infantile spasms on a 24-hour video-EEG, exhibited an average of one spasm per day and could not be spasm-free for 3 consecutive days. Eleven patients (mean age of 24 months at study entry) received an initial TPM dose of 25 mg in addition to their current AED therapy. A "rapid-dose" titration schedule was devised such that TPM dosage was increased by 25 mg every 2 to 3 days over a 4-week period until either a maximal tolerated dose was reached, spasms were controlled, or a maximal dose of 24 mg/kg/day was achieved. During this study, five patients (45%) became spasm-free with absence of infantile spasms and either classic or modified hypsarrhythmia proven by repeat 24-hour video-EEG. A total of nine patients (82%) achieved at least 50 percent spasm reduction. Overall, spasms decreased in frequency from a mean of 25.6 ± 19.3 spasms per day to 6.9 ± 5.9 spasms per day. Seven of the 11 patients (64%) were able to achieve TPM monotherapy, while the others were able to reduce their intake of concomitant AEDs.

Topiramate Monotherapeutic Substitution in Children

A single-center, open-label pilot study was initiated to evaluate the effects of TPM as monotherapy in children (14,62). Patients between the ages of 3 and 12 years old were chosen for study if they had partial-onset seizures that were controlled using one AED but still experienced intolerable side effects. Before TPM substitution, patients had to be seizure-free for at least 1 month. Two different titration schedules were used to study five enrolled patients. In three patients, 1 mg/kg/day TPM was added concomitantly to their background AED regimen, and then the dose was increased at weekly intervals to 3 mg/kg/day and then to 6 mg/kg/day. The two other patients received an initial dose of 1 mg/kg/day TPM, which was increased at weekly intervals to 2 mg/kg/day and then to 3 mg/kg/day. For both schedules, the background AED could eventually be withdrawn if seizures were still controlled and the maximum TPM dose was tolerated. Among the three patients on the first, more rapid, titration schedule, one patient was discontinued after 22 days because of cognitive and behavioral adverse experiences, and the other two patients had not yet achieved monotherapy at the time of a preliminary report. The two patients on the slower titration schedule have achieved TPM monotherapy and have remained seizure-free, with one patient having mild to moderate behavioral difficulties. Thus, preliminary

results indicate that with the slower titration schedule TPM monotherapy can be achieved with efficacy and an acceptable tolerability in children with partial seizures.

Topiramate Side-Effect Profile in Children

The safety profile of TPM in children is similar to that seen in adults (Table 36-3) (R. Reife, personal communication). Results of placebo-controlled trials using TPM as adjunctive therapy in children 16 years of age or younger indicate that the most commonly reported adverse events were somnolence, anorexia, fatigue, and nervousness. The slower rate of TPM titration (i.e., increases at 2-week intervals) used in some of these pediatric studies may have resulted in a lower frequency of adverse events compared to the higher frequency observed with a more rapid rate of titration used in many of the adult studies. During the double-blind portion of the placebo-controlled studies

Table 36-3. Incidence of the Most Common Treatment-Emergent Adverse Events During a Double-blind Study in Children with Partial-Onset Seizures

Body system/Adverse Event	Placebo ($N = 45$)	Topiramate ($N = 41$)
Respiratory system Upper respiratory tract infection	36	41
Sinusitis	27	17
Coughing	11	15
Gastrointestinal system Diarrhea	22	10
Neuropsychiatric Somnolence	13	12
Anorexia	11	12
Emotional lability	4	12
Difficulty with concentration or attention	2	12
Mood problems	11	10
Aggressive reaction	7	10
Nervousness	7	10
Resistance mechanism Infection viral	4	15
Otitis media	11	10
Skin and appendages Rash	9	12
Platelet, bleeding and clotting Purpura	4	15
Body as a whole Fever	24	29
Injury	9	20
Fatigue	7	15

*Reported by <10 percent of the patients in the topiramate group
Source: From Elterman R, Glauser TA, Wyllie E, Reife R, Wu S-C. A trial of topiramate as adjunctive therapy in children with partial-onset seizures. *Neurology* 1999; 52:1338–1344, with permission.

involving children, the use of TPM did not result in any discontinuations due to an adverse event. In placebo-controlled trials involving children receiving a target dose of approximately 6 mg/kg/day, the most commonly reported adverse events compared with controls were (in addition to fatigue, somnolence, anorexia, and nervousness) difficulty with concentration and attention, difficulty with memory, aggressive reaction, and weight decrease.

TIPS FOR SUCCESSFUL USE OF TOPIRAMATE

Based on the aforementioned clinical trials of TPM in children, TPM has been shown to be effective for drop attacks (tonic or atonic seizures) associated with Lennox-Gastaut syndrome and in partial-onset seizures. In addition, TPM has been demonstrated to be effective in the treatment of adults and children with GTC seizures of nonfocal origin and has shown efficacy in pilot studies in West syndrome and as monotherapy. Based on these trials and my experience both as an investigator in most of these studies and with over 300 children in my clinical practice receiving topiramate, I present here a few tips that may increase the effectiveness and tolerability of TPM use (63).

The initial dose of TPM, subsequent titration rates, and the maintenance regimen are important (63). At our institution, an initial dose ranges from 0.5 to 1 mg/kg/day with subsequent weekly increments of 0.5 to 1 mg/kg. This "start low, go slow" approach has generally been well tolerated. If adverse experiences do occur, titration can be slowed; on the other hand, titration can be more rapid if the suppression of seizures is urgently needed. Based on the double-blind studies, 6 mg/kg/day is effective as adjunctive therapy. Based on pharmacokinetic studies indicating that clearance is 50 percent higher in pediatric patients than in adult patients with epilepsy (48), TPM concentrations are expected to be approximately 33 percent lower in children than in adults. Thus, the 6 mg/kg/day dose in children may be equivalent to a dose of only 200 to 300 mg/day in adults, a minimally effective dose. In fact, the efficacy of TPM improved in open-label extensions of the double-blind trials as the dose of TPM increased. For example, in the double-blind phase of the trial in children with Lennox-Gastaut syndrome (10), 28 percent of patients had at least 50 percent decrease in drop attacks with a median average maintenance dose of 5.8 mg/kg/day; while in the open-label extension, 58 percent of patients had at least 50 percent decrease in drop attacks with a mean dose of 11 mg/kg/day (61). A similar effect was noted in the studies of children with partial-onset seizures (11,60).

With slow titration, tolerability may be increased. In particular, the CNS adverse events that occurred with TPM may be less frequently observed. For example, in the study in patients with Lennox-Gastaut syndrome (10), a 3-week titration period resulted in much higher frequencies of adverse experiences than were observed in the study in patients with partial-onset seizures with an 8-week titration period (11). In the study with the more rapid titration, the incidence of somnolence, anorexia, nervousness, behavioral problems, fatigue, dizziness, and weight loss were 10 percent or more frequent in the TPM group than in the placebo group. If these adverse events were observed in the study with slower titration, they were at much lower frequencies and only purpura, injury and viral infection as a resistance mechanism were more frequent by at least 10 percent among the TPM patients than among the placebo patients.

In our practice, the response to a given dose of TPM is variable with some patients responding to doses lower than 6 mg/kg/day and others requiring 15 mg/kg/day or more to achieve a response. As with all AEDs, TPM should be titrated until there is a response (either seizure control without intolerable adverse events or persisting seizures with intolerable side effects). In patients showing some seizure reduction without intolerable adverse events, the dose of TPM should be increased further. High doses (we have used doses up to 60 mg/kg/day) may be well tolerated, particularly in the presence of a concomitant enzyme-inducing AED such as carbamazepine.

With the slow rates of titration that we recommend, it may take 6 to 8 weeks to begin to see efficacy, and it is important to explain this time frame to the parents of the patient to avoid undue anxiety and frustration.

In our patient population, a small subset of patients (1–3%) appear unable to tolerate even the lowest doses of TPM. In these cases, we discontinue TPM for 2 or more weeks and then suggest a retry. If side effects occur again at extremely low doses, then TPM is discontinued and another medication is substituted. The vast majority of our patients, however, are able to tolerate the "start low, go slow" approach.

CONCLUSION

Topiramate is a promising new agent for the treatment of a variety of seizure types seen in children. It exhibits a favorable pharmacokinetic profile, including rapid absorption, long duration of action, and minimal interaction with other AEDs. Among its mechanisms of action are a state-dependent blockade of Na^+ channels, potentiation of GABA-mediated (inhibitory) neurotransmission, and antagonism of glutamate (excitatory) receptors of the kainate (non-NMDA) subtype.

Its unique chemical structure and multiple mechanisms of activity in laboratory tests suggest that TPM has a broad spectrum of clinical activity and may be effective in patients with epilepsy previously resistant to treatment. In adult studies, TPM was effective and well-tolerated as adjunctive therapy in patients with refractory partial-onset seizures with and without secondary generalization. TPM also showed efficacy and safety as monotherapy in patients with refractory partial-onset seizures and as adjunctive therapy in adults and children with generalized tonic-clonic seizures of nonfocal origin. In children, TPM doses of 5 to 9 mg/kg/day were effective and well tolerated in partial-onset seizures and drop attacks associated with Lennox-Gastaut syndrome. Results of a pilot study in patients with West syndrome indicate that TPM may be effective and safe in this population. Overall, TPM has emerged as a valuable new AED in the field of pediatric epilepsy.

REFERENCES

1. Sharief M, Viteri C, Ben-Menachem E, et al. Double-blind, placebo-controlled study of topiramate in patients with refractory partial epilepsy. *Epilepsy Res* 1996; 25:217–224.

2. Tassinari CA, Michelucci R, Chauvel P, et al. Double-blind, placebo-controlled trial of topiramate (600 mg daily) for the treatment of refractory partial epilepsy. *Epilepsia* 1996; 37:763–768.

3. Ben-Menachem E, Henriksen O, Dam M, et al. Double-blind, placebo-controlled trial of topiramate as add-on therapy in patients with refractory partial seizures. *Epilepsia* 1996; 37:539–543.

4. Faught E, Wilder BJ, Ramsay RE, et al. Topiramate placebo-controlled dose-ranging trial in refractory partial epilepsy using 200-, 400-, and 600-mg daily dosages. *Neurology* 1996; 46:1684–1690.

5. Privitera M, Fincham R, Penry J, et al. Topiramate placebo-controlled dose-ranging trial in refractory partial epilepsy using 600-, 800-, and 1,000-mg daily dosages. *Neurology* 1996; 46:1678–1683.

6. Reife R, Pledger G, Lim P, Karim R. Topiramate: pooled analysis of six placebo-controlled trials. *Epilepsia* 1996; 37(Suppl 4):74.

7. Rosenfeld WE, Sachdeo RC, Faught RE, Privitera M. Long-term experience with topiramate as adjunctive therapy and as monotherapy in patients with partial onset seizures: retrospective survey of open-label treatment. *Epilepsia* 1997; 38(Suppl 1):S34–S36.

8. Sachdeo RC, Reife RA, Lim P, Pledger G. Topiramate monotherapy for partial onset seizures. *Epilepsia* 1997; 38:294–300.

9. Reife R. Topiramate: a novel antiepileptic agent. In: Shorvon S, Dreifuss F, Fish D, Thomas D, eds. *Treatment of Epilepsy.* Oxford, U.K.: Blackwell Science, 1996.

10. Sachdeo RC, Glauser TA, Ritter F, Reife R, Lim P, Pledger G. A double-blind, randomized trial of topiramate in Lennox-Gastaut syndrome. Topiramate YL Study Group. *Neurology* 1999; 52:1882–1887.

11. Elterman R, Glauser TA, Wyllie E, Reife R, Wu S-C. A trial of topiramate as adjunctive therapy in children with partial-onset seizures. *Neurology* 1999; 52:1338–1344.

12. Biton V, Montouris GD, Ritter F, et al. A randomized, placebo-controlled study of topiramate in primary generalized tonic-clonic seizures. Topiramate YTC Study Group. *Neurology* 1999; 52:1330–1337.

13. Glauser TA, Clark PO, Strawsburg R. A pilot study of topiramate in the treatment of infantile spasms. *Epilepsia* 1998; 39:1324–1328.

14. Glauser TA. Topiramate. *Semin Ped Neurol* 1997; 4:34–42.

15. Shank RP, Gardocki JF, Vaught JL, et al. Topiramate: preclinical evaluation of a structurally novel anticonvulsant. *Epilepsia* 1994; 35:450–460.

16. Maryanoff BE, Nortey SO, Gardocki JF, Shank RP, Dodgson SP. Anticonvulsant *O*-alkyl sulfamates. 2,3:4,5-*bis-O*-(1-methylethylidene)-*β*-D-fructopyranose sulfamate and related compounds. *J Med Chem* 1987; 30:880–887.

17. Coulter DA, Sombati S, DeLorenzo RJ. Selective effects of topiramate on sustained repetitive firing and spontaneous bursting in cultured hippocampal neurons. *Epilepsia* 1993; 34 (Suppl 2):123.

18. White HS, Brown SD, Woodhead JH, Skeen GA, Wolf HH. Topiramate enhances GABA-mediated chloride flux and GABA-evoked chloride currents in murine brain neurons and increases seizure threshold. *Epilepsy Res* 1997; 28:167–179.

19. Brown SD, Wolf HH, Swinyard EA, Twyman RE, White HS. The novel anticonvulsant topiramate enhances GABA-mediated chloride flux. *Epilepsia* 1993; 34(Suppl 2):122–123.

20. White HS, Brown SD, Skeen GA, Twyman RE. The investigational anticonvulsant topiramate potentiates GABA-evoked currents in mouse cortical neurons. *Epilepsia* 1995; 36 (Suppl 4):34.

21. Severt L, Coulter DA, Sombati S, De Lorenzo RJ. Topiramate selectively blocks kainate currents in cultured hippocampal neurons. *Epilepsia* 1995; 36(Suppl 4):38.

22. White HS. Clinical significance of animal seizure models and mechanism of action studies of potential antiepileptic drugs. *Epilepsia* 1997; 38(Suppl 1):S9–S17.

23. Rogawski MA, Porter RJ. Antiepileptic drugs: pharmacological mechanisms and clinical efficacy with consideration of promising developmental stage compounds. *Pharmacol Rev* 1990; 42:223–286.

24. Wauquier A, Zhou S. Topiramate: a potent anticonvulsant in the amygdala-kindled rat. *Epilepsy Res* 1996; 24:73–77.

25. Nakamura J, Tamura S, Kanta T, et al. Inhibition by topiramate of seizures in spontaneously epileptic rats and DBA/2 mice. *Eur J Pharmacol* 1994; 254:83–89.

26. Edmonds H, Jiang D, Zhang YP, Vaught JL. Topiramate in rat model of post traumatic epilepsy. *Epilepsia* 1991; 32 (Suppl 3):15.

27. Kimishima K, Wang Y, Tanabe K. Anticonvulsant activities and properties of topiramate. *Japan J Pharmacol* 1992; 58(Suppl 1):211.

28. Hersey SJ, High WL. On the mechanism of acid secretory inhibition by acetazolamide. *Biochim Biophys Acta* 1971; 233:604–609.

29. Cho CH, Chen SM, Chen SW, et al. Pathogenesis of gastric ulceration produced by acetazolamide in rats. *Digestion* 1984; 29:5–11.

30. Ryberg B, Bishop AE, Bloom SR, et al. Omeprazole and ranitidine, antisecretagogues with different modes of action, are equally effective in causing hyperplasia of enterochromaffin-like cells in rat stomach. *Regul Peptides* 1989; 2:235–246.

31. Molon-Noblot S, Boussiquet-Leroux C, Owen RA, et al. Rat urinary bladder hyperplasia induced by oral administration of carbonic anhydrase inhibitors. *Toxicol Pathol* 1992; 20:93.

32. Hirsch KS, Scott WJ, Hurley LS. Acetazolamide teratology: The presence of carbonic anhydrase during the sensitive stage of rat development. *Teratology* 1973; 17:38A.

33. Scott WJ, Hirsch KS, DeSesso JM, Wilson JG. Comparative studies on acetazolamide teratogenesis in pregnant rats, rabbits, and rhesus monkeys. *Teratology* 1981; 24:37–42.

34. Nakatsuka T, Komatsu T, Fujii T. Axial skeletal malformations induced by acetazolamide in rabbits. *Teratology* 1992; 45:629–636.

35. Doose DR, Walker SA, Gisclon LG, Nayak RK. Single-dose pharmacokinetics and effect of food on the bioavailability of topiramate, a novel antiepileptic drug. *J Clin Pharmacol* 1996; 36:884–891.

36. Nayak RK, Gisclon LG, Curtin CA, Benet LZ. Estimation of the absolute bioavailability of topiramate in humans without intravenous data. *J Clin Pharmacol* 1994; 34:1029.

37. Easterling DE, Zakszewski T, Moyer MD, Margul BL, Marriott TB, Nayak RK. Plasma pharmacokinetics of topiramate, a new anticonvulsant in humans. *Epilepsia* 1988; 29:662.

38. Johannessen SI. Pharmacokinetics and interaction profile of topiramate: review and comparison with other newer antiepileptic drugs. *Epilepsia* 1997; 38(Suppl 1):S18–S23.

39. Gisclon LG, Riffitts JM, Sica DA, Gehr T, Ruddley J. The pharmacokinetics (PK) of topiramate (T) in subjects with renal impairment (RI) as compared to matched subjects with normal renal function (NRF). *Pharm Res* 1993; 10(Suppl 10):S397.

40. Wu WN, Heebner JB, Streeter AJ, et al. Evaluation of the absorption, excretion, pharmacokinetics and metabolism of the anticonvulsant topiramate in healthy men. *Pharm Res* 1994; 11(Suppl 10):S336.

41. Perucca E. Pharmacokinetic profile of topiramate in comparison with other new antiepileptic drugs. *Epilepsia* 1996; 37(Suppl 2):S8–S13.

42. Gisclon LG, Curtin CR, Kramer LD. The steady-state (SS) pharmacokinetics (PK) of phenytoin (Dilantin®) and topiramate (Topamax™) in epileptic patients on monotherapy, and during combination therapy. *Epilepsia* 1994; 35 (Suppl 8):54.

43. Sachdeo RC, Sachdeo SK, Walker SA, et al. Steady-state pharmacokinetics of topiramate and carbamazepine in patients with epilepsy during monotherapy and concomitant therapy. *Epilepsia* 1996; 37:774–780.

44. Rosenfeld WE, Liao S, Kramer LD, et al. Comparison of the steady-state pharmacokinetics of topiramate and valproate in patients with epilepsy during monotherapy and concomitant therapy. *Epilepsia* 1997; 38:324–333.

45. Doose DR, Walker SA, Pledger G, Lim P, Reife RA. Evaluation of phenobarbital and primidone/phenobarbital (primidone's active metabolite) plasma concentrations during administration of add-on topiramate therapy in five multicenter, double-blind, placebo-controlled trials in outpatients with partial seizures. *Epilepsia* 1995; 36(Suppl 3):S158.

46. Rosenfeld WE, Doose DR, Walker SA, Nayak RK. Effect of topiramate on the pharmacokinetics of an oral contraceptive containing norethindrone and ethinyl estradiol in patients with epilepsy. *Epilepsia* 1997; 38:317–323.

47. Liao S, Palmer M. Digoxin and topiramate drug interaction study in male volunteers. *Pharm Res* 1993; 10(Suppl 10):S405.

48. Rosenfeld WE, Doose DR, Walker SA, Baldassarre JS, Reife RA. A study of topiramate pharmacokinetics and tolerability in children with epilepsy. *Pediatr Neurol* 1999; 20:339–344.

49. Glauser TA, Miles MV, Tang P, Clark P, McGee K, Doose DR. Topiramate pharmacokinetics in infants. *Epilepsia* 1999; 40:788–791.

50. Reife R, Pledger G, Lim P, Karim R. Patients achieving 75 percent and 100 percent seizure reductions in double-blind trials of topiramate. *Epilepsia* 1997; 38(Suppl 3):59.

51. Reife R, Pledger G, Wu SC. Topiramate as add-on therapy: pooled analysis of randomized controlled trials in adults. *Epilepsia* 2000; 41:S66–S71.

52. Chadwick DW. An overview of the efficacy and tolerability of new antiepileptic drugs. *Epilepsia* 1997; 38(Suppl 1):S59–S62.

53. Marson AG, Kadir ZA, Chadwick DW. New antiepileptic drugs: a systematic review of their efficacy and tolerability. *Br Med J* 1996; 313:1169–1174.

54. Elferink AJ, Van Zwieten-Boot BJ. Analysis based on number needed to treat shows differences between drugs studied. *Br Med J* 1997; 314:603.

55. Shorvon SD. Safety of topiramate: adverse events and relationships to dosing. *Epilepsia* 1996; 37(Suppl 2):S18–S22.

56. Wasserstein AG, Rak I, Reife RA. Nephrolithiasis during treatment with topiramate. *Epilepsia* 1995; 36(Suppl 3):S153.

57. Edwards KR, Kamin M, Topiramate TPS-TR Study Group. The beneficial effect of slowing the initial titration rate of topiramate. *Neurology* 1997; 48(Suppl 2):A39.

58. Hauser WA. Seizure disorders: the changes with age. *Epilepsia* 1992; 33(Suppl 4):S6–S14.

59. O'Donohoe NV. *Epilepsies of Childhood*. 3rd ed. Oxford: Butterworth-Heineman, 1994: 1–5.

60. Ritter F, Glauser TA, Elterman RD, Wyllie E. Effectiveness, tolerability, and safety of topiramate in children with partial-onset seizures. Topiramate YP Study Group. *Epilepsia* 2000; 41:S82–S85.

61. Glauser TA, Levisohn PM, Ritter F, Sachdeo RC. Topiramate in Lennox-Gastaut syndrome: open-label treatment of patients completing a randomized controlled trial. Topiramate YL Study Group. *Epilepsia* 2000; 41:S86–S90.

62. Glauser TA, Olberding L, Clark P, et al. Topiramate monotherapy substitution in children with partial epilepsy. *Epilepsia* 1996; 37(Suppl 4):98.

63. Glauser TA. Topiramate use in pediatric patients. *Can J Neurol Sci* 1998; 25:S8–S12.

CHAPTER 37

Tiagabine

Shlomo Shinnar M.D., Ph.D., and Kenneth W. Sommerville, M.D.

In the last few years a new generation of antiepileptic drugs (AEDs) has been developed (1,2) with much interest in drugs that work on the gamma-aminobutyric acid (GABA) system. GABA is the primary inhibitory neurotransmitter in the mammalian nervous system (3,4). Increasing the effects of the GABA system is thought to prevent seizures. This has already been shown with the barbiturates and benzodiazepines that act on the GABA receptor. Valproate, a GABA analogue, is an effective AED against a variety of seizure disorders, although its precise mechanism of action is unclear (5,6). Recent attempts to utilize the GABA system have focused on GABA metabolism and have resulted in the development of two new drugs. One drug, vigabatrin, which is widely available in much of the world but still experimental in the United States, is an irreversible inhibitor of GABA transaminase (1,5,7). By blocking degradation, levels of GABA are raised. The second drug, tiagabine (Gabitril), was approved by the U.S. Food and Drug Administration for the adjunctive treatment of partial seizures in adults and adolescents in 1997.

Tiagabine was developed as a designer drug to block GABA uptake by presynaptic neurons and glial cells (1,3,8–13). This should result in an increase in GABA concentration in the synapse, resulting in longer duration of action in the synaptic cleft without substantially altering total brain GABA levels. Tiagabine has undergone extensive clinical trials in adults with intractable partial seizure disorders (14–19). Less information is available on the use of tiagabine in children, although clinical trials in children are ongoing (20–23). In this chapter we review the available data on tiagabine with an emphasis on its use in the pediatric age group. Because tiagabine is a new drug, some of these data, particularly those relevant to children, have only been presented in abstract form and have not yet been published in peer-reviewed journals. Although every effort has been made to review the data in detail, much of the pediatric safety and efficacy data must be regarded as preliminary at this point.

PHYSICOCHEMICAL CHARACTERISTICS

Tiagabine hydrochloride is a whitish, odorless crystalline powder with the chemical name (−)-(R)-1-[4,4-bis(3-methyl-2-thienyl)-3-butenyl] nipecotic acid hydrochloride. The chemical formula is $C_{20}H_{25}NO_2S_2HCl$, and the structure is shown in Figure 37-1. It is 3 percent soluble in water and is insoluble in hexane. The nipecotic acid moiety of the molecule has an asymmetric carbon, and the R(−) enantiomer is four times more potent that the S(+) enantiomer. The name *tiagabine* refers to the R(−) enantiomer, which consists of nipecotic acid joined to a lipophilic anchor.

Animal experiments demonstrated that nipecotic acid was anticonvulsant and could preferentially block glial and neural GABA uptake in mice (24). However, nipecotic acid had to be injected intracerebrally in

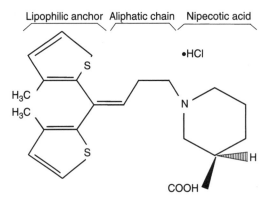

Figure 37-1. Chemical structure of tiagabine HCl.

animals because there was no penetration through the blood–brain barrier. The addition of a lipophilic anchor to nipecotic acid allowed passage across the brain barrier and maintained the desired property of blocking GABA uptake. This compound is tiagabine hydrochloride and is referred to as tiagabine.

MECHANISM OF ACTION

Tiagabine increases the amount of GABA available in the extracellular space by preventing GABA uptake into presynaptic neurons (Figure 37-2). The increased GABA enhances inhibitory effects on receptors of post-synaptic cells. This was confirmed in hippocampal rat slices in which tiagabine prolongs GABA-mediated inhibitory postsynaptic potentials (25).

In vitro work in adult rats has shown that tiagabine blocks GABA uptake by binding in a stereospecific and saturable fashion to the GABA recognition sites in neurons and glial cells (26). Tiagabine binds to a class of high affinity binding sites that most likely represent the GABA transporter GAT-1 (27).

The action of tiagabine is confined to blocking GABA uptake. Tiagabine is not itself taken into neurons or glia. It is highly selective for the GABA system and does not affect other neurotransmitters. It weakly binds to the benzodiazepine and H_1 receptors, but only at concentrations 20 to 400 times those required to inhibit GABA uptake (26). This binding is unlikely to be clinically relevant.

Tiagabine is an anticonvulsant in a variety of animal models of epilepsy including pentylenetetrazol-induced (PTZ) seizures (11), methyl 6,7-dimethoxy-4-ethyl-beta-carboline-3-carboxylate (DMCM)-induced seizures (8), and, at high doses, seizures induced by maximal electroshock (11). DMCM is a proconvulsant that is an inverse agonist of the benzodiazepine receptor.

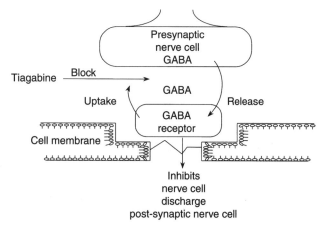

Figure 37-2. Tiagabine inhibits the uptake of gamma-amino butyric acid (GABA) in the synaptic cleft.

Tiagabine has shown other anticonvulsant activity in animal models. It suppresses amygdala-kindled seizures in rats (8) and is effective in treating convulsive status epilepticus in cobalt-lesioned rats (28). It also has moderate efficacy in the genetically determined generalized epilepsy in photosensitive baboons. It may have the same proconvulsant effect as other AEDs. Spike and wave discharges were noted after control of motor status at doses of more than 5 mg/kg in both lesioned and normal rats (28). In a genetically epilepsy-prone strain of rats (WAG/Rij), which is considered an animal model of generalized nonconvulsive absence epilepsy, type II spike and wave discharges were increased at a dose of 3 mg/kg and 10 mg/kg but not at doses of 1 mg/kg, which is closer to the therapeutic range (29). In these epilepsy-prone rats, the increase in spike and wave discharges was not correlated with any behavioral abnormalities. These data suggest that tiagabine may exacerbate absence seizures. However, tiagabine is effective in blocking pentylenetetrazol-induced seizures, which often predicts efficacy against generalized seizures.

The adult animal data suggest that tiagabine may have efficacy in treating some types of both partial and generalized seizure disorders. Data on the effects of tiagabine on experimental seizure models in the developing brain of animals are lacking. This is unfortunate because some AEDs have age-dependent effects on seizures (30–32) but this is a common problem with all AEDs in early clinical usage.

METABOLISM AND PHARMACOKINETICS

Animal studies have shown that tiagabine is rapidly absorbed and has a short half-life of 1 to 3 hours in rats and 1 to 2 hours in dogs. Bioavailability is 25 percent in dogs and 50 percent to 75 percent in rats (9). Like many other AEDs, tiagabine is metabolized by the hepatic cytochrome P-450 system (33). Metabolites include 5-oxo-tiagabine, which is excreted in the urine. Tiagabine is also conjugated with glucuronic acid and metabolites are excreted via urine and feces through the biliary system (9).

Studies in adult volunteers have shown that tiagabine is rapidly absorbed from the gastrointestinal tract, and peak plasma concentrations (C_{max}) are achieved within 2 hours. Absorption is linear and independent of the dose (34). The rate but not the extent of absorption is reduced by food. The time to peak plasma concentration (T_{max}) after a meal is more than twice that in the fasting state. However, while the C_{max} is lower, the area under the curve (AUC) is similar (35). Clinical trials were therefore performed with patients taking tiagabine after a meal as this reduces the possible peak-related toxicities without altering the total amount of drug absorbed.

In normal volunteers, the mean half-life of tiagabine is 4 to 9 hours and is independent of the dose. Because tiagabine is metabolized by the hepatic cytochrome P-450 system, patients taking drugs that induce that system such as barbiturates, carbamazepine, and phenytoin will have a shorter tiagabine half-life (36). Tiagabine does not appear to induce or inhibit hepatic microsomal enzyme systems when given in single or multiple doses (34,37).

Tiagabine is extensively metabolized by the hepatic microsomal system because less than 2 percent is excreted unchanged in the urine (34,38,39). Radiolabeled [^{14}C] tiagabine studies in human volunteers showed that 25 percent was excreted in the urine and 63 percent in the feces (40). Tiagabine has no identified active metabolites (40). It does not appear to accumulate appreciably in plasma with multiple dosing. In phase I studies of healthy volunteers given daily doses over a 5-day period, both the peak levels and the AUC increased proportionally with the dose, as would be expected in a drug with linear pharmacokinetics (34). The therapeutic half-life as distinct from the serum half-life is unclear. Microdialysis studies in patients given oral tiagabine demonstrated that extracellular GABA levels in the brain rise within about an hour after oral dosing (41) but are not sustained more than a few hours and do not completely correlate with the serum concentrations (40). The duration of the antiepileptic activity, which presumably is mediated by these changes in GABA, remains unclear and has not been precisely studied.

Tiagabine is heavily protein bound, although it does not appear to either displace or be displaced by most of the commonly used drugs (42,43). In vitro studies showed tiagabine is more than 95 percent protein bound, primarily to albumin and a glycoprotein.

Tiagabine pharmacokinetics were studied in patients with epilepsy who were taking tiagabine as add-on therapy. Steady-state tiagabine doses ranged from 24 to 80 mg/day in four divided doses (44). All patients were taking enzyme-inducing concomitant AEDs. Results showed that tiagabine had linear kinetics in this population and a linear dose-response curve for C_{max} and the AUC. Although the kinetics remained linear, the half-life of tiagabine was shorter in patients taking AEDs that induce the cytochrome P-450 system than for those on monotherapy or taking noninducing AEDs (36). This is what one would expect and explains why the doses used in this study were considerably higher than those tolerated by healthy volunteers who were not taking enzyme-inducing AEDs. The dose ranges in this study exceeded the upper doses of 56 mg/day used in the randomized clinical trials described subsequently.

The most important drug interaction of tiagabine to date is the effect of enzyme-inducing AEDs. The half-life of tiagabine was shorter and the AUC smaller for the same dose in patients receiving enzyme-inducing AEDs (carbamazepine, phenytoin, phenobarbital, primidone) than in those on tiagabine monotherapy (9,36,45). The pharmacokinetics of tiagabine in patients taking a non–enzyme-inducing AED such as valproate were similar to those in healthy volunteers. Doses of tiagabine need to be substantially higher in patients taking concurrent enzyme-inducing AEDs than with monotherapy or noninducing AEDs. Similar guidelines have been suggested for lamotrigine (46,47). Although the half-life of tiagabine is shortened by the concurrent use of enzyme-inducing AEDs, it is not prolonged by the concurrent use of valproate, as is the case with lamotrigine and phenobarbital (46–49).

Tiagabine has little effect on other AEDs. It does not appear to affect the kinetics of carbamazepine or phenytoin (42). However, tiagabine did reduce the C_{max} and the AUC of valproate by approximately 10 percent (49). This reduction is expected to be of little or no clinical importance. Because tiagabine is metabolized by the 3A-isoform subfamily of the hepatic cytochrome P450 system (33), there is potential for interaction with other drugs with similar metabolism including other AEDs, cimetidine, theophylline, warfarin, and digoxin. However, no clinically significant interactions have been found between tiagabine and these drugs (43). A recent study showed no interaction with erythromycin (50).

Oral contraceptives are also metabolized by the cytochrome P-450 system. In one study, tiagabine, given at a dose of 8 mg/day as monotherapy to healthy young women did not affect the metabolism of oral contraceptives (37,43). Higher doses of tiagabine would not be expected to have an interaction because it is neither an inducer nor an inhibitor of the cytochrome P-450 system, but data are lacking to confirm this impression.

Tiagabine pharmacokinetics behave predictably in hepatic and renal disease (51,52). There is no effect from renal impairment, and there is reduced clearance and a longer half-life with hepatic impairment. Patients with hepatic disease require lower doses than healthy subjects to attain similar concentrations.

Single-dose tiagabine pharmacokinetics have been studied in children (20). In this study, 25 children aged 3 to 10 years with complex partial seizures who were taking one AED were given a single dose of 0.1 mg/kg of tiagabine, and plasma concentrations were checked over the next 24 hours. The mean half-life of tiagabine was 3.2 hours in the 17 children on enzyme-inducing concomitant AEDs (carbamazepine or phenytoin) and 5.7 hours for the 8 children on valproate (noninducing AED). This is comparable to the adult data. Clearance rates, C_{max}, and AUC of tiagabine were affected by the concurrent AEDs in a manner similar to that in adults. The clearance of tiagabine was twice as high in children than in uninduced adults with epilepsy when adjusted for body weight. However, when adjusted according to body surface area, clearance rates of tiagabine in children were 1.5 times higher than those in uninduced adults with epilepsy. The results indicate that tiagabine pharmacokinetics in children aged 2 years and older are similar to those seen in adults, including the effects of concurrent AEDs. Tiagabine pharmacokinetics have not been studied in infants.

HUMAN ADULT EFFICACY DATA

Add-On Therapy in Adults with Partial Seizures

The clinical data regarding the efficacy of tiagabine as add-on therapy come from five placebo-controlled clinical trials in patients with intractable partial seizures. In all five trials, tiagabine was statistically significantly more effective than placebo in the treatment of one or more partial seizure types (53). Two of the studies were crossover trials and three were parallel-group studies. Most of the patients were aged 18 to 75 years, but adolescents starting at age 12 were also included. Efficacy data are available in this age group, although in a relatively small number of patients. Pediatric trials in younger children are in progress, and the available data are discussed separately.

The first phase II multicenter study was a crossover design performed in Europe with 94 patients 18 to 65 years of age with refractory complex partial seizures (14). The study had an "enrichment" design. Patients started with an 8 mg/day dose of tiagabine and the dose was titrated either to reduce seizures sufficiently or to produce unacceptable adverse events with a maximum dose of 52 mg/day. Patients who improved in this phase were then enrolled in a double-blind trial. Of the 94 patients enrolled, 20 discontinued participation during the open-label phase and another 28 failed to qualify for the double-blind phase for lack of sufficient reduction in seizures. The average total daily dose of tiagabine in the 42 patients in the double-blind phase was 33 mg/day, and most were receiving a concomitant enzyme-inducing AED. Even with this relatively small sample size, the frequency of complex partial seizures only and partial seizures with secondary generalization was significantly reduced when the tiagabine and placebo phases were compared. Details of the second crossover trial have not yet been published, but the results were similar to those of the first study (53).

The three randomized phase III multicenter, placebo-controlled, double-blind, parallel-group studies in adults included two in the United States and one in Europe. All of these studies showed tiagabine to be significantly superior to placebo as adjunctive treatment of partial seizures.

The first U.S. study (15) was a dose-response study with patients receiving placebo or 16, 32, or 56 mg/day

of tiagabine in addition to their regular stable AED regimen. Tiagabine was significantly better than placebo at both 32 and 56 mg for median change from baseline and proportion of patients achieving at least 50 percent reduction in complex partial seizures (p in both ≤ 0.03). Tiagabine was effective for both median change from baseline and proportion with at least 50 percent reduction in the 16, 32, and 56 mg groups for simple partial seizures.

Partial seizures with secondary generalization were reduced compared with placebo, but this did not reach significance, possibly because there were fewer patients and numbers of seizures. A clear dose response was present in this study. The minimum effective dose of tiagabine necessary to achieve a 50 percent reduction in complex partial seizure frequency was 32 mg/day, with the 56-mg/day group showing a better response. Doses above 56 mg were not studied in this trial. The patients in this study and in the other two randomized studies were all taking one to three concurrent AEDs, at least one of which was required to be an enzyme inducer of the cytochrome P-450 system. Therefore, the doses required in monotherapy or with a single concomitant noninducer such as valproate may be substantially smaller. The patients in this study were by and large a very refractory group with a median duration of epilepsy of 20 years and had failed to respond to a median of seven AEDs before study entry.

The second U.S. multicenter, randomized, double-blind, placebo-controlled, parallel-group trial compared placebo to 32 mg/day of tiagabine as add-on therapy in 318 patients (16). In this dose-frequency trial, the tiagabine patients received a total of 32 mg/day as 16 mg twice a day or as 8 mg four times a day. Both groups were superior to placebo ($p < 0.001$) in the number of patients achieving at least 50 percent reduction in complex partial seizures. Both groups were also superior to placebo for simple partial seizures for either reduction from baseline or proportion with at least 50 percent reduction in seizures. Taken together with the prior study, the data suggested that the add-on dose of 32 mg/day was likely to be in the low therapeutic range for enzyme-induced patients.

The multicenter, European double-blind, parallel-group study was the only adjunctive trial to evaluate tiagabine given three times daily (54). Tiagabine was given as 10 mg three times daily or 8 mg three times daily if 30 mg/day was not tolerated. There were 154 patients randomized to tiagabine ($n = 77$) or placebo ($n = 77$). The tiagabine-treated group had a significant reduction in the number of both complex and simple partial seizures.

Tiagabine consistently demonstrated efficacy against partial seizures in these trials, but the dose ranges chosen were probably too low in enzyme-induced patients to establish its upper therapeutic range and maximum efficacy. These trials included 67 adolescents aged 12 to 18 years and therefore can be regarded as demonstrating efficacy and safety for this age group was well.

These placebo-controlled trials showed that tiagabine is superior to placebo. The challenge for the practicing clinician is to determine where a new AED belongs in the treatment of patients for whom there are a number of other AEDs to consider. Tiagabine has been compared with add-on carbamazepine or phenytoin in a double-blind multicenter study. Placebo and active drug were given in a double-dummy design to patients on baseline carbamazepine who received add-on tiagabine or phenytoin, or to patients on baseline phenytoin who received add-on tiagabine or carbamazepine. Patients were allowed to titrate to their best-tolerated dose within a wide range to mimic clinical practice.

Preliminary results of the patients taking baseline carbamazepine were recently reported (55). There was no difference in efficacy between the tiagabine group ($n = 106$) and the phenytoin group ($n = 100$) for any partial seizure type in the intent-to-treat analysis. However, phenytoin patients had greater discontinuations for adverse events (17%) than those receiving tiagabine (10%). Overall, discontinuation rates also favored tiagabine (31% vs. 22%). These results suggested that tiagabine may have similar efficacy to phenytoin and is better tolerated when added to carbamazepine. Further detail and analysis of these data are needed, but this preliminary report suggests that tiagabine should be considered for early adjunctive therapy with carbamazepine.

Monotherapy Trials

There have been three studies of tiagabine monotherapy in adults with partial seizures (56,57). The first was a double-blind randomized pilot study of 11 patients in whom AEDs were discontinued during monitoring for presurgical evaluation (57). Patients receiving tiagabine had fewer seizures than those receiving placebo during the treatment period. In the second study (56), which was an open-label dose-ranging study, 19 (61%) of 31 patients successfully converted to tiagabine monotherapy. In the third study, which included 198 randomized patients with partial seizures, patients were randomized to daily doses of tiagabine of either 6 or 36 mg/day. Baseline AEDs were discontinued after tiagabine was added on. Seizure frequency was reduced in both the low- and high-dose groups with the high-dose group having a significantly higher proportion of patients who experienced at least 50 percent reduction in seizure frequency (56). Open-label pediatric data discussed next have also been promising (22).

HUMAN PEDIATRIC EFFICACY DATA

A U.S. add-on, multicenter, double-blind trial with a parallel design is under way. Results of this study should be available in the near future. Preliminary data from the open-label extension study were reported recently and suggest that children do well on tiagabine (58). A total of 152 children took tiagabine in doses of 4 to 66 mg/day (average 23.5 mg/day). Seventeen (11%) were on monotherapy at least 10 weeks; 23 (15%) were seizure-free at least 8 weeks; 12 (8%) were seizure-free on monotherapy (average of 44.8 weeks seizure-free, 60.2 weeks on monotherapy). At present, preliminary data are available from two other nonrandomized pediatric trials.

In a pilot open-label study (22), 25 children with refractory complex partial seizures from a single-dose pharmacokinetics study (20) were enrolled in an open-label, long-term study. Children were initially taking a dose of 0.1 mg/kg/day of tiagabine. They were also continuing a baseline concomitant AED. The dosage was increased every 2 weeks by 0.1 mg/kg/day until clinical efficacy or toxicity was reached. The results of this study have been encouraging for the use of tiagabine in children. This trial ended in November 1998 when a compassionate use study was available. A total of 21 of the original 25 children completed the study. Two were lost to follow-up, and two discontinued for lack of efficacy. Eighteen of the 21 completers were receiving tiagabine monotherapy on the last day of the trial. The 18 children had been on monotherapy an average of 1,270 days (range 986–1,417 days). (Data on file, Abbott Laboratories).

The other pediatric study was a dose-ranging, multicenter, add-on study of 52 children aged 2 to 15 years with epilepsy with a variety of seizure types and epilepsy syndromes refractory to other AEDs; it was conducted at three European sites (21). Unfortunately, the results are difficult to interpret because of the heterogeneous nature of the epilepsy disorders in the study. Twenty-two of the children had generalized epilepsies including Lennox-Gastaut syndrome, other myoclonic seizures disorders, infantile spasms, or childhood absence epilepsy. Before entry into the trial, more than 80 percent of the children had been unsuccessfully tried on 3 to 16 other AEDs, including carbamazepine, valproate, and vigabatrin.

This study differed from the U.S. open-label study. After a 3-week placebo lead-in period, tiagabine was given at more rapid escalating doses (0.25 mg/kg/day up to 1.5 mg/kg/day) than in the U.S. study. Dose escalation in the U.S. study was by 0.1 mg/kg/day at no more than weekly intervals. Patients who completed this phase either entered a long-term extension study or were withdrawn from tiagabine. Of the 53 patients enrolled, 47 entered the tiagabine dosing phase. Of these, 20 completed the trial and 16 withdrew for lack of efficacy, 3 for adverse events, and one for other reasons. Seven were still in the dosing phase at the time the preliminary report was published (21). Seventeen of 20 patients completing the study entered the long-term extension.

Tiagabine was generally well tolerated (see subsequent discussion of safety). The study showed no improvement for children with generalized epilepsy, whereas those with partial seizures improved at doses ranging from 0.37 to 1.25 mg/kg/day, but the results of this small-scale trial in a very refractory population did not demonstrate a statistically significant effect. These results suggest even more strongly that a controlled trial is necessary to determine the place of tiagabine in treating children with partial seizures. The results from the open-label U.S. experience are encouraging but need further confirmation.

An open-label pilot study in children under the age of 12 years with epilepsy and spasticity was also favorable (59). Three of 14 had better than 50 percent improvement by a modified Ashworth scale. Doses started at 0.1 to 0.2 mg/kg/day and could be taken to 1.1 mg/kg/day/ Further investigation in this area appears warranted.

SAFETY

Animal Safety Data

In the preclinical animal studies of tiagabine, there was a large therapeutic window because doses producing sedation were 2.5- to 30-fold greater than the doses treating seizures (60). Other studies in animals have shown no evidence of abnormalities relevant to humans or of carcinogenicity, mutagenicity, or teratogenicity (9).

Adult Data

Phase I studies in healthy volunteers showed that multiple doses of tiagabine were well tolerated up to 10 mg/day (39) and that side effects greater than placebo were noted when the initial dose reached 12 mg/day (61). The side effects included difficulty concentrating, light-headedness, impaired visual perception, and confusion; side effects increased at higher initial doses. These doses may be lower than that which might be tolerated by patients taking enzyme-inducing concomitant AEDs with which the clearance of tiagabine is greater.

Clinical trials of tiagabine therapy in patients with epilepsy have shown a favorable adverse-event profile comparable to many of the current AEDs. The most common adverse events involved the central nervous

system (CNS) and usually are mild to moderate and transient. In the U.S. multicenter, dose-response trial, adverse events sufficient to require discontinuation of the drug occurred twice as often in the groups receiving 32 mg (15%) and 56 mg (16%) per day of tiagabine as in the groups receiving placebo (8%) or 16 mg (7%) of tiagabine (15). The side effects significantly more frequent in tiagabine-treated patients were dizziness, tremor, and difficulty concentrating or mental lethargy. Adverse events in the second U.S. study, which used a 32-mg/day dose regimen, either twice a day or four times a day, were similar to those seen in the first study, although they were milder (16). Again, the percentage of patients withdrawn from the study because of adverse events was higher in the combined tiagabine groups (10%) than in the placebo group (7%). Nervousness, difficulty with immediate recall (amnesia), and emotional lability were other CNS events significantly greater with tiagabine. Abdominal pain, vomiting, and other pain were also significantly increased but usually were not attributed to tiagabine. Myalgia was increased with placebo compared with tiagabine given four times a day.

Three monotherapy studies again showed that CNS-related adverse events were the most common (56). These studies may have used higher doses of tiagabine than may be necessary for clinical practice. One study was a small inpatient presurgical population; one was an open-label pilot study with titration to the maximally tolerated dose; and the third was a controlled high-dose versus low-dose conversion to monotherapy study. The conversion study enabled an evaluation of dose-related side effects in which dizziness, trouble concentrating, nervousness, and paresthesias were significantly increased in the high-dose (36 mg/day) group. A key finding for safety in the open-label pilot study was that patients converting to monotherapy from enzyme-inducing AEDs experienced deinduction of tiagabine clearance. The dose of tiagabine may need to be reduced once monotherapy is reached because tiagabine concentrations will rise without an increase in dose when the inducing AED is discontinued. This does not occur if the concomitant AED is a single noninducer such as valproate.

Neuropsychological testing has been performed in add-on studies and in the controlled conversion to monotherapy study (18,19,62). Compared with placebo, tiagabine had no adverse effects on neuropsychological test scores in both an add-on Finnish study using 30 mg/day (18) and in the multicenter U.S. dose-response study using 16, 32, and 56 mg/day (19). The multicenter U.S. high-dose versus low-dose conversion to monotherapy study showed results related to both dose and whether monotherapy was attained (62). Patients achieving monotherapy improved in mood in the low-dose group, whereas abilities improved in the high-dose group. There was worse performance for mood in the high-dose group if monotherapy was not reached. The reasons for improvement did not correlate with control of seizures and may have been from benefits of withdrawing the baseline concomitant AED and/or better tolerance of tiagabine.

Long-term safety data from the open-label studies have also been reassuring. There have been no clinically relevant changes in laboratory values for hematological or hepatic function. The most commonly reported adverse events were dizziness, somnolence, accidental injury, asthenia (lack of energy), and headache, which are similar to those in the randomized studies (17). Accidental injury and headache are common in populations with severe epilepsy. These adverse events were usually mild and transient and did not require discontinuation of tiagabine therapy. In the long-term, open-label clinical trials of tiagabine in the United States, 220 of 1,437 patients (15%) have discontinued therapy for adverse events (63).

There have been reports of possible nonconvulsive status epilepticus associated with tiagabine therapy (64,65). The most recent report described two patients with confusion and reduced consciousness and simultaneous generalized spike-wave discharges on electroencephalogram (EEG) (65). The authors suggested that this reaction may be from $GABA_B$ receptor agonism and that frontal lobe foci (present in both patients) may be a risk factor. The reports, however, did not confirm that the patients had nonconvulsive status epilepticus or that tiagabine was the cause. The first patient improved slightly after receiving intravenous diazepam and then spontaneously improved 3 hours later. The second patient deteriorated 5 days after a 25 percent reduction in tiagabine dose, suggesting that the possible nonconvulsive status was precipitated by a dose reduction.

An additional 13 cases of possible spike-wave discharges and impaired mental status associated with tiagabine therapy have been intensively reviewed (66). The medical histories and pretreatment EEGs were located and reviewed by an advisory panel. Eight of the cases were thought to have preexisting generalized spike-wave abnormalities that worsened with poorly tolerated increases in tiagabine dose. These patients improved with dose reductions and usually continued on tiagabine at lower doses. Three patients had nonconvulsive status epilepticus that could be attributed to their underlying condition. The remaining two patients either improved with a higher tiagabine dose or did not have spike-wave discharges.

The panel concluded that the evidence so far is that tiagabine does not cause spike-wave discharges but that an exacerbation of preexisting spike-wave patterns was possible in association with poorly tolerated doses. Further study of the rates of nonconvulsive status epilepticus in controlled clinical trials showed similar rates for placebo and tiagabine. Similar rates of all forms of status epilepticus were also found when comparing long-term rates in clinical trials to four external cohorts of patients with epilepsy followed up long-term (67). These findings suggest that tiagabine does not cause nonconvulsive status epilepticus but is associated with confusional states and possible worsening of spike-wave patterns at excessive doses for the individual patient. These reactions are reversible with dose adjustment and do not prohibit the continued use of tiagabine for the patient at a lower dose.

Recently, peripheral visual field loss has been reported in patients treated with vigabatrin (68). Theoretically, this is a concern for all GABAergic drugs including tiagabine. However, the mechanism of action of tiagabine is different than that of vigabatrin. Tiagabine does not cause total brain GABA to rise and is only associated with a transient rise in extracellular GABA concentrations (41). Review of the tiagabine safety database and a study of visual fields by Novo Nordisk have found no comparable visual abnormalities attributable to tiagabine therapy to date (72). Extensive visual field testing by Kalviainen and colleagues was recently reported on 20 patients receiving tiagabine as initial monotherapy for an average of 28 months and on 15 other patients converted to tiagabine monotherapy and exposed an average of 29 months (70,71). No defects attributable to tiagabine have been found.

Safety data have also been published on tiagabine overdose (72,73). There were 22 overdoses in clinical trials as of the end of 1996 with the highest single dose of 800 mg. The most common symptoms were ataxia, confusion, somnolence, agitation, hostility, speech difficulty, weakness, impaired consciousness, and myoclonus. All patients completely recovered. One adolescent had generalized tonic-clonic status epilepticus from a 400-mg overdose and recovered after treatment with phenobarbital. Only supportive care is generally recommended. These findings suggest that the margin of safety with tiagabine is large.

The experience in pregnancy is limited to 21 cases from clinical trials as of October 1996 (74). There were nine carried to term. Eight infants were healthy and one had a hip displacement attributed to a breech presentation. There were five elective abortions, four patients had miscarriages, one had a blighted ovum, and another had a salpingectomy for an ectopic pregnancy. The remaining patient drowned in a bathtub during a seizure after discontinuing tiagabine 3 months earlier. Postmortem examination showed a healthy fetus of 5 months.

Pediatric Safety Data

The safety data in children have also been reassuring. Children in the U.S. open-label pharmacokinetics trial tolerated the drug well in single doses of 0.1 mg/kg (20). Nine of 25 children (36%) reported adverse events, with somnolence being the most common ($n = 7$). One other patient reported a headache, and another had pain at the site of the heparin lock used for sampling blood. All adverse events were mild in severity and resolved without treatment. These children have also tolerated tiagabine very well in a subsequent open-label, long-term study (22). The study was completed in November 1998; 21 of the 25 children completed the study, and there were no discontinuations for adverse events. No safety issues were found in the long-term extension study in children (58).

The data from the European pediatric study, which used higher doses and a more rapid titration, were also comparable to adult data (20). Three of 47 children were withdrawn from tiagabine for adverse events including ataxia ($n = 2$), somnolence ($n = 1$), and depression ($n = 1$). Two additional children had been hospitalized, and both had complete recoveries and were discharged on the same dose of tiagabine. The common adverse events were CNS-related and were similar to those seen in adults. Most were mild to moderate in severity and resolved without requiring discontinuation of the drug.

The pilot study of epilepsy and spasticity in children showed that the drug was well tolerated (59). None of the 14 children treated for spasticity discontinued for adverse events.

CONCLUSIONS

To date, tiagabine has been given to over 3,000 patients and subjects in clinical trials, and postmarketing experience is just beginning to accumulate. Results in multiple controlled trials have consistently shown tiagabine to be an effective AED for patients with partial seizures. The side-effect profile appears to be favorable. Pediatric data are being gathered but are limited so far except for pharmacokinetics data, although a U.S. multicenter, controlled, add-on trial is in progress. The data suggest that tiagabine is effective in partial seizures disorders in adults and children. As the National Institutes of Health consensus conference has pointed out, pediatric seizure disorders are not always the same in adults (32). Myoclonic epilepsies of childhood are likely to be different from myoclonic seizures in adults, and it is unclear whether tiagabine might be of benefit in this area. The preliminary data from open-label pediatric trials in children with myoclonic epilepsy were negative (21), but tiagabine does have efficacy in some

models of genetically mediated myoclonus in animals, and further trials are needed to explore this possibility.

At this time tiagabine has received regulatory approvals in the United States, Australia, New Zealand, and most of western Europe, including France, Germany, and the United Kingdom. As of March 1999, approximately 85,000 patients have been exposed to tiagabine (Data on file, Abbott Laboratories). Tiagabine has great theoretical appeal as a "designer drug" that enhances the availability of GABA at the postsynaptic membrane without interfering with overall GABA metabolism or altering brain GABA levels. Tiagabine has a number of favorable characteristics including a spectrum of efficacy in animal models, a relatively high therapeutic index, and a relative lack of sedation or changes in neuropsychological testing, which make it an exciting new drug. It is still too early to state whether this profile translates into clinical advantages for large numbers of patients.

The role of tiagabine in the treatment of epilepsy will ultimately be determined by the efficacy in treating patients with a variety of seizure disorders including less refractory ones and by the side-effect profile compared with standard AEDs. The early data on tiagabine versus phenytoin suggest that tiagabine may have advantages as adjunctive therapy. Patients with less refractory seizures treated with monotherapy may differ in their tolerance for tiagabine. Idiosyncratic side effects may still occur as the number of exposures increases. In the case of some drugs such as carbamazepine, early concerns about aplastic anemia have diminished with time, and it has become a first-line drug for partial seizures in all age groups (48). In the case of other drugs such as felbamate, concerns about these serious adverse effects have limited its use to patients with refractory epilepsy (75). There is so far no evidence that tiagabine has unique toxicity with long-term treatment, but caution is suggested until more data have accumulated.

Although it is too early to know the precise role tiagabine will have, physicians caring for patients with seizures can add tiagabine or one of several other promising new AEDs. It is gratifying to have these choices after a long hiatus. This will undoubtedly improve our ability to care for children and adults with seizures.

REFERENCES

1. Dichter MA, Brodie MJ. New antiepileptic drugs. *N Engl J Med* 1996; 334:1583–1590.

2. Wyllie E, ed. New developments in antiepileptic drug therapy. *Epilepsia* 1995; 36(Suppl 2):S1–S118.

3. Suzdak PD, Jansen JA. A review of the preclinical pharmacology of tiagabine: A potent and selective anticonvulsant GABA uptake inhibitor. *Epilepsia* 1995; 36:612–626.

4. Meldrum B. Pharmacology of GABA. *Clin Neuropharmacol* 1982; 5:293–316.

5. MacDonald RL, Kelly KM. Antiepileptic drug mechanisms of action. *Epilepsia* 1995; 36(Suppl 2):S2–S12.

6. Farriello RG, Varasi M, Smith MC. Valproic acid: mechanisms of action. In: Levy RH, Mattson RH, Meldrum BS, eds. *Antiepileptic Drugs*. 4th ed. New York: Raven Press, 1995:581–588.

7. Ben-Menachem E. Vigabatrin. *Epilepsia* 1995; 36(Suppl 2):S95–S104.

8. Giardina WJ. Anticonvulsant action of tiagabine, a new GABA-uptake inhibitor. *J Epilepsy* 1994; 7:161–166.

9. Ostergaard LH, Gram L, Dam M. Potential antiepileptic drugs: tiagabine. In: Levy RH, Mattson RH, Meldrum BS, eds. *Antiepileptic Drugs*. 4th ed. New York: Raven Press, 1995:1057–1061.

10. Mengel HB. Tiagabine. *Epilepsia* 1994; 35(Suppl 5): S81–S84.

11. Neilsen EB, Suzdac PD, Andersen KE, et al. Characterization of tiagabine (NO-328), a new potent and selective GABA uptake inhibitor. *Eur J Pharmacol* 1991; 196:257–266.

12. Andersen KE, Braestrop C, Gronwald FC, et al. The synthesis of novel GABA uptake inhibitors. 1. Elucidation of the structure-activity studies leading to the choice of (R)-1-[4,4-bis(3-methyl-2-thienyl)-3-butenyl]-3-piperidinecarboxylic acid (tiagabine) as an anticonvulsant drug candidate. *J Med Chem* 1993; 36:1716–1725.

13. Thompson SM, Gähwiler BH. Effects of the GABA uptake inhibitor tiagabine on inhibitory synaptic potentials in rat hippocampal slice cultures. *J Neurophysiol* 1992; 67:1698–1701.

14. Richens A, Chadwick D, Duncan J, et al. Adjunctive treatment of partial seizures with tiagabine: a placebo-controlled trial. *Epilepsy Res* 1995; 21:37–42.

15. Uthman BM, Rowan AJ, Ahmann PA, et al. Tiagabine for complex partial seizures: a randomized, add-on, dose-response trial. *Arch Neurol* 1998; 55:56–62.

16. Sachdeo R, Leroy R, Krauss G, et al. Tiagabine therapy for complex partial seizures: a dose-frequency study. *Arch Neurol* 1997; 54:595–601.

17. Leppik IE. Tiagabine: the safety landscape. *Epilepsia* 1995; 36(Suppl 6):S10–S13.

18. Kalviainen R, Salmenpera T, Aikia M, et al. Tiagabine monotherapy in newly diagnosed partial epilepsy: follow-up with cognitive tests, EEG, quantitative MRI, and CSF amino acids. *Epilepsia* 1994; 35(Suppl 7):74.

19. Dodrill CB, Arnett JL, Sommerville KW, et al. Cognitive and quality of life effects of differing doses of tiagabine in epilepsy. *Neurology* 1997; 48:1025–1031.

20. Gustavson LE, Boellner SW, Granneman GR, et al. A single-dose study to define the tiagabine pharmacokinetics in pediatric patients with complex partial seizures. *Neurology* 1997; 48:1–6.

21. Uldall P, Bulteau C, Pederson SA, et al. Single-blind study of safety, tolerability, and preliminary efficacy of tiagabine as adjunctive treatment of children with epilepsy. *Epilepsia* 1995; 36(Suppl 3):S147.

22. Boellner S, McCarty J, Mercante D, et al. Pilot study of tiagabine in children with partial seizures. *Epilepsia* 1996; 37(Suppl 4):92.

23. Biton V, Alto G, Pixton G, Sommerville K. Tiagabine monotherapy in adults and children in a long-term study. *Epilepsia* 1996; 37(Suppl 5):1–7.

24. Croucher MJ, Meldrum BS, Krogsgaard-Larsen P. Anticonvulsant activity of GABA uptake inhibitors and their prodrugs following central or systemic administration. *Eur J Pharmacol* 1983; 89:217–228.

25. Rekling JC, Jahnsen H, Laursen AM. The effect of two lipophilic gamma-aminobutyric acid uptake blockers in CA1 of the rat hippocampal slice. *Br J Pharmacol* 1990; 99:103–106.

26. Braestrup C, Nielsen EB, Sonnewald U, et al. (R)-N-[4,4-bis(3-methyl-2-thienyl)but-3-en-1-yl]ninecotic acid binds with high affinity to the brain gamma-aminobutyric acid uptake carrier. *J Neurochem* 1990; 54:639–647.

27. Borden LA, Murali Dhar TG, Smith KE, et al. Tiagabine, SKF 89976-A, CI-966 and NNC-711 are selective for the cloned GABA transporter GAT-1. *Eur J Pharmacol* 1994; 269:2219–224.

28. Walton NY, Gunawan S, Treiman DM. Treatment of experimental status epilepticus with the GABA uptake inhibitor, tiagabine. *Epilepsy Res* 1994; 19:237–244.

29. Coenen AM, Blezer EH, van Luijtelaar EL. Effects of the GABA uptake inhibitor tiagabine on electroencephalogram, spike-wave discharges and behaviour of rats. *Epilepsy Res* 1995; 21:89–94.

30. Velíšek L, Veliskova J, Ptachewich Y, Shinnar S, Moshe SL. Effects of MK-801 and phenytoin on flurothyl-induced seizures during development. *Epilepsia* 1995; 36:179–185.

31. Velíšek L, Veliskova J, Ptachewich Y, et al. Age-dependent effects of gamma-aminobutyric acid agents on flurothyl seizures. *Epilepsia* 1995; 36:636–643.

32. Sheridan PH, Jacobs MP. Conference Review. The development of antiepileptic drugs for children: report from the NIH workshop, Bethesda, Maryland, February 17–18, 1994. *Epilepsy Res* 1996; 23:87–92.

33. Bopp BA, Nequist GE, Rodrigues AD. Role of the cytochrome P450 3A subfamily in the metabolism of [^{14}C] tiagabine in human hepatic microsomes. *Epilepsia* 1995; 36(Suppl 3):S159.

34. Gustavson LE, Mengel HB. Pharmacokinetics of tiagabine, a gamma-aminobutyric acid-uptake inhibitor, in healthy subjects after single and multiple doses. *Epilepsia* 1995; 36:605–611.

35. Mengel HB, Gustavson LE, Soerensen HJ, et al. Effect of food on the bioavailability of tiagabine HCl. *Epilepsia* 1991; 32(Suppl 3):6.

36. Richens A, Gustavson LE, McKelvy JF, et al. Pharmacokinetics and safety of single-dose tiagabine HCl in epileptic patients chronically treated with four other antiepileptic drug regimens. *Epilepsia* 1991; 32(Suppl 3):12.

37. Mengel HB, Houston A, Back DJ. An evaluation of the interaction between tiagabine and oral contraceptives in female volunteers. *J Pharm Med* 1994; 4:141–150.

38. Gustavson LE, Mengel HB, Pierce MW, Chu S-Y. Tiagabine, a new gamma-aminobutyric acid uptake inhibitor

antiepileptic drug: pharmacokinetics after single oral doses in man. *Epilepsia* 1990; 31:642.

39. Mengel HB, Pierce M, Mant T, Gustavson L. Tiagabine, a GABA-uptake inhibitor: safety and tolerance of multiple dosing in normal subjects. *Acta Neurol Scand* 1990; 82(Suppl 133):35.

40. Bopp BA, Gustavson LE, Johnson MK, et al. Disposition and metabolism of orally administered ^{14}C-tiagabine in humans. *Epilepsia* 1992; 33(Suppl 3):83.

41. During M, Mattson R, Scheyer R, et al. The effect of tiagabine HCl on extracellular GABA levels in the human hippocampus. *Epilepsia* 1992; 33(Suppl 3):83.

42. Gustavson LE, Cato A, Boellner SW, et al. Lack of pharmacokinetics drug interactions between tiagabine and carbamazepine or phenytoin. *Am J Therapeutics* 1998; 5:9–16.

43. Mengel HB, Jansen JA, Sommerville K, et al. Tiagabine: evaluation of the risk of interaction with theophylline, warfarin digoxin, cimetidine, oral contraceptives, triazolam, or ethanol. *Epilepsia* 1995; 36(Suppl 3):S160.

44. So EL, Wolff D, Graves NM, et al. Pharmacokinetics of tiagabine as add-on therapy in patients taking enzyme-inducing drugs. *Epilepsy Res* 1995; 22:221–226.

45. Brodie MJ. Tiagabine pharmacology in profile. *Epilepsia* 1995; 36(Suppl 6):S7–S9.

46. Messenheimer JA. Lamotrigine. *Epilepsia* 1995; 36(Suppl 2):S87–S94.

47. Yuen AWC. Lamotrigine: interaction with other drugs. In: Levy RH, Mattson RH, Meldrum BS, eds. *Antiepileptic Drugs*. 4th ed. New York: Raven Press, 1995:883–888.

48. Dodson WE. Principles of antiepileptic drug therapy. In: Shinnar S, Amir N, Branski D, eds. *Childhood Seizures*. Basel: S Karger, 1995:78–92.

49. Gustavson LE, Sommerville KW, Cato A, et al. Lack of a clinically significant pharmacokinetics drug interaction between tiagabine and valproate. *Online J Curr Clin Trials* February 18, 1997; document 203.

50. Thompson MS, Groes L, Schwietert HR, et al. An open label sequence listed two period crossover pharmacokinetics trial evaluating the possible interaction between tiagabine and erythromycin during multiple administration to healthy volunteers. *Epilepsia* 1997; 38(Suppl 3):64.

51. Cato A, Gustavson LE, Qian J, et al. Effect of renal impairment on the pharmacokinetics and tolerability of tiagabine. *Epilepsia* 1998; 39(Suppl 1):43–47.

52. Lau AH, Gustavson LE, Sperelakis R, et al. Pharmacokinetics and safety of tiagabine in subjects with various degrees of hepatic function. *Epilepsia* 1997; 38:445–451.

53. Ben-Menachem E. International experience with tiagabine add-on therapy. *Epilepsia* 1995; 36(Suppl 6):S14–S21.

54. Schachter SC, Sommerville KW. Tiagabine. A potent new drug for partial seizures. Presented at Third Eilat conference on new antiepileptic drugs, May 28–29, 1996, Eilat, Israel.

55. Vasquez B, Sachdeo RC, Chang, et al. Tiagabine or phenytoin as first add-on therapy for complex partial seizures. *Neurology* 1998; 50(Suppl 4):A199.

56. Schachter SC. Tiagabine monotherapy in the treatment of partial epilepsy. *Epilepsia* 1995; 36(Suppl 6):S2–S6.

57. Alarcon G, Binnie CD, Elwes RDC, Polkey CE. Monotherapy antiepileptic drug trials in patients undergoing presurgical assessment: Methodological problems and possibilities. *Seizure* 1995; 4:293–301.

58. Collins SD, Fugate J., Sommerville KW. Long term use of Gabitril (tiagabine HCl) monotherapy in pediatric patients. *Neurology* 1999; 52(Suppl 2):A392.

59. Holden KR, Titus O. Effect of tiagabine on spasticity in children with intractable epilepsy. *Neurology* 1999; 52(Suppl 2):A21.

60. Pierce MW, Suzdak PD, Andersen KE, et al. Tiagabine. In: Pisani F, Perucca E, Avansini A, eds. *New Antiepileptic Drugs*. Amsterdam: Elsevier, 1991:157–160.

61. Mengel HB, Mant TGK, McKelvy JM, Pierce MW. Tiagabine: phase I study of safety and tolerance following single oral doses. *Epilepsia* 1990; 31:642–643.

62. Dodrill CE, Arnett JL, Shu V, et al. Effects of tiagabine monotherapy on abilities, adjustment, and mood. *Epilepsia* 1998; 39:33–42.

63. Gabitril™ prescribing information, Abbott Laboratories, 1997.

64. Schapel G, Chadwick D. Tiagabine and non-convulsive status epilepticus. *Seizure* 1996; 5: 153–156.

65. Eckardt KM, Steinhoff BJ. Non-convulsive status epilepticus in two patients receiving tiagabine treatment. *Epilepsia* 1998; 39: 671–674.

66. Shinnar S, Berg AT, Sommerville KW, et al. Evaluation of spike and wave discharges and complex partial status epilepticus in association with tiagabine therapy. *Neurology* 1997; 48:A39.

67. Shinnar S, Berg AT, Hauser WA, et al. Evaluation of the incidence of status epilepticus in association with tiagabine therapy. *Epilepsia* 1997; 38(Suppl 3):65.

68. Eke T, Talbot JF, Lawden MC. Severe persistent visual field constriction associated with vigabatrin. *BMJ* 1997; 314:180–181.

69. Collins SD, Brim S, Kirstein YG., Sommerville KW. Absence of visual defects in patients taking tiagabine (Gabitril). *Epilepsia* 1998; 38(Suppl 6):146.

70. Kalviainen R, Nousiainen I, Mantyjarvi M. Absence of concentric visual field defects in patients with initial tiagabine monotherapy. *Epilepsia* 1999; 40(Suppl 2):259.

71. Kalviainen R, Salmenpera T, Jutila L, Aikia M, Nousiainen I. Tiagabine monotherapy in chronic partial epilepsy. *Epilepsia* 1999; 40(Suppl 2):258.

72. Parks BR, Flowers WG, Dostrow VG, et al. Experience with clinical overdoses of tiagabine. Antiepileptic drug treatment: state of the art and further perspectives. Biedefeld, Germany, April 24–27, 1997.

73. Leach JP, Stolarek I, Brodie MJ. Deliberate overdose with the novel anticonvulsant tiagabine. *Seizure* 1995; 4:155–157.

74. Collins SD, Sommerville KW, Donnelly J, et al. Pregnancy and tiagabine exposure. *Neurology* 1997; 48(Suppl 2):A38.

75. Leppik IE. Felbamate. *Epilepsia* 1995; 36(Suppl 2): S66–S72.

CHAPTER 38

Vigabatrin

Günter Krämer, M.D.

Gamma-aminobutyric acid (GABA) is the major inhibitory neurotransmitter in the mammalian brain. Vigabatrin (γ-vinyl-GABA, 4-amino-5-hexenoic acid; VGB) was synthesized in 1974 as structural GABA-analogue with a vinyl appendage. The aim was to achieve an enzyme-activated inhibition of GABA catabolism (1). It has been regarded as a prime example of a drug developed on a rational scientific basis for treatment of a disease (2). VGB was first marketed for adults in the United Kingdom in 1989 and thereafter in most European countries (3). The application was extended in 1990 to the use of VGB in children with refractory epilepsy and later to its use as monotherapy for infantile spasms. Although VGB has been approved for use in more than 65 countries worldwide, its use has currently declined after the detection of persistent peripheral visual field defects (VFD) in up to 40 percent of patients.

PHARMACOLOGY AND MECHANISM OF ACTION

Pharmacology

Vigabatrin is a white to off-white crystalline amino acid; it is highly water-soluble and only slightly soluble in ethanol and methanol. The molecular weight is 129.16, and the conversion factor is 7.75 (mg/L × 7.75 = μmol/L). VGB exists as a racemic mixture of S(+)- and R(−)-enantiomers in equal proportions. The S(+)-enantiomer is responsible for the pharmacologic action, and the R(−)-enantiomer is inactive (4,5). The only available forms of VGB are oral formulations (tablets and sachets containing 500 mg).

Mechanism of Action

Vigabatrin acts by replacing GABA as a substrate of GABA-transaminase (GABA-T) (6). However, because VGB possesses an inert appendage at the γ-position, it prevents the transamination of GABA to form succinic acid semialdehyde by irreversible and covalent binding to GABA-T, causing its permanent inactivation (7,8). This results in prolonged elevation of brain GABA levels without any major influence on other enzymes involved in GABA synthesis and metabolism. The effect is maximal 3 to 4 hours after administration and maintained for at least 24 hours. Thus, the major pharmacologic effects of VGB are determined not by the pharmacokinetic half-life of the drug itself but by that of GABA-T. Restoration of normal enzyme activity by resynthesis after withdrawal of VGB takes several days (9). In addition, VGB significantly reduces the activity of the plasma alanine aminotransferase (ALAT) by 20 percent to 100 percent (10,11).

In patients with epilepsy, a dose-related (up to 3 g/day) elevation of free GABA, total GABA, and homocarnosine (a dipeptide of GABA) cerebrospinal fluid (CSF) levels could be demonstrated (12). ^{1}H-MR spectroscopy has shown that the brain GABA content in the occipital region of patients with epilepsy increased two- to threefold (13–15). Increasing VGB dose from 3 to 6 g/day did not result in a further increase in brain GABA concentrations, most probably because of a feedback inhibition of glutamic acid decarboxylase (GAD), the GABA synthesizing enzyme, at high GABA concentrations.

PHARMACOKINETICS AND DRUG INTERACTIONS

Pharmacokinetics

Adults

Vigabatrin is rapidly and almost completely absorbed from the gastrointestinal (GI) tract. Food does not influence absorption (16), and peak plasma concentrations

(c_{max}) are reached within 0.5 to 2 hours after single doses (17). Areas under the plasma concentration time curve (AUC) and c_{max} indicate linear pharmacokinetics over the dose range of 0.5 to 4 g. VGB is widely distributed in the body with a volume of distribution of 0.8 L/kg; levels in the CSF are approximately 10 percent of those in the blood (18). It is not bound to proteins and neither does it influence the protein binding of other drugs or cytochrome P-450–dependent enzymes. Elimination is primarily renal, with a renal clearance of unchanged drug accounting for 60 percent to 70 percent of the total clearance, which indicates an oral bioavailability of at least that magnitude. The elimination half-life ($t_{1/2}$) is between 5 and 7 hours, but in patients taking hepatic enzyme-inducing drugs slightly shorter half-life values of 4 to 6 hours have been observed (18,19). Because approximately 60 percent of the drug is removed from the blood during hemodialysis, VGB should be administered thereafter (20). The passage of both enantiomers of VGB across the human placenta is slow, and the concentration ratio in breast milk compared to plasma for the active S(+) enantiomer is below 0.5 (21).

Children and Infants

Following single oral doses of 125 mg VGB racemate in six neonates, the mean values of c_{max} and AUC were significantly lower for the active S(+) enantiomer, whereas no difference was found for the time to reach peak plasma concentrations (t_{max}). Repeated administration of 125 mg twice daily over 4 days was without evidence of accumulation of either enantiomer (22). A pharmacokinetic study after administration of a single 50 mg/kg VGB dose in six infants (5–24 months) and six children (4–14 years) with intractable epilepsy showed results comparable to those in adults, mainly with regard to the elimination of the active S(+) enantiomer, which seems to be age-independent. In contrast to adults, in whom t_{max} of the inactive R(−)-enantiomer is about twice that of the active S(+)-enantiomer, no differences were found for t_{max} of the two allosteric forms in children. However, the mean AUC of the R(−)-enantiomer was also significantly greater. In addition, the AUC values for both isomers were significantly lower in infants than in children, which in turn were lower than in adults. Despite lower AUC values in children, age appears to have only little influence on the pharmacokinetics of VGB, and VGB accumulation during multiple dose administration (5 days) did not occur (23). No studies of GABA levels in CSF during VGB treatment have been performed, and GABA levels in brain have not been measured by magnetic resonance (MR) spectroscopy in young children.

Drug Interactions

Vigabatrin has no effect on the plasma concentrations of valproate (VPA) (24) or felbamate (FBM) (25). There usually is also no effect on carbamazepine (CBZ) levels, but an increase of up to 39 percent has been described by one group (26) as well as a decrease of about 50 percent by other investigators (27). After a latency of some weeks VGB reduces phenytoin (PHT) levels by about 25 percent without altered absorption (28) or plasma protein binding (29). In children with epilepsy, the drop of PHT levels can be even more pronounced (30). Serum levels of phenobarbital and primidone can also be slightly reduced by VGB (19). VPA has no effect on VGB plasma levels (24), and this has also been described for the other established AEDs (31), although a shorter half-life of VGB in patients receiving enzyme-inducing drugs has been observed (18,19). FBM leads to a slight increase of the active S(+)-enantiomer (25). Regarding drugs other than AEDs, VGB has no effect on oral steroid contraceptives (32), and there is no information about effects of other drugs on VGB (33).

Drug Monitoring

Vigabatrin can be determined in biological fluids by high-performance liquid chromatography (HPLC) and gas chromatography-mass spectroscopy (34). A sensitive HPLC method for the simultaneous determination of VGB and gabapentin in serum and urine has been described (35). The value of plasma level determinations of VGB for therapeutic drug monitoring is limited, mainly because of its mechanism of action with irreversible enzyme inhibition resulting in a biological half-life of several days. Consequently, in 16 children with refractory epilepsy there was no strong correlation between VGB dosages, plasma concentrations, and clinical efficacy (36).

ANIMAL STUDIES

The anticonvulsant effect of VGB has been demonstrated in numerous animal models. Whereas it is inactive in models such as maximal electroshock or pentylenetetrazol, it protects against bicuculline-induced myoclonic activity, strychnine-induced tonic seizures, isoniazid-induced generalized seizures, audiogenic seizures in mice, light-induced seizures in the baboon, and amygdala-kindled seizures in the rat (37).

The usual preclinical safety studies carried out in rats, mice, dogs, and monkeys demonstrated no significant adverse effects on the liver, kidney, lung, heart, or GI tract. Studies revealed no evidence of mutagenic or carcinogenic effects. However, in the brain, microvacuolation has been observed in white matter tracts of rats, mice, and dogs at doses of 30 to 50 mg/kg/day. These lesions were minimal or equivocal in the monkey. This effect is caused by a separation of the outer lamellar sheath of myelinated fibers, a change that is characteristic of intramyelinic edema. In both rats and dogs the intramyelinic edema was reversible upon discontinuation of VGB, and even with continued treatment histologic regression was observed. Minor residual changes consisting of swollen axons and mineralized microbodies have been observed in rodents (38,39).

Vigabatrin-associated retinotoxicity has been observed in albino rats but not in pigmented rats, dogs, or monkeys. The retinal changes in albino rats were characterized as focal or multifocal disorganization of the outer nuclear layer with displacement of nuclei into the rod and cone area. The other layers of the retina were not affected. Although the histologic appearance of these lesions was similar to that found in albino rats following excessive exposure to light, the retinal changes may also represent a direct drug-induced effect (38).

Although there is no evidence of intramyelinic edema in humans, the U.S. Food and Drug Administration halted clinical studies with VGB because of these findings for 5 years between 1983 and 1988. Tests done to confirm lack of significant adverse effect on neurologic function include evoked potentials, computed tomography (CT) and magnetic resonance imaging (MRI) scans, CSF analyses, and, in a small number of cases, neuropathological examinations of brain specimens (39,40).

Further animal experiments have shown that VGB has no negative influence on fertility or pup development. No teratogenicity was seen in rats at doses up to 150 mg/kg (three times the human dose) or in rabbits in doses up to 100 mg/kg. However, a slight increase in the incidence of cleft palate at doses of 150 to 200 mg/kg was seen in rabbits. Therefore, the use of VGB is presently not recommended for women with childbearing potential (41).

CLINICAL STUDIES

Adults

Clinical studies with VGB have included over 2,000 patients. After initial open and single-blind dose-finding studies, several randomized, double-blind, placebo-controlled crossover studies in adult patients with refractory partial epilepsies and add-on therapy with VGB were conducted.

An Australian study in 97 patients with uncontrolled partial seizures comparing 2 g/day and 3 g/day showed a similar efficacy with 42 percent of the patients experiencing a 50 percent or greater reduction of their seizure frequency in comparison to placebo (= responders). In addition, the number of seizure-free days and the longest seizure-free period were significantly longer during VGB administration, and more patients had less severe and shorter seizures (42).

In addition to the crossover studies, several double-blind, placebo-controlled, parallel group studies were carried out. The therapeutic efficacy of VGB add-on in treatment-resistant epilepsy, assessed as the percentage of patients having at least a 50 percent reduction in seizure frequency, was quite similar across the studies, with about 40 percent of patients being responders (for review of the earlier studies see 43–45). In the first of more recent studies from the United States, 92 patients received VGB 3 g/day add-on and were compared with 90 patients in the placebo group (46). Significantly more patients receiving VGB were responders with 50 percent to 99 percent reduction of seizure frequency (37% vs. 18%) or seizure freedom (6% vs. 1%). The second study examined three different VGB daily doses (1, 3, or 6 g) in 174 patients (47). Whereas only 7 percent in the placebo group were responders, the corresponding figures for the VGB groups were 24 percent, 51 percent, and 54 percent.

A double-blind, double-dummy substitution trial comparing add-on VGB (2–4 g daily) and valproate (1–2 g daily) in CBZ-resistant partial epilepsy, allowing withdrawal of CBZ in responders, showed similar percentages of responders (53% vs. 51%) and maintenance of alternative monotherapy (27% vs. 31%) (48).

Two open, single-center, randomized monotherapy studies using CBZ as comparator included 100 patients (49) and 51 patients (50), respectively. Both studies failed to show differences in efficacy but demonstrated a more favorable side-effect profile of VGB (before the knowledge of VFD related to VGB). In addition, several open, long-term studies on the add-on use of VGB in adult patients with treatment-resistant partial epilepsy have been reported. The length of follow-up varied between 9 and 78 weeks. Most of the patients included had a favorable initial response to VGB, which was maintained in 22 percent to 75 percent of the patients.

More recently, a larger randomized, double-blind, parallel-group study has been carried out to compare the efficacy of VGB as monotherapy with CBZ in newly diagnosed epilepsy. Fifty-three percent of the 229 patients receiving 2 g VGB daily and 57 percent of the 230 patients receiving 600 mg CBZ daily achieved a 6-month period of remission. However, significantly more patients receiving VGB withdrew because of lack of efficacy than with CBZ, and time to first seizure after the first 6 weeks from randomization also showed CBZ to be more effective. It was concluded that VGB cannot be recommended as a first-line drug for monotherapy of newly diagnosed partial epilepsies (51).

In most double-blind trials in adults, the daily dose of VGB was 2 to 3 g. Initial studies suggested that 1 g might also have some therapeutic efficacy, and there are patients who benefit from doses of 4 g or more. In the U.S. study comparing daily doses of 1, 3, and 6 g, no improvement in efficacy was observed in patients given 6 g versus 3 g, but side effects increased substantially (47). Although VGB is usually administered twice daily, a double-blind pilot study in 50 patients comparing once-daily versus twice-daily add-on administration demonstrated no statistical difference (52).

During long-term treatment with VGB, development of tolerance after an initially beneficial effect is observed in about one-third to one-half of patients (53).

Children and Infants

The approval of VGB in childhood refractory epilepsies in several countries has been granted on the basis of several open studies and compassionate experience (54). Since the efficacy of VGB had been demonstrated in adults and the safety profile was reassuring in adults, it was not deemed necessary to repeat those studies in children. Nevertheless, the pediatric file was supplemented with two single-blind, placebo-controlled, run-in dose-ranging studies (55,56) and one additional open dose-ranging study (57). These studies also allowed for a better definition of the profile of activity of VGB in different types of resistant epilepsies, including the epileptic syndromes specific to childhood, and for the assessment of the tolerability of VGB in children.

The two dose-response studies performed in a total of 86 children with refractory epilepsy (55,56) demonstrated an optimal efficacy at the first dose step (40–80 mg/kg/day, mean: 60 mg/kg/day), which is higher than in adults (35–65 mg/kg/day). Further dose increases in nonresponders, although well-tolerated, did not result in a higher number of patients being controlled.

On the basis of pharmacokinetic and dose-response studies, the following dose regimen for children was recommended and approved: starting dose: 40 mg/kg/day, increasing to 80 to 100 mg/kg/day, depending on response. Children with partial seizures seemed to show similar benefits to those seen in adults with difficult-to-control partial epilepsy. Greater than 50 percent seizure suppression was seen in 38 percent to 54 percent of patients in three studies (54,57–59) but in more than 80 percent of the patients in the study of Herranz and coworkers (56). VGB was effective against both simple and complex partial seizures and secondary generalization. Among different epilepsies, the best efficacy was seen in localization-related

epilepsies with symptomatic or cryptogenic etiology. Anecdotal case reports described favorable effects in neonatal seizures due to Ohtahara syndrome (60) or Sturge-Weber syndrome (61).

Two double-blind, placebo-controlled, parallel design, efficacy/safety studies in pediatric patients with treatment-resistant complex partial seizures with or without secondary generalization were recently completed in the United States. There were four arms in protocol 118, placebo and three fixed-dose VGB groups, at 20, 60, and 100 mg/kg/day, respectively. All patients had uncontrolled seizures. VGB (or placebo) was administered as add-on treatment. VGB exhibited a linear dose-response trend in reducing mean seizure frequency ($p = 0.057$). Although reductions in mean seizure frequency occurred in all VGB treatment groups, only the 100 mg/kg/day dose was statistically significantly more effective than placebo (median change in mean seizures frequency −5.00 vs. −2.75 for placebo; $p < 0.05$). In the 100 mg/kg/day group, therapeutic success rate was 56 percent versus 31 percent for placebo ($p < 0.05$), and both caregiver and investigator evaluations showed more improvement in VGB patients than in placebo patients ($p < 0.05$). Adverse events occurred somewhat more frequently in the 100 mg/kg/day VGB group than placebo but were mostly mild or moderate in severity and did not result in patient withdrawal from the study (62).

Study 221 was a two-arm parallel trial with placebo and VGB administration in variable doses between 1.5 and 4.0 g/day, primarily dependent on body weight. The therapeutic success rate (defined as % of responders) was 50 percent with VGB and 27 percent with placebo ($p < 0.01$). Change in seizures-free days (number/28 days) was greater with VGB than placebo ($p < 0.01$), and caregiver evaluations showed improvement in significantly more patients receiving VGB than receiving placebo ($p < 0.05$) (62).

There are several further add-on, open-label studies of VGB in the treatment of uncontrolled epilepsies in children, the results of which have been published mostly as abstracts. A single-blind, dose-increasing study in 46 children with refractory partial seizures demonstrated a decrease of the average monthly seizure rate from 97 during placebo add-on to 21, 12, and 9 after 2, 4, and 6 months of VGB treatment, respectively (30). The study of Chiron and coworkers (63) was a randomized withdrawal study of placebo versus VGB in children who had responded earlier to VGB. In these studies, over 50 percent decreases in seizure frequency were observed in 40 percent to 64 percent of the children. There were no differences in efficacy between children with simple or complex partial seizures and children with secondarily generalized seizures. Ten percent to 40 percent of the children became seizure-free.

Long-term efficacy data of VGB treatment in children who have been followed up to 6 years have been published. The findings in one of these studies (follow-up 1.5–5.5 years) of a cohort of 196 children with drug-resistant epilepsy and VGB as add-on therapy were as follows (64):

- Increase of seizure frequency occurred in only 10 percent of patients, with half occurring during the first month of treatment. Patients with atypical absences had the highest incidence of increase in seizure frequency (38%) compared with less than 8 percent of those with partial seizures. Nonprogressive myoclonic epilepsy and Lennox-Gastaut syndrome (LGS) showed the greatest increase in seizure frequency, 38 percent and 29 percent, respectively.

- Loss of efficacy was reported in 12 mostly of children who were receiving VGB (25–50% of responders, some of whom had been seizure-free). Three-quarters of these patients had never had their seizures controlled before the introduction of VGB. Loss of efficacy was not connected to any specific seizure type except atypical absences and clonic seizures. The average time to reported loss of efficacy was 7 months. In 38 percent, the loss of efficacy was consecutive to an attempt to decrease concomitant antiepileptic medication.

- Eleven percent of the children developed new seizure types, mainly myoclonus and new partial seizures, after a quite variable time lag. Partial seizures were better tolerated than the initial seizure type and had little impact on the patient's overall clinical development.

The satisfying results obtained with VGB in children with drug-resistant epilepsy have prompted some investigators to use it as first-line therapy in partial epilepsy. Preliminary uncontrolled data show trends in favor of a disappearance of seizures in approximately 50 percent of patients, with similar reported side effects as in add-on therapy. However, no controlled study has been implemented so far to confirm these data. In addition, uncontrolled trials of VGB monotherapy after successful add-on effect have usually been disappointing (60,65).

Infantile Spasms (West Syndrome)

There are three controlled studies of VGB in infantile spasms (IS). Only one study was blinded; the other two studies were open-label. All studies used cessation of IS by caregiver observation as the primary efficacy endpoint. Initial doses of VGB varied between 50 and 150 mg/kg/day, but in all studies the dose was titrated up to 150 mg/kg/day.

In the blinded study in 40 children with newly diagnosed IS comparing VGB and placebo over 5 days (66), VGB showed only a slight and not statistically significant advantage over placebo using a 2-hour intensive monitoring period. However, using a 24-hour window based on observation of nursing staff or parents, VGB showed a large significant difference in seizure reduction. This difference was also supported by the investigator's overall assessment, which noted a marked or moderate improvement in 80 percent of VGB patients compared with 15 percent of placebo patients. Other efficacy measures (complete cessation of IS on the final treatment day and disappearance of hypsarrhythmia in the EEG) showed a trend toward advantage of VGB but did not reach statistical significance (66).

The second randomized, prospective study compared VGB (100–150 mg/kg/day) with adrenocorticotropic hormone (ACTH; 10 IU/day) as first-line therapy in 42 infants with IS (67). In nonresponders (within 20 days) or in case of intolerance to the initial therapy, the alternative drug was administered. Contrary to the other two studies, only 4 of 42 patients had symptomatic IS due to tuberous sclerosis, in which VGB has its best efficacy (45). Cessation of IS was observed in 48 percent (11 of 23) under VGB and 74 percent (14 of 19) under ACTH. The response to VGB was seen within 14 days. Follow-up data for up to 44 months showed only one relapse. In the ACTH group, in which treatment was stopped after 40 to 45 days and replaced with a benzodiazepine, six patients had a relapse.

The third prospective, randomized, multicenter monotherapy study in 22 newly diagnosed patients (63) with an optional crossover for nonresponders showed a highly significant difference between oral hydrocortisone (15 mg/kg/day) and VGB (150 mg/kg/day) both before and after crossover, with 100 percent (11 of 11) of patients on VGB but less than half (5 of 11) on hydrocortisone responding. All seven patients crossed from hydrocortisone to VGB (6 for inefficacy, 1 for adverse events) also became totally controlled. In addition, there was a statistically significant difference for the mean time to disappearance of IS favoring VGB (3.5 days vs. 13 days), and side effects were less common.

In addition to these controlled studies, there have been many reports on VGB treatment in newly diagnosed or refractory IS. Most of the reports have been published either as an abstract or as a letter to the editor, and they included different patient groups regarding symptomatic or cryptogenic etiology. In the fully published reports, the percentage of complete control of IS without relapse seemed to be comparable for newly diagnosed patients (68,69) and refractory patients (70,71).

In a retrospective survey, analyses were conducted of the safety and efficacy data from IS patients treated initially with VGB monotherapy at 59 European centers (72). The dose of VGB in the evaluable patients ranged from 20 to 400 mg/kg/day (mean dose, 99 mg/kg/day) and the duration of therapy ranged from 0.2 to 28.6 months. Complete disappearance of IS was reported in 131 of 192 (68%) patients. Treatment with VGB did not result in any improvement in 24 (12.5%) patients, and one patient deteriorated. Of the subgroups of IS types, patients with tuberous sclerosis had the highest response rate (27 of 28 = 97%), and VGB was least effective in patients with dysplasia (45%). Of the 131 patients who demonstrated a complete initial response to VGB, 28 (21.3%) relapsed.

A prospective U.S. study of VGB as initial therapy in newly diagnosed IS was designed as a randomized, open-label comparison of low-dose (18–36 mg/kg/day) and high-dose (up to 150 mg/kg/day) VGB. Preliminary efficacy data are available before a cut-off date of June 30, 1997, for 62 patients, 29 in the high-dose group and 33 in the low-dose group. In the first 2-week period of the study, 13 of 62 were free from IS by caregiver observation and EEG criteria. Five of 33 (15%) low-dose patients and 8 of 29 (28%) high-dose patients responded. The 62 patients were then also evaluated by caregiver report only (not to include EEG criteria). The total number of patients that were IS-free, including both new responders and continuing responders, was 5 of 61 (8%) at 2 weeks, 19 of 58 (33%) at 1 month, 20 of 47 (43%) at 2 months, and 26 of 43 (61%) at 3 months (52).

In an open-label, prospective, add-on study in 45 infants with refractory IS (range, 2 months–13 years of age, most (2 years) VGB was titrated up to 105 mg/kg/day and treatment duration was up to 23 months. Two patients discontinued the study prematurely due to adverse events and were not included in the efficacy evaluation. At the end of the initial evaluation phase (mean duration of therapy, 3.8 months), 20 of 43 (47%) patients included in the efficacy analysis were seizure-free. Of the 8 patients with tuberous sclerosis, 6 patients (75%) were seizure-free. Of the 33 patients with adequate response to VGB who were entered into a long-term phase, decreased frequency of IS was maintained in 22 patients (52).

The efficacy of a protocol using VGB as the first agent and ACTH or VPA as the second drug was studied in the patients with newly diagnosed IS in a population-based design. Only total disappearance of IS for a minimum duration of 1 month was accepted as treatment success, and the response was confirmed by video-EEG. Altogether 42 infants, 10 with cryptogenic and 32 with symptomatic etiology, were treated. Eleven patients (26%) responded to VGB, 5 patients (50%) with cryptogenic etiology and 6 patients (19%) with symptomatic etiology. Ninety-one percent of infants responded to a dose of 50 to 100 mg/kg/day and 82 percent of them within 1 week. ACTH was given in combination with VGB to 22 infants and VPA to 4 infants who failed VGB. Eleven patients responded to ACTH and one to VPA. In total, 26 (62%) infants responded to the treatment protocol; all (100%) with cryptogenic etiology and 16 (50%) with symptomatic etiology. ACTH treatment was associated with more severe side effects than VGB or VPA. Only one infant relapsed after a spasm-free period on VGB of more than 4 months but none after ACTH was combined to VGB (73).

Lennox-Gastaut Syndrome

Results have been controversial in the treatment of children with Lennox-Gastaut syndrome (LGS). In a first European add-on clinical study, 26 children with LGS were included. Good seizure response was observed in less than 30 percent of children (55). Only a small number of children with LGS were included in other studies, and most of them have not been regarded as treatment successes. A good response rate to VGB was observed in only one open study (74). Twenty children aged 2 to 20 years with refractory LGS were first treated with high-level VPA monotherapy and after that for 12 months with add-on VGB. Eighty-five percent experienced more than 50 percent seizure reduction and 40 percent became seizure-free. A decrease by at least 50 percent was observed in all seizure types (tonic, atonic, atypical absences, tonic-clonic, and complex partial seizures), except myoclonic seizures, which increased by 5 percent. VGB may therefore play a limited role as add-on treatment in the management of LGS but not in case of myoclonic seizures as the main seizure type.

The precipitation or exacerbation of myoclonic seizures, absence seizures, and nonconvulsive status have also been reported (75,76). Therefore, the prescription of VGB in idiopathic generalized epilepsies is not recommended and has been mentioned as a contraindication in some countries.

ADVERSE EVENTS

Side effects during VGB treatment are usually mild and well tolerated, even with high doses. In adults and older children fatigue, drowsiness, dizziness, nystagmus, agitation, amnesia, abnormal vision, ataxia, weight increase, confusion, depression, and diarrhea were most often reported (47). In children and infants receiving VGB, drowsiness, insomnia, hyperexcitability, hypotension, weight gain, and hypertonia or hypotonia were the most frequently reported adverse events

(40,59,77). A VGB-induced encephalopathy with stupor, confusion, and EEG slowing has been described (78,79). A fatal hepatotoxicity in a child treated with VGB (80) was later attributed most likely to an undetected metabolic disorder (81).

An adverse event possibly related to the GABA-ergic mechanism of action is an increased incidence of psychosis (82), sometimes as forced normalization. A retrospective survey of behavior disorders in 81 patients identified 50 patients meeting the criteria for either psychosis ($n = 28$) or depression ($n = 22$). A comparison with psychotic events in epilepsy patients never treated with VGB revealed an increased risk for more severe epilepsies, right-sided EEG focus, and suppression of seizures (83). A formal testing of mood disturbances in 73 adult patients with refractory epilepsy before and during treatment with VGB revealed that mood problems were the main reason for discontinuation (84). Repeated testing with a series of eight cognitive measures in a double-blind, placebo-controlled, parallel group, dose-response study in patients with difficult-to-control focal seizures detected a decreased performance in only one cognitive test (Digit Cancellation Test) (85).

A recent review of U.S. and non-U.S. double-blind, placebo-controlled trials of VGB as add-on therapy for refractory partial epilepsy in a total of 717 patients revealed a significantly higher incidence of depression and psychosis without differences between treatment groups for aggressive reactions, manic symptoms, agitation, emotional lability, anxiety, or suicide attempt (86). Depression and psychosis were usually observed during the first 3 months. Depression was usually mild, and psychosis was reported to respond to reduction or discontinuation of VGB or to treatment with neuroleptics.

As a secondary effect of treatment with VGB a significant increase of γ-aminoadipic acid in plasma and urine occurs, which may mimic γ-aminoadipic aciduria, a known rare metabolic disease. Therefore, when a genetic metabolic disease is suspected, amino acid chromatography should be performed before initiation of VGB treatment (87). In addition, VGB can interfere with urinary amino acid analysis because of inhibition of catabolism of beta-alanine (88).

In 1997 three patients with severe, symptomatic, persistent visual field defects (VFD) associated with the use of VGB were described (89). In the meantime, it has been demonstrated that VFD are a very common side effect of VGB, at least in adults, associated with retinal cone system dysfunction (90). The most important data for adult patients are from a randomized monotherapy trial in newly diagnosed patients comparing VGB and CBZ (91). Of 32 patients on long-term VGB monotherapy, 13 patients (40%) had concentric VFD. The main reason it took almost a decade to detect this neurotoxicity is that the vast majority of even severe defects are asymptomatic. Because VGB is often administered during different developmental stages at even higher doses (related to the body weight), and formal visual field testing in younger children and infants is difficult or impossible, the risk of VGB-induced VFD is a major challenge for pediatric patients with epilepsy. Whereas a recent placebo-controlled series found no VFD after 3 months of VGB treatment (92), case reports have confirmed at least the possibility of their occurrence in childhood (93). Regardless of age, an ophthalmologic examination is recommended before initiation of VGB and periodically thereafter.

In addition to the persistent VFDs, discrete nonhemorrhagic focal lesions in the splenium of the corpus callosum have been described in six patients with epilepsy treated with VGB and/or PHT. In two of the patients, the lesions disappeared on follow-up MRI after withdrawal of VGB and/or PHT (94).

CONCLUSIONS

Vigabatrin is an effective treatment in the management of children with a variety of uncontrolled epilepsies, mainly partial epilepsies with or without secondary generalization. The maintenance of VGB efficacy over time in most children, the low potential for exacerbation of seizures, the good tolerability and unproblematic use in association with other AEDs provide evidence of the therapeutic benefit of VGB in children, in whom a good control of the epilepsy is particularly important to minimize the negative impact of epilepsy on their learning and mental abilities.

Vigabatrin is indicated in combination with other AEDs for patients with drug-resistant partial epilepsy with or without secondary generalization, that is, where all other appropriate drug combinations have proven inadequate or have not been tolerated, and for monotherapy in the treatment of IS. Where available, VGB remains for the majority of child neurologists the drug of choice for the treatment of IS in spite of the high incidence of VFD. It has been argued that ACTH, one of the alternative drugs for IS, is more toxic than VGB and might not be approved by the FDA if it were reviewed now (95). Nevertheless, earlier risk-benefit assessments for VGB (96) have to be modified, and new guidelines for prescription are necessary (97).

REFERENCES

1. Bey P. Mechanism-based enzyme inhibitors as an approach to drug design. In: Palfreyman MG, McCann PP,

Lovenberg W, Temple JR Jr, Sjoedsma A, eds. *Enzymes as Targets for Drug Design*. San Diego: Academic Press, 1989:59–83.

2. Cereghino JJ. New antiepileptic drugs. In: Dodson WE, Pellock JM, eds. *Pediatric Epilepsy: Diagnosis and Therapy*. New York: Demos, 1993:343–355.

3. Krämer G, Schmidt D, eds. *Vigabatrin, Pharmakologie — Wirksamkeit — Verträglichkeit*. Berlin: Springer, 1994.

4. Ben-Menachem E. Vigabatrin. Chemistry, absorption, distribution, and elimination. In: Levy RH, Mattson RH, Meldrum BS, eds. *Antiepileptic Drugs*. 4th ed. New York: Lippincott-Raven, 1995:915–923.

5. Richens A. Pharmacology and clinical pharmacology of vigabatrin. *J Child Neurol* 1991; 6(Suppl 2):2S7–2S10.

6. Lewis P. Introduction. Vigabatrin: a new antiepileptic drug. *Br J Clin Neuropharmacol* 1989; 27(Suppl 1):1S.

7. Lippert B. Metcalf BW, Jung MJ, Casar P. 4-amino-hex-5-enoic acid, a selective catalytic inhibitor of 4-aminobutyric-acid aminotransferase in mammalian brain. *Eur J Biochem* 1977; 74:441–445.

8. Patsalos PN, Duncan JS. The pharmacology and pharmacokinetics of vigabatrin. *Rev Contemp Pharmacother* 1995; 6:447–456.

9. Jung MJ, Palfreyman MG. Vigabatrin. Mechanisms of action. In: Levy RH, Mattson RH, Meldrum BS, eds. *Antiepileptic Drugs*. 4th ed. New York: Raven Press, 1995:903–913.

10. Foletti GB, Delisle M-C, Bachmann C. Reduction of plasma alanine aminotransferase during vigabatrin treatment. *Epilepsia* 1995; 36:804–809.

11. Richens A, McEwan JR, Deybach JC, Mumford JP. Evidence for both in vivo and in vitro interaction between vigabatrin and alanine transaminase. *Br J Clin Pharmacol* 1997; 43:163–168.

12. Schechter PJ, Hanke NFJ, Grove J, Huebert N, Sjoerdsma A. Biochemical and clinical effects of *gamma*-vinyl GABA in patients with epilepsy. *Neurology* 1984; 34:182–186.

13. Mattson RH, Petroff O, Rothman D, Behar K. Vigabatrin: effects on human brain GABA levels by nuclear magnetic resonance spectroscopy. *Epilepsia* 1994; 35(Suppl 5):S29–S31.

14. Petroff OAC, Rothman DL, Behar RL, Mattson RH. Human brain GABA levels rise after initiation of vigabatrin therapy but fail to rise further with increasing dose. *Neurology* 1996; 46:1459–1463.

15. Petroff OAC, Hyder F, Collins T, Mattson RH, Rothman DL. Acute effects of vigabatrin on brain GABA and homocarnosine in patients with complex partial seizures. *Epilepsia* 1999; 40:958–964.

16. Frisk-Holmberg M, Kerth P, Meyer P. Effect of food on the absorption of vigabatrin. *Br J Clin Pharmacol* 1889; 27(Suppl):23S–25S.

17. Haegele KD, Schechter PJ. Kinetics of the enantiomers of vigabatrin after an oral dose of the racemate or the inactive S-enantiomer. *Clin Pharmacol Ther* 1986; 40:581–586.

18. Ben-Menachem E, Persson LI, Schechter PJ, et al. Effects of single doses of vigabatrin on CSF concentrations

of GABA, homocarnosine, homovanillic acid and 5-hydroxyindoleacetic acid in patients with complex partial epilepsy. *Epilepsy Res* 1988; 2:96–101.

19. Browne TR, Mattson TH, Penry JK, et al. Vigabatrin for refractory complex partial seizures: multicenter single-blind study with long-term follow-up. *Neurology* 1987; 37:184–189.

20. Bachmann D, Ritz R, Wad N, Haefeli E. Vigabatrin dosing during haemodialysis. *Seizure* 1996; 5:239–242.

21. Tran A, O'Mahoney T, Rey E, et al. Vigabatrin: placental transfer in vivo and excretion into breast milk of the enantiomers. *Br J Clin Pharmacol* 1998; 45:409–411.

22. Vauzelle-Kervroëdan F, Rey E, Pons G, et al. Pharmacokinetics of the individual enantiomers of vigabatrin in neonates with uncontrolled seizures. *Br J Clin Pharmacol* 1996; 42:779–781.

23. Rey E, Pons G, Richard MO, et al. Pharmacokinetics of the individual anantiomers of vigabatrin (gamma-vinyl-GABA) in epileptic children. *Br J Clin Pharmacol* 1990; 30:253–257.

24. Armijo JA, Arteaga R, Valdizán EM, Herranz JL. Coadministration of vigabatrin and valproate in children with refractory epilepsy. *Clin Neuropharmacol* 1992; 15:459–469.

25. Reidenberg P, Glue P, Banfield CR, et al. Pharmacokinetic interaction studies between felbamate and vigabatrin. *Br J Clin Pharmacol* 1995; 40:157–160.

26. Jedrzejczak J, Dtaivichowska E, Owczarek K, Majkowski K. Effect of vigabatrin addition on carbamazepine blood serum levels in patients with epilepsy. *Epilepsy Res* 2000; 49:115.

27. Sánchez-Alcarez A, Quintana B, Rodriguez I, López E. Plasma concentrations of vigabatrin in epileptic patients. *J Clin Pharm Ther* 1996; 21:393–398.

28. Gatti G, Bartoli A, Marchiselli R. Vigabatrin-induced decrease in phenytoin concentration does not involve a change in phenytoin bioavailability. *Br J Clin Pharmacol* 1993; 36:603–606.

29. Rimmer EM, Richens A. Interaction between vigabatrin and phenytoin. *Br J Clin Pharmacol* 1989; 27:27S–33S.

30. Dalla Bernadina B, Fontana E, Vigevano F, et al. Efficacy and tolerability of vigabatrin in children with refractory partial seizures: a single-blind dose-increasing study. *Epilepsia* 1995; 36:687–691.

31. Szylleyko OJ, Hoke JF, Eller MG, et al. A definitive study evaluating the pharmacokinetic of vigabatrin in patients with epilepsy. *Epilepsia* 1993; 34(Suppl 6):41–42.

32. Bartoli A, Gatti G, Cipolla G, et al. A double-blind, placebo-controlled study on the effect of vigabatrin on in vivo parameters of hepatic microsomal enzyme induction and on the kinetics of steroid oral contraceptives in healthy female volunteers. *Epilepsia* 1997; 38:702–707.

33. Krämer G. Pharmacokinetic interactions of new antiepileptic drugs. In: Stefan H, Krämer G, Mamoli B, eds. *Challenge Epilepsy — New Antiepileptic Drugs*. Berlin: Blackwell Science, 1998:87–103.

34. Rey E, Pons G, Olive G. Vigabatrin. Clinical pharmacokinetics. *Clin Pharmacokinet* 1992; 23:267–278.

35. Wad N, Krämer G. Sensitive high-performance liquid chromatographic method with fluorometric detection for the simultaneous determination of gabapentin and vigabatrin in serum and urine. *J Chromatography* 1998; 705:154–158.

36. Arteaga R, Herranz JL, Valdizan EM, Armilo JA. Gamma-vinyl-GABA (vigabatrin): relationship between dosage, plasma concentrations, platelet GABA-transaminase inhibition, and seizure reduction in children. *Epilepsia* 1992; 33:923–931.

37. Ben-Menachem E, French J. Vigabatrin. In: Engel J Jr, Pedley TA, eds. *Epilepsy. A Comprehensive Textbook.* Philadelphia: Lippincott-Raven, 1997:1609–1618.

38. Butler WH. The neuropathology of vigabatrin. *Epilepsia* 1989; 30(Suppl 3):S15–S17.

39. Cannon DJ, Buttler WH, Mumford JP, Lewis PJ. Neuropathologic findings in patients receiving long-term vigabatrin therapy for chronic intractable epilepsy. *J Child Neurol* 1991; 6(Suppl 2):2S17–2S24.

40. Fisher RS, Kerrigan JF III. Vigabatrin. Toxicity. In: Levy RH, Mattson RH, Meldrum BS, eds. *Antiepileptic Drugs.* 4th ed. New York: Raven Press, 1995:931–939.

41. Morrell MJ. The new antiepileptic drugs and women: efficacy, reproductive health, pregnancy, and fetal outcome. *Epilepsia* 1996; 37(Suppl 6):S34–S44.

42. Beran RG, Berkovic SF, Buchanan N, et al. A double-blind, placebo-controlled crossover study of vigabatrin 2 g/day and 3 g/day in uncontrolled partial seizures. *Seizure* 1996; 5:259–265.

43. Grant SM, Heel RC. Vigabatrin. A review of its pharmacodynamic and pharmacokinetic properties, and therapeutic potential in epilepsy. *Drugs* 1991; 41:889–926.

44. Ferrie CD, Panayiotopoulos CP. The clinical efficacy of vigabatrin in adults. *Rev Contemp Pharmacother* 1995; 6:457–468.

45. Ferrie CD, Robinson RO. The clinical efficacy of vigabatrin in children. *Rev Contemp Pharmacother* 1995; 6:469–476.

46. French JA, Mosier M, Walker S, Sommerville K, Sussmann N, and the Vigabatrin Protocol 024 Investigative Cohort. A double-blind, placebo-controlled study of vigabatrin three g/day in patients with uncontrolled complex partial seizures. *Neurology* 1996; 46:54–61.

47. Dean C, Mosier M, Penry K. Dose-response study of vigabatrin as add-on therapy in patients with uncontrolled complex partial seizures. *Epilepsia* 1999; 40:74–82.

48. Brodie MJ, Mumford JP, 012 study group. Double-blind substitution of vigabatrin and valproate in carbamazepine-resistant partial epilepsy. *Epilepsy Res* 1999; 34:199–205.

49. Kälviäinen R, Äikiä M, Saukkonen AM, Mervaala E, Riekkinen PJ Sr. Vigabatrin vs carbamazepine monotherapy in patients with newly diagnosed epilepsy. A randomized, controlled study. *Arch Neurol* 1995; 52:989–996.

50. Tanganelli P, Regesta G. Vigabatrin vs. carbamazepine monotherapy in newly diagnosed focal epilepsy: a randomized response conditional cross-over study. *Epilepsy Res* 1996; 25:257–262.

51. Chadwick D, for the Vigabatrin European Monotherapy Study Group. Safety and efficacy of vigabatrin and carbamazepine in newly diagnosed epilepsy: a multicentre randomised double-blind study. *Lancet* 1999; 354:13–19.

52. Zahner B, Stefan H, Blankenhorn V, et al. Once-daily versus twice-daily vigabatrin: is there a difference? The results of a double-blind pilot study. *Epilepsia* 1999; 40:311–315.

53. Michelucci R, Veri L, Passarelli D, et al. Long-term follow-up study of vigabatrin in the treatment of refractory epilepsy. *J Epilepsy* 1994; 7:88–93.

54. Livingston JH, Beaumont D, Arzimanoglou A, Aicardi J. Vigabatrin in the treatment of epilepsy in children. *Br J Clin Pharmacol* 1989; 27(Suppl 1):109–112.

55. Herranz JL, Arteaga R, Farr IN, et al. Dose-response study of vigabatrin in children with refractory epilepsy. *J Child Neurol* 1991; 6(Suppl 2):2S45–2S51.

56. Luna D, Dulac O, Pajot N, Beaumont D. Vigabatrin in the treatment of childhood epilepsies: a single-blind placebo-controlled study. *Epilepsia* 1989; 30:430–437.

57. Uldall P, Alving J, Gram L, Beck S. Vigabatrin in pediatric epilepsy—an open study. *J Child Neurol* 1991; 6(Suppl 2):2S38–2S44.

58. Dulac O, Chiron C, Luna C, et al. Vigabatrin in childhood epilepsy. *J Child Neurol* 1991; 6(Suppl 2):2S38–2S44.

59. Uldall P, Alving J, Gram L, Hogenhaven H. Vigabatrin in childhood epilepsy: a 5-year follow-up study. *Neuropediatrics* 1995; 26:253–256.

60. Baxter PS, Gardner-Medwin D, Barwick DD, et al. Vigabatrin monotherapy in resistant neonatal seizures. *Seizure* 1995; 4:57–59.

61. Buchanan N, Kearney B. Vigabatrin in Sturge-Weber syndrome. *Med J Aust* 1993; 158:652.

62. Aventis (formerly Hoechst Marion Roussel). Data on file, 1999.

63. Chiron C, Dumas C, Jambaqué I, Mumford J, Dulac O. Randomized trial comparing vigabatrin and hydrocortisone in infantile spasms due to tuberous sclerosis. *Epilepsy Res* 1997; 26:389–395.

64. Lortie A, Chiron C, Dumas C, Mumford JP, Dulac O. Optimizing the indication of vigabatrin in children with refractory epilepsy. *J Child Neurol* 1997; 12:253–259

65. Nabbout RC, Chiron C, Mumford J, Dumas C, Dulac O. Vigabatrin in partial seizures in children. *J Child Neurol* 1997; 12:172–177.

66. Appleton RE, Peters ACB, Mumford JP, Shaw DE. Randomised, placebo-controlled study of vigabatrin as first-line treatment of infantile spasms. *Epilepsia* 1999; 40:1627–1633.

67. Vigevano F, Cilio MR. Vigabatrin versus ACTH as first-line treatment for infantile spasms: a randomized, prospective study. *Epilepsia* 1997; 38:1270–1274.

68. Wohlrab G, Boltshauser E, Schmitt B. Vigabatrin as a first-line drug in West syndrome: clinical and electroencephalographic outcome. *Neuropediatrics* 998; 29:133–136.

69. Covanis A, Theodorou V, Lada C, Skiadas K, Loli N. The first-line use of vigabatrin to achieve complete control of seizures. *J Epilepsy* 1998; 11:265–269.

70. Chiron C, Dulac O, Beaumont D, et al. Therapeutic trial of vigabatrin in refractory infantile spasms. *J Child Neurol* 1991; 6(Suppl 2):2S52–2S59.

71. Siemes H, Brandl U, Spohr HL, Völger S, Weschke B. Long-term follow-up study of vigabatrin in pretreated children with West syndrome. *Seizure* 1998; 7:293–297.

72. Aicardi J, Sabril IS investigator and peer review groups, Mumford J, Dumas C, Wood S. Vigabatrin as initial therapy for infantile spasms: a European retrospective survey. *Epilepsia* 1996; 37:638–642.

73. Granström ML, Gaily E, Liukkonen E. Treatment of infantile spasms: results of a population-based study with vigabatrin as the first drug for spasms. *Epilepsia* 1999; 40:950–957.

74. Feucht M, Brantner-Inthaler S. γ-vinyl-GABA (vigabatrin) in the therapy of Lennox-Gastaut syndrome: an open study. *Epilepsia* 1994; 35:993–998.

75. Appleton RE. Vigabatrin in the management of generalized seizures in children. *Seizure* 1995; 4:45–48.

76. Vogt H, Krämer G. Vigabatrin und Lamotrigin. Erfahrungen mit zwei neuen Antiepileptika an der Schweizerischen Epilepsie-Klinik. *Schweiz Med Wochenschr* 1995; 125:125–132.

77. Gherpelli JLD, Guerreiro MM, da Costa JC, et al. Vigabatrin in refractory childhood epilepsy. The Brazilian multicenter study. *Epilepsy Res* 1997; 29:1–6.

78. Sälke-Kellermann A, Baier H, Rambeck B, Boenigk HE, Wolf P. Acute encephalopathy with vigabatrin. *Lancet* 1993; 342:185.

79. Sharif MK, Sander JWA, Shorvon SD. Acute encephalopathy with vigabatrin. *Lancet* 1993; 342:619.

80. Kellermann K, Soditt V, Rambeck B, Klinge O. Fatal hepatotoxicity in a child treated with vigabatrin. *Acta Neurol Scand* 1996; 93:380–381.

81. Kellermann K. Personal communication, 1999.

82. Sander JWAS, Hart YM, Trimble MR, Shorvon SD. Vigabatrin and psychosis. *J Neurol Neurosurg Psychiatry* 1991; 54:435–439.

83. Thomas L, Trimble M, Schmitz B, Ring H. Vigabatrin and behaviour disorders: a retrospective survey. *Epilepsy Res* 1996; 25:21–27.

84. Aldenkamp AP, Vermeulen J, Mulder OG, et al. γ-vinyl GABA (vigabatrin) and mood disturbances. *Epilepsia* 1994; 35:999–1004.

85. Dodrill CB, Arnett JL, Sommerville KW, Sussman NM. Effects of differing dosages of vigabatrin (Sabril) on cognitive abilities and quality of life in epilepsy. *Epilepsia* 1995; 36:164–173.

86. Levinson DF, Devinsky O. Psychiatric adverse events during vigabatrin therapy. *Neurology* 1999; 53:1503–1511.

87. Vallat C, Rivier F, Bellet H, et al. Treatment with vigabatrin may mimic γ-aminoadipic aciduria. *Epilepsia* 1996; 37:803–805.

88. Preece MA, Sewell IJ, Taylor JA, Green A. Vigabatrin-interference with urinary amino acid analysis. *Clin Chimica Acta* 1993; 218:113–116.

89. Eke T, Talbot JF, Lawdon MC. Severe persistent visual field constriction associated with vigabatrin. *Br Med J* 1997; 314:180–181.

90. Krauss GL, Johnson MA, Miller NR. Vigabatrin-associated retinal cone system dysfunction. Electroretinogram and ophthalmologic findings. *Neurology* 1998; 50:614–618.

91. Kalviäinen R, Nousiainen I, Mäntyjärvi M, et al. Vigabatrin, a gabaergic antiepileptic drug, causes concentric visual field defects. *Neurology* 1999; 53:922–926.

92. Duckett T, Brigell MG, Ruckh S. Electroretinographic changes are not associated with loss of visual function in pediatric epileptic patients following treatment with vigabatrin. *Invest Ophthalmol Vis Sci* 1998; 39(Suppl 4):S973.

93. Vanhatalo S, Pääkkönen L. Visual field constriction in children treated with vigabatrin. *Neurology* 1999; 52:1713–1714.

94. Kim SS, Chang K-H, Kim ST, et al. Focal lesion of the splenium of the corpus callosum in epileptic patients: antiepileptic drug toxicity? *Am J Neuroradiol* 1999; 20:125–129.

95. Sankar R, Wasterlain CG. Is the devil we know the lesser of the evils? Vigabatrin and visual fields. *Neurology* 1999; 52:1537–1538.

96. Srinivasan J, Richens A. A risk-benefit assessment of vigabatrin in the treatment of neurological disorders. *Drug Safety* 1994; 10:395–405.

97. Appleton RE. Guidelines may help in prescribing vigabatrin. *Br Med J* 1998; 317:1322.

CHAPTER 39

Zonisamide

Robert S. Fisher, M.D., Ph.D., John F. Kerrigan III, M.D., and John M. Pellock, M.D.

Zonisamide (ZNS; 1,2-benzisoxazole-3methanesulfonamide; AD-810, CI-912) is a derivative of the sulfonamide class (1,2), with a structural similarity to serotonin (3). ZNS exerts actions on ion channels, blocking sodium channel recovery (4), blocking T-type calcium current (5,6), and binding to a chloride channel associated with the gamma-aminobutyric acids (GABA) receptor (7). ZNS has mild carbonic anhydrase activity, but that probably is not a major mechanism of its action (8).

Shimizu has reviewed the actions of ZNS in animal models of the epilepsies (9). ZNS has good efficacy against maximal electroshock (MES) seizures and weaker efficacy against pentylenetetrazol (PTZ) (13) and 4-aminopyridine (11) seizures. Seizures produced by focal tungstic acid (12) and conjugated estrogens in cat thalamus (12) respond to ZNS.

Zonisamide is absorbed well when taken orally (12). Delivery of ZNS can also be accomplished by rectal suppository (10). Therapeutic serum levels are not firmly established, but clinical studies have found efficacy in the range of 10 to 40 mg/L (1,13,14). ZNS is about 50 percent bound to plasma proteins (15). Metabolism of ZNS is principally hepatic, with renal excretion (16). Half-life in monotherapy is 24 to 60 hours (17) and is shorter in the presence of medications that induce the cytochrome P-450 system. ZNS is metabolized by the cytochrome P-450 3A4 system (18). Inducers of this system, such as phenytoin, carbamazepine, and phenobarbital, therefore lower serum levels of ZNS (19,20). ZNS itself has no effect on metabolism of phenytoin, carbamazepine, or valproic acid (18), but it inhibits metabolism of carbamazepine to its epoxide (20).

Zonisamide originated in Japan (21), but early pilot studies were accomplished in the United States by Sackellares and coworkers (22) and Wilensky and associates (14). Although these pilot studies consisted of only 18 adult patients, they suggest effectiveness against partial seizures at doses of 5 to 12.5 mg/kg/day. These findings were confirmed by studies in South Korea and Japan (23). A multicenter, randomized study (24) was initiated in the United States but was stopped when 11 patients of 152 enrolled in the trial developed renal stones. Studies continued in Europe (25) and Japan (26), with infrequent emergence of renal stones.

In the U.S. study 152 patients received ZNS or placebo as add-on therapy for 12 weeks. Seizures were reduced a mean of 30 percent, and approximately 30 percent of patients were "responders" with at least a 50 percent seizure reduction compared to baseline. The European ZNS multicenter study (25) enrolled 139 patients and found similar success rates. Two randomized studies of patients with intractable partial seizures in Japan (2) compared ZNS with carbamazepine for a 12-week course ($n = 123$), and with valproic acid ($n = 32$ children less than age 15) for an 8-week course. In each of these studies ZNS showed efficacy equivalent to the older drug.

Zonisamide appears to be effective for a broad spectrum of seizure types, including primarily generalized seizures (23), absence seizures (27), infantile spasms (28), and myoclonic seizures (29). Response in myoclonic seizures associated with Baltic myoclonus (syndrome of Unverricht and Lundborg) can sometimes be dramatic (29). A summary of the efficacy in the Japanese experience is noted in Table 39-1 (30).

Zonisamide is usually well tolerated. Among 1,008 patients enrolled in phase II and III trials in Japan, 51 percent reported adverse events and 18 percent withdrew because of them (2). Among 55 patients receiving ZNS monotherapy, the most common complaints were drowsiness (9%), loss of appetite (7%), gastrointestinal (GI) symptoms (7%), weight loss (6%), decreased spontaneity (6%), headache (6%), and rash (6%). In the European trial, 59 percent of patients receiving ZNS

Table 39-1. Seizure Improvement Rate Among Patients Classified by Seizure Type

Seizure Type (n)	% Patients				
	Seizure-Free	Markedly Improved	Improved	No change	Worse
Partial (1172)	43.4	10	17.1	23.5	6
Tonic-clonic (122)	42.6	11.5	13.9	28.7	3.3
Tonic (128)	18.8	7	17.2	43.8	13.3
Clonic (24)	62.5	0	12.5	20.8	4.2
Atonic (37)	24.3	13.5	18.9	32.4	10.8
Myoclonic (56)	19.6	14.3	17.9	46.4	1.8
Typical absence (8)	50	12.5	25	12.5	0
Atypical absence (54)	14.8	5.6	25.9	51.9	1.9
Other (30)	16.7	13.3	13.3	43.3	13.3
Total (1631)	39	9.9	17.1	27.7	6.3

Source: Yamauchi T, Efficacy of Zonisamide ... our experience. *Epilepsia* 1999 (in press).

and 28 percent of those receiving placebo reported adverse effects (25). ZNS can reduce sweating and hyperthermia (31) and suppress immunoglobulin synthesis (32). A few children taking ZNS have developed behavioral disturbance (33) or mania (34). Approximately 2 percent of patients receiving ZNS, almost all on polypharmacy, experienced episodes of psychosis (35). The symptoms usually appeared from several days to several months after starting or incrementing ZNS. In the U.S. multicenter study, 14 percent in the ZNS group and 1 percent in the placebo group discontinued treatment because of side effects. Renal stones, composed of calcium oxalate or calcium citrate, occurred in about 2 percent of participants in the U.S. and European multicenter trials. The majority of these patients had a history of renal stones or urinary tract manipulations (1). Incidence of stones in Japanese patients has been much lower, in the range of 0.2 percent (36), perhaps because of differences in genetic predisposition, or diet.

A recent study including 928 children and 584 adults (age 1 month–79 years) with localization-related and generalized epilepsy found that 31.5 percent reported at least one adverse event. Adverse events occurred in 21 percent of patients treated with monotherapy versus 35.6 percent using polypharmacy. The rate of reported side effects in children was lower, both for monotherapy and polypharmacy, being 18.9 percent in children versus 29.4 percent in adults for monotherapy and 30.4 percent in children versus 419 percent in adults for polypharmacy. The total incidence of adverse effects overall was lower in children at 26.2 percent versus adults at 39.9 percent. Side effects included psychiatric symptoms (19.38%), GI symptoms (8.73%), central and peripheral neurologic symptoms (5.82%), hepatic dysfunction (2.38%), skin lesions (2.18%), and visual disturbances (1.42%). It was thought that toxicity qualitatively particular to ZNS included impairment of higher mental function, motivation, or volition, and

hypohidrosis among the skin symptoms. Calculi in the urinary tract were detected in only two patients (0.13%) (37). Of particular interest to those treating children is a condition of hypohidrosis in which decreased sweating is associated with fever and frequently occurs in the summer. This symptom appears to be confined to children, particularly infants, and severely handicapped individuals. The functional suppression of sweat glands by ZNS is believed to be the mechanism behind this adverse effect (37).

Early trials of ZNS used doses in excess of 8 mg/kg/day, but this is now considered too high for most adults. The incidence of cognitive problems rises at high doses or serum levels above 30 mg/L. (38). To minimize problems, ZNS should be started at no more than 100 mg/day and increased by 100 mg every 1 to 3 weeks up to approximately 200 to 400 mg or 4 to 8 mg/kg/day (39). The drug usually is administered in a single daily dose. Seino and Ito (2) recommend a maximum dose of 600 mg/day for adults and 12 mg/kg/day for children.

Dosing in children appears to be best tolerated when ZNS is initiated at approximately 1 to 2 mg/kg/day and gradually increased to 8 mg/kg/day in increments of 1 to 2 mg/kg/day every 2 weeks. Adjustments are made dependent on the efficacy and observed adverse effects to a maximum of 12 mg/kg/day (40). At the maintenance dose of 8 mg/kg/day, blood levels of 27.0 ± 9.4 mcg/mL, at the trough state, with only minor differences from peak to trough levels (41). When carbamazepine was combined with ZNS, plasma levels decreased from 35.4 ± 10 mcg/mL to 22.2 ± 9.8 mcg/mL, whereas plasma levels of carbamazepine and its 10–11 epoxide were unaffected. As with all new antiepileptic drugs (AEDs), the risk of teratogenicity from ZNS is not known. However, a preliminary study by Kondo and coworkers (42) followed up a cohort of women who gave birth to 26 offspring from 1989 to 1994. Malformations occurred in two babies — one with anencephaly and one with an atrial septal defect. This 7 percent incidence is similar to that associated with other AEDs.

Zonisamide is one of the few new drugs to have been specifically evaluated in the pediatric population. In one unblinded study of 65 children with refractory partial or generalized epilepsies (2), 91 percent of the children responded with at least a 50 percent reduction in seizures. Oguni and colleagues (43) randomized 32 children to add either ZNS or valproic acid (VPA) to their regimen of AEDs. All children had an average of more than four various types of seizures per month. Generalized tonic-clonic seizures were reduced a mean of 81 percent for ZNS and 67 percent for VPA compared to baseline. Three of 10 children with Lennox-Gastaut syndrome responded with nearly complete seizure control when given ZNS (44). The overall impact of ZNS monotherapy on pediatric epilepsy was assessed in 77 children aged 8 months to 15 years; 82 percent became seizure-free with cryptogenic or symptomatic partial epilepsy. Of 11 patients with cryptogenic and symptomatic generalized epilepsy, 91 percent (10 patients) became seizure-free and the remaining patient experienced no change. Efficacy in the treatment of encephalopathic epilepsy and infantile spasms has been less robust (40,45).

Recent randomized, multicenter trials in the United States have been reported (46). A cohort of 203 patients with intractable partial epilepsy were given either placebo, ZNS 100 mg/day, or 200 mg/day in addition to their stable regimen of baseline AEDs for 5 weeks. At week 7, both ZNS groups were increased to 400 mg/day. At week 12, placebo patients were crossed over to ZNS. Median seizure frequencies for the ZNS and placebo groups, respectively, were 100 mg (25% vs. 8.3%), 200 mg (20% vs. 4%), and week 12 cohort (41% vs. 9%). The conclusion was that 100- and 200-mg doses of ZNS showed some efficacy, but efficacy was better at 400 mg/day. ZNS is registered in Japan and South Korea. U.S. pivotal trials have been accomplished, and the drug has been approved by regulatory authorities.

CONCLUSION

Zonisamide has proven a useful drug in the treatment of partial and generalized epilepsy in both children and adults. The drug may be particularly effective in patients with syndrome of progressive myoclonus. A syndrome of hypohidrosis and hyperthermia has been reported rarely in young children and mentally retarded individuals. Reports suggest, however, that it is fairly well tolerated in most patients. Its eventual use still needs to be defined.

REFERENCES

1. Seino M, Naurto S, Ito T, Miyazaki H. Other antiepileptic drugs: zonisamide. In: Levy RH, Mattson RH, Meldrum BD, eds. *Antiepileptic Drugs.* 4th ed. New York: Raven Press, 1995:1011–1023.

2. Sino M, Ito T. Zonisamide. In: Engel J Jr, Pedley TA, eds. *Epilepsy: A Comprehensive Textbook.* Philadelphia: Lippincott-Raven, 1997:1619–1626.

3. Seino M, Miyazaki H, Ito T. Zonisamide. *Epilepsy Res* 1991; 3(Suppl):169–174.

4. Rock DM, Macdonald RL, Taylor CP. Blockade of sustained repetitive action potentials in cultured spinal cord neurons by zonisamide (AD 810, CI 912), a novel anticonvulsant. *Epilepsy Res* 1989; 3:138–143.

5. Kito M, Maehara M, Watanabe K. Mechanisms of T-type calcium channel blockade by zonisamide. *Seizure* 1996; 5:115–119.

6. Suzuki S, Kawakami K, Nishimura S, et al. Zonisamide blocks T-type calcium channel in cultured neurons of rat cerebral cortex. *Epilepsy Res* 1992; 21:21–37.

7. Mimaki T, Tanoue H, Matsunaga Y, Miyazaki H, Mino M. Regional distribution of 14C- zonisamide in rat brain. *Epilepsy Res* 1994; 17:233–236.

8. Masuda Y, Noguchi H, Karasawa T. Evidence against a significant implication of carbonic anhydrase inhibitory activity of zonisamide in its anticonvulsive effects. *Arzneimittel-Forschung* 1994; 44:267–269.

9. Shimizu M, Uno H, Ito T, Masuda Y, Kurokawa M. [Research and development of zonisamide, a new type of antiepileptic drug]. *Yakugaku Zasshi* 1996; 116:533–547.

10. Yamaguchi S, Rogawski MA. Effects of anticonvulsant drugs on 4-aminopyridine-induced seizures in mice. *Epilepsy Res* 1992; 11:9–16.

11. Ito T, Hori M, Kadokawa T. Effects of zonisamide (AD-810) on tungstic acid gel-induced thalamic generalized seizures and conjugated estrogen-induced cortical spike-wave discharges in cats. *Epilepsia* 1986; 27:367–374.

12. Peters DH, Sorkin EM. Zonisamide. A review of its pharmacodynamic and pharmacokinetic properties, and therapeutic potential in epilepsy. *Drugs* 1993; 45:760–787.

13. Nagatomi A, Mishima M, Tsuzuki O, Ohdo S, Higuchi S. Utility of a rectal suppository containing the antiepileptic drug zonisamide. *Biol Pharm Bull* 1997; 20:892–896.

14. Wilensky AJ, Friel PN, Ojemann LM, et al. Zonisamide in epilepsy: a pilot study. *Epilepsia* 1985; 26:212–220.

15. Perucca E, Bailer M. The clinical pharmacokinetics of the newer antiepileptic drugs. Focus on topiramate, zonisamide and tiagabine. *Clin Pharmacokinet* 1996; 31:29–46.

16. Stiff DD, Robicheau JT, Zemaitis MA. Reductive metabolism of the anticonvulsant agent zonisamide, a 1,2-benzisoxazole derivative. *Xenobiotica* 1992; 22:1–11.

17. Hammond EJ, Perchalski RJ, Wilder BJ, McLean JR. Neuropharmacology of zonisamide, a new antiepileptic drug. *Gen Pharmacol* 1987; 18:303–307.

18. Buchanan RA, Page JG, French JA, Leppik IE, Padgett CS. Zonisamide drug interactions. *Epilepsia* 1997; **VOL:** 38–107.

19. Ojemann LM, Shastri RA, Wilensky AJ, et al. Comparative pharmacokinetics of zonisamide (CI-912) in epileptic patients on carbamazepine or phenytoin monotherapy. *Ther Drug Mon* 1986; 8:293–296.

20. Shinoda M, Akita M, Hasegawa T, Nabeshima T. The necessity of adjusting the dosage of zonisamide when coadministered with other anti-epileptic drugs. *Biol Pharm Bull* 1996; 19:1090–1092.

21. Uno H, Kurokawa M, Natsuka K, Yamato Y, Nishimura H. Studies on 3-substituted 1,2 -benzisoxazole derivatives. 1. *Chem Pharm Bull* 1976; 24:632–643.

22. Sackellares JC, Donofrio PD, Wagner JG, Abou-Khalil B, Berent S. Pilot study of zonisamide (1,2-benzisoxazole-3-methanesulfonamide) in patients with refractory partial seizures. *Epilepsia* 1985; 26:206–211.

23. Kumagai N, Seki T, Yamawaki H, et al. Monotherapy for childhood epilepsies with zonisamide. *Japan J Psychiatry Neurol* 1991; 45:357–359.

24. Leppik IE, Willmore LJ, Homan RW, et al. Efficacy and safety of zonisamide: results of a multicenter study. *Epilepsy Res* 1993; 14:165–173.

25. Schmidt D, Jacob R, Loiseau P, et al. Zonisamide for add-on treatment of refractory partial epilepsy: a European double-blind trial. *Epilepsy Res* 1993; 15:67–73.

26. Shimizu A, Ikoma R, Shimizu T. Effects and side effects of zonisamide during long-term medication. *Curr Ther Res* 1998; 47:696–706.

27. Kotani H, Hirai K, Nishiki T, et al. Zonisamide monotherapy against absence attacks: report of two cases. *No to Hattatsu* 1994; 26:349–354.

28. Kamei A, Ichinohe S, Ito M, Fujowara T. A case of infantile spasms: epileptic apnea as partial seizures at onset. *Brain Dev* 1996; 18:239–241.

29. Henry TR, Leppik IE, Gumnit RJ, Jacobs M. Progressive myoclonus epilepsy treated with zonisamide. *Neurology* 1988; 38:928–931.

30. Yamauchi T, Efficacy of zonisamide . . . our experience. *Epilepsia* 1999 (in press).

31. Shimizu T, Yamashita Y, Satoi M, et al. Heat stroke-like episode in a child caused by zonisamide. *Brain Dev* 1997; 19:366–368.

32. Maeoka Y, Hara T, Dejima S, Takeshita K. IgA and IgG2 deficiency associated with zonisamide therapy: a case report. *Epilepsia* 1997; 38:611–613.

33. Kimura S. Zonisamide-induced behavior disorder in two children. *Epilepsia* 1994; 35:403–405.

34. Charles CL, Stoesz L, Tollefson G. Zonisamide-induced mania. *Psychosomatics* 1990; 31:214–217.

35. Matsuura M, Trimble MR. Zonisamide and psychosis. *J Epilepsy* 1997; 10:52–54.

36. Yagi K, Seino M. Methodological requirements for clinical trials in refractory epilepsies — our experience with zonisamide. *Prog Neuropsychopharmacol Biol Psychiatry* 1992; 16:79–95.

37. Ohtahara — Safety of zonisamide therapy: prospective follow up survey.

38. Berent S, Sackellares JC, Giordani B, et al. Zonisamide (CI-912) and cognition: results from preliminary study. *Epilepsia* 1987; 28:61–67.

39. Wilder BJ, French JA, Ramsey ER, Bergen DC, Padgett CS. Zonisamide introduction and tolerance. *Epilepsia* 1997; **VOL:** 38–108.

40. Seki T, Kumagai N, Maezawa M: Effects of zonisamide monotherapy on epileptic children.

41. Miura H. Zonisamide monotherapy with once daily dosing in children with cryptogenic localization related epilepsy: clinical effects and pharmacokinetic studies.

42. Kondo T, Kaneko S, Amano Y, Egawa I. Preliminary report on teratogenic effects of zonisamide in the offspring of treated women with epilepsy. *Epilepsia* 1996; 37:1242–1244.

43. Oguni H, Hayashi K, Fukuyama Y. Phase III study of a new antiepileptic, AD-810, zonisamide in childhood epilepsy. *Jpn J Pediatr* 1988; 41:439–450.

44. Yamatogi Y, Ohtahara S. Current topics of treatment. In: Ohtahara S, Roget J, eds. *Proceedings of the International Symposium. New Trends in Pediatric Epileptology.* 1990;:136–148.

45. Iinuma K. Clinical efficacy of zonisamide in childhood epilepsy after long-term treatment — a post marketing multi institutional survey 46.

46. Padgett CS, Ayala R, Montouris GD, Ascher S, Buchanan RA. Zonisamide efficacy and dose response. *Epilepsia* 1997; 38:107.

CHAPTER 40

Other New Antiepileptic Drugs

Robert S. Fisher, M.D., Ph.D., and John F. Kerrigan III, M.D.

A distressing irony of epilepsy, which is one of the most prevalent neurologic disorders in children, is that it is treated by medications that are predominantly designed for and tested in adults. Nevertheless, the introduction of new antiepileptic medications provides opportunities for therapy in the pediatric population. No antiepileptic drug (AED) to date has been used exclusively in adults, and none probably will ever be excluded in practice from use for children.

Antiepileptic drug therapy has developed a long way from the era of treatment with hippopotamus testicles, crocodile feces, plasters of pigeon dung, and blood from a recently stabbed gladiator (1). Table 40-1 illustrates one representation of the eras of AED development.

The initial era may be considered the time of "wrong theory." In this era bromides were introduced under the mistaken theory that epilepsy resulted from excess sexual drive (2). Salts of bromide did turn out to be effective and have been used until recent years as medications of last resort. The introduction of phenobarbital

Table 40-1. Antiepileptic Drug Eras

Decade	Era	Mechanism	Example
1850	Wrong theory	Reduced sex drive	Bromides
1910	Serendipity	Sedatives	Phenobarbital
1930	Imitation	Barbiturates	Primidone
1940	Screening	MES	Phenytoin
		PTZ	Ethosuximide
		Other models	
1990	Physiochemistry	GABA	Tiagabine, vigabatrin
		Glutamate	Remacemide
		Channels	Several
2000	Genetics	Replace gene product	?
		Repair gene	

in 1912 ushered in the era of serendipity. Phenobarbital was introduced as a sleeping medication but was found to be an effective antiseizure medication. Following this discovery was the era of imitation, in which barbiturates and other drugs based on the barbiturate formula were tried as antiepileptic medications. In 1938 Merritt and Putnam (3) introduced phenytoin, the first nonsedating antiepileptic medication. Phenytoin was also the first drug developed by systematic screening of compounds from industry and academia in laboratory models of the epilepsies. Two important more recent drugs, carbamazepine and valproic acid, were developed by "informed serendipity," a marker of the earlier era. Carbamazepine is related to the tricyclic medications and was used by people suffering from depression. Some of these depressed individuals also had chronic pain syndromes, such as trigeminal neuralgia, for which carbamazepine was effective. Reasoning that trigeminal neuralgia was a type of "seizure" (or at least uncontrolled rapid neuronal firing) in the trigeminal ganglion, carbamazepine was evaluated in other types of seizures. Valproic acid (propyl acetic acid) was a solvent used to dissolve a variety of test compounds. All compounds dissolved in the propyl acetic acid had antiepileptic activity, an unlikely circumstance. The solvent itself was found to be the effective medication.

After the introduction of valproic acid in the United States in 1978, no additional major new categories of medications were released for 15 years. Since that time we have been engaged in an era of designing antiepileptic medications by physiochemistry. This strategy requires an understanding of the function of ion channels and neurotransmitters in networks of the brain (4). Gabapentin, tiagabine, and vigabatrin enhance the function of the inhibitory neurotransmitter gamma-aminobutyric acid (GABA). Lamotrigine, among other mechanisms, inhibits release of the excitatory amino acid transmitter glutamate. Felbamate and several of the older medications such as phenytoin and carbamazepine inhibit activity-dependent sodium channels and therefore suppress excessive neuronal firing.

Future generations of medications are likely to arise during the era of genetics. Advances in molecular biology will allow us to identify genetic flaws that predispose one to epileptic seizures. Particular progress has been made in understanding molecular defects in the hereditary epilepsies. As an example, in some forms of autosomal dominant nocturnal frontal lobe epilepsy, the defective gene (the gene encoding the α4 subunit of the neuronal nicotinic acetylcholine receptor) contains a single base pair substitution, resulting in the change of an amino acid residue within a critical domain of the ion channel. The altered conduction properties of this ion channel act to lower the seizure threshold, resulting in epilepsy for those who inherit the gene (5). With this type of knowledge, we can potentially design medications to counteract these disorders and perhaps eventually to replace the defective gene with a functional gene. When we have accomplished these tasks, we will have created true antiepileptic treatments instead of misnamed "antiepileptic" medications that do not affect the process of epilepsy but only suppress seizures.

The rapid pace of new drug development is evident from reviewing this chapter by James Cereghino (6) in the previous edition of this book. Among the new drugs not yet on the market mentioned in the 1993 chapter, felbamate, gabapentin, lamotrigine, topiramate, and zonisamide are on the market at the time of this writing. These new medications are useful because they offer something else to try that may be effective in individuals whose seizures are not controlled by any existing medications, and because the side-effect profile of the new medications is in many cases superior to that of older medications (7). It is, nonetheless, clear that the ideal antiepileptic medication has not yet been invented, so the search continues for better medications. This need remains substantial. Approximately 1 percent of children will develop epilepsy. If we assume that approximately 65 percent of this group is adequately controlled with existing medications, the number of uncontrolled patients is still larger than the sum total of those with brain tumors, muscular dystrophies, neurodegenerative disorders, and many other serious neurologic illnesses of childhood.

Several recent texts (8–11) and articles (12–19) have reviewed the subject of new AEDs. In the following section, we consider a few of the drugs that are not discussed elsewhere in this volume that may have future applicability to the treatment of children with epilepsy: ganaxolone, loreclezole, losigamone, ralitoline, remacemide, rufinamide, and stiripentol. We also discuss levetiracetam, which has recently been approved for use in the U.S. market, specifically as adjunctive therapy for adult patients with partial onset seizures. Several other medications are in very early stages of investigation and are deferred for future reviews.

For most of these medications, the investigational experience demonstrating safety and effectiveness in children is very limited. For several of these medications, drug trials are currently under way in children, including populations that are of particular importance in pediatric epilepsy, such as those with infantile spasms and Lennox-Gastaut syndrome. The willingness of the pharmaceutical industry to conduct controlled trials of new drugs for children with epilepsy should be supported. The cooperation of parents who enroll their children in investigational trials, accepting the uncertainty that comes with such studies, must also be acknowledged and respected.

GANAXOLONE

Ganaxolone (GNX: 3alpha-hydroxy-3beta-methyl-5alpha-pregnan-20-one) is a novel neuroactive steroid, in a new class of drugs called epalons, which was under development by CoCensys, Inc. It was developed as a synthetic analogue of progesterone metabolites after these naturally occurring metabolites were found to have activity against seizures (20). It has been found to have any glucocorticoid, mineralocorticoid, or sex steroid activity and consequently does not appear to have side effects in these areas. Ganaxolone is a positive allosteric modulator of the GABA$_A$ receptor, binding specifically to a novel neurosteroid binding site, distinct from the benzodiazepine binding site (21). It acts by potentiating the effect of GABA as GABA binds to its receptor-ionophore complex. Animal studies have shown that GNX is effective against pentylenetetrazol (PTZ), bicuculline, and kindled seizures but minimally effective against maximal electroshock seizures (MES) (21,22). Like several other GABA-related agents, GNX may exacerbate seizures in animal models of absence epilepsy (23).

Early clinical work with GNX in 96 adult volunteers was reported by Monaghan and colleagues (24). Insoluble in water, GNX therefore is administered as a complex with 2-hydroxypropyl-β-cyclodextrin to facilitate oral absorption. Single doses of 50 to 1500 mg were well tolerated. Serum half-life ranged from 18 to 28 hours with single dosing but increased to a terminal half-life of 40 to 65 hours with multiple dosing. In open-label studies with daily doses up to 1500 mg, GNX produced only occasional instances of mild gastrointesinal (GI) upset, light-headedness, tiredness, somnolence, and headache.

Several clinical studies have now been presented in abstract form. GNX has been studied as monotherapy in adult patients with intractable partial epilepsy who are hospitalized for presurgical evaluation. After withdrawal of other AEDs, patients were randomized to either placebo or GNX at 1875 mg/day. Preliminary data demonstrate a trend toward efficacy in prevention of reaching the exit criteria of four complex partial seizures (or three secondarily generalized seizures) (25).

An open-label pilot study has been conducted in children and adolescents (ages 5–15 years), with poorly controlled seizures, either partial or generalized. Ganaxolone was given in doses up to 36 mg/kg/day with other preexisting AEDs. No serious adverse events were reported. Mild to moderate adverse events included somnolence, sleep disturbance, nervousness, constipation, and change in seizure type. Six of 15 patients (40%) showed at least a 50 percent improvement in seizure frequency (26).

An open-label study has also been conducted in children with intractable seizures and a history of infantile spasms. GNX was given in doses up to 36 mg/kg/day in addition to preexisting AEDs. Of the 16 patients completing the study, 15 had infantile spasms that were resistant to conventional therapy at the time of enrollment. In this open-label study, 5 of 15 patients (33%) had at least a 50 percent improvement in spasm frequency, and an additional 5 patients (33%) experienced some improvement (25–50% reduction in spasm frequency). GNX was well tolerated, and no patient withdrew from the study because of medication side effects (27).

LEVETIRACETAM

Levetiracetam (LEV, ucb LO59, [S]-a-ethyl-2-oxopyrrolidine acetamide) is a new AED chemically related to the nootropic (cognition-enhancing) agent piracetam. In high doses, piracetam suppresses myoclonic jerks (28); therefore, similar drugs were evaluated for efficacy against seizures. Levetiracetam was developed by UCB S.A. Pharma Sector, Chemin du Foriest, Braine-I'Alleud, Belgium, and Smyrna, Georgia. The mechanism of action of LEV remains uncertain. It has little effect on global brain GABA levels or the activity of glutamic acid decarboxylase (GAD) or GABA transaminase (GABA-T) (29). However, a novel brain binding site for Levetiracetam (30) may affect GABA turnover in key regions of the brain, such as the substantia nigra (31).

Levetiracetam suppresses seizures and EEG spike-wave activity in genetically prone animal models for audiogenic and absence seizures with a wide therapeutic margin (32). In contrast, piracetam showed little beneficial effect in these models. Levetiracetam is also useful in the tetanus toxin model of subacute hippocampal seizures (33) and in the prevention of development of kindled seizures (34).

Levetiracetam is well absorbed orally and achieves peak levels within an hour. Approximately 50 percent of the drug is excreted unchanged in the urine, and serum half-life is 4 to 11 hours (35,36). Levetiracetam may increase serum levels of concurrently administered phenytoin, phenobarbital, valproate, primidone, or clobazam, but not carbamazepine (36).

Levetiracetam underwent pilot studies in Europe with 29 adult patients receiving four ascending dose levels of LEV in the range of 1000 to 4000 mg/day. The French arm was open-label; the British arm was single-blinded. At 1000 mg/day, 5 patients became seizure-free for the 4-week trial. At 4000 mg/day, 7 of 27 patients became seizure-free. The responder rate for at least 50 percent seizure reduction compared with baseline was 60 percent. Adverse events, consisting mainly of somnolence and fatigue were dose-related (37,38). Single 750- to 1000-mg doses of LEV significantly reduced photoparoxysmal EEG responses in 9 of 12 patients with photosensitivity (35).

The results of a multicenter, randomized, placebo-controlled trial of LEV have recently been published (38a). Adult patients (age range 16–70 years) with poorly controlled partial seizures were randomized to either placebo, LEV 1000 mg/day, or LEV 3000 mg/day as add-on therapy, after a baseline period. The responder rate (at least 50% improvement in seizure frequency) was 10.8 percent for placebo, 33.0 percent for patients treated with LEV 1000 mg/day, and 39.8 percent for those treated with LEV 3000 mg/day. Complete cessation of seizures during the 14-week treatment period was seen in 5.5 percent of the LEV-treated patients and in none of the controls. Side effects more likely to occur in the LEV groups included dizziness, fatigue, headaches, upper respiratory tract infections, and somnolence. Most of these treatment-emergent adverse events were rated as mild to moderate.

The preliminary adverse-event profile for LEV raises the hope that it may spare patients some of the cognitive problems so common with other old and new AEDs (39). LEV appears to have a beneficial impact on epilepsy-related quality of life when used an add-on therapy in a short-term study (40). Not surprisingly, patients with improved seizure control reported more robust improvement in the quality of life scales.

Limited information is available with respect to the use of LEV in children. Body clearance of the drug appears to be somewhat more rapid in children as compared with adults (40a). A multicenter, open-label, pilot trail of LEV in 23 children with poorly controlled partial onset seizures, added to preexisting monotherapy, determined that 12 children (52%) had at least a 50 percent reduction in seizure frequency (40b). A multicenter, randomized, placebo-controlled, add-on trial in children with intractable partial epilepsy is currently under way.

Levetiracetam was approved for release in the U.S. market in November 1999, with an indication for adjunctive use in adult patients with partial-onset seizures.

LORECLEZOLE

Loreclezole (LRC, Z-1-12-chloro-2-2,4 dichlorophenyl-ethenyl-1H-1,2,4-triazole, R72063) is under development by Janssen Research Foundation in Beerse, Belgium (41). This triazole derivative is similar in some ways to the barbiturate class of drugs and may present some advantages over the older AEDs.

Loreclezole increases GABA-mediated inhibition in feed-forward collateral circuits of the hippocampus (42). It may directly activate the chloride channel in the GABA-A receptor complex, even in the absence of GABA (43–45). Work with recombinant GABA-A receptor subunits demonstrates that LRC acts at a site distinct from that of benzodiazepines, barbiturates, and neurosteroids (46,47) and may act to allosterically modulate the GABA-A receptor at a unique site on one of the membrane spanning domains (48).

Loreclezole exerts a broad spectrum of antiseizure activity in animal models. It suppresses PTZ seizures in adults (49) and developing (50) rats with a profile similar to that of phenytoin and carbamazepine. Unlike phenytoin and carbamazepine, however, LRC antagonizes clonic components of convulsions. Spike-wave electroencephalogram (EEG) discharges in rats that are genetically prone to absence seizures were reduced by LRC (51). Loreclezole also reduces ictal-like patterns in hippocampal slices produced by low magnesium perfusion (52).

Loreclezole is well absorbed by the oral route and exhibits a very long half-life, on the order of 1 to 4 weeks (41). This long half-life may present some challenges to clinical care. One clinical trial observed an effect of LRC to decrease concurrent carbamazepine serum levels, with no change in the ratio of carbamazepine to its epoxide (53). In contrast, several patients experienced an increase in phenytoin levels.

The clinical efficacy of LRC initially was tested in patients with photosensitive EEG responses. Single doses of LRC, 100 to 150 mg, decreased photosensitivity in all patients (54). Rentmeester and colleagues (55) conducted a randomized, placebo-controlled, add-on trial in 62 adult patients with uncontrolled partial seizures. Six of 32 patients (19%) in the treatment group and none of the 30 in the placebo group experienced at least a 50 percent reduction in their seizures. Serum LRC levels ranged from 1 to 2 mg/L. After the randomized trial, 56 patients continued into an open-label study (53) with serum levels increased to 5 to 6 mg/L. At these levels, 22 of 56 patients (39%) achieved at least

a 50 percent reduction in seizures compared with their initial baseline rate. Nine patients carried forward from prior LRC studies were weaned to LRC monotherapy; seven of these patients were able to maintain LRC as a single drug at last follow-up (56).

Although LRC acts on the GABA receptor, its different site of action from benzodiazepines and barbiturates indicates that it may spare patients the usual sedative and depressant side effects of these older agents. In rats LRC does, in fact, preserve learning in comparison to diazepam-like drugs (57). Cognitive-sparing in patients has yet to be established, but so far LRC has been very well tolerated. The long-term study of 56 adults (53) reported side effects including weight loss, drowsiness, and fatigue. Serum laboratory values were not significantly altered. Pediatric studies are not available.

LOSIGAMONE

Losigamone (LSG, 5-α-2-chlorophenyl-hydroxymethyl-4-methoxy-5H-furanone, ADD-137022, AO-33), which was developed by Dr. Willmar Schwabe Pharmaceuticals, Karlsruhe, Germany, and the Epilepsy Branch of the National Institutes of Health, is a tetronic acid derivative with antiseizure properties (58). LSG reduced hippocampal firing to depolarizing neuronal currents and slightly reduced excitatory postsynaptic potential (EPSP) amplitudes (59). In contrast, inhibitory postsynaptic potential (IPSP) amplitudes were unaffected. Dimpfel and associates (60) concurred that LSG did not affect binding of GABA or benzodiazepines but argued that the drug could directly increase chloride influx, which should have an inhibitory effect on neurons. LSG can partially reverse the excitation produced by the potassium-channel blocker 4-aminopyridine (61,62) and block hippocampal slice cellular bursting produced by low magnesium perfusates (63) and low calcium perfusates (64). Analysis of miniature synaptic potential kinetics suggests that LSG exerts its actions mainly on presynaptic sodium channels (65). In higher doses, calcium currents are also reduced by LSG (66). Losigamone presents a therapeutic ratio superior to that of phenytoin in MES testing and shows good efficacy against PTZ, bicuculline, and picrotoxin seizures, but not strychnine seizures (67).

Losigamone is a racemate of two enantiomers, AO-242 (S-(+)-LSG) and AO-294 (R-(−)-LSG). Seizure susceptibility in audiogenic seizure-prone mice (DBA/2 mice), as well as selected in vitro studies, suggests that the S-(+)-LSG enantiomer is pharmacologically active (68).

Pharmacokinetics of LSG were tested in four phase I studies in 52 normal adult volunteers (69). For single doses, the dose-serum relationship was linear over the range 100 to 1000 mg. Doses of 1500 mg/day produce serum levels around 2 mg/L (67). The serum half-life was approximately 4 hours. LSG is approximately 80 percent bound to serum proteins (58).

A U.S. study of nine adults with intractable partial seizures has been reported by Morris (70). Doses of LSG were escalated weekly to 2100 mg/day in three divided doses. Seizure frequency was reduced 39 percent overall, and three patients became seizure-free. Adverse events, reported in order of decreasing frequency, were dizziness, headache, somnolence, abnormal thinking, and insomnia. Two patients experienced more than a twofold increase in serum ALT (SGPT). Interactions with other AEDs were not significant. A multicenter trial of LSG at a total daily dose of 1500 mg was completed in Europe (71). Preliminary analysis of data from 198 patients revealed a 21 percent responder rate (at least 50% improvement in seizure frequency) in the treatment arm, lack of significant interaction with other AEDs, no laboratory abnormalities, and good tolerability. Studies in children are not available.

RALITOLINE

Ralitoline (RLT, N-(2-chloro-6-methyl-phenyl)-2-(3-methyl-4-oxo-2-thiazolidinylidene) is a thiazolidine derivative developed at the Godecke AG, Research Institute, Freiburg, Germany (72). RLT is a state-dependent blocker of voltage-sensitive sodium channels (73) and has a profile in epilepsy models (74) similar to that of phenytoin and carbamazepine, except that RLT has slightly more action against clonic seizures (75). The drug is weakly effective in PTZ and strychnine models of epilepsy (76). RLT does not affect responses to applied glutamate nor GABA (77).

Little clinical information on ralitoline has been published so far. The drug is very potent in MES testing, with effective 50 percent doses of 3.5 mg/kg intraperitoneally (compared with phenytoin at 11.5, phenobarbital at 24, and diazepam at 23 mg/kg) (79), but the rotorod ataxia test is positive at only 5.8 mg/kg. This relatively narrow therapeutic window and a short half-life for the drug may pose problems in the clinical arena. RLT has also demonstrated significant teratogenic potential in Sprague-Dawley rats at maternal doses of 120 mg/kg and above (78).

REMACEMIDE

Remacemide (REM, 2-amino-N-(1-methyl-1,2-diphenylethyl)-acetamide monochloride) was originally developed by Fisons Pharmaceuticals and is now under further development by Astra-Merck (80).

Remacemide is a noncompetitive NMDA-associated ion channel blocker and serves as a prodrug for the des-glycine metabolite, FPL12495. REM blocks repetitive firing in hippocampal neurons from depolarizing pulses (81,82). FPL12495 inhibits veratridine-stimulated release of excitatory amino acids (83). The blocking action of REM on the NMDA-associated channel is relatively weak, with 68 μM required for a 50 percent inhibitory concentration (84). The affinity for the NMDA-associated channel is lower than that for MK-801 or phencyclidine (85), which may account for its favorable side-effect profile relative to older NMDA antagonists.

Remacemide is effective against MES seizures in rats (86), with a therapeutic ratio of 28, compared with 5 to 10 for traditional AEDs (87). The drug is also effective against audiogenic seizures in rats and seizures produced by NMDA (87). REM is not effective in PTZ seizures or in preventing the development of kindling. REM and FPL12495 block spike-wave discharges in the WAG/Rij rat (88), a reasonable predictor of efficacy against clinical absence epilepsies. In most of the animal epilepsy models REM is effective in the dose range of 6 to 60 mg/kg (85).

Remacemide is soluble in water and is mildly lipophilic. It is absorbed orally and rapidly distributed to the brain. The drug is metabolized by the hepatic P-450 system to at least four active metabolites by a combination of oxidation, glucuronidation, and removal of a glycine group. REM penetrates the blood–brain barrier by passive diffusion and is deglycinated to FPL12495 within the brain (89). The des-glycine metabolite is more potent and specific for NMDA-associated channel blockade than is the parent compound (90). In normal adult volunteers, half-life after acute oral dosing is 3 to 4 hours. REM is approximately 75 percent protein-bound, and its FPL12495 metabolite is approximately 90 percent protein-bound (84).

Pharmacokinetic interactions of AEDs and REM are complex. Hepatic enzyme inducers such as phenobarbital, phenytoin, and carbamazepine induce more rapid clearance of REM and FPL12495. REM increases serum levels of phenytoin (91) and carbamazepine (92) by approximately 20 percent to 25 percent. This probably results from inhibition of metabolic enzymes for these drugs by REM. Remacemide has little effect on the carbamazepine epoxide (92) and little interaction with valproic acid (93).

A primary concern with an NMDA-channel blocker is the possible effect on learning known to be associated with this category of compounds. So far data on REM have been relatively reassuring. In an operant learning paradigm in rats, REM produced less disruption of learning in animal models than did MK-801, clonazepam, phenobarbital, phenytoin, carbamazepine, or felbamate (94).

Published clinical studies of REM, even in adults subjects, are limited. A placebo-controlled, double-blind, add-on, crossover study in 28 adult patients with refractory epilepsy demonstrated a 50 percent reduction in seizure frequency in 33 percent of those taking REM and 9 percent of those taking placebo. Four patients were seizure-free while taking REM. Most patients in this study had more than one seizure type (95). A larger series of 327 patients in a multicenter, placebo-controlled trial, has also been reported in abstract form (96). This study compared three different doses of REM and placebo in patients with refractory epilepsy and determined a responder rate (at least 50% improvement in seizure frequency) in 31 percent of those taking REM at 800 mg/day. Side effects included worsening of seizures, dizziness, somnolence, ataxia, anxiety, and depression. Studies in children are not available.

Because of its potential role as a neuroprotective agent, remacemide is also being studied in a wide variety of other neurologic disorders, including stroke (97), neuroprotection during cardiopulmonary bypass surgery (97a), Huntington's disease (98), and Parkinson's disease (99). REM has also been investigated in an animal model as a possible cerebral protectant against neuronal damage caused by seizure activity, specifically in rats with status epilepticus provoked by perforant pathway stimulation (100). Pretreatment with REM, but not posttreatment, resulted in decreased pyramidal cell damage in the CA1 and CA3 regions of hippocampus, as well as in parahippocampal regions, in comparison to control animals.

RUFINAMIDE

Rufinamide (RUF; 1-(2,6-diflurophenyl)-1H-1,2,3-triazole-4-carboxamide; CGP 33101) is a structurally novel compound developed by Novartis Pharmaceuticals. At least part of its mechanism of action involves blockade of sodium channels (101). It is active against MES and chemical convulsant seizures with an unusually favorable therapeutic-to-toxic ratio (101). Rufinamide is metabolized by hydrolysis into inactive metabolites (102) and has an elimination half-life of 8 to 12 hours.

Rufinamide has undergone trials in Europe, but details have not yet been published. Palhagen and associates reported results of a multicenter study in abstract form (101). Fifty patients, ages 20 to 60 years, were given RUF 400 to 1600 mg/day in a randomized, placebo-controlled, double-blind, add-on trial. Study subjects had intractable partial seizures, with or without secondarily generalized seizures. After a baseline, subjects were assigned to placebo therapy or to weekly escalation of 400 mg RUF to a maximum of 1600 mg/day. Median seizure frequency was

decreased 42 percent in the RUF group and increased 52 percent in the placebo group. The 50 percent responder rate was 39 percent for RUF and 16 percent for placebo, but differences were not statistically significant. Two patients discontinued because of adverse events. The rate of adverse events for RUF versus placebo were headache 20 percent vs. 12 percent; tiredness 20 percent vs. 4 percent; tremor 12 percent vs. 0 percent. Multicenter, randomized, placebo-controlled, add-on trials in adults with intractable partial-onset seizure have recently been completed, but results are pending at this time.

A report regarding open-label use of RUF in nine children (age range 4–16 years) with intractable partial epilepsy has recently been published in abstract form (102a). Four of nine patients (45%) experienced at least a 50 percent reduction in seizure frequency, compared with baseline, during a brief period of open-label treatment. No adverse effects were observed.

A multicenter, randomized, placebo-controlled, double-blind, add-on trial for children with intractable partial seizures has recently been completed, but results are pending at this time. A similar trial in children and adults with intractable seizures associated with Lennox-Gastaut syndrome is currently under way.

STIRIPENTOL

Stiripentol (STP; 4,4-dimethyl-1-[(3,4-methylenedioxy)phenyl]-1-penten-3-ol) is an alcohol derivative (103, 104) that has been under investigation for approximately 15 years, sponsored by Biocodex Laboratories. STP has two enantiomers, with the (+) form showing greater potency against seizures (105). It inhibits both uptake and metabolism of GABA (106), although it is not known whether this is the primary mode of action.

Stiripentol is effective against PTZ (107), strychnine, and bicuculline-induced chemical seizures (106) and spiking produced by alumina gel in monkeys (108).

Stiripentol is well absorbed by the oral route. Almost 99 percent of the circulating STP is bound to serum proteins (109). STP, like phenytoin, reaches a metabolic saturation point in the clinically relevant range, such that serum levels may increase dramatically with a small dose increment (104). Target serum levels in clinical trials were in the range of 17 to 22 mg/L (110). Stiripentol metabolism is extremely complex, with at least 13 metabolites resulting from glucuronidation, oxidation, o-methylation, and other pathways (111).

Stiripentol interacts in multiple ways with antiepileptic medications (112), raising serum levels of carbamazepine, phenytoin, and phenobarbital by 25 percent to 50 percent (113). Addition of STP increases the carbamazepine-to-epoxide ratio (114,115). Some researchers have suggested that these interactions open up the possibility of rational polypharmacy with STP and the older AEDs (116). When used in polypharmacy, STP paradoxically may protect against phenytoin-induced teratogenesis in rats (117), possibly by inhibiting the ability of the cytochrome P-450 system to produce teratogenic oxidative metabolites of phenytoin. STP may also protect patients receiving valproic acid (VPA) against formation of the potentially toxic 4-ene-VPA metabolite (118).

Vincent (110) first reported the benefit of 1800 to 3000 mg of STP in 26 patients with partial seizures. Several other open-label studies of adult patients with partial seizures suggested efficacy (113,119,120). The early trials are difficult to interpret because they were add-on studies and efficacy could have been the result of stiripentol-induced increases in serum levels of concurrent AEDs.

Farwell and colleagues conducted an open-label study of STP, 1000 to 3000 g/per day in three divided doses for 20 weeks in 10 children, ages 6 to 16 years, with atypical absence seizures (121). Serum levels of other AEDs were stabilized as much as possible by dose adjustments. The frequency of atypical absence seizures was reduced by a mean of 70 percent compared with baseline rates. A second open-label add-on study has also been completed in children, ages 9 months to 17 years, with intractable epilepsy of either partial or generalized type (122). This study investigated doses up to 80 to 100 mg/kg/day and determined a responder rate (at least 50% improvement in seizure frequency) of up to 37 percent. Children with partial epilepsy did particularly well.

More recently, Perez has reported a series of 108 children with intractable epilepsy enrolled in a single-blind, placebo-controlled, add-on study design (age range 9 months to 20 years) (123). This was a heterogeneous group with respect to seizure type and epilepsy syndrome: approximately half the patients were characterized as having localization-related epilepsy. Patients were treated with doses of STP up to 100 mg/kg/day for three months after a one-month single-blind, placebo-controlled baseline. At three months, 49 percent had responded with at least a 50 percent reduction in seizure frequency. Patients with partial-onset seizures were more likely to respond, as were patients taking carbamazepine as their preexisting medication (plasma concentrations of carbamazepine increased with STP treatment).

Perez also examined the tolerability of STP in a total of 206 children by combining the population of the study noted above with additional patients treated on an open-label basis (123). Forty-eight percent reported at least one adverse event, including drowsiness (16.5%), anorexia (15.0%), nausea/vomiting (5.8%),

ataxia (5.3%), and insomnia (5.3%). Most adverse events occurred during the first few days of STP therapy and were successfully managed by reducing the dose of concomitant medications. Although one-third of the adverse events were reported to be "severe," only two patients withdraw from STP treatment.

CONCLUSION

The wave of testing and release of new AEDs that began in 1993 so far continues with vigor. The continued pursuit of new agents is justified by the high prevalence of intractable epilepsy and by the limitations of all existing medical therapies for seizures. Nevertheless, researchers and pharmaceutical companies recognize that a drug must have a potential advantage over older agents to justify the large cost and effort of development. The new medications discussed in this chapter may possess such advantages.

Ganaxolone is the first tested AED based on neurosteroid hormones. Levetiracetam is based on drugs that enhance cognition, raising the possibility that this drug may avoid some of the cognitive impairment produced by most of the older AEDs. Loreclezole is a broad-spectrum drug that acts at an interesting new site on the $GABA_A$ receptor complex. It may provide some of the advantages of the barbiturates without their full degree of sedation and depression. Losigamone is in early testing, with promising but still inconclusive results. Remacemide is a (weak) NMDA-associated channel blocker, with little suggestion so far of the psychotomimetic side effects that have limited use of previous NMDA blockers. It may hypothetically be useful both in blocking excitation leading to seizures and for tissue neuroprotection during status epilepticus. Rufinamide is in early stages of testing. Although similar in antiepileptic profile to phenytoin and carbamazepine, early results with rufinamide suggest a particularly favorable therapeutic-to-toxic ratio. Stiripentol provides unique pharmacokinetic advantages in polypharmacy, allowing reduction of concurrent drug dose and possibly some protection against toxic or teratogenic metabolites of other drugs.

Several of these agents are undergoing controlled study in groups of children with partial seizures and in those with Lennox-Gastaut syndrome. Hopefully, as more experience is gained with these drugs, indications for pediatric use will emerge. The result should be a wider variety of choice for those children currently failing medical management because of either poor seizure control or difficulties with medication side effects.

REFERENCES

1. Temkin O. *The Falling Sickness: A History of Epilepsy from the Greeks to the Beginnings of Modern Neurology.* Baltimore: The Johns Hopkins Press, 1971.

2. Friedlander WJ. Who was 'the father of bromide treatment of epilepsy'? *Arch Neurol* 1986; 43:505–507.

3. Merritt HH, Putnam TJ. A new series of anticonvulsant drugs tested by experiments on animals. *Arch Neurol Psych* 1938; 39:1003–1015.

4. Meldrum BS. Update on the mechanism of action of antiepileptic drugs. *Epilepsia* 1996; 37(Suppl 6):S4–S11.

5. Berkovic SF. Epilepsy genes and the genetics of epilepsy syndromes: the promise of new therapies based on genetic knowledge. *Epilepsia* 1997; 39(Suppl 9):S32–S36.

6. Cereghino JJ. New antiepileptic drugs. In: Dodson WE, Pellock JM, eds. *Pediatric Epilepsy.* New York: Demos, 1993, Chapter 32:343–355.

7. Bauer J, Elger CE. Anticonvulsive drug therapy. Historical and current aspects. *Nervenarzt* 1995; 66:403–411.

8. Engel J Jr, Pedley TA, eds. *Epilepsy: A Comprehensive Textbook.* Philadelphia: Lippincott-Raven, 1997.

9. Levy RH, Mattson RH, Meldrum BS, Penry JK, eds. *Antiepileptic Drugs.* 4th ed. New York: Raven Press, 1995.

10. Shorvon SD, Dreifuss FE, Fish DE, Thomas DGT, eds. *The Treatment of Epilepsy.* Oxford, U.K.: Blackwell Scientific Publications, 1996.

11. Wyllie E, ed. *The Treatment of Epilspsy: Principles and Practice.* 2nd ed. Philadelphia: Lea & Febiger, 1996.

12. Blum DE. New drugs for persons with epilepsy. *Adv Neurol* 1998; 76:57–87.

13. Sander JW. New drugs for epilepsy. *Curr Opin Neurol* 1998; 11(2):141–148.

14. Bourgeois BF. New antiepileptic drugs. *Arch Neurol* 1998; 55(9):1181–1183.

15. Ben-Menachem E. The role of new antiepileptic drugs. *Adv Neurol* 1999; 81:317–321.

16. Bialer M, Johannessen SI, Kupferberg HJ, et al. Progress report on new antiepileptic drugs: a summary of the fourth Eilat conference (EILAT IV). *Epilepsy Res* 1999; 34(1):1–41.

17. Cramer JA, Fisher R, Ben-Menachem E, et al. New antiepileptic drugs: comparison of key clinical trials. *Epilepsia* 1999; 40(5):590–600.

18. Pellock JM. Managing pediatric epilepsy syndromes with new antiepileptic drugs. *Pediatrics* 1999; 104(5):1106–1116.

19. Morton LD, Pellock JM. Overview of childhood epilepsy and epileptic syndromes and advances in therapy. *Curr Pharm Des* 2000; 6(8):879–900.

20. Craig CR. Antiepileptic activity of steroids: separability of antiepileptic from hormonal effects. *J Pharmacol Exp Ther* 1966; 153:337–343.

21. Carter RB, Wood PL, Wieland S, et al. Characterization of the anticonvulsant properties of ganaxolone (CCD 1042; 3alpha-hydroxy-3beta-methyl-5alpha-pregnan-20-one), a selective, high-affinity, steroid modulator of the gamma-aminobutyric acid (A) receptor. *J Pharmacol Exp Ther* 1997; 280:1284–1295.

22. Gasior M, Carter RB, Goldberg SR, Witkin JM. Anticonvulsant and behavioral effects of neuroactive steroids alone and in conjunction with diazepam. *J Pharmacol Exp Ther* 1997; 282:543–553.

23. Snead OC. Ganaxolone, a selective high-affinity steroid modulator of the gamma-aminobutyric acid-A receptor, exacerbates seizures in animal models of absence. *Ann Neurol* 1998; 44(4):688–691.

24. Monaghan EP, Navalta LA, Shum L, Ashbrook DW, Lee DA. Initial human experience with ganaxolone, a neuroactive steroid with antiepileptic activity. *Epilepsia* 1997; 38:1026–1031.

25. Monaghan EP, Harris S, Blum D, et al. Ganaxolone in the treatment of complex partial seizures: a double-blind, presurgical design. *Epilepsia* 1997; 38:179.

26. Lechtenberg R, Villeneuve N, Monaghan EP, et al. An open-label dose-escalation study to evaluate the safety and tolerability of ganaxolone in the treatment of refractory epilepsy in pediatric patients. *Epilepsia* 1996; 37(Suppl 5):204.

27. Kerrigan JF, Shields WD, Nelson TY, et al. Ganaxolone for treating intractable infantile spasms: a multicenter, open-label, add-on trial. *Epilepsy Res* 2000, in press.

28. Brown P, Steiger MJ, Thompson PD, et al. Effectiveness of piracetam in cortical myoclonus. *Mov Dis* 1993; 8:63–68.

29. Sills GJ, Leach JP, Fraser CM, et al. Neurochemical studies with the novel anticonvulsant levetiracetam in mouse brain. *Eur J Pharmacol* 1997; 325:35–40.

30. Noyer M, Gillard M, Matagne A, Henichart JP, Wulfert E. The novel antiepileptic drug levetiracetam (ucb L059) appears to act via a specific binding site in CNS membranes. *Eur J Pharmacol* 1995; 286:137–146.

31. Löscher W, Honack D, Bloms-Funke P. The novel antiepileptic drug levetiracetam (ucb L059) induces alterations in GABA metabolism and turnover in discrete areas of rat brain and reduces neuronal activity in substantia nigra pars reticulata. *Brain Res* 1996; 735:208–216.

32. Gower AJ, Hirsch E, Boehrer A, Noyer M, Marescaux C. Effects of levetiracetam, a novel antiepileptic drug, on convulsant activity in two genetic rat models of epilepsy. *Epilepsy Res* 1995; 22:207–213.

33. Doheny HC, Whittington MA, Jefferys JGR, Patsalos PN. Levetiracetam in a chronic limbic model of epilepsy. *Epilepsia* 1997; 38:30.

34. Klitgaard H, Matagne A, Löscher W, Gobert J, Wulfert E. Levetiracetam (ucb LO59) protects selectively against kindled seizures and reveals powerful antiepileptogenic properties in rodents. *Epilepsia* 1997; 38:44.

35. Kasteleijn-Nolst Trenite DG, Marescaux C, Stodieck S, Edelbroek PM, Oosting J. Photosensitive epilepsy: a model to study the effects of antiepileptic drugs. Evaluation of the piracetam analogue, levetiracetam. *Epilepsy Res* 1996; 25:225–230.

36. Sharief MK, Singh P, Sander JWAS, Patsalos PN, Shorvon SD. Efficacy and tolerability study of ucb LO59

in patients with refractory epilepsy. *J Epilepsy* 1996; 9:106–112.

37. Chevalier Y, Grant R, Sander JWAS, Hiersemenzel R, Debrabandere L. Twelve-week add-on, increasing dose (1000–4000 mg/d) multicenter pilot study of ucb LO59 in epileptic patients. *Epilepsia* 1995; 36:S153.

38. Shorvon SD. Comparative evidence on efficacy and safety of different dosages of levetiracetam in add-on treatment of partial epilepsy. *Epilepsia* 1997; 38(Suppl 3):78.

38a. Cereghino JJ, Biton V, Abou-Khalil B, et al. Levetiracetam for partial seizures: results of a double-blind, randomized clinical trial. *Neurology* 2000; 55(2):236–242.

39. Lîscher W, Hînack D. Profile of ucb LO59, a novel anticonvulsant drug, in models of partial and generalized epilepsy in mice and rats. *Eur J Clin Pharmacol* 1993; 232:147–158.

40. Cramer JA, Arrigo C, Van Hammee G, et al. Effect of levetiracetam on epilepsy-related quality of life. N132 Study Group. *Epilepsia* 2000; 41(7):868–874.

40a. Pellock J, Glauser T, Bebin M, et al. Single-dose pharmacokinetics of levetiracetam in pediatric patients with partial seizures. *Epilepsia* 1999; 40(Suppl 7):124.

40b. Glauser T, Bebin M, Ritter F, et al. Open-label efficacy and safety of levetiracetam in pediatric patients with partial onset seizures. *Epilepsia* 1999; 40(Suppl 7):161.

41. de Beukelaar F, Tritsmans L. Loreclezole. *Epilepsy Res* 1991; 3 (Suppl):125–128.

42. Ashton D, Willems R. In vitro studies on the broad spectrum anticonvulsant loreclezole in the hippocampus. *Epilepsy Res* 1992; 11:75–88.

43. Ghiani CA, Tuligi G, Maciocco E, et al. Biochemical evaluations of the effects of loreclezole and propofol on the GABAA receptor in rat brain. *Biochem Pharmacol* 1996; 51:1527–1534.

44. Sanna E, Murgia A, Casula A, et al. Direct activation of GABAA receptors by loreclezole, an anticonvulsant drug with selectivity for the beta-subunit. *Neuropharmacology* 1996; 35:1753–1760.

45. Zhong Y, Simmonds MA. Interactions between loreclezole, chlormethiazole and pentobarbitone at GABA-A receptors: functional and binding studies. *Br J Pharmacol* 1997; 121:1392–1396.

46. Wafford KA, Bain CJ, Quirk K, et al. A novel allosteric modulatory site on the GABA$_A$ receptor beta subunit. *Neuron* 1994; 12:775–82.

47. Wingrove PB, Wafford KA, Bain C, Whiting PJ. The modulatory action of loreclezole at the gamma-aminobutyric acid type A receptor is determined by a single amino acid in the beta 2 and beta 3 subunit. *Proc Natl Acad Sci USA* 1994; 91:4569–4573.

48. Fisher JL, Hinkle DJ, Macdonald RL. Loreclezole inhibition of recombinant alpha1beta1gamma2L GABA(A) receptor single channel currents. *Neuropharmacology* 2000; 39(2):235–245.

49. Green AR, Misra A, Murray TK, Snape MF, Cross AJ. A behavioural and neurochemical study in rats of the pharmacology of loreclezole, a novel allosteric

50. Pohl M, Mares P. Effects of loreclezole on metrazol-induced phenomena in developing rats. *Arch Int Pharmacodyn Ther* 1990; 305:163–71:163–171.

51. Ates N, van Luijtelaar EL, Drinkenburg WH, Vossen JM, Coenen AM. Effects of loreclezole on epileptic activity and on EEG and behaviour in rats with absence seizures. *Epilepsy Res* 1992; 13:43–48.

52. Zhang CL, Heinemann U. Effects of the triazole derivative loreclezole (R72063) on stimulus induced ionic and field potential responses and on different patterns of epileptiform activity induced by low magnesium in rat entorhinal cortex-hippocampal slices. *Naunyn Schmiedebergs Arch Pharmacol* 1992; 346:581–587.

53. Rentmeester T, Janssen A, Hulsman J, et al. Long-term evaluation of the efficacy and safety of loreclezole as add-on therapy in patients with uncontrolled partial seizures: a 1-year open follow-up. *Epilepsy Res* 1991b; 9:65–70.

54. Overweg J, de Beukelaar F. Single-dose efficacy evaluation of loreclezole in patients with photosensitive epilepsy. *Epilepsy Res* 1990; 6:227–233.

55. Rentmeester T, Janssen A, Hulsman J, et al. A double-blind, placebo-controlled evaluation of the efficacy and safety of loreclezole as add-on therapy in patients with uncontrolled partial seizures. *Epilepsy Res* 1991a; 9:59–64.

56. Rentmeester TW, Hulsman JA. Loreclezole monotherapy in patients with partial seizures. *Epilepsy Res* 1992; 11:141–145.

57. Raffa RB, Vaught JL, Setler PE. The novel anticonvulsant loreclezole (R 72063) does not produce diazepam-like anterograde amnesia in a passive avoidance test in rats. *Naunyn Schmiedebergs Arch Pharmacol* 1990; 342:613–615.

58. Stein U, Klessing K, Chatterjee SS. Losigamone. *Epilepsy Res* 1991; 3(Suppl):129–133.

59. Schmitz D, Gloveli T, Heinemann U. Effects of losigamone on synaptic potentials and spike frequency habituation in rat entorhinal cortex and hippocampal CA1 neurones. *Neurosci Lett* 1995; 200:141–143.

60. Dimpfel W, Chatterjee SS, Noldner M, Ticku MK. Effects of the anticonvulsant losigamone and its isomers on the GABA$_A$ receptor system. *Epilepsia* 1995; 36:983–989.

61. Kapetanovic IM, Yonekawa WD, Kupferberg HJ. The effects of anticonvulsant compounds on 4-aminopyridine-induced de novo synthesis of neurotransmitter amino acids in rat hippocampus in vitro. *Epilepsy Res* 1995; 20:113–120.

62. Yonekawa WD, Kapetanovic IM, Kupferberg HJ. The effects of anticonvulsant agents on 4-aminopyridine induced epileptiform activity in rat hippocampus in vitro. *Epilepsy Res* 1995; 20:137–150.

63. Zhang CL, Chatterjee SS, Stein U, Heinemann U. Comparison of the effects of losigamone and its isomers on maximal electroshock induced convulsions in mice and on three different patterns of low magnesium induced

epileptiform activity in slices of the rat temporal cortex. *Naunyn Schmiedebergs Arch Pharmacol* 1992; 345:85–92.

64. Kohr G, Heinemann U. Effects of the tetronic acid derivatives AO33 (losigamone) and AO78 on epileptiform activity and on stimulus-induced calcium concentration changes in rat hippocampal slices. *Epilepsy Res* 1990; 7:49–58.

65. Draguhn A, Jungclaus M, Sokolowa S, Heinemann U. Losigamone decreases spontaneous synaptic activity in cultured hippocampal neurons. *Eur J Pharmacol* 1997; 325:245–251.

66. Kelly KM, Macdonald RL. Losigamone (AO-33) reduces high-threshold calcium currents in rat dorsal root ganglion neurons. *Epilepsia* 1993; 34(Suppl 6):118.

67. Stein U. Potential antiepileptic drugs. Losigamone. In: Levy RH, Mattson RH, Meldrum BS (eds.). *Antiepileptic drugs.* 4th ed. New York, Raven Press, 1995:1025–1034.

68. Jones FA, Davies JA. The anticonvulsant effects of the enantiomers of losigamone. *Br J Pharmacol* 1999; 128(6):1223–1228.

69. Biber A, Dienel A. Pharmacokinetics of losigamone, a new antiepileptic drug, in healthy male volunteers. *Int J Clin Pharmacol Ther* 1996; 34:6–11.

70. Morris G III, Collins S, Bell W, et al. Losigamone: a putative antiepileptic drug. *J Epilepsy* 1997; 10:62–66

71. Elger CE, Stefan H, Runge U, Dienel A, and the Losigamone Study Group. Losigamone, double-blind study of 1500 mg/day versus placebo in patients with focal epilepsy. *Epilepsia* 1996; 37:64.

72. Bartoszyk GD, Dooley D-J, Fritschi E, Satzinger G. Ralitoline: a thiazolidinone. In: Meldrum BS, Porter RJ, eds. *New Anticonvulsant Drugs.* London, John Libbey, 1986:309–311.

73. Wagner B, Strumpf G, Bartoszyk GD. Similar effects of ralitoline and phenytoin on papillary muscle action potentials: evidence for sodium antagonistic activity. *Pharmacol Res Commun* 1987; 19:591–596.

74. Satzinger G. Ralitoline. *Drugs Fut* 1985; 10:920–921.

75. Bartoszyk GD, Hamer M. The genetic animal model of reflex epilepsy in the Mongolian gerbil: differential efficacy of new anticonvulsive drugs and prototype antiepileptics. *Pharmacol Res Commun* 1987; 19:429–440.

76. Fischer W, Bodewei R, Satzinger G. Anticonvulsant and sodium channel blocking effects of ralitoline in different screening models. *Naunyn Schmiedebergs Arch Pharmacol* 1992; 346:442–452.

77. Rock DM, McLean MJ, Macdonald RL, Catterall WA, Taylor CP. Ralitoline (CI-946) and CI-953 block sustained repetitive sodium action potentials in cultured mouse spinal cord neurons and displace batrachotoxinin A 20-alpha-benzoate binding in vitro. *Epilepsy Res* 1991; 8:197–203.

78. Dostal LA, Anderson JA. Developmental toxicity study in rats treated with the anticonvulsant, ralitoline. *Teratology* 1995; 51(1):11–19.

79. Löscher W, von Hodenberg A, Nolting B, Fassbender C-P, Taylor C. Ralitoline: a reevaluation of anticonvulsant profile and determination of "active" plasma concentrations in comparison with prototype antiepileptic drugs in mice. *Epilepsia* 1991; 32:560–568.

80. Muir KT, Palmer GC. Remacemide. *Epilepsy Res* 1991; 3(Suppl):147–152.

81. Norris SK, King AE. Electrophysiological effects of the anticonvulsant remacemide hydrochloride and its metabolite ARL 12495AA on rat CA1 hippocampal neurons in vitro. *Neuropharmacology* 1997; 36:951–959.

82. Wamil AW, Cheung H, Harris EW, McLean MJ. Remacemide HCl and its metabolite, FPL 12495AA, limit action potential firing frequency and block NMDA responses of mouse spinal cord neurons in cell culture. *Epilepsy Res* 1996; 23:1–14.

83. Srinivasan J, Richens A, Davies JA. The effect of the desglycinyl metabolite of remacemide hydrochloride (FPL 12495AA) and dizocilpine (MK-801) on endogenous amino acid release from mouse cortex. *Br J Pharmacol* 1995; 116:3087–3092.

84. Palmer GC, Jamieson V, Jones T. Remacemide. In: Engel J Jr, Pedley TA, eds. *Epilepsy: A Comprehensive Textbook.* Philadelphia: Lippencott-Raven, 1997:1659–1663.

85. Davies JA. Remacemide hydrochloride: a novel antiepileptic agent. *Gen Pharmacol* 1997; 28: 499–502.

86. Garske GE, Palmer GC, Napier JJ, et al., Preclinical profile of the anticonvulsant remacemide and its enantiomers in the rat. *Epilepsy Res* 1991; 9:161–174.

87. Stagnitto ML, Palmer GC, Ordy JM et al. Preclinical profile of remacemide: a novel anticonvulsant effective against maximal electroshock seizures in mice. *Epilepsy Res* 1990; 7:11–28.

88. van Luijtelaar EL, Coenen AM. Effects of remacemide and its metabolite FPL 12495 on spike-wave discharges, electroencephalogram and behaviour in rats with absence epilepsy. *Neuropharmacology* 1995; 34:419–425.

89. Heyn H, McCarthy DJ, Curry SH, Eisman MS, Anders MW. Brain uptake and biotransformation of remacemide hydrochloride, a novel anticonvulsant. *Drug Metab Dispos* 1994; 22:443–446.

90. Subramaniam S, Donevan SD, Rogawski MA. Block of the *N*-methyl-*D*-aspartate receptor by remacemide and its des-glycine metabolite. *J Pharmacol Exp Ther* 1996; 276:161–168.

91. Leach JP, Girvan J, Jamieson V, et al. Mutual interaction between remacemide hydrochloride and phenytoin. *Epilepsy Res* 1997; 26:381–388.

92. Leach JP, Blacklaw J, Jamieson V, et al. Mutual interaction between remacemide hydrochloride and carbamazepine: two drugs with active metabolites. *Epilepsia* 1996; 37:1100–1106.

93. Leach JP, Girvan J, Jamieson V, et al. Lack of pharmacokinetic interaction between remacemide hydrochloride and sodium valproate in epileptic patients. *Seizure* 1997; 6:179–184.

94. Hudzik TJ, Palmer GC. Effects of anticonvulsants in a novel operant learning paradigm in rats: comparison of remacemide hydrochloride and FPL 15896AR to other anticonvulsant agents. *Epilepsy Res* 1995; 21:183–193.

95. Crawford P, Richens A, Mawer G, et al. A double-blind placebo controlled cross-over study of remacemide hydrochloride as adjunctive therapy in pateints with refractory epilepsy. *Seizure* 1992; 1:7–13.

96. Jones MW, Blume W, Guberman A, et al. Remacemide hydrochloride (300 mg, 600 mg, 800 mg/day) efficacy and safety versus placebo in patients with refractory epilepsy. *Epilepsia* 1996; 37(Suppl 5):166.

97. Dyker AG, Lees KR. Remacemide hydrochloride: a double-blind, placebo-controlled, safety and tolerability study in patients with acute ischemic stroke. *Stroke* 1999; 30(9):1796–1801.

97a. Arrowsmith JE, Harrison MJ, Newman SP, et al. Neuroprotection of the brain during cardiopulmonary bypass: a randomized trial of remacemide during coronary artery bypass in 171 patients. *Stroke* 1998; 29(11):2357–2362.

98. Kieburtz K, Feigin A, McDermott M, et al. A controlled trial of remacemide hydrochloride in Huntington's disease. *Mov Disord* 1996; 11(3):273–277.

99. Parkinson Study Group. A multicenter randomized controlled trial of remacemide hydrochloride as monotherapy for PD. *Neurology* 2000; 54(8):1583–1588.

100. Halonen T, Nissinen J, Pitkanan A. Neuroprotective effect of remacemide hydrochloride in a perforant pathway stimulation model of status epilepticus in the rat. *Epilepsy Res* 1999; 34(2-3):251–269.

101. Palhagen S, Canger R, Henriksen O, van Parys JA, Karolchyk MA. Efficacy and safety of rufinamide in patients with refractory epilepsy. *Epilepsia* 1997; 38(Suppl 8):207.

102. Rouan MC, Souppart C, Alif L, et al. Automated analysis of a novel anti-epileptic compound, CGP 33, 101, and its metabolite, CGP 47,292, in body fluids by high-performance liquid chromatography and liquid-solid extraction. *J Chromatogr Biomed Appl* 1995; 667:307–313.

103. Loiseau P, Duché B, Tor J. Stiripentol in absence seizures. An open study updated. *Epilepsia* 1989; 30:639.

104. Vincent JC. Stiripentol. *Epilepsy Res* 1991; 3(Suppl): 153–156.

105. Arends RH, Zhang K, Levy RH, Baillie TA, Shen DD. Stereoselective pharmacokinetics of stiripentol: an explanation for the development of tolerance to anticonvulsant effect. *Epilepsy Res* 1994; 18:91–96.

106. Poisson M, Huguet F, Savattier A, Bakri-Logeais F, Narcisse G. A new type of anticonvulsant, stiripentol. Pharmacological profile and neurochemical study. *Arzneimittel-Forschung.* 1984; 34:199–204.

107. Shen DD, Levy RH, Moor MJ, Savitch JL. Efficacy of stiripentol in the intravenous pentylenetetrazol infusion seizure model in the rat. *Epilepsy Res* 1990; 7:40–48.

108. Lockard JS, Levy RH, Rhodes PH, Moore DF. Stiripentol in acute/chronic efficacy tests in monkey model. *Epilepsia* 1985; 26:704–712.

109. Loiseau P, Duché B. Potential antiepileptic drugs: stiripentol. In: Levy RH, Mattson RH, Meldrum BS, eds. *Antiepileptic Drugs.* 4th ed. New York: Raven Press, 1995:1045–1056.

110. Vincent JC. Stiripentol. In: Meldrum BS, Porter RJ, eds. *New Anticonvulsant Drugs.* London: John Libbey, 1986:255–263.

111. Moreland TA, Astoin J, Lepage F, et al. The metabolic fate of stiripentol in man. *Drug Metab Disp.* 1986; 14:654–662.

112. Levy RH, Loiseau P, Guyot M, et al. Stiripentol kinetics in epilepsy: nonlinearity and interactions. *Clin Pharmacol Ther* 1984; 36:661–669.

113. Loiseau P, Strube E, Tor J, Levy RH, Dodrill C. Neurophysiological and therapeutic evaluation of stiripentol in epilepsy. Preliminary results. *Rev Neurol (Paris)* 1988; 144:165–172.

114. Kerr BM, Martinez-Lage JM, Viteri C, et al. Carbamazepine dose requirements during stiripentol therapy: influence of cytochrome P-450 inhibition by stiripentol. *Epilepsia* 1991; 32:267–274.

115. Tran A, Vauzelle-Kervroedan F, Rey E, et al. Effect of stiripentol on carbamazepine plasma concentration and metabolism in epileptic children. *Eur J Clin Pharmacol* 1996; 50:497–500.

116. Lockard JS, Levy RH. Carbamazepine plus stiripentol: is polytherapy by design possible? *Epilepsia* 1988; 29:476–481.

117. Finnell RH, Kerr BM, van Waes M, Steward RL, Levy RH. Protection from phenytoin-induced congenital malformations by coadministration of the antiepileptic drug stiripentol in a mouse model. *Epilepsia* 1994; 35: 141–148.

118. Levy RH, Rettenmeier AW, Anderson GD, et al. Effects of polytherapy with phenytoin, carbamazepine, and stiripentol on formation of 4-ene-valproate, a hepatotoxic metabolite of valproic acid. *Clin Pharmacol Ther* 1990; 48:225–235.

119. Martinez-Lage M, Loiseau P, Levy RH, et al. Clinical antiepileptic efficacy of stiripentol in resistant partial epilepsies. *Epilepsia* 1984; 25:673.

120. Rascol O, Squalli A, Montastruc JL, et al. A pilot study of stiripentol, a new anticonvulsant drug, in complex partial seizures uncontrolled by carbamazepine. *Clin Neuropharmacol* 1989; 12:119–123.

121. Farwell JR, Anderson GD, Kerr BM, Tor JA, Levy RH. Stiripentol in atypical absence seizures in children: an open trial. *Epilepsia* 1993; 34:305–311.

122. Chiron C, Renard F, Musial C, Tor JA, Dulac O. Single-blind add-on trial of stiripentol in epileptic children. *Epilepsia* 1993; 34(Suppl 6):74.

123. Perez J, Chiron C, Musial C, et al. Stiripentol: efficacy and tolerability in children with epilepsy. *Epilepsia* 1999; 40(11):1618–1626.

CHAPTER 41

ACTH and Steroids

Katherine M. Martien, M.D., and O. Carter Snead III, M.D.

HISTORY

The first report of the therapeutic efficacy of adreno-corticotropic hormone (ACTH) therapy in childhood seizures was in 1950, when Klein and Livingston (1) observed a beneficial effect of ACTH treatment in four of six children ranging in age from 4.5 to 16 years who were suffering from a variety of seizure types intractable to standard medical therapy. In 1958 Sorel and Dusaucy-Bauloye (2) reported a dramatic response to ACTH therapy in a series of children with infantile spasms (IS) who showed control of seizures and an improvement in the EEG after treatment with the drug. This finding was confirmed the following year (3–5).

The effect of oral steroids on the convulsive state was first reported in 1942, when McQuarrie and coworkers (6) observed the exacerbation of seizures by deoxycorticosterone. The benefit of oral steroids in IS was established soon after that of ACTH (3,7). Since that time ACTH and steroids have been used to treat a number of epilepsy syndromes. The main indication for the use of these drugs has been IS; however, they also have been reported to be effective in Ohtahara's syndrome, Lennox-Gastaut syndrome and other myoclonic epilepsies, Landau-Kleffner syndrome, opsoclonus-myoclonus, and Rasmussen's encephalitis (8).

In the first report on the use of ACTH in treating IS, Sorel and Dusaucy-Bauloye (2) described regression in developmental behavior in their patients before ACTH treatment, which showed improvement after treatment with ACTH and coincident with the control of spasms. The importance of these initial observations is reflected by the fact that the natural history of virtually all the epilepsy syndromes in which ACTH and steroids are effective is characterized by a narrow age-related onset during a critical period of brain development. Furthermore, those epilepsy syndromes that respond uniquely

to ACTH and steroid therapy are associated with both a regression or plateau of acquired milestones and a poor mental outcome. There is increasing evidence that, in addition to positively affecting the convulsive state, ACTH and/or steroids may improve the short-term developmental trajectory and the long-term prognosis for language and cognitive development in at least some patients with these epilepsy syndromes (9–13).

ACTH AND STEROIDS IN INFANTILE SPASMS

Infantile spasms were first described by West in 1841 in his son as "a peculiar form of infantile convulsions" (14). It later became clear that IS often were associated with the sequelae of severe mental deficiency. The electroencephalogram (EEG) manifestations of IS were described by Gibbs and Gibbs in 1952 when they termed the high-voltage, chaotic slowing with multifocal spikes and marked asynchrony of this disorder *hypsarrhythmia* (15). Thus arose the definition of West syndrome: a triad of IS, hypsarrhythmia, and psychomotor regression and mental retardation.

With the advent of EEG video-telemetry monitoring, IS and their associated EEG manifestations have been well characterized (16); however, the psychomotor regression associated with the spasms and subsequent developmental outcome have been less well investigated. Most of the studies that have addressed the therapeutic efficacy of various treatment regimens on IS have used outcome measures related to control of seizures, improvement of the EEG, and incidence of later epilepsy. Although a broad spectrum of cognitive outcomes and outcome predictors have been described in the literature, few studies have systematically examined the effect of different treatment protocols on developmental trajectory and long-term cognitive outcome. Similarly, while numerous studies on the efficacy of ACTH and corticosteroids in IS have been published, there is great variability of study design, which clouds the process of arriving at research-based recommendations for optimal treatment of this condition. Further complicating this process is the advent of newer antiepileptic drugs (AEDs), particularly vigabatrin (17,18), which are effective in IS. Vigabatrin, although not without side effects, is generally considered to be a safer drug than either ACTH or corticosteroids, and its role in treating IS and the sequelae of this disorder deserves further investigation. Finally, a new group of synthetic neurosteroids, the prototype of which is ganaxalone (19), may be promising in the treatment of IS.

There are only a few accepted caveats for the medical treatment of IS.

1. The cumulative spontaneous remission rate over the first 12 months of seizures is approximately 25 percent (20).

2. Seizures are almost always intractable to treatment with standard anticonvulsant drugs, with the exception of certain benzodiazepines, valproic acid, and vigabatrin.

3. Either ACTH or oral steroid therapy should result in a significant reduction of seizures in 50 percent to 75 percent of patients.

4. Natural ACTH is preferable to the synthetic form of the drug because it has fewer side effects.

5. There is probably an age window between 4 and 12 months in which the prognosis for a treatment response is best (9,11,21–23).

6. The ultimate prognosis in these patients is dismal for most and depends heavily on the etiology of the spasm, the preexisting neurologic and developmental status, the presence or absence of other seizures that occur concomitantly with the spasms, and the age of the patient at the onset of seizure (9,10,21,24–27).

In summary, the child with the best prognosis is one who is older than 4 months but less than 8 months of age and neurologically normal at the onset of the spasms, who has no other kind of seizures, who does not lose visual following during the course of the seizures, and who lacks a demonstrable etiology for the spasms.

The controversial questions concerning the treatment of IS outnumber those that engender agreement.

1. Which is the most effective therapy for IS: ACTH, oral steroids, valproic acid, benzodiazepines, pyridoxine, vigabatrin, a combination of some or all of these, or some other treatment?

2. What is the impact of the treatment of IS with ACTH versus steroids versus anticonvulsants on long-term outcome in terms of recurrence of spasms, evolution of other forms of intractable epilepsy, and cognitive and/or behavioral function?

3. Does it make any difference in the long-term outcome in terms of cognitive and/or behavioral functioning and the development of intractable epilepsy in a patient with preexisting mental retardation and a clearly defined structural abnormality of brain whether the spasms are treated at all?

4. What is the optimal dose of these drugs, and how long should the patient be treated once the spasms are brought under control?

5. Does it make a difference in the long-term outcome in terms of cognitive and/or behavioral function and the development of intractable epilepsy whether the patient is treated early or late after onset of IS?

6. Is the therapeutic efficacy of ACTH in the treatment of IS dependent on the formulation used, i.e., biologic versus synthetic or depot versus short-acting?

Table 41-1 lists the natural and synthetic formulations of ACTH that have been used in the treatment of IS. The biologic activity, expressed in international units (IU), is intended to provide a basis for comparison of potency of these compounds; however, the stated biologic activity represents the relative potency of the peptide in its ability to stimulate the adrenals and may not reflect its ability to affect brain function either directly or indirectly. In addition, the biologic activity of natural ACTH in the brain may differ from that of synthetic ACTH (9) as a result of the presence of ACTH fragments and possibly other pituitary hormones with neurobiologic activity in the brain in the pituitary extracts. These compounds could conceivably

Table 41-1. Available Preparations of ACTH

Corticotropin (ACTH 1–39) — porcine pituitary extract (short-acting)		
Acthar gel 80 IU/mL	100 IU* = 0.72 mg	
Acthar lyophylised powder	100 IU* = 0.72 mg	
Cosyntropin/Tetracoscatin (ACTH 1–24) — synthetic (short-acting)		
Cortrosyn	100 IU* = 1.0 mg	
Cosyntropin/Tetracoscatin (ACTH 1–24) — synthetic (long-acting)		
Synacthen depot(CIBA)	100 IU* = 2.5 mg	
Cortrosyn-Z(Organon)	100 IU* = 2.5 mg	

*Commercial preparations are described in international units (IU) based on a potency assay in hypophysectomized rats in which depletion of adrenal ascorbic acid is measured after subcutaneous ACTH injection.

further enhance the therapeutic efficacy of the natural ACTH preparation (28). In addition, pituitary extracts may have fewer associated side effects than synthetic ACTH at comparable doses (29). Any differences in the biologic effects of sustained levels of ACTH provided by the depot formulations compared with those of the short-acting preparations are not known.

STUDIES OF ACTH AND STEROIDS IN THE TREATMENT OF INFANTILE SPASMS

Most of the studies comparing the efficacy of ACTH and steroids in controlling the acute manifestations of IS have been retrospective (7,9–11,13,21,30–32), but there are a few published prospective studies available for review (25,33–39). The majority of published studies support the hypothesis that ACTH is more effective than prednisone in the treatment of IS as defined by cessation of seizures and resolution of the hypsarrhythmic EEG. However, the most effective dose of ACTH is a controversial issue.

Prednisone has been shown to stop spasms in 25 percent to 59 percent of patients (9,32,33–35). In uncontrolled studies, 75 percent to 80 percent of children treated with low-dose ACTH (2.5–30 IU/day or 8–90 IU/m^2/day) showed cessation of spasms (30,36); however, prospective studies have demonstrated response rates that range from 42 percent to 58 percent (35,37). Treatment of IS with high-dose ACTH (40–80 IU/day or 110–200 IU/m^2/day) has been reported by some authors to be effective in 86 percent to 97 percent of children in terms of stopping the seizures and normalizing the EEG (32,34,38).

The difficulty in interpreting the literature on the treatment response of IS to various therapeutic regimens is that cohort size is quite small in some cases. In addition, the proportion of cryptogenic to symptomatic patients varies from study to study, as does the proportion of patients with long lag time between onset of spasms and initiation of treatment. Treatment protocols also vary greatly from study to study, as do the preparations of ACTH used. For example, Hrachovy and coworkers (36), in an open trial, reported an 80 percent response rate to a regimen of short-term, low-dose ACTH therapy for IS in a cohort of five patients. The same authors, in a subsequent prospective, randomized trial with larger cohorts (24 patients receiving ACTH in each of two studies), reported response rates of 42 percent to 58 percent using the same protocol that had shown an 80 percent response rate in the open trial (35,37). Ito and colleagues (30) reported a 75 percent response to "low-dose" ACTH, using a long-acting, synthetic depot formulation of ACTH (1–24) compared with the short-acting, pituitary extract formulation of ACTH (1–39) used by North American

investigators. The findings of Ito and colleagues raise the possibility that lower amounts of the long-acting, depot preparations may be more equivalent to high doses of the short-acting preparations of ACTH.

Some consistency is conferred on many of the studies of high-dose ACTH therapy by the use of natural ACTH (1–39). The 1989 study by Snead and coworkers (38) consisted of an open, prospective trial of ACTH initiated at 150 IU/m^2/day in a cohort of 15 patients, most of whom had symptomatic spasms. All of these children were treated less than 2 months after onset of spasms, and half of them were receiving concomitant anticonvulsants, principally phenobarbital. The therapeutic efficacy of 90 percent obtained in this study is consistent with that demonstrated in a previous retrospective study by the same group (32) and with the response rate of 87 percent obtained in the prospective, randomized study by Baram and colleagues (34) in which high-dose ACTH was compared with prednisone therapy.

Singer (31) reported a lower efficacy rate with high-dose ACTH (74%). However, when one examines the 31 patients treated within 1 month of the onset of spasms, the response rate in the Singer study rises to 87 percent. By comparison, patients in that study who were treated after 1 or more months from the onset of spasms achieved a 58 percent response rate despite a long course of ACTH. These data suggest that the maximal beneficial response to high-dose therapy of IS may depend on a short lag time to treatment.

In a prospective study done in 1983, Lombroso (9) demonstrated a cessation of seizures in 49 percent of infantile spasm patients treated with high-dose ACTH. These data appear to be at odds with those from other published studies, both retrospective and prospective (31,32,34,38). However, there are some differences between the studies that may explain the discrepancy between these trials.

1. The dose used in the Lombroso study was lower (110 IU/m^2/day vs. 150 IU/m^2/day).
2. Response rates in the Lombroso study were reported for an endpoint 10 months after initiation of therapy, reflecting response minus relapses over that 10-month period rather than initial response.
3. None of Lombroso's patients received a second course of ACTH.
4. None of Lombroso's patients were receiving anticonvulsant therapy, a situation that has been advocated by some as decreasing relapse after ACTH treatment (40).
5. Seventy-one percent of the cryptogenic patients in the Lombroso study had ACTH treatment begun more than 1 month after the onset of IS. This

characteristic of the treatment trial alone has the potential to bias that study toward decreased response rates and outcome. Indeed, Lombroso reported a difference in outcome of the treatment of IS with ACTH relative to lag time from onset of spasms to initiation of treatment. The long-term rates of epilepsy in cryptogenic patients treated beyond 1 month of onset was 67 percent versus 33 percent in those treated within 1 month of onset of spasms.

Hrachovy and colleagues investigated high-dose versus low-dose ACTH in the treatment of IS in a randomized, prospective study (37) in which no difference between the two regimens was found. The relatively low responses in the high-dose (50%) and low-dose (58%) groups were surprising because there was a relatively high proportion of cryptogenic patients in whom one would predict a positive response. It is conceivable that the low response rate in this study may be the result of differing causes among the symptomatic patients; different responses of various etiologic subgroups to treatment regimens for IS are beginning to emerge in the literature (40,41).

Relapse of IS after treatment is not an infrequent occurrence. Relapse rates in the high-dose ACTH studies have ranged from 36 percent to 47 percent. However, in those studies many patients who relapsed during or after a defined course of ACTH subsequently were recontrolled with a second course of ACTH, yielding long-term response rates of 73 percent to 80 percent. Hrachovy and colleagues reported lower rates of relapse in the prospective high-dose versus low-dose ACTH study. However, a second course of ACTH apparently was not used to reestablish control in relapsers. When one compares the rates of response to high-dose ACTH after first relapse in Snead's studies (53% and 60%) and Lombroso's studies (42%) with that reported by Hrachovy (42%), there is little difference. It therefore appears that the initial use of high-dose ACTH, although important in controlling the acute manifestations of IS, must be accompanied in relapsers by a second course of ACTH to obtain the best long-term results.

In two other significant studies of the treatment of IS with ACTH and steroids the authors took a stepwise approach to treatment. In the first study by Schlumberger and Dulac in 1994 (40), patients were initially treated with a combination of hydrocortisone (15 mg/kg/day) and valproic acid (40 mg/kg/day). If a treatment response had been obtained by the end of the second week, the patients were weaned off hydrocortisone over the ensuing 2 weeks, but valproate was continued until the age of 12 to 18 months. If a treatment response to hydrocortisone was not observed, the patient was changed to high-dose synthetic ACTH

(1–25) (tetracoscatin 0.1 mg/kg/day = 10 IU/kg/day) for 2 weeks, followed by a tapering dose of hydrocortisone over 1 month while continuing valproate to 18 months of age. Seventy-five percent of patients responded to this regimen in the first 2 weeks. Fifteen patients relapsed within 1 month or failed the initial course of treatment and went on to receive ACTH. Nine of these ACTH-treated patients showed a complete response, yielding a combined response rate of 84 percent. Seventy-five percent of these remained spasm-free in the long term and 64 percent remained seizure-free. Relapse after ACTH treatment in this study did not result in a second course of ACTH. Although a second course of ACTH in relapsers might have improved the long-term response rates, Schlumberger and coworkers have demonstrated that the use of valproic acid, steroids, and ACTH in a stepwise fashion in selected patients with IS is as effective as has been reported using high-dose ACTH therapy in this disorder.

The second study applying a stepwise approach to the treatment of IS used only depot (long-acting) synthetic ACTH (42). Patients were tapered off all standard AEDs and begun on ACTH at 3 IU/kg/day. If a complete response was obtained at the end of 2 weeks and the spasms were cryptogenic, ACTH was rapidly tapered. If the spasms were symptomatic and a response was obtained at the end of 2 weeks, the dose was continued for an additional 2 weeks and then rapidly tapered. If no therapeutic response was observed in the initial 2-week period, the dose of ACTH was doubled to 6 IU/kg/day for an additional 2 weeks. The same strategy was employed at the 4-week point, responders being tapered off and nonresponders being increased to 12 IU/kg/day for 2 weeks. At the end of the 6 weeks, any patients still not responding were tapered off and other anticonvulsant therapy was instituted. Spasms were controlled initially in 65 percent of patients with a very high relapse rate. In this study population 40 percent of patients had a treatment lag of more than 1 month after the onset of spasms. Seven percent of the patients had experienced IS for close to 1 year before ACTH treatment was started. The long lag to treatment, without the use of any other anticonvulsants, and the decision to forgo a second course of ACTH in relapsers may have contributed to the relatively low response rate reported in this study. Nevertheless, these two studies provide a basis for a stepwise approach to the treatment of IS in which the dose of drug is predicated on treatment response rather than being determined empirically.

The relative efficacy of vigabatrin in IS compared with that of ACTH and steroids is not clear. In 1991 vigabatrin was shown to be useful in the treatment of IS refractory to steroids (17). Subsequent studies have validated the initial observation of efficacy but were all open label trials (43–46) and showed a high incidence of relapse of spasms in children treated with vigabatrin (47). Chiron and coworkers (17) found that vigabatrin was more effective in controlling symptomatic spasms than cryptogenic spasms in a group of patients with spasms refractory to steroids and other anticonvulsants. Also, vigabatrin has been found to be significantly more effective than hydrocortisone in tuberous sclerosis patients with IS (41).

The only prospective trial of vigabatrin versus ACTH published to date (18) used a depot formulation of ACTH in a dose of 10 IU/day in a small number of patients with little follow-up. This low dose of ACTH is comparable to the dose of depot ACTH used by Ito and coworkers (30). The initial response rate for ACTH-treated patients was 74 percent versus 48 percent in the vigabatrin group. Despite post-ACTH treatment with benzodiazepines, ACTH-treated patients had a higher relapse rate after tapering than did those children who continued receiving vigabatrin. The resulting response rates after relapse were 42 percent and 43 percent associated with ACTH and vigabatrin, respectively. No second course of ACTH was instituted. Vigabatrin appeared to be more effective in controlling spasms in symptomatic patients with cerebral malformations; however, the data were insufficient to determine whether vigabatrin was superior to ACTH in the treatment of spasms that resulted from tuberous sclerosis. ACTH was found to be more effective in symptomatic patients whose spasms were secondary to perinatal hypoxic-ischemic encephalopathy, a finding consistent with that of Dulac and colleagues (17,40,41). There also was a trend toward a superior efficacy of ACTH in the cryptogenic population, and ACTH was noted to normalize the EEG more rapidly than vigabatrin, regardless of etiology. This last observation is very important in view of the fact that normalization of the EEG during the course of treatment of IS is a powerful predictor of favorable outcome (10).

Effects of Treatment on Long-Term Cognitive Outcome After Infantile Spasms

Impairment of cognitive development in most symptomatic and many cryptogenic IS patients appears to be inevitable based on the cognitive sequelae of the original insult to the brain, identified or not. Although the severity of the inciting insult certainly dictates the minimum severity of mental impairment, the question remains unanswered whether further impairment of cognitive development is associated with the phenomenon of ongoing IS and, if so, whether treatment of the spasms will affect the long-term cognitive outcome. The latter question was addressed by Sher and Sheikh (11) in a group of children with symptomatic spasms. These authors examined the cognitive

level of symptomatic patients at the time of onset of spasms and at a mean follow-up of 3 years. Sixty-seven percent of patients who failed to respond to ACTH treatment were shown to have a deterioration in developmental level. Conversely, of those patients who responded to ACTH with complete cessation of spasms, only 17 percent deteriorated, 65 percent maintained their developmental level, and 17 percent of patients improved their developmental level. This is an important study because developmental data were collected *before* initiation of treatment of the spasms and at follow-up. The data from this study suggest that patients with existing mental retardation do suffer further cognitive decline during the course of IS. In addition, the data suggest that treatment that stops the spasms also benefits cognitive outcome.

Two prospective studies in the literature have examined long-term cognitive outcome in ACTH-treated and steroid-treated patients. Glaze and coworkers (39) reported that there was no difference in long-term cognitive or seizure outcome between prednisone (2 mg/kg/d) or low-dose ACTH (20–30 IU/day), but the study population was rather small. Lombroso (9) reported outcome data in a larger group of patients with cryptogenic IS treated with ACTH or steroids. This study showed that 55 percent of patients treated with high-dose ACTH (110 IU/m^2/day) had normal development at 6-year follow-up versus 12 percent normal outcome in prednisone-treated patients (2 mg/kg/day). Taken together, these two studies raise the possibility that moderate to high-dose ACTH results in a better long-term developmental outcome than low-dose ACTH or steroids, at least in the cryptogenic group. This conclusion is supported by the retrospective study of Lerman and Kivity (13), who found that ACTH doses of either 80 IU/day of ACTH gel or 40 IU/day of depot-synthetic ACTH (tetracoscatrin) resulted in a normal cognitive outcome in 100 percent of cryptogenic patients treated within 1 month of the onset of IS, whereas smaller amounts of ACTH resulted in normal cognitive outcome in only 60 percent of cryptogenic patients treated early.

The superiority of high-dose versus low-dose ACTH in terms of a better long-term cognitive outcome in patients with symptomatic IS is supported by the retrospective study of Sher and Sheikh (11). They demonstrated that children with symptomatic spasms treated with high doses of ACTH (>80 IU/m^2/day) begun within 1 month of the onset of the spasms showed better response rates and better long-term cognitive outcome than those children who were treated at a similar early time in the course of the spasms with lower doses of ACTH.

Two retrospective studies have examined the effect of low-dose and high-dose ACTH on outcome after IS in cohorts that combined cryptogenic and symptomatic patients. The majority of patients in these two cohorts suffered from symptomatic spasms. Ito and coworkers (30) reported a long-term follow-up study in one of these cohorts, 90 percent of whom were symptomatic. Those patients in this study who were treated with the highest dose used, 50 IU/m²/day, had a better mental outcome than those children treated with smaller doses of ACTH. The other combined cohort, 86 percent of whom were symptomatic, was reported by Riikonen (21), who found that only 5 percent of the children treated with *very* high-dose ACTH (120–140 IU/day or 400 + IU/m²/day) had normal cognitive outcomes versus 17 percent with normal cognitive outcome in the group treated with "low-dose" ACTH (20–40 IU/day or 80–120 IU/m²/day). The high-dose regimen employed by Riikonen is three times higher than the highest doses used by other investigators and was a long-acting, depot formulation. The low-dose ACTH regimen in this study was in a range considered high-dose by most investigators. Some authors have suggested that the poor outcomes reported by Riikonen among those patients whose IS were treated with very high-dose ACTH may reflect an adverse influence of supramaximal doses of ACTH on brain development (30).

The effect of treatment lag on cognitive outcome has been examined prospectively by both Lombroso (9) and Glaze and colleagues (39). Lombroso examined cryptogenic patients treated with ACTH within 1 month of onset of the spasms and found a normal IQ in 52 percent of patients at 6-year follow-up compared with 27 percent of children with a normal IQ in the group in which treatment was instituted more than 1 month after the onset of spasms. The conclusion from that study was that delay in treatment has an adverse effect on cognitive outcome in children with cryptogenic IS. Glaze and colleagues, however, reached the opposite conclusion: that time from onset of spasms to the beginning of treatment makes no difference in the ultimate prognosis in children with IS. However, an examination of data from the limited number of cryptogenic patients in the Glaze study suggests an alternative conclusion that comports more with that derived from the Lombroso study. All of the children with cryptogenic spasms in the Glaze study who responded to treatment began their therapy within 5 weeks of the onset of IS, but there were only four children in this group. Two of these children had a normal outcome, whereas the other two showed moderate cognitive impairment; however, of those children with cryptogenic spasms in this study who were nonresponders, 75 percent were treated more than 5 weeks after the onset of spasms. None of the children who were treated relatively late had normal development, and three were severely to profoundly retarded. Thus

one might reasonably conclude from the Glaze study that treatment delay in children with cryptogenic IS may have the potential to decrease response rates to therapy and thereby lead to a poorer cognitive outcome than that seen in children treated within 1 month of onset of spasms.

Although the response rates of symptomatic patients to either low-dose ACTH or prednisone were not significantly different in the study by Glaze and colleagues whether treatment was instituted early or late, 70 percent of the patients with symptomatic spasms were treated late. Better response rates might have been achieved if more intensive and early treatment were given to this more difficult to treat population. Among the symptomatic responders, severe to profound impairment occurred in 54 percent of patients treated early. In contrast, 78 percent of responding patients treated late had an outcome characterized by severe to profound impairment. Among the symptomatic nonresponders, no difference in cognitive outcome could be demonstrated between those treated early or late. In fact, no patient — cryptogenic or symptomatic — who failed to respond to treatment had a normal or even mildly impaired outcome. One would reasonably conclude from the Glaze data that cognitive outcome is optimized among children with IS who respond to early steroid treatment. The same conclusion was formed from the retrospective study of Sher and Sheikh and is supported by other authors (10,21,48–51).

The optimal dose of ACTH required to enhance cognitive outcome remains to be established; however, relatively high doses given early in the course of the disease appear to be indicated. Some investigators have suggested that better cognitive outcomes are achieved in cryptogenic patients when high-dose ACTH is used even though spasm control may be achieved in similar patients with smaller doses of ACTH or even with anticonvulsants alone (13).

Finally, little work has been done to examine the effect of the treatment of IS on behavioral outcomes. There is one retrospective report that suggests there may be a beneficial effect of ACTH on behavioral outcome in cryptogenic IS, particularly with respect to autistic features (52). Oral corticosteroids have not been studied in this regard.

Recommended Protocols for the Treatment of Infantile Spasms

Although there clearly is a lack of consensus for the best way to treat IS, an aggressive approach in which high-dose ACTH used as soon as the diagnosis is made is most consistently supported by the literature. Whether adjuvant anticonvulsant therapy is of added value remains unclear. In patients with tuberous sclerosis and those with cerebral malformations, the choice of vigabatrin as a first-line drug has some support in the literature, but more study of vigabatrin versus ACTH with long-term follow-up is needed before any conclusions can be made. The high-dose ACTH regimen described next (32,38), with which we have had a very good success rate in more than 500 children, is currently recommended for all IS patients.

ACTH

If the decision is made to use ACTH to treat IS, the child should be admitted to the hospital or a day-care unit to begin the ACTH; monitor blood pressure, urine, and electrolytes; and teach the parents to give the injection, measure urine glucose three times daily with Chemstix, and recognize spasms so they can keep an accurate seizure calendar. In addition, any diagnostic workup indicated by clinical circumstances is carried out during this initial evaluation. An endocrine profile, complete blood count (CBC), urinalysis, electrolytes, baseline renal function, calcium, phosphorus, and serum glucose are obtained before starting the ACTH. The drug is not begun if any of these studies are abnormal.

Diagnostic neuroimaging is indicated before the initiation of ACTH or steroid therapy in IS because of the propensity of the therapy to be associated with ventriculomegaly (see "Side Effects of ACTH and Steroids"). The neuroimaging procedure of choice is a magnetic resonance imaging (MRI) study because this procedure is more likely than a computed tomography (CT) scan to detect cortical dysplasias and other migrational abnormalities. It is very important to make the appropriate diagnosis of such a structural abnormality because it places the child into the symptomatic category of IS with the poorer prognosis that implies.

The recommended initial dose of ACTH is 150 IU/m^2/day of ACTH gel, 80 IU/mL, intramuscularly in two divided doses for 1 week. The second week the dose is 75 IU/m^2/day in one daily dose for 1 week. The third week the dose is 75 IU/m^2 every other day for 1 week. The ACTH is gradually tapered over the next 6 weeks. The lot number of the ACTH gel is carefully recorded. A treatment response usually is seen within the first 7 days, but if no response is seen in 2 weeks, the lot is changed.

When the patient is sent home from day care or from the hospital (day 2), arrangements must be made for daily blood pressure measurement at home the first week, then three times weekly after that. If hypertension occurs, attempts are made to control it with salt restriction and diuretic therapy rather than stopping the ACTH. The patient is followed up in the outpatient clinic weekly for the first month and then biweekly. A waking and sleeping EEG is obtained at 1, 2, and 4 weeks after the start of ACTH to determine the

treatment response. It has been suggested (36,53) that the only way to determine such a therapeutic response is by remonitoring the patient with EEG-video telemetry because the parents do not recognize the spasms. However, it would appear that because the treatment response is usually all or none (36,53), a positive treatment response is suggested when parents trained to recognize spasms observe no seizures in a child in whom the waking and sleeping EEG has normalized.

Using this regimen, a high relapse rate (50%) during the tapering period has been reported, particularly in the symptomatic patients. When this occurs, the dose may be increased to the previously effective dose for 2 weeks and then another taper begun. If the seizures continue in the face of such a dose increase, the dose may be increased to 150 units/m^2/day and the regimen begun again.

Prednisone

If one wishes to use prednisone because of the ease of oral administration and the lower incidence of serious side effects, the same pretreatment laboratory evaluation is recommended. The initial dose is 3 mg/kg/day in four divided doses for 2 weeks, followed by a 10-week taper (32). The reason for the multiple daily dose regimen is that children treated with the high-dose ACTH protocol have been shown to have sustained elevations of plasma cortisol rather than the usual peaks and valleys (36,38). Because of the short half-life of prednisone, the best way to produce a sustained plasma level of the steroid is to give frequent daily doses.

Side Effects of ACTH and Steroids

ACTH and steroids are dangerous medications, particularly at the high doses recommended. However, the morbidity and mortality reported by Riikonen and Donner (54) with ACTH seem exceptionally high, perhaps because synthetic ACTH was used. The side effects undoubtedly are more frequent and pronounced with ACTH than with steroids. Virtually all children develop cushingoid features. Most show extreme irritability early in the course, and a few develop hypertension. One should be constantly alert for sepsis, glucosuria, metabolic abnormalities involving electrolytes, calcium, and phosphorus (55–57), and congestive heart failure (58,59).

An additional side effect of ACTH is cerebral ventriculomegaly (60–66), which is not always reversible (65) and has the potential to lead to subdural hematoma (67,68). The cause of the apparent cerebral atrophy is obscure, but this phenomenon emphasizes the importance of performing diagnostic neuroimaging in children with IS before initiation of ACTH.

Hypothalamic-pituitary or adrenocortical dysfunction may occur as a result of ACTH therapy (69,70), so one must always use caution when withdrawing these children from ACTH. While tapering ACTH, one should monitor A.M. levels of cortisol and treat any medical stress with high-dose steroids (71). Treatment with either ACTH or steroids can cause immunosuppression, which may be associated with many infectious complications, perhaps because of impairment of polymorphonuclear leukocyte function (72). The practical ramifications of this side effect is that both ACTH and steroids are contraindicated in the face of a serious bacterial or viral infection such as varicella or cytomegalovirus. Finally, ACTH rarely may make seizures worse (73,74).

The Vigabatrin Alternative

If one wishes to use vigabatrin because immunosuppression is contraindicated in the face of congenital or acquired infection or because tuberous sclerosis or cerebral malformations are present, a dose of 100–150 mg/kg/day for 12 to 18 months is recommended (41). Vigabatrin is significantly better tolerated than ACTH; however, it also has behavioral side effects that consist of somnolence, hypotonia, and extreme irritability and agitation (18). Of greater concern are recent reports of permanent visual field cuts in patients treated with vigabatrin (75,76). There currently are seven such case reports in adult patients in the literature. The incidence of this side effect is about 30 percent. The problem is further complicated by the fact that there is no way to monitor for this complication in infants.

USE OF ACTH AND STEROIDS IN SEIZURES OTHER THAN INFANTILE SPASMS

Although the therapeutic efficacy of ACTH and steroids in controlling seizures in IS is well documented, the benefit of these medications in other types of seizures is less well substantiated. Two such syndromes, Ohtahara's syndrome and Lennox-Gastaut syndrome, are considered by many to represent early and later manifestations of a spectrum of infantile epileptic encephalopathies that includes IS (77–79). Evolution of Ohtahara's syndrome into IS followed by Lennox-Gastaut syndrome is not uncommon (80). The evolution of IS patients into Lennox-Gastaut syndrome occurs in 30 percent of patients (81).

Landau-Kleffner syndrome also may benefit from ACTH or steroid treatment. This syndrome is now also viewed by many as part of a spectrum of disorders in which cognitive and behavioral regressions are associated with evolving abnormalities of the waking and/or sleep EEG, with or without

clinical seizures (82,83). The spectrum includes continuous spike and wave in slow-wave sleep (CSWS) in which electrographic abnormalities during sleep are similar to those in Landau-Kleffner syndrome and Lennox-Gastaut syndrome (83). This raises the possibility that Ohtahara's syndrome, IS, Lennox-Gastaut syndrome, Landau-Kleffner syndrome, and related disorders may be parts of an even larger spectrum of disorders of brain development with variable clinical manifestations based on age at onset, maturational changes of the brain, degree of severity, and underlying pathoetiologic abnormalities. This possibility is supported by the fact that all these conditions often respond poorly to traditional anticonvulsant therapies but do, in some cases, respond well to the same spectrum of AEDs that are used in IS (i.e., ACTH, steroids, benzodiazepines, and valproic acid). The limited study of vigabatrin in these conditions suggests that it also may belong on this list (17,84,85).

Opsoclonus-myoclonus and Rasmussen's encephalitis are two other epileptic syndromes in which ACTH and steroids have been used. Both of these syndromes are characterized by intractable and malignant seizures as well as neurologic and cognitive impairment. The pathophysiologic mechanisms that underlie these disorders are not known but have been speculated to be immunologically mediated, either postinfectious or parainfectious or, in the case of opsoclonus-myoclonus, paraneoplastic. Therefore, in these two disorders the therapeutic benefit of prednisone and ACTH may be related to the immunosuppressive effects of these drugs. Alternatively, some have suggested that ACTH may have a direct brain stem effect in opsoclonus-myoclonus (86). Tolerance to ACTH with reemergence of the myoclonic symptoms in these patients has been associated with high anti-ACTH antibodies despite preserved cortisol responsiveness to the antibody-bound ACTH (86). Such an antimyoclonic action of ACTH could be implicated in its efficacy in Rasmussen's encephalitis as well.

Ohtahara's Syndrome

Ohtahara's syndrome, which is also known as early infantile epileptic encephalopathy (EIEE), is characterized by the onset of spasms often within the first week of life associated with burst-suppression on the EEG. The etiology may be cryptogenic (87), but symptomatic causes are often similar to those described for IS and include cerebral dysgenesis in particular (77,88). Seizures may be intractable to all modes of AED therapy, including ACTH and steroids. The infants manifest severe developmental delays, and their prognosis is grave, with most evolving to profound mental retardation or death (84,89). Although there are isolated reports of improvement of spasms and EEG after treatment with ACTH (89) and vigabatrin (84), the long-term prognosis is generally unchanged by any treatment. If used in the treatment of Ohtahara's syndrome, ACTH should be administered using the regimen previously described for IS.

Lennox-Gastaut Syndrome and Related Seizure Disorders

ACTH and steroids have been found to be useful in younger children with multiple seizure types that are severe and intractable, particularly those with atypical absence, myoclonic, tonic, and atonic seizures in varying combinations (1,32,90–95). This includes the Lennox-Gastaut syndrome, a disorder characterized by mental retardation, generalized slow spike-and-wave discharges, intractable atypical absence, myoclonus, and frequent ictal falls (96). Several uncontrolled, retrospective studies suggest that ACTH is superior to oral steroids against these types of seizures (32,90–92). The same regimen for ACTH or prednisone described previously is recommended for the treatment of the severe multiple seizure types in Lennox-Gastaut syndrome. ACTH and steroids are drugs of last resort when used in this fashion and should be employed only after an aggressive, logical trial of other, more standard anticonvulsant drugs has been attempted and found wanting. Usually the best one can hope for with ACTH or steroids in this situation is temporary relief because 70 percent to 90 percent of patients with multiple seizure types suffer a relapse of seizures during the tapering process (32).

Landau-Kleffner Syndrome and Related Disorders

Landau-Kleffner syndrome (LKS), which was first described in 1957 (97), is also known as *acquired epileptic aphasia* and is characterized by a regression in receptive and expressive language associated with epileptic seizures. Children with this disorder usually present between the ages of 2 and 8 years. Clinical seizures may precede or be coincident with language deterioration in 40 percent to 50 percent of patients; however, 20 percent to 30 percent of patients with LKS develop seizures months after the onset of language loss, and up to 25 percent of children with language loss and epileptiform EEGs never develop clinical seizures (98). In addition to language regression, affected children frequently exhibit a behavioral disturbance that ranges from hyperactivity and aggressivity to autism and global cognitive deterioration. Although some children with LKS display sustained agnosia and mutism, others show a waxing and waning course that parallels the changes on EEG. Still others resolve spontaneously. The typical EEG of LKS shows 1 to 3 Hz spikes and spike-and-slow waves of high amplitude. These may be unilateral, bilateral, unifocal, or multifocal but often include the temporal region with or without parietal and occipital involvement. These features are enhanced during sleep and, features of continuous spike and wave are seen to occupy large parts of the sleep record early in the course of the disorder (98).

Although valproate and benzodiazepines may be effective in controlling clinical seizures in LKS, the effect of these drugs on the EEG abnormalities that accompany this syndrome may be partial and transient (99,100). The beneficial effect of ACTH on seizures, language regression, and behavioral changes in LKS was first reported by McKinney and McGreal in 1974 (101). Of nine patients described in this retrospective study, three were treated with ACTH and all had rapid normalization in language comprehension and speech with no further seizures. The other six patients were treated with anticonvulsants alone and in one case temporal lobectomy. Five of the six became seizure-free on anticonvulsants, but language normalized in only one.

No controlled prospective trials of ACTH or steroids in LKS have been published; however, several additional reports on the utility of these compounds in LKS are in the literature. In two isolated case reports, improvement was seen in both seizures and language after treatment with prednisone or prednisolone, although both authors believed this effect was likely the result of coincidental remission of the disorder (102,103). In the studies by Marescaux, Hirsch, and coworkers (99,100), a series of five patients with LKS were described, three of whom were treated with prednisone or hydrocortisone in combination with valproate. All three steroid-treated patients had resolution of their language and seizure disorders; however, the two children whose treatment was begun more than 2 years from the onset of speech arrest had residual deficits. The two remaining patients treated with anticonvulsants alone both responded transiently to clobazam and valproate and then relapsed.

Lerman and colleagues (104) reported four children with LKS, one treated with ACTH (80 IU/day) and three treated with corticosteroids (prednisone 60 mg/day or dexamethasone 4 mg/day). All patients showed resolution of the seizure disorder and normalization of language, although the response was fastest in those treated shortly after the onset of language regression. In two cases relapse of aphasia occurred: in one on tapering of steroids, and in the other 2 years after ACTH was discontinued. Both patients responded to retreatment with steroids with subsequent sustained language normalization.

The most recent report on steroid use in LKS is from Guerreiro and colleagues (105), who published results on four children treated with prednisone (20–40 mg/day). Seizure control and language improvement were obtained in all patients, but language normalized in none. All four patients had single photon emission computed tomography (SPECT) scans showing abnormalities in the left temporal lobes, which improved minimally (3%) after treatment. The poorer outcomes in this study may reflect treatment with lower doses of corticosteroids.

At the present time, the use of ACTH or corticosteroids in patients with Landau-Kleffner syndrome appears justified; however, further study of dose and duration of therapy is warranted, as is exploration of the newer anticonvulsants in the treatment of this condition. We currently would recommend high-dose ACTH or prednisone as outlined in the section on IS with consideration given to incorporating longer tapering schedules and the use of concomitant valproic acid. Further study is necessary before steroids can be recommended for children with acquired aphasia with focal cortical abnormalities on functional imaging who do not show EEG abnormalities consistent with Landau-Kleffner syndrome.

Opsoclonus-Myoclonus

Opsoclonus-myoclonus (OM), also known as dancing eyes syndrome, is a movement disorder characterized by chaotic, nonconjugate, rapid eye movements often accompanied by myoclonic seizures and ataxia as well as deterioration in cognitive and behavioral functioning. Up to one half of patients have an occult neuroblastoma. The remainder of children with opsoclonus-myoclonus have a viral or postinfectious etiology. Resection of the neuroblastoma generally does not affect any of the neurologic manifestations in the paraneoplastic patients (106). Treatment with ACTH has been beneficial in suppressing the neurologic symptoms acutely in 80 percent to 90 percent of patients with opsoclonus-myoclonus (107); however, symptoms may persist long-term in up to 15 percent of patients (106). Although some improvement in the acute cognitive and behavioral manifestations of opsoclonus-myoclonus may occur over time on ACTH therapy, up to 90 percent of children are left with motor delays and specific cognitive and behavioral deficits (106,108–110). Other agents used in the treatment of opsoclonus-myoclonus include prednisone, intravenous immunoglobulin G (IgG), valproic acid, and propranolol, but ACTH is the drug of choice (107). The ACTH regimen recommended for opsoclonus-myoclonus is the same as that for IS; however, relapse rates of up to 90 percent (110) have been reported, and repeated courses with quite prolonged tapering are required in some patients to maintain control of the neurologic manifestations.

Rasmussen's Encephalitis

Rasmussen's encephalitis is a focal progressive inflammatory condition of the brain of unclear etiology. There is growing evidence that the disease is immunologically mediated, in some cases through an autoantibody response against the GluR3 glutamate receptor subunit in the brain (111–113) and may be either postinfectious or parainfectious (114). Rasmussen's encephalitis is characterized by malignant, progressive, and intractable partial seizures with a high incidence of epilepsia partialis continua. The progressive nature of Rasmussen's encephalitis ultimately leads to involvement of the entire affected hemisphere, with specific and invariably severe cognitive and motor impairments related to the dominance of the involved hemisphere. Treatments advocated for Rasmussen's encephalitis include anticonvulsants, high-dose steroids, ACTH, intravenous IgG, plasmapheresis antiviral agents, or hemispherectomy (115). Two studies support the use of steroids in Rasmussen's encephalitis. In 1992 Dulac (116) reported the results of intravenous high-dose methylprednisolone (400 mg/m^2), followed by oral prednisone, in seven Rasmussen's patients with epilepsia partialis continua. Six of the seven patients showed an improvement in seizure control, which was variably sustained over a 2-year follow-up period. Hart (117) reported a benefit of steroids in Rasmussen's encephalitis with 10 of 17 patients showing a reduction of 25 percent to 75 percent in seizure frequency.

THE NEUROSTEROIDS

A new class of neurosteroids with anticonvulsant activity are derivatives of progesterone and are termed *epalons* (118). These compounds are synthesized in the brain, have been reproduced pharmacologically, and have been shown to have both convulsant and anticonvulsant properties in animal models of epilepsy. Epalons are capable of rapidly altering the excitability of neurons by direct actions on ligand-gated ion channels, particularly the GABA$_A$ receptor complex (119,120). One such epalon, ganaxalone, underwent clinical trials to determine its therapeutic effect on epilepsy in humans; however, the role of these compounds in the treatment of epilepsy in children remains to be established, and the development of ganaxalone came to a halt because of insufficient evidence if efficacy in early double-blind testing.

MECHANISMS OF ACTION OF ACTH AND STEROIDS

The basic pathogenesis of IS and therefore the mechanisms of action of ACTH and steroids in alleviating this disorder are not known. ACTH is not generally anticonvulsant in most animal models of epilepsy, although little work has been done on this during critical periods of brain development (107). Rather, ACTH has proconvulsant (excitatory) effects, particularly in adrenalectomized, developing animal models (121,122). One of the major reasons for our lack of knowledge concerning the actions of ACTH and steroids in IS is that there is no known animal model for this disorder. Until a specific animal model of IS is found, the underlying abnormality and thus the mechanisms of action of ACTH, steroids, and other AEDs effective in this disorder can only be speculated.

To formulate hypotheses of the mechanism of action of ACTH and steroids in IS, one must reconcile the known biologic properties of these compounds with what is known of the pathogenesis of IS. Any theory of pathogenesis of IS must reconcile the following observations:

- IS is a disorder of very young children with a narrow window of age of onset.
- IS appear to be self-limited in time; that is, they either disappear or evolve into other types of seizures as the child grows older.
- There is associated massive myoclonus.
- There is an association with a hypsarrhythmic EEG.
- There is a marked decrease in rapid eye movement (REM) sleep in children with IS, yet the EEG abnormalities disappear during REM sleep.
- IS may respond to steroid and ACTH therapy and to AEDs that seem to act by GABAergic mechanisms.
- IS may result from a wide variety of anatomic abnormalities of brain or may have no apparent cause. Yet not all children with disorders associated with IS (e.g., tuberous sclerosis) are afflicted with spasms.
- There is very high morbidity in terms of subsequent cognitive delay and the development of autism.

The nature of the anticonvulsant effect of ACTH and corticosteroids seems to differ from that of conventional AEDs in IS because the effect of steroids in stopping seizures and normalizing the EEG in IS is frequently an all-or-none phenomenon. Moreover, in contrast to traditional AEDs, which have little or no effect on the natural history of epilepsy (123), the steroid-induced seizure-free state, when achieved, frequently is sustainable and long-lasting even when the drug is withdrawn shortly after efficacy has been established. These observations have led to the hypothesis that, within a very narrow developmental window, ACTH and steroids are capable of resetting a deranged homeostatic mechanism(s) in the brain, thereby decreasing the convulsive tendency and improving the developmental trajectory.

Mechanisms of Action of ACTH and the Melanocortins in the Brain

ACTH may play an indirect role in the development and function of the brain through its ability to stimulate adrenocorticosteroid production; however, there is strong evidence that ACTH and its peptide fragments, the melanocortins, also have a direct effect on the brain. ACTH could exert its anticonvulsant effects in IS through such an extraadrenal mechanism. In support of this hypothesis are the data previously cited, which suggest that ACTH is more effective than steroids in the treatment of IS as well as reports that ACTH is effective against IS in adrenal suppressed patients (94,124,125).

To date, no receptor for intact ACTH (1–39) has been found in the brain, which raises the possibility that the peptide may not have direct neuronal activity. However, the reason for the inability to identify a high affinity ACTH receptor site may be a technical one because radioactive labeling of the peptide may cause it to lose biologic activity and receptor affinity (107). In spite of the absence of evidence for a stereospecific, high affinity binding site for ACTH in the brain, there are now substantial physiologic and pharmacologic data to support the hypothesis that ACTH has a direct neurobiologic effect on brain function. These actions include increasing dendrite outsprouting in immature animals (107); stimulating myelination (126); modulating the regulation of synthesis, release, uptake, and metabolism of a number of neurotransmitters such as dopamine, norepinephrine, acetylcholine, serotonin, and γ-aminobutyric acid (GABA); and regulation of binding at glutamatergic, serotoninergic, muscarinic type 1, opiate, and dopaminergic receptors (127,128). In addition, ACTH has been shown to alter neuronal membrane lipid fluidity, permeability, and signal transduction (107). All these neurobiologic effects of ACTH have the potential to impact synaptic function and neurotransmission.

In some instances the ability of ACTH to exert these protean neurobiologic effects in the brain may reside in fragments of the peptide that are devoid of corticotrophic activity, further supporting the hypothesis that the direct effect of ACTH on neuronal function is independent of its corticotrophic action. Three CNS melanocortin receptors, MC3, MC4, and MC5, have been identified that show a high affinity for α-MSH, an ACTH fragment (ACTH 1–13) (129). Although ACTH-derived peptides, principally α-MSH, and analogues have been shown to have both pro- and anticonvulsant effects experimentally (107), these compounds have had no demonstrable therapeutic benefit when administered to children with IS (130,131).

Mechanisms of Action of Corticosteroids in the Brain

The direct anticonvulsant effects of corticosteroids appear to be limited (132). Recently, however, interest has been focused on the putative role of corticotrophin-releasing hormone (CRF) in the pathogenesis of IS. This peptide has been shown to be a potent convulsant (133–135). Furthermore, patients with IS have been shown to have low levels of ACTH and cortisol in the cerebrospinal fluid (CSF) (136,137). Thus, derangements of CRF synthesis and release have been postulated to play a role in the pathogenesis of IS, as have similar derangements of ACTH and steroids and hence their feedback on CRF production (138). However, it remains unclear what events might precipitate these endocrinologic abnormalities.

Pharmacologic manipulation of the hypothalamo-pituitary-adrenocortical (HPA) axis, circulating corticosteroid levels, and neurosteroids by treatment with exogenous ACTH, corticosteroids, or epalons would be expected to produce both specific and nonspecific alterations of neuronal function. Currently, however, it is completely unknown which changes affected by these treatment modalities in IS might explain their therapeutic efficacy in this disorder. In the absence of an animal model of IS, the answer to this question is unlikely to be forthcoming.

ACKNOWLEDGMENT

This work was supported in part by the Bloorview Children's Hospital Foundation

REFERENCES

1. Klein R, Livingston S. The effect of adrenocorticotropic hormone in epilepsy. *J Pediatr* 1950; 37:733–742.

2. Sorel L, Dusaucy-Bauloye A. A propos de cas d'hypsarythmia de Gibbs: son traitement spectaculaire par l'ACTH. *Acta Neurol Belg* 1958; 58:130–141.

3. Dumermuth G. Über die Blitz-Nick-Salaam-Krämpfe und ihre Behandlung mit ACTH und Hydrocortison. *Mitteilung Helv Ped Acta* 1959; 14:250–270.

4. Gastaut H, Salfiel J, Raybaud C, Pitot M, Meynadier AA. A propos du traitement par l'ACTH des encéphalities myoclonique de la première enfance avec majeure — (Hypsarythmia). *Pediatrie* 1959; 14:35–45.

5. Stamps FW, Gibbs EL, Rosenthal IM, Gibbs FA. Treatment of hypsarrhythmia with ACTH. *JAMA* 1959; 171:408–411.

6. McQuarrie I, Anderson JA, Ziegler RR. Observations on the antagonistic effects of posterior pituitary and cortico-adrenal hormones in the epileptic subject. *J Clin Endocrinol* 1942; 2:406–410.

7. Low NL. Infantile spasms with mental retardation: I. Treatment with cortisone and adrenocorticotropin. *Pediatrics* 1958; 22:1165–1169.

8. Hrachovy RA. ACTH and steroids. In: Engel J, Pedley TA, eds. *Epilepsy: A Comprehensive Textbook.* Philadelphia: Lippincott-Raven, 1997:1463–1473.

9. Lombroso CT. A prospective study of infantile spasms: clinical and therapeutic correlations. *Epilepsia* 1983; 24:135–158.

10. Koo B, Hwang P, Logan W, Hunjan A. Infantile spasms: outcome and prognosis factors of cryptogenic and symptomatic groups. *Neurology* 1993; 43:2322–2327.

11. Sher PK, Sheikh MR. Therapeutic efficacy of ACTH in symptomatic infantile spasms with hypsarrhythmia. *Pediatr Neurol* 1993; 9:451–456.

12. Marescaux C, Hirsch E, Finck S, et al. Landau-Kleffner syndrome. *Epilepsia* 1990; 31:768–777.

13. Lerman P, Kivity S. The efficacy of corticotropin in primary infantile spasms. *J Pediatr* 1982; 101:294–296.

14. West WJ. On a peculiar form of infantile convulsions. *Lancet* 1841; 1:724–725.

15. Gibbs FA, Gibbs EL. *Atlas of Electroencephalography.* Vol. 2: *Epilepsy.* Cambridge: Addison-Wesley, 1952.

16. Kellaway PR, Hrachovy RA, Frost JD, Zion TE. Precise characterization and quantification of infantile spasms. *Ann Neurol* 1079; 6:214–218.

17. Chiron C, Dulac O, Beaumont D, et al. Therapeutic trial of vigabatrin in refractory infantile spasms. *J Child Neurol* 1991; 6:(Suppl 2):S52–S59.

18. Vigevano F, Cilio MR. Vigabatrin versus ACTH as first-line treatment for infantile spasms: a randomized, prospective study. *Epilepsia* 1997; 38:1270–1274.

19. Carter RB, Wood PL, Weiland S, et al. Characterization of the anticonvulsant properties of ganaxalone 9CCD 1042: (3a-hydroxy-3B-methyl-5a-preganan-20-one), a selective, high-affinity, steroid modulator of the gamma-aminobutyric acid A receptor. *J Pharmacol Exp Ther* 1997; 280:1284–1295.

20. Hrachovy RA, Glaze DG, Frost JD. A retrospective study of spontaneous remission and long-term outcome in patients with infantile spasms. *Epilepsia* 1991; 32:212–214.

21. Riikonen R. A long-term follow-up study of 214 children with the syndrome of infantile spasms. *Neuropediatrics* 1982; 13:14–23.

22. Chevrie J, Aicardi J. Le prognostic psychique des spasms infantiles traites par l'ACTH ou les cortocoides. Analyse statistique de 78 cas suivis plus d'un an. *J Neurol Sci* 1971; 12:351–368.

23. Jeavons PM, Bower BD, Dimitrakoudi M. Long term prognosis of 150 cases of "West syndrome." *Epilepsia* 1973; 14:153–164.

24. Pollack MA, Zion TE, Kellaway PR. Long term prognosis of patients with infantile spasms following ACTH therapy. *Epilepsia* 1979; 20:255–260.

25. Nolte R, Christen HJ, Doerrer J. Preliminary report of a multi-center study on the West syndrome. *Brain Dev* 1988; 10:236–242.

26. Dulac O, Plouin P, Jambaque I, Motte J. Benign epileptic infantile spasms. *Rev Electroencephalogr Neurophysiol Clin* 1986; 16:371–382.

27. Favata I, Leuzzi V, Curalto P. Mental outcome in West syndrome: prognostic value of some clinical factors. *J Ment Defic Res* 1987; 31:9–15.

28. Snead OC, Chiron C. Medical treatment. In: Dulas O, Chugani HT, Dalla Bernardina B, eds. *Infantile Spasms and West Syndrome*. London: WB Saunders, 1994:244–256.

29. Snead OC III. Other antiepileptic drugs: adrenocorticotropic hormone (ACTH). In: Levy R, Mattson R, Meldrum B, Penry JK, Dreifuss FE, eds. *Antiepileptic Drugs*. New York: Raven Press, 1989:905–912.

30. Ito M, Okuno T, Fujii T, et al. ACTH therapy in infantile spasms: relationship between dose of ACTH and initial effect or long-term prognosis. *Ped Neurol* 1990; 6:240–244.

31. Singer WD, Rabe EF, Haller JS. The effect of ACTH therapy on infantile spasms. *J Pediatr* 1980; 96:485–489.

32. Snead OC, Benton JW, Myers GJ. ACTH and prednisone in childhood seizure disorders. *Neurology* 1983; 33:966–970.

33. Hrachovy RA, Frost JD, Kellaway PR, Zion TE. A controlled study of prednisone therapy in infantile spasms. *Epilepsia* 1979; 20:403–407.

34. Baram, TZ, Mitchell WG, Tournay A, et al. High-dose corticotrophin (ACTH) versus prednisone for infantile spasms: a prospective, randomized, blinded study. *Pediatrics* 1996; 97:375–379.

35. Hrachovy RA, Frost JD, Kellaway PR, Zion TE. Double-blind study of ACTH vs. prednisone therapy in infantile spasms. *J Pediatr* 1983; 103:641–645.

36. Hrachovy RA, Frost JD, Kellaway PR, Zion TE. A controlled study of ACTH therapy in infantile spasms. *Epilepsia* 1980; 21:631–636.

37. Hrachovy RA, Frost JD Jr, Glaze DG. High dose/long duration vs low dose/short duration corticotropin therapy in infantile spasms: A single blind study. *J Pediatr* 1994; 124: 803–806.

38. Snead OC, Benton JW, Hosey LC, et al. Treatment of infantile spasms with high dose ACTH: efficacy and plasma levels of ACTH and cortisol. *Neurology* 1989; 39:1027–1030.

39. Glaze DG, Hrachovy RA, Frost JD, Kellaway PR, Zion TE. Prospective study of outcome of infants with infantile spasms treated during controlled studies of ACTH and prednisone. *J Pediatr* 1988; 112:389–396.

40. Schlumberger E, Dulac O. A simple, effective and well-tolerated treatment regime for West syndrome. *Dev Med Child Neuro* 1994; 36:863–872.

41. Chiron C, Dumas C, Jambaque I, Mumford J, Dulac O. Randomized trial comparing vigabatrin and hydrocortisone in infantile spasms due to tuberous sclerosis. *Epilepsy Res* 1997; 26:389–395.

42. Heiskala H, Riikonen R, Santavuori P, et al. West syndrome: individualized ACTH therapy. *Brain Dev* 1996; 18:456–460.

43. Livingston JH, Beaumont D, Arzimanoglou A. Vigabatrin in the treatment of epilepsy in children. *Br J Clin Pharmacol* 1989; 27:S109–S112.

44. Vles BIS, Van der Heyden AMHG, Ghils A, Troost J. Vigabatrin in the treatment of infantile spasms. *Neuropediatrics* 1993; 24:230–231.

45. Aicardi J, Mumford JP, Dumas C, Wood S. Vigabatrin as initial therapy for infantile spasms: a European retrospective survey. Sabril IS. Investigator and Peer Review Groups. *Epilepsia* 1996; 37:638–642.

46. Kwong L. Vigabatrin as first-line therapy in infantile spasms: review of seven patients. *J Ped Child Health* 1997; 33:121–124.

47. Appleton ER. The role of vigabatrin in the management of infantile epileptic syndromes. *Neurology* 1993; 43(Suppl 5):S21–S23.

48. Singer WD, Haller JS, Sullivan LR, et al. The value of neuroradiology in infantile spasms. *J Pediatr* 1982; 100:47–50.

49. Matsumoto A, Watanabe K, Negoro T, et al. Prognostic factors of infantile spasms from the etiological viewpoint. *Brain Dev* 1981; 3:361–364.

50. Matsumoto A, Kumagai T, Takeuchi T, Miyazaki S, Watanabe K. Clinical effects of thryotropin-releasing hormone for severe epilepsy in childhood: a comparative study with ACTH therapy. *Epilepsia* 1987; 28:49–55.

51. Fois A, Malandrini F, Balestri G, Giorgi D. Infantile spasms—Long term results of ACTH treatment. *Eur J Pediatr* 1984; 142:51–55.

52. Martien KM, Banwell B, Hwang PA, Roberts W. ACTH treatment in cryptogenic infantile spasms: effects on later autistic features. *Epilepsia* 1997; 38(Suppl 8):184.

53. Kellaway PR, Frost JD, Hrachovy RA. Infantile spasms. In: Morselli PL, C Pippenger C, Penry JK, eds. *Antiepileptic Drug Therapy in Pediatrics*. New York: Raven Press, 1983:115–136.

54. Riikonen R, Donner M. ACTH therapy in infantile spasms: side effects. *Arch Dis Child* 1980; 55:664–672.

55. Riikonen R, Simell O, Jääskeläinen J, Rapola J, Perheentupa J. Disturbed calcium and phosphate homeostasis during treatment with ACTH of infantile spasms. *Arch Dis Child* 1986; 61:671–676.

56. Rausch HP. Medullary nephrocalcinosis and pancreatic calcifications demonstrated by ultrasound and CT in infants after treatment with ACTH. *Radiology* 1984; 153:105–107.

57. Hanefeld F, Sperner J, Rating D, Rausch H, Kaufmann HJ. Renal and pancreatic calcification during treatment of infantile spasms with ACTH. *Lancet* 1984; 1:901.

58. Alpert BS. Steroid-induced hypertrophic cardiomyopathy in an infant. *Pediatr Cardiol* 1984; 5:117–118.

59. Tacke E, Kupferschmid C, Lang D. Hypertrophic cardiomyopathy during ACTH treatment. *Klin Padiatr* 1983; 195:124–128.

60. Deona T, Voumard C. Reversible cerebral atrophy and corticotropin. *Lancet* 1979; 2:207.

61. Lagenstein I, Willig RP, Kuhne D. Cranial computed tomography (CCT) findings in children treated with ACTH and dexamethasone: first results. *Neuropädiatrie* 1979; 10:370–384.

62. Maekawa K, Ohta H, Tamai I. Transient brain shrinkage in infantile spasms after ACTH treatment. Report of two cases. *Neuropadiatrie* 1980; 11:80–84.

63. Lyen KR, Holland IM, Lyen YC. Reversible cerebral atrophy in infantile spasms caused by corticotropin. *Lancet* 1979; 2:237–238.

64. Howitz P, Neergaard K, Pedersen H. Cranial computed tomography in infantile spasms. Primary findings related to long-term mental prognosis. *Acta Paediatr Scand* 1990; 79:1087–1091.

65. Glaze DG, Hrachovy RA, Frost JD, Zion TE, Bryan RN. Computed tomography in infantile spasms: effects of hormonal therapy. *Pediatr Neurol* 1986; 2:23–27.

66. Konishi Y, Yasujima M, Kuriyama M, et al. Magnetic resonance imaging in infantile spasms: effects of hormonal therapy. *Epilepsia* 1992; 33:304–309.

67. Hara K, Watanabe K, Miyazaki S, et al. Apparent brain atrophy and subdural hematoma following ACTH therapy. *Brain Dev* 1981; 3:45–49.

68. Okuno T, Ito M, Konishi Y, Yoshioka M, Nakano Y. Cerebral atrophy following ACTH therapy. *J Comput Assist Tomogr* 1980; 4:20–23.

69. Rao JK, Willis J. Hypothalamo-pituitary-adrenal function in infantile spasms: effects of ACTH therapy. *J Child Neurol* 1987; 2:220–223.

70. Ross DL. Suppressed pituitary ACTH response after ACTH treatment of infantile spasms. *J Child Neurol* 1986; 1:34–37.

71. Perheentupa J, Riikonen R, Dunkel L, Simell O. Adrenocortical hyporesponsiveness after treatment with ACTH of infantile spasms. *Arch Dis Child* 1986; 61:750–753.

72. Colleselli P, Milani M, Drigo P, et al. Impairment of polymorphonuclear leucocyte function during therapy with synthetic ACTH in children affected by epileptic encephalopathies. *Acta Paediatr Scand* 1986; 75:159–163.

73. Rutledge SL, Snead OC, Kelly DR, et al. Pyruvate carboxylase deficiency: acute exacerbation after ACTH treatment of infantile spasms. *Pediatr Neurol* 1989; 5:201–206.

74. Kanayama M, Ishikawa T, Tauchi A, et al. ACTH-induced seizures in an infant with West syndrome. *Brain Dev* 1989; 11:329–331.

75. Eke T, Talbot JF, Lawden MC. Severe persistent visual field constriction associated with vigabatrin. *Br Med J* 1997; 314:180–181.

76. Kramer G, Scollo-Lavizzari G, Jallon P, et al. Vigabatrin-associated bilateral concentric visual field defects in four patients. *Epilepsia* 1997; 38:179 (5.035).

77. Yamatogi Y, Ohtahara S. Age dependent epileptic encephalopathy: a longitudinal study. *Folia Psych Neurol Jap* 1981; 35 (3):321–332.

78. Donat JF. The age dependent epileptic encephalopathies. *J Child Neurol* 1992; 7:7–21.

79. Martinez BA, Roche C, Lopez-Martin V, Pascual Castroviejo I. Early infantile epileptic encephalopathy. *Rev Neurol* 1995; 23:297–300.

80. Chakova L. On a rare form of epilepsy in infancy: Ohtahara syndrome. *Folia Medica* 1996; 38:69–73.

81. Tuchman RF. Epilepsy, language and behavior. *J Child Neurol* 1994; 9:95–102.

82. Gross-Selbeck G. Treatment of "benign" partial epilepsies of childhood, including atypical forms. *Neuropediatrics* 1995; 26:45–50.

83. Deonna TW. Acquired epileptiform aphasia in children (Landau Kleffner syndrome). *J Clin Neurophys* 1991; 8:288–298.

84. Baxter PS, Gardner-Medwin D, Barwick DD, et al. Vigabatrin monotherapy in resistant neonatal seizures. *Seizure* 1995; 4:57–59.

85. Appleton R, Hughes A, Beirne M, Acomb B. Vigabatrin in the Landau-Kleffner syndrome. *Dev Med Child Neurol* 1993; 35:456–459.

86. Pranzetelli MR, Kao PC, Tate ED, et al. Antibodies to ACTH in opsoclonus-myoclonus. *Neuropediatrics* 1993; 24:131–133.

87. Clarke M, Gill J, Noronha M, McKinlay I. Early infantile epileptic encephalopathy with burst suppression: Ohtahara syndrome. *Dev Med Child Neurol* 1987; 29:520–528.

88. Ogahara M, Kinoue K, Takamiya H, et al. A case of early infantile epileptic encephalopathy (EIEE) with anatomical cerebral asymmetry and myoclonus. *Brain Dev* 1993; 15:133–139.

89. Campistol J. Garcia-Garcia JJ, Lobera E, et al. The Ohtahara syndrome: a special form of age dependent epilepsy. *Rev Neurol* 1997; 25: 212–214.

90. Dobbs JM, Baird HW. The use of corticotropin and a corticosteroid in patients with minor motor seizures. *Am J Dis Child* 1960; 100:584–585.

91. Lagenstein I, Willig RP, Iffland E. Behandlung fruhkindlicher Anfalle mit ACTH und Dexamethasone unter standardisierten Bedingungen. I. *Klinische Ergebnisse. Mschr Kindreheilk* 1978; 126:492–499.

92. Lagenstein I, Willig RP, Iffland E. Behandlung fruhkindlicher Anfalle mit ACTH und Dexamethasone unter standardisierten Bedingungen. II. *Elektrocencephalographische Beobachtungen. Mschr Kindreheilk* 1978; 126:500–506.

93. Paul L, O'Neal R, Ybanez M, Livingston S. Minor motor epilepsy. Treatment with corticotropin (ACTH) and steroid therapy. *JAMA* 1960; 172:1408–1412.

94. Willig RP, Lagenstein I, Iffland E. Cortisoltagesprofile unter ACTH und Dexamethason-Therapie fruhkindlicher Anfalle (BNS- und Lennox-Syndrom). *Mschr Kindreheilk* 1977; 126:191–197.

95. Kurakawa T, Nagahide G, Fukuyama Y, et al. West syndrome and Lennox-Gastaut syndrome: a survey of natural history. *Pediatrics* 1980; 65:81–88.

96. Snead OC. Pharmacology of epileptic falling spells. *Clin Neuropharm* 1987; 10:205–214.

97. Landau W, Kleffner FR. Syndrome of acquired aphasia with convulsive disorder in children. *Neurology* 1957; 7:523–530.

98. Appleon RE. The Landau Kleffner syndrome. *Arch Dis Child* 1995; 72:386–387.

99. Marescaux C, Hirsch E, Finck S, et al. Landau-Kleffner syndrome: a pharmacologic study of five cases. *Epilepsia* 1990; 31:768–777.

100. Hirsch E, Marescaux C, Finck S, et al. Landau-Kleffner syndrome: a clinical and EEG study of five cases. *Epilepsia* 1990; 31:756–767.

101. McKinney W, McGreal DA. An aphasic syndrome in children. *Can Med Asso J* 1974; 110:637–639.

102. Kellerman K. Recurrent aphasia with subclinical bioelectic status epilepticus during sleep. *Eur J Ped* 1978; 128:207–212.

103. Van der Sandt-Koenderman WME, Smit IAC, Van Dongen HR, Van Hest JBC. A case of acquired aphasia and convulsive disorder. Some linguistic aspects of recovery and breakdown. *Brain Lang* 1984; 21:174–183.

104. Lerman P, Lerman-Sagie T, Kivity S. Effect of early steroid therapy for Landau-Kleffner syndrome. *Dev Med Child Neurol* 1991; 33:257–266.

105. Guerreiro MM, Carmargo EE, Kato M, et al. Brain single photon emission computed tomography imaging in Landau-Kleffner syndrome. *Epilepsia* 1996; 37:60–67.

106. Koh P, Raffensperger JG, Berry S, et al. Long-term outcome in children with opsoclonus-myoclonus and ataxia and coincident neuroblastoma. *J Peds* 1994; 125 (5 Pt 1):712–716.

107. Pranzetelli MR. On the molecular mechanism of adrenocorticotropic hormone in the CNS: neurotransmitters and receptors. *Exp Neurol* 1994; 125:142–161.

108. Papero PH, Pranzatelli MR, Margolis LJ, et al. Neurobehavioral and psychosocial functions of children with opsoclonus-myoclonus. *Dev Med Child Neurol* 1995; 37:915–932.

109. Russo C, Cohn SL, Petruzzi MJ, de Alarcon PA. Long-term neurologic outcome in children with opsoclonus-myoclonus associated with neuroblastoma: A report from the Pediatric Oncology Group. *Med Ped Oncol* 1997; 28:284–288.

110. Hammer MS, Larsen Mb, Stack CV. Outcome of children with opsoclonus-myclonus regardless of etiology. *Ped Neurol* 1995; 13:21–24.

111. Rodgers SW, Andrews PI, Gahring LC, et al. Autoantibodies to glutamate receptor GluR3 in Rasmussen's encephalitis. *Science* 1994; 265:648–651.

112. Andrews PI, McNamara JO. Rasmussen's encephalitis: an autoimmune disorder? *Curr Opin Neurol* 1996; 9:141–145.

113. Twyman RE, Gahring LC, Spiess J, Rogers SW. Glutamate receptor antibodies activate a subset of receptors and reveal an agonist binding site. *Neuron* 1995: 14:755–762.

114. Jay V, Becker LE, Otsubo H, et al. Chronic encephalitis and epilepsy (Rasmussen's encephalitis): Detection of cytomegalovirus and herpes simpex virus 1 by the polymerase chain reaction and in situ hybridization. *Neurology* 1995; 45:108–117.

115. Dulac O. Rasmussen's syndrome. *Curr Opin Neurol* 1996; 9:75–77.

116. Dulac O, Chinchilla D, Plouin P, et al. Follow-up of Rasmussen's syndrome treated by high dose steroids. *Epilepsia* 1992; 33:128.

117. Hart YM, Cortez M, Andermann F, et al. Medical treatment of Rasmussen's syndrome (chronic encephalitis and epilepsy): Effect of high dose steroids or immunoglobulin in 19 patients. *Neurology* 1994; 44:1030–1036.

118. Gee KW, McCauley LD, Lan NC. A putative receptor for neurosteroids on the GABA A receptor complex: the pharmacologic properties and therapeutic potential of epalons. *Crit Rev Neurobiol* 1995; 9:207–227.

119. Gasior M, Carter RB, Goldberg, SR Witkin JM. Anticonvulsant and behavioral effects of neuroactive steroids alone and in conjunction with neuroactive steroids. *J Pharm Exp Ther* 1997; 282:543–553.

120. Kokate TG, Cohen AL, Karp E, Rogawski MA. Neuroactive steroids protect against pilocarpine- and kainic acid–induced limbic seizures and status epilepticus in mice. *Neuropharm* 1996; 35:1049–1056.

121. Torda C, Wolff G. Effects of various concentrations of adrenocorticotropic hormone on electrical activity of brain and on sensitivity to convulsion inducing agents. *Am J Physiol* 1952; 168:406–413.

122. Wasserman MJ, Neville BS, Belton R, Millichamp JG. The effect of corticotropin (ACTH) on experimental seizures. *Neurology* 1965; 15:1136–1141.

123. Shinnar S, Berg AT. Does antiepileptic drug therapy prevent the development of "chronic" epilepsy? *Epilepsia* 1996; 37:701–708.

124. Crosley CJ, Richman RA, Thorpy MJ. Evidence for cortisol-independent anticonvulsant activity of adrenocorticotropic hormone in infantile spasms. *Ann Neurol* 1980; 8:220.

125. Farwell J, Milstein J, Opheim K, Smith E, Glass S. Adrenocorticotropic hormone controls infantile spasms independently of cortisol stimulation. *Epilepsia* 1984; 25:605–608.

126. Palo J, Savolainen H. The effect of high dose synthetic ACTH on rat brain. *Brain Res* 1974; 70:313–320.

127. Kendall DA, McEwen BS, Enne SJ. The influence of ACTH and corticosterone on $^3[H]GABA$ receptor binding in rat brain. *Brain Res* 1982; 236:365–374.

128. Pranzatelli MR. In vivo and in vitro effects of adrenocorticotropic hormone on serotonin receptors in neonatal rat brain. *Dev Pharmacol Ther* 1989; 12:49–56.

129. Adan RAH, van der Kraan M, Doornbos RP, et al. Melanocortin receptors mediate alpha-MSH induced stimulation of neurite outgrowth in Neuro 2A cells. *Mol Brain Res* 1996; 36:37–44.

130. Pentella K, Bachman DS, Sandman CA. Trial of an ACTH 4-9 analog (ORG 2766) in children with intractable seizures. *Neuropediatrics* 1982; 13:59–62.

131. Willig RP, Lagenstein I. Use of ACTH fragments in children with intractable seizures. *Neuropediatrics* 1982; 13:55–58.

132. Joels M. Steroid hormones and excitability in the mammalian brain. *Front Neuroendo* 1997; 18:2–48.

133. Ehlers CL, Henriksen SJ, Wang M, et al. Corticotrophin releasing factor produces increase in brain excitability and convulsive seizures in rats. *Brain Res* 1983; 278:332–336.

134. Marrosu F, Fratta W, Carcangiu P, Giagheddu M, Gessa GL. Localized epileptiform activity induced by murine CRF in rats. *Epilepsia* 1988; 29:369–373.

135. Baram TZ, Schultz L. Corticotropin-releasing hormone is a rapid and potent convulsant in the infant rat. *Dev Brain Res* 1991; 61:97–101.

136. Baram TZ, Mitchell WG, Snead OC 3rd, Horton EJ, Saito M. Brain-adrenal axis hormones are altered in the CSF of infants with massive infantile spasms. *Neurology* 1992; 42:1171–1175.

137. Baram TZ, Mitchell WG, Hanson RA, Snead OC 3rd, Horton EJ. Cerebral fluid corticotropin and cortisol are decreased in infantile spasms. *Ped Neurol* 1995; 13:108–110.

138. Baram TZ. Pathophysiology of massive infantile spasms: perspective on the putative role of brain adrenal axis. *Ann Neurol* 1993; 33:231–236.

Vitamins, Dietary Considerations, and Alternative Antiepileptic Drugs

Philip H. Sheridan, M.D.

Previous chapters have outlined the process of arriving at a correct seizure diagnosis and the guidelines for determining which patients require treatment (1). When medication is required, the use of one or two appropriate major antiepileptic drugs (AEDs) will control the seizures in the majority of patients.

This chapter discusses vitamin supplementation and dietary considerations for children with epilepsy (except for the ketogenic diet, which is presented in Chapter 42). It also reviews the use of two AED treatments (acetazolamide and bromides) that remain useful alternative therapies in certain children when first-line medications are not successful in fully controlling seizures without producing unacceptable side effects.

DIETARY CONSIDERATIONS

Families who ask about the usefulness of special diets to aid the management of their children's seizures should be cautioned against faddish diets and encouraged to give their children the same well-balanced diet that any child requires. A daily multivitamin tablet containing the usual recommended daily doses for age is a reasonable suggestion for many children who may not be eating a full spectrum of foods. As discussed subsequently, routine folate supplementation in adolescent girls and in women of child-bearing potential is recommended to reduce the incidence of birth defects. Children on the ketogenic diet require more extensive vitamin and mineral supplementation. The use of specific vitamins is addressed in a subsequent section. A consultation with a dietitian is useful for children who are overweight or underweight. Their antiepileptic medication may be contributing to the problem (e.g.,

valproate may lead to inappropriate weight gain and felbamate or topiramate to weight loss).

The sedative effects of many AEDs may encourage overuse of caffeine in soft drinks, tea, or coffee. Patients should be cautioned that this excessive caffeine could increase their tendency to seizures either primarily (2) or secondarily by disrupting their sleep patterns. The disrupted sleep patterns could cause a vicious cycle of exacerbated daytime sleepiness leading to further excessive ingestion of caffeine. A similar caution would apply to the stimulant effects of cigarette smoking; of course, there obviously are sufficient other adverse effects from cigarette smoking (pulmonary, cardiovascular, etc.) for their use by anyone to be discouraged. Moderate use of caffeine or nicotine does not significantly alter the metabolism of currently marketed AEDs.

A common question for adolescent patients is whether they can drink alcoholic beverages. Although alcohol abuse and withdrawal can lower seizure thresholds, moderate use of alcohol usually does not have a significant effect on seizure control. Patients and their families should be cautioned about the additive adverse sedative effects of alcohol and antiepileptic medication. The complex interrelation of seizures, alcohol, and epilepsy merits further research (3).

The total absorption of most AEDs is not significantly influenced by a meal or protein load, but the time course of absorption may be affected. In general, patients should be encouraged to take their medication in a consistent relationship to meals to avoid this potential source of variability in seizure protection or fluctuating adverse effects (e.g., double vision or sedation). Mealtimes can also serve as a reminder that it is time for a medication dose. Grapefruit juice (but not orange juice) increases the oral bioavailability of certain drugs (such as carbamazepine) by inhibiting metabolism by a P-450 isozyme (CYP3A4) in the wall of the small intestine. This inhibition can last for a full day and may lead to clinically significant increases in medication drug level and effect (4).

VITAMINS AND SUPPLEMENTS

The role of vitamin toxicity, vitamin deficiency, and vitamin dependency (inborn errors of metabolism requiring pharmacologic rather than physiologic amounts of vitamin supplementation) in clinical syndromes affecting the central and peripheral nervous system was recently reviewed (5). The following discussions concern those vitamins and dietary supplements particularly relevant to seizure disorder management. Several of the syndromes discussed are metabolic disorders that may present as acute or chronic seizures of the neonate, infant, or child and that may respond to vitamin therapy. Prompt diagnosis and treatment may be required to prevent permanent neurologic damage.

Pyridoxine (Vitamin B6)

Vitamin B6 is formed by three pyridine derivatives (pyridoxine, pyridoxamine, and pyridoxal); its active form in the human body is pyridoxal phosphate. Vitamin B6 is a cofactor for many enzymatic reactions in the metabolism of amino acids and neurotransmitters [dopamine, serotonin, norepinephrine, and gamma-aminobutyric acid (GABA)] (6). Pyridoxine deficiency or dependency probably increases seizure susceptibility as a result of reduced GABA synthesis.

Neonatal seizures that do not respond to AEDs may be due to pyridoxine dependency, a rare metabolic disorder (7). Exceptionally, the seizures of pyridoxine dependency may not occur until as late as the second year of life. Possible seizure types include persistent partial seizures, recurrent status epilepticus, generalized myoclonic and atonic seizures, and infantile spasms. Electroencephalogram (EEG) findings may also vary from the characteristic generalized bursts of bilateral, asynchronous, high-voltage 1–4 Hz waves intermixed with spikes or sharp waves to other epileptiform patterns such as focal or multifocal spikes, generalized delta wave bursts, and paroxysmal sharp and slow wave complexes. Therefore, any neonate or infant presenting with repeated idiopathic seizures resistant to medication should receive a test dose of 50 to 100 mg of intravenous pyridoxine during a seizure to see if a response (EEG improvement or seizure resolution) occurs over minutes to hours (8). Because of the unlikely but possible danger of circulatory collapse after the initial dose of pyridoxine, this first dose

should be given in a clinical setting with facilities for emergency resuscitation (9). Children who respond to pyridoxine should be maintained on pyridoxine supplementation to achieve ongoing seizure control and normal development (10,11).

In contrast to the few patients presenting with infantile spasms who have been found to have pyridoxine deficiency or dependency responsive to pyridoxine supplementation (12), patients who have infantile spasms from other etiologies have had a variable response to high-dose pyridoxal phosphate, which has been proposed as an alternative to adrenocorticotropic hormone (ACTH) or steroids (13,14). Better results are reported from the combination of lower doses of pyridoxal phosphate (40–50 mg/kg/day) and low-dose ACTH (0.4 IU/kg/day), although the efficacy of pyridoxal phosphate for this indication is not firmly established (15).

Biotin (Vitamin H)

Biotin is an essential cofactor for a number of carboxylation reactions involved in gluconeogenesis, fatty acid synthesis, and leucine metabolism (5). Biotinidase deficiency may present in infancy with seizures (generalized tonic-clonic, infantile spasms, or myoclonic seizures) that are resistant to drug therapy (16). Other manifestations include an erythematous rash, alopecia, ataxia, developmental delay, OPHC atrophy, hearing loss, and lactic acidosis. Diagnosis is made by serum enzyme assay. Oral biotin therapy (5–10 mg daily) is effective in stopping seizures and preventing neurologic damage if begun before damage is permanent.

Folate (Vitamin M)

Various interconvertible forms of folate cofactors are essential for the one-carbon transfer reactions of DNA synthesis. Adequate maternal folate stores reduce the incidence of fetal neural tube defect (NTD). AEDs can reduce the absorption of folate causing a folate deficiency.

Routine folic acid supplementation is recommended for adolescent girls and women of child-bearing potential because supplementation should begin well before conception and the timing of a pregnancy is not always planned.

In 1998 the American Academy of Neurology published a practice parameter (17) regarding women with epilepsy (WWE) on AEDs, which stated:

Treatment with some AEDs, including phenytoin, carbamazepine, and barbiturates, can impair folate absorption, and there is a substantial scientific basis for the recommendation of prepregnancy and early pregnancy supplementation of folic acid for WWE during reproductive years. There is little information in the literature concerning the use of folic acid supplementation specifically referable to WWE who take AEDs. Recommendations for WWE draw on the literature regarding supplementation for the general population. Studies have confirmed that folic acid supplementation reduces primary and secondary risk of neural tube defects in infants of women who do not take AEDs. Optimal dosage is not clear because study supplementation has varied between 0.36 and 5 mg/d.

The 1996 *American College of Obstetricians and Gynecologists Educational Bulletin on Seizure Disorders in Pregnancy* recommended a dose of 4 mg/day of folic acid before conception and in the first trimester for all patients who have had a prior pregnancy affected by a NTD and stated that a similar dose appears to be appropriate for women receiving AEDs (16).

Folate-dependency syndromes are rare. The most common is methylene tetrahydrofolate reductase deficiency. Its clinical presentation is varied and ranges from infancy to adolescence. Seizures are most likely in the infantile form, which presents with seizures (generalized myoclonic and atonic, infantile spasms, and partial seizures), developmental regression, and acquired microcephaly. The biochemical profile is mild to moderate homocystinuria and homocystinemia; decreased enzyme activity in cultured fibroblasts is diagnostic. The response to high-dose folate or folinic acid (which can be supplemented with betaine, methionine, and vitamin B6) is variable. Treatment is probably more effective if started promptly after early diagnosis. (5,19).

Cobalamin (Vitamin B12)

Vitamin B12 is a microbially derived vitamin naturally found in meat, eggs, and dairy products. The classic neurologic presentation of vitamin B12 deficiency caused by malabsorption is subacute combined degeneration, a syndrome that does not include seizures.

Recurrent acute episodes of vomiting, ketoacidosis, and lethargy precipitated by infection or a high protein load may be a manifestation of a methylmalonic acidemia resulting from methylmalonyl-CoA deficiency. These episodes may result in seizures, neurologic deficits, or death. Some of these patients respond to vitamin B12 administration (intramuscular 1000 µg of hydroxycobalamin continued on a weekly or biweekly basis). Measurement of urinary organic acids during a metabolic crisis helps to establish the diagnosis (5).

Cholecalciferol (Vitamin D)

Vitamin D is a secosteroid produced from 7-dehydrocholesterol in the skin when exposed to ultraviolet radiation. Vitamin D is involved in calcium, phosphate, and hormonal metabolism. Children and adults who suffer from or who are at risk for osteomalacia or rickets (e.g.,

homebound, institutionalized, malnourished, or malabsorption syndrome patients) may require vitamin D and calcium supplementation, especially when chronic antiepileptic medication is required for seizure management. Published reports suggest that phenytoin, carbamazepine, phenobarbital, and valproate may produce mild vitamin D deficiency responsive to low-dose vitamin D therapy (20). Otherwise healthy epileptic children who are receiving antiepileptic medication but who have a regular diet and environment would not usually require routine calcium and vitamin D supplementation. A recent National Institutes of Health (NIH) consensus conference reviewed current recommendations for calcium and vitamin D supplementation (21).

Phytonadione and Menaquinone (Vitamin K)

Vitamin K1 (phytonadione, from leafy green vegetables) and vitamin K2 (menaquinone, synthesized by bacteria colonizing the human intestine) are fat-soluble and require bile salts for absorption. Vitamin K is required for the biologic activity of prothrombin and factors II, VII, IX, and X of the coagulation cascade (22). Maternal AEDs may cross the placenta and induce hepatic microsomal enzymes in the fetal liver. This would promote the fetal degradation of vitamin K, resulting in neonatal vitamin K deficiency (hemorrhagic disease of the newborn).

In 1998 the American Academy of Neurology (17) published the following recommendation on the prevention of hemorrhagic disease of the newborn caused by vitamin K deficiency in babies born to WWE on AEDs:

Vitamin K, 10 mg per day, should be prescribed in the last month of pregnancy to WWE taking enzyme-inducing AEDs. If this has not been done, parenteral vitamin K-1 should be administered to women with epilepsy as soon as possible after the onset of labor. Note: This recommendation does not supplant the ACOG/AAP recommendation for the administration of 1 mg vitamin K-1 to the neonate.

Carnitine

Carnitine is a naturally occurring amino acid found mostly in skeletal muscle and liver. Carnitine acts as a carrier of long-chain fatty acids across the mitochondrial membrane to allow mitochondrial oxidation and fatty acid metabolism. Numerous inborn errors of metabolism can produce primary or secondary carnitine deficiency. Secondary carnitine deficiency can also be associated with acquired medical conditions (extreme prematurity, cirrhosis, chronic renal disease, malnutrition, malabsorption) or iatrogenic states (hemodialysis, parenteral nutrition, adverse drug effect) (23).

Chronic therapy with valproic acid causes cellular depletion of carnitine in some patients, presumably by interfering directly with the active transport of carnitine across the plasma membrane; valproate may also cause carnitine deficiency by increasing excretion of acylcarnitine or by exacerbating preexisting metabolic disorders and acquired medical conditions that cause secondary carnitine deficiency. The relationship of the rare but serious adverse effects of valproic acid (life-threatening hepatotoxicity, Reye-like syndrome, and pancreatitis) to carnitine homeostasis is unclear. Carnitine supplementation does not appear to alter the efficacy or concentration of valproic acid (23).

In November 1996 a panel of pediatric neurologists updated a consensus statement on L-carnitine supplementation in childhood epilepsy (24):

The panelists agreed that intravenous L-carnitine supplementation is clearly indicated for valproate (VPA)-induced hepatotoxicity, overdose, and other acute metabolic crises associated with carnitine deficiency. Oral supplementation is clearly indicated for the primary plasmalemmal carnitine transporter defect. The panelists concurred that oral L-carnitine supplementation is strongly suggested for the following groups as well: patients with certain secondary carnitine-deficiency syndromes, symptomatic VPA-associated hyperammonemia, multiple risk factors for VPA hepatotoxicity, or renal-associated syndromes; infants and young children taking VPA; patients with epilepsy using the ketogenic diet who have hypocarnitinemia; patients receiving dialysis; and premature infants who are receiving total parenteral nutrition. The panel recommended an oral L-carnitine dosage of 100 mg/kg/day, up to a maximum of 2 g/day. Intravenous supplementation for medical emergency situations usually exceeds this recommended dosage.

ALTERNATIVE ANTIEPILEPTIC DRUGS

Acetazolamide

Acetazolamide (5-acetamido-1,3,4-thiadiazole-2-sulfonamide, Diamox) is an unsubstituted sulfonamide that inhibits the enzyme carbonic anhydrase. It has both systemic and central nervous system effects.

Acetazolamide has some effectiveness against most seizure types, although it has been used primarily against absence seizures. It usually is not effective when given on a chronic basis because of the development of tolerance. Administered intermittently, it may be useful in treating catamenial seizures, although it is not recommended if pregnancy may occur (25). To prevent menstrual exacerbation of seizures, it may be given 10 days before anticipated menstruation and then continued until termination of bleeding (26). One series reported acetazolamide to be effective in the chronic therapy of juvenile myoclonic epilepsy patients who are not fully responsive to valproic acid (27).

Acetazolamide is thought to act by inhibiting carbonic anhydrase. Carbonic anhydrase catalyzes the synthesis of bicarbonate from carbon dioxide and water. Acetazolamide inhibits carbonic anhydrase in myelin, cytoplasm, and glial cell membranes. The resultant carbon dioxide accumulation in brain blocks the spread of seizure activity and elevates seizure threshold. Chronic exposure to acetazolamide induces carbonic anhydrase synthesis and proliferation of glial cells, which result in tolerance to the drug. Very high doses of acetazolamide can increase neural excitability by blocking carbonic anhydrase–dependent glial uptake of chloride and bicarbonate (25).

The clinical pharmacology of acetazolamide is summarized in Table 42-1. Acetazolamide is absorbed from the stomach and upper intestines and reaches peak plasma concentrations within 2 to 3 hours after oral administration. It is 90 percent protein bound, the free portion distributing with total body water. However, penetration into the brain and cerebrospinal fluid (CSF) occurs more slowly and depends on the CSF flow, permeability of the blood–brain barrier, and rate of active transport out of the CSF. Brain and CSF concentrations are lower than plasma concentrations.

Within 24 hours, almost all of the drug in tissue is bound to tissue carbonic anhydrase to form the enzyme-inhibitor complex. Although the renal elimination half-life is 10–15 hours, the enzyme-inhibitor complex has a slow dissociation constant. The drug is released slowly from the tissues as it is excreted in the urine. Acetazolamide thus has an effective half-life of several days. Most of the bound drug in the body is found in red blood cells, which contain a large amount of carbonic anhydrase (25).

The recommended daily dose of acetazolamide is 10–20 mg/kg/day given two to three times daily, which usually produces a plasma level of 10–14 μg/mL

Table 42-1. Acetazolamide

Pharmacokinetics:
　Oral absorption: rapid and complete in normal dose range
　Protein binding: 90%
　Elimination half-life: 10–15 h (effective half-life longer because of binding to enzyme)
　PKa: 7.4
　Time to steady state: 40–48 h
　Excretion: renal
How supplied: Diamox 125- and 250-mg tablets, 500-mg sustained-release capsule, and parenteral vial
Maintenance dose: 10–20 mg/kg/day in two to three divided doses PO
Therapeutic range: 10–14 μg/mL
Common side effects: drowsiness, paresthesias, loss of appetite
Severe side effects: confusion, acidosis, renal calculi, polyuria, hypersensitivity reaction, hepatic insufficiency, gastrointestinal disturbance paralysis, convulsions

(25,28). When adding acetazolamide to other AEDs, the starting dose should be approximately one-third of the maintenance dose to minimize the possibility of the acetazolamide enhancing the side effects of the other AEDs. The dose can subsequently be increased as tolerated over several weeks.

Acetazolamide is one of the least toxic of the AEDs. Side effects include paresthesias, slight alteration of taste sensation, and transient drowsiness. A sulfonamide hypersensitivity reaction is possible (fever, rash, thrombocytopenia, leukopenia, hemolytic anemia, and agranulocytosis) (28). Acetazolamide reduces urinary citrate, which could lead to calculus formation and ureteral colic. In hepatic cirrhosis, episodic disorientation may be induced apparently as a result of alkalinization of the urine, which reduces ammonia clearance. Other rare side effects include abdominal distention, polyuria, transient myopia, melena, hematuria, glycosuria, hepatic insufficiency, flaccid paralysis, and convulsions (25,28).

Given the systemic activity of acetazolamide, there are many theoretical possibilities for drug interactions, but few have been observed. Induction or inhibition of hepatic enzymes by other AEDs does not affect acetazolamide because it is not metabolized by the liver. Acetazolamide increases the concentration of weak acids in tissues. Because most AEDs are weak acids, the addition of acetazolamide to an AED regimen may allow an increased brain concentration of the other AEDs to be achieved at lower doses with possibly fewer side effects (25). For example, one series reported that concomitant acetazolamide allowed reduction of carbamazepine dose with consequent reduction of side effects and better long-term seizure control than could have been achieved by simply raising the carbamazepine dose (29,30).

One recent report suggested that acetazolamide therapy produces a sufficient metabolic acidosis to cause growth suppression in children (31). Acetazolamide should be discontinued 2 weeks before initiating the ketogenic diet to avoid a potentially dangerous metabolic acidosis. Acetazolamide is not recommended for women in early pregnancy because teratogenic effects have been described in experimental animals (25).

Bromides

The anticonvulsant efficacy of bromides was described by Locock in 1857 (32). Bromides have rarely been prescribed since the discovery of phenobarbital and other AEDs, but they may be useful for certain patients.

Bromides have a broad spectrum of activity and are effective against both partial and generalized seizures. One recent series found that generalized convulsive seizures responded best to bromide therapy but that complex partial seizures and absence seizures were less responsive (33). Another series reported bromides to be effective in intractable childhood epilepsy characterized by early-onset, predominantly generalized tonic-clonic seizures (34). In a third study, most children with intractable focal epilepsy or Lennox-Gastaut syndrome had sustained improvement with the addition of bromide to their drug regimens, which usually also included valproate (35). Bromides are useful for patients who are allergic to standard AEDs. Bromide therapy is also one of the few antiepileptic agents that can safely be used in porphyria (36).

Bromide is a simple inorganic ion rapidly absorbed after oral administration (Table 42-2). Body tissues do not distinguish between chloride and bromide ions, so bromide's volume of distribution is similar to that of chloride. Bromide is not protein bound. The concentration in CSF and in brain is approximately one-third that in plasma. Bromide is eliminated by renal excretion in competition with chloride. The plasma half-life is quite long, approximately 12 days (37). Its resemblance to chloride may allow it to enhance GABA-mediated neuronal inhibition (37,38).

Therapy is usually administered as triple bromide elixir containing 1200 mg bromide salt per 5 mL prepared with equal quantities of potassium, sodium, and ammonium salts. The elixir can be mixed with other liquids to make it palatable. Therapy can be initiated at 10 mg bromide salt/kg daily in two to three divided doses and increased gradually (35). In children under 6 years of age, the dose ranges from 300 mg twice a day to 600 mg three times a day. In children over 6 years of age, the dose ranges from 300 mg to 1 g given three times a day. The therapeutic blood

Table 42-2. Bromides

Pharmacokinetics:
   Oral absorption: rapid and complete
   Protein binding: none
   Plasma half-life: 12 days
   Time to steady state: 50 days
   Excretion: renal
How supplied: triple bromide elixir (1200 mg bromide salt/5 mL)
Initiating dose: 10 mg bromide salt/kg/day in two to three divided doses
Maintenance dose:
   Under age 6 years: 300 mg bid–600 mg tid PO
   Over age 6 years: 300–1000 mg tid PO
Therapeutic range: 75–125 mg/100 mL (10–15 mEq/L)
Common side effects: intoxication as a result of chronic accumulation (weakness, mental disturbance, loss of appetite, skin rash)
Severe side effects: headache, dementia, sedation, incoordination, anorexia, dry mucous membranes, vasomotor disturbance, gastrointestinal disturbance

concentration is 75 to 125 mg/100 mL (10–15 mEq/L) (37). Careful monitoring of blood levels can avoid toxic effects, which usually do not occur until levels exceed 150 mg/100 mL (35,37).

Bromide intoxication (bromism) develops gradually over a prolonged period because of the slow excretion of bromide from the body. Chronic bromism is more common in elderly patients, particularly if renal function is impaired. Mild bromism manifests as weakness, fatigue, mental disturbances, and loss of appetite. More severe bromism includes restlessness, headache, disorientation, and increasing dementia. Incoordination, loss of pupillary reflexes, dry mucous membranes, anorexia, vasomotor disturbances, and emaciation also may occur. Skin rashes are frequently found in younger patients, although they are not always present. An acneiform rash erupting on the face and spreading over the neck, chest, and arms is the most common form. A nodular rash, vesicles, or pustules also may occur. Bromide intoxication is rare with blood levels below 200 mg/100 mL. Treatment of bromism consists of stopping the medication and increasing urinary excretion by administering large amounts of fluid. Because bromide displaces chloride in extracellular fluid, about 40 percent of chloride may have been replaced by bromide as bromide intoxication developed. Therefore, infusion of sodium chloride (or ammonium chloride if sodium chloride is contraindicated because of heart failure) may be necessary. Hemodialysis rapidly lowers the bromide level (37).

Because bromide is not metabolized by the liver and is not protein bound, it does not interact with standard AEDs. Blood levels should be monitored periodically to avoid chronic accumulation (35,37). Because bromides cross the placenta and can cause fetal hypotonia and neurologic depression, use of bromide therapy during pregnancy is contraindicated (35).

CONCLUSION

This chapter has addressed some dietary and nutritional issues for pediatric seizure management as well as two alternative drug treatments. As is the case for most antiepileptic therapies, these treatments were usually developed for adults, and much of the available information is based on testing and experience with adults.

Children are not simply "little adults." A recent NIH workshop (39) emphasized the need for further preclinical studies and clinical trials targeting pediatric epileptic syndromes and addressing age-related issues (including brain development, cognition, and systemic growth and maturation). It is hoped that the results from such research will be included in future editions of this book.

REFERENCES

1. Aicardi J. Clinical approach to the management of intractable epilepsy. *Dev Med Child Neurol* 1988; 30:429–440.

2. Gasior M, Borowicz K, Buszewicz G, Kleinrok Z, Czuczwar SJ. Anticonvulsant activity of phenobarbital and valproate against maximal electroshock in mice during chronic treatment with caffeine and caffeine discontinuation. *Epilepsia* 1996; 37(3):262–263.

3. Hauser WA, Ng SK, Brust JC. Alcohol, seizures, and epilepsy. *Epilepsia* 1988; 29(Suppl 2):S66–S78.

4. Fuhr U. Drug interactions with grapefruit juice. Extent, probable mechanism and clinical relevance. *Drug Safety* 1998; 18:251–272.

5. Berman PH. Vitamins. In: Berg BO, ed. *Principles of Child Neurology*. New York: McGraw-Hill, 1996.

6. Prensky AL. Nutritional deficiency and the nervous system. In: Berg BO, ed. *Principles of Child Neurology*. New York: McGraw-Hill, 1996.

7. Clarke TA, Saunders BS, Feldman B. Pyridoxine-dependent seizures requiring high doses of pyridoxine for control. *Am J Dis Child* 1979; 133:963–965.

8. Goutieres F, Aicardi J. Atypical presentations of pyridoxine-dependent seizures: a treatable cause of intractable epilepsy in infants. *Ann Neurol* 1985; 17:117–120.

9. Tanaka R, Okumura M, Arima J, Yamakura S, Momoi T. Pyridoxine-dependent seizures: report of a case with atypical clinical features and abnormal MRI scans. *J Child Neurol* 1992; 7:24–28.

10. Mikati MA, Trevathan E, Krishnamoorthy KS, Lombroso CT. Pyyridoxine-dependent epilepsy: EEG investigations and long-term follow-up. *Electroencephalogr Clin Neurophysiol* 1991; 78:215–221.

11. Bankier A, Turner M, Hopkins IJ. Pyridoxine-dependent seizures — a wider clinical spectrum. *Arch Dis Child* 1983; 58:415–418.

12. French JH, Grueter BB, Druckman R, O'Brien D. Pyridoxine and infantile myoclonic seizures. *Neurology* 1965; 15:101–113.

13. Blennow G, Starck L. High dose B₆ treatment in infantile spasms. *Neuropediatrics* 1986; 17:7–10.

14. Pietz J, Benninger C, Schäfer H, et al. Treatment of infantile spasms with high-dose vitamin B₆. *Epilepsia* 1993; 34:757–763.

15. Takuma Y. ACTH therapy for infantile spasms: a combination therapy with high-dose pyridoxal phosphate and low-lose ACTH. *Epilepsia* 1998; 39(Suppl.5):42–45.

16. Salbert BA, Pellock JM, Wolf B. Characterization of seizures associated with biotinidase deficiency. *Neurology* 1993; 43:1351–1355.

17. Quality Standards Subcommittee of the American Academy of Neurology. Management issues for women with epilepsy (summary statement). *Neurology* 1998; 51:944–948.

18. ACOG educational bulletin. Seizure disorders in pregnancy. Number 231, December 1996. Committee on Educational Bulletins of the American College of Obstetricians and Gynecologists. *Int J Gynaecol Obstet* 1997; 56:279–286.

19. Garcia-Alvarez M, Nordli DR, DeVivo DC. Inherited metabolic disorders. In: Engel J Jr., Pedley TA, eds. *Epilepsy: A Comprehensive Textbook*. New York: Lippincott-Raven, 1997:2553–2559.

20. Offermann G. Chronic antiepileptic drug treatment and disorders of mineral metabolism. In: *Antiepileptic Therapy: Chronic Toxicity of Antiepileptic Drugs*. New York: Raven Press, 1983:175–184.

21. NIH consensus statement. Optimal calcium intake. 1994; 12:1–31. Also published in *Nutrition* 1995; 11:409–417.

22. O'Reilly RA, Drugs used in disorders of coagulation. In: Katzung BG, ed. *Basic and Clinical Pharmacology*. 7th ed. Stamford, CT: Appleton and Lange, 1998:547–562.

23. Pons R, DeVivo DC. Primary and secondary carnitine deficiency syndromes. *J Child Neurol* 1995; 10(Suppl 2):S8–S24.

24. DeVivo DC, Bohan TP, Coulter DL, et al. L-carnitine supplementation in childhood epilepsy: current perspectives. *Epilepsia* 1998; 39:11216–11225.

25. Resor SR Jr, Resor LD, Woodbury DM, Kemp JW. Acetazolamide In: Levy RH, Mattson RH, Meldrum BS, eds. *Antiepileptic Drugs*. 4th ed. New York: Raven Press, 1995:969–985.

26. Newmark ME, Penry JK. Catamenial epilepsy: a review. *Epilepsia* 1980; 21:281–300.

27. Resor SR Jr, Resor LD. Acetazolamide in the treatment of juvenile myoclonic epilepsy. *Neurology* 1985; 35(Suppl 1):285.

28. Browne TR. Paraldehyde, acetazolamide, trimethadione, paramethadione, and phenacemide. In: Brown TR, Feldman RG, eds. *Epilepsy, Diagnosis and Management*. Boston: Little, Brown, 1983:247–258.

29. Aicardi J. *Epilepsy in Children*. 2nd ed. New York: Raven Press, 1994.

30. Forsythe WI, Owens JR, Toothill C. Effectiveness of acetazolamide in the treatment of carbamazepine-resistant epilepsy in children. *Dev Med Child Neurol* 1981; 17:743–748.

31. Futagi Y, Otani K, Abe J. Growth suppression in children receiving acetazolamide with antiepileptic drugs. *Pediatr Neurol* 1996; 15:323–326.

32. Locock C Discussion of paper by E. H. Sieveking: analysis of 52 cases of epilepsy observed by author. *Lancet* 1857; 1:527.

33. Dreifuss FE, Bertram EH. Bromide therapy for intractable seizures. *Epilepsia* 1986; 27:593.

34. Ernst JP, Doose H, Baier WK Bromides were effective in intractable epilepsy with generalized tonic-clonic seizures and onset in early childhood. *Brain Dev* 1988; 10:385–388.

35. Woody RC. Bromide therapy for pediatric seizure disorder intractable to other antiepileptic drugs. *J Child Neurol* 1990; 5:65–67.

36. Engel J Jr. *Seizures and Epilepsy*. Philadelphia: FA. Davis, 1989.

37. Dreifuss FE. How to use bromides. In: Morselli PL, Pippenger CE, Penry JK, eds. *Antiepileptic Drug Therapy in Pediatrics*. New York: Raven Press, 1983:281–282.

38. Dreifuss FE. Bromides In: Levy RH, Mattson RH, Meldrum BS, eds. *Antiepileptic Drugs*. 4th ed. New York: Raven Press, 1995: 949–951.

39. Sheridan PH, Jacobs MP. The development of antiepileptic drugs for children: report from the NIH workshop. *Epilepsy Res* 1996; 23:87–92.

CHAPTER 43

The Ketogenic Diet

Douglas R. Nordli, Jr., M.D., and Darryl C. De Vivo, M.D.

The ketogenic diet is a high-fat, low-carbohydrate, and low-protein regimen. It has been used for more than 70 years on thousands of patients. It is effective and safe, but, like any medical treatment for epilepsy, it must be judiciously applied and carefully monitored.

There are biblical references of the salutary effects of starvation on seizure control, but the earliest scientific reports emerged in the 1920s. Geyelin at the Presbyterian Hospital carefully studied the beneficial effects of starvation on seizures (1). Shortly thereafter Wilder proposed a high-fat diet to mimic the effects of starvation (2). At the time it was known that ketone bodies, produced when fatty acids are oxidized, could be found in the urine of patients with diabetes. This led to the notion that ketone bodies were undesirable by-products of fatty acid degradation. Because this high-fat diet increased the production of ketone bodies, the regimen became known as a keto or ketogenic diet. Its anticonvulsant effect was attributed to a sedative effect of the ketone bodies on the nervous system, and it is easy to understand this notion because the available anticonvulsants of that era, bromides and phenobarbital, were both sedatives.

In the 1950s, however, it was discovered that a separate pathway synthesized the ketone bodies, acetoacetate and 3-hydroxybutyrate, and in 1961 Krebs suggested that ketone bodies were fuels for respiration. In 1967 Owen proved that ketone bodies were the major fuel for brain metabolism during starvation (3). Appleton and De Vivo later showed in experimental animals that the utilization of ketone bodies during starvation alters brain metabolites and increases cerebral energy reserves (4). Huttenlocher showed that the level of ketosis correlated with efficacy (5).

There are several different variations of the ketogenic diet, but the most widely used regimen uses long-chain triglycerides (LCT) in the form of heavy cream, butter, and meat fat. We review here the scientific basis, efficacy, and safety of the LCT diet.

SCIENTIFIC BASIS OF THE DIET

Appleton and De Vivo developed an animal model to permit study of the effect of the ketogenic diet on cerebral metabolism (4). Adult male albino rats were placed on either a high-fat diet containing (by weight) 38 percent corn oil, 38 percent lard, 11 percent vitamin-free casein, 6.8 percent glucose, 4 percent U.S.P. salt mixture, and 2.2 percent vitamin diet fortification mixture, or a high-carbohydrate diet containing (by weight) 50 percent glucose, 28.8 percent vitamin-free casein, 7.5 percent corn oil, 7.5 percent lard, 4 percent U.S.P. salt mixture, and 2.2 percent vitamin diet fortification mixture. Parallel studies were conducted to evaluate electroconvulsive shock responses and biochemical alterations. These studies revealed that the mean voltage necessary to produce a minimal convulsion remained constant for 12 days before the high-fat diet was started and for about 10 days after beginning the feedings (69.75 ± 1.88 volts). About 10 to 12 days after starting the high-fat diet, the intensity of the convulsive response to the established voltage decreased, necessitating an increase in voltage to reestablish a minimal convulsive response. Approximately 20 days after beginning the high-fat diet, a new convulsive threshold was achieved (81.25 ± 2.39 volts) ($p < 0.01$). When the high-fat fat diet was replaced by the high-carbohydrate diet, a rapid change in response to the voltage was observed. Within 48 hours the animal exhibited a maximal convulsion to the electrical stimulus, which had previously produced only a minimal convulsion, and the mean voltage to produce a minimal convulsion returned to a value similar to prestudy (70.75 ± 1.37 volts).

Blood concentrations of beta-hydroxybutyrate, acetoacetate, chloride, esterified fatty acids, triglycerides, cholesterol, and total lipids increased in the rats fed on the high-fat diet. Brain levels of beta-hydroxybutyrate and sodium were significantly increased in the fat-fed rats.

Subsequently, De Vivo and coworkers reported the changes in cerebral metabolites in chronically ketotic rats (6). No changes in brain-water content, electrolytes, and pH were found. As expected, fat-fed rats had significantly lower blood glucose concentrations and higher blood beta-hydroxybutyrate and acetoacetate concentrations. More importantly, the brain concentrations of adenosine triphosphate (ATP), glycogen, glucose-6-phosphate, pyruvate, lactate, beta-hydroxybutyrate, citrate, alpha-ketoglutarate, and alanine were higher and the brain concentrations of fructose-1,6-diphosphate, aspartate, adenosine diphosphate (ADP), creatine, cyclic nucleotides, acid-insoluble coenzyme A(CoA) and total CoA were lower in the fat-fed group. Cerebral energy reserves were significantly higher in the fat-fed rats (26.4 ± 0.6) compared with controls (23.6 ± 0.2) ($p < 0.005$). Many of these changes in metabolites could be explained by the higher energy state of the brain cells in the fat-fed group, specifically by the ratio of ATP to ADP. In addition, the normal oxaloacetate, elevated alpha-ketoglutarate, and decreased succinyl-CoA imply maximal TCA cycle activity — quite contrary to the metabolite profile seen with anesthetic-sedative agents. Elevated alpha-ketoglutarate raises the possibility of increased flux through the gamma-aminobutyric acid (GABA) shunt. Al-Mudallal and coworkers recently showed that in adult male rats fed a high-fat ketogenic diet neither cerebral pH nor total cerebral GABA levels were altered when compared with controls (7). Although the whole brain GABA concentrations are unchanged during chronic ketosis, regional differences may well occur. Finally, it is worth speculating about possible GABA mimetic effects of ketosis given the chemical structural similarities of GABA, beta-hydroxybutyrate, and acetoacetate.

These observations suggest that the ketogenic diet favorably influences cerebral energetics and that increased cerebral energy reserves and increased GABA shunt activity may be important factors bestowing an increased resistance to seizures in ketotic brain tissue (8).

INITIATION OF THERAPY

Before the initiation of the diet, a nutrition support team or registered dietitian (RD) performs a comprehensive assessment. The nutritionist or dietitian asks if there have been any gastrointestinal problems, food allergies, or feeding difficulties, such as problems with sucking, swallowing, or chewing. They also note the patient's weight, height, usual weight, weight pattern since birth, and head circumference. Next, weight-for-age and height-for-age are plotted, and ideal body weight-for-height is determined. Laboratory data are used as another tool for nutritional assessment of the patient, and we routinely obtain serum protein, lipid profile, electrolytes, free and total carnitine, hemoglobin, hematocrit, and red blood indices.

The nutritionist or dietitian reviews the method of delivery of the diet, taking into consideration factors such as the patient's age, stage of development, and expected tolerance of the regimen. In the usual case, the diet is offered in a normal, enteral fashion with the expectation being that the child will eat and drink as is appropriate for his or her developmental stage. The consistency of the diet can be altered to adjust for any feeding difficulties. The nutritional support team may recommend the use of a feeding tube in very rare circumstances.

Patients should be hospitalized for the initiation of the ketogenic diet. Close observation is important because a child with an occult underlying inborn error of metabolism, particularly one that interferes with utilization of ketone bodies, could quickly decompensate (9). The hospitalization also provides the opportunity for family members to be instructed on the maintenance of the diet.

The first step is to promote ketosis by a fast. This can be done by fasting the patient after dinner (6 PM) on the evening of admission and continuing the fast until breakfast at 8 AM on the third day (38 hours). This allows metabolic adaptation to the state of ketosis and an opportunity to screen the child for any severe hypoglycemic predisposition. During the first few days, it is typical to see a transient hypoglycemia which does not require treatment unless the child demonstrates symptoms. Treatment of asymptomatic hypoglycemia delays the metabolic adaptation of the child to the state of chronic ketosis. During the fast, the patient is offered water, sugar-free beverages, and unsweetened gelatin.

The diet is begun when the urine reveals medium to large ketones. The LCT diet consists of three or four parts fat to one part nonfat (carbohydrate and protein) calculated on the basis of weight. It is computed to provide 75 to 100 kcal/kg body weight and 1 to 2 g dietary protein per kg of body weight per day. Caloric requirements are adjusted to minimize weight gain and maximize ketonemia. If a 3:1 (fat-to-nonfat) ratio is insufficient to produce the required ketosis, a ratio of 4:1 is used.

THE CONVENTIONAL KETOGENIC DIET OR LONG-CHAIN TRIGLYCERIDE DIET

Before initiating the conventional ketogenic or LCT diet, a dietary prescription is made. Calculation of this prescription is straightforward. For example, if a 10-kg child is to be started on a 3:1 diet, one begins by estimating the calorie requirements of the child:

$$10 \text{ kg} \times 100 \text{ kcal/day} = 1000 \text{ kcal/day}$$

Alternatively, this figure can be derived by consulting a table of recommended daily allowances (RDA). In either case, it may require adjustment based on the child's individual metabolic needs.

The 3:1 ratio of the diet stipulates that 4 g of food must contain 3 g of fat and 1 g of nonfat. The nonfat consists of both carbohydrate and protein. One gram of fat has the calorie equivalent of 9 calories, whereas 1 g of protein or carbohydrate has the calorie equivalent of approximately 4 calories. Four g of food (arbitrarily referred to as one unit here) on a 3:1 diet is then equal to 31 calories:

1 g fat = 9 calories × 3 = 27 calories

1 g protein and CHO = 4 calories × 1 = 4 calories

Total calories = 27 + 4 = 31 calories per unit

To calculate the daily fat intake, one first divides the daily requirements of calories by this figure of 31 calories/unit, which generates the number of units required for the day:

1000 calories/day/31 calories/unit = 32.25 units/day

Next, multiplying by 27 calories of fat/unit provides the daily fat requirement:

32.26 units/day × 27 calories of fat/unit = 871

calories of fat per day, which is equivalent to 96 g

The protein requirement is 10 kg × 2 g/kg or 20 g/day (80 calories). Alternatively, one may consult the RDA table to determine the protein requirement.

So far, the combination of 871 calories of fat and 80 calories of protein leaves only 49 calories (1000 − 951) not accounted for in the daily allowance. The carbohydrate intake is then calculated to supply the necessary remaining calories (49 calories), which here is approximately 12 g.

The diet prescription for this 10-kg patient on a 3:1 LCT diet is then:

Fat: 96 g per day or 32 g per meal

Protein: 20 g per day or 6.6 g per meal

Carbohydrate: 12 g per day or 4 g per meal

Although the calculation of the calorie requirements is straightforward, the generation of the actual food prescription requires more time and effort. The approach may vary from institution to institution. In our institution, the nutrition support team does this, and to provide a successful regimen, the constituents are customized to fit the individual's preferences and special needs. In so doing, the various elements of the diet may be "juggled" to conform to the nutritional requirements. A food substitution approach may be used, analogous to that used for diabetic diets. This approach is simple to implement and increases the flexibility of the diet (10).

LIQUID KETOGENIC DIET

The ketogenic diet can be adapted to a liquid form for infants who are bottle-fed or older children who are tube-fed. The ingredients are readily available, and the preparation is simple for parents to learn. A formula manufactured by Ross Laboratories (Columbus, Ohio), Ross Carbohydrate Free (RCF), is a soy-based protein formula that provides all the vitamins and minerals found in formula made for normal infants. RCF contains 20 g of protein/L, 36 g of fat/L, and no carbohydrate. In addition, each liter supplies 700 mg of calcium, 300 mg sodium, 710 mg of potassium, and 1.5 mg of iron.

The liquid ketogenic diet must be formulated to include a sufficient quantity of RCF formula to provide 2 g protein/kg/day. If this formula is used in combination with food, RCF should contribute approximately 50 percent of the patient's total protein needs, with the remaining 50 percent coming from food sources. Polycose or granulated sugar is added to the formula in the amount required by the prescribed diet's protein to carbohydrate ratio. Additional fat is supplied in the form of Microlipid made by Sherwood Medical Inc. (St. Louis, MO) to provide either 3:1 or 4:1 ratio. This microlipid consists of a safflower oil emulsion that provides 1 g fat per 2 mL. The mixture is blenderized and refrigerated. It is then used as the entire intake for the child for the next 24 hours. Water may be given between feedings but usually is not needed. The formula can be given in scheduled feedings or as a continuous drip tube feeding if indicated.

The additional fat may also be added to the formula in the form of medium-chain triglycerides (MCT) or corn oil. In this case, the amount added is based on MCT percentage of calories (as in the previous MCT example). The advantage of the microlipid is that it is an emulsion and therefore blends better with the formula; however, its expense and availability may be mitigating factors against its use.

MAINTENANCE OF THERAPY

After initiation of the diet, the patient remains in the hospital for another 3 to 4 days. This time is used to carefully instruct the parents or caretakers on the techniques of providing the diet, weighing the food, providing food substitutions, and monitoring ketosis. Patients on the ketogenic diet are often supplemented with calcium, iron, folate, and multivitamins, including vitamin D, to provide the RDA requirements. Protein requirements are carefully monitored and increased on an individual basis to allow for weight gain and growth.

After discharge from the hospital, the child is initially seen on a monthly basis by the nutrition support team or RD. The child's height, weight, and head circumference are charted at each visit. Serum electrolytes, liver function tests, serum lipids and proteins, and a complete blood count (CBC) are periodically checked. On average, the calorie and nutritional needs are readjusted monthly for infants and every 6 to 12 months for children.

RESULTS

Livingston reported extensive (41-year) experience with the diet in the treatment of myoclonic seizures of childhood (11). He stated that it completely controlled seizures in 54 percent of his patients and markedly improved control in another 26 percent. Only 20 percent of patients did not respond. In Livingston's experience, the diet was ineffective in controlling either true "petit mal" or temporal lobe epilepsy, although others have found the diet helpful in a wide variety of different seizures types (12).

Other investigators using both the "classic" diet and its variants have reported results similar to those of Livingston. In 63 diet trials conducted by Schwartz in 55 patients and coworkers, a total of 51 diet trials (81%) showed a greater than 50 percent reduction in seizure frequency regardless of the type of diet used (12). Others, however, have found that the MCT diet is slightly less efficacious, with 44 percent of patients achieving greater than 50 percent reduction in the number of seizures (13). A corn oil ketogenic diet was found to be equally beneficial compared with the MCT diet (14). Seizure control appears to be inconsistently accompanied by electroencephalographic improvement (12,15).* In addition to improved seizure control, the diet may have a calming effect on behavior.

---

* In 150 consecutive patients treated with the diet at Johns Hopkins, 32 percent had a greater than 90 percent decrease in seizures at 6 months and 27 percent had a greater than 90 percent decrease at year (16).

INDICATIONS FOR USE

Primary Therapy

The ketogenic diet is first-line therapy for the treatment of seizures in association with glucose transporter protein deficiency and pyruvate dehydrogenase deficiency (17,18). In both cases, the diet effectively treats seizures while providing essential fuel for brain metabolic activity. In this manner, the diet is not only an anticonvulsant treatment but also a treatment for the other nonepileptic manifestations of these diseases.

Secondary Treatment

The ketogenic diet may be considered as an alternate treatment, usually after the failure of valproate, for generalized epilepsies, particularly those with myoclonic seizures including early myoclonic epilepsy (EME), early infantile epileptic encephalopathy (EIEE), and myoclonic-absence epilepsy. Given the effectiveness of the diet in the treatment of myoclonic epilepsies, it could be considered as first-line treatment for patients with very severe epileptogenic encephalopathies that are notoriously difficult to control with medications: Lennox-Gastaut syndrome, myoclonic-astatic epilepsy, and severe infantile myoclonic epilepsy. In our experience, however, most parents prefer the convenience of a medication, and it is unusual to try the ketogenic diet before at least one or two AEDs have failed. The ketogenic diet can be beneficial in infants with West syndrome who are refractory to corticosteroids and other medications (19). Based on Keith's data and our own experience, the ketogenic diet may also be useful in the treatment of children with refractory absence epilepsy without myoclonus (20).

FURTHER POSSIBLE INDICATIONS

Partial Seizures

It is very difficult to determine the efficacy of the diet in the treatment of partial seizure disorders. Livingston stated that the diet was not effective in treating patients with partial seizures. Keith did not classify his patients in a manner that allows one to determine the effectiveness in partial seizures. In current use, the diet is usually prescribed for children with other forms of refractory epilepsy. In a recent scientific study of the efficacy of the diet in kindled animals, the diet was shown to have at least transient anticonvulsant properties (21). This bolsters the consideration of its use in children with refractory partial epilepsy. Nevertheless, while the diet may be considered in this group, there are no compelling clinical data to favor its use. Children with refractory partial seizures, therefore, should be evaluated to determine if they are candidates for focal resective surgery. If they are, then surgery need not be delayed to institute a trial of the ketogenic diet. On the other hand, if drugs have failed and the patient is deemed to be a poor surgical candidate, the diet should be considered. It would seem inappropriate to treat children with otherwise benign seizure disorders, such as febrile seizures, benign rolandic epilepsy, benign occipital epilepsy, and benign familial neonatal convulsions, with the ketogenic diet.

PRECAUTIONS

The ketogenic diet may be lethal in certain circumstances in which cerebral energy metabolism is deranged. An example of this is pyruvate carboxylase deficiency in which patients may present early in life with refractory myoclonic seizures (9).

Mitochondrial/disorders or diseases that involve the respiratory chain, such as myoclonus epilepsy with ragged red fibers (MERRF), mitochondrial encephalomyopathy–latic acidosis–and strokelike symptoms (MELAS), and cytochrome oxidase deficiency, would also probably be contraindications for use of the ketogenic diet because of the increased stress on respiratory chain and tricarboxylic acid (TCA) cycle function. Patients with fatty acid oxidation problems would also be adversely affected by the ketogenic diet, but such patients do not, as a rule, present with seizures.

COMPLICATIONS

Patients on the ketogenic diet exhibit a significantly reduced quantity of bone mass, which improves in response to vitamin D supplementation (5000 ID/day) (22). Renal calculi may develop but are rarely seen. Lipemia retinalis developed in two of Livingston's patients (23). Bilateral optic neuropathy has been reported in two children who were treated with a 4:1 "classic" ketogenic diet. These patients were not originally given vitamin B supplements. Vision was restored in both after administration of vitamin B supplements. Thinning of hair and, rarely, alopecia may occur. Cardiovascular complications have not been seen in those adults examined (23). A recent report does describe some cardiac complications in children (24). Prolonged QT interval and dilated cardiomyopathy were described.

STOPPING THE KETOGENIC DIET

The ketogenic diet should be tapered and stopped gradually. A sudden stop of the diet or sudden administration of glucose may aggravate seizures and precipitate status epilepticus (25). Livingston advocates

maintaining the diet at a ratio 4:1 for 2 years and, if successful, weaning to a 3:1 diet for 6 months, followed by 6 months of a 2:1 diet (23). At this point a regular diet is begun. We have not used such a rigorous protocol.

POTENTIAL ADVERSE DRUG INTERACTIONS

Carbonic anhydrase inhibitors such as acetazolamide and topiramate should be avoided, particularly in the early stages of treatment with the ketogenic diet. Valproate (VPA) is an inhibitor of fatty acid oxidation and a mitigator of hepatic ketogenesis. When possible, therefore, we avoid use of this agent.

Carnitine supplementation is complex. It is often used to supplement the diet of patients with various metabolic derangements whose defects allow a buildup of undesirable intermediates. It is also not uncommon in patients who need the ketogenic diet that a metabolic disorder of this sort is either suspected or confirmed (another reason to avoid VPA if possible). Carnitine supplementation may be desirable for these patients. These factors must be weighed in each patient, and the decision to use the supplementation should be individualized.

CONCLUSIONS

It is remarkable that 80 years and scores of drugs later, the ketogenic diet retains a role in the modern treatment of children with refractory epilepsy, however, even with our new pharmacologic armamentarium, there remain patients whose epilepsy is resistant to the effects of antiepileptic drugs (AEDs). Indeed, once several AEDs with multiple different mechanisms of action have failed, it is unlikely that another AED will demonstrate good efficacy. In a sense, these patients may be declaring that they are not candidates for drugs and that they require alternate forms of treatment such as the ketogenic diet or surgery. Yet, it is still difficult to determine who these patients are at the onset, and the only reliable way to determine the refractory nature of their epilepsy is by trying treatment with various AEDs. Improvements in the classification of epilepsy, animal models, clinical studies, and deeper insights into the basic pathogenesis of refractory epilepsy will most likely provide useful information. In the meantime, the physicians caring for the child with epilepsy must still carefully weigh the known risks and benefits of all forms of treatment and use their best clinical judgment to arrive at the optimal regimen for the patient.

REFERENCES

1. Geyelin HR. Fasting as a method for treating epilepsy. *Medical Record* 1921; 99:1037–1039.

2. Wilder RM. Effects of ketonuria on the course of epilepsy. *Mayo Clin Bull* 1921; 2:307–314.

3. Owen OE, Morgan AP, Kemp HG, et al. Brain metabolism during fasting. *J Clin Invest* 1967; 46:1589–1595.

4. Appleton DB, DeVivo DC. An animal model for the ketogenic diet. *Epilepsia* 1974; 15:211–227.

5. Huttenlocher PR. Ketonemia and seizures: metabolic and anticonvulsant effects of two ketogenic diets in childhood epilepsy. *Pediatr Res* 1976; 10:536–540.

6. DeVivo DC, Leckie MP, Ferrendelli JS, McDougal DB. Chronic ketosis and cerebral metabolism. *Ann Neurol* 1978; 3:331–337.

7. Al-Mudallal AS, LaManna JC, Lust WD, Harik SI. Diet-induced ketosis does not cause cerebral acidosis. *Epilepsia* 1996; 37:258–561.

8. Nordli DR, De Vivo DC. The ketogenic diet revisited: back to the future. *Epilepsia* 1997; 38:743–749.

9. DeVivo DC, Haymond MW, Leckie MP, et al. The clinical and biochemical implications of pyruvate carboxylase deficiency. *Clin Endocrinol Metab* 1977; 45:1281–1296.

10. Carroll J, Koenigsberger D. The ketogenic diet: a practical guide for caregivers. *J Am Diet Assoc* 1998; 98:316–321.

11. Livingston S, Pauli LL, Pruce I. Ketogenic diet in the treatment of childhood epilepsy. *Dev Med Child Neurol* 1977; 19:833–834.

12. Schwartz RH, Eaton J, Bower BD, Aynsley-Green A. Ketogenic diets in the treatment of epilepsy: short-term clinical effects. *Dev Med Child Neurol* 1989; 31(2):145–51.

13. Sills MA, Forsythe WI, Haidukewych D, MacDonald A, Robinson M. The medium chain triglyceride diet and intractable epilepsy. *Arch Dis Child* 1986; 61:1168–1172.

14. Woody RC, Brodie M, Hampton DK, Fiser RH Jr. Corn oil ketogenic diet for children with intractable seizures. *J Child Neurol* 1988; 3:21–24.

15. Janaki S, Rashid MK, Gulati MS, et al. A clinical electroencephalographic correlation of seizures on a ketogenic diet. *Indian J Med Res* 1976; 64:1057–1063.

16. Freeman FM, Vining EP, Pillas DF, Pyzik PL, Casey FC, Kelly LM. The efficacy of the ketogenic diet—1998: a prospective evaluation of intervention in 150 children. *Pediatrics* 1998; 102:1358–1363.

17. DeVivo DC, Trifiletti RR, Jacobson RI, et al. Defective glucose transport across the blood-brain barrier as a cause of persistent hypolycorrhachia, seizures, and developmental delay. *N Engl J Med* 1991; 325:713–721.

18. Wexler ID, Hemalatha SG, McConnell J, et al. Outcome of pyruvate dehydrogenase deficiency treated with ketogenic diets. Studies in patients with identical mutations. *Neurology* 1997; 49:1655–1661.

19. Nordli DR, Koenigsberger D, Carroll J, DeVivo DC. Successful treatment of infants with the ketogenic diet. *Ann Neurol* 1995; 38:523. Abstract.

20. Keith HM. *Convulsive Disorders in Children: With Reference to Treatment with Ketogenic Diet.* Boston: Little, Brown, 1963.

21. Hori A, Tandon P, Holmes GL, Stafstrom C. Ketogenic diet: effects on expression of kindled seizures and behavior in adult rats. *Epilepsia* 1997; 38:750–758.

22. Hahn TJ, Halstead LR, DeVivo DC. Disordered mineral metabolism produced by ketogenic diet therapy. *Calcif Tissue Int* 1979; 28:17–22.

23. Livingston S. *Comprehensive Management of Epilepsy in Infancy, Childhood and Adolescence.* Springfield, IL: Charles C Thomas, 1972.

24. Best TH, Franz DN, Gilbert DL, Nelson DP, Epstein MR. Cardiac complications in pediatric patients on the ketogenic diet. *Neurology* 2000; 54:2328–2330.

25. Nordli DR, Koenigsberger D, Schroeder J, DeVivo DC. Ketogenic diets. In: Resor S, Kutt H, eds. *The Medical Treatment of Epilepsy.* New York: Marcel Dekker, 1992:455–472.

CHAPTER 44

Drug Interactions

Jamie T. Gilman, Pharm.D.

In the ever-growing field of pharmacotherapy, understanding the fundamentals of drug interactions has become increasingly important. This is especially true in epileptology, in which patients are receiving chronic agents that have a high potential for drug interactions. The antiepileptic drugs (AEDs) as a therapeutic class have the propensity to exhibit interactions the magnitude of which often require dosage modifications. The unfortunate consequence of these interactions is often loss of seizure control, failure to attain optimal therapeutic effects, or adverse drug reactions.

The advancement of biotechnology, molecular biology, and medical research has enabled the development and release of an unprecedented number of new therapeutic modalities. It has consequently become almost an impossibility to remain current on all potential drug interactions. This chapter does not aim to discuss each agent that may interact with the AEDs but rather focuses on mechanisms of these interactions. This understanding should equip clinicians with the ability to predict interactions as new products are marketed. Tables 44-1 and 44-2 are provided as a reference for some common AED interactions.

TYPES OF INTERACTIONS

The actions of xenobiotics administered into biological systems are usually described in terms of pharmacokinetics and pharmacodynamics. Pharmacokinetics can have considerable interpatient variability, while pharmacodynamics typically does not. Pharmacokinetics describes the time course of the drug's concentration in the blood, which encompasses drug protein binding, renal excretion, gastrointestinal absorption, and metabolism. Pharmacodynamics describes the pharmacologic response resulting from these pharmacokinetic processes. While distinctly different, the two are intricately interrelated.

A mechanism that has gained the focus of attention in the drug interaction arena is drug biotransformation. Although similar, the terms *drug biotransformation* and *drug metabolism* are not synonymous (1). The pharmacokinetic term *drug metabolism* typically refers to the total fate of a drug in the body, whereas *biotransformation* particularly describes its chemical transformation, usually by enzyme-catalyzed reactions. Although drug biotransformation is a facet of drug metabolism, it is discussed separately because of its complexity and the heightened understanding of this process.

Drug interactions can occur at any phase: pharmacokinetic, pharmacodynamic, or biotransformation processes. Of the three, changes in hepatic drug biotransformation pathways elicit the most serious interactions. Therapeutic agents most likely to be affected are those whose rate-limiting step for elimination is biotransformation, particularly those dependent on a single biotransformation pathway.

CONSEQUENCES OF INTERACTIONS

Drug interactions typically present themselves by creating unexpected pharmacologic actions that may be in the form of an exaggerated response, lack of desired effect, or toxicity. The alteration of protein binding or receptor responsiveness may elicit exaggerated pharmacologic responses despite low serum drug concentrations or low doses. Serum drug concentrations may be unexpectedly high because of biotransformation inhibition. Drug interactions may also be responsible for pharmacotherapeutic failures, as sufficient serum concentrations may be hindered by poor oral drug absorption or increased elimination. Drug-drug interactions also may potentiate some of the serious toxicities documented in epileptic patients such as the increased incidence of valproic acid hepatotoxicity and

Table 44-1. Select Interactions Between Antiepileptic Drugs AEDs and Other Therapeutic Categories

Drug Class	AED	Clinical Interaction
ADRENERGIC BLOCKERS Alprenolol Metoprolol Propranolol	PB	PB increases metabolism; dosage of adrenergic blockers may need to be increased.
ANALGESICS Acetaminophen	CBZ, LTG, PB, PHT	Patients on enzyme inducers such as CBZ, PHT, and PB may be at greater risk of hepatotoxicity following acetaminophen overdose. Acetaminophen appears to slightly increase the elimination of LTG.
Narcotics	CBZ, PB, PHT	Enzyme inducers (CBZ, PHT, PB) increase the toxicity and decrease the efficacy of meperidine by increasing the conversation to normeperidine.
Propoxyphene	CBZ	Propoxyphene inhibits CBZ elimination and may lead to CBZ toxicity. Propoxyphene should be avoided if possible.
Salicylates	PHT, VPA	High-dose salicylates displace PHT and VPA from protein-binding sites and may decrease VPA elimination.
ANTIARRYTHMICS Disopyramide	PB, PHT	PB and PHT may increase hepatic metabolism of disopyramide and require dosage adjustments.
Mexiletine	CBZ, PB, PHT	Enzyme inducers can substantially decrease mexiletine serum concentrations.
Quinidine	PB, PHT	Enzyme inducers decrease serum concentrations of quinidine.
ANTICOAGULANTS Warfarin	CBZ, PB, PHT	Inducers increase warfarin metabolism and decrease hypoprothrombinemic effect.
ANTIDEPRESSANTS Tricyclics	CBZ, PB	Induction of tricyclic metabolism. Dosage may require adjustment.
ANTIDIABETIC AGENTS Tolazamide Tolbutamide Acetohexamide Glibenclamide	CBZ, PB, PHT	Enzyme inducers increase elimination and decrease hypoglycemic effects.
ANTIMICROBIAL AGENTS Ciprofloxacin	PHT	Ciprofloxacin increases serum PHT concentrations probably by decreasing phenytoin elimination.
Erythromycin	CBZ, BZD, VPA	Erythromycin decreases biotransformation and can markedly increase serum concentrations.
ANTIFUNGAL Fluconazole	PHT	Fluconazole decreases biotransformation of PHT and can result in marked increase in serum concentrations.
ANTINEOPLASTICS	PHT	Cytotoxic agents appear to decrease oral absorption of PHT with marked reductions in serum PHT concentrations.
ANTITUBERCULOUS AGENTS Isoniazid	CBZ, PHT, VPA	Isoniazid decreases CBZ, PHT, and VPA elimination and may lead to toxicity.
Rifampin	BZD, PHT, VPA	Rifampin increases elimination, dosage adjustments may be necessary.
CARBONIC ANHYDRASE INHIBITORS Acetazolamide Dichlorphenamide Methazolamide	TPM	Concomitant use may lead to increased risk of nephrolithiasis.

(continued overleaf)

Table 44-1. (*Continued*)

Drug Class	AED	Clinical Interaction
CORTICOSTEROIDS		
Dexamethasone	CBZ, PB, PHT	Enzyme inducers increase metabolism of steroids and decrease efficacy. Decreased PHT absorption and subsequent decrease in serum concentrations.
Hydrocortisone		
Methylprednisolone		
Prednisone		
MISCELLANEOUS		
Cimetidine	CBZ, PHT, BZD, ESM	Cimetidine decreases biotransformation of CBZ and PHT and may lead to toxicity.
Clozapine	CBZ	May result in increased risk of bone marrow suppression.
Enteral feedings	PHT	Decreased PHT absorption and marked decreased in serum concentration.
Nafimidone	CBZ, PHT	May result in CBZ toxicity.
Ritonavir	BDZ, ESM	Ritonavir decreases biotransformation of BDZ and ESM and may lead to toxicity.
SELECTIVE SEROTONIN REUPTAKE INHIBITORS		
Fluoxetine	CBZ	Fluoxetine has been reported to result in CBZ toxicity by inhibiting CYP 3A3/4.

BDZ = benzodiazepines; CBZ = carbamazepine; LTG = lamotrigine; PB = phenobarbital; PHT = phenytoin; PRM = primidone; VPA = valproic Acid; ESM = ethosuximide; TPM = topiramate; MSM = methsuximide.
Source: McInnes GT, Brodie MJ. Drug interactions that matter—a critical reappraisal. *Drugs* 1988; 36:83–110.

death in young children comedicated with hepatic enzyme inducers, especially phenobarbital. Although the number of potential interactions with antiepileptic agents is substantial, most, fortunately, have little clinical relevance (2).

PATIENTS AT RISK

Patients at the greatest risks for drug interactions are usually those who are the most severely ill (3). This includes patients in the intensive care unit, geriatric patients, premature neonates, and young children with immature organ function. As the number of concomitant medications increases, so does the likelihood of drug interactions. The most refractory epilepsy patients are consequently more likely to encounter problems with drug interactions related to concomitant AED therapy than their controlled counterpart. A drug interaction check should be considered standard care in patients with pharmacoresistant seizures.

PHARMACOKINETIC INTERACTIONS

Gastrointestinal Absorption

The primary variables that have been identified to elicit interactions involving AED gastrointestinal absorption have been limited primarily to food, antacids, and enteral feedings. The interaction between phenytoin and enteral feedings has been recognized and documented since the early 1980s (4–6). Because the elimination half-life of phenytoin is concentration-dependent, the half-life shortens and serum concentrations decline even further when absorption is impeded. Maintaining adequate serum concentrations with concurrent enteral feedings and oral-enteral phenytoin can become difficult. It generally is recommended that the administration of feedings and oral phenytoin be spaced at least 2 hours apart (4). This practice may not always be practical, especially in young children or infants who may require continuous feedings. If serum phenytoin concentrations fail to rise after several attempts at optimizing absorption, it probably is better to seek treatment

Table 44-2. Interactions Between Antiepileptic Drugs (AEDs) (26)

Agent	Interacts With	Clinical Interaction
Barbiturates (PB PRM)	PHT	Decrease in serum concentration of PB
	ESM	Increase in serum concentration of PB and ESM
	VPA	
Benzodiazepines (Clobazam, Diazepam, Midazolam)	PHT, CBZ	Increased clearance of benzodiazepine parent drug and decreased effect
Carbamazepine	ESM	May result in decreased ESM serum concentrations
	LTG	Increase in elimination of LTG and decrease in serum concentration
	PHT	Decrease in serum concentration of CBZ and increase in concentration of CBZ-10,11-epoxide
	TPM	May result in decreased TPM serum concentrations
	VPA	Increase in serum CBZ concentrations and decrease in serum VPA concentration
Felbamate	CBZ, PHT, VPA	FBM increases VPA and PHT serum concentration and decreases CBZ serum concentrations
Lamotrigine	PB, CBZ, PHT, PRM	Enzyme inducers increase LTG elimination and decrease serum concentrations
	VPA	Decrease LTG elimination and increases serum concentration
Phenytoin	GBP, MSM	May lead to phenytoin toxicity
	LTG	Increase in LTG elimination and decrease in LTG serum concentration
	VPA	Decrease in VPA concentration and increase in unbound PHT concentration
Tiagabine	CBZ, PB, PHT, PRM	May result in decreased TGB levels and efficacy
	VPA	May result in increased risk of TGB adverse effects
Topiramate	PHT	May result in altered serum concentrations of either agent
	VPA	May result in decreased serum concentrations of TPM or VPA
Valproic Acid	LTG	Decrease in LTG elimination and increase in serum concentration
	TGB	May result in increased TGB toxicity
	TPM	May result in decreased TPM or VPA serum concentrations

CBZ = carbamazepine; LTG = lamotrigine; PB = phenobarbital; PHT = phenytoin; PRM = primidone; VPA = valproic Acid; ESM = ethosuximide; TPM = topiramate; TGB = tiagabine; MSM = methsuximide; GBP = gabapentin.
Source: McInnes GT, Brodie MJ. Drug interactions that matter—a critical reappraisal. *Drugs* 1988; 36:83–110.

with a different AED. Although this is not well documented, it probably is also advisable to avoid simultaneous administration of any AED with infant formulas.

Food has been documented to delay the time to attain peak concentrations of valproate by approximately 5 hours. Fisher and coworkers (7) demonstrated a significant effect on the pharmacokinetic profile when valproate was taken with food. The extent of absorption was unaffected, but peak concentrations of valproate were not reached until approximately 8 hours after the dose (7). Serum concentrations obtained before a dose are likely to yield peak values instead of the traditional trough values in patients who are medicated three times daily and take their medications with meals.

Role of Protein Binding

Protein binding displacement interactions among the AEDs usually do not lead to serious adverse effects. Only agents with at least 90 percent protein binding can be displaced enough to create a clinical concern.

Among the AEDs, this applies only to valproic acid and phenytoin. When these two agents are administered in tandem, unbound phenytoin concentrations are higher than expected and effective total concentrations are lower (8). It usually is not necessary to monitor unbound concentrations as long as the treating physician realizes that lower total concentrations are still therapeutic. In most instances, when unbound concentrations begin to rise, clinical toxicity manifests, which signals that a dosage reduction is in order. When adding agents in other therapeutic categories to a phenytoin regimen, it is always prudent to check for protein binding affinity of the added agent. High-dose salicylates are known displacing agents from protein binding sites. The displacement of valproic acid usually is not problematic.

Drug Elimination

Pharmacokinetic interactions affecting drug elimination are any actions between two agents that affect the time course for drug excretion from the body.

This could entail a change in renal excretion, hepatic metabolism, or any other change that alters the ordinary fate of the drug in the body. The greatest impact of this interaction occurs if the target agent has only one route of elimination. Most of the AEDs are hepatically metabolized, and their interactions consequently are more related to biotransformation. Interactions strictly involving drug biotransformation are considered in the section "Biotransformation Interactions." Although unclear, the interaction between vigabatrin and phenytoin may prove to be a drug elimination interaction (9).

Clinical Significance

Pharmacokinetic interactions usually can be predicted with a working knowledge of each drug's disposition properties. The extent of the interaction, however, is more difficult to anticipate because of marked interindividual variability. Fortunately, only a small percentage of patients experience significant clinical repercussions from pharmacokinetic interactions with the AEDs.

BIOTRANSFORMATION INTERACTIONS

Advances in molecular biology in the 1990s have enabled a better understanding of drug biotransformation pathways. Biotransformation reactions create three distinct mechanisms that affect a drug's pharmacologic effect: (1) conversion of an inactive precursor or prodrug to a pharmacologically active compound; an example of this is the conversion of fosphenytoin to phenytoin; (2) extension of pharmacologic effect through the transformation of the active parent compound to an active metabolite; an example of this is the biotransformation of diazepam to one of its many active metabolites, and oxcarbazepine to the active 10-monohydroxy derivative (MHD); and (3) inactivation of the active parent compound to an inactive metabolite such as seen with phenytoin.

Most important drug biotransformations occur in the liver, although they can occur in almost any body tissue and at various subcellular sites within the tissues. An example of this is the transformation of fosphenytoin to phenytoin, which can occur almost anywhere in the body. These reactions have been classified into phase I and phase II reactions. Reactions involving microsomal enzymes are phase I reactions and include drug oxidation, reduction, and hydrolysis reactions. Phase II reactions are extramolecular changes that may be catalyzed by microsomal, mitochondrial, and/or cytoplasmic enzymes. The one most thoroughly studied, with probably the most impact on the AEDs, is the phase I cytochrome P-450 mixed-function oxidase system (1).

Cytochrome P-450 System

The enzymes of this system exist in the highest concentration in the liver but are found in virtually all tissues. There have been at least 12 cytochrome P-450 gene families and 31 functional cytochrome P-450 gene products identified in humans along with 5 pseudogenes (nonfunctional). Individual cytochromes are distinguished based on their molecular and spectral properties and can have several different epitopes. Cytochromes are included in the same family if their sequence identity is greater than 40 percent and in the same subfamily with greater than 55 percent homology (10).

Cytochrome P-450 nomenclature was established by the P-450 Nomenclature Committee and is based on similarities in amino acid sequences (11). This permits the identification of not only the enzyme family and subfamily but also the individual enzyme. "CYP" identifies the cytochrome P-450 group, which is followed by an Arabic number indicating the enzyme family, followed by a capital letter designating the subfamily, and finally ending with an Arabic number representing the individual enzyme (e.g., CYP 2D6) (10,11). The majority of drug biotransformation in humans occur in the CYP1, CYP2, and CYP3 families (12). With respect to drug interactions, the most important isoenzymes identified at this time include CYP1A2, CYP2D6, and CYP3A3/4. Phenytoin and phenobarbital increase the activity of CYP1A2, which is the isoenzyme that catalyzes theophylline, warfarin, and caffeine metabolism. The isoenzyme CYP2D6 exhibits polymorphism, which leads to clinical phenotypes and mediates the metabolism of some psychotropic agents such as amitriptyline, desipramine, and nortriptyline (10). CYP3A3/4 is found in the highest concentration in intestinal tract enterocytes and can cause a significant first-pass metabolism (13). Of the 36 identified gene families, only three are significantly pertinent to AEDs (CYP2C9/10, CYP2C19, and CYP3A4) (10).

CYP-Mediated Interactions

Agents that either undergo biotransformation or are capable of changing the rate of cytochrome P-450 transformation either by induction or by inhibition are susceptible to interactions in this category. Drugs or foods that fit this description are categorized into groups called accomplice agents or substrates. Agents that are accomplices are those that either inhibit or induce CYP isoenzymes, while substrates are those whose serum concentrations are affected by accomplice isoenzyme alterations. For a drug interaction to occur, an accomplice needs a substrate. A knowledge of the specific biotransformation isoform for drug catabolism enables the prediction of these interactions as new AEDs are introduced into clinical practice. These reactions are enzyme-specific and substrate-independent.

All substrates metabolized to a significant degree by the specific isoform affected exhibit the interaction regardless of their chemical structure and pharmacologic and therapeutic activity. As a result, a wide array of agents can be substrates for the same isoform (14,15).

Table 44-3 depicts selected accomplices and substrates for isoforms important for AED biotransformation. For isoenzymes in which the AEDs act as accomplices, the substrate list is expanded to include agents that may be used concomitantly in children and adolescents.

Table 44-3. Selected Cytochrome P-450 Isoforms That Impact Antiepileptic Drugs (AEDs). Interactions Occur Between Accomplices (inducers and inhibitiors) and Substrates. No Interaction Occurs Between Inhibitors and Inducers

Cyp Isoform	Substrate	Inhibitors	Inducers
2C9/10	Phenytoin	Sulfaphenazole Fluconazole Miconazole	Rifampin
2C19	Diazepam S-Mephenytoin Phenytoin (minor pathway)	Cimetidine Omeprazole Ketoconazole Diazepam Tranylcypromine Imipramine Fluoxetine	
3A 3/4	*ANTICONVULSANTS* Carbamazepine Ethosuximide Phenytoin	*ANTIDEPRESSANTS* Fluoxetine Fluvoxamine Sertraline	*ANTICONVULSANTS* Carbamazepine Phenobarbital Phenytoin Primidone
	ANTIDEPRESSANTS Amitriptyline Doxepin Imipramine Sertraline Nafazodine Venlafaxine	*AZOLES* Fluconazole Itraconazole Ketoconazole	*ANTITUBERCULINS* Rifampin
	MISCELLANEOUS Acetaminophen Corticosteroids Codeine Oral contraceptives Retinoic acid Rinonavir Theophylline Warfarin	*FOOD* Grapefruit juice	
	BENZODIAZEPINES Alprazolam Diazepam Midazolam Triazolam	*MACROLIDES* Clarithromycin Erythromycin	*MISCELLANEOUS* Clotrimazole Dexamethasone Griseofulvin Phenylbutazone
		MISCELLANEOUS Cimetidine Diltiazem Ethinylestradiol Grestodene Omeprazole Ritonavar Indinavir Tacrolimus Valproic acid	

Source: Reference 10,12,20.

Inhibition

Interactions with inhibitor accomplice agents usually result in increases in blood substrate concentrations with increased drug response and/or toxicity. Because of these potential effects, biotransformation inhibition is the most important drug interaction mechanism. If the substrate happens to be a prodrug with the metabolite as the active pharmacologic component, the therapeutic effect of the substrate is diminished. This reaction begins within the first two doses of the accomplice and can be either competitive or noncompetitive (16). In a competitive interaction, the accomplice agent binds tightly to the heme moiety of the isoenzyme. The CYP isoform is incapable of biotransformation of the substrate as long as this site is occupied by the accomplice. The extent of the inhibition is dependent on the affinity of the accomplice to the isoenzyme (17). An example of this is the interaction between the accomplice macrolide antibiotics (erythromycin, clarithromycin) and carbamazepine (substrate) (18). A noncompetitive inhibition occurs when the accomplice incapacitates the isoenzyme by destroying, inactivating, or allosterically changing it (10,17).

Substrates are capable of having multiple pathways for biotransformation. If minor pathways are altered, only minimal serum concentration changes occur (e.g., isoform 2C19, which is a minor pathway for phenytoin). However, when the major pathway is inhibited, (e.g., 2C9/10 for phenytoin), dramatic changes in serum concentration are possible. A mathematical model has been proposed to assist in the prediction of inhibitory interactions (19).

Because of the bioflavonoids, grapefruit juice is an inhibitor accomplice for the isoform CYP3A/4. This isoenzyme performs oxidation reactions in the gastrointestinal wall. Inhibition seems maximal if grapefruit juice is ingested 30 to 60 minutes before drug administration (20,21). Patients should be advised that it is not good practice to take medications with grapefruit juice. Orange juice apparently is devoid of bioflavonoids.

Induction

Unlike inhibition, enzyme induction is a gradual process because the onset depends on synthesis of new enzymes and accumulation of the accomplice. The offset of induction is also gradual because of the dependence on the decay of both the increased enzyme stores and the induction agent. Enzyme induction is noted for diminishing serum concentrations of the substrate drug and subsequent decline of therapeutic effect. If the substrate metabolite is active, however, this interaction could actually increase therapeutic effect. There have been several molecular mechanisms identified for enzyme induction, the most common of which is increased DNA transcription. Posttranscriptional mechanisms have also been identified and include RNA processing, mRNA stabilization, translational efficiency, protein stabilization, and decreased heme degradation (10,17).

Carbamazepine, phenobarbital, and phenytoin are inducer accomplices for CYP3A. This creates an interaction with the benzodiazepines clobazam, diazepam, and midazolam. Clobazam serum concentrations have been reported to decrease by 61 percent with concomitant administration of carbamazepine (22). Concomitant use of these agents with diazepam usually does not diminish therapeutic effect because diazepam metabolites are active. These agents have the potential to lead to oral contraceptive failure because some estrogens are metabolized by CYP3A3/4. Parkinson additionally reports the precipitation of porphyria crises related to enzyme induction by anticonvulsants and alcohol. This reaction is related to the increased demand for heme and accumulation of heme intermediates (23).

Physiologic and Environmental Influences

Many factors contribute to the interpatient variability in drug biotransformation, but the most pronounced is genetically regulated polymorphic biotransformation. The isoform CYP2C19, S-mephenytoin hydroxylase, exhibits polymorphism, with 5 percent of whites and 20 percent of Asians exhibiting poor metabolism. CYP2D6 (debrisoquine/sparteine hydroxylase) also exhibits genetic polymorphism with 5 percent to 10 percent of whites and 1 percent of Asians demonstrating slow metabolism (12). Polymorphic N-acetyltransferase, of which clonazepam is a substrate, has also been extensively described (24).

Environmental influences have also been described to act as accomplices of drug biotransformations. A diet that is high in protein, charcoal-broiled beef consumption, and cigarette smoking induce oxidative biotransformation, while a high-carbohydrate diet slows down this reaction (25).

PHARMACODYNAMIC INTERACTIONS

Pharmacodynamic interactions are harder to predict than those that are dependent on pharmacokinetic or biotransformation mechanisms. These reactions are evidenced by the production of a synergism or antagonism between two agents that leads to unexpected adverse or therapeutic effects. This reaction is more than additive, is unrelated to a change in serum concentrations, and presumably occurs at the receptor site (26). An example of this is enhanced cerebellar dysfunction observed when lamotrigine is added to existing carbamazepine therapy. Neither carbamazepine nor carbamazepine 10, 11-epoxide serum concentrations change significantly under controlled conditions. These symptoms usually resolve when carbamazepine doses are lowered (27).

SUMMARY

Patients treated for epilepsy with chronic AEDs frequently require treatment with other therapeutic agents. Table 44-1 lists some interactions between the AEDs and other therapeutic agents. This list is by no means complete but highlights selected agents that have documented interactions. Patients with pharmacoresistant epilepsy may require multiple AEDs, and Table 44-2 is provided for interactions among the AEDs. The most important variable, however, in the recognition of drug interactions is an acute awareness of their occurrence potential and a basic knowledge of possible mechanisms.

REFERENCES

1. Kalant H. Drug biotransformation. In: Kalant H, Roschiau W, eds. *Principles of Medical Pharmacology*. 5th ed. Lewiston, NY: BC Decker, 1989:35–48.

2. Pisani F, Perucca G, DePerri R. Clinically relevant antiepileptic drug interactions. *J Int Med Res* 1990; 18:1–15.

3. Brodie MJ, Feely J. Adverse drug interactions. *Br Med J* 1988; 296:845–849.

4. Bauer LA. Interference of oral phenytoin absorption by continuous nasogastric feedings. *Neurology* 1982; 32:570–572.

5. Krueger KA, Garnett WR, Comstock TJ, et al. Effect of two administration schedules of an enteral nutrient formula on phenytoin bioavailability. *Epilepsia* 1987; 28:706–712.

6. Nishimura LY, Armstrong EP, Plezia PM, et al. Influence of enteral feedings on phenytoin sodium absorption from capsules. *Drug Intell Clin Pharm* 1988; 22:130–133.

7. Fischer JH, Barr AN, Paloucek FP, Dorociak JV, Spunt AL. Effect of food on the serum concentration profile of enteric-coated valproic acid. *Neurology* 1988; 38:1319–1322.

8. Mattson RH, Cramer JA, Williamson PD, et al. Valproic acid in epilepsy: clinical and pharmacological effects. *Ann Neurol* 1978; 3:20–25.

9. Rimmer EM, Richens A. Interaction between vigabatrin and phenytoin. *Br J Clin Pharmacol* 1989; 27:27S–33S.

10. Riddick DS. Drug biotransformation. In: Kalant H, Roschlau W, eds. *Principles of Medical Pharmacology*. 6th ed. New York: Oxford University Press, 1997:38–54.

11. Nelson DR, Kamataki T, Waxman DJ, et al. The P450 superfamily: update on new sequences, gene mapping accession numbers, early trivial names of enzymes, and nomenclature. *DNA Cell Biol* 1993; 12:1–51.

12. Slaughter RL, Edwards DJ. Recent advances: the cytochrome P450 enzymes. *Ann Pharmacother* 1995; 29:619–624.

13. Watkins PB. Drug metabolism by cytochromes P450 in the liver and small bowel. *Gastroenterol Clin North Am* 1992; 21:511–526.

14. Mather GG, Levy RH. Pharmacokinetics of polypharmacy: prediction of drug interactions. *Epilepsy Res* 1996; 11 (Suppl):113–121.

15. Shapiro L, Singer M, Shear NH. Pharmacokinetic mechanisms of drug-drug and drug-food interactions in dermatology. *Curr Opin Dermatol* 1997; 4:25–31.

16. Andersen WK, Feingold DS. Adverse drug interactions clinically important for the dermatologist. *Arch Dermatol* 1995; 131:468–473.

17. Timbrell JA. *Principles of Biochemical Toxicology*. 2nd ed. London: Taylor and Francis, 1991.

18. Murray M. P450 enzymes: inhibition mechanisms, genetic regulation and effects of liver disease. *Clin Pharmacokinet* 1992; 23:132–146.

19. Von Moltke LL, Breenblatt DJ, Duan SX, Harmatz JS, Shader RI. In vitro prediction of the terfenadine-ketoconazole pharmacokinetic interaction. *J Clin Pharmacol* 1994; 34:1222–1227.

20. Gibaldi M. Drug interactions. Part II. *Ann Pharmacother* 1992; 26:829–834.

21. Benton R, Honig P, Zamani K, Cantilena L, Woosley R. Grapefruit juice alters terfenadine pharmacokinetics, resulting in prolongation of repolarization of the electrocardiogram. *Clin Pharmacol Ther* 1996; 59:383–388.

22. Levy RH, Lane EA, Guyot M, et al. Analysis of parent drug-metabolite relationship in the presence of an inducer. Application to the carbamazepine-clobazam interaction in normal man. *Drug Metab Dispos* 1983; 11:286–294.

23. Parkinson A. Biotransformation of xenobiotics. In: Klaassen CD, ed. *Casarett and Doull's Toxicology: The Basic Science of Poisons*. 5th ed. New York: McGraw-Hill, 1996:113–186.

24. Evans DAP, White TA. Human acetylation polymorphism. *J Lab Clin Med* 1964; 63:395.

25. Chandler MHH, Blouin RA. Dietary influences on drug disposition. In: Evans WE, Schentag JJ, Jusko WJ, eds. *Applied Pharmacokinetics Principles of Therapeutic Drug Monitoring*. 3rd ed. Vancouver, WA: Applied Therapeutics, Inc.:12.1–12.17.

26. McInnes GT, Brodie MJ. Drug interactions that matter—a critical reappraisal. *Drugs* 1988; 36:83–110.

27. Gilman JT. Lamotrigine: an antiepileptic agent for the treatment of partial seizures. *Ann Pharmacother* 1995; 29:144–151.

28. Moore LL, Rumack BH, eds. *Drug-Reax(R) System*. Englewood, CO: Micromedex, Inc., June 1998.

CHAPTER 45

Combination Drug Therapy (Monotherapy Versus Polytherapy)

Blaise F.D. Bourgeois, M.D.

Over the past two decades, the medical management of patients with epilepsy has been characterized by a trend toward a reduction in the number of antiepileptic drugs (AEDs) prescribed simultaneously to any given patient. In particular, monotherapy has been strongly advocated (1). The proponents of monotherapy have based their recommendation on several observations that a reduction in the number of AEDs frequently diminishes the severity or number of side effects with little or no loss in seizure control (2–6), and that the beneficial effect of adding a second drug when the first has failed is rather modest (7). Patients undergoing a temporal lobe resection were randomized to ongoing polytherapy or to reduction to carbamazepine monotherapy (8). The seizure recurrence rate was the same for both groups, but drug-related side effects were more common in the polytherapy group (30%) than in the monotherapy group (10%). Nevertheless, for as long as single-drug therapy fails to control every patient with epilepsy, AED combinations will be used. The advantages and disadvantages of AED combinations, therefore, must be assessed and weighed carefully, and potentially beneficial specific drug combinations must be identified.

DISADVANTAGES OF COMBINATION DRUG THERAPY

Pharmacokinetic Interactions

Adding a drug to the treatment regimen may alter the established relationship between dose and blood level of drugs already in use. In general, pharmacokinetic interactions make more frequent drug level determinations and dosagee readjustments necessary. Several newer AEDs have a lower potential for interactions, and some have virtually none. Pharmacokinetic interactions are reviewed in detail in Chapter 44. Rarely, pharmacokinetic interactions can be beneficial. For instance, phenobarbital can have an advantageous effect on phenytoin kinetics by rendering its kinetics more linear. In most instances, however, pharmacokinetic interactions are at best nondetrimental if they are anticipated or recognized early. Valproate levels are particularly sensitive to comedication with enzyme inducing drugs, especially in children. Even at very high doses of more than 100 mg/kg/day, some children cannot achieve therapeutic levels of valproate when in combination therapy with enzyme-inducing drugs (9). The carbamazepine dose-to-level ratio can also be markedly affected by inducing drugs, and the increased dose requirement is associated with an increase in the concentration of the active metabolite carbamazepine-10,11-epoxide. The accelerated biotransformation of such drugs as valproate and carbamazepine usually shortens their half-life and lowers their concentration, causing larger fluctuations in blood levels between doses. Larger fluctuations may increase the risk of seizures just before the dose or increase the risk of toxic side effects at the time of the peak level. Inversely, the inhibition of lamotrigine elimination by valproate increases the level-to-dose ratio of lamotrigine and is likely to be responsible for an increase in the incidence of rashes associated with lamotrigine (10).

Cumulative Toxicity

Experimental data on the pharmacodynamic interactions of AEDs suggest that neurological toxicity is mostly additive (11). This finding implies that two drugs with a concentration in the recommended therapeutic range are more likely to cause side effects than each drug alone at the same concentration. Correspondingly, in several clinical studies in which polypharmacy was reduced, there was an associated decrease in side effects, especially a reduction in sedation (2,3,5,6). This increased alertness was especially apparent after withdrawal of barbiturates or benzodiazepines (4). Controlled monotherapy trials with some of the newer AEDs have demonstrated a lower incidence of side effects than in the corresponding add-on trials with the same drug. The notion of cumulative toxicity becomes particularly important if one considers the fact that toxicity is often subtle and can be associated with chronic impairment of cognitive function (12).

In addition to cumulative toxicity, when two or more drugs are prescribed together, there is a greater likelihood that one of the drug concentrations will eventually be in the toxic range. In a longitudinal study of children with epilepsy, the number of children with one or more drug levels in the toxic range increased with the numbers of drugs prescribed (13). Toxic levels occurred in 14 percent of those taking one drug, 50 percent of those taking two drugs, and 100 percent of those taking three or more drugs. Therefore, polytherapy is likely to increase the frequency of dose-related side effects. It also increases the probability of idiosyncratic adverse effects and organ toxicity. Deckers and coworkers (14) recently reviewed the literature to reassess the relationship between AED polytherapy and adverse effects. They found some evidence suggesting that the toxicity of polytherapy may be related to total drug load, that is, total dose, rather than to the number of drugs. In other words, one drug at a relatively high dose may cause more adverse effects than two drugs at low doses.

Differences in Therapeutic Range

The therapeutic range is a statistical compromise based on studies of groups of patients. It provides loose guidelines with regard to the minimal effective concentration and the concentration at which side effects become frequent. Based on the experimental evidence for additive interactions between AEDs, it is unlikely that the therapeutic range of a drug will be the same when it is taken alone as when it is taken in combination with other drugs. Polytherapy is more likely to be associated with toxicity when drug levels are within the therapeutic range. Clinical observations indeed suggest that toxicity from carbamazepine or phenytoin (15) and from valproate (16) appears at higher levels when these drugs are taken alone. Therefore, when side effects occur at a certain level of a drug during combination therapy, this finding does not necessarily imply that the side effects will recur at similar levels in monotherapy in the same patient.

Interpretation of Drug Effect

Among patients on polytherapy, it may be difficult to determine which drug has caused a reduction in seizure frequency and which drug is responsible for side effects. Idiosyncratic toxic reactions do not necessarily appear promptly after the introduction of a new drug; therefore, they may not necessarily be caused by the last drug added to the regimen. These problems are confounded by frequent dose changes and short periods of observation. A carry-over effect or delayed maximal efficacy of a drug contribute to confusion when several drugs are prescribed simultaneously.

Idiosyncratic Toxic Reactions

Idiosyncratic adverse side effects of drugs are not dose-related. Certain idiosyncratic reactions are more likely to occur when two drugs are taken in combination. As mentioned earlier, valproate can increase the incidence of rashes associated with lamotrigine. Also, the combination of valproate with other AEDs can result in a dramatic encephalopathic state, which does not result from toxic drug levels or from a pharmacokinetic interaction (16,17). This is characterized by alteration of consciousness, usually a stuporous state, and by sudden and pronounced slowing of the background activity in the electroencephalogram. It is important to recognize the cause of these stuporous episodes because they are rapidly reversible upon discontinuation of valproate or of the last introduced drug. The mechanism of this encephalopathy has not been elucidated, but it does not appear to be related to hyperammonemia. Finally, one of the disadvantages of taking two or more drugs is the higher cost. For patients who are prescribed multiple drugs for several years, this is a tangible factor and there needs to be some evidence that the higher cost is associated with an increased benefit.

POTENTIAL ADVANTAGES OF COMBINATION DRUG THERAPY

Compared with single-drug therapy there are two potential advantages of combination drug therapy: namely, better seizure control or a similar degree of seizure control with fewer dose-related side effects. For any combination of AEDs to fulfill either of these criteria, the particular combination must have either a wider antiepileptic spectrum or a better therapeutic index than either drug alone. For example, a patient with both primarily generalized tonic-clonic seizures and absence seizures who failed to respond to both valproate and lamotrigine, or cannot tolerate either drug, might take phenytoin and ethosuximide. Although neither phenytoin nor ethosuximide alone is expected to control both seizure types, together they may be effective and have a wider antiepileptic spectrum than either one alone. In another hypothetical case, consider a patient whose partial seizures were not controlled by the maximal tolerated doses of either phenytoin alone or carbamazepine alone, leading to both drugs being prescribed together. If the seizures can be controlled by the combination of phenytoin and carbamazepine at doses tolerated by the patient, a superior therapeutic index for the combination of phenytoin and carbamazepine would have been demonstrated. Unfortunately, there are very few data in the clinical literature demonstrating a better therapeutic index for any combination of AEDs. On the other hand, a great deal of information is available on the pharmacokinetic interactions between AEDs, while less is known about pharmacodynamic interactions—interactions that occur in the central nervous system. However, increasing attention is being paid to the theoretical, experimental, and clinical background for the practice of combining AEDs.

A supraadditive pharmacodynamic interaction (potentiation or synergism) between two drugs with regard to their protective effect against seizures has often been used as supportive evidence that these two drugs represent a superior combination. However, this antiepileptic interaction in itself has little meaning unless the neurotoxic effects are also evaluated. If toxicity is also supraadditive to a same or greater extent as the antiepileptic effect, the therapeutic index of the combination is equal to or inferior to the therapeutic index of each drug alone. In other words, at the same level of neurotoxicity, the drug combination does not provide more seizure protection than either of the two drugs alone. Clinically, it is very difficult to study the individual and combined therapeutic index of AEDs because both seizure protection and neurotoxic side effects of single drugs and of combinations of drugs must be assessed quantitatively in a homogeneous population of patients with epilepsy. Therefore, most of the available information on the pharmacodynamic effect of combining AEDs has been obtained from animal experiments (11).

Experimental Studies

Table 45-1 summarizes the results of studies on antiepileptic and neurotoxic interactions between most of the established AEDs, including interactions between drugs and their active metabolites (18–25). All results in these studies are based on the analysis of brain drug concentrations in mice. Seizure protection was assessed by maximal electroshock or with pentylenetetrazol. Neurotoxicity was assessed by the rotorod test, which is a measure of motor incoordination. Although this is a rough assessment of dose-related neurotoxicity, there is no reliable animal model that reflects the scope of dose-related neurotoxicity of AEDs. The methods used

Table 45-1. Summary of Pharmacodynamics Interactions Between Antiepileptic Drugs in Mice

Drug pair	Interaction Antiepileptic	Interaction Neurotoxic	Reference
PHT + PB	Additive	Infraadditive	(18)
PHT + CBZ	Additive	Additive	(19)
CBZ + PB	Additive	Additive	(20)
VPA + ESM	Additive	Infraadditive	(21)
VPA + PB	Additive	Additive	(22)
VPA + CBZ	Additive	Infraadditive	(22)
VPA + PHT	Supraadditive	Additive	(23)
CBZ + CBZ-E	Additive	Additive	(24)
PRM + PB	Supraadditive	Infraadditive	(25)
PB + PEMA	Supraadditive	Supraadditive	(25)

Abbreviations: CBZ = carbamazepine; CBZ-E = carbamazepine-epoxide; CZP = clonazepam; ESM = ethosuximide; PB = phenobarbital; PEMA = phenyl-ethyl-malonamide; PHT = phenytoin; PRM = primidone; VPA = valproate; (Modified from Bourgeois BFD, Dodson WE. Antiepileptic and neurotoxic interactions between antiepileptic drugs. In: Pitlick WH, ed. *Antiepileptic Drug Interactions.* New York: Demos, 1989:209–218 by permission.)

for the quantitative assessment of the pharmacodynamic drug interactions were either the isobolographic analysis or the fractional effective concentration index or both (18,20,21).

The majority of the neurotoxic interactions are additive or infraadditive, but not supraadditive. Thus, neurotoxicity of AEDs does not seem to be potentiated when they are combined. Inversely, antiepileptic interactions are either additive or supraadditive, never infraadditive. Drug pairs with supraadditive antiepileptic interactions can be advantageous even when the neurotoxic interaction is additive. When the antiepileptic interaction is additive, only combinations with an infraadditive neurotoxic interaction can have a better protective index than the single drug. Five pairs of drugs appear advantageous in this model: phenobarbital with phenytoin, phenobarbital with primidone, valproate with ethosuximide, valproate with carbamazepine, and valproate with phenytoin. Because of the relatively low therapeutic index of phenobarbital, the therapeutic index of combinations involving phenobarbital is still relatively low, even when the neurotoxicity of the combination is infraadditive. When carrying out such studies of pharmacodynamic interactions, drug concentrations and not doses must be used because of the effect of possible pharmacokinetic interactions. For example, earlier studies of the antiepileptic interaction between phenytoin and phenobarbital, based on the analysis of doses administered, suggested a supraadditive interaction. A purely additive interaction was found when brain levels were measured in two independent studies (18,26). Indeed, an acute elevation of the phenytoin level-to-dose ratio in the presence of phenobarbital could be demonstrated (18).

The combinations of clonazepam with valproate and clonazepam with ethosuximide were also tested in mice (27). Nonprotective and nontoxic doses of clonazepam increased the protective effect and the neurotoxicity of valproate and ethosuximide, indicating supraadditive effects. The two drug combinations had a better protective index than each drug alone despite supraadditive neurotoxicity. Using a similar model, Gordon and coworkers (28) studied pharmacodynamic interactions between felbamate and phenytoin, carbamazepine, valproate, and phenobarbital. They found that nonprotective doses of the latter four drugs decreased the median effective dose (ED_{50}) values of felbamate against maximal electroshock seizures. However, neurotoxicity was not potentiated and the protective index of felbamate was more than doubled by the addition of either one of the four drugs. Although the analysis was based on doses, the authors did measure plasma drug levels and demonstrated the absence of pharmacokinetic interaction.

Clinical Studies

There have been very few clinical studies of AED combinations based on systematic comparisons between the effect of two drugs administered both in monotherapy and their effect in combination. Comparing the effect of adding a second drug with the result of monotherapy with the first drug is not sufficient to demonstrate the superiority of the combination. In 30 adult patients who had failed to respond to the maximal tolerated dose of carbamazepine, phenytoin, phenobarbital, or primidone, a second drug (carbamazepine, phenytoin, phenobarbital, primidone, valproic acid, clonazepam, or clobazam) was added, if necessary up to the maximal tolerated dose (7). A reduction in seizure frequency by 75 percent or more was observed in four patients (13%). However, no patient became seizure-free, and three patients (10%) experienced an increase in seizure frequency by more than 100 percent. Among the drugs used in the treatment of absence seizures, one clinical study suggests that the combination of valproate and ethosuximide is possibly beneficial. Five patients with absence seizures that had remained refractory to ethosuximide or to sodium valproate alone (or to both) became seizure-free when the two drugs were combined (29). The experimental evidence discussed earlier also suggests that valproate with ethosuximide is one of the combinations with a favorable protective index. Schapel and coworkers (30) evaluated the combination of vigabatrin with lamotrigine in 42 patients with intractable epilepsy. On the combination, the median seizure frequency was reduced by 18 percent when vigabatrin was added to lamotrigine ($N = 27$) and by 24 percent when lamotrigine was added to vigabatrin ($N = 15$).

However, this study does not document superiority of the combination. Because patients did not receive both drugs in monotherapy before the combination, the results may just reflect the effect of the second drug added, not of the combination. Brodie and Yuen (31) found evidence suggestive of a synergism between lamotrigine and valproate in a lamotrigine substitution study. In 347 uncontrolled patients on monotherapy with valproate, carbamazepine, phenytoin, or phenobarbital, lamotrigine was added. An attempt was made to withdraw the first drug in patients with a 50 percent or greater seizure reduction. A synergism between lamotrigine and valproate was suggested on the basis of two observations: (1) a significantly better response after adding lamotrigine to valproate than to carbamazepine or phenytoin ($p < 0.001$), both for partial seizures ($p < 0.02$), and for generalized tonic-clonic seizures (not statistically significant), and (2) a poorer response after valproate was withdrawn.

HOW SHOULD ANTIEPILEPTIC DRUG COMBINATIONS BE SELECTED?

Considering the fact that there are no definitive clinical studies documenting the superiority of any specific drug combination, selecting a combination of two AEDs remains at the present time an educated guess at best. The choice may be based on several considerations that include the mechanisms of action, the clinical spectrum of activity, and pharmacokinetic interactions.

The mechanism of action of AEDs has been suggested as a consideration for rational combinations (32,33) based on the concept that drugs to be combined should have different mechanisms of action that could be complementary. This is an elegant hypothesis, which has never been proved experimentally or clinically. For the time being, choosing a drug combination based on the mechanisms of action remains purely hypothetical, and no specific drug pair can be recommended.

When a patient has two or more seizure types that cannot be controlled by one drug alone, two drugs can be selected according to their spectrum of efficacy. For each seizure type, the most effective and best tolerated drug should be selected. An example of epilepsy with multiple seizure types is the Lennox-Gastaut syndrome. Valproate has long been the drug of choice in patients with Lennox-Gastaut syndrome, but three drugs have now been shown in double-blind studies to be effective: felbamate (34), lamotrigine (35), and topiramate (36). Combinations between these four drugs might be more effective in reducing drop attacks as well as atypical absences and tonic seizures than only one drug alone. Inversely, phenytoin and carbamazepine usually are not effective and can even exacerbate certain seizures in these patients (37).

The absence of pharmacokinetic interactions between two drugs certainly makes it easier to use them together. However, pharmacokinetic interactions are known and predictable, and it is the physician's responsibility to make appropriate dosage adjustments, either as a corrective measure or preferably as a preventive measure. Therefore, pharmacokinetic interactions should not be a reason to avoid a drug combination that could be beneficial to the patient. Primidone is a drug that should probably not be given in combination with enzyme-inducing drugs. The amount of derived phenobarbital is increased by the presence of phenytoin and carbamazepine in particular. The serum phenobarbital/primidone concentration ratio at steady-state is 1.55 on primidone monotherapy and 5.48 in the presence of carbamazepine and/or phenytoin (38). Thus, in the latter case, primidone therapy becomes virtually identical to therapy with phenobarbital alone. Primidone is prescribed under the assumption that, because primidone itself has antiepileptic activity, therapy with primidone may differ from therapy with phenobarbital. Therefore, it appears to be meaningless to use primidone rather than phenobarbital, when carbamazepine or phenytoin is prescribed simultaneously. Other combinations to be avoided are those between drugs with similar side effects such as barbiturates and benzodiazepines or barbiturates and topiramate (sedation) or acetazolamide and topiramate (nephrolithiasis).

Finally, opposed to the classic concept of "high-dose monotherapy" (15), a concept of "low-dose polytherapy" could be advocated. The rationale would be that AEDs share their antiepileptic effect but do not always share their adverse effects. Therefore, if a patient has a good seizure response to two drugs in monotherapy, but with side effects, the two drugs might achieve the same seizure reduction together, at lower doses that could be below the clinical threshold for their side effects. An example would be a child with absence seizures who has thrombocytopenia or tremor at effective doses of valproate, and persisting gastrointestinal side effects at effective doses of ethosuximide. The same seizure control without the side effects might be achieved with the two drugs at lower doses. Any two drugs with different side effects but efficacy against the same seizure type could be combined according to this concept. This concept is supported by the experimental pharmacodynamic interaction studies described earlier. These studies have demonstrated that the neurotoxic pharmacodynamic interaction often does not parallel the antiepileptic pharmacodynamic interaction (Table 45-1).

In conclusion, in view of the known disadvantages of combination therapy, the benefit of a given drug combination must be well documented in every patient if the combination is to be maintained. To quote Meinardi (39), "at present, however, there are too many gaps in our knowledge to make theoretical planning of [combination] drug therapy more promising than an empirical approach." Drug combinations are best chosen by selecting the best drugs known to be effective against the patient's seizure type or seizure types. Rational polytherapy cannot be predicted and must be documented for every patient according to the following definition: when the patient does better in terms of seizure control versus side effects while taking drugs A and B together (at any dose) than the patient had done on drug A alone *and* on drug B alone at their respective optimal doses. There may be instances in which it would be appropriate to maintain a drug combination even when the above definition is not met. For instance, a patient may respond partially to a first drug and experience further improvement after addition of the second drug, or the patient becomes seizure-free after addition of the second drug, despite lack of response to the first drug. In such cases, it is understandable that one may be reluctant to make any change.

REFERENCES

1. Reynolds EH, Shorvon SD. Single drug or combination therapy for epilepsy? *Drugs* 1981; 21:374–382.

2. Fischbacher E. Effect of reduction of anticonvulsants on well-being. *Br Med J* 1982; 285:423–424.

3. Bennett HS, Dunlop T, Ziring P. Reduction of polypharmacy for epilepsy in an institution for the retarded. *Dev Med Child Neurol* 1983; 25:735–737.

4. Theodore WH, Porter RJ. Removal of sedative-hypnotic antiepileptic drugs from the regimen of patients with intractable epilepsy. *Ann Neurol* 1983; 13:320–324.

5. Albright P, Bruni J. Reduction of polytherapy in epileptic patients. *Arch Neurol* 1985; 42:797–799.

6. Schmidt D. Reduction of two-drug therapy in intractable epilepsy. *Epilepsia* 1983; 24:368–376.

7. Schmidt D. Two antiepileptic drugs for intractable epilepsy with complex-partial seizures. *J Neurol Psychiatry* 1982; 45:1119–1124.

8. Kuzniecky R, Rubin ZK, Faught E, Morawetz R. Antiepileptic drug treatment after temporal lobe epilepsy surgery: a randomized study comparing carbamazepine and polytherapy. *Epilepsia* 1992; 33:908–912.

9. Henriksen O, Johannessen SI. Clinical and pharmacokinetic observations on sodium valproate—a 5-year follow-up study in 100 children with epilepsy. *Acta Neurol Scand* 1982; 65:504–523.

10. Besag FMC, Wallace SJ, Dulac O, et al. Lamotrigine for the treatment of epilepsy in childhood. *J Pediatr* 1995; 127:991–997.

11. Bourgeois BFD, Dodson WE. Antiepileptic and neurotoxic interactions between antiepileptic drugs. In: Pitlick WH, ed. *Antiepileptic Drug Interactions*. New York: Demos, 1989:209–218.

12. Trimble MR, Thompson PJ. Anticonvulsant drugs, cognitive function, and behaviour. *Epilepsia* 1983; 24(Suppl):S55–S63.

13. Bourgeois BFD. Problems of combination drug therapy in children. *Epilepsia* 1988; 29:S20–S24.

14. Deckers CLP, Hekster YA, Keyser A, Meinardi H, Renier WO. Reappraisal of polytherapy in epilepsy: a critical review of drug load and adverse effects. *Epilepsia* 1997; 38:570–575.

15. Lesser RP, Pippinger CE, Lüders H, Dinner DS. High-dose monotherapy in the treatment of intractable seizures. *Neurology* 1984; 34:707–711.

16. Sackellares JC, Lee SI, Dreifuss FE. Stupor following administration of valproic acid to patients receiving other antiepileptic drugs. *Epilepsia* 1979; 20:697–703.

17. Marescaux C, Warter JM, Micheletti G, et al. Stuporous episodes during treatment with sodium valproate: report of seven cases. *Epilepsia* 1982; 23:297–305.

18. Bourgeois BFD. Antiepileptic drug combinations and experimental background: the case of phenobarbital and phenytoin. *Naunyn-Schmiedeberg's Arch Pharmacol* 1986; 333:406–411.

19. Morris JC, Dodson WE, Hatlelid JM, Ferrendelli JA. Phenytoin and carbamazepine alone and in combination: anticonvulsant and neurotoxic effects. *Neurology* 1987; 37:1111–1118.

20. Bourgeois BFD, Wad N. Combined administration of carbamazepine and phenobarbital: effect on anticonvulsant activity and neurotoxicity. *Epilepsia* 1988; 29:482–487.

21. Bourgeois BFD. Combination of valproate and ethosuximide: antiepileptic and neurotoxic interaction. *J Pharmacol Exp Ther* 1988; 237:1128–1132.

22. Bourgeois BFD. Anticonvulsant potency and neurotoxicity of valproate alone and in combination with carbamazepine or phenobarbital. *Clin Neuropharmacol* 1988; 11:348–359.

23. Chez MG, Bourgeois BFD, Pippinger CE, Knowles WD. Pharmacodynamic interactions between phenytoin and valproate: Individual and combined antiepileptic and neurotoxic actions in mice. *Clin Neuropharmacol* 1994; 17:32–37.

24. Bourgeois BFD, Wad N. Individual and combined antiepileptic and neurotoxic activity of carbamazepine and carbamazepine-10,11-epoxide in mice. *J Pharmacol Exp Ther* 1984; 231:411–415.

25. Bourgeois BFD, Dodson WE, Ferrendelli JA. Primidone, phenobarbital and PEMA: II. Seizure protection, neuro-toxicity and therapeutic index of varying combinations in mice. *Neurology* 1983; 33:291–295.

26. Leppik IE, Sherwin AL. Anticonvulsant activity of phenobarbital and phenytoin in combination. *J Pharmacol Exp Ther* 1977; 200:570–575.

27. Bourgeois BFD, VanLente F. Effect of clonazepam on antiepileptic potency, neurotoxicity and therapeutic index of valproate and ethosuximide in mice. *Epilepsia* 1994; 35(Suppl 8):142.

28. Gordon R, Gels M, Wichman J, Diamantis W, Sofia RD. Interaction of felbamate with several other antiepileptic drugs against seizures induced by maximal electroshock in mice. *Epilepsia* 1993; 34:367–371.

29. Rowan AJ, Binnie CD, Warfield CA, Meinardi H, Meijer JWA. The delayed effect of sodium valproate on the photoconvulsive response in man. *Epilepsia* 1979; 20:61–68.

30. Schapel GJ, Black AB, Lam EL, Robinson M, Dollman WB. Combination vigabatrin and lamotrigine therapy for intractable epilepsy. *Seizure* 1996; 5:51–56.

31. Brodie MJ, Yuen AW. Lamotrigine substitution study: evidence for synergism with sodium valproate? 105 Study Group. *Epilepsy Res* 1997; 26:423–432.

32. Perucca E. Pharmacological principles as a basis for polytherapy. *Acta Neurol Scand* 1995; 162(Suppl):31–34.

33. Macdonald RL. Is there a mechanistic basis for rational polypharmacy? *Epilepsy Res* 1996; 11:79–93.

34. The Felbamate Study Group in Lennox-Gastaut Syndrome. Efficacy of felbamate in childhood epileptic encephalopathy (Lennox-Gastaut syndrome). *N Engl J Med* 1993; 328:29–33.

35. Motte J, Trevathan E, Arvidsson JF, et al. Lamotrigine for generalized seizures associated with the Lennox-Gastaut syndrome. *N Engl J Med* 1997; 337:1807–1812.

36. Glauser TA, Sachdeo RC, Ritter FJ, et al. Topiramate as adjunctive therapy in Lennox-Gastaut syndrome. *Epilepsia* 1997; 38(Suppl 8):207.

37. Snead OC, Hosey LC. Exacerbation of seizures in children by carbamazepine. *N Engl J Med* 1985; 313:916–921.

38. Bourgeois BFD. Primidone: chemistry and biotransformation. In: Levy RH, Mattson RH, Meldrum BS, eds. *Antiepileptic Drugs*. 4th ed. New York: Raven Press, 1995:449–457.

39. Meinardi H. Use of combined antiepileptic drug therapy. In: Levy RH, Mattson RH, Meldrum BS, eds. *Antiepileptic Drugs*. 4th ed. New York: Raven Press, 1995:91–97.

CHAPTER 46

Costs of Pediatric Epilepsy

John F. Annegers, Ph.D., and Charles E. Begley, M.D.

The cost of epilepsy and other diseases has received considerable attention in recent years. This interest has been generated by the need to assess and control medical care cost, allocate research funds, and justify therapies or systems of health care delivery. There are two fundamental types of cost studies: cost of illness and cost-benefit.

Cost of illness studies attempt to measure the total cost of epilepsy to society. They are used by advocacy groups to promote research funding and private foundations. Some cost of illness studies also determine the distribution of cost by items such as drug costs, physician costs, and costs attributable to excess unemployment and excess mortality. Cost of illness studies may also determine cost by patient characteristics such as intractable epilepsy versus remitting epilepsy. These studies can assist in resource allocation and can be a basis for cost-benefit studies.

In contrast to cost of illness studies, which measure total cost by item or by disease characteristics, cost-benefit studies evaluate the impact of specific measures in diagnosis, therapy, or clinical practice. The main objective of cost-benefit studies is to allow comparisons of specific therapies or systems of health care delivery in terms of their relative benefits and costs. Cost-benefit studies are dependent on a thorough understanding of the detailed cost of illness. The following are examples:

1. A new drug or device with additional costs, more or less adverse side effects, more or less need for monitoring, but some gain in efficacy. What are the costs and benefits of the new therapy versus the old therapy?
2. In health care delivery, what is the benefit of a neurologist versus a general practitioner evaluation of first-seizure patients and at what additional cost? The cost-benefit evaluation would

apply to the diagnostic procedures and patient outcomes, including adverse affects.
3. What are the costs and benefits of specific tests such as magnetic resonance imaging (MRI) versus computed tomography (CT) scans?

Economic studies of epilepsy are largely in the developmental stage. Cost of illness studies face unresolved issues of the range of case definition, attribution, and methodologies for determining indirect costs. Cost-benefit studies lack standardized measures of treatment outcomes. In cost of illness studies, direct cost and indirect cost are estimated. Direct cost includes three broad categories:

1. The cost of medical care, including professional services, laboratory tests, medications, hospital care, medical supplies, and equipment.
2. Nonmedical direct cost, including social services and resources related to special education, transportation, and modifications to the residence. It also includes imputed costs of caregivers' time devoted to accessing care or providing care.

Indirect cost is measured by comparing unemployment rates, sick days, reduced productivity at home and at work, and mortality for people with epilepsy compared with the general population. National age- and sex-specific earnings data, available from the U.S. Bureau of the Census and the Bureau of Labor Statistics are used to estimate lost earnings. Indirect costs of illness include:

1. Loss of earnings associated with reduced employment.
2. Reduced earnings because of illness or reduced productivity on the job.
3. The lost value of household production when people are unable to conduct household work.

4. The lost earnings because of productive years of life lost from increased mortality attributable to epilepsy. Productive years are usually defined as ages 18 through 64. Although the pediatric ages are not included, childhood-onset epilepsy may have an impact on the productive years of life as adults.

Cost studies vary in time perspective. Cross-sectional studies present annual costs for prevalent cases. Longitudinal studies estimate the cost borne throughout the life span for incident cases. The longitudinal perspective is necessary if the full evaluation of a new treatment or delivery system change is to be conducted. For example, to evaluate the direct and indirect effects of a treatment, one must include the lifetime effects on relapse seizures, side effects of medications, future employment, and mortality.

HOW THE COST OF EPILEPSY IS MEASURED

Because the total direct and indirect cost of illness includes many components, one must combine data from several sources to estimate these costs. Direct medical cost typically is determined from utilization and billing records on groups of patients (1,2), from national population surveys (3), or simulated from a disease prognosis model (4,5). Nonmedical direct cost is more difficult to measure but can be obtained for pediatric epilepsy through interviews with caregivers of a representative sample of patients. The indirect cost related to differences in employment and wages can also be made from national survey data comparing people with epilepsy with the general population. Age-specific person years of productive life lost can be determined from studies that measure the excess mortality in individuals with epilepsy.

CASE DEFINITION FOR PEDIATRIC COST STUDIES

Cost of illness estimates are strongly influenced by the case definition used. If cases of epilepsy are restricted to patients with recurrent unprovoked seizures, almost 1 percent of children will be affected by their 18th birthday (see Chapter 7). However, should single unprovoked seizures, which occur in approximately 0.3 percent of children, be included in cost of epilepsy studies? The first seizure, if the patient is identified at that time, is when the major diagnostic workup occurs and is a significant direct medical cost. For this reason, a practical definition would include all cost from the first recognized seizure, even if there is only one.

Cost related to the diagnosis and treatment of febrile convulsions have not been included in the cost of epilepsy. Even though the direct and indirect cost per febrile seizure case usually are low, the large number, 2 percent to 3 percent of all children who have such seizures, would greatly increase the pediatric cost of epilepsy including febrile convulsions. Approximately 0.5 percent of all children experience acute symptomatic seizures—seizures related to transient central nervous system insults, the most common of which in children are traumatic brain injury, encephalitis, and perinatal insults. The cost of these seizures is not included in the cost of epilepsy studies and is more appropriately considered part of the cost of the underlying causes. In addition to children found to have had epilepsy or seizures, there are many who have symptoms suggestive of seizures and incur direct medical cost as a result. Cost of epilepsy studies have ignored this sizable population.

SEPARATING THE COST OF EPILEPSY FROM THAT OF OTHER ILLNESSES

Some pediatric epilepsy patients have severe comorbidities, especially cerebral palsy and/or mental retardation, that contribute to their direct medical and indirect cost because of potential unemployment and excess mortality. If the cost of epilepsy is to be separated from that of other illnesses, one must determine what proportion should be reasonably attributed to epilepsy. In cases of severe neurologic deficits, presumably from birth (i.e., preceding the epilepsy), only the cost related to the seizure disorder should be attributed to epilepsy. If all the direct and indirect costs in children with severe neurologic deficits and epilepsy are attributed to epilepsy, the total cost of pediatric epilepsy is greatly inflated in the portion of cost incurred by children with neurologic deficit (3). To avoid this problem, only the direct cost related to the management of seizures in these children is attributed to epilepsy in a recent simulation study (4). Likewise, in cases of postnatal acquired epilepsy, mainly traumatic brain injury, central nervous system infections, and intracranial tumors in children, only those components of direct cost related to seizures should be included. There is a small but, in terms of cost, very important group of children with catastrophic epilepsy of childhood in whom the other disabilities may be a product of epilepsy.

STUDIES OF THE COST OF EPILEPSY

A number of recent studies have estimated the direct and/or indirect cost of epilepsy in people of all ages. No study has provided separate cost estimates for children. Table 46-1 indicates a range for direct cost of $2,750 to $9,400 per person in 1995 dollars. Estimates

Table 46-1. Prevalence-Based Estimates of the Annual Cost of Epilepsy

Author	Country	Year	Population	Cost Measures	Data Sources	Cost per Person 1995 US$	Cost per Person 1995 US$
Banks, et al.; Beren & Banks	Australia	1992	All "epilepsy," age 5+	Direct medical, some indirect	Provider and population surveys	2,751	3,381
Gessner, et al.	Switzerland	1990	Patients on anticonvulsants	Direct medical, nonmedical some medical	Provider and population surveys	9,400	5,130
Cockerrell, et al.	U.K.	1990	Active and inactive epilepsy patients on anticonvulsants	Direct medical, nonmedical, some indirect	Administrative records	2,600	5,989
Murray, et al.	U.S.A	1994	Adult refractory epilepsy patients	Direct medical, some indirect	Disease model	2.971	9,418
CCEC	U.S.A.	1975	Active and inactive epilepsy patients	Direct medical, nonmedical, some indirect	Provider and population surveys	4,407	4,284

of indirect cost range from $3,380 to $9,418 per person. The relative amount of direct and indirect cost varies widely, with researchers attributing 35 percent to 75 percent of the total cost to indirect cost.

A simulation was conducted to estimate the direct and indirect cost of epilepsy (4). A model was constructed that considered the annual number of cases, the variable prognosis of epilepsy in six categories, the use of services and medications by prognostic group and time from the diagnosis, and estimates of relative unemployment and mortality for indirect costs. For this chapter, that model has been modified in two respects. First, cases are confined to pediatric-onset epilepsy (age 0–17 years), although cost is projected throughout the lifetime. Second, an additional category, group 0, has been included to expand the definition to all initial diagnoses of unprovoked seizures, even if they do not progress to epilepsy. All future costs were discounted to 1990 using a 5 percent discount rate. The estimated U.S. lifetime cost, based on 1990 incidence cases, was $805 million; the total direct cost was $354 million; and the total indirect cost was $451 million.

DIRECT COST BY SERVICE

The distribution of the direct cost by type of service is presented in Table 46-2. These include emergency services, inpatient hospitalizations, outpatient visits, electroencephalogram (EEG), CT, and MRI. Table 46-3 presents the estimated number of cases by prognostic group and the total and per capita direct and indirect costs. The largest direct item is antiepileptic drugs (AEDs), which account for almost 37 percent of the cost of epilepsy. Outpatient physician cost accounted for almost 20 percent, and inpatient cost accounted for approximately 18 percent.

COST BY PROGNOSTIC CATEGORY

To capture the dynamics and heterogeneity of epilepsy, six prognostic categories for epilepsy and one for isolated unprovoked seizure were constructed (4). The natural history and number of individuals in each of these categories in the United States were based on epidemiological studies of seizure disorders. The utilization of medical services was based on a panel, and indirect cost of unemployment and excess mortality was based on estimates from the literature. The prognostic groups and group criteria are depicted in Figure 46-1 and Table 46-2, and the estimated number in the United States in 1990 is shown in Table 46-3.

Group 0 represents the large number of individuals with isolated seizures. Whether they go on to develop recurrent seizures does not affect the initial diagnostic workup but largely affects AED use. The direct cost for pediatric single seizures is estimated at over $43 million, or approximately $2,700 per person. Group 1 consists of individuals who have recurrent seizures but respond after initial diagnosis and treatment. Direct cost is $3,594 per person, but because of the large number in this category the total direct cost exceeds $100 million, while the indirect cost is small.

Group 2 consists of those patients with initial treatment but who relapse on later AED withdrawal. The average direct cost is higher in this group—almost $15,000—while indirect cost remains small. Group 3 consists of patients who continue to have seizures after initial diagnosis but who achieve remission within a year or two with the appropriate medication if not simply by natural history. In this group, the average direct cost is $7,100 and indirect cost is $1,360. Group 4 consists of patients who continue to have seizures but less then one per month, often less than

Table 46-2. Direct Costs by Cost Category and Group

Category of direct cost	Group 0*	Percentage of group cost	Group 1*	Percentage of group cost	Group 2*	Percentage of group cost	Group 3*	Percentage of group cost	Group 4*	Percentage of group cost	Group 5*	Percentage of group cost	Group 6*	Percentage of group cost	Total cost	Percentage of total cost
Emergency services	2,568,424	5.9	4,734,660	4.4	717,435	1.5	671,102	3.3	1,635,991	4.4	3,984,244	4.2	33,746	0.9	14,345,602	4.0
Inpatient hospital (not included: drug reactions, surgical workup, and operation)	13,928,610	32.1	25,786,022	24.2	3,854,449	7.9	2,463,334	12.1	1,798,381	4.8	15,765,600	16.8	158,867	4.4	63,755,263	18.0
Outpatient physician visits	11,246,802	25.9	20,712,345	19.4	5,919,420	12.2	4,180,433	20.5	8,807,584	23.4	17,750,635	18.9	536,595	14.7	69,153,814	19.5
EEG services	3,762,411	8.7	6,937,778	6.5	4,351,255	8.9	1,938,989	9.5	1,975,434	5.3	5,532,242	5.9	368,533	10.1	24,866,642	7.0
CT scan/MRI	3,215,891	7.4	5,925,349	5.6	799,248	1.6	944,907	4.6	1,470,214	3.9	2,364,203	2.5	34,381	0.9	14,754,193	4.2
Serum level tests (not included: drug reactions)	565,474	1.3	1,042,401	1.0	886,834	1.8	361,697	1.8	523,475	1.4	761,884	0.8	98,290	2.7	4,240,055	1.2
Drug reaction costs (including hospitalization)	3,284,132	7.6	6,054,005	5.7	1,377,664	2.8	897,705	4.4	924,308	2.5	1,133,274	1.2	174,493	4.8	13,845,581	3.9
Drug treatment costs	4,827,245	11.1	35,302,317	33.1	30,787,702	63.2	8,956,996	43.9	20,472,087	54.4	27,112,938	28.8	2,239,148	61.4	129,698,433	36.6
Surgical workup	0		0		0		0		0		13,156,537	14.0	0		13,156,537	3.7
Operation	0		0		0		0		0		6,459,704	6.9	0		6,459,704	1.8
TOTAL DOLLARS	43,398,989		106,494,877		48,694,007		20,415,163		37,607,474		94,021,261		3,644,053		354,275,824	

*Cost in dollars

EEG = electroencephalogram; CT = computed tomography; MRI = magnetic resonance imaging.

Table 46-3. Costs by Prognostic Group

Group	Projected Cases	Direct Total Cost	Direct Cost per Capita	Indirect Total Cost	Indirect Cost per Capita	Total Total Cost	Total Cost per Capita
0	16,075	43,398,988.54	2,699.85	3,734,702.00	232.34	47,133,690.54	2,932.18
1	29,632	106,494,877.37	3,593.91	6,884,569.00	232.34	113,379,4466.37	3,826.25
2	3,311	48,694,007.00	14,706.74	3,302,139.00	997.32	51,996,146.00	15,704.06
3	2,860	20,415,163.00	7,138.17	9,684,016.00	3,386.02	30,099,179.00	10,524.19
4	2,107	37,607,474.00	17,848.82	103,958,994.00	49,339.82	141,566,468.00	67,1888.64
5	2,078	94,021,261.00	45,246.04	323,254,485.00	155,560.39	417,275,746.00	200,806.42
6	176	3,644,053.00	20,704.85	0.00	0.00	3,644,053.00	20,704.85
TOTAL	56,239	354,275,823.91	6,299.51	450,818,905.00	8,016.18	805,094,728.91	14,315.70

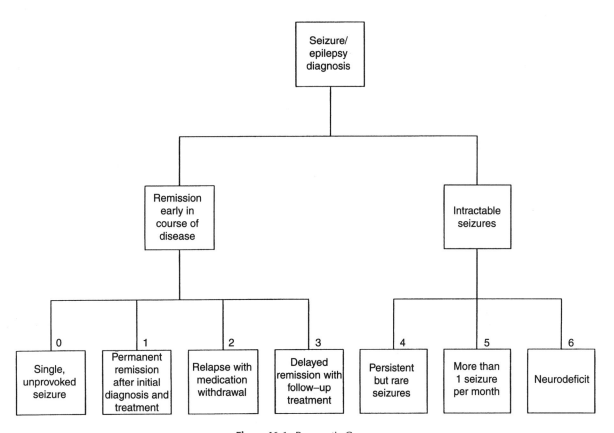

Figure 46-1. Prognostic Groups

one per year. Here the average direct cost increases to $17,800 per patient and indirect cost, because of the long-term impact on employment, greatly exceeds the direct cost. Group 5 would have the usual definition of intractable seizures, in being frequent, more than one per month, and persistent. In this group, the average direct cost is $45,250 because of long-term management of their seizure disorders; the indirect cost is greatly increased because of long-term changes in employment and excess mortality. Group 6 represents those with cerebral palsy and/or mental retardation. This group has been treated separately because the elimination of their seizures would not greatly change

the indirect cost related to the underlying deficit such as unemployment, greatly excessive mortality, and institutionalization. The average direct cost for Group 6 is $20,705.

CONCLUSIONS

The total cost of all pediatric epilepsy and unprovoked seizure cases in the United States in 1990 is estimated to be approximately $805 million, of which $355 million was direct medical cost. The cost per case was $14,316, but this varied from $2,932 for single seizures to $200,806 for intractable epilepsy. These represent the first lifetime estimates developed for children with epilepsy. They are based on hypothetical modeling of prognosis, assumptions about future treatment patterns, and wage and employment effects inferred from the literature.

Compared with cross-sectional studies, these estimates appear to be conservative. Presumably, this difference is largely due to two or three factors. First, the model consists of all incidence cases of unprovoked seizures, while a prevalence sample is weighted toward long-duration, intractable epilepsy. Second, the model strives to include only those direct and indirect costs that can reasonably be attributed to epilepsy rather than comorbidities.

ACKNOWLEDGMENT

The authors acknowledge Tom Reynolds and Sharon Coan for their assistance in preparation of this chapter.

REFERENCES

1. Banks GK, Regan KJ, Beran RG. The prevalence and direct costs of epilepsy in Australia. In: Beran RG, Pachlatko C, eds. *Cost of Epilepsy: Proceedings of the 20th International Epilepsy Congress.* Baden, Germany: Ciba-Geigy Verlag; 1995:39–48.

2. Cockerell OC, Hart YM, Sander JW, Shorvon SD. The cost of epilepsy in the United Kingdom: an estimation based on the results of two population-based studies. *Epilepsy Res* 1994; 18:249–260.

3. Commission for the Control of Epilepsy and Its Consequences, Economic Cost of Epilepsy. *Plan for Nationwide Action on Epilepsy, Vol. IV. DHEW Publication No. 78-279.* Washington, D.C., (NIH). 1978; 117–148.

4. Begley CE, Annegers JF, Lairson DR, Reynolds TF, Hauser WA. Cost of epilepsy in the United States: a model based on incidence and prognosis. *Epilepsia* 1994; 35: 1230–1243.

5. Murray MI, Halpern MT, Leppik IE. Cost of refractory epilepsy in adults in the USA. *Epilepsy Res* 1996;23:139–48.

CHAPTER 47

Surgical Evaluation

Michael Duchowny, M.D.

Epilepsy surgery is becoming increasingly common as a treatment for children with medically resistant seizures. Successful surgical therapy offers hope for reversing long-standing medical and psychosocial disability and for achieving a more productive and independent life (1).

Identifying appropriate pediatric surgical candidates and evaluating their seizure patterns is rarely a straightforward exercise, as children manifest a wide range of seizure types with polymorphous clinical presentations. When electroencephalogram (EEG) findings are nonspecific, a comprehensive battery of investigations is often performed to assist in seizure localization. This chapter reviews the indications and special features of epilepsy surgery in the pediatric population, emphasizing currently available procedures for determining surgical candidacy.

CANDIDATE IDENTIFICATION AND SELECTION

Refractory Seizures

Partial seizures are a common form of epilepsy. Their incidence in the Danish registry is 135 cases per 100,000 unselected patients (2) accounting for 60 percent of the cumulative lifetime prevalence of all epileptic seizures (3,4). Fortunately, most patients can be controlled medically, but there is still a large pool of individuals who have recurrent seizures and are at risk for personal injury, diminished quality of life, and occasionally, death. For the 5 percent to 10 percent of chronic epilepsy patients who are disabled by their disorder, surgery is a justifiable option (5).

To establish intractability, it is necessary to first show that appropriate antiepileptic drugs (AEDs) are ineffective. Serum concentrations should optimally be administered to achieve high therapeutic levels, and polytherapy must be chosen judiciously. While there are many new and investigational AEDs for partial seizure disorders, most children who do not respond to traditional agents are unlikely to go into remission.

Special factors in children may compromise the goal of complete remission. Medication noncompliance in the adolescent population and parental anxiety are two common concerns. At the same time, physician factors such as medication omissions and dosing errors can undermine otherwise successful treatment efforts and allow seizures to persist indefinitely (6).

Nonepileptic disorders and psychogenic seizures affect approximately 10 percent of adolescent and adult epilepsy patients and are a common cause of "pseudo-intractability" (7). Mimickers of epilepsy are particularly common in children and show a diverse clinical spectrum (8). Two common pitfalls are mistaking complex partial seizures for primary absence epilepsy and failing to identify precipitating factors such as sleep deprivation. Neurodegenerative disorders, inborn errors of metabolism, and indolent gliomas are occasionally associated with refractory seizures.

Surgical referral is indicated for patients with partial seizures that do not respond to conventional AEDs and the ketogenic diet and that interfere with daily functioning. Family dynamics and perceptions of well-being often influence referral patterns.

Gilman and coworkers (6) reexamined the diagnosis of medical intractability in 21 children referred for epilepsy surgery who had significant treatment omissions such as nonutilization of a first- or second-line AED or absence of therapeutic drug level. Correcting these omissions did not benefit 19 children (90%), whereas 2 improved on high-dose AED monotherapy. This experience suggests that although a few medically intractable patients respond to further therapeutic manipulations, definitive remission is unlikely in most instances.

Pediatric Risk Factors

Several seizure-related factors are associated with medical intractability (9). Frequent seizures (daily or weekly), clustering (10), and early seizure onset (particularly in infancy) favor seizure persistence (11). Infantile hemiconvulsive status epilepticus is linked to later temporal lobe epilepsy in some individuals (12–14). Motor convulsions in nonconvulsive disorders worsen prognosis in direct proportion to the overall number of convulsive episodes (15). Children with brain damage are particularly prone to persistent seizures (10,16), with the greatest risk in more severely damaged patients (17).

The negative consequences of medically uncontrolled childhood epilepsy were starkly revealed by an early prospective cohort study begun shortly after World War II of 100 children with temporal lobe epilepsy (18). When seizures persisted into adolescence, patients regressed behaviorally and cognitively, and few symptomatic individuals ever led functionally independent lives. Psychosocial disturbance was most troublesome, and less than 5 percent of the children with significant psychopathology ever functioned normally if their schooling was interrupted (18).

Deleterious Effects of Repeated Seizure Activity

While psychosocial and intellectual deterioration are not uniformly associated with chronic epilepsy, seizures are deleterious to the developing nervous system. Recurrent seizures induce both transient and long-lasting disruptions of neural circuitry and permanent memory dysfunction (19). Kainic acid exposure increases binding sites in fascia dentata and the CA_3 regions of the hippocampus (20), while even brief seizures are capable of inducing mossy fiber sprouting, synaptic reorganization, long-lasting alterations in gene expression, and potentiated neural excitability (21,22). Similar findings are noted in anterior temporal lobectomy specimens (23,24) emphasizing that regulatory disturbance of neural excitation and abnormal cellular architecture accompany human epilepsy as well. Hippocampal damage identical to that seen in chronic temporal lobe epilepsy is also seen in patients with dementia (25).

Other factors predispose children to limbic dysfunction and cellular change. Prolonged early febrile seizures are a recognized antecedent of hippocampal sclerosis (HS) and temporal lobe epilepsy (26). Developmental staging is critical because older individuals are less likely to be damaged (27). Bacterial meningitis and viral encephalitis only predispose children to hippocampal sclerosis after infections before 4 years of age (28,29).

Hippocampal sclerosis, the predominant histopathologic feature of adults with temporal lobe epilepsy, is also prevalent in childhood. In a study of 53 children with chronic temporal lobe seizures who underwent detailed MRI evaluations, 30 demonstrated either hippocampal sclerosis or abnormal hippocampal signal without evidence of a mass lesion (14). Hippocampal sclerosis was subsequently confirmed pathologically in 11 of 13 patients treated surgically.

Syndromes Associated with Medically Intractable Epilepsy

Epilepsy syndromes were included in the 1989 International League Against Epilepsy classification (30), and that classification is presently in widespread use to categorize epileptic seizures (31). Identification of specific epilepsy syndromes helps define long-term prognosis, assist genetic analysis, and facilitate surgical referral.

Sturge-Weber Syndrome

Sturge-Weber syndrome is a neurocutaneous disorder manifested by venous angiomas of the leptomeninges and ipsilateral facial angiomatosis (port wine stain, nevus flammeus), which are associated with varying degrees of mental deficiency, ocular defects including glaucoma and buphthalmos, and epilepsy (32). Partial seizures are particularly common (33), and patients often have uncontrolled seizures and deteriorate clinically. Depressed glucose metabolism on positron emission tomography (PET) (34) and decreased regional blood flow on ^{133}Xenon single photon emission computed tomography (SPECT) (35) confirm severe functional derangement of cerebral cortex underlying the angioma.

Tuberous Sclerosis

Tuberous sclerosis is a phakomatous disorder causing multiorgan dysfunction, severe psychomotor delay, hypopigmentary skin lesions, adenoma sebaceum, and shagreen patches. Eighty-five percent of patients have infantile spasms and partial epilepsy (36), a high proportion of which are drug-resistant. Excisional procedures designed to remove cortical tissue in proximity to the epileptogenic tuber successfully induces seizure remission (37). Multiple tubers are not a surgical contraindication as sustained seizure relief is still possible (38).

Cortical Dysplastic Lesions (CDLs)

Dysplasias of the cerebral cortex represent abnormal patterns of neuronal migration and cellular morphogenesis and are an important cause of intractable

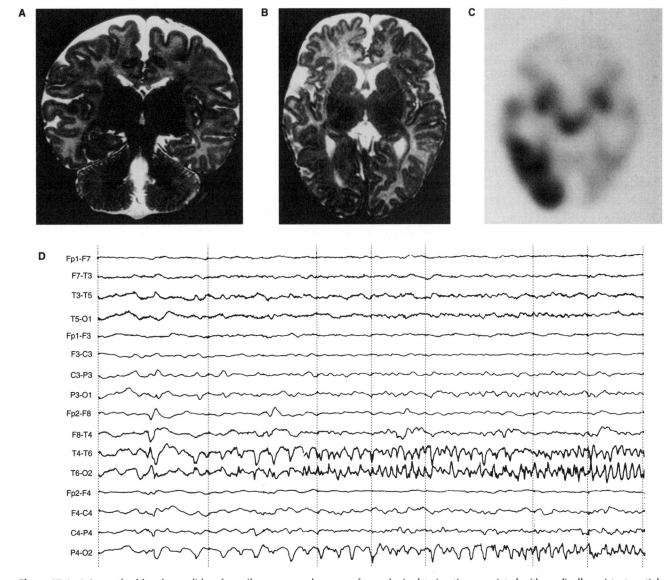

Figure 47-1. A 3-month-old male candidate for epilepsy surgery because of neurologic deterioration associated with medically resistant partial seizures and infantile spasms. **A.** T2-weighted coronal MR image. There is asymmetric thickening of the cortex in the right parahippocampal and occipitotemporal gyri consistent with cortical dysplasia. **B.** T2-weighted axial MR image. There is asymmetric increased myelin deposition in the right occipital and posterior temporal lobes as indicated by the hypointense white matter signal (in comparison to the normal hyperintensity of cerebral white matter in a 3-month-old patient). Areas of hypermyelination are known to occur in conjunction with cortical dysplasia. **C.** Axial Tc99m HMPAO ictal SPECT. There is increased activity in the right occipital and posterior temporal lobes corresponding to the regions of abnormality on MR images. **D.** Ictal EEG recorded during injection for SPECT study demonstrating repetitive rhythmic sharp waves in the right temporooccipital region. The electrographic discharge was accompanied by contraversive eye deviation and facial grimacing.

childhood epilepsy. High–field strength magnetic resonance (MR) and functional imaging can detect subtle abnormalities in cryptogenic disorders (Figure 47-1). While the generalized dysplasias such as lissencephaly and band heterotopia are rarely amenable to excisional procedures, focal lesions often merit surgical consideration (39,40).

Very young patients with intractable partial seizures have a high proportion of CDLs and are prone to severe developmental deterioration. Dysplastic changes in infants with catastrophic seizures are often multilobar and show a predilection for the posterior hemispheres

(41,42) Treatment with multilobar excision or hemispherectomy is often required for full seizure control.

Hemimegalencephaly

Hemimegalencephaly is a rare disorder of brain growth in which one cerebral hemisphere undergoes striking enlargement in conjunction with gyral thickening and accelerated myelination. Histologic analysis reveals bizarre giant neurons and heterotopias similar to tuberous sclerosis and high-grade cortical dysplasia (43). Fulminant hemiconvulsive seizures and mental deterioration lead to early death in some affected individuals (44), whereas others experience a more benign course (45).

Chronic Focal (Rasmussen's) Encephalitis

First described by Rasmussen in 1958 (46), chronic focal encephalitis is a rare but striking cause of epilepsia partialis continua and progressive hemiplegia and characteristically is drug-resistant. Serial neuroimaging reveals progressive atrophy associated with nonspecific focal inflammatory changes in brain tissue and cerebral vasculature (47,48). A viral etiology has not been established despite repeated attempts to culture an agent (49). Acquired autoimmune dysfunction is suggested by the partial resolution of symptoms after immunotherapy and the recent identification of antibodies to the GluR3 receptor in some patients. Hemispherectomy prevents progression in patients with unilateral hemispheric involvement (48).

West Syndrome

West syndrome, a disorder of brief clonic or tonic spasms, developmental delay, and EEG hypsarrhythmia, is a catastrophic early-onset epilepsy that is often drug-resistant. Treatment with corticosteroids and vigabatrin induce remission in approximately one-half of affected individuals, leaving a sizable proportion with continuing seizures.

The occurrence of spasms in patients with confirmed structural lesions or evidence of localized functional derangement often leads to consideration of excisional surgery (42,50). The ability to induce surgical remission in an apparently generalized disorder implies that the spasms are a form of secondarily generalized epilepsy. PET abnormalities in dysplastic cortical regions (34) and the cessation of generalized and partial epileptic seizures support this hypothesis (51,51).

Surgery in Infancy

Despite compelling evidence that very young patients can deteriorate rapidly, surgery is often postponed until later childhood or adolescence (52,53). Rapid deterioration is especially common in infants with exceptionally frequent seizures. Hemispherectomy is indicated when there is hemispheric damage and widespread unilateral epileptic involvement (54). Approximately 85 percent of hemispherectomy patients achieve seizure-freedom. Smaller resections are restricted to patients with localized ictal patterns and convergent neuroimaging findings (55,56). In an early report, three of five infants with partial epilepsy undergoing resections became seizure-free, two

improved significantly, and none deteriorated (57). The favorable experience has been confirmed in larger series of infants undergoing excisional procedures (58,59).

Surgical Contraindications

Degenerative and Metabolic Disorders

Metabolic and degenerative disorders are important surgical contraindications. Most present in the first decade of life and are occasionally associated with partial seizures.

Benign Focal Epilepsies

Syndromes of benign partial epilepsy resolve by the end of the second decade. Benign rolandic epilepsy and benign focal epilepsy of childhood with occipital spikes are relatively common and easily diagnosed by their distinctive clinical and EEG features (60,61).

Medication Noncompliance

Noncompliance is usually established by the referring physician and rarely surfaces as an issue during the preoperative evaluation. Noncompliant patients are unsuitable surgical candidates.

Psychosis

The occurrence of psychotic symptoms in children with partial seizures is controversial and rarely reported. Chronic thought disorders in the adult are rarely improved after surgery, and periictal disturbances generally remit with seizure control (62). It is not known whether psychotic symptoms can be prevented by early surgical intervention.

Mental Retardation

Patients with chronic epilepsy manifest variable cognitive impairment, but surgery is rarely withheld if patients can comply with the preoperative evaluation. Retarded individuals clearly benefit from seizure-freedom.

Dysfunctional Families

Cooperation with epilepsy surgery team members is fundamental to the success of elective surgery. Psychodynamically dysfunctional families are rarely comfortable during intensive or prolonged hospitalizations and may not be able to objectively evaluate the risks and benefits of surgery. Dysfunctional families require psychological and social intervention and support before surgical workup.

PREOPERATIVE EVALUATION

Neuropathologic Considerations

Disorders of cortical development underlie the majority of intractable seizures in childhood, while acquired lesions (i.e., atrophic and/or sclerotic) are less common. Extensive resections (hemispherectomy or multilobar excision) prove necessary because developmental lesions are associated with widespread anatomic and functional derangement. While temporal lobectomy is frequently used to treat adults, pediatric patients are prone to extratemporal seizures and catastrophic presentations (1,63). Direct comparisons of children and adults with cortical dysplasia and epilepsy reveal that younger age of seizure onset is associated with a higher incidence of developmental delay, gross structural lesions, and frequent seizures (64).

Not unexpectedly, seizures from a developmentally abnormal cortex are more difficult to characterize by scalp EEG; high field–strength MR imaging can assist localization by detecting subtle dysplastic lesions. Even so, many low-grade dysplastic lesions and neuronal heterotopias remain undetected (65). Functional localization using PET and SPECT can identify epileptogenic regions through abnormal metabolism or ictal blood flow (66–69).

Clinical Seizure Semiology

Frontal Lobe Epilepsy (FLE)

The clinical and electrographic manifestations of FLE are extremely heterogeneous. Frontal lobe seizures are typically brief (<5 minutes) and stereotyped. Clustering and sleep onset are common, while prolonged seizure episodes and auras are unusual. Patients may experience brief nonspecific fears or sensations immediately before seizure onset.

Motor seizures of frontal lobe origin may be tonic or clonic, reflecting involvement of Brodmann areas 6 or 4. Seizures arising in motor strip produce contralateral clonic activity with or without Jacksonian spread to adjacent cortical areas. Very young children are more prone to secondary generalization. Tonic contraversive arm, head, or eye movements suggest involvement of dorsolateral frontal cortex anterior to motor strip. Tonic version is commonly the result of secondary spread of epileptic activity to the frontal cortex.

Ictal head version is a common frontal lobe seizure manifestation and occurs when the sternocleidomastoid muscle is activated. This muscle has two heads (sternal and clavicular), which rotate the head and neck in opposite trajectories (contralateral turning versus ipsilateral tilting) (70). Either or both heads may become active, resulting complex ictal movement patterns.

Stereotyped psychomotor patterns are more typical of seizures arising in the premotor cortex. Symptoms include bicycling movements, repetitive arm postures and gestures, and disturbances of phonation including speech arrest and vocalization (71,72). Activation of anterior and orbitofrontal cortexes are associated with prominent automatisms and complex behavioral sequences. Truncal postural change is not unusual, and patients often appear frightened or agitated. Seizures are typically nocturnal, with frequent arousals that, together with the lack of epileptiform discharges, have suggested paroxysmal nocturnal dystonia.

Supplementary motor area (SMA) seizures often begin in childhood (73); they cause bilateral proximal tonic limb posturing with fully preserved consciousness. The routine EEG may be normal or nondiagnostic, yielding a false impression of psychogenic seizures. Intracortical propagation of SMA discharges may falsely localize seizure onset to the dorsolateral convexity.

Temporal Lobe Epilepsy (TLE)

Seizures of temporal lobe origin are common in childhood. Although well-characterized in adolescents and adults, the manifestations of TLE are less well documented in infants and children. Many features are seen in adults, but diagnostic pitfalls abound.

Complex partial seizures of temporal lobe origin impair or distort consciousness. Auras are common although rarely described by the preverbal or nonverbal patient. Automatisms typically consist of gestural or oroalimentary movements in infancy, while verbal and complex behavioral automatisms are characteristic of older patients (74).

Secondary motor seizures occur frequently in infants and may be the only seizure manifestation. Their incidence declines with advancing age, while behavioral arrest and stereotyped automatisms increasingly predominate. Video-EEG is often required to diagnose secondary motor phenomena (74,75).

Parietal Lobe Epilepsy (PLE)

Seizures of parietal lobe origin are relatively uncommon, and their true incidence is probably underestimated because symptoms arise only after extraparietal spread. Two clinically distinct propagation patterns are recognized: motor convulsions with spread to the frontal lobes and complex partial seizures with temporal lobe involvement (76–78). Both patterns may occur in the same patient (78). Panic attacks may be the sole manifestation of right parietal lobe seizures (79).

The EEG is often silent or subtly abnormal. Ictal SPECT may confirm anterior parietal seizure origin in patients with sensorimotor symptoms; psychoparetic symptoms arise posteriorly (78).

Occipital Lobe Epilepsy (OLE)

Occipital seizures produce visual symptomatology including hallucinations, amaurosis, visual field deficits, and forced eye and eyelid movement (76). Seizure activity may spread frontally or, more rarely, to the temporal lobe and produce regional symptoms. Many children with OLE have benign syndromes that are easily controlled and remit during adolescence (80,81).

Scalp EEG

The EEG evaluation remains the single most useful tool for evaluating pediatric epilepsy surgery patients. Experienced pediatric EEG personnel should evaluate the EEG because the interpretation of pediatric seizure patterns is complex (82). Although patients referred for surgery usually have had extensive EEG evaluations, electroclinical diagnoses should always be reconfirmed by careful review of prior EEG recordings. Video-EEG is essential for documenting seizure manifestations. The appearance of electrographic discharges before clinical seizure onset suggests remote seizure onset (82).

Ictal patterns in the childhood epilepsies are more often regional than localized, and children display a wide variety of artifacts that obscure EEG interpretation. There is a close relationship between ictal and interictal electrographic findings, but less than half of all interictal spikes are detected at the scalp (82). Pediatric surgical candidates often manifest bilaterally synchronous or multifocal discharges. Regionalization serves as a basis for planning further invasive studies. MR and functional imaging may help confirm equivocal electrophysiologic data.

Structural Imaging

Magnetic resonance imaging is the modality of choice for evaluating pediatric epilepsy surgery candidates. Its high specificity and sensitivity provide clues to the pathologic basis of many developmental disorders including cortical dysplastic lesions, migrational disturbances, and developmental tumors (i.e., dysembryoplastic neuroepithelial tumors, gangliogliomas, and so forth).

MRI presently detects a pathologic substrate in over 80 percent of children with intractable partial epilepsy (65). Thirty of 98 children and adolescents with partial epilepsy undergoing both computed tomography (CT) and MRI investigations had lesions responsible for their epilepsy detected by MRI but noy by CT (83).

MRI studies also reveal a high incidence of HS in childhood. In a study of 53 children with TLE undergoing detailed MRI investigations, 30 children showed either HS or regions of abnormal signal in the absence of a mass lesion (84). Hippocampal volume loss can also be documented (85). One developmentally delayed infant with a normal MRI reportedly developed a unilaterally increased signal in the hippocampus within 24 hours of an episode of status epilepticus (86). Cortical dysgenesis was identified in the temporal lobe specimen.

Neuroimaging of pediatric epilepsy surgery candidates should employ techniques to maximize yield. T1-weighted data are optimally acquired in an oblique coronal orientation, orthogonal to the long axis of the hippocampi (87). Sequencing should include thin (1–1.5 mm) images without gaps, especially through the hippocampal regions. Further sequences such as fluid attenuated inversion recovery (FLAIR) help to detect subtle abnormalities. We routinely perform MRI after video-EEG monitoring to facilitate more detailed examination of the candidate seizure region.

Functional Imaging

Functional imaging of the epileptogenic region may help define the seizure focus, especially when other modalities yield equivocal or divergent findings. Several techniques are presently available.

Positron Emission Tomography (PET)

PET utilizes radioactive tracers with short half-lives linked to cerebral blood flow. ^{18}Fluorodeoxyglucose (FDG) is a marker of the interictal focus, correlating with the epileptogenic region, usually the temporal lobe, in approximately 80 percent of adult cases (88). Ictal capture is unlikely and should not be induced by convulsant agents because of technical limitations of the scanning process.

The requirement for sedation and the higher proportion of extratemporal seizures limits the clinical utility of PET in children. Newer isotopes that bind to receptor-specific compounds such as ^{11}C-flumazenil, which is linked to the benzodiazepine receptor, hold promise for enhanced localization (89).

Single Photon Emission Computerized Tomography

Imaging with SPECT utilizes isotopes such as hexylmethylpropylene amineoxine (HMPAO) for qualitative measures of regional cerebral perfusion (rCP). Early studies were performed in the interictal state, but ictal injections are acknowledged to yield more accurate localization of the epileptogenic region (90). The high yield of ictal SPECT has supplanted PET in the functional evaluation of pediatric epilepsy surgery candidates (91).

Proton Magnetic Resonance Spectroscopy (MRS)

MRS studies in epilepsy use *N*-acetyl aspartate (NAA), creatine, and phosphocreatine-containing compounds, as several lines of evidence indicate that NAA is primarily intraneuronal and an indicator of neuronal well-being (92). ^{1}H-MRS can be added to routine imaging and provides important lateralizing information, especially in temporal lobe epilepsy (93). Recent MRS studies document neuronal dysfunction in neocortical dysplastic lesions, and correction of metabolic derangement at mirror temporal foci improve after successful surgery (94).

Functional MR Imaging (FMRI)

FMRI is based on noninvasive detection of small regions of increased cerebral blood flow through decreases in deoxyhemoglobin concentration. Three applications are especially promising for patients with epilepsy: delineation of ictal events, localization of the primary epileptogenic region, and identification of a functionally critical cortex (95).

At present, pediatric applications of FMRI are limited. Subjects must be awake, fully cooperative, and not easily distracted. As many candidates are developmentally delayed and behaviorally and/or motorically handicapped, FMRI data is not easily acquired. It is likely that FMRI will play an increasingly important role as technological hurdles are resolved.

Neurobehavioral and Psychsocial Assessment

Candidate Selection

Neurobehavioral and psychosocial disabilities are common in pediatric epilepsy surgical candidates. A high proportion display mental handicap, short attention span, or high activity level (53,96). There is a clear link between brain damage and the presence of these features, with the most damaged patients showing earlier seizure onset and a higher frequency of recurrence (10). Older children and adolescents with TLE may develop psychotic thought disorders, especially with left-sided seizure origin (62); adults may experience hyposexuality and personality disturbances (97).

The high incidence of psychosocial and behavioral problems makes baseline assessment of these areas of functioning critical to the preoperative evaluation. However, level of cooperation is often poor, and cognitive deficits may not permit standardized testing.

There is also greater difficulty lateralizing and localizing function in the immature nervous system. Whereas neuropsychological assessment in adults can lateralize dysfunction, similar procedures are rarely successful in children. The frontal lobes are not fully mature until the second decade, and temporal lobe

findings are often nonspecific. Developmental lesions may produce widespread functional disturbance.

The contribution of psychosocial assessment to pediatric epilepsy surgery is more realistically directed in two ways. First, preoperative baseline level of function can be documented for future comparisons. Second, psychosocial assessment provides a descriptor of overall maturational brain status.

Testing Protocol

There is no single neurobehavioral protocol for children being worked up for epilepsy surgery. At the Palm Desert II Epilepsy Surgery Conference, 82 centers completed detailed questionnaires about neuropsychological testing (98). Forty-two (52.4%) included information about pediatrics, although children were often a small minority. Most centers employed adult test batteries with pediatric norms rather than devising their own batteries. There was uniformity of testing for intelligence and certain measures of cognition but a striking diversity in tests of certain verbal skills and nondominant hemisphere function. The Wisconsin Card Sorting Test and the Controlled Oral Word Association Test (FAS Fluency) were most commonly used. A more complete listing of tests is found elsewhere (99).

Invasive EEG Studies

Intracranial EEG Recording

In children, as anomalous development occurs throughout the neocortex (100) and is frequently in proximity to eloquent cortex, even seizures of temporal lobe origin are rarely evaluated properly by adult evaluation paradigms (101,102).

Several additional factors in children explain the higher incidence of more complex workups and higher rates of electrode implantation. Electrocorticographic (ECoG) monitoring, the only tool for physiologically assessing seizure foci intraoperatively, is performed under general anesthesia and frequently is nondiagnostic (82). Electrographically active regions may extend beyond known anatomic boundaries (103), are particularly extensive in infants and very young children, (100,104,105), and are more likely to involve eloquent cortical regions (106,107). Dysplastic tissue is rarely visible in the operating room, making visually guided surgery problematic.

Depth electrodes, which are used primarily to sample temporolimbic structures, have limited utility for neocortical foci. Subdural electrodes provide more comprehensive coverage and are well tolerated, even in very young children and infants (107,108).

Indications for Implanting Electrodes

There are no universal criteria for invasive EEG monitoring in pediatric patients. Invasive monitoring is often indicated for nonlesional cases (109), whereas scalp EEG, in conjunction with imaging and ECoG, is usually sufficient to evaluate seizures associated with gross structural lesions. Excisional procedures have been performed in patients undergoing only intraoperative ECoG monitoring and PET (42).

Possible indications for invasive EEG recording include:

1. *Partial seizures with normal or nonlocalizing imaging data.* Nonlesional epilepsy patients become seizure-free only if the ictal onset zone and interictal abnormalities are completely resected. Subdural recording helps define the limits of the epileptogenic region, as depth electrodes cannot sample wide regions of epileptogenic cortex.

2. *Epileptogenic zone larger than the structural lesion.* The true physiologic limits of the epileptic focus in patients with developmental lesions require careful documentation (110). Invasive recording assists surgical planning (111). In 42 children with lesional epilepsy, 90 percent were seizure-free after complete excision of the lesion and entire epileptogenic region, whereas half were seizure-free with lesion removal and incomplete resection of electrophysiologically abnormal tissue (112).

3. *Noncongruence of data.* Defining the epileptogenic zone with noncongruent seizure semiology, interictal-ictal EEG, and imaging data may not be possible. Invasive EEG recording can help resolve incongruities.

4. *Multiple lesions and/or multifocal interictal epileptiform activity.* Children with multiple structural lesions and/or multifocal interictal spike discharges are surgical candidates when seizures arise from a single operable epileptogenic zone (38,113,114). Multiple epileptogenic regions can exert complex ictal interactions, rendering localization difficult from scalp EEG data alone.

5. *Involvement of regions subserving eloquent cortical function.* Regions of eloquent cortex that are contiguous to the epileptic focus require mapping with subdural electrodes. Sensory cortex may be identified intraoperatively by median nerve stimulation. In children, language function is optimally defined extraoperatively.

Functional Cortical Stimulation

The high incidence of extratemporal and multilobar epilepsy in children requires definition of cortical function in many surgical candidates. The standard adult paradigm whereby baseline stimulation is increased in 0.5 to 1.0 mA steps until an afterdischarge, functional response or 15 mA ceiling is obtained is rarely successful in younger patients (115,116). Electrical responsiveness increases in direct proportion to age, while threshold for functional responsiveness decreases until adolescence (116).

Cortical responses are more reliably elicited in children by increasing both stimulus intensity and duration in a stepwise fashion (116). Increasing both domains rather than intensity alone causes the stimulus to converge toward the chronaxie on the strength-duration curve. Responses obtained at the chronaxie are elicited at the lowest possible expenditure of energy, a clear advantage when working in immature cortex. In comparison to the adult paradigm, only dual stimulation successfully evokes both afterdischarges and functional responses in patients 4 years of age and younger (116).

Sensorimotor Mapping

Dual stimulation mapping of sensorimotor responses in pediatric epilepsy surgery candidates reveals anatomic representation of cortical function similar to that in the adult. Despite the similarities, however, there are several important maturational features (117). Children under the age of 4 years have predominantly tonic rather than clonic movements, and movement of the tongue is unusual. Below the age of 6 years, hand movement but not individual finger movement is observed. As a rule, tonic finger movements appear earlier than clonic movements, a developmental sequence that mirrors the ontogenetic expression of motor seizure patterns in childhood (74,118).

Below the age of 2 years, facial motor responses may be bilateral (117), resembling a grimace that lasts several seconds. Bilateral facial movement is absent in older children, suggesting that bilateral facial innervation is a postnatal pattern that predates axonal and/or synaptic elimination (119,120). Ipsilateral lower facial innervation is gradually lost with maturation. Bilateral facial movement is supported by the observation of facial sparing in congenital but not acquired hemiplegia (121).

Patients with aberrant cortical development exhibit unexpected anomalies of the motor homunculus (117). A hand region superior to primary shoulder region and double shoulder region above and below hand and finger cortex have been described. Aberrant cortical motor organization is more common in patients with other anomalies of cortical development (122). Experimental studies in the primate brain indicate that prenatal lesions are capable of inducing anomalous cortical sulci and functional reorganization at remote cortical sites in both cerebral hemispheres (123,124).

Language Mapping

Much of our knowledge of the organization of primary language cortex in the child comes from studies of recovery from childhood aphasia (125). Complete or near-complete recovery is possible based on age at which the lesion occuerred and size and location of the damage (126). Recovery involves interhemispheric reorganization and a switch to right-hemisphere dominance. Language recovers well after early postnatal lesions, but deficits in nonlinguistic skills suggest that recovery is rarely complete or predictable (127).

While postnatal lesions of the dominant hemisphere in early childhood lead to significant reorganization of language cortex, there is little information about language representation in children with partial seizures and anomalous cortical development. Clarification has obvious implications when seizures originate within or adjacent to language cortex (128).

A recent investigation of electrical stimulation of language cortex in 34 predominantly pediatric patients with implanted subdural grid electrodes, identified 28 with MRI and/or histologic evidence of developmental pathology (107). Patients with developmental lesions had language cortex in frontal and temporal sites anatomically similar to the adult. The "adult" representation has been documented in an epilepsy patient as young as 4 years old and a 2-year-old being mapped for tumoral surgery. The actual amount of square surface area of cortex devoted to language (based on the number of subdural electrodes showing language representation) is also similar to that of the adult (106,129), which suggests that language sites are designated in early life and conserved anatomically over the lifespan. The increasing language competence of the child is therefore not attributable to increased cortical surface area.

The relatively fixed position of language cortex in children with anomalous disorders of cortical development contrasts sharply with the relocation of language following early peri- or postnatally acquired lesions (130). Relocation of language sites occurs if language cortex is destroyed before the age of 6 years. By contrast, developmental lesions do not ablate language cortex and therefore do not lead to relocation. Epileptic bombardment also does not displace language cortex from predetermined sites.

Preoperative Predictors of Seizure Outcome

Clinical, EEG, imaging, and neurospsychological features have been used to predict outcome of adults selected for temporal lobectomy (1), and multivariate algorithms for predicting success have been described (131). Children exhibit more diverse causes for intractable seizures, making extrapolation from the adult experience difficult. Pediatric candidates with a well-circumscribed interictal EEG focus, localized seizure pattern on monitoring, and tumoral epilepsy have a greater likelihood of seizure-freedom (132). Although younger age at surgery is not associated with reduced chances of success, younger patients more often manifest poorly localized EEG patterns (132), and completeness of resection of the epileptogenic area (1) may not be possible.

Studies of preoperative factors for pediatric temporal lobectomy have not identified specific predictors of seizure outcome (133). The absence of statistically significant adult variables such as duration of epilepsy, daily seizures, motor convulsions, and mental retardation suggests caution before excluding potential candidates, and directly contrasts with the adult experience. The lower predictive power of preoperative variables in pediatric epilepsy surgical candidates suggests that all children with surgically amenable intractable seizures are potential surgical candidates.

REFERENCES

1. Engel JJ. Epilepsy surgery. *Curr Opin Neurol* 1994; 7:140–147.

2. Juul Jensen P, Foldspang A. Natural history of epileptic seizures. *Epilepsia* 1983; 24: 297–312.

3. Hauser WA, Annegers JF, Kurland LT. Prevalence of epilepsy in Rochester, Minnesota: 1940–1980. *Epilepsia* 1991; 32:429–445.

4. Hauser WA. Recent developments in the epidemiology of epilepsy. *Acta Neurol Scand* 1995; 162 (Suppl):17–21.

5. Panel NC. Consensus conference on surgery for epilepsy. *JAMA* 1990; 264:729–733.

6. Gilman JT, Duchowny M, Jayakar P, Resnick TJ. Medical intractability in children evaluated for epilepsy surgery. *Neurology* 1994; 44:1341–1343.

7. Desai BT, Porter RJ, Penry JK. Psychogenic seizures. A study of 42 attacks in six patients, with intensive monitoring. *Arch Neurol* 1982; 39:202–209.

8. Sassower K, Duchowny M. Psychogenic seizures and nonepileptic phenomena in childhood. In: Devinsky O, Theodore W, eds. *Epilepsy and Behavior*. New York: Wiley-Liss, 1991:223–235.

9. Chevrie JJ, Aicardi J. Convulsive disorders in the first year of life: persistence of epileptic seizures. *Epilepsia* 1979; 20: 643–649.

10. Aicardi J. Epilepsy in brain-injured children. *Dev Med Child Neurol* 1990; 32:191–202.

11. Lindsay J, Ounsted C, Richards P. Long-term outcome in children with temporal lobe seizures. IV: Genetic factors, febrile convulsions and the remission of seizures. *Dev Med Child Neurol* 1980; 22: 429–439.

12. Gastaut H, Poirier F, Payan H, et al. HHE syndrome, hemiconvulsions, hemiplegia, epilepsy. *Epilepsia* 1959; 1: 418–447.

13. Cendes F, Andermann F, Dubeau F, et al. Early childhood prolonged febrile convulsions, atrophy and sclerosis of mesial structures, and temporal lobe epilepsy: an MRI volumetric study. *Neurology* 1993; 43: 1083–1087.

14. Harvey AS, Grattan Smith JD, Desmond PM, Chow CW, Berkovic SF. Febrile seizures and hippocampal sclerosis: frequent and related findings in intractable temporal lobe epilepsy of childhood. *Pediatr Neurol* 1995; 12: 201–206.

15. Emerson R, D'Souza BJ, Vining EP, et al. Stopping medication in children with epilepsy. Predictors of outcome. *N Engl J Med* 1981; 304:1125–1129.

16. Huttenlocher PR, Hapke RJ. A follow-up study of intractable seizures in childhood [see comments]. *Ann Neurol* 1990; 28:699–705.

17. Hadjipanayis A, Hadjichristodoulou C, Youroukos S. Epilepsy in patients with cerebral palsy. *Dev Med Child Neurol* 1997; 39:659–663.

18. Ounsted C, Lindsay J, Norman R. *Biological Factors in Temporal Lobe Epilepsy*. Philadelphia: Lippincott, 1966. Clinics in Developmental Medicine, no. 22. London: SIMP with Heinemann Medical.

19. Ben Ari Y. Activity-dependent forms of plasticity. *J Neurobiol* 1995; 26:295–298.

20. Represa A, Niquet J, Pollard H, Ben Ari Y. Cell death, gliosis, and synaptic remodeling in the hippocampus of epileptic rats. *J Neurobiol* 1995; 26: 413–425.

21. Represa A, Ben Ari Y. Molecular and cellular cascades in seizure-induced neosynapse formation. *Adv Neurol* 1997; 72:25–34.

22. Sloviter RS. Hippocampal pathology and pathophysiology in temporal lobe epilepsy. *Neurologia* 1996; 4: 29–32.

23. Sutula T, Cascino G, Cavazos J, et al. Mossy fiber synaptic reorganization in the epileptic human temporal lobe. *Ann Neurol* 1989; 26:321–330.

24. Houser CR. Granule cell dispersion in the dentate gyrus of humans with temporal lobe epilepsy. *Brain Res* 1990; 535:195–204.

25. Bloom JC, Sabbagh MN, Bondi MW, Hansen L, Alford MF, Masliah E, Thal LJ. 1997. Hippocampal sclerosis contributes to dementia in the elderly. *Neurology* 1997; 48:154–160.

26. Verity CM, Ross EM, Golding J. Outcome of childhood status epilepticus and lengthy febrile convulsions: findings of national cohort study. *Br Med J* 1993:225–228.

27. Sagar HJ, Oxbury JM. Hippocampal neuron loss in temporal lobe epilepsy: correlation with early childhood convulsions. *Ann Neurol* 1987; 22:334–340.

28. Ounsted C, Glaser GH, Lindsay J, Richards P. Focal epilepsy with mesial temporal sclerosis after acute meningitis. *Arch Neurol* 1985; 42:1058–1060.

29. Marks DA, Kim J, Spencer DD, Spencer SS. Characteristics of intractable seizures following meningitis and encephalitis. *Neurology* 1992; 42:1513–1518.

30. Commission on Classification and Terminology of the International League Against Epilepsy. Proposal for classification of epilepsies and epileptic syndromes. *Epilepsia* 1985; 26:268–278.

31. Duchowny M, Harvey AS. Pediatric epilepsy syndromes: an update and critical review. *Epilepsia* 1996; 37:S26–S40.

32. Alexander GL, Norman R. *The Sturge-Weber syndrome.* Bristol: Wright and Son, 1960.

33. Peterman AF, Hayles AB, Dockrty MD, Love JG. 1958. Encephalotrigeminal angiomatosis (Sturge-Weber disease): clinical study of thirty-five cases. *JAMA* 1958; 67:2169–2176.

34. Chugani HT, Mazziotta JC, Phelps ME. Sturge-Weber syndrome: a study of cerebral glucose utilization with positron emission tomography. *J Pediatr* 1989; 114:244–253.

35. Vaernet K. 1983. Temporal lobotomy in children and young adults. In: Parsonage M, ed. *XIVth Epilepsy International Symposium*. Raven Press, New York.

36. Monaghan HP, Krafchik B, Mac Gregor D, Fitz C. Tuberous sclerosis complex in children. *Am J Dis Child* 1981; 135:912–917.

37. Perot P, Weir B, Rasmussen T. Tuberous sclerosis. Surgical therapy for seizures. *Arch Neurol* 1966; 15:498–506.

38. Erba G, Duchowny MS. 1990. Partial epilepsy and tuberous sclerosis: indications for surgery in disseminated disease. In: Duchowny MS, Resnick TJ, Alvarez LA, eds. *Pediatric Epilepsy Surgery*. New York: Demos, 1990:315–322.

39. Guerrini R, Canapicchi R, Zifkin BG, et al. *Dysplasias of Cerebral Cortex and Epilepsy*. Philadelphia: Lippincott-Raven, 1996.

40. Duchowny M. Epilepsy surgery in children. *Curr Opin Neurol* 1995; 8:112–116.

41. Guerrini R, Dubeau F, Dulac O, et al. Bilateral parasagittal parietooccipital polymicrogyria and epilepsy. *Ann Neurol* 1997; 41:65–73.

42. Chugani HT, Shields WD, Shewmon DA, et al. Infantile spasms: I. PET identifies focal cortical dysgenesis in cryptogenic cases for surgical treatment [see comments]. *Ann Neurol* 1990; 27:406–13.

43. Robain O, Chiron C, Dulac O. Electron microscopic and Golgi study in a case of hemimegalencephaly. *Acta Neuropathol Berl* 1989; 77:664–666.

44. King M, Stephenson JB, Ziervogel M, Doyle D, Galbraith S. Hemimegalencephaly—a case for hemispherectomy? *Neuropediatrics* 1985; 16:46–55.

45. Vigevano F, Fusco L, Holthausen H, Lahl R. The morphological spectrum and variable clinical picture in children with hemimegalencephaly. In: Tuxhorn I, Holthausen H, Boenigk H. eds. *Pediatric Epilepsy Syndromes and Their Surgical Treatment*. London: John Libbey & Company, 1997:377–391.

46. Rasmussen T, McCann W. Clinical studies of patients with focal epilepsy due to "chronic encephalitis." *Trans Am Neurol Assoc* 1968; 93:89–94.

47. Andermann F. Clinical indications for hemispherectomy and callosotomy. *Epilepsy Res* 1992; Suppl 5:189–199.

48. Rasmussen T, Andermann F. Update on the syndrome of "chronic encephalitis" and epilepsy. *Cleve Clin J Med* 1989; 56:S181–S184.

49. Rasmussen T, Olszewski J, Lloyd-Smith D. Focal seizures due to chronic localized encephalitis. *Neurology* 1958; 8:435–445.

50. Chugani HT. Infantile spasms. *Curr Opin Neurol* 1995; 8:139–144.

51. Shields WD, Shewmon DA, Chugani HT, Peacock WJ. The role of surgery in the treatment of infantile spasms. *J Epilepsy* 1990: S321–S324.

52. Duchowny MS. 1989. Surgery for intractable epilepsy: issues and outcome. *Pediatrics* 1989; 84:886–894.

53. Shields WD, Peacock WJ, Roper SN. Surgery for epilepsy. Special pediatric considerations. *Neurosurg Clin N Am* 1993; 4:301–310.

54. Peacock WJ. Hemispherectomy for the treatment of intractable seizures in childhood. *Neurosurg Clin N Am* 1995; 6:549–563.

55. Wyllie E, Comair YG, Kotagal P, Raja S, Ruggieri P. Epilepsy surgery in infants. *Epilepsia* 1996; 37:625–637.

56. Duchowny M, Jayakar P, Resnick T, et al. Epilepsy surgery in patients under age 3 years. *Ann Neurol* 1996; 40:286.

57. Duchowny MS, Resnick TJ, Alvarez LA, Morrison G. Focal resection for malignant partial seizures in infancy. *Neurology* 1990; 40:980–984.

58. Wyllie E. Surgery for catastrophic localization-related epilepsy in infants. *Epilepsia* 1998; 39:737–743.

59. Duchowny M, Jayakar P, Resnick T, et al. Epilepsy surgery in the first three years of life. *Epilepsia* 1998; 39:737–743.

60. Heijbel J, Blom S, Bergfors PG. Benign epilepsy of children with centrotemporal EEG foci. A study of incidence rate in outpatient care. *Epilepsia* 1975; 16:657–664.

61. Gastaut H. A new type of epilepsy: benign partial epilepsy of childhood with occipital spike-waves. *Clin Electroencephalogr* 1982; 13:13–22.

62. Trimble M. Behavioural complications of limbic epilepsy: implications for an understanding of the emotional motor system in man. *Prog Brain Res* 1996; 107:605–616.

63. Duchowny M, Harvey AS, Jayakar P, et al. The preoperative evaluation of pediatric temporal lobe epilepsy. In: Tuxhorn I, Holthausen H, and Boenigk H, eds. *Pediatric Epilepsy Syndromes and Their Surgical Treatment.* London: John Libbey, 1997:261–273.

64. Wyllie E. Children with seizures: when can treatment be deferred? *J Child Neurol* 1994; 2:8–13.

65. Kuzniecky R, Murro A, King D, et al. Magnetic resonance imaging in childhood intractable partial epilepsies: pathologic correlations. *Neurology* 1993; 43:681–687.

66. Harvey AS, Berkovic SF. Functional neuroimaging with SPECT in children with partial epilepsy. *J Child Neurol* 1994; 9:S71–S81.

67. Chugani HT. The use of positron emission tomography in the clinical assessment of epilepsy. *Semin Nucl Med* 1992; 22:247–253.

68. Cross JH, Gordon I, Jackson GD, et al. Children with intractable focal epilepsy: ictal and interictal 99TcM HMPAO single photon emission computed tomography. *Dev Med Child Neurol* 1995; 37:673–681.

69. Cross JH, Gordon I, Connelly A, et al. Interictal 99Tc(m) HMPAO SPECT and 1H MRS in children with temporal lobe epilepsy. *Epilepsia* 1997; 38:338–345.

70. Jayakar P, Duchowny M, Resnick T, Alvarez L. Ictal head deviation: lateralizing significance of the pattern of head movement. *Neurology* 1992; 42:1989–1992.

71. Salanova V, Morris HH, Van Ness P, Kotagal P, Wyllie E, Luders H. Frontal lobe seizures: electroclinical syndromes. *Epilepsia* 1995; 36:16–24.

72. Riggio S, Harner RN. Repetitive motor activity in frontal lobe epilepsy. *Adv Neurol* 1995; 66: 153–164.

73. Bass N, Wyllie E, Comair Y, et al. Supplementary sensorimotor area seizures in children and adolescents. *J Pediatr* 1995; 126:537–544.

74. Jayakar P, Duchowny MS. Complex partial seizures of temporal lobe origin in early childhood. In: Duchowny MS, Resnick TJ, Alvarez LA, eds. *Pediatric Epilepsy Surgery.* New York: Demos, 1990:41–46.

75. Duchowny MS. Complex partial seizures of infancy. *Arch Neurol* 1987; 44:911–914.

76. Williamson PD, Boon PA, Thadani VM, et al. Parietal lobe epilepsy: diagnostic considerations and results of surgery. *Ann Neurol* 1992; 31:193–201.

77. So NK. Atonic phenomena and partial seizures. A reappraisal. *Adv Neurol* 1995; 67:29–39.

78. Ho SS, Berkovic SF, Newton MR, et al. Parietal lobe epilepsy: clinical features and seizure localization by ictal SPECT. *Neurology* 1994; 44:2277–2284.

79. Alemayehu S, Bergey GK, Barry E, et al. Panic attacks as ictal manifestations of parietal lobe seizures. *Epilepsia* 1995; 36:824–830.

80. Fois A, Tomaccini D, Balestri P, et al. Intractable epilepsy: etiology, risk factors and treatment. *Clin Electroencephalogr* 1988; 19:68–73.

81. Panayiotopoulos CP. Benign childhood epilepsy with occipital paroxysms: a 15-year prospective study. *Ann Neurol* 1989; 26:51–56.

82. Jayakar P, Duchowny M, Resnick TJ, Alvarez LA. Localization of seizure foci: pitfalls and caveats. *J Clin Neurophysiol* 1991; 8:414–431.

83. Resta M, Dicuonzo PF, Spagnolo P, et al. Imaging studies in partial epilepsy in children and adolescents. *Epilepsia* 1994; 35:1187–1193.

84. Grattan Smith JD, Harvey AS, Desmond PM, Chow CW. Hippocampal sclerosis in children with intractable temporal lobe epilepsy: detection with MR imaging. *Am J Roentgenol* 1993; 161:1045–1048.

85. Kuks JB, Cook MJ, Fish DR, Stevens JM, Shorvon SD. Hippocampal sclerosis in epilepsy and childhood febrile seizures [see comments]. *Lancet* 1993; 342:1391–4.

86. Nohria V, Lee N, Tien RD, et al. Magnetic resonance imaging evidence of hippocampal sclerosis in progression: a case report. *Epilepsia* 1994; 35: 1332–1336.

87. Duncan JS. Imaging and epilepsy. *Brain* 1997; 120:339–377.

88. Engel JJ. PET scanning in partial epilepsy. *Can J Neurol Sci* 1991; 18:588–592.

89. Savic I, Thorell JO, Roland P. [^{11}C]flumazenil positron emission tomography visualizes frontal epileptogenic regions. *Epilepsia* 1995; 36:1225–1232.

90. Duncan R, Patterson J, Roberts R, Hadley DM, Bone I. Ictal/postictal SPECT in the pre-surgical localisation of complex partial seizures. *J Neurol Neurosurg Psychiatry* 1993; 56:141–148.

91. Harvey AS, Bowe JM, Hopkins IJ, Shield LK, Cook DJ, Berkovic SF. Ictal 99mTc-HMPAO single photon emission computed tomography in children with temporal lobe epilepsy. *Epilepsia* 1993; 34:869–877.

92. Connelly A, Jackson GD, Duncan JS, King MD, Gadian DG. Magnetic resonance spectroscopy in temporal lobe epilepsy. *Neurology* 1994; 44: 1411–1417.

93. Gadian DG, Connelly A, Duncan JS, et al. ^{1}H magnetic resonance spectroscopy in the investigation of intractable epilepsy. *Acta Neurol Scand* 1994; 152 (Suppl):116–121.

94. Cendes F, Andermann F, Dubeau F, Matthews PM, Arnold DL. Normalization of neuronal metabolic dysfunction after surgery for temporal lobe epilepsy, evidence from proton MR spectroscopic imaging. *Neurology* 1997; 49: 1525–1533.

95. Connelly A. Ictal imaging using functional magnetic resonance. *Magn Reson Imaging* 1995; 13:1233–1237.

96. Holmes GL, King DW. Epilepsy surgery in children. *Wien Klin Wochenschr* 1990; 102:189–97.

97. Lindsay J, Ounsted C, Richards P. Long-term outcome in children with temporal lobe seizures. III: Psychiatric aspects in childhood and adult life. *Dev Med Child Neurol* 1979; 21: 630–636.

98. Jones-Gotman M, Smith ML, Zatorre RJ. Neuropsychological testing for localizing and lateralizing the epileptogenic region. In: Engel J, ed. *Surgical Treatment of the Epilepsies*. New York: Raven Press, 1993.

99. Levin B, Feldman E, Duchowny M, Brown M. Neuropsychological assessment of children with epilepsy. *Int Pediatr* 1991; 6:214–219.

100. Wyllie E. Developmental aspects of seizure semiology: problems in identifying localized-onset seizures in infants and children [editorial]. *Epilepsia* 1995; 36:1170–1172.

101. Duchowny M, Levin B, Jayakar P, et al. Temporal lobectomy in early childhood. *Epilepsia* 1992; 33:298–303.

102. Duchowny M, Jayakar P, Resnick T, Levin B, Alvarez L. Posterior temporal epilepsy: electroclinical features. *Ann Neurol* 1994; 35:427–431.

103. Farrell MA, DeRosa MJ, Curran JG, et al. Neuropathologic findings in cortical resections (including hemispherectomies) performed for the treatment of intractable childhood epilepsy. *Acta Neuropathol Berl* 1992; 83:246–259.

104. Mischel PS, Nguyen LP, Vinters HV. Cerebral cortical dysplasia associated with pediatric epilepsy. Review of neuropathologic features and proposal for a grading system. *J Neuropathol Exp Neurol* 1995; 54:137–153.

105. Adelson PD, Peacock WJ, Chugani HT, et al. Temporal and extended temporal resections for the treatment of intractable seizures in early childhood. *Pediatr Neurosurg* 1992; 18:169–178.

106. DeVos KJ, Wyllie E, Geckler C, Kotagal P, Comair Y. Language dominance in patients with early childhood tumors near left hemisphere language areas. *Neurology* 1995; 45:349–356.

107. Duchowny M, Jayakar P, Harvey AS, et al. Language cortex representation: effects of developmental versus acquired pathology. *Ann Neurol* 1996; 40:31–38.

108. Kramer U, Riviello JJ, Carmant L, et al. Morbidity of depth and subdural electrodes: children and adolescents versus young adults. *J Epilepsy* 1994; 7:7–10.

109. Wyllie E, Luders H, Morris HH, et al. Subdural electrodes in the evaluation for epilepsy surgery in children and adults. *Neuropediatrics* 1988; 19:80–86.

110. Palmini A, Andermann F, Olivier A, Tampieri D, Robitaille Y. Focal neuronal migration disorders and intractable partial epilepsy: results of surgical treatment. *Ann Neurol* 1991; 30:750–757.

111. Jayakar P, Duchowny M, Resnick TJ. Subdural monitoring in the evaluation of children for epilepsy surgery. *J Child Neurol* 1994; 2:61–66.

112. Jayakar P, Duchowny M, Alvarez L, Resnick T. Intraictal activation in the neocortex: a marker of the epileptogenic region. *Epilepsia* 1994; 35:489–494.

113. Bebin EM, Kelly PJ, Gomez MR. Surgical treatment for epilepsy in cerebral tuberous sclerosis. *Epilepsia* 1993; 34:651–657.

114. Bye AM, Matheson JM, Tobias VH, Mackenzie RA. Selective epilepsy surgery in tuberous sclerosis. *Aust Paediatr J* 1989; 25:243–245.

115. Alvarez LA, Jayakar P. 1990. Cortical stimulation with subdural electrodes: special considerations in infancy and childhood. *J Epilepsy* 1990; 3(Suppl):125–130.

116. Jayakar P, Alvarez LA, Duchowny MS, Resnick TJ. A safe and effective paradigm to functionally map the cortex in childhood. *J Clin Neurophysiol* 1992; 9:288–293.

117. Duchowny M, Jayakar P. Functional cortical mapping in children. *Adv Neurol* 1993; 63:149–154.

118. Brockhaus A, Elger CE. Complex partial seizures of temporal lobe origin in children of different age groups. *Epilepsia* 1995; 36:1173–1181.

119. Innocenti GM, Caminitti R. Postnatal shaping of callosal connections from sensory areas. *Brain Res* 1980; 38: 381–394.

120. Rakic P, Bourgeois JP, Eckenhoff MF, Zecevic N, Goldman-Rakic PS. Concurrent overproduction of

synapses in diverse regions of the primate cerebral cortex. *Science* 1986; 232:231–232.

121. Lenn NJ, Freinkel AJ. Facial sparing as a feature of prenatal-onset hemiparesis. *Pediatr Neurol* 1989; 5:291–295.

122. Maegaki Y, Yamamoto T, Takeshita K. Plasticity of central motor and sensory pathways in a case of unilateral extensive cortical dysplasia: investigation of magnetic resonance imaging, transcranial magnetic stimulation, and short-latency somatosensory evoked potentials. *Neurology* 1995; 45:2255–2261.

123. Goldman PS. Neuronal plasticity in primate telencephalon: anomalous projections induced by prenatal removal of frontal cortex. *Science* 1978; 202:767–768.

124. Goldman PS, Galkin TW. Prenatal removal of frontal association cortex in the fetal rhesus monkey: anatomical and functional consequences in postnatal life. *Brain Res* 1978; 152:451–485.

125. Rapin I. Acquired aphasia in children. *J Child Neurol* 1995; 10:267–270.

126. Woods BT, Carey S. Language deficits after apparent clinical recovery from childhood aphasia. *Ann Neurol* 1979; 6:405–409.

127. Alajouanine TH, Lhermitte F. Acquired aphasia in children. *Brain* 1965; 88:653–662.

128. Berger MS, Kincaid J, Ojemann GA, Lettich E. Brain mapping techniques to maximize resection, safety, and seizure control in children with brain tumors. *Neurosurgery* 1989; 25:786–792.

129. Lesser RP, Luders H, Dinner DS. The location of speech and writing functions in the frontal language area: results of extraoperative cortical stimulation. *Brain* 1985; 107:275–291.

130. Basser LS. Hemiplegia of early onset and the faculty of speech with special reference to the effects of hemispherectomy. *Brain* 1962; 85:427–460.

131. Dodrill C, Wilkus R, Ojemann G. Multidisciplinary prediction of seizure relief from cortical resection surgery. *Ann Neurol* 1986; 20:2–12.

132. Vossler DG, Wilkus RJ, Ojemann GA. Preoperative EEG correlates of seizure outcome from epilepsy surgery in children. *J Epilepsy* 1995; 8:236–245.

133. Goldstein R, Harvey AS, Duchowny M, et al. Preoperative clinical, EEG, and imaging findings do not predict seizure outcome following temporal lobectomy in childhood. *J Child Neurol* 1996; 11:445–450.

CHAPTER 48

Surgical Treatment: Surgery and Outcome

Jeffrey G. Ojemann, M.D., and T.S. Park, M.D.

Surgical treatment of epilepsy is an effective therapy for medically intractable seizures. Extending this therapy to the pediatric population has only recently become widely accepted, although authors have argued for earlier intervention for some time. Because the etiology of pediatric epilepsy is often different from the cause of epilepsy in the adult population, the surgical interventions that are considered also differ. For example, mesial temporal sclerosis is less common than in adults, often not seen until later adolescence. However, focal lesions do exist and are amenable to treatment. Seizures secondary to neoplasm, developmental lesions, and hamartomatous lesions can also be treated surgically. Other seizure disorders discussed are the diffuse syndromes that may involve entire hemispheres or may not be localized at all. Even children with such syndromes may benefit from certain surgical interventions.

Other considerations are involved in surgery in children. Surgical resections often encroach on critical areas of cortex, such as motor or language areas, which must be identified before resection. In the cooperative adult, language cortex can be identified by direct stimulation during an awake surgery. This requires a great deal of cooperation and is more difficult in older children and impossible in younger children. Other issues involved in the preservation of function include the often more extensive resections required in certain pediatric surgeries, especially in the younger children and infants, and the increased plasticity of function relative to adults that this same group may show if certain cortical regions are removed. Finally, although outcome data exist for all the major surgeries performed on children, the most definitive data for outcome in most operations come from adult or mixed populations.

The most common surgeries performed in children are those for invasive monitoring for diagnostic purposes, temporal lobectomy, extratemporal resection (including multilobar resection), hemispherectomy, and corpus callosotomy. Both surgical technique and outcome are specific to the clinical situation. Different epilepsy syndromes call for different surgeries with special consideration for the localization of a specific seizure focus and preservation of function.

INVASIVE MONITORING

Often in the evaluation of epileptic syndromes, surgical placement of invasive electrical monitoring is considered before any surgical treatment. After initial evaluation with interictal electroencephalogram (EEG), video-EEG, magnetic resonance imaging (MRI) and other imaging modalities such as single photon emission computed tomography (SPECT) and/or positron emission tomography (PET), further localization of seizure onset may require the use of invasive electrodes, such as depth electrodes, grid electrodes, or strip electrodes (1–6). In some cases, a lesion is identified and seizure foci are nearby, but it is unclear how the seizure focus relates to the lesion. Invasive monitoring can define this relationship. In other cases, no definitive focus can be found and invasive monitoring may help lateralizing, for example, in the setting of temporal lobe epilepsy with typical clinical symptoms but evidence for bilateral onset from noninvasive monitoring. Finally, invasive monitoring may be necessary when a lesion is identified, but the presence of dual pathology in both the lesion and the medial temporal structures is suspected. In this latter case, invasive monitoring of both the lesion and mesial temporal structures may be desirable.

There are several techniques for invasive monitoring, all of which rely on placement of electrodes as close as possible to the surface of the regions of interest. Grid electrodes (GEs) (Figure 48-1) can cover a large area of

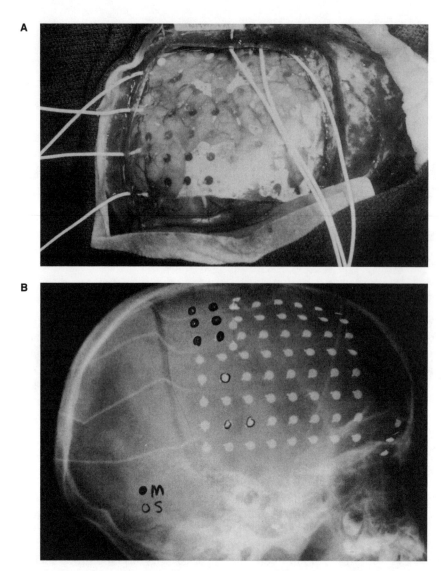

Figure 48-1. A. Intraoperative photograph of grid electrode placement. Electrode leads exit to the (right) are tunneled through the scalp to allow recording of the leads. The underlying (frontal) lobe is visible through the transparent silastic grid. **B.** Postoperative skull radiograph of grid electrode placement. Darkened and circled leads indicate location of motor and sensory function, respectively, as determined by extraoperative mapping.

cortex. Placement of GEs can be particularly helpful when seizures must be localized within a particular lobe (6,7). GEs can provide detailed information about seizure focus in relation to a structural lesion. Alternatively, if noninvasive testing suggests involvement of a particular hemisphere or lobe, GEs can cover these extensive areas to help in defining more focal areas.

Grid electrodes are also useful for functional mapping (2,7–9). Cortex can be stimulated through the same electrodes used for monitoring. This allows for mapping of motor, sensory, and even language function outside the operating room (10,11). This is particularly important for children in whom language mapping would be difficult using traditional methods such as awake craniotomy. Motor mapping by applying current to the cortical surface may not work in children younger than 5 years old (2,12). In these

cases, monitoring of somatosensory evoked potentials may be more helpful in localizing the central sulcus. Similar information can be gained using epidural electrodes (2,12). This technique uses the same GEs but involves placing the grid in the epidural space rather than subdurally.

Strip electrodes are also used (4,5,10,11,13,14), especially in monitoring areas other than the lateral cortical surface. Similar to GEs, monitoring leads are spaced in a single row within a flexible strip that can be passed safely along the brain. When passed along the undersurface of the temporal lobe, the distal electrode sits just over the parahippocampal gyrus, providing good monitoring of mesial temporal lobe structures (6). These strips also can be passed interhemispherically to monitor mesial frontal lobe regions or inferiorly to monitor orbitofrontal cortex.

Similar information may be obtained with depth electrodes. Several centers (15,16) use this method, which involves placement of a narrow probe directly into the region of interest. Depth electrodes are helpful in lateralizing seizure foci, and direct hippocampal recording is possible (10), although the region that can be recorded is limited. These various electrodes can be used in combination (17).

The safety and effectiveness of these techniques has been described several times, and they have received wide acceptance (5,14,18,19). The most common complications are cerebrospinal fluid (CSF) leakage, low-grade fever, and, less commonly, infection. Complication rates have been reviewed and appear to be 1 percent for strip electrodes and 4 percent for GEs. Historically, strip electrodes have had lower complication rates than depth electrodes (4,6,10). Prophylactic antibiotics are given when placing the electrodes, although the necessity for prolonged antibiotic administration has been questioned (20). CSF leakage and infection is minimized by careful closure of the dura, tunneling of the leads through the scalp, and pursestring closure of the sites where the grid leads exit the scalp (21). Rarely, grids can be associated with mass effect and local irritation that may respond to steroids. Exceptionally, grids may need to be removed if patients show signs of elevated intracranial pressure. Although low-grade fever is common when the grids are in place, suspicion should remain high for the development of meningitis, especially after prolonged grid placement. In our experience, the grids are typically left in place 7 days or less; however, the risk of infection from prolonged invasive monitoring is balanced with the ability to observe enough ictal events to adequately determine seizure foci and obtain functional mapping.

TEMPORAL LOBECTOMY

Temporal lobectomy covers a broad category of surgeries including resections for mesial temporal lobe pathology (e.g., mesial temporal sclerosis), lesions within the medial or lateral temporal lobe, or resections of lateral, neocortical temporal lobe (22). Pediatric series differ as the spectrum of pathology is different in children. Structural lesions may be present in as many as half of the temporal lobectomies performed for intractable seizures (18,23).

For mesial temporal lobe pathology, a variety of surgical techniques have been used in adults and children, focusing on resecting mesial temporal structures, including hippocampus, parahippocampus, and amygdala, with variable resection of temporal lobe neocortex (24). These are the most common surgeries in adults, and surgical resection for mesial temporal sclerosis is similar in children and in adults. Falconer (25) first advocated extending the operation to children, and

earlier surgical intervention may reduce the behavioral, cognitive, and social sequelae of continued seizures through late adolescence and early adulthood (22).

The anatomic relationship between the hippocampus and the rest of the temporal lobe (Figure 48-2, A) allows for various surgical approaches. A standardized anterior temporal lobectomy involves resection of the lateral aspect of the anterior temporal lobe, entering the temporal horn deep to the temporal gyri (22,24,26). The ventricle forms the roof of the hippocampus, which is visible once the ventricle is entered. The hippocampus is then resected posteriorly, at least 1.5 to 3.5 cm posterior from the pes, or anterior portion, of the hippocampus (27).

Several variants on the standard anterior temporal lobectomy have been developed. In particular, a tailored resection has been advocated by several groups, tailoring the resection for both epileptic foci and language function (24). Language mapping can be performed when surgery is done under local anesthesia (28). Short-acting agents are used to sedate the patient during the exposure of the dura; the patient is then allowed to awaken (24). Sites critical to language function are determined by stimulating the cortex while the patient performs an object-naming task. These areas are then avoided in planning the temporal lobe resection. Electrocorticography can also be used to tailor the resection. Placement of electrodes on the temporal lobe surface can identify lateral cortex with interictal spike activity, although the significance of this activity remains controversial (24,29). Additionally, electrical recordings directly from the hippocampus can be used to guide the extent of hippocampal resection.

Selective amygdalohippocampectomies can be achieved through small cortical resections that enter the ventricle directly, without extensive lateral resections (30,31). The hippocampus and amygdala can then be resected through this exposure. Alternatively, mesial temporal structures can be reached using a subtemporal approach (30). The temporal lobe is gently retracted superiorly, and the mesial and inferior region of the temporal lobe are reached directly (Figure 48-2, B). Another approach to the mesial temporal lobe is superiorly through the sylvian fissure (31). Although this approach requires working around the middle cerebral artery and its branches, the mesial temporal lobe structures can be reached without resecting lateral temporal lobe structures. Finally, seizure control can be achieved with hippocampal resection that spares the amygdala (32).

The outcomes from anterior temporal lobectomy and amygdalohippocampectomy are well documented for the general surgical population (Table 48-1). Similar outcomes have been reported in pediatric series of temporal lobectomy (33–36). The outcome from temporal lobectomy cannot be immediately determined in

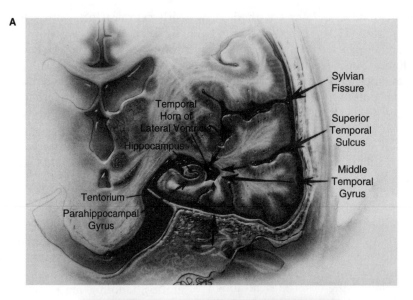

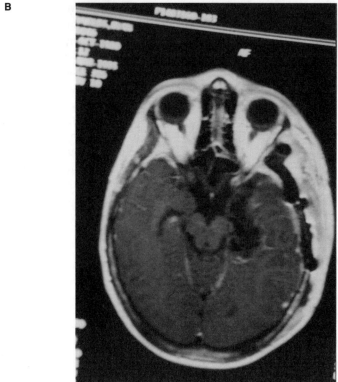

Figure 48-2. A. Coronal cross section demonstrating the relationship of lateral and mesial temporal lobe structures. **B.** Postoperative MRI demonstrating localized resection of mesial temporal lobe structures following selective amygdalohippocampectomy.

a given patient. As with all seizure surgery, outcome should be measured at least 1 year postoperatively as seizure control changes over time (37), even over several years. Additionally, seizures in the immediate postoperative period do not predict long-term seizure control (38), although a recurrence of seizures within the first postoperative year carries a worse prognosis (37,39).

Certain neuropsychological complications can arise following temporal lobe resections. Some degree of superior quadranatanopsia is very common in temporal lobe resection as Meyer's loop fibers pass from the lateral geniculate body to the occipital lobe via the temporal lobe white matter (40–42). Anterior temporal lobectomies open the ventricle wall, probably damaging visual fibers at that point. Such deficits, however, are rarely noticed by patients or identifiable on bedside exam (43). In dominant temporal lobe resections, transient anomias may result from postoperative swelling, especially if resections are close

Table 48-1. Temporal Lobectomy

Indications	Medial temporal focus
	Temporal lobe lesion
	Neocortical temporal lobe focus
Procedures	Anterior temporal lobectomy
	Selective amygdalohippocampectomy
Outcome (37)	Anterior temporal lobectomy: 68% seizure-free, 24% improved, 8% not improved
	Amygdalohippocampectomy: 69% seizure-free, 22% improved, 9% not improved

Table 48-2. Extratemporal Resection

Indications	Lesion
	Cortical focus
Procedures	Lobectomy
	Topectomy
	Resection of lesion
Outcome (37)	45% seizure-free, 35% improved, 20% not improved
	Outcome for lesion resections are better, with 67% or more seizure-free for resections of lesions and seizure foci (57).

to language areas (43–46). Many series have reported a small incidence of significant verbal performance loss after dominant temporal lobectomy (41,47,48), although this usually resolves (45). Additionally, injury to vascular structures can lead to hemiparesis; manipulation of vessels may be the cause of the transient hemiparesis that has been reported historically in 2 percent to 5 percent of cases (41,45).

The mortality of anterior temporal lobectomy is less than 1 percent (41). As with any cranial surgery, infection, CSF leak and hemorrhage are known risks. In addition to damage to visual and language function previously discussed, the medial aspect of the temporal lobe resection puts other structures at risk, including cranial nerve III and the cerebral peduncle, which lies immediately medial to the temporal lobe. The incidence of damage to these structures appears to be quite low (41). The risk of infection also is low, probably less than 0.5 percent for major infection (45).

Similar surgical approaches can be used when seizure foci are identified in lateral temporal cortex (33,49). Often mesial temporal structures are also involved and can be removed along with lateral temporal cortex foci. Lesions, such as neoplasms, located in the temporal lobe commonly cause seizure activity. When seizure foci are identified separate from a lesion, resection of the lesion only can give good results, with the best outcome achieved by resection of both lesion and foci (50–52). Resection of only the foci gives the worst outcome. These principles must be balanced with the desire to avoid significant neurologic morbidity. Carrying lateral temporal lobe resections too far posteriorly can lead to significant postoperative aphasia. Mapping of language function, either intraoperatively with cortical stimulation or extraoperatively with GEs, may permit more extensive resections of regions found not to be critical for language function.

EXTRATEMPORAL RESECTIONS

Seizure foci can arise in any portion of cortex. Extratemporal foci are more common in children than in adults,

with frontal lobe being the most common extratemporal location for seizure foci, followed by parietooccipital regions (53). Within the frontal lobe, foci are restricted to orbitofrontal, dorsolateral frontal, and medial frontal supplementary motor area (SMA) regions. Multilobar resections may also be performed if foci are found in multiple regions. Even some cases of seizure disorders in infants may benefit from focal resections (54).

Identification of lesions by MRI and epileptic foci by EEG or invasive monitoring can guide surgical resection (18). These lesions, such as neoplasms, are often sources of seizure foci. Resection of the lesion and adjacent epileptic foci has been advocated (55,56) by means of intraoperative corticography (55,57). The problem of "dual pathology" must be considered, in which patients have seizures originating from both a lesion and temporal lobe structures (58,59). In these cases, seizure control results from either lesionectomy or temporal lobectomy but is maximized when both procedures are performed (57).

Once the seizure focus has been identified, surgery to excise the focus must also limit functional impairment (60). Identification of motor cortex is particularly important in frontal and parietal resections. Generally, in focal resections, motor and language cortex is avoided because the morbidity of paralysis or aphasia may exceed any benefit in seizure control. As with temporal lobe resections, functional mapping can be performed intraoperatively or extraoperatively, the latter often being more appropriate for language mapping in the younger child.

Surgical technique can minimize damage to nonepileptogenic regions. The pial surface is coagulated and divided in a small, relatively avascular region. The resection of a gyrus is then carried out in a subpial fashion. This allows vessels within the pia that might supply other nonresected tissue to remain undamaged. By following the cortex along the crown and depths of a gyrus with a resection — a so-called "topectomy" — excessive disruption of white matter fibers can be avoided (Figure 48-3).

The technique of multiple subpial transection may be used when an epileptic focus is within an area of critical function, (61,62). This method involves making

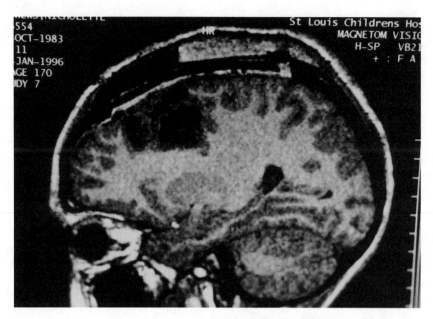

Figure 48-3. Postoperative MRI of a frontal topectomy. The resection is carried out along the cortex but spares underlying white matter.

small cuts in the cortex perpendicular to the long axis of the gyrus. This is thought to disrupt seizure spread without disrupting the propagation of information. Especially when lesionectomy or resection of most of a seizure focus can be performed, multiple subpial transection appears to be a useful adjuvant to deal with residual seizure foci that lie within critical areas of cortex (62). This procedure has yet to gain wide acceptance.

In some cases localization implicates multiple regions and a multilobar resection is appropriate. Particular syndromes, such as hemimegalencephaly (63), Sturge-Weber syndrome, and chronic (Rasmussen's) encephalitis (64), often involve multiple cortical regions. Topectomies or lobectomies can be performed in multiple lobes, although the risk of neurologic deficit naturally increases the greater the resection. When the cortical resection is extensive enough, the patient may be best served by a form of hemispherectomy, which is discussed in the next section.

In addition to the potential complications inherent in any cortical resection, such as infection or hemorrhage, resection in a given cortical region carries its own specific risks of neurologic injury. Frontal lobe resections can lead to motor and language deficits. Especially transiently, frontal lobe syndromes including apathy and abulia can occur following unilateral frontal resections. Medial frontal lobe resections can cause so-called SMA-syndromes, which, on the dominant side, may include mutism and motor apraxia (65). These syndromes typically are transient. Parietal resections may lead to neglect syndromes or sensory deficits, and visual deficits are predictable after occipital lobe resections. As a general rule, children appear to recover better functionally following cortical resection (66). Some benefit to neurologic function can often be

demonstrated from resection (66,67), presumably secondary to decreasing the adverse effect of seizures on function.

HEMISPHERECTOMY

In some cases seizures can be localized only to a particular hemisphere. This may be true in several conditions (Table 48-3), including Sturge-Weber syndrome (in which vascular malformations involve entire hemispheric surfaces) (68), encephalitis (64), infantile spasm (69), and infantile hemiplegia (70). The latter may include cortical dysplasias, hemimegalencephaly (63), and ischemic injury (68). When seizures originate diffusely but within one hemisphere, seizure control can often be obtained either by disconnection or by resection of the entire hemisphere. A combination of resection and disconnection typically is performed in a hemispherectomy. The ideal candidate for a hemispherectomy also would have significant loss of function from that hemisphere. In particular, the hemiplegic patient may suffer little additional morbidity from hemispherectomy. In the setting of

Table 48-3. Hemispherectomy

Indications	Pathology localized to one hemisphere
	Chronic (Rasmussen's) encephalitis
	Infantile hemiplegia
	Sturge-Weber syndrome
Procedures	Anatomic hemispherectomy (not used)
	Functional hemispherectomy
	Hemispherotomy
Outcome (37)	67% seizure-free, 21% improved, 12% not improved

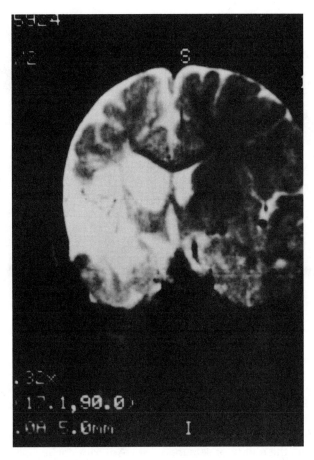

Figure 48-4. Postoperative MRI of hemispherotomy. The cortical structures have been spared, but underlying connections have been disconnected.

long-standing seizures, hemisphere removal may even lead to improved cognition (71).

Early uses of hemispherectomy for intractable seizures involved the so-called anatomic hemispherectomy (69). This surgery involved resection of the frontal, parietal, and occipital cortices along with a complete temporal lobectomy and insular resection. The subcortical structures of the basal ganglia and thalamus were spared. This method led to the severe, delayed complication of superficial siderosis and other hemorrhagic complications (45), presumably as a result of microtrauma sustained by the residual brain within a larger cranial vault. The procedure was modified, as a functional hemispherectomy, such that the anterior frontal and posterior occipital lobes were left intact while a central resection and temporal lobectomy were performed. The remaining cortex was completely disconnected by resecting the corpus callosum. Thus the frontal and occipital lobes were structurally present but functionally disconnected from the remainder of the brain (72). The incidence of delayed complications dropped with this method (73,74).

Delayed development of postoperative hydrocephalus may occur with hemispherectomy. The surgery itself can lead to extensive blood loss, which is poorly tolerated by small children (41). Hemispherectomy is effective in seizure control, with two-thirds of patients seizure-free (37).

Recent modifications of the hemispherectomy require less extensive resection. Several variations, termed a *hemispherotomy* (74) or a *hemispheric deafferentation* (75), involve a temporal lobectomy followed by a functional disconnection of the remainder of the cortex. Insular resection may be carried out directly. By entering the ventricular system, following temporal lobectomy, white matter projections from frontal, parietal, and occipital lobes can be disconnected (74,75). This provides for functional isolation of the entire cortex, accomplishing the goal of the hemispherectomy. This technique is particularly suited for children with enlarged ventricular systems (74) or enlarged perisylvian space, such as a child with porencephaly secondary to ischemia. The enlarged access to the ventricular system allows cortical disconnection with minimal trauma in a child with little residual function in that hemisphere (Figure 48-4).

CORPUS CALLOSOTOMY

Unlike the surgeries discussed so far, corpus callosotomy is primarily a palliative procedure. Candidates

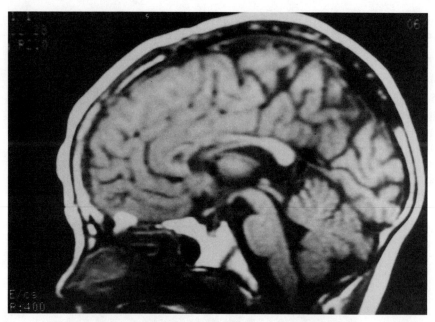

Figure 48-5. Postoperative MRI following resection of the anterior two-thirds of the corpus callosum. The remaining corpus callosum was later resected because adequate seizure reduction was not maintained after an initial 6 months of reduced seizure frequency.

for callosotomy are patients with drop attacks or other generalized seizures (72,76–79). Atonic seizures ("drop attacks") seem to be especially amenable to reduction with this surgery (76,80,81). By partially or completely disrupting the corpus callosum, the ability of seizures to spread bilaterally is diminished. This can lead to a reduction in the frequency of generalized seizures. Although it may have little or no effect on partial seizures, it can reduce the incidence of secondary generalization (Table 48-4).

Typically, when a child is determined to be a candidate for corpus callosotomy, the procedure performed is resection of the anterior two-thirds of the corpus callosum (Figure 48-5). In many cases limiting the resection provides significant seizure reduction and may avoid some of the cognitive complications that may arise from complete corpus callosotomy. The resection is performed by approaching the corpus callosum superiorly, usually along the medial border of the right hemisphere. The brain is gently retracted laterally, with care to avoid excessive disruption of bridging veins draining into the superior sagittal sinus.

Table 48-4. Corpus Callosotomy

Indications	Diffuse or bilateral seizure foci Primary or secondarily generalized seizures Astatic seizures ("drop attacks")
Procedures	Anterior two-thirds of corpus callosum Total resection of corpus callosum
Outcome (37)	8% seizure-free, 61% improved, 31% not improved

The corpus callosum is then visible, often with the pericollosal arteries lying over the white fibers. Resection in the midline is then carried out and extended well anterior to the splenium.

Anterior corpus callosotomy is less likely to lead to significant cognitive difficulties—the so-called split-brain phenomenon—than larger resections (76,78). More extensive corpus callosum resections can disrupt the cross-hemispheric communication of visual information and may lead to more noticeable neuropsychological sequelae (82). All divisions likely cause some deficit (81), and acute transient problems are common, especially in total resections (45). Nevertheless, when anterior corpus callosotomy fails to provide significant seizure reduction, some patients may benefit from a second procedure that resects the remaining posterior one-third of the corpus callosum. Some authors have advocated extending the resection posteriorly but sparing the splenium itself (82).

The goal of these procedures is seizure reduction, not cure. Accordingly, reduction in seizures to a certain percentage is used as a measure of success. Overall outcome has been reported as 8 percent seizure-free, 61 percent improved, and 31 percent not improved (37). In children who undergo corpus callosotomy, quality-of-life measures improved with seizure reduction, even in the absence of seizure-free status (83).

CONCLUSIONS

The goal of all epilepsy surgery is to improve the quality of life of the children who suffer from seizure disorders and their families. Several studies have demonstrated that measures of quality of life improve after seizure reduction, with seizure cure being the most important factor (35,84,85). In addition to selecting operations that maximize seizure reduction, the benefit of earlier intervention should be emphasized. Many of the quality-of-life measures demonstrate that reduction of seizures later in life, after various social, economic, and intellectual development has already occurred, suggest less benefit in some aspects of the patient's life, such as employment (85). Earlier surgical intervention for intractable seizures may help intellectual and behavioral development (66,86–88) and may prove critical in providing quality-of-life benefits from seizure reduction.

REFERENCES

1. Engel J Jr, Henry TR, Risinger MW, et al. Presurgical evaluation for partial epilepsy: relative contributions of chronic depth-electrode recordings versus FDG-PET and scalp-sphenoidal ictal EEG. *Neurology* 1990; 40:1670–1677.

2. Goldring S, Gregorie EM. Surgical management of epilepsy using epidural recordings to localize the seizure focus: review of 100 cases. *J Neurosurg* 1984; 40:447–466.

3. Jayakar P, Duchowny M, Resnick TJ. Subdural monitoring in the evaluation of children for epilepsy. *J Child Neurol* 1994; 9(Suppl 2):61–66.

4. Spencer SS. Depth versus subdural electrode studies for unlocalized epilepsy. *J Epilepsy* 1989; 2:123–127.

5. Wyler AR, Ojemann GA, Lettich E, Ward AA Jr. Subdural strip electrodes for localizing seizure foci in children. *J Neurosurg* 1984; 60:1195–1200.

6. Wyler AR, Wilkus RJ, Blume WT. Strip electrodes. In: Engel J Jr, ed. *Surgical Treatment of the Epilepsies*. 2nd ed. New York: Raven Press, 1993.

7. Sutherling WW, Risinger MW, Crandall PH, et al. Focal functional anatomy of dorsolateral frontocentral seizures. *Neurology* 1990; 40:87–98.

8. Lesser RP, Lüders H, Klem G, et al. Extraoperative cortical functional localization in patients with epilepsy. *J Clin Neurophysiol* 1987; 4:27–53.

9. Ojemann GA, Sutherling WW, Lesser RP, et al. Cortical stimulation. In: Engel J Jr, ed. *Surgical treatment of the epilepsies*. 2nd ed. New York: Raven Press, 1993.

10. Adelson PD, O'Rourke DK, Albright AL. Chronic invasive monitoring for identifying seizure foci in children. *Neurosurg Clin North Am* 1995; 6:491–504.

11. Morrison G, Duchowny M, Resnick T, et al. Epilepsy surgery in children. A report of 79 patients. *Pediatr Neurosurg* 1992; 18:291–297.

12. Goldring S. A method for surgical management of focal epilepsy, especially as it relates to children. *J Neurosurg* 1978; 49:344–356.

13. Rosenbaum TJ, Laxer KD, Vessely M, Sarth WB. Subdural electrodes for seizure focus localization. *Neurosurgery* 1986; 19:73–81.

14. Wyler AR, Walker G, Richey ET, Hermann BP. Chronic subdural strip electrode recordings for difficult epileptic problems. *J Epilepsy* 1988; 1:71–78.

15. Olivier A, Gloor P, Andermann F, Quesney LF. The place of stereotactic depth electrode recording in epilepsy. *Appl Neurophysiol* 1985; 48:395–399.

16. Smith JR, Flanigan HF, King DW, et al. Analysis of a four-year experience with depth electrodes and a two-year experience with subdural electrodes in the evaluation of ablative seizure surgery candidates. *Appl Neurophysiol* 1987; 50:380–385.

17. Spencer SS, Spencer DD, Williamson PD, Mattson R. Combined depth and subdural electrode investigation in uncontrolled epilepsy. *Neurology* 1990; 40:74–79.

18. Shields WD, Peacock WJ, Roper SN. Surgery for epilepsy: special pediatric considerations. *Neurosurg Clin North Am* 1993; 4:301–310.

19. Swartz BE, Rich JR, Dwan PS, et al. The safety and efficacy of chronically implanted subdural electrodes: a prospective study. *Surg Neurol* 1996; 46:87–93.

20. Wyler AR, Walker G, Somes G. The morbidity of long-term seizure monitoring using subdural strip electrodes. *J Neurosurg* 1991; 74:734–737.

21. Arroyo S, Lesser RP, Awad IA, et al. Subdural and epidural grids and strips. In: Engel J Jr, ed. *Surgical Treatment of the Epilepsies*. 2nd ed. New York: Raven Press, 1993

22. Adelson PD, Black PMcL. Temporal lobe resections in children. *Neurosurg Clin North Am* 1995; 6:521–532.

23. Kotagal P, Lüders HO. Recent advances in childhood epilepsy. *Brain Dev* 1994; 16:1–15.

24. Silbergeld DL, Ojemann GA. The tailored temporal lobectomy. *Neurosurg Clin North Am* 1993; 4(2): 273–281.

25. Falconer MA. Significance of surgery for temporal lobe epilepsy in childhood and adolescence. *J Neurosurg* 1970; 33:233–252.

26. Spencer DD, Spencer SS, Mattson RH, Williamson PD, Novelly RA. Access to the posterior medial temporal lobe structures in the surgical treatment of temporal lobe epilepsy. *Neurosurgery* 1984; 15:667–671.

27. Spencer DD, Ojemann GA. Overview of therapeutic procedures. In: Engel J Jr, ed. *Surgical Treatment of the Epilepsies*. 2nd ed. New York: Raven Press, 1993

28. Ojemann GA, Ojemann JG, Lettich E, Berger M. Cortical language localization in left, dominant hemisphere. An electrical stimulation mapping investigation in 117 patients. *J Neurosurg* 1989; 71:316–326.

29. Schwartz TH, Bazil CW, Walczak TS, et al. The predictive value of intraoperative electrocorticography in resections for limbic epilepsy associated with mesial temporal sclerosis. *Neurosurgery* 1997; 40:302.

30. Park TS, Bourgeois BF, Silbergeld DL, Dodson WE. Subtemporal transparahippocampal amygdalohippocampectomy for surgical treatment of mesial temporal lobe epilepsy. *J Neurosurg* 1996; 85:1172–1176.

31. Wieser HG, Yasargil MG. Selective amygdalahippocampectomy as a surgical treatment of mediobasal limbic epilepsy. *Surg Neurol* 1982; 17:445–457.

32. Goldring S, Edwards I, Harding GW, et al. Results of anterior temporal lobectomy that spares the amygdala with complex partial seizures. *J Neurosurg* 1992; 77:185–193.

33. Duchowny M, Levin B, Jayakar P, Resnick TJ. Neurobiologic considerations in early surgery for epilepsy. *J Child Neurol* 1994; 9(Suppl 2):42–49.

34. Guldvog B, Loyning Y, Hauglie-Hanssen E, Flood S. Bjornaes H. Surgical treatment for partial epilepsy among Norwegian children and adolescents. *Epilepsia* 1994; 35: 554–565.

35. Keene DL, Higgins MS, Ventuneyra ECG. Outcome and life prospects after surgical management of medically intractable epilepsy in patients under 18 years of age. *Childs Nerv Sys* 1997; 13:530–535.

36. Meyer FB, Marsh WR, Laws ER Jr, Sharbrough FW. Temporal lobectomy in children with epilepsy. *J Neurosurg* 1993; 64:371–376.

37. Engel J Jr, Van Ness PC, Rasmussen TB, and Ojemann LM. Outcome with respect to epileptic seizures. In: Engel J Jr, ed. *Surgical Treatment of the Epilepsies.* 2nd ed. New York: Raven Press, 1993.

38. Ojemann GA, Bourgeois BF. Early postoperative management. In: Engel J Jr, ed. *Surgical Treatment of the Epilepsies.* 2nd ed. New York: Raven Press, 1993.

39. Armon C, Radtke RA, Friedman AH, Dawson DV. Predictors of outcome of epilepsy surgery: Multivariate analysis with validation. *Epilepsia* 1996; 37:814–821.

40. Marino R, Rasmussen T. Visual field changes after temporal lobectomy in man. *Neurology* 1968; 18:825–835.

41. Pilcher WH, Roberts DW, Flanigin HF, et al. Complications of epilepsy surgery. In: Engel J Jr, ed. *Surgical Treatment of the Epilepsies.* 2nd ed. New York: Raven Press, 1993.

42. Van Buren JM, Baldwin M. The architecture of the optic radiation in the temporal lobe of man. *Brain* 1958; 81:15–40.

43. Wyllie, Lüders H, Morris H, et al. Clinical outcome after complete or partial cortical resections for intractable epilepsy. *Neurology* 1987; 37:1634–1641.

44. Haglund MM, Berger MS, Shamselden M, Lettich E, Ojemann GA. Cortical localization of temporal lobe language sites in patients with gliomas. *Neurosurgery* 1994; 34:567–576.

45. Pilcher WH and Rusyniak WG. Complications of epilepsy surgery. *Neurosurg Clin North Am* 1993; 4:311–325.

46. Stafiniak P, Saykin AJ, Sperling MR, et al. Acute naming deficits following dominant temporal lobectomy: prediction by age at first risk for seizures. *Neurology* 1990; 40:1509–1512.

47. Crandall PH. Postoperative management and criteria for evaluation. In: Purpura DP, Penry JK, Walter RD, eds. *Neurosurgical Management of the Epilepsies.* New York: Raven Press, 1975:265–279 (Advances in Neurology, vol. 8).

48. Hermann BP, Wyler AR, Sones G, Clement L. Dysnomia after left anterior temporal lobectomy without functional mapping: frequency and correlates. *Neurosurgery* 1994; 35:52–56.

49. Adelson PD, Peacock WJ, Chugani HT, et al. Temporal and extended temporal resections for the treatment of intractable seizures in early childhood. *Pediatr Neurosurg* 1992; 18:169–178.

50. Clarke DB, Olivier A, Anderman F, Fish D. Surgical treatment of epilepsy: the problem of lesion/focus incongruence. *Surg Neurol* 1996; 46:579–585.

51. Montes JL, Rosenblatt B, Farmer JP, et al. Lesionectomy of MRI detected lesions in children with epilepsy. *Pediatr Neurosurg* 1995; 22:167–173.

52. Vossler DG, Wilkus RJ, Ojemann GA. Preoperative EEG correlates of seizure outcome from epilepsy surgery in children. *J Epilepsy* 1995; 8:236–245.

53. Prats AR, Morrison G, Wolf AL. Focal cortical resections for the treatment of extratemporal epilepsy in children. *Neurosurg Clin North Am* 1995; 6:533–540.

54. Duchowny MS, Resnick TJ, Alvarez LA, Morrison G. Focal resection for malignant partial seizures in infancy. *Neurology* 1990; 40:980–984.

55. Berger MS, Ghatan S, Haglund MM, Dobbins J, Ojemann GA. Low-grade gliomas associated with intractable epilepsy: seizure outcome utilizing electrocorticography during tumor resection. *J Neurosurg* 1993; 79:62–69.

56. Zentner J, Hufnagel A, Wolf HK, et al. Surgical treatment of neoplasms associated with medically intractable epilepsy. *Neurosurgery* 1997; 41:378–386.

57. Weber JP, Silbergeld DL, and Winn HR. Surgical resection of epileptogenic cortex associated with structural lesions. *Neurosurg Clin North Am* 1993; 4:327–336.

58. Levesque MF, Nakasato N, Vinters HV, Babb TL. Surgical treatment of limbic epilepsy associated with extrahippocampal lesions: the problem of dual pathology. *J Neurosurg* 1991; 75:364–370.

59. Li LM, Cendes F, Watson C, et al. Surgical treatment of patients with single and dual pathology: relevance of lesion and of hippocampal atrophy to seizure outcome. *Neurology* 1997; 48: 437–444.

60. Rasmussen T. Tailoring of cortical excisions for frontal lobe epilepsy. *Can J Neurol Sci* 1991; 18(Suppl 4):606–610.

61. Morrell F, Whisler WW, Bleck TP. Multiple subpial transection: a new approach to the surgical treatment of focal epilepsy. *J Neurosurg* 1989; 70:231–239.

62. Wyler AR, Wilkus RJ, Rostad SW, Vossler DG. Multiple subpial transections for partial seizures in sensorimotor cortex. *Neurosurgery* 1995; 37:1122–1127.

63. Vigevano F, Bertin E, Boldrini R, et al. Hemimegalencephaly and intractable epilepsy: benefits of hemispherectomy. *Epilepsia* 1989; 30:833–843.

64. Rasmussen T, Olszewski J, Lloyd-Smith D. Focal seizures due to chronic localized encephalitis. *Neurology* 1958; 8:435–455.

65. Rostomily RC, Berger MS, Ojemann GA, et al. Postoperative deficits and functional recovery following removal of

tumors involving the dominant hemisphere. *J Neurosurg* 1991; 75:62–68.

66. Duchowny M, Levin B, Jayakar P, Resnick TJ. Neurobiologic considerations in early surgery for epilepsy. *J Child Neurol* 1994; 9(Suppl 2):42–49.

67. Beckung E, Uvebrant P, Hedstrom A, Rydenhag B. The effects of epilepsy surgery on the sensorimotor function of children. *Dev Med Child Neurol* 1994; 36:893–901.

68. Peacock WJ. Hemispherectomy for the treatment of intractable seizures in childhood. *Neurosurg Clin North Am* 1995; 6:549–563.

69. Krynaw RW. Infantile hemiplegia treated by removing one cerebral hemisphere. *J Neurol Neurosurg Psychiatry* 1950; 13:243–267.

70. Wilson PJE Cerebral hemispherectomy for infantile hemiplegia. *Brain* 1970; 93: 147–180.

71. Caplan R, Guthrie D, Shields WD, et al. Early onset intractable seizures: nonverbal communication after hemispherectomy. *J Dev Behav Pediatr* 1992; 13:348–355.

72. Rasmussen T. Hemispherectomy for seizures revisited. *Can J Neurosci* 1983; 10:71–78.

73. Davies KG, Maxwell RE, French LA. Hemispherectomy for intractable seizures: long-term results in 17 patients followed for up to 38 years. *J Neurosurg* 1993; 78:733–740.

74. Villemure J-G, Mascott CR. Peri-insular hemispherotomy: surgical principles and anatomy. *Neurosurgery* 1995; 37:975–981.

75. Schramm J, Behrens E, Entzien W. Hemispheric deafferentation: an alternative to functional hemispherectomy. *Neurosurgery* 1995; 36:509–515.

76. Carmant L, Holmes GL. Commissurotomies in children *J Child Neurol* 1994; 9(Suppl 2):50–60.

77. Madsen JR, Carmant L, Holmes GL, Black PMcL. Corpus callosotomy in children. *Neurosurg Clin North Am* 1995; 6(3):541–548.

78. Makai GS, Holmes GL, Murro AM, et al. Corpus callosotomy for the treatment of intractable epilepsy in children. *J Epilepsy* 1989; 2:1–7.

79. Sawhney IMS, Robertson IJA, Polkay CE, Binnie CD, Elwes RDC. Multiple subpial transection: a review of 21 cases. *J Neurol Neurosurg Psychiatry* 1995; 58:344–349.

80. Rossi GF, Colicchio G, Marchese E, Pompucci A. Callosotomy for severe epilepsies with generalized seizures: outcome and prognostic factors. *Acta Neurochirurgica* 1996; 138:221–227.

81. Roberts DW. The role of callosal section in surgical treatment of epilepsies. *Neurosurg Clin North Am* 1993; 4:293–300, 1993.

82. Cendes F, Ragazzo PC, da Costa V, Martins LF. Corpus callosotomy in treatment of medically resistant epilepsy: preliminary results in a pediatric population. *Epilepsia* 1993; 34:910–917.

83. Yang TF, Wong TT, Kwan S, et al. Quality of life and life satisfaction in families after a child has undergone corpus callosotomy. *Epilepsia* 1996; 37:76–80.

84. Mihara T, Inoue Y, Matsuda K, et al. Recommendation of early surgery from the viewpoint of daily quality of life. *Epilepsia* 1996; 37(Suppl 3): 33–36.

85. Vickrey BG, Hays RD, Hermann BP, Bladin PF, Batzel LW. Outcomes with respect to quality of life. In: Engel J Jr, ed. *Surgical Treatment of the Epilepsies.* 2nd ed. New York: Raven Press, 1993.

86. Davidson S, Falconer MA. Outcome of surgery in 40 children with temporal-lobe epilepsy. *Lancet* 1975; 1:1260–1263.

87. Rausch R, Babb TL, Engel JE. Memory following intracarotid amobarbital injection contralateral to hippocampal damage. *Arch Neurol* 1989; 46:783–788.

88. Resnick TJ, Duchowny M, Jayakar P. Early surgery for epilepsy: redefining candidacy. *J Child Neurol* 1994; 9(Suppl 2):36–41.

CHAPTER 49

Quality of Life in Children with Epilepsy

Joan K. Austin, D.N.S., R.N., and Nancy Santilli, R.N., P.N.P., M.N.

Recent changes in health care have led to an increased emphasis on documenting outcomes of care. In childhood epilepsy, the goal of care has traditionally been optimal seizure control. Recently, however, with the increased recognition of the importance of quality-of-life outcomes in the treatment of chronically ill children (1), there has been an impetus to assess the quality of life in children with epilepsy. This chapter provides a general introduction to health-related quality-of-life (HRQOL) assessment in children and adolescents with epilepsy.

Although references to HRQOL are relatively new in the field of pediatric epilepsy, there has been long-standing interest in quality-of-life issues. For example, the adjustment problems experienced by children with epilepsy and their parents have always been a concern to clinicians, and adjustment problems are important components of quality of life in these children. Moreover, a clinician's asking "How are you doing?" can be viewed as an attempt, albeit unrefined, to assess quality of life in the clinical setting (2). The recent emphasis on quality-of-life outcomes, however, has led to a need for more formal or systematic approaches to the assessment of quality of life in children with epilepsy. A formal approach to HRQOL is the focus in this chapter. Major areas addressed are core dimensions, quality-of-life problems, and measurement of quality of life in the clinical setting.

HEALTH-RELATED QUALITY OF LIFE

Core Dimensions

Although health-related quality of life is inconsistently defined, there is general agreement that it refers to a person's state of functioning and well-being across multiple health dimensions (3,4). These dimensions most commonly include those related to physical status and functioning, psychological functioning, social relationships, and economic status (5). There also is general consensus that, in the measurement of HRQOL, information should be included that is disease-specific and addresses both the impact of the condition and the effects of treatment for the condition. The few studies that focus on quality of life in children with epilepsy are consistent with these recommendations in that both used a multidimensional approach and included information specific to epilepsy. For example, Austin and colleagues (6,7) conceptualized quality of life around functioning in four dimensions: physical, psychological, social, and school. Information on seizure frequency was included in their measurement of the physical dimension (6). In another study of quality of life in children with epilepsy, Hoare and Russell (8) conceptualized quality of life somewhat differently but also in four areas: impact of epilepsy and its treatment on the child, impact on the child's development and adjustment, impact on parents, and impact on the family. In a final study Wildrick and colleagues (9) conceptualized quality of life in children with epilepsy in five domains: self-concept, home life (e.g., family relationships), school life, social activities, and medication (e.g., compliance).

For the purposes of this chapter, five dimensions relevant to health-related quality of life in children with epilepsy are presented in Table 49-1 and described in the next section. The domains presented here are based on the literature on quality of life in epilepsy as well as in other chronic conditions and, although independent, are highly interrelated. The five core dimensions represent a broad-based conceptualization of HRQOL in pediatric epilepsy. The first four domains focus on aspects of child functioning. Because the family environment is integral to child functioning, the final

Table 49-1. Suggested Quality of Life Dimensions for Pediatric Epilepsy

Functioning Related to Epilepsy and Treatment
Neurologic functioning
Cognitive functioning
    Attention, memory, abstract reasoning, psychomotor
        functioning
Epilepsy syndrome
Seizure severity
    Seizure type, seizure frequency, resulting physical
        injury
Antiepilepsy medication effects
    Physical, cognitive, and behavior side effects

Psychological Functioning
Emotional status
    Happiness and satisfaction
    Anxiety, depression, behavioral problems, and
        psychiatric disturbance
    Self-esteem
Feelings about epilepsy
    Concerns and fears
    Attitude toward having epilepsy
    Perceptions of stigma

Social Functioning
Completion of age-appropriate psychosocial
    developmental tasks
Satisfaction with family relationships
Peer relationships
Engagement in activities
    Sports, clubs, hobbies, teams, organizations

School Functioning
Academic achievement
Learning problems
Adaptive characteristics
    Works hard, behaves appropriately

Family Functioning Related to Epilepsy
Seizure-management skills
Psychological adjustment to epilepsy
    Concerns and fears
    Attitude toward epilepsy in child
    Perceptions of stigma
    Supervision of child's activities
Leisure activity participation

domain focuses on family adjustment related to the child's epilepsy.

Neurologic and Cognitive Functioning Related to Epilepsy and Treatment

Assessment in this domain addresses disease-specific information, including neurologic and cognitive functioning and information on the nature of the epilepsy. General information on physical functioning is not included because children with epilepsy should not have physical limitations as a result of their seizure condition. Much of this data would be routinely obtained in a clinical setting because assessment of information specific to the condition is a basic component of medical care. Assessments made in establishing a diagnosis generally include a complete neurologic examination that provides information about possible neurologic deficits. Moreover, in the diagnosis and classification of the epilepsy syndrome, information on the nature of the seizure condition and its possible physical effects is collected. Once medications are prescribed, any side effects also are regularly assessed. In this domain it is only the information related to cognitive functioning, such as attention, memory, abstract reasoning, and psychomotor functioning, that may not be routinely assessed in all children with epilepsy.

Psychological Functioning

Two areas are covered in this assessment domain: the common adjustment problems experienced by children who have any chronic physical condition and those specific to epilepsy. Children with chronic neurologic conditions, such as epilepsy, are more likely to experience emotional problems than children with non–brain-related physical chronic conditions (10,11); therefore, it is critical that this domain include negative aspects of emotional status (e.g., anxiety, depression, behavioral problems, and psychiatric disturbances). Based on Ware's (12) recommendation that the full range of the health state be included in an assessment, positive aspects of psychological functioning (e.g., happiness, satisfaction, and self-esteem) are also included. The second area relates to the feelings associated with having epilepsy. To what extent are children concerned and fearful about having epilepsy? Do they have negative feelings or a negative attitude about having epilepsy? Do they perceive a stigma associated with epilepsy to the point that it negatively affects their behavior?

Social Functioning

Assessment of social functioning is included because children with neurologic conditions have poorer social competence than children with other chronic conditions (6,7,13). An important component of social functioning is the accomplishment of developmental tasks. Because children with epilepsy show delay in some of these tasks, such as the development of independence (14), their assessment is included in this domain. Information on social functioning in both family relationships and peer relationships also is included. The final information included in this domain relates to the child's engagement in age-appropriate activities, including participation in sports, clubs, hobbies, teams, and organizations.

School Functioning

Success at school is important to successful employment in adulthood. One general population sample of parents identified learning and remembering school work as one of six most important areas of quality of life (15). Functioning at school is especially important to measure in children with epilepsy because they have high rates of learning problems (16), poorer academic achievement than would be expected based on intelligence (17), and high rates of school failure (18). Because success at school is partially dependent on behaviors that enhance success at school, such as working hard, school adaptive characteristics also are included in this domain.

Family Adjustment to Epilepsy

Assessment of the family is important for two major reasons. First, children are not independent beings, and it is the persons in their immediate environment who are in a position to influence their quality of life (19). There is a close relationship between family adjustment to the epilepsy and the child's functioning. Second, a chronic condition in a child has been found to negatively affect the adjustment of other family members, especially the mother (20). Included in this domain are factors related to the parents' ability to manage the epilepsy and their psychological adjustment to the epilepsy. Do parents feel competent in their ability to handle future seizures? Are parents overly concerned and fearful about their child's condition? Are siblings unduly worried? Do family members have an optimistic attitude toward the epilepsy? Are family members unduly concerned about a stigma being associated with epilepsy? Is parents' supervision of the child's activities appropriate for the child's age? Finally, information on the participation of the family in leisure activity is included in this domain because of the importance of such participation in relation to family interaction and cohesion (21). Are family activities being overly restricted because of the epilepsy?

QUALITY-OF-LIFE PROBLEMS

Few studies have been carried out that measured more than one or two quality-of-life domains in children with epilepsy. Austin and colleagues (6) compared differences in four domains of quality of life (physical, psychological, social, and school) between 136 children with epilepsy and 134 children with asthma aged 8 to 13 years. Results indicated that children with epilepsy had a higher quality of life in the physical domain and a poorer quality of life in the psychological, social, and school domains. A 4-year follow-up study again

comparing quality of life in these two samples indicated that those with epilepsy were still experiencing a poorer quality of life than those with asthma, even though substantially more of the epilepsy sample had inactive conditions. When the epilepsy sample was grouped by severity (inactive, low severity, and high severity), those with the most severe seizures were faring the worst, especially in the social domain. In the psychological domain, girls had more anxiety, less happiness, and more negative feelings about having epilepsy than boys (7). Another study focused on the quality of life of children in Japan (22). In this study quality of life was studied in two environments, home and school, and included the assessment of problems as perceived by the children themselves, their families, and their schoolteachers. The main concerns of children were related to medication and seizures. Parents were most concerned about their child's future, their seizures, and their child's school performance. The most common problems experienced at school were difficulty in keeping up with learning and problems in developing friendships.

A review of the literature indicates that functioning in one domain is often related to functioning in other domains. Because information on the assessment and treatment of the child's epilepsy is covered in other chapters in this book, the focus here is on quality-of-life problems experienced by the child and family in the other four domains.

Psychological Functioning

The literature provides strong evidence that children with epilepsy are at risk for poor psychological functioning. Epidemiologic studies indicate that children with epilepsy are 4.7 (23) to 4.8 times (11) more likely to have mental health problems than children from the general population. Studies of behavioral problems in children with epilepsy from clinical populations indicate that approximately 50 percent have behavior problem scores in the at-risk range based on standardized scales (24,25). These problems range from minor problems in daily living to psychosis. Most commonly found are behavioral problems, poor self-concept, social isolation, depression, and other psychiatric disturbances (11,26–28).

The psychological problems found in children with epilepsy do not appear to be solely from having a chronic illness because the prevalence rate of problems is higher in children with epilepsy than for children with other chronic physical conditions (11,16,29). In a major epidemiologic study Rutter, Graham, and Yule (11) found that for children with idiopathic epilepsy the prevalence of psychiatric disorders was approximately 2.5 times higher than for children with other physical disorders. Long and Moore (30) found children with epilepsy to have significantly poorer self-esteem scores, more social isolation, and poorer reading skills than their healthy siblings.

Few studies have focused on children's perceptions and coping responses related to epilepsy. A study investigating the relationship between coping responses and mental health outcomes in youth with epilepsy found that coping responses of competence, optimism, compliance, and seeking support were associated with fewer behavioral problems and a positive self-concept. In contrast, coping responses of irritability, feeling different, and social withdrawal were related to more behavioral problems and a poorer self-concept (31). Austin and Huberty (32) found children's negative attitudes toward epilepsy to be related to poor self-concept and more behavioral problems. In another recent study children's attitudes toward having epilepsy, locus of control, and satisfaction with family relationships were significantly associated with symptoms of depression in youth with epilepsy (33).

Some have hypothesized that mental health problems are caused by underlying neurologic dysfunction that causes both the seizures and the behavioral problems, and some empirical studies support this hypothesis. Children with epilepsy who have accompanying deficits in neurologic functioning seem to be at increased risk for mental health problems (34,35). Moreover, higher rates of psychiatric disorder are found in children with chronic conditions involving the brain than in children with chronic conditions that do not involve the brain (10,11,29). In addition, a recent study of children with new-onset seizures found 24 percent of them had been at risk for behavioral problems *before* the onset of their seizures (36).

Social Functioning

For optimal social development, children need an environment in which they can develop autonomy and initiative. There is empirical evidence that children with epilepsy have problems with developing independence. For example, children with epilepsy have been found to be more dependent than children with tonsillectomies (14). Hoare (37) studied child dependency on the mother in four groups: children with newly diagnosed epilepsy, children with chronic epilepsy, children with newly diagnosed diabetes, and children with chronic epilepsy. Results comparing these groups with population-based norms indicated that children with either newly diagnosed or chronic epilepsy were significantly more dependent on their mothers in three of four areas. In contrast, no differences were found between the norms and children with newly diagnosed diabetes. Finally, children with chronic diabetes differed from norms in only one dependency area.

Studies investigating factors related to social functioning have led to inconsistent results. Austin and colleagues (7) found youth with the most severe epilepsy to be faring the worst socially. In contrast, Camfield and colleagues (18) did not find epilepsy-related variables (e.g., age of onset, seizure type) to be related to social functioning. Furthermore, in that study remission of epilepsy did not predict social functioning. There is some support in the literature that the social functioning of children might be influenced by parenting behaviors. In an early descriptive study of 12 families, Mulder and Suurmeijer (38) found a relationship between parental control and dependency in children with epilepsy. Long and Moore (30) hypothesized that parents might have different expectations for a child with epilepsy than for a healthy sibling, which might lead to more restrictive parenting practices and subsequently more adaptation problems in the child with epilepsy. In a study of 19 families, Long and Moore (30) found that parents had different expectations for their children with epilepsy than for their healthy children. For example, they expected children with epilepsy to have more emotional problems, to be more unpredictable, and to be more "high-strung" than their siblings. Moreover, in this study parents perceived themselves as being more restrictive in parenting their children with epilepsy than the healthy brothers and sisters. Lothman, Pianta, and Clarson (39) studied parenting behaviors of children with epilepsy through observing mother–child interactions and found praise to be related to child competence and positive affect. In contrast, intrusive and overcontrolling parenting behaviors were related to less autonomy and confidence in these children.

School Functioning

School problems are overrepresented in children with epilepsy. Research comparing academic achievement across different chronic childhood conditions consistently indicates that children with epilepsy are one of the most vulnerable groups. For example, a comparison study of 270 children with 1 of 11 different conditions showed that children with epilepsy, sickle cell disease, or spina bifida were doing the poorest (40). Academic performance in children with epilepsy has consistently been found to be poorer than would be expected by intellectual ability (17). In a classic study teachers rated 53 percent of children with epilepsy in regular classrooms to be functioning below grade level (41). Moreover, one large epidemiologic study found that children with uncomplicated epilepsy were, on average, about 1 year delayed in overall reading ability and that approximately 20 percent demonstrated severe deficits (42). More recent studies indicate that children with epilepsy make less academic progress than would be expected for their age and intelligence level in arithmetic, reading, comprehension, and word recognition (43). In another study on children with epilepsy who had intelligence in the normal range, 39.7 percent had repeated at least one grade in school (44). When academic achievement on school-administered tests was compared between children with epilepsy and those with asthma, children with epilepsy had significantly lower scores than children with asthma in reading, mathematics, language, and vocabulary (45). In this study boys with the most severe seizure conditions were found to be faring the worst.

The relationship between seizures and academic functioning is unclear. Some studies have found that seizure type and frequency are related to academic achievement (46). In addition, Westbrook and colleagues (47) found that adolescents with mild idiopathic epilepsy had more problems with academic functioning than would be expected. In a recent study however, academic underachievement was not related to any seizure variables or medication variables (48). Moreover, in that study youth who were newly diagnosed with epilepsy and had not been treated with medication already were showing problems in academic achievement.

Neurologic dysfunction has been identified as a potential cause of academic achievement problems in children with epilepsy. It is hypothesized that neurologic dysfunction leads to cognitive impairments, which in turn lead to academic problems. Even though broad intellectual abilities are stable and normal in the majority of children with epilepsy, these same children often perform below expected levels in the classroom. Although some studies have shown neurologic variables to be related to some of the academic problems observed (43), they appear to account for only a small part of the academic picture (48).

Family Adjustment

Few studies have investigated the adjustment of family members of children with epilepsy. Hoare (49) studied the prevalence of psychiatric disorder in parents and school-aged siblings of children with either newly diagnosed or chronic epilepsy. Results indicated that children with newly diagnosed epilepsy were significantly more disturbed than their siblings. The siblings' scores, however, did not differ from population norms. In contrast, the siblings of the children with chronic epilepsy were significantly more disturbed than both siblings of children newly diagnosed with epilepsy and population norms. In this study there was an association between psychiatric disturbance in the child with chronic epilepsy and psychiatric disturbance in their mothers. This relationship was not found in the sample of children with newly diagnosed epilepsy. Hoare (49)

hypothesized that chronic epilepsy leads to stress that can negatively affect the mental health of other family members.

Two studies have investigated the concerns of parents whose children have seizures. Ward and Bower (50) studied the parents of 81 children with epilepsy, 30 of whom were newly diagnosed. These parents reported many concerns and fears related to the nature of the seizure, effects of medications, causes of seizures, injury, effects on intelligence, brain damage, mental health problems, and social problems. Austin and colleagues (51) studied 100 parents of children within 4 months of their first seizure to identify concerns and fears. Concerns and fears focused on two broad areas: epilepsy and treatment (e.g., effect of seizures on the brain, on the child's mental health, and on the child's future life) and management of the epilepsy (e.g., handling future seizures, negative responses of others, lifestyle changes, and preventing mental health problems). Suurmeijer (52) found that families imposed fewer restrictions on their child with epilepsy when the parents perceived that the information given to them about their child's condition was adequate. In that study he also found parents to report that they would more easily accept, would be less frightened about, and would know how to better deal with the epilepsy if they received adequate information about the condition.

The few empirical studies exploring the relationship between family environment variables and adaptation problems in children with epilepsy support a relationship between them. For example, Hoare and Kerley (25) found family stress, epilepsy variables, medication variables, and socioeconomic status to be associated with child behavioral problems. Austin, Risinger, and Beckett (24) also found family stress, high seizure frequency, lack of family social support, and low family mastery and control to be associated with behavioral problems in children with epilepsy. Pianta and Lothman (53) found family stress to be associated with child behavioral problems even after epilepsy factors and child characteristics were statistically controlled. Both negative parental attitudes and perceptions of stigma associated with epilepsy may contribute to poor child adaptation. Relationships have been found between negative parental attitudes and poor parent adaptation to the epilepsy (54) and between negative parental attitudes and poor child adaptation (55).

MEASURING HEALTH-RELATED QUALITY OF LIFE

Measurement of HRQOL has received less attention in children and adolescents than in adults. One of the reasons instrument development has lagged behind in pediatrics is the diversity of the many developmental periods experienced by children as they mature from infancy through middle childhood, adolescence, and late adolescence. In deciding how to assess quality of life in children with epilepsy, much depends on the purpose. If the purpose is research-related, measurements should be made with the goal of answering the research questions in the most valid and reliable manner. In a clinical trial, measurement would be targeted to the specific quality-of-life domains most likely to be affected by the treatment under study. One advantage in a research study is that children and families expect to spend a significant amount of time being interviewed or completing instruments.

When HRQOL is measured in the clinical setting, the goal is to select the method that provides the best data to guide treatment decisions. It is these decisions that are the focus of the issues addressed here. The two most common methods used in the clinical setting are structured interview and self-report questionnaire. Advantages of the interview are that the interviewer is available to explain things that are not clear, answer questions, and make sure that all questions are answered. Interviews can be conducted either in person or by telephone. Moreover, information on quality of life can be part of history-taking by the clinician. Advantages of using self-report questionnaires are flexibility in relation to when they are completed and the fact that no interviewer is needed. Disadvantages include questions being skipped and the lack of opportunity for children and families to ask questions if something is unclear.

The information that follows focuses on issues related to the use of self-report questionnaires in the clinical setting. The criteria for evaluating instruments, practical considerations, selection of respondent, and selection of scales are addressed.

Criteria for Evaluating Instruments

Criteria for evaluating data collection instruments relate to psychometric properties and clinical standards. The best instruments are those that have excellent psychometric properties and meet clinical standards.

The two major criteria related to the theory of measurement (psychometrics) are reliability and validity. Reliability refers to the consistency or the extent to which a measuring instrument yields similar results over repeated administrations. Stability reliability demonstrates consistency over time, and internal consistency reliability refers to the homogeneity of the items measuring the concept. Validity, which is the extent to which an instrument measures what it is supposed to measure, is commonly of three types: content validity, criterion validity, and construct validity. Content validity answers the question "Do the items measure what they are supposed to?" Criterion validity refers to the extent that the score on an instrument is systematically

related to some external criterion. Construct validity refers to the extent that scores on an instrument are logically related to other measures.

An instrument that meets clinical standards differentiates between different levels of severity within the condition. Recently, there has been an emphasis on the extent to which a scale is sensitive or responsive to change. Responsiveness refers to the instrument's ability to detect anticipated clinical change over time (56). An instrument must be able to detect even small improvements in a condition if it is going to be used to show effects of treatment.

Practical Considerations

There also are practical considerations when selecting instruments. Length of time for collecting information must be considered because time is especially important in the clinical setting. Are the instruments easily administered in the clinical setting? Are there norms based on age and gender? Because of the large differences across the different ages, one must use well-developed scales with norms based on age of the child. In addition, because of the different trajectories of boys and girls at different ages, the scales must have norms based on gender.

The complexity of the scoring also is an important practical consideration. Clinical staff may need to be made available to assist children and families to complete the instruments. The staff must use instruments that are easily scored and interpreted so the information can be used immediately. Unfortunately, most scales that can be used for a wide age range because they have norms for age and gender also have complex scoring; however, most of these scales have computer scoring programs that are easy to use.

Staff cooperation and training and an infrastructure for collecting data, scoring instruments, and incorporating the information into treatment are necessary. The assessment must take place in a manner that best fits with clinical practice. Will children and families be asked to complete instruments before, during, or after office visits? More time is available for completion of scales if they are done outside the clinical setting before the clinic visit. The scale or questionnaire can be sent out with an appointment reminder to bring it to the visit with them. When there is only a short period of time available for measurement or completing a questionnaire (e.g., while waiting to see the doctor), decisions must be made whether to do a comprehensive assessment on a few HRQOL dimensions, screen for functioning in all areas, or a combination of the two.

Other questions that must be considered relate to frequency and timing of assessment. Will all children be screened at every visit? Will more complete assessments be carried out on new patients? Will different dimensions be targeted for the different age groups? An assessment of HRQOL could also be triggered by critical events that occur in the child's life such as:

- Age-related changes (e.g., beginning school, transition into adolescence);
- Health-related changes (e.g., seizures increase, medication change);
- Social-related changes (e.g., new school, parent divorce, new sibling).

Selection of Respondent

An important decision focuses on who should provide the data. Generally, it is ideal to obtain both objective data and subjective data from multiple sources (parents, children, and teachers). According to Landfraf and Abetz (56), children as young as 5 years old can provide reliable information on very concrete concepts such as pain. Austin and colleagues have obtained reliable information on abstract concepts from children with epilepsy as young as 8 years of age (31,32). As a general rule, parents should provide most of the information when the children are younger than 7 years old. Even when the children are age 8 or older, the decision about who should provide information is not an easy one to make. Cognitive development and the ability to understand abstract concepts must be considered. For example, children may have a good understanding of and can report on how they feel today, but have trouble conceptualizing usual health (57). Children who have had seizures from a very young age also may not be able conceptualize what life would be without epilepsy and would have trouble answering questions about their life compared with the best possible life.

Even when children are able to understand the content of the question being asked, other factors must be considered when interpreting results. For example, children under 12 years of age tend to endorse negatively worded items more than children aged 12 years and older (57). Differences should be expected when data are collected from both parents. For example, mothers tend to rate children as having more problems than do fathers (56). Moreover, children's assessments of certain areas consistently differ from those of their parents. There tends to be more agreement on concepts related to physical functioning (e.g., activities and chores) and less agreement on abstract concepts such as interpersonal relationships with peers (57). For example, Austin and colleagues found that adolescents with epilepsy rated themselves to have fewer behavioral problems than their mothers, fathers, and teachers did (58). Parents' reports on children's mental health problems, however, have been found to be more valid than children's reports (59).

The fact that parents, children, and teachers rate things differently does not mean that one viewpoint is better than the other, just that they provide different perspectives. Some information is only available from

Table 49-2. Selected Instruments to Measure Quality of Life

Scales	Description
Multiple Domain Instruments	
Child Health Questionnaire (62)	A generic scale for children ages 5 and older. There are three parent-completed versions of differing lengths that measure 14 concepts and one child-completed version with 12 concepts. Has good psychometric properties and norms.
Quality of Life in Epilepsy — Adolescent (63)	A general epilepsy scale for adolescents 11 to 17 years. The scale has 48 items that measure effects of epilepsy and medicine, stigma, feelings about self, and general HRQOL concepts of family, friends, activities, mood, cognition and memory.
Single Domain Instruments	
Child Behavior Checklist, Teacher's Report Form, and Youth Self-Report (64)	A group of instruments that measure child psychological and social functioning. There are versions for parents, teachers, and youth (age 11–18) to complete. The scales have 118 behavior items and 28 social competence items. Has good psychometric properties and norms.
Child Attitude Toward Illness Scale (32)	A 13-item self-report scale for children age 8 and older. The scale measures children's feelings about having epilepsy. Has good psychometric properties.
Family APGAR (65) and Revised Family APGAR (66)	Two 5-item scales that measure satisfaction with family relationships. Parents and children 11 and older complete Family APGAR. The Revised Family APGAR is for children age 8 and older. Has good psychometric properties.
Children's Concern Scale (67)	A 13-item scale for children 8–15 years to report their concerns and fears about having seizures.

Table 49-3. Questions to Assess HRQOL in the Clinical Setting

Assessment Questions for Parents

Functioning related to epilepsy and treatment
- What concerns do you have about your child's seizure condition or treatment?
- What concerns do you have about handling your child's seizures?

Psychological functioning
- What concerns do you have about your child's ability to cope with seizures?
- Do you think your child is unduly worried or sad about having seizures?

Social functioning
- Compared to other children, how well does your child get along with others?
- Compared to other children, how involved in activities is your child?

School functioning
- What concerns do you have about handling your child's seizures at school?
- Is your child having any problems with school?

Family functioning related to epilepsy
- Are any members of your family having problems coping with the seizures?
- Is your family avoiding any activities because of the seizures?

Assessment Questions for Older Children and Adolescents

Functioning related to epilepsy and treatment
- What questions do you have about your seizure condition?
- What questions do you have about your medication?

Psychological functioning
- Have you been feeling sad or down in the dumps about having seizures?
- What kinds of things worry you about having seizures?

Social functioning
- How well do you get along with other kids?
- What things are you not doing because of seizures?

School functioning
- Do you feel you have to work harder on school work than other kids?
- Are you having any trouble paying attention in school?

Family functioning related to epilepsy
- Do your brothers and sisters treat you differently because of the seizures?
- Do your parents treat you differently because of the seizures?

---

the child. It also is important to consider that only children can report their emotional feelings, so if this information is desired, it must be obtained from children.

Selection of Scales

It is important to use both general and disease-specific scales in a comprehensive assessment of HRQOL (60). The use of general scales allows for comparing across samples, although a disadvantage of using general scales is that they often contain questions irrelevant for epilepsy. For example, questions about physical functioning are not relevant for children with epilepsy. Decisions relate to the selection of instruments that would provide the best data to guide treatment decisions. Foremost, the clinician must consider what to do with the information once it has been collected. For example, a screening survey could be administered first and then followed with more specific information on areas in which there are problems identified on the screening. The purpose for carrying out the HRQOL assessment should guide decisions regarding whether to use one general scale that assesses a large number of dimensions, a battery approach in which several well-developed scales are used to measure each dimension, or a combination of the two.

Clinical Application of HRQOL Assessment

Incorporating HRQOL information into the clinical care of children with epilepsy can improve the quality of care provided, and therefore it is critical that a strategy for HRQOL assessment be developed that can be efficiently incorporated into the office routine. Assessments can identify children who are at risk for problems so preventive efforts can be initiated at the earliest opportunity. Assessments also can improve clinical decision making by increasing the clinician's understanding of the quality-of-life problems experienced by children with epilepsy and their families. Finally, information from assessment of HRQOL over time can be used to document treatment outcomes (61).

Unfortunately, strategies to facilitate the application of HRQOL assessment in the clinical setting are noticeably absent in the literature. Furthermore, recent changes in health care delivery leading to shorter visits do not always make it practical to administer questionnaires in outpatient settings, although they should be considered if at all possible. Table 49-2 describes a few of the available instruments that could be used to measure different aspects of quality of life.

If the use of a formal HRQOL assessment instrument is deemed to be impractical, suggestions for key questions to assess needs or concerns in each of the five HRQOL domains are presented in Table 49-3. These questions could be incorporated into an office visit. Moreover, because it often is difficult to obtain all the necessary information in one encounter, carrying the questions around on a pocket card or providing blank forms to be completed by the child or parent at the time of clinic registration could increase the likelihood that the questions would be regularly assessed. Other suggestions are to include an adapted version of the questions on the back of letters or appointment reminders that are routinely sent to patients, so that the parents could think ahead about the areas and be prepared with questions and answers. Because the back side of letters is not generally used, this would be an efficient way to incorporate the assessment into established routines.

SUMMARY

Quality of life in people with health problems is strongly linked to the quality of their care. In the treatment of a chronic condition such as childhood epilepsy, the clinician is not so much concerned with "cure" but with preventing adverse consequences of the condition and optimizing the child's functioning. When the outcome is narrowly conceptualized to be optimal seizure control, care is based on assessment of seizures and treatment to reduce seizures. When the outcome is conceptualized to also include the child's quality of life, care is based on the assessment of the five core dimensions and treatment to improve the child's functioning in each of five areas. A focus on quality of life as the primary outcome leads to the provision not only of the very important optimal seizure control but also of comprehensive care for the child and family that includes assessment and interventions in each of the quality-of-life domains. Optimal seizure control should be only one of many goals.

REFERENCES

1. Drotar D, Levi R, Palermo TM, et al. Clinical applications of health-related quality of life assessment for children and adolescents. *Measuring Health-Related Quality of Life in Children and Adolescents*. Mahwah, N.J.: Lawrence Erlbaum, 1998.

2. Hoffman LG, Rouse MW, Brin BN. Quality of life: a review. *J Am Optom Assn* 1995; 66:281–289.

3. Croog SH. Current issues in conceptualizing and measuring quality of life. *Quality of Life Assessment* 1990; 3:11–21.

4. Fallowfield L. *The Quality of Life*. London: Souvenir Press, 1990.

5. Spilker B. *Quality of Life Assessments in Clinical Trials*. New York: Raven Press, 1990.

6. Austin JK, Smith MS, Risinger MW, McNelis AM. Childhood epilepsy and asthma: comparison of quality of life. *Epilepsia* 1994; 35:608–615.

7. Austin JK, Huster GA, Dunn DW, Risinger MW. Adolescents with active or inactive epilepsy or asthma: a comparison of quality of life. *Epilepsia* 1996; 37:1228–1238.

8. Hoare P, Russell M. The quality of life of children with chronic epilepsy and their families: preliminary findings with a new assessment measure. *Dev Med Child Neurol* 1995; 37:689–696.

9. Wildrick D, Parker-Fisher S, Morales A. Quality of life in children with well-controlled epilepsy. *J Neurosci Nurs* 1996; 28:192–198.

10. Howe GW, Feinstein C, Reiss D, Molock S, Berger K. Adolescent adjustment to chronic physical disorders — I. Comparing neurological and non-neurological conditions. *J Child Psychol Psychiat* 1993; 34:1153–1171.

11. Rutter M, Graham P, Yule W. *A Neuropsychiatric Study in Childhood*. Philadelphia: JB Lippincott, 1970.

12. Ware JE. Evaluating measures of general health concepts for use in clinical trials. *Quality of Life Assessment* 1990; 6:51–63.

13. Nassau JH, Drotar D. Social competence among children with central nervous system-related chronic health conditions: a review. *J Ped Psychol* 1997; 22:771–793.

14. Hartlage LC, Green JB. The relation of parental attitudes to academic and social achievement in epileptic children. *Epilepsia* 1972; 13:21–26.

15. Rosenbaum PL, Saigal S. Measuring health-related quality of life in pediatric populations: conceptual issues. In: Spilker B, *Quality of Life and Pharmacoeconomics in Clinical Trials*. Philadelphia: Lippincott-Raven, 1996.

16. Kim WJ. Psychiatric aspects of epileptic children and adolescents. *J Am Acad Child Adolesc Psychiatry* 1991; 30:874–886.

17. Seidenberg M, Berent S. Childhood epilepsy and the role of psychology. *Am Psychol* 1992; 47:1130–1133.

18. Camfield C, Camfield P, Smith B, Gordon K, Dooley J. Biological factors as predictors of social outcomes of epilepsy in intellectually normal children: a population-based study. *J Pediatr* 1993; 122:869–873.

19. Pal DK. Quality of life assessment in children: a review of conceptual and methodological issues in multidimensional health status measures. *Epidemiology and Community Health* 1996; 50:391–396.

20. Eiser C. Psychological effects of chronic disease. *J Child Psychol Psychiat* 1990; 31:85–98.

21. Orthner DK, Mancini JA. Leisure impacts on family interaction and cohesion. *J Leisure Res* 1990; 22:125–137.

22. Hanai T. Quality of life in children with epilepsy. *Epilepsia* 1996; 37(Suppl 3):28–32.

23. McDermott S, Mani S, Krishnaswami S. A population-based analysis of specific behavior problems associated with childhood seizures. *J Epilepsy* 1995; 8:110–118.

24. Austin JK, Risinger MW, Beckett LA. Correlates of behavior problems in children with epilepsy. *Epilepsia* 1992; 33:1115–1122.

25. Hoare P, Kerley S. Psychosocial adjustment of children with chronic epilepsy and their families. *Dev Med Child Neurol* 1991; 33:201–215.

26. Hoare P. The development of psychiatric disorder among schoolchildren with epilepsy. *Dev Med Child Neurol* 1984; 26:3–13.

27. Margalit M, Heiman T. Anxiety and self-dissatisfaction in epileptic children. *Dev Med Child Neurol* 1983; 29:220–224.

28. Matthews WS, Barabas G, Ferrari M. Emotional concomitants of childhood epilepsy. *Epilepsia* 1982; 23:671–681.

29. Breslau N. Psychiatric disorder in children with physical disabilities. *J Am Acad Child Adolesc Psychiatry* 1985; 24:87–94.

30. Long CG, Moore JR. Parental perceptions for their epileptic children. *J Child Psychol Psychiatry* 1979; 20:299–312.

31. Austin JK, Patterson JM, Huberty TJ. Development of the coping health inventory for children. *J Pediatr Nurs* 1991; 6:166–174.

32. Austin JK, Huberty TJ. Development of the child attitude toward illness scale. *J Pediatr Psychol* 1993; 18:467–480.

33. Dunn DW, Austin JK, Huster GA. Symptoms of depression in children with epilepsy. *J Child Adolesc Psychiatr* 1999; 38:1132–1138.

34. Hermann BP. Deficits in neuropsychological functioning and psychopathology in persons with epilepsy: a rejected hypothesis revisited. *Epilepsia* 1981; 22:161–167.

35. Hermann BP. Neurological functioning and psychopathology in children with epilepsy. *Epilepsia* 1982; 22:703–710.

36. Dunn DW, Austin JK, Huster GA. Behaviour problems in children with new-onset epilepsy. *Seizure* 1997; 6:283–287.

37. Hoare P. Does illness foster dependency? A study of epileptic and diabetic children. *Dev Med Child Neurol* 1984; 26:20–24.

38. Mulder HC, Suurmeijer TPBM. Families with a child with epilepsy: a sociological contribution. *J Biosoc Sci* 1977; 9:13–24.

39. Lothman DJ, Pianta RC, Clarson SM. Mother-child interaction in children with epilepsy: relations with child competence. *J Epilepsy* 1990; 3:157–163.

40. Fowler MG, Johnson MP, Atkinson SS. School achievement and absence in children with chronic health conditions. *J Pediatr* 1985; 106:683–687.

41. Holdsworth L, Whitmore K. A study of children with epilepsy attending ordinary schools. II: Information and attitudes held by their teachers. *Dev Med Child Neurol* 1974; 16:746–758.

42. Yule W. Educational achievement. In: Kulig BM, *Epilepsy and Behavior*. Lisse, The Netherlands: Swets and Zeitlinger, 1980.

43. Seidenberg M, Beck N, Geisser M, et al. Academic achievement of children with epilepsy. *Epilepsia* 1986; 27:753–759.

44. Huberty TJ, Austin JK, Risinger MW, McNelis AM. Relationship of selected seizure variables in children with epilepsy to performance on school-administered achievement tests. *J Epilepsy* 1992; 5:10–16.

45. Austin JK, Huberty TJ, Huster GA, Dunn DW. Academic achievement in children with epilepsy or asthma. *Dev Med Child Neurol* 1998; 40:248–255.

46. Seidenberg M. Academic achievement and school performance of children with epilepsy. In: *Childhood Epilepsies: Neuropsychological, Psychosocial and Intervention Aspects*. Chichester: John Wiley & Sons, 1989.

47. Westbrook LE, Silver EJ, Coupey SM, Shinnar S. Social characteristics of adolescents with idiopathic epilepsy: a comparison to chronically ill and nonchronically ill peers. *J Epilepsy* 1991; 4:87–94.

48. Mitchell WG, Chavez JM, Lee H, Guzman BL. Academic underachievement in children with epilepsy. *J Child Neurol* 1991; 6:65–72.

49. Hoare P. Psychiatric disturbance in the families of epileptic children. *Dev Med Child Neurol* 1984; 26:14–19.

50. Ward F, Bower BD. A study of certain social aspects of epilepsy in childhood. *Dev Med Child Neurol* 1978; 20:1–50.

51. Austin JK, Oruche UM, Dunn DW, Levstek DA. New-onset childhood seizures: parents' concerns and needs. *Clinical Nursing Practice in Epilepsy* 1995; Winter:8–10.

52. Suurmeijer PBM. Quality of care and quality of life from the perspective of patients and parents. *Internat J Adolesc Med Health* 1994; 7:290–302.

53. Pianta RC, Lothman DJ. Predicting behavior problems in children with epilepsy: child factors, disease factors, family stress, and child-parent interaction. *Child Dev* 1994; 65:1415–1428.

54. Austin JK, McBride AB, Howard DW. Parental attitude and adjustment to childhood epilepsy. *Nurs Research* 1984; 32:92–96.

55. Austin JK, Smith MS, Risinger MW. Predictors of adaptation in children with epilepsy or asthma. *American Epilepsy Society Proceedings. Epilepsia* 1992; 33(Suppl 6):24.

56. Landgraf JM, Abetz LN. Measuring health outcomes in pediatric populations: issues in psychometrics and application. In: Spilker B, *Quality of Life and Pharmacoeconomics in Clinical Trials*. Philadelphia: Lippincott-Raven, 1996.

57. Pantell RH, Lewis CC. Measuring the impact of medical care on children. *J Chron Dis* 1987; 40(Suppl 1):99S–108S.

58. Austin JK, Dunn DW, Huster GR. Differences in quality of life ratings among adolescents, parents, and teachers.

The 21st *International Epilepsy Congress Proceedings. Epilepsia* 1995; 36(Suppl 3):190.

59. Dadds MR. *Families, Children, and the Development of Dysfunction.* Thousand Oaks, Calif.: Sage, 1995.

60. Shumaker SA, Moinpour CM, Aaronson NK, et al. Design and implementation issues. *Quality of Life Assessment* 1990; 5:27–46.

61. Levi R, Drotar D. Critical issues and needs in health-related quality of life assessment of children and adolescents with chronic health conditions. In: Drotar D, ed. *Measuring Health-Related Quality of Life in Children and Adolescents.* Mahwah, NJ: Lawrence Erlbaum, 1998.

62. Landgraf JM, Abetz L, Ware JE. *Child Health Questionnaire (CHQ): A User's Manual.* Boston: The Health Institute, New England Medical Center, 1996.

63. Cramer J, Westbrook L, Devinsky O, et al. Development of the Quality of Life in Epilepsy Inventory for Adolescents: The QOLIE-AD-48. *Epilepsia* 1999; 8:1114–1121.

64. Achenbach TM. *Integrative Guide for the 1991 CBCL.4-18, YSR, and TRF Profiles.* Burlington: University of Vermont Department of Psychiatry, 1991.

65. Smilkstein G. The family APGAR: a proposal for a family function test and its use by physicians. *J Fam Prac* 1978; 6:1231–1239.

66. Austin JK, Huberty TJ. Revision of the family APGAR for use by 8-year-olds. *Family Systems Medicine* 1989; 7:323–327.

67. Austin JK, Dunn DW. Assessing children's concerns about epilepsy. *Clinical Nursing Practice in Epilepsy* 1996; 3:11–12.

CHAPTER 50

Epilepsy, Cerebral Palsy, and IQ

W. Edwin Dodson, M.D.

In all cultures children with epilepsy exhibit a disproportionately high share of problems with learning and behavior (1–5). As a group, children with epilepsy have an average IQ that is 10 points below normal, resulting in a three-fold increased risk of mental retardation (4,6). (Figure 50-1). Even those children who are not retarded are at increased risk for academic underachievement or school failure and maladjustment in later life (3, 7–10). Pazzaglia and coworkers (11) found that among children with epilepsy in Cesena, Italy, only half had normal scholastic records. One-third were in special classes; 17 percent were one or more grades behind. Behaviorally, children with epilepsy have an increased risk of being described as fidgety, restless, irritable, inattentive, not liked, worrisome, solitary, disobedient, fussy, destructive, and are more likely to tell lies and fight with other children (12). They also are more likely to have temper tantrums, tics, sleep difficulties, poor appetite, loss of bowel control, lisping, stuttering, and headaches.

The specific component(s) of cognitive function that account for the problems of patients with epilepsy are not well defined. Studies in epileptic children who were not taking medications suggest that perceptual problems and attention are major factors (7). In adults with intractable seizures, verbal and comprehension problems contribute more to variability in their IQs than attention or perceptual issue (3).

Academic underachievement is more prevalent in boys than girls, a trend that persists among children with epilepsy. In the study summarized in Table 50-1, boys did worse in spelling than girls. Many factors were associated with underachievement in arithmetic. These included older age, generalized versus partial seizures, an earlier age of onset, and more seizures.

It is often difficult to determine the cause when children with epilepsy have academic or behavioral complaints. Parents and teachers tend to blame the epilepsy and/or the medication for the child's every imperfection. Isolating a cause is always complicated

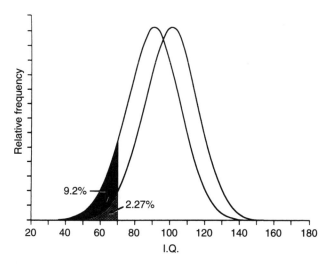

Figure 50-1. Frequency distribution of IQ in normal children and children with epilepsy. Adapted from Ellenberg JH, Hirtz D, Nelson KB. Do seizures cause intellectual deterioration? *N Engl J Med* 1986; 314:1085–1088.

Table 50-1. Academic Achievement among Children with Epilepsy Measured by the Wide Range Achievement Test (WRAT)

WRAT Subtest	Percent Underachieving	
	Boys	Girls
Word recognition	10.5	10.1
Spelling	33.3	15.9
Arithmetic	28.1	31.9
Reading comprehension	22.8	13.0

Source: Adapted from Seidenberg M, Beck N. Geisser M, et al. Academic achievement of children with epilepsy. *Epilepsia* 1986; 27:753–759

because numerous factors affect learning and behavior simultaneously. These factors include temperament, intrinsic developmental capability, associated brain disease, parent–child interactions, socioeconomic level, seizures, and medication-induced side effects. Some investigators have emphasized the importance of epilepsy or uncontrolled seizures, whereas others have highlighted the importance of other factors, especially drug therapy. Relatively few studies have considered the confounding effects of socioeconomic level. Among the many factors that influence a child's academic achievement in the population overall, socioeconomic status has the most pervasive influence (14,15).

Do seizures and epilepsy impair global intellectual ability? They usually do not. A majority of children with epilepsy develop normally and enjoy normal cognitive ability. Aside from immediate ictal and postictal interruptions of awareness, seizures usually do not impair cognition permanently; however, relationships between seizures, motor handicap, and intellectual impairment can be complex. Although etiology has the most powerful effect on intellectual outcome, other seizure-related variables are influential as well, and there are exceptions in which childhood epilepsy and cognitive impairment progress simultaneously, resulting in permanent encephalopathy.

In exploring the relationship between epilepsy and cognitive function, a sequential approach helps to clarify the issues. First, factors that are not related to epilepsy are considered. Next, epilepsy-related factors such as etiology, comorbid conditions, seizure type, frequency, age of onset, and duration are discussed. In Chapter 51 Professor Aldenkamp discusses the effects of drug therapy. Degenerative disorders in which neurologic deterioration is the primary feature are not discussed here. Throughout this chapter the reader should remember that seizures, like mental retardation and cerebral palsy, are symptoms of abnormal brain function.

TERMINOLOGY AND DEFINITIONS

The *intelligence quotient* or IQ has been defined as an individual's mental age divided by chronological age times 100. In determining IQ, many tests such as the Wechsler Adult Intelligence Scale (WAIS) do not require the actual calculation of a mental age but instead determine IQ based on standardized scale scores. The IQ is normally distributed in the general population with a mean of 100 and a standard deviation (SD) of 15 (Figure 50-2). Thus, by definition, approximately 2.3 percent of the population has an IQ that is equal to or less than 70, the IQ value that is two SDs below the mean.

Most investigators who have studied the relationship between epilepsy and IQ report IQ values as

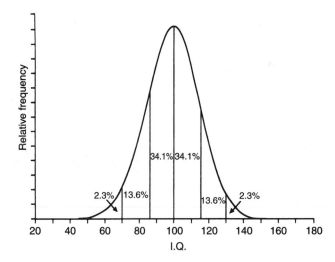

Figure 50-2. The distribution of IQ scores showing standard deviations and percent of the population in each group.

group means and SDs. In such situations it is important to translate these values into terms that allow one to discern the magnitude of increased risk of mental retardation that is shared by group members. For example, if a particular group has an IQ of 90 with a SD of 20, 16.5 percent of those groups are expected to have an IQ of 70 or less. In this example, even though most group members have normal intellect, the risk of mental retardation is increased sevenfold among group members. Although groups of patients with epilepsy who have been studied with IQ measurements do not necessarily have normally distributed values, for purposes of comparison in this chapter I have assumed that all group values are distributed normally.

Mental retardation implies that an individual's global intellect and adaptation to the problems of living are defective and that these abnormalities have been present during development. This definition encompasses more than an IQ criterion; however, the IQ score is one dimension of adaptive ability that is measured objectively, and it predicts academic performance. The IQ score also is weighed heavily in the diagnosis of mental retardation. Thus, for purposes of this chapter, an IQ score of 70 or less is considered to indicate mental retardation.

Developmental disabilities are legally defined on a state-by-state basis. Nonetheless, federal legislation defined the condition as functional limitation in three or more major life activities. The major categories of activities include self-care, understanding and use of language, learning, mobility, self-direction, and capacity for independent living (16). The diagnosis of being developmentally disabled qualifies the child for important educational and rehabilitative benefits. Although disabled children between the ages of 3 and 20 years have federal guarantees of access to educational and rehabilitative services, the authority to determine eligibility and the responsibility for providing services is vested in the states. Disability determinations are not categorical by diagnosis but rather depend on the child's functional ability. Thus, seizures may or may not be handicapping depending on their frequency, severity, and time of occurrence.

Cerebral palsy encompasses a group of nonprogressive motor impairment syndromes secondary to lesions or brain abnormalities that arise early in development. The prevalence is 1.5 to 2.5 per 1,000 live births. The most common forms of cerebral palsy include hemiplegia (right side twice as frequent as left), spastic diplegia, and spastic quadriplegia. Less common forms include ataxic and athetoid disorders. Cerebral palsy, mental retardation, and epilepsy are often simultaneous manifestations of diffuse brain lesions that were acquired prenatally.

Definitions of *learning disability* vary depending on the source, but generally the term implies that an individual's actual performance on measures of academic skills such as reading or arithmetic is substantially inferior to what would be predicted from that individual's global cognitive ability measured by the IQ. Most investigators designate an individual as learning disabled when that individual's IQ and measured academic skills differ by 1 SD or more. School systems in the United States have more complex definitions of learning disability such that individuals with lower IQ scores require less statistical discrepancy between IQ and measures of scholastic skills to qualify for special remedial help than individuals with normal or above average IQ scores.

Studies of learning disabilities are more difficult to compare than studies of global cognitive ability because of the many issues that are involved in learning disabilities, including inconsistent definitions of the condition (17,18). In studying learning disabilities, various investigators have different theoretical orientations and use different technical approaches. Although the role of factors such as strategic orientation, cognitive style, and motivation have been emphasized in the past, current theory points to defective auditory processing as the seminal abnormality in dyslexia, the most common learning disability (9).

For these reasons, I focus this chapter on studies that reported IQ scores. Similarly, cognitive functioning is emphasized more than behavior here because the studies are more homogeneous and allow conclusions to be drawn.

NON–EPILEPSY-RELATED VARIABLES

Associated disease and social class are important background factors that interact with epilepsy and with antiepileptic therapy to influence behavior and cognitive ability in individual patients (14,15). Although many variables affect IQ, most of the determinants of IQ cannot be defined in large-scale investigations. In these types of studies, the largest determinant of IQ is socioeconomic class.

Socioeconomic Status

The National Collaborative Perinatal Project evaluated the relationship between various health-related and social factors and IQ measured at 7 years. Overall, the strongest determinants of intellect were socioeconomic class and related variables such as maternal education. However, considering all predictor variables, the investigators could account for only 25 percent to 28 percent of the variance in IQ among whites and 15 percent to 17 percent among blacks (10). The highest correlation ($r = 0.38$) was found between socioeconomic index and IQ. This value yields a coefficient of determination of approximately 8 percent, indicating that 8 percent of the variability in IQ is linked to socioeconomic class. The correlation between the mother's nonverbal IQ and the child's IQ was lower ($r = 0.28$). The effects of socioeconomic factors are manifest in various ways. For example, 20.2 percent of children from families in the lowest socioeconomic class failed a test of language comprehension at age 8 years, as compared with only a 2 percent failure rate for those from the highest social class (20).

Studies of epilepsy and IQ that considered socioeconomic variables have confirmed that the influence of socioeconomic class on IQ is universal. The findings have been similar in India and in western countries (11). Furthermore, sociocultural context plays a major role in the attitudes and behaviors about epilepsy (12).

The nature and quality of the parent–child interaction is also an important contributor to the child's cognitive development and behavior. Whereas seizure-related variables heavily influence medical outcome, sociocultural differences and the quality of the parent–child interactions exert the preponderant effects on the child's behavioral outcome and statistically have a more far reaching influence than disease-related factors (22,23). Furthermore, even after seizures are controlled, flawed early psychosocial development can continue to thwart the maturation of skills necessary for productive, independent functioning (24).

EPILEPSY-RELATED VARIABLES AND IQ

The etiology of a child's epilepsy is the best predictor of cognitive functioning. Unfortunately, in a majority of patients the etiology cannot be identified.

Instead of having an etiological or lesional diagnosis, the diagnosis is descriptive by seizure type or by epileptic syndrome. When the etiology is identified, the relationship between the epilepsy and intellect is usually clear-cut. As the diagnosis of epilepsy becomes more descriptive, that is, by epileptic syndrome or by seizure type, the situation is less predictable.

Specific Etiologies

Among all epilepsy-related variables, the etiology of the epilepsy has the most pervasive effect on cognitive ability (Table 50-2). In most cases in which people with epilepsy are impaired intellectually or behaviorally, underlying brain disease, not epilepsy, is the major contributor to the difficulties.

Studies from the National Collaborative Perinatal Project indicate that associated brain disease, not seizures, is the most important contributor to subnormal intellect among children with epilepsy. In population-based studies of epilepsy and IQ, there is no evidence that epilepsy causes intellectual deficit. Rather, the antecedent conditions that cause epilepsy are associated with lowered group IQ. Among youngsters who began to have seizures between the ages of 4 and 7 years, the group IQ was similar to that of well-matched controls (4) (Table 50-3). By and large, the appearance of seizures in otherwise normal children does not predict reduced IQ.

When patients with symptomatic versus idiopathic epilepsy are compared, the symptomatic group have

Table 50-2. Examples of Etiologies of Symptomatic Epilepsy that also Affect Global Cognitive Function

Perinatal asphyxia
Symptomatic neonatal hypoglycemia
Neurocutaneous disorders
   Tuberous sclerosis
   Neurofibromatosis
   Hypomelanosis of Ito
Chromosomal disorders
   Down's syndrome
   Fragile X syndrome
   Microdeletion syndromes
      Angelman's syndrome
      Prader-Willi syndrome
Inborn errors of metabolism (untreated)
Rett's syndrome
Progressive myoclonus epilepsies
   Unverricht-Lundborg disease
   Lafora body disease
   Northern epilepsy syndrome
Central nervous system infections
   Meningitis
   Encephalitis
   Subacute sclerosing panencephalitis (SSPE)

Table 50-3. Effect of Epilepsy on IQ at Age 7 Years from the National Collaborative Perinatal Project

	EPILEPSY		CONTROLS	
	n	IQ	n	IQ
All children	368	90.0(13)	—	102.9(13)
Sibling comparison	98	91.5(20.9)	98	95.3(15.1)
Normal early evaluation	59	99.8(14.9)	59	98.0(13)
Onset between age 4 and 7 years	62	94.5	4,154	96.5

Values shown are means and standard deviations.
Source: Ellenberg JH, Hirtz D, Nelson KB. Do seizures cause intellectual deterioration? *N Engl J Med* 1986; 314:1085–1088.

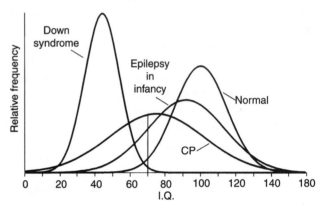

Figure 50-3. IQ distributions for people affected by disorders associated with epilepsy. Developed from information in Broman SH, Nichols PL, Kennedy WA. *Preschool IQ Prenatal and Early Developmental Correlates.* Hillsdale, N.J.: Lawrence Erlbaum Associates, Publishers, 1975.

lower IQs. For example, in a prospective study of children with new-onset epilepsy, the mean IQ for the symptomatic group was 89.1 (SD 29.6) compared to 102.5 (SD 16.1) for the idiopathic group (2) (Figure 50-3). Differences of this magnitude lead to approximately a 10-fold increased chance of mental retardation among children with symptomatic epilepsy (25.8% vs. 2.3%).

Symptomatic epilepsy caused by a cerebral lesion heightens the chance of cognitive impairment even when the cause of the lesion is not known. The impact of structural brain abnormalities varies with the location of the lesion and the timing of its intrusion on brain circuitry as well as the intensity and frequency of the seizures that the lesion causes.

Brain malformations can cause both epilepsy and mental impairment. Malformations range from being subtle and localized in the case of focal cortical dysplasia to pervasive and dramatic in the case of lissencephaly. Recently recognized cerebral malformations such as double cortex, frontal opercular syndrome, and congenital bilateral perisylvian syndrome have variably severe adverse effects on cognition (25–27). Despite improvements in imaging, specific brain malformations such as bilateral parasagittal polymicrogyria can still be difficult to detect on imaging tests, and it can cause a spectrum of cognitive problems plus epilepsy that begins in childhood (28). The range of cognitive impairments linked to bilateral parasagittal polymicrogyria extends from normal functioning to mild retardation and includes subtle problems such as normal intelligence with slow mental processing.

Since the first edition of this book was published, the proportion of epilepsy that is recognized as symptomatic of brain lesions has increased because of the vast improvements in imaging techniques. These advances have allowed visualization of increasingly subtle brain lesions that can produce severe epilepsy despite their inconspicuous appearance. Contemporary magnetic resonance imaging (MRI) procedures allow visualization of mesial temporal lobe and other brain structures that previously were obscure. Consequently, variations in these structures are being linked to cognitive differences among people with epilepsy. For example, Strauss and coworkers found that among a group of people with epilepsy, the size of the posterior corpus callosum correlated positively with IQ (29). As more neurons connect to each other via the corpus callosum, the corpus callosum enlarges.

Chromosomal disorders illustrate how a particular etiology can produce both seizures and mental retardation independently. Among patients with Down's syndrome the average IQ is 43.5 (SD 10.1), resulting in a 99 percent chance that patients with this disorder will be mentally retarded, independent of epilepsy (30). Angelman's "happy puppet" syndrome

and Prader-Willi syndrome are both caused by a microdeletion of a portion of the long arm of chromosome 15 (31). Seizures are an invariable component of Angelman's syndrome but occur in only 20 percent of children with Prader-Willi syndrome; however, subnormal intellect is a major feature of both disorders.

X-linked mental retardation is the most common inherited cause of mental subnormality. Associated with fragile X chromosome in 25 percent to 50 percent of cases, mental handicap is a uniform feature of this disorder. Although seizures occur in 20 percent of patients, they have a negligible relationship to intellect (32,33).

In some instances of symptomatic seizures, both the etiology and the actual occurrence of seizures affect the cognitive outcome. The various causes of neonatal seizures help to illustrate how these relationships operate. Certain etiologies of neonatal seizures are benign, whereas others have grave consequences for intellectual outcome.

For example, hypocalcemia in the context of late neonatal tetany can cause dramatic and numerous seizures, but it does not increase the risk of mental retardation unless there are additional complications. On the other hand, neonatal hypoglycemia that causes seizures approximately doubles the risk of mental handicap compared with symptomatic neonatal hypoglycemia that does not cause seizures (34). Asymptomatic hypoglycemia only slightly increases the risk of subsequent cognitive impairment. Therefore, etiology can influence the cognitive consequences of the seizures. In certain etiologies such as hypoglycemia, however, the actual occurrence of seizures is a critical step in the pathogenesis of the adverse intellectual outcome.

In pyridoxine dependency, the number and duration of seizures contributes to the adverse cognitive outcome in children who otherwise would be normal if treated with vitamin B6. Mental retardation occurs mainly in those individuals who have numerous seizures as a result of pyridoxine dependency but usually not in those who have only a few (20–23). Pyridoxine dependency can be difficult to identify. It initially was believed that pyridoxine dependency caused only neonatal seizures and neonatal status epilepticus. Subsequently, pyridoxine dependency was found to cause other types of seizures, including epileptic syndromes that are associated with cognitive decline. Those patients who experience the worst seizures in terms of seizure types, seizure frequency, and duration of epilepsy have a high risk of irreversible cognitive impairment. To make the condition all the more difficult to diagnose, the seizures caused by pyridoxine dependency are partially responsive to antiepileptic drugs like other forms of epilepsy.

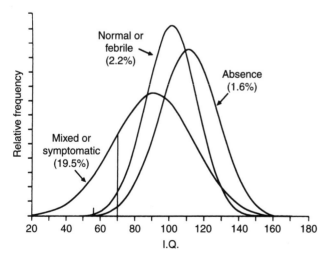

Figure 50-4. Frequency distributions of IQ scores among children with various seizure types. The percentage values shown in parentheses indicate the proportion of the group that is expected to have an IQ of 70 or less. The average and standard deviations (SD) for the groups are febrile 100.7 (SD 24.0), mixed 91.2 (SD 22.7), and generalized absence 109.7 (SD 16.4).

Perinatal asphyxia causes a distinctive combination of cerebral palsy, mental retardation, and epilepsy. Findings from the National Collaborative Perinatal Project revealed that when perinatal asphyxia in full-term newborns caused later epilepsy, it also caused cerebral palsy (30). In the absence of cerebral palsy, no relationship was found between various measures of perinatal asphyxia and the occurrence of epilepsy in later childhood (38). Among 87 newborns who had Apgar scores of 0 to 3 at 10 minutes and who did not develop cerebral palsy, none developed epilepsy during the 7-year follow-up period.

Similar to the relationship between etiology and cognitive impairment, the underlying brain disease, more so than seizure-related variables, increases the risk of behavior disorders. Beran and Flanagan (39) compared adults who had posttraumatic versus idiopathic epilepsy of comparable severity using the Washington Psychosocial Seizure Inventory. There were differences across eight measures that indicated that the extent of brain dysfunction correlated with psychosocial dysfunction more than the severity of the epilepsy. Corbett and coworkers (40) concluded that among children with epilepsy, brain damage and dysfunction were of greater importance in causing behavioral problems than medication. Deb (41) studied the relationship between epilepsy and psychopathology among mentally retarded people and found that the underlying brain damage was more influential in producing behavioral symptoms than seizures.

Associated Neurological Symptoms — Comorbidities

The linkage between mental retardation, epilepsy and cerebral palsy is well established. Historically, one-third of children with cerebral palsy developed epilepsy. However, as obstetrical and perinatal medical care has improved, the distribution of different forms of cerebral palsy have changed and the incidence of epilepsy in cerebral palsy also has changed (42). In various series, epilepsy has been most likely to occur in hypotonic and spastic hemiplegic or tetraplegic forms of cerebral palsy (43,44). It is less common with spastic diplegia (44). Cerebral palsy has also been linked to the onset of epilepsy in the first year of life, to neonatal seizures, and to a high incidence of mental retardation (45). Among infants with hypotonia, the mean IQ is 80 (SD 24.9), leading to a 34.6 percent risk of mental retardation (20). Among children with cerebral palsy as defined in the National Collaborative Perinatal Project, the mean IQ was 74.8 (SD 27.2), resulting in a 43.5 percent risk of mental retardation (20). Cerebral palsy is the most important single risk factor for severe epilepsy among young children (46,47).

In the presence of mental retardation the risk of epilepsy increases with the severity of the mental handicap (Table 50-4). The lower the IQ, the more likely that

Table 50-4. Occurrence of Epilepsy Among Various Intellectual Categories

Intellectual Category	Prevalence of Epilepsy
Normal IQ	1%
Mild mental retardation (IQ 50–70)	15%
Severe mental retardation (IQ < 50)	47%

Source: Adapted from Susser M. Hauser WA, Kiely JL, et al. Quantitative estimates of prenatal and perinatal risk factors for perinatal mortality, cerebral palsy, mental retardation and epilepsy. In: Freeman J, ed. *Prenatal and Perinatal Factors Associated with Brain Disorders*. NIH Publication No. 85-1149, 1985; 359–439.

the child will also have epilepsy and the less likely that the seizures will respond to treatment. Conversely, among children who are mentally retarded, those who also have epilepsy are more severely retarded (48). Chelune and coworkers (49) reported that among people with IQ of 75 or less, the chance of failure of surgical treatment was fourfold greater than when the IQ was higher. The concurrence of multiple neurologic handicaps has an adverse compounding effect on the child's overall functionality, with the combined deficits having multiplicative rather than additive impact on the child's functioning (50). A majority of severely retarded children have definable brain abnormalities that are known to heighten the risk of epilepsy. For example, in one series the causes of severe retardation (IQ < 50) included the following: chromosomal abnormalities (36%), congenital malformations (20%), perinatal complications or infections (12%), and single locus genetic diseases (7%). Only 3 percent had postnatal causes, and the unknown/other category accounted for 22 percent ().

Studies conducted since the completion of the National Collaborative Perinatal Project have provided more refined information about the interrelationship between epilepsy, mental retardation, and cerebral palsy (51). Ignoring whether the mental retardation is associated with cerebral palsy, the overall risk of epilepsy among mentally retarded people is 15 percent. Among mentally retarded children without cerebral palsy, the risk of developing epilepsy by age 22 years is substantially lower (5.2%). Mental retardation plus cerebral palsy increases the risk of developing epilepsy by age 22 approximately sixfold to 38 percent. Mental retardation that has been acquired as a result of postnatal causes carries an even higher risk of also developing epilepsy (66%).

Other manifestations of brain disease and epilepsy are interrelated in children who are neurologically abnormal (Table 50-5). In young infants coincidental congenital disorders that do not seem to affect the nervous system directly nonetheless can be adversely

Table 50-5. Associations of Comorbid Neurologic Handicaps in Children from the National Collaborative Perinatal Project (NCPP)

	Dependent Variable			
	CP	**SZ**	**MMR**	**SMR**
Independent Variable				
CP	33.9%	30%	30%	
CP and MR		38%		
Hemiplegia		50%		
Quadriplegia		27%		75%
SZ	19%		27%	
MR	20%	13–22%		
Postnatal MR	66%			
SMR	20%	47%		
Autism		25%		

CP = cerebral palsy; SZ = seizures; MMR = mild mental retardation; SMR = severe mental retardation; MR = mental retardation. Independent variables are listed in the left most column. (30,51,93,94).

related to IQ. For example, congenital heart disease is associated with a 10-point reduction in mean IQ from 100 to 90.4 (SD 23.5), resulting in a 19.8 percent risk of having an IQ below 70 (30). The mechanisms by which such associated conditions reduce IQ are undefined. Most of these patients have static, nonprogressive intellectual deficits unless additional insults to brain occur.

Among youngsters with congenital neurologic abnormalities the symptoms of mental retardation, motor disability, and epilepsy are tightly intertwined. These associations notwithstanding, the etiology of the brain dysfunction remains the principal determinant of IQ.

EPILEPTIC SYNDROMES

Approximately 50 percent of children who have epilepsy can be categorized into one of the epileptic syndromes. Epileptic syndromes are descriptive phenotypic groupings and nonspecific in regard to etiology. A given syndrome can result from many causes and be either symptomatic or idiopathic (primary). In most instances the idiopathic cases have the better prognosis for control with medication, eventual remission, and intellectual outcome.

The appeal of epileptic syndromes types of epilepsy as diagnostic groups is rooted in the need for a descriptive diagnostic terminology that is more informative than seizure type. Several clinical elements define the various syndromes. These include seizure type(s), precipitating factors, electroencephalogram (EEG) patterns (both ictal and interictal), the age of onset, response to various medications, natural history, and associated clinical features such as whether the patient has

Table 50-6. Examples of Epileptic Syndromes and Prognosis for Cognitive Function

Unfavorable Cognitive Development
  West syndrome (infantile spasms)
  Lennox-Gastaut syndrome
  Doose's syndrome
  Landau-Kleffner syndrome
  Rett's Syndrome
Favorable Cognitive Development
  Febrile seizures
  Childhood absence epilepsy (petit mal, pyknolepsy)
  Benign partial epilepsy of childhood (rolandic epilepsy)
  Juvenile myoclonic epilepsy

encephalopathy (52). The last two features, the natural history and the presence or absence of encephalopathy, are central to this discussion because syndromic groupings usually imply an intellectual prognosis. For example, the encephalopathic epilepsies, such as West syndrome, Lennox-Gastaut syndrome, and Doose's syndrome, are regularly associated with cognitive impairment. In other syndromes, such as childhood absence epilepsy, the prognosis is benign, including the intellectual outcome (Table 50-6). Therefore, by including associated clinical features such as encephalopathy in the diagnostic criteria, epileptic syndromes are self-fulfilling in relation to predicting cognitive deficits.

ENCEPHALOPATHIC EPILEPSIES

Epileptic encephalopathy (or encephalopathic epilepsy) is a term that has been used to describe the development of mental impairment that is apparently caused by a high frequency of uncontrolled seizures. The usual progression of events is stagnation of development, which causes the affected child to be left behind developmentally. Less often the child actually regresses developmentally because of the loss of previously acquired skills and knowledge.

The epilepsies that lead to the progressive encephalopathy are poorly understood. The major ones, West syndrome and Lennox-Gastaut syndrome, are both characterized by early childhood onset, high seizure frequencies, and multiple types of seizures. The disorders are interrelated in that many of the infants who develop infantile spasms later evolve a clinical pattern of Lennox-Gastaut syndrome. West syndrome consists of infantile spasms, an EEG pattern of hypsarrhythmia, and developmental arrest. Lennox-Gastaut syndrome includes multiple seizure types, especially tonic, astatic, partial, and atypical absence seizures; developmental arrest; and a slow spike-wave pattern on EEG. Doose's syndrome is idiopathic and shares features of Lennox-Gastaut syndrome. Normal intellect can be preserved if seizures can be controlled in Doose's syndrome, but mental impairment accrues if seizures rage on.

Other epilepsies in which encephalopathy is a consistent and integral feature include acquired epileptic aphasia (the Landau-Kleffner syndrome), a disorder of epileptic seizures with electrical status epilepticus in slow-wave sleep (ESES), and Rett's syndrome, a degenerative condition that has its onset in girls in the first or second year of life. Whereas Landau-Kleffner and ESES are reversible in some cases, Rett's syndrome is usually relentlessly degenerative in nature. Encephalopathy is a dominant clinical feature in these disorders (see Chapter 15).

SEIZURE TYPE

Generalized seizures and generalized epileptiform patterns on the EEG have been linked to greater degrees of cognitive impairment than partial seizures. One comparison of neuropsychological test results for people with partial seizures and those with partial secondarily generalized seizures found that those with secondarily generalization perform less well on tests of concentration and mental flexibility (53). Moreover, these differences were present before drug therapy was initiated. In another study that looked at the effects of partial versus partial secondarily generalized seizures, patients with only partial seizures did better than those with secondary generalization on subtests of arithmetic, digit span, digit symbol, block design, and object assembly (54). Wilkus and Dodrill (55) found that on 11 of 15 Halstead-Reitan measures patients with generalized EEG discharges did worst, patients with focal EEG discharges did intermediate, and patients with no epileptiform EEG discharges did best.

Table 50-7. Seizure Types and Average IQ Among Children 6–15 Years Old

Seizure Type	Group Average IQ
Minor motor	70
Atypical absence	74
Partial and generalized	96
Partial only	98
Generalized tonic-clonic	99
Classic absence and generalized tonic-clonic	106

Source: Farwell JR, Dodrill CB, Gatzel LW. Neuropsychological abilities of children with epilepsy. *Epilepsia* 1985; 26:305–400.

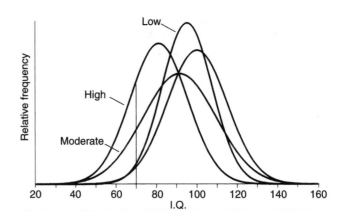

Figure 50-5. Effect of seizure frequency on full-scale IQ among people having seizure frequencies that were low (3 or fewer seizures per year), moderate (4–12 seizures per year) or high (12 or more seizures per year). Adapted from Dikmen S, Matthews CG, Harley JP. Effect of early versus late onset of major motor epilepsy on cognitive-intellectual performance: further considerations. *Epilepsia* 1977; 18:31–36.

Data from Farwell and coworkers (3) (Table 50-7) and from Bourgeois and colleagues (2) (Figure 50-5) illustrate how the patient's predominant seizure type correlates with IQ. For example, generalized absence seizures are a feature of many epileptic syndromes, some benign and some ominous. Absence seizures that occur in petit mal epilepsy bear a substantially better prognosis than atypical absence seizures that are coupled with other types of generalized seizures such as astatic seizures or drop attacks. Atypical absence seizures and astatic or drop seizures have been labeled collectively as minor motor seizures; these seizures have a poor prognosis for mental development and functioning. Groups of children with classic absence seizures have a mean IQ that is above average. These youngsters probably have childhood absence epilepsy (petit mal epilepsy, pyknolepsy) whereas those patients with classic absence and generalized tonic-clonic seizures most likely have juvenile myoclonic epilepsy, both of which are genetically determined and are linked to normal or superior intellect. However, absence seizures, especially atypical absence seizures, are linked to some of the worst cognitive outcomes when they occur in children with encephalopathic epilepsy such as infantile spasms or Lennox-Gastaut syndrome. Consistent with these relationships, hospital-based studies of children have found that nonconvulsive absence seizures are associated with lower cognitive scores than convulsive seizures (56).

The major drawback with trying to relate seizure type to intellectual outcome is that the classification of seizure types provides only limited information. Seizure type alone is nonspecific in relation to either etiology or epileptic syndrome because individual seizure types occur in several different syndromes.

Therefore, attempts to correlate seizure types with cognitive ability usually fall short because the groupings invariably encompass diverse etiologies and syndromes.

LOCALIZATION OF PARTIAL SEIZURES

Along with seizure type, seizure frequency, and epileptic syndrome the localization of partial seizures is sometimes related to difficulty with learning and cognition (57,58). However, these relationships tend to be inconsistent from one patient to the next, possibly because of inaccuracy in reliably locating the epileptic focus. Fixed cerebral lesions and neurologic deficits produce more consistent clinical pictures, whereas interictal EEG epileptic foci tend to wander over time. Moreover, the types of abnormality found in repeated recordings from the same individuals can fluctuate over time, switching from focal to generalized epileptiform patterns and vice versa (59). Furthermore, localized discharges also vary in their distant effects on other brain regions that play key roles in cognition. Positron emission tomography (PET) scans have demonstrated depressed cerebral metabolic activity in areas that are remote from EEG-defined epileptic foci (60). These mechanisms of distant neuronal suppression appear to impair cognitive processing more so than memory.

Nonetheless, many investigators have tried to relate the cerebral lateralization of focal seizures to cognitive and behavioral outcomes. The results of this line of research generally support the theory that left-sided lesions are prone to interfere with verbal cognitive functions (61). Muszkat and coworkers compared 26 children with partial epilepsy with 61 children who did not have epilepsy. Overall, the children with epilepsy did less well than the control group. Furthermore, right hemisphere EEG spike lateralization was linked to lower scores on measures of spatial ability and nonverbal attention. Left hemisphere spike lateralization was linked to low scores on only digit span. Mitchell and coworkers found that children with epilepsy tend to have slower reaction time and more variable performance, and make more errors of omission, but not commission, than normal control children (62).

Hermann and colleagues (63) compared patients with left versus right temporal lobe EEG foci. Subjects with left EEG foci did worse than either patients with right temporal foci or control subjects on verbal learning ability, immediate memory, and retrieval of verbal material from memory. Patients with left temporal lobe foci also had more problems with semantic organization, whereas the group with right temporal abnormalities did as well as controls. In another study, adult patients with left, but not right, temporal lobe

EEG foci had reduced recognition of symbols presented tachistoscopically in their right visual fields. However, epileptic patients as a group had worse retention (memory) for the symbols than controls (64). In yet other studies, left-sided lateralization of the epileptic focus was linked to loss of verbal abilities, whereas right-sided lateralization was linked to loss of nonverbal cognitive functions (65). Verbal-manual tasks used to assess cerebral organization for language indicate those children with left, but not right, hemisphere EEG foci have atypical patterns of hemispheric dominance such as bihemispheric dominance (66).

Whereas linkages between cognitive difficulties and the laterality of EEG foci tend to be inconsistent, structural hemispheric lesions that produce hemiplegia have more dependable relationships to cognitive outcome. Sussova and coworkers reported that among children with hemiplegic cerebral palsy, 80 percent had paroxysmal EEG features, although less than half actually had seizures (67). In these children, the presence of epilepsy, not simply EEG abnormalities, was linked to lower IQ scores. Interestingly, in this particular study, right hemisphere lesions were more often linked to low IQ than left hemisphere lesions. In a different study, left hemispheric dysfunction producing right hemiplegia and epilepsy was linked to reduced IQ scores (14).

In children with tuberous sclerosis, the higher the number of lesions on MRI, the lower the IQ, the worse the behavior, and the more severe the epilepsy (68). There are also relationships between the age of onset and cognitive outcome in tuberous sclerosis. Epileptic foci in the left hemisphere have been linked to behavior disturbances, too. Corbett and coworkers (40) found that patients whose seizures originated in the left hemisphere were more likely to have behavioral problems, including destruction of property, worrying, irritability, fussiness, and being resentful and aggressive. Overall, however, in comparisons of the influence of various epilepsy-related variables on cognitive outcome, laterality of the epileptic seizure has been a less powerful covariable than age of onset (69).

INTERRELATIONSHIPS OF EPILEPSY-RELATED VARIABLES

Epilepsy-related variables that are linked to cognitive ability tend to be interrelated and often occur simultaneously. As seen in the sections that follow, age of onset and duration of epilepsy are closely intertwined. Collectively, these variables seem to relate in a loose manner to the overall intensity of the epileptic disorder. Dikmen and Matthews (70) evaluated 14 measures from the Halstead-Reitan Battery in adults who were categorized on the basis of seizure frequency, age of onset, and duration of epilepsy. Seizure frequency was directly related to reductions on 7 of 14 measures. Specifically, the average full-scale IQ declined from 95 to 81 as seizure frequency increased from 3 or less per year to more than 12 per year (Figure 50-5). When these investigators combined all three risk factors and compared the 12 patients with lowest risk and the 12 who had the highest risk, most cognitive measures were worse in the highest risk group—those patients who had the earliest onset, longest duration, and highest seizure frequency.

AGE OF ONSET OF EPILEPSY

Many investigations have found relationships between the age of onset of seizures and IQ (2,3,71,75). In the study by Farwell and coworkers (3), the correlation between age of onset and full-scale IQ was 0.30: the older the age of onset, the higher the IQ. Overall, the onset of epilepsy in the first year of life has an ominous prognosis (72,73). A long-term prospective study of 133 children whose epilepsy began in the first year found that 11 percent died before reaching age 7 years, 40 percent were severely retarded, and only 40 percent had an IQ of greater than 70 (74). The prognosis was the same regardless of whether the child had infantile spasms or another type of epilepsy.

In the National Collaborative Perinatal Project, epilepsy in the first year of life was associated with an average IQ of 91.8 (SD 22.0), which would result in 16.7 percent of this group being mentally retarded (4). In clinic-based studies, the variables of age of onset and duration of epilepsy are usually interrelated. For example, Dikmen and coworkers (71) found that among adults with persistent epilepsy that began in childhood, the average group IQ declines in relation to the age of onset, the younger age of onset the lower the IQ score (Table 50-8). In addition, the early-onset group did worse on all 10 WAIS subtests, with statistically significant differences occurring on information, comprehension, arithmetic, and object assembly.

Seizure-related variables can interact simultaneously with etiology and the location of cerebral lesions to contribute to the child's cognitive capabilities. For example, in tuberous sclerosis the age of onset of seizures correlates with IQ: the earlier the onset of seizures, the lower the IQ (75) (Figure 50-6). Whereas most people with tuberous sclerosis are mentally retarded, virtually all mentally retarded people with tuberous sclerosis also have epilepsy. Finally, the location of the cerebral lesion(s) in tuberous sclerosis plays a pivotal role in determining the overall clinical picture (68).

Table 50-8. Age of Seizure Onset and IQ Among Adults Who Had Childhood Onset of Epilepsy that Lasted for 4 or More Years[a]

	Age of Onset	
	Early (0–5)	Late (10–15)
Number of subjects	22	22
Duration (years)	22.28 (10.4)	23.6 (9.68)
Verbal IQ	81.04 (13.45)	91.00 (17.37)[b]
Performance IQ	78.14 (15.25)	88.41 (16.22)[b]
Full-scale IQ	78.5 (14.1)	89.36 (17.22)[b]
Fraction retarded	28.5%	13.7%

[a] Values in parenthesis are standard deviations.
[b] $P < 0.01$
Source: Adapted from Dikmen S, Matthews CG, Harley JP. Effect of early versus late onset of major motor epilepsy on cognitive-intellectual performance: further considerations. *Epilepsia* 1977; 18:31–36.

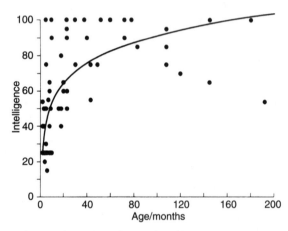

Figure 50-6. Relationship of age onset of seizures to IQ scores in children with tuberous sclerosis. Reproduced with permission from Gomez MR. *Tuberous Sclerosis.* 2nd ed. New York, Raven Press, 1988.

SEIZURE FREQUENCY

Seizure control usually results in improved cognitive function (75–78). Farwell and coworkers found that among children whose seizures were controlled, the mean IQ was 99.6 compared with 87.0 for the group with continuing seizures (3). Improved seizure control leads to improved neuropsychological performance (79) (Table 50-9). Among those patients whose seizure frequency declined, there were overall improvements in IQ plus improvements on 8 of 11 subtests. By contrast, only the performance IQ and object assembly score improved among those whose seizure frequency remained the same or increased. Although the severity of the epilepsy has been linked to the degree of mental handicap, the severity of mental handicap does not preclude good seizure control (80).

In benign partial epilepsy of childhood (rolandic epilepsy) spike frequency, not seizure frequency or

Table 50-9. Effect of Improved Seizure Control Among Young Adults with Epilepsy[a]

IG	Test	Retest
Verbal	91.96 (12.51)	95.55 (12.02)
Performance	86.09 (12.51)	96.32 (16.41)
Full Scale	88.78 (12.12)	95.64 (13.76)

[a] Values shown are means and standard deviations.
Source: Adapted from Seidenberg M, O'Leary DS, Berent S, Boll T. Changes in seizure frequency and test-retest scores on the Wechsler Adult Intelligence Scale. *Epilepsia* 1981; 22:75–83.

lateralization of the focus, has been linked to reduced IQ and other measures of cognition (81). Compared with control children, rolandic spikes led to impaired IQ, defective visual perception, short-term memory disturbance, and deteriorated psychiatric status and fine motor performance. However, the cognitive impediments usually resolve after rolandic epilepsy remits (82).

Intuitively, seizure frequency would seem to be associated with cognitive impairment because of the extremely high seizure frequency among children with encephalopathic epilepsies. In practice this association has been difficult to document, especially when the seizure frequency is moderate to low. For example, among children with febrile seizures, neither the number of seizures nor the duration of individual seizures was associated with a reduction in IQ among patients compared with siblings. In the National Collaborative Perinatal Project, among 36 children who had three or more febrile seizures, the full-scale IQ was 95.9 (SD 10.8) versus 95.9 (SD 11.6) in control siblings (83).

DURATION OF EPILEPSY

In most studies, the duration of epilepsy is related to the age of onset in that an early age of onset tends to be followed by a prolonged duration of the disorder. Thus, both of these factors are associated with reductions in group IQ scores. In some studies, the duration of epilepsy has been inversely correlated with IQ in children with a correlation coefficient of −0.40 (3). When adjusted for duration of seizure-free years, the correlation has been even stronger (−0.62).

Factors that predict persistent seizures are also linked to adverse cognitive outcomes for children with epilepsy. These include frequent seizures, an early age of onset, secondary generalization, symptomatic epilepsy as a result of structural brain lesions and abnormal neurologic status (84). When clinic-based groups of children who have partial seizures have been followed up for long periods, those who have

these features are at high risk for cognitive and social morbidity and seizure-related death (85,86).

Although population-based studies do not provide evidence that cognitive decline occurs in people with epilepsy, studies from institutions and referral centers indicate that severe epilepsy is occasionally followed by declining IQ scores. Corbett and coworkers (40) found that 15.7 percent of patients at Lingfield Hospital experienced a reduction in IQ of 15 or more points. Factors that were associated with decreased IQ included higher levels of primidone and phenytoin and lower folate levels but not the severity of EEG abnormalities or the seizure frequency. In a prospective clinic-based study of children with epilepsy, decreasing IQ scores were associated with earlier age of onset, more difficult to control seizures, having drug levels in toxic range, and having more drugs that caused toxicity (2). However, the mean IQ for the group as a whole did not decline. Whereas IQ scores declined in 11.1 percent, they increased in 16.7 percent.

Long-term follow-up of children with temporal lobe epilepsy indicate that a high percentage encounter academic failure if seizures continue unabated for years. In the series reported by Lindsay and coworkers, there were four seizure-related deaths before age 16 years. Ten of 58 children who were candidates for epilepsy surgery died. Among those whose seizures persisted and who were not treated surgically, only 25 of 45 completed regular school and 16 of 45 experienced early cognitive deterioration (85). Only 4 of the 45 members of this group were employable, and only 6 obtained driver's licenses.

EPILEPSY AND NEUROPSYCHIATRIC ADAPTION

Although adults with epilepsy have a greater risk of neuropsychiatric problems, the nature and extent of these problems is difficult to characterize. In the Veterans Administration Collaborative Study, 118 patients were compared with normal controls before therapy (53). Patients with epilepsy had significantly worse scores on 14 of 18 neuropsychological measures before medication was started. However, the risk of neuropsychological compromise among adult patients with epilepsy seems to be the same as among patients with other chronic neurologic ailments. Hermann and coworkers (87) found no differences as a result of seizure type or age of onset on Minnesota Multiphasic Personality Inventory (MMPI) measures of psychopathology, but epilepsy per se was associated with a greater risk of problems. After an extensive analysis of MMPI profiles from the literature, other investigators have concluded that, compared to people without epilepsy, patients with epilepsy are at higher risk for psychopathology, but the risk associated with epilepsy is similar to chronic disease in general (88). In a later report, Dodrill and Batzel (89) reiterated that patients with epilepsy are at greater risk than normal but argued that the risk of psychopathology for people with epilepsy is the same as for people with other neurologic disease; both of the neurologic disease groups, epileptic and nonepileptic, have higher risk than patients with chronic, nonneurologic diseases. The excess of psychopathology among people with neurologic disease is manifest primarily as a high prevalence of psychotic MMPI profiles for both epileptic and other neurologic groups.

Studies in adults that relate seizure type to distinctive personality profiles are controversial. Although some investigators have suggested that adults with temporal lobe epilepsy have distinctive personalities, others have been unable to confirm it (88,89). Thus, a majority of investigators conclude that temporal lobe epilepsy is no worse than any other type of epilepsy in this regard. Dodrill and Batzel (89), in reviewing this issue, also criticized the item content of the MMPI as being inappropriate for people with epilepsy. In general, when adults with epilepsy have psychopathology, it tends to be severe (88). Depression is a particularly common problem (90).

Psychological tests in teenagers do correlate with overall adjustment later in adulthood. Dodrill and Clemmons (91) followed up patients with epilepsy 5.9 (SD 1.86) years after their original evaluations during adolescence. The patients were rated on vocational adjustment (unemployed to full-time employment—four categories) and on daily life functioning (fully dependent to independent—three categories). The MMPI did not predict either vocational adjustment or daily life functioning. Predictive measures of being fully functional (adequate in both vocational and independence measures) included the Halstead Impairment Index, Seashore Rhythm, Aphasia Screening (total errors), and verbal, performance, and full-scale IQ. Discriminant function analysis indicated that vocational adjustment related best to the Halstead Impairment Index, whereas independence in living was predicted by Seashore Rhythm and Thematic Perception Test (memory). Language skills were especially important. In a separate study, marital adjustment among adults with epilepsy was more related to emotional adjustment, whereas living independently was related to mental ability (92).

CONCLUSIONS

Although most children with epilepsy are developmentally and behaviorally normal, as a group children with epilepsy have an average IQ that is approximately 10 points lower than in children without epilepsy. Learning disabilities are also more prevalent among children

with epilepsy. Boys are at higher risk than girls. The lower IQ found among groups of epileptic children is largely a consequence of antecedent etiologically specific neurologic abnormalities rather than a consequence of seizures or antiepileptic drug therapy.

Although seizures do not cause intellectual decline in most cases, certain exceptional encephalopathic epileptic syndromes are associated with abnormal development and intellectual decline. These severe epilepsies are so rare that they are not encountered to a meaningful extent in most population-based studies. Among all epileptic syndromes, childhood absence epilepsy (pyknolepsy or petit mal epilepsy) alone is associated with an above average IQ.

The risk of associated mental retardation in patients with epilepsy is increased when epilepsy begins at an early age, when the duration of epilepsy is prolonged, when there are multiple seizure types—especially minor motor seizures—and when multiple drugs in high doses are required for seizure control.

REFERENCES

1. Addy DP. Cognitive function in children with epilepsy. *Dev Med Child Neurol* 1987; 29:394–397.

2. Bourgeois BFD, Prensky AL, Palkes HS, et al. Intelligence in epilepsy: a prospective study in children. *Ann Neurol* 1983; 14:438–444.

3. Farwell JR, Dodrill CB, Batzel LW. Neuropsychological abilities of children with epilepsy. *Epilepsia* 1985; 26:395–400.

4. Ellenberg JH, Hirtz D, Nelson KB. Do seizures cause intellectual deterioration? *N Engl J Med* 1986; 314:1085–1088

5. Sturniolo MG, Galletti F. Idiopathic epilepsy and school achievement. *Arch Dis Child* 1994; 70:424–428.

6. Pestana EM, Trujillo C, Sardinas N, Hernandez M. Intellectual achievements of the epileptic child in primary school. *Rev Neurol* 1996; 24:1513–1515.

7. Epir S, Renda Y, Baser N. Cognitive and behavioral characteristics of children with idiopathic epilepsy in a low-income area of Ankara, Turkey. *Dev Med Child Neurol* 1984; 26:201–207.

8. Seidenberg M, Beck N, Geisser M, et al. Academic achievement of children with epilepsy. *Epilepsia* 1986; 27:753–759.

9. Jennekens-Schinkel A, Linschooten-Duikersloot EM, Bouma PA, et al. Spelling errors made by children with mild epilepsy: writing to dictation. *Epilepsia* 1987; 28:555–563.

10. Jalava M, Sillanpaa M, Camfield C, Camfield P. Social adjustment and competence 35 years after onset of childhood epilepsy: a prospective controlled study. *Epilepsia* 1997; 38:708–715.

11. Pazzaglia P, Franke-Pazzaglia L. Record in grade school of pupils with epilepsy: an epidemiological study. *Epilepsia* 1976; 17:361–366.

12. Kurokawa T, Matsuo M, Yoshida K, et al. Behavioral disorders in Japanese epileptic children. *Folia Psychiatr Neurol Jpn* 1983; 37:259–265.

13. Bornstein RA, Drake ME Jr, Pakalnis A. WAIS R factor structure in epileptic patients. *Epilepsia* 1988; 29:14–18.

14. Glosser G, Cole LC, French JA, et al. Predictors of intellectual performance in adults with intractable temporal lobe epilepsy. *J Int Neuropsychol Soc* 1997; 252–259.

15. Mitchell WG, Chavez JM, Lee H, et al. Academic underachievement in children with epilepsy. *J Child Neurol* 1991; 6:65–72.

16. Hauser WA, Hesdorffer DC. *Epilepsy: Frequency, Causes and Consequences.* New York: Demos, 1990:120.

17. Feagans L. A current review of learning disabilities. *J Pediatr* 1983; 102:487–493.

18. Hammill DD. On defining learning disabilities: an emerging consensus. *J Learn Disabil* 1990; 23:74–84.

19. Shaywitz BA, Fletcher JM, Shaywitz SE. Defining and classifying learning disabilities and attention-deficit/hyperactivity disorder. *J Child Neurol* 1995; 10(Suppl 1):S50–S57.

20. Broman SH, Nichols PL, Kennedy WA. *Preschool IQ Prenatal and Early Developmental Correlates.* Hillsdale, N.J.: Lawrence Erlbaum Associates, Publishers, 1975.

21. Singhi PD, Bansal U, Singhi S, Pershad D. Determinants of IQ profile in children with idiopathic generalized epilepsy. *Epilepsia* 1992; 33:1106–1114.

22. Mitchell WG, Scheier LM, Baker SA. Psychosocial, behavioral, and medical outcomes in children with epilepsy: a developmental risk factor model using longitudinal data. *Pediatrics* 1994; 94:471–477.

23. Pianta RC, Lothman DJ. Predicting behavior problems in children with epilepsy: child factors, disease factors, family stress, and child-mother interaction. *Child Dev* 1994; 65:1415–1428.

24. Chovaz CJ, McLachlan RS, Derry PA, Cummings AL. Psychosocial function following temporal lobectomy: influence of seizure control and learned helplessness. *Seizure* 1994; 3:171–176.

25. Kuzniecky R, Andermann F. The congenital bilateral perisylvian syndrome: imaging findings in a multicenter study. CBPS Study Group. *Am J Neuroradiol* 1994; 15:139–144.

26. Gleeson JG, Allen KM, Fox JW, et al. Doublecortin, a brain-specific gene mutated in human X-linked lissencephaly and double cortex syndrome, encodes a putative signaling protein. *Cell* 1998; 92:63–72.

27. Ono J, Mano T, Andermann E, et al. Band heterotopia or double cortex in a male: bridging structures suggest abnormality of the radial glial guide system. *Neurology* 1997; 48:1701–1703.

28. Guerrini R, Dubeau F, Dulac O, et al. Bilateral parasagittal parietooccipital polymicrogyria and epilepsy. *Ann Neurol* 1997; 41:65–73.

29. Strauss E, Wada J, Hunter M. Callosal morphology and performance on intelligence tests. *J Clin Exp Neuropsychol* 1994; 16:79–83.

30. Susser M, Hauser WA, Kiely JL, et al. Quantitative estimates of prenatal and perinatal risk factors for perinatal mortality, cerebral palsy, mental retardation and epilepsy. In: Freeman JM, ed. *Prenatal and Perinatal Factors Associated with Brain Disorders.* NIH Publication No 85-1149, 1985:359–439.

31. Schnizel A. Microdeletion syndromes, balanced translocations, and gene mapping. *J Med Genet* 1988; 25:454–462.

32. Hagerman RJ. Fragile X syndrome. *Curr Probl Pediatr* 1987; 17:621–674

33. Wisniewski KE, French JH, Fernando S, et al. Fragile X syndrome: associated neurological abnormalities and developmental disabilities. *Ann Neurol* 1985; 18:665–669.

34. Fluge G. Neurological findings at follow-up in neonatal hypoglycemia. *Acta Paediat Scand* 1975; 62:629.

35. Goutieres F, Aicardi J. Atypical presentations of pyridoxine-dependent seizures: a treatable cause of intractable epilepsy in infants. *Ann Neurol* 1985; 17:117–120.

36. Bankier A, Turner M, Hopkins IJ. Pyridoxine dependent seizures — a wider clinical spectrum. *Arch Dis Child* 1983; 58:415–418.

37. Stephenson JB, Byrne KE. Pyridoxine responsive epilepsy: expanded pyridoxine dependency? *Arch Dis Child* 1983; 58:1034.

38. Nelson KB, Ellenberg JH. An epidemiologic approach to the problems of cerebral palsy. In: Fukuyama F, Arima M, Maekawa, Yamaguchi K, eds. *International Congress Series No. 579: Child Neurology.* Amsterdam: Excerpta Medica, 1981:341–350.

39. Beran RG, Flanagan PJ. Psychosocial sequelae of epilepsy: the role of associated cerebral pathology. *Epilepsia* 1987; 28:107–110.

40. Corbett JA, Trimble MR, Nichol TC. Behavioral and cognitive impairments in children with epilepsy: the long-term effects of anticonvulsant therapy. *J Am Acad Child Psychiatry* 1985; 24:17–23

41. Deb S. Mental disorder in adults with mental retardation and epilepsy. *Comp Psychiatry* 1887; 38:179–84.

42. Hagberg B, Hagberg G, Olow I, van Wendt L. The changing panorama of cerebral palsy in Sweden. VII. Prevalence and origin in the birth year period 1987–90. *Acta Paediatr* 1996; 85:954–960.

43. Kaushik A, Agarwal RP, Sadhna. Association of cerebral palsy with epilepsy. *J Indian Med Assn* 1997; 95:552–554.

44. Hadjipanayis A, Hadjichristodoulou C, Youroukos S. Epilepsy in patients with cerebral palsy. *Dev Med Child Neurol* 1997; 39:659–663.

45. Kwong KL, Wong SN, So KT. Epilepsy in children with cerebral palsy. *Pediatr Neurol* 1998; 19:31–36.

46. Aksu F. Nature and prognosis of seizures in patients with cerebral palsy [see comments]. *Dev Med Child Neurol* 1990; 32:661–668.

47. Eriksson K, Erila T, Kivimaki T, Koivikko M. Evolution of epilepsy in children with mental retardation: five-year experience in 78 cases. *Am J Ment Retard* 1998; 102:464–472.

48. Forsgren L, Edvinsson SO, Blomquist HK, et al. Epilepsy in a population of mentally retarded children and adults. *Epilepsy Res* 1990; 6:234–248.

49. Chelune GJ, Naugle RI, Hermann BP, et al. Does presurgical IQ predict seizure outcome after temporal lobectomy? Evidence from the Bozeman Epilepsy Consortium. *Epilepsia* 1998; 39:314–318.

50. Beckung E, Uvebrant P. Motor and sensory impairments in children with intractable epilepsy. *Epilepsia* 1993; 34:924–929.

51. Goulden KJ, Shinnar S, Koller H, et al. Epilepsy in children with mental retardation: a cohort study. *Epilepsia* 1991; 32:690–697.

52. Roger J, Dravet C, Bureau M, et al. *Epileptic Syndromes in Infancy, Childhood, and Adolescence.* London: John Libbey, 1985.

53. Prevey ML, Delaney RC, Cramer JA, Mattson RH. Complex partial and secondarily generalized seizure patients: cognitive functioning prior to treatment with antiepileptic medication. VA Epilepsy Cooperative Study 264 Group. *Epilepsy Res* 1998; 30:1–9.

54. Giordani B, Sackellares JC, Miller S, et al. Improvement in neuropsychological performance in patients with refractory seizures after intensive diagnostic and therapeutic intervention. *Neurology* 1983; 33:489–493.

55. Wilkus RJ, Dodrill CB. Neuropsychological correlates of the electroencephalogram in epileptics: I. Topographic distribution and average rate of epileptiform activity. *Epilepsia* 1976; 17:89–100.

56. Mandelbaum DE, Burack GD. The effect of seizure type and medication on cognitive and behavioral functioning in children with idiopathic epilepsy. *Dev Med Child Neurol* 1997; 39:731–735.

57. Berent S, Giordani B, Sackellares JC, et al. Cerebrally lateralized epileptogenic foci and performance on a verbal and visual graphic learning task. *Percept Mot Skills* 1983; 56:991–1001.

58. Mungas D, Ehlers C, Walton N, et al. Verbal learning differences in epileptic patients with left and right temporal lobe foci. *Epilepsia* 1985; 26:340–345.

59. Camfield P, Gordon K, Camfield C, et al. EEG results are rarely the same if repeated within six months in childhood epilepsy. *Can J Neurol Sci* 1995; 2:297–300.

60. Jokeit H, Seitz RJ, Markowitsch HJ, et al. Prefrontal asymmetric interictal glucose hypometabolism and cognitive impairment in patients with temporal lobe epilepsy. *Brain* 1997; 120:2283–2294.

61. Trimble MR, Thompson PJ. Neuropsychological and behavioral sequelae of spontaneous seizures. *Ann NY Acad Sci* 1986; 462:284–292.

62. Mitchell WG, Zhou Y, Chavez JM, Guzman BL. Reaction time, attention, and impulsivity in epilepsy. *Pediatr Neurol* 1992; 8:19–24.

63. Hermann BP, Wyler AR, Richley ET, Rea JM. Memory function and verbal learning ability in patients with complex partial seizures of temporal lobe origin. *Epilepsia* 1987; 28:547–554.

64. Masui K, Niwa SI, Anzai N, et al. Verbal memory disturbances in felt temporal lobe epileptics. *Cortex* 1984; 20:361–368.

65. Gadian DG, Isaacs EB, Cross JH, et al. Lateralization of brain function in childhood revealed by magnetic resonance spectroscopy. *Neurology* 1996; 46:974–977.

66. Piccirilli M, D'Alessandro P, Tiacci C, et al. Language lateralization in children with benign partial epilepsy. *Epilepsia* 1988; 29:19–25.

67. Sussova J, Seidl Z, Faber J. Hemiparetic forms of cerebral palsy in relation to epilepsy and mental retardation. *Dev Med Child Neurol* 1990; 32:792–795.

68. Jambaque I, Cusmai R, Curatolo P, et al. Neuropsychological aspects of tuberous sclerosis in relation to epilepsy and MRI findings. *Dev Med Child Neurol* 1991; 33:698–705.

69. Strauss E, Loring D, Chelune G, et al. Predicting cognitive impairment in epilepsy: findings from the Bozeman epilepsy consortium. *J Clin Exp Neuropsychol* 1995; 7:909–917.

70. Dikmen S, Matthews CG. Effect of major motor seizure frequency upon cognitive-intellectual functions in adults. *Epilepsia* 1977; 18:21–29.

71. Dikmen S, Matthews CG, Harley JP. Effect of early versus late onset of major motor epilepsy on cognitive-intellectual performance: further considerations. *Epilepsia* 1977; 18:31–36

72. Chevrie JJ, Aicardi J. Convulsive disorders in the first year of life: persistence of epileptic seizures. *Epilepsia* 1979; 20:643–649.

73. Chevrie JJ, Aicardi J. Convulsive disorders in the first year of life: neurological and mental outcome and mortality. *Epilepsia* 1978; 19:67–74.

74. Czochanska J, Langner-Tyszka B, Losiowski Z, Schmidt-Sidor B. Children who develop epilepsy in the first year of life: a prospective study. *Dev Med Child Neurol* 1994; 36:345–350.

75. Gomez MR. *Tuberous Sclerosis.* 2nd ed. New York, Raven Press, 1988.

76. Gilliam F, Wyllie E, Kashden J, et al. Epilepsy surgery outcome: comprehensive assessment in children. *Neurology* 1997; 48:1368–1374.

77. Czochanska J, Langner-Tyszka B, Losiowski Z, Schmidt-Sidor B. Children who develop epilepsy in the first year of life: a prospective study. *Dev Med Child Neurol* 1994; 36:345–350.

78. Gordon K, Bawden H, Camfield P, et al. Valproic acid treatment of learning disorder and severely epileptiform EEG without clinical seizures. *J Child Neurol* 1996; 11:41–43.

79. Seidenberg M, O'Leary DS, Berent S, Boll T. Changes in seizure frequency and test-retest scores on the Wechsler Adult Intelligence Scale. *Epilepsia* 1981; 22:75–83.

80. Marcus JC. Control of epilepsy in a mentally retarded population: lack of correlation with IQ, neurological status, and electroencephalogram. *Am J Ment Retard* 1993; 98(Suppl):47–51.

81. Weglage J, Demsky A, Pietsch M, Kurlemann G. Neuropsychological, intellectual, and behavioral findings in patients with centrotemporal spikes with and without seizures. *Dev Med Child Neurol* 1997; 39:646–651.

82. D'Alessandro P, Piccirilli M, Tiacci C, et al. Neuropsychological features of benign partial epilepsy in children. *Ital J Neurol Sci* 1990; 11:265–269.

83. Ellenberg JH, Nelson KB. Febrile seizures and later intellectual performance. *Arch Neurol* 1978; 35:17–21.

84. Duchowny MS, Levin B, Jayakar P et al. Temporal lobectomy in early childhood. *Epilepsia* 1992; 33:298–303.

85. Lindsay J, Glaser G, Richards P, Ounsted C. Developmental aspects of focal epilepsies of childhood treated by neurosurgery. *Dev Med Child Neurol* 1984; 26:574–587.

86. Lindsay J, Ounsted C, Richards P. Long-term outcome in children with temporal lobe seizures, IV: Genetic factors, febrile convulsions and the remission of seizures. *Dev Med Child Neurol* 1980; 22:429–440.

87. Hermann BP, Schwartz MS, Karnes WE, et al. Psychopathology in epilepsy: relationship of seizure type to age at onset. *Epilepsia* 1980; 21:15–23.

88. Whitman S, Hermann BP, Gordon AC. Psychopathology in epilepsy: how great is the risk? *Biol Psychiatry* 1984; 19:213–236.

89. Dodrill CB, Batzel LW. Interictal features of patients with epilepsy. *Epilepsia* 1986; 27(Suppl 2):S64–S76.

90. Robertson MM, Trimble MR, Townsend HRA. Phenomenology of depression in epilepsy. *Epilepsia* 1987; 28:364–372.

91. Dodrill CB, Clemmons D. Use of neuropsychological tests to identify high school students with epilepsy who later demonstrate inadequate performances in life. *J Consult Clin Psychol* 1984; 52:520–527.

92. Batzel LW, Dodrill CB. Neuropsychological and emotional correlates of marital status and ability to live independently in individuals with epilepsy. *Epilepsia* 1984; 25:594–598.

93. Olsson I, Steffenburg S, Gillberg C. Epilepsy in autism and autisticlike conditions. *Arch Neurol* 1988; 45:666–668.

94. Wellesley DG, Hockey KA, Montgomery PD, et al. Prevalence of intellectual handicap in Western Australia: a community study. *Med J Aust* 1992; 156:94–96.

CHAPTER 51

Cognitive Side Effects of Antiepileptic Drugs

Albert P. Aldenkamp, Ph.D., and Jan Vermeulen

Antiepileptic drug (AED) treatment is usually necessary for several years but may last a lifetime in a large group of patients (1). During such long treatment periods, a variety of AED-induced side effects may occur. A number of these side effects appear immediately after the start of drug exposure but are relatively benign because they show habituation (2). Other side effects are reversible upon reduction of the dose. *Chronic side effects*, however, have an insidious onset and emerge only after extended periods of treatment. Multitudes of such chronic side effects have been documented (3). These include effects on metabolism, bone and connective tissue, and the endocrine system; however, the most common effects concern the central nervous system (CNS).

This chapter reviews our knowledge about a specific subgroup of such chronic CNS-related side effects, that is, the *cognitive side effects* such as drug-induced impairments of memory, attention, and mental speed. These cognitive side effects are generally reported to be mild to moderate in magnitude compared with most of the other types of side effects. Nonetheless, a number of studies have claimed that drug-induced cognitive impairment may have a much greater impact on function and daily living than hitherto suspected (4–6). Examples of how these might effect daily life include potential impact on critical functions such as learning in children (5), driving skills in adults, which require responses in the milliseconds range, or vulnerable functions such as memory in the elderly. Moreover, because the cognitive side effects represent long-term consequences of AED therapy, the effects may accumulate with prolonged treatment and have a negative impact on daily functioning, especially among children with refractory epilepsy (6).

The interest in cognitive side effects of antiepileptic treatment dates back to the early 1970s (7,8). Most of the early studies compared phenytoin (PHT) with the newcomer at that time, carbamazepine (CBZ). The fact that both drugs were targeted to localization-related epilepsy may well have stimulated the cognitive research on these agents. During the later 1970s and 1980s the emphasis on treatment and drug trials gradually shifted from mere seizure count to a more comprehensive evaluation that balanced both drug efficacy and tolerability, including attention for full range of adverse effects (9–12). Consequently, from 1972 through 1996 there were 1,357 studies on the cognitive effects of AEDs. Unfortunately, this large literature base, although impressive, is not easily interpretable because it contains substantial controversies about the type and severity of drug-induced cognitive impairment. There are several reasons for such controversies, including differences among the studies with respect to the type of subjects investigated and the designs that have been used to detect drug effects. Some of these controversies are highlighted in this chapter.

For example, the summary in a recent authoritative review suggests that PHT has serious adverse effects on cognitive function, whereas CBZ has a more favourable profile (13). This conclusion, however, has been debated when other studies have failed to reproduce the adverse cognitive effects of PHT after serum concentrations were controlled (14–17). Dodrill and Troupin (18) revisited their original pioneering study of adverse effects of PHT. Based on the reevaluation of the original data, they concluded that some of the differences that they had reported between CBZ and PHT actually were due to artifacts, such as difference in relative drug concentrations (18). Moreover, some studies suggested that subject selection bias also influenced the results, as there was evidence that in some countries PHT had been administered to different types of patients than CBZ. Circumstances that promote different administration patterns include the fact that in many parts of the world PHT is less expensive and it can be administered once daily, which is more convenient than CBZ (19). The differences that were observed between the groups after PHT and CBZ treatment therefore may reflect differences in patient characteristics rather than drug effects. Finally, it has been suggested that the adverse effects of PHT on cognitive function may be due to a confounding factor of motor speed. In one study motor slowing appeared to be the only factor that discriminated between PHT and CBZ (20). Whereas almost all cognitive tests depend on motor output, peripheral motor effects may have been interpreted erroneously as central or cognitive effects. This example illustrates that a critical review of the literature is useful for both future research and the proper interpretation of existing data because cognitive function remains a highly relevant issue in clinical practice.

With respect to the type of cognitive impairment that may be induced by antiepileptic treatment, most reports show that AEDs do not cause entirely new areas of cognitive dysfunction; rather they seem to depress the capacity of the information-processing system by producing slowing. As a result, they can decrease the input of working memory and decrease mental flexibility. Some investigators have reduced these three areas to one major problem: the slowing of central information processing or mental slowing (13,21–26). These three areas of impairment have been reconfirmed in three consensus meetings: the International Workshop "Cognitive Effects of the Newer Antiepileptic Drugs" organized during the International Epilepsy Conference in Sydney, 1995 (22) and the unpublished consensus meetings organized by Cilag Janssen/Ortho McNeil in New York City and by Glaxo-Wellcome in Raleigh-Durham, both in 1996.

LITERATURE REVIEW

Identification of potentially relevant studies was accomplished through computerized searches of the English language literature published between January 1970 and December 1994 (29). This included a computerized search of several databases and reviews of the topics (11,12,15–17,23–26,27–29).

One criterion for papers to be selected was that the data be published in a peer-reviewed journal in the English language. In order to be included, the studies also must have reported psychometrically assessed cognitive function, not just clinical observations. This chapter deals only with drugs that are currently in use and does not focus on investigational agents. Finally, only studies that were primarily concerned with patients with epilepsy are included; other patient groups such as psychiatric patients or patients with chronic pain are not included. However, drug administration to healthy volunteers is considered because

it controls the effects of seizures and helps isolate the absolute cognitive effects of the drugs.

Starting with 1,284 titles (29), newly published papers through 1996 were also included, expanding the database to 1,357 titles. Scanning these articles one at a time, it soon became clear that the results could not be compiled simply as written because of discrepancies in the validity of the conclusions. Problems that were encountered were not simply minor annoyances; their impact on the validity of the conclusions that had been drawn were substantial. In some reports an otherwise useful AED might be portrayed as having such severe adverse effects on cognitive functioning as to label it as harmful, while in practice the actual cognitive effects might be inconspicuous.

Illustrating the need for careful interpretation of the published data stems from complications that arise from conclusions drawn about studies with negative findings or "no significant differences." In general, nonsignificant results tend to be regarded as disappointing; however, research on adverse drug effects is an area in which one seeks nonsignificance because this outcome indicates an absence of harmful cognitive effects. This follows from the tendency to compare a new drug with an established drug that has a presumed favorable cognitive profile. However, this "equivalence approach" may be flawed depending on the statistical power of the study. Conclusions that there is no difference between two drugs only make sense if the study has a reasonable a priori chance (80% or better) of detecting a cognitive side effect when, in fact, one is present. This probability, that is, the statistical power, is heavily dependent on the sample size and the magnitude of the difference between the groups that are being compared. For example, to attain a power of 0.80, which is to have an 80 percent chance of detecting small, medium, and large difference differences between two groups, the necessary sample size gets smaller as a magnitude of difference between the two groups increases. When the expected difference is "medium" (often a half standard deviation difference) (30), the number of subjects necessary to detect a difference with 5 percent significance would be 64. This number increases for "small differences" (i.e., of a magnitude of one-fifth of a standard deviation), yielding a necessary sample size of 393 subjects (30). Most of the authorities who have reviewed this area have claimed that although the long-term impact of AEDs on daily functioning may be considerable, the cognitive effects as assessed by cognitive testing are generally small to medium in magnitude and thus require relatively large samples sizes of 64 or more subjects to be detected. Nonetheless, smaller sample sizes of usually 20 patients or fewer have been used in a majority of studies that claim "no effect results." In reality, these studies could have detected only cognitive effects that are very large, large enough to be obvious to the clinician without psychological testing. Therefore, when "no-effect reports" are encountered, it is worth checking whether these results might not reflect inadequate statistical power. Overlooking these types of issues opens the door to the possibility of false-negative conclusions.

Methodological issues must be evaluated because of the extent to which they can erode the validity of this type of research. In weighing the evidence from these studies, the approach that is taken here has been to exclude those studies that contain potential deficiencies based on the following criteria.

1. *Statistical detail and power.* In some studies the description of the methods appear to be below acceptable standards of scientific communication. Many studies did not even report the number of subjects included. Therefore, only studies were included that describe the design, number of subjects, and outcome measures in sufficient detail to evaluate the power of the investigation. Subsequently, power calculations were carried out, and studies that did not reach an acceptable of power (set, according to the conventions proposed by Cohen, at 0.80) (30) were not included. The aforementioned examples illustrate that studies with insufficient power may *underestimate* the cognitive effects of AEDs.

2. *Duration of drug exposure.* Another important consideration is drug exposure duration. An insufficient period of drug administration is a limiting problem in some studies that investigated normal volunteers. Studies of volunteers offer the best opportunity to evaluate the absolute cognitive effects of AEDs. These types of studies have the ability to implement powerful crossover designs that allow random assignment to AEDs or placebos. However, many of these studies suffer because the period of drug exposure is too limited to adapt to short-term, transient side effects. There is evidence that with most AEDs the early cognitive side effects that develop during the first days or weeks of therapy subsequently abate because of the development of tolerance or habituation (32). Although little is known about how tolerance to these adverse effects develops, failure to accommodate the development of tolerance may lead to an *overestimation* of the negative impact of drugs on cognition (12). This important point must be considered in studies of healthy volunteers who are typically given AEDs for only a few weeks. Some studies used very short periods of exposure, often no longer than one day. For these reasons, studies that exposed subjects to drug for one day or less were not included in our review.

3. *Drug interactions and polytherapy.* Typically, cognitive effects of AEDs have been studied in add-on studies in which a new drug is added to a multidrug regimen resulting in polytherapy (31). Polytherapy induces critical complications in identifying what is actually causing the observed cognitive changes. Pharmacokinetic interactions that affect drug concentrations can alter therapeutic efficacy and cognitive functioning (32). Moreover, because polytherapy is usually administered to patients with severe or refractive epilepsy, the threat of the seizure frequency being a confounding variable is ever-present. It is thus unwise to base inferences about cognitive side effects of AEDs in these types of studies. In general, add-on polytherapy studies tend to *underestimate* cognitive effects of AEDs when the cognitive benefits that result from improved seizure control offset adverse drug effects on cognition.

For these reasons we excluded studies if (1) they did not provide sufficient statistical detail or they do not reach acceptable power, (2) they were too brief without sufficient drug exposure of at least more than one day, or (3) they were based on studies performed during polytherapy. The remaining studies are used to draw some conclusions about the cognitive side effects per drug.

ESTABLISHED DRUGS

The cognitive effects for the most commonly used AEDs are summarized in Table 51-1. The sections that follow focus on key studies that have been conducted on these agents.

Phenobarbital

The single study by McLeod and coworkers (33) compared the effects of phenobarbital to a nondrug condition and found impairment of memory in subjects with epilepsy. Differences between phenobarbital (PHB) and other AEDs were identified in three other studies among patients with epilepsy (16,34,35). One study revealed greater impairment with PHB than phenytoin (PHT) or carbamazepine (CBZ) on visual motor and memory tests (35), whereas another showed lower intelligence scores after long-term PHB treatment in comparison with valproate (VPA) (34). However, Meador and coworkers (16) did not detect differences between PHB, PHT, or CBZ. In the balance, the majority of these studies provide evidence for a PHB-induced cognitive impairment. There are no studies available that evaluated the effect of dose.

Phenytoin

Five studies have documented PHT-induced cognitive impairment in the areas of attention, memory, and especially mental speed compared with a nondrug condition (21,36–39). All of these studies were conducted in normal volunteers, opening the possibility that these

Table 51-1. Results of Investigated Studies. Summary of the Cognitive Side Effects of Antiepileptic Drugs

	Type of Impairment	Number of Subjects (e = epilepsy; nv = volunteers)
Phenobarbitone (PHB)		
Absolute effects (versus nondrug)	Short-term memory	19(e)(33)
	Memory/visual-motor functions	29(e)(35)
	Intelligence	21(e)(34)
Relative effects (versus other drugs)	No difference with PHT/CBZ	15(e)(16)
Dose relation		
no studies		
Phenytoin (PHT)		
Absolute effects	Memory/mental speed	10(nv)(36)
(versus nondrug)	Memory	8(nv)(37)
	Memory/attention/mental speed	8(nv)(38)
	Attention/mental speed	21(nv)(21)
	Impairment of memory	15(nv)(29)
Relative effects	Intelligence and memory	29(e)(35)
(versus other drugs)	No difference with CBZ/PHB	21(nv) 15(nv) 15(e)(16,21,39)
Dose relation	No dose effects	107(nv)(40)
Carbamazepine (CBZ)		
Absolute effects	No impairment	8(nv)(37)
(versus nondrug)	Mental speed/attention	21(nv)(21)
	Impairment of memory	15(nv)(39)
	No impairment	56(e)(43)
Relative effects	More favorable profile compared with PHT & PHB	9(e)(35)
(versus other drugs)	No differences with PHT & PHB	15(nv) 21(nv) 15(e)(16,21,39)
Dose relation	Variability at peak levels	11(e)(42)
	Improvement at higher doses	50(e)(43)
Valproate (VPA)		
Absolute effects		
(versus nondrug)	Mental speed	10(nv)(44)
Relative effects	Visuomotor and memory compared with CBZ	29(e)(35)
(versus other drugs)	Higher scores on intelligence compared with PHB	21(e)(34)
Dose relation	No dose effects	46(e)(46)

effects represent short-term drug actions. However, this possibility was not substantiated in other studies that compared PHT with other AEDs. Studied in long-term treatment and after withdrawal of therapy, the findings of PHT effects on patients were similar to those in normal volunteers (35,41). To the contrary, however, studies by Meador and coworkers (16,17,39) did not detect differences between PHT, CBZ, or PHB. These discrepant results raise the possibility of a "center bias." No relationship between dose and type of cognitive impairment has been identified (40).

Carbamazepine

Evaluated in normal volunteers and people with epilepsy, CBZ had a favorable profile when compared with PHT, PHB, and VPA (35,37,41). The exception to this has been the work of Meador and colleagues in the United States, who found different results (16,21). Although no consensus has been reached about the effect of increasing dose, both cognitive impairment

and increased variability in performance have been observed in higher serum concentrations (42,43).

Valproate

One study demonstrated that VPA produces mild to moderate impairment of mental speed (44). When compared with other drugs, VPA lowered performance of memory and visual motor function tests compared with CBZ (35) and had a more favorable profile than PHB (34). Cognitive impairment associated with VPA has not been linked to dose (45).

REMAINING ESTABLISHED DRUGS

After applying methodological criteria, no studies were available regarding clonazepam and clobazam, two drugs that are commonly used. Clinical reports suggest that cognitive impairment may be caused by clonazepam because of its tendency to produce irritability and reduce attention. On the other hand, clobazam is widely considered to have a more favorable cognitive profile.

NEWER ANTIEPILEPTIC DRUGS

When applying the aforementioned criteria, data available regarding the cognitive effects of established AEDs are quite meager despite their long use. This illustrates how long it takes to begin to define the adverse cognitive effects of AEDs. Based on this experience, it is not surprising that little or no reliable data are available regarding the AEDs that have been introduced in the 1990s, including vigabatrin, lamotrigine, oxcarbazepine, tiagabine, gabapentin, and topiramate. Furthermore, most of the information available was gleaned in add-on polytherapy designs that were intended to establish drug efficacy. Investigations in normal volunteers are not available for any of these drugs. Nonetheless, we attempt to give some overview, based, however, mainly on clinical experience and anecdotal information. Most of the information that is presented here draws on the exchange of information between researchers, clinicians, and pharmaceutical industries that took place during the International Workshop on "Cognitive Effects of Neuro Anti-Epileptic Drugs" that was held during the International Epilepsy Congress in Sydney Australia in 1995 (22).

Vigabatrin

Although an absence of cognitive side effects has been claimed from vigabatrin, the data are limited and come from a single center (46,47). Furthermore, these studies had only limited power to detect differences and therefore entail a risk of underestimating the cognitive side effects. Although other studies have been published (49–52), these studies did not pass our criteria for inclusion because they were conducted in polytherapy designs. Moreover, mood disorders linked with this drug may secondarily lead to lower cognitive scores in some patients (53–57).

Lamotrigine

Clinical studies assert that lamotrigine does not impair cognition and in fact may benefit mental performance in some patients (58). This is consistent with the claimed psychotropic effect. Unfortunately, there are no data from controlled cognitive studies to support this claim. A few communications have opened the possibility of "speeding effects" possibly related to euphoria that could have a secondary impact on cognitive productivity.

Oxcarbazepine

It has been claimed that oxcarbazepine has no cognitive effects (59,60). One group of investigators reported improved cognitive functioning in the areas of speed compared with a nondrug condition, but they did not control for the beneficial cognitive effects of improved seizure control. Other studies did not pass our methodological screening criteria for inclusion (31,61). A number of questions remain regarding the effects of this agent in children and the elderly. Unfortunately, the pharmaceutical sponsor of the drug stopped investigations in these age groups before they were completed. No studies are under way at the time of this writing.

Tiagabine

A favorable cognitive profile has been reported for tiagabine. However, only anecdotal clinical reports support it; no systematic studies are available. Studies that were initiated were curtailed at the end of 1997, when the development of this drug was transferred from one company to another.

Gabapentin

Gabapentin appears to have a favorable cognitive profile despite the disadvantage that all controlled studies have been performed in a limited number of centers in the United States. In light of the discrepancies that have been found between studies conducted in the United States and Europe regarding CBZ and PHT, the results of these studies should be reviewed cautiously until they are confirmed more widely.

Topiramate

Topiramate is being investigated, but currently there is no information available from controlled studies regarding its effects on cognitive function. The World Health Organization (WHO)-ART rating for adverse events during four clinical dose-ranging studies showed that CSN-related side effects are the dominant subjective patient complaints (Cilag International, Product Information, 1995). These reports point to slowing of mental speed and attention that appears to be dose-related and possibly linked to the rate of dose escalation when the medication is being started. Two studies of topiramate and cognitive function are under way, one in Europe and one in the United States, and are reviewing topiramate as a first-line add-on drug. The randomized studies have sample sizes that exceed 80 subjects.

Investigational Drugs

The information is limited for AEDs that are still investigational. However, rufinamide (CGP 33.101) has been linked to improved scores on reaction timed tests at lower doses but impairment of short-term memory at higher doses. Although these data have not yet been released by the company, the study had an impressive sample size of more than 200 subjects (62). Although a nootropic effect has been claimed for levetiracetam, the data are based on a small pilot study that does not allow conclusions to be drawn (63).

REFERENCES

1. Overweg J. Withdrawal of antiepileptic drugs in seizure-free adult patients. Amsterdam: University of Amsterdam, 1985. Thesis.

2. Kulig B, Meinardi H. Effects of antiepileptic drugs on motor activity and learned behavior in the rat. In: Meinardi H, Rowan AJ, eds. *Advances in Epileptology.* Amsterdam: Swets & Zeitlinger, 1977:98–104.

3. Reynolds EH. Chronic antiepileptic toxicity: a review. *Epilepsia* 1975; 16:319–352.

4. Trimble MR. Anticonvulsant drugs: mood and cognitive function. In: Trimble MR, Reynolds EH, eds. *Epilepsy, Behaviour and Cognitive Function.* Chichester: John Wiley & Sons, 1987:135–145.

5. Aldenkamp AP. Cognitive side effects of antiepileptic drugs. In: Aldenkamp AP, Dreifuss FE, Renier WO, eds. *Epilepsy in Children and Adolescents.* Boca Raton: CRC Press, 1995:161–183.

6. Committee on Drugs. Behavioral and cognitive effects of anticonvulsant therapy. *Pediatrics* 1985; 76:644–647.

7. Ideström CM, Schalling D, Carlquist U, et al. Behavioral and psychological studies: acute effects of diphenylhydantoin in relation to plasma levels. *Psych Med* 1972; 2:111–120.

8. Dodrill CB, Troupin AS. Psychotropic effects of carbamazepine in epilepsy: a double-blind comparison with phenytoin. *Neurology* 1977, 27:1023–1028.

9. Parnas J, Flachs H, Gram L. Psychotropic effect of antiepileptic drugs. *Acta Neurol Scand* 1979; 60:329–343.

10. Parnas J, Gram L, Flachs H. Psychopharmacological aspects of antiepileptic treatment. *Prog Neurobiol* 1980; 15:119–138.

11. Dodrill CB. Behavioral effects of antiepileptic drugs. In: Smith D, Treiman D, Trimble M, eds. *Advances in Neurology.* New York: Raven Press, 1991; 55:213–224.

12. Dodrill CB. Problems in the assessment of cognitive effects of antiepileptic drugs. *Epilepsia* 1992; 33(S6):29–32.

13. Evans RW, Gualtieri CT. Carbamazepine: a neuropsychological and psychiatric profile. *Clin Neuropharmacol* 1985; 8:221–241.

14. Smith DB, Mattson RH, Cramer JA, et al. Results of a nationwide Veterans Administration Cooperative Study comparing the efficacy and toxicity of carbamazepine, phenobarbital, phenytoin, and primidone. *Epilepsia* 1987; 28(S3):50–58.

15. Smith DB. Cognitive effects of antiepileptic drugs. In: Smith D, Treiman D, Trimble M, eds. *Advances in Neurology.* New York: Raven Press, 1991; 55:197–212.

16. Meador KJM, Loring DW, Huh K, et al. Comparative cognitive effects of anticonvulsants. *Neurology* 1990; 40:391–394.

17. Meador KJ, Loring DW. Cognitive effects of antiepileptic drugs. In: Devinski O, Theodore W, eds. *Epilepsy and Behavior.* New York: Wiley-Liss, 1991:151–170

18. Dodrill CB, Troupin AS. Neuropsychological effects of carbamazepine and phenytoin: a reanalysis. *Neurology* 1991; 41:141–143.

19. Wilder BJ, Rangel RJ. Phenytoin, clinical use. In: Dreifuss FE, Mattson RH, Meldrum BS, et al., eds. *Antiepileptic Drugs.* 3rd ed. New York: Raven Press, 1989:233–241.

20. Dodrill CB, Temkin NR. Motor speed is a contaminating factor in evaluating the "cognitive" effects of phenytoin. *Epilepsia* 1989; 30:453–457.

21. Meador KJM, Loring DW, Allen ME, et al. Comparative cognitive effects of carbamazepine and phenytoin in healthy adults. *Neurology* 1991; 41:1537–1540.

22. Aldenkamp AP, Trimble MR. Cognitive side effects of antiepileptic drugs: fact or fiction? *Epilepsia* 1996: 37:82. Abstract.

23. Trimble MR, Thompson PJ. Memory, anticonvulsant drugs and seizures. *Acta Neurol Scand* 1981; 64:31–41.

24. Trimble MR, Thompson PJ. Anticonvulsant drugs, cognitive function and behaviour. *Epilepsia* 1983; 24(Suppl 1):S55–S63.

25. Trimble MR. Anticonvulsant drugs and psychosocial development: phenobarbitone, sodium valproate, and benzodiazepines. In: Morselli PL, Pippenger CE, Penry JK, eds. *Antiepileptic Drug Therapy in Pediatrics.* New York: Raven Press, 1983:201–217.

26. Trimble MR. Anticonvulsant drugs and cognitive function: a review of the literature. *Epilepsia* 1987; 28(Suppl 3): 37–45.

27. Novelly RA, Schwartz MM, Mattson RH, et al. Behavioral toxicity associated with antiepileptic drugs: concepts and methods of assessment. *Epilepsia* 1986; 27:331–340.

28. Trimble MR, Cull C. Children of school age: the influence of antiepileptic drugs on behavior and intellect. *Epilepsia* 1988; 29(Suppl 3):S15–S19.

29. Vermeulen J, Aldenkamp AP. Cognitive side-effects of chronic antiepileptic drug treatment: a review of 25 years of research. *Epilepsy Res* 1995; 22:65–95.

30. Cohen J. *Statistical Power Analysis for the Behavioral Sciences.* New York: Academic Press, 1978.

31. McKee PJW, Blacklaw J, Forrest G, et al. A double-blind placebo-controlled interaction study between oxcarbazepine and carbamazepine, sodium valproate and phenytoin in epileptic patients. *Br J Clin Pharmacol* 1994; 37:27–32.

32. Brown SW. Clinical aspects of antiepileptic treatment. In: Aldenkamp AP, Dreifuss FE, Renier WO, et al., eds. *Epilepsy in Children and Adolescents.* New York: CRC Press, 1994:98–112.

33. MacLeod CM, Dekaban AS, Hunt E. Memory impairment in epileptic patients: selective effects of phenobarbital concentration. *Science* 1978; 202:1102–1104.

34. Vining EP, Mellitis ED, Dorsen MM, et al. Psychologic and behavioral effects of antiepileptic drugs in children:

a double-blind comparison between phenobarbital and valproic acid. *Pediatrics* 1987; 80:165–74.

35. Gallassi R, Morreale A, Di Sarro R, et al. Cognitive effects of antiepileptic drug discontinuation. *Epilepsia* 1992; 33:41–44.

36. Smith WL, Lowrey JB. Effects of diphenylhydantoin on mental abilities in the elderly. *J Am Geriatr Soc* 1975; 23:207–211.

37. Thompson PJ, Huppert F, Trimble MR. Anticonvulsant drugs, cognitive function and memory. *Acta Neurol Scand* 1980; (Suppl 80):75–80.

38. Thompson PJ, Huppert FA, Trimble MR. Phenytoin and cognitive functions: effects on normal volunteers and implications for epilepsy. *Br J Clin Psychol* 1981; 20:155–162.

39. Meador KJM, Loring DW, Abney OL, et al. Effects of carbamazepine and phenytoin on EEG and memory in healthy adults. Epilepsia, 1993; 34(1):153–157.

40. Stevens JH, Schaffer JW, Brown CC. A controlled comparison of the effect of diphenylhydantoin and placebo on mood and psychomotor functioning in normal volunteers. *J Clin Pharmacol* 1974; 14:543–551.

41. Aldenkamp AP, Alpherts WCJ, Blennow G, et al. Withdrawal of antiepileptic medication — effects on cognitive function in children — the results of the multicentre 'Holmfrid' study. *Neurology* 1993; 43:41–51.

42. Aldenkamp AP, Alpherts WCJ, Moerland MC, et al. Controlled release carbamazepine: cognitive side effects in patients with epilepsy. *Epilepsia* 1987; 28:507–514.

43. Amman MG, Werry JS, Paxton JW, et al. Effects of carbamazepine on psychomotor performance in children as a function of drug concentration, seizure type and time of medication. *Epilepsia* 1990; 31:51–60.

44. Thompson PJ, Trimble MR. Sodium valproate en cognitive functioning in normal volunteers. *Br J Clin Pharmacol* 1981; 12:819–824.

45. Amman MG, Werry JS, Paxton JW, et al. Effect of sodium valproate on psychomotor performance in children as a function of dose, fluctuations in concentration and diagnosis. *Epilepsia* 1987; 28:115–124.

46. Riekkinen PJ, Kalviasinen R, Aikia M, et al. Cognitive and electrophysiological effects of vigabatrin and carbamazepine. *Epilepsia* 1990; 31:620.

47. Mervaala E, Partanen J, Nousiainen U, Sivenius J, Riekinnen P. Electrophysiological effects of gamma-vinyl GABA and carbamazepine. *Epilepsia* 1989; 30:189–193.

48. Gram L, Klosterskov P, Dam M. Gamma-vinyl-GABA: a double blind placebo controlled trial in partial epilepsy. *Ann Neurol* 1985; 17:262–266.

49. Saletu B, Grunberger J, Linzmayer L, et al. Psychophysiological and psychometric studies after manipulating the GABA system by vigabatrin, a GABA-transaminase inhibitor. *Int J Psychophysiol* 1986; 4:63–80.

50. McGuire AM, Duncan JS, Trimble MR. Effects of vigabatrin on cognitive function and mood when used as add-on therapy in patients with intractable epilepsy. *Epilepsia* 1992; 33:128–134.

51. Gilham RA, Blacklaw J, Mckee PJW, et al. Effects of vigabatrin on sedation and cognitive function in patients with refractory epilepsy. *J Neurol Neurosurg Psychiatry* 1993; 56:1271–1275.

52. Dodrill CB, Arnett JL, Sommerville KW, et al. Evaluation of the effects of vigabatrin on cognitive abilities and quality of life in epilepsy. *Neurology* 1993; 43:2501–2507.

53. Lambert PA, Chabannes JP, Cantiniaux P, Schechter PJ, Tell GP. Effets du gamma-vinyl-GABA per os dans cinq cas de schizophrenie hebephreno-catatonique. *Encephale* 1983: 9:145–149

54. Ring HA, Reynolds EH. Vigabatrin and behavior disturbance. *Lancet* 1990; 335:970.

55. Robinson MK, Richens A, Oxley R. Vigabatrin and behaviour disturbances. *Lancet* 1990; 336:8713.

56. Sander JW, Hart YM, Trimble MR, Shorvon SD. Vigabatrin and psychosis. *J Neurol Neurosurg Psychiatry* 1991: 54:435–439

57. Aldenkamp AP, Vermeulen J, Mulder OG, et al. τ-Vinyl GABA (Vigabatrin) and mood disturbances. *Epilepsia* 1994: 35:999–1004.

58. Aldenkamp AP, Mulder OG, Overweg J. Cognitive effects of lamotrigine as first-line add-on in patients with localized related (partial) epilepsy. *J. Epilepsy* 1994; 10:117–121.

59. Aikiae M, Kaelviaeinen R, Sivenius J, et al. Cognitive effects of oxcarbazepine and phenytoin monotherapy in newly diagnosed epilepsy: one year follow-up. *Epilepsy Res* 1992; 11:199–203.

60. Curran HV, Java R. Memory and psychomotor effects of oxcarbazepine in healthy human volunteers. *Eur J Clin Pharmacol* 1993; 44:529–533.

61. Zaccara G, Gangemi PF, Messori A, et al. Effects of oxcarbazepine and carbamazepine on the central nervous system: computerized analysis of saccadic and smooth-pursuit eye movements. *Acta Neurol Scand* 1992; 85:425–429.

62. Aldenkamp AP. The cognitive profile of the experimental antiepileptic drug CGP 33.101. Basel, Presentation at the Final Investigators Meeting, March 14, 1996.

63. Neyens LGJ, Alpherts WCJ, Aldenkamp AP. Cognitive effects of a new pyrrolidine derivative (Levetiracetam) in patients with epilepsy. *Prog Neuropsychopharmacol Biol Psychiatry* 1995; 19:411–419.

Index

Note: Boldface numbers indicate illustrations; italicized *t* indicates a table.